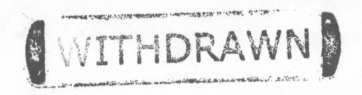

BRAD W. NEVILLE, D.D.S.

Professor and Director
Division of Oral Pathology
Department of Stomatology
College of Dental Medicine
Medical University of South Carolina
Charleston, South Carolina

DOUGLAS D. DAMM, D.D.S.

Professor of Oral Pathology
College of Dentistry
University of Kentucky
Lexington, Kentucky

CARL M. ALLEN, D.D.S., M.S.D.

Associate Professor and Director
Oral Pathology
Section of Oral and Maxillofacial Surgery and Pathology
College of Dentistry
The Ohio State University
Columbus, Ohio

JERRY E. BOUQUOT, D.D.S., M.S.D.

Director of Research
The Maxillofacial Center for Diagnostics and Research
Morgantown, West Virginia

Senior Visiting Scientist
Department of Research and Epidemiology
Mayo Clinic
Rochester, Minnesota

Consultant in Pediatric Oral Pathology
Department of Dentistry
Pittsburgh Children's Hospital
Pittsburgh, Pennsylvania

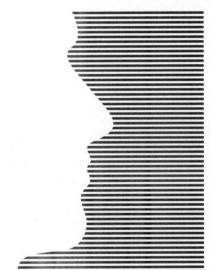

Oral
& Maxillofacial
Pathology

W.B. SAUNDERS COMPANY
A Division of Harcourt Brace & Company
Philadelphia   London   Toronto   Montreal   Sydney   Tokyo

W.B. SAUNDERS COMPANY
A Division of Harcourt Brace & Company

The Curtis Center
Independence Square West
Philadelphia, Pennsylvania 19106

Library of Congress Cataloging-in-Publication Data

Neville, Brad W
  Oral and maxillofacial pathology / Brad W. Neville [et al.] — 1st ed.
     p.   cm.
  Includes index.
  ISBN 0-7216-6695-7
  1. Mouth—Diseases. 2. Teeth—Diseases. 3. Maxilla—Diseases. I. Neville, Brad W. [et al.]
     [DNLM: 1. Mouth Diseases—pathology. 2. Tooth Diseases—pathology.
  3. Maxillofacial Injuries—pathology.   WU 140 06168 1995]
  RK307.073 1995
  617.5′22—dc20
  DNLM/DLC   94-20442

ORAL AND MAXILLOFACIAL PATHOLOGY   ISBN 0-7216-6695-7

Last digit is the print number: 9   8   7   6   5   4   3   2

This book is dedicated to three of our mentors:

CHARLES A. WALDRON
WILLIAM G. SHAFER
ROBERT J. GORLIN

in appreciation for all that they have taught us
and
in recognition of their contributions to the field of
Oral and Maxillofacial Pathology

List of Contributors

Edward E. Herschaft, D.D.S., M.A., F.A.C.D.

Professor of Oral Pathology and Forensic Dentistry
Department of Stomatology
College of Dental Medicine
Medical University of South Carolina
Charleston, South Carolina

Diplomate, American Boards of Forensic Odontology and Oral Medicine
Past Vice President and Fellow, American Academy of Forensic Sciences
Past President, American Society of Forensic Odontology
Consultant in Forensic Odontology, Charleston County Medical Examiner's Office
South Carolina State Law Enforcement Division (SLED)
University of South Carolina School of Law
Director, South Carolina Forensic Dental Network

Forensic Dentistry

Charles A. Waldron, D.D.S., M.S.D.

Professor Emeritus
Division of Head and Neck Pathology
Department of Pathology
Emory University School of Medicine
Atlanta, Georgia

Bone Pathology; Odontogenic Cysts and Tumors

Preface

Oral and maxillofacial pathology is the specialty of dentistry and pathology that deals with the nature, identification, and management of diseases affecting the oral and maxillofacial regions. As such, it occupies a unique position in the health care community for both the dental and medical professions. Naturally, members of the dental profession (including general practitioners, specialists, and dental hygienists) must have a good knowledge of the pathogenesis, clinical features, treatment, and prognosis for oral and paraoral diseases. Likewise, such knowledge is also important for the medical profession, especially those who specialize in such areas as otolaryngology, dermatology, and pathology.

The purpose of this text is to provide the reader with a comprehensive discussion of the wide variety of diseases that may affect the oral and maxillofacial region. The book has been organized to serve as a primary teaching text, although it should also be useful as a reference source for the practicing clinician. Chapters have been created that include disease processes of a similar source (e.g., "Bacterial Infections," "Salivary Gland Pathology," "Bone Pathology," "Dermatologic Diseases"), because the basic understanding of pathology is facilitated by discussing diseases of a similar nature at the same time. It is only after attaining this basic understanding that the clinician can tackle the difficult task of clinical diagnosis and treatment. With this in mind, a comprehensive Appendix is included at the end of the book to help the clinician with the differential diagnosis of oral and maxillofacial disease processes.

It is impossible to write a book that perfectly matches the requirements of every reader. Because all of the authors are involved in teaching, the choice of subjects selected for inclusion within this text primarily reflects what is taught in courses on Oral and Maxillofacial Pathology. Although dental caries is undeniably a common and important disease affecting the oral cavity, it is usually not taught in an Oral and Maxillofacial Pathology course but elsewhere in most dental schools' curricula. Therefore, we have not included a chapter on dental caries. Likewise, our discussion on common gingivitis and periodontitis is limited in scope, although more indepth discussion is provided for other conditions that affect the periodontium. In other areas, the text may be greater in detail than necessary for some primary courses in Oral and Maxillofacial Pathology. However, because this book is also intended as a reference source for the practicing clinician, this additional material has been included.

This book obviously could not have been accomplished without the help of many other individuals. We were most fortunate to have Dr. Charles Waldron (one of the persons to whom this book is dedicated) write two outstanding chapters on areas of his special interest and expertise, "Bone Pathology" and "Odontogenic Cysts and Tumors." We also thank Dr. Edward Herschaft, who wrote an excellent chapter, "Forensic Dentistry."

Special thanks and praise go to Mr. Thomson Rast for his many hours of hard work to prepare most of the illustrations for the book. We are also indebted to many of our colleagues who shared cases with us, and they have been credited in the legends of the illustrations. Although the list is too numerous to cite here, one person in particular, Dr. George Blozis, deserves special recognition for his generosity in sharing his excellent teaching collection. We have attempted to be as thorough as possible in listing credit for all of the cases shared with us. However, if someone's name has been inadvertently omitted, please accept our apologies.

We express our sincere appreciation to several drug companies that provided financial help for this project: Pfizer, Inc.; Miles, Inc.; Chemex Pharmaceuticals, Inc.; and Schering Laboratories. Their aid enabled us to expand the number of color illustrations that we have included in the book.

We also would like to thank the people at the W.B. Saunders Company for their work in making this book a success—especially Larry McGrew, Dolores Meloni, and Ray Kersey. They were instrumental in keeping us on schedule, answering questions, fixing our mistakes, and taking care of innumerable details to make our task easier.

Finally, our deepest thanks must go to our families for their support during the writing of this book. They have had to endure our neglect during the long hours of work, and this project could never have been completed without their love and encouragement.

BRAD W. NEVILLE

DOUGLAS D. DAMM

CARL M. ALLEN

JERRY E. BOUQUOT

Contents

13

14

15

Color Plates

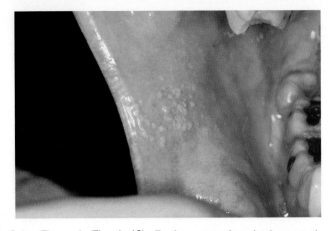

Color Figure 1 (Fig. 1–10). **Fordyce granules**. Lesions at the commissure.

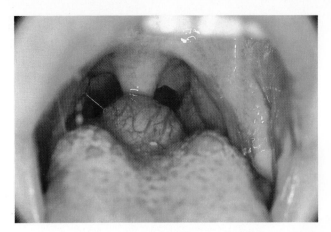

Color Figure 4 (Fig. 1–20). **Lingual thyroid**. Nodular mass of the posterior dorsal midline of the tongue in a 4-year-old girl.

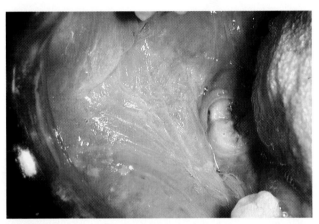

Color Figure 2 (Fig. 1–13). **Leukoedema**. Diffuse white appearance of the buccal mucosa.

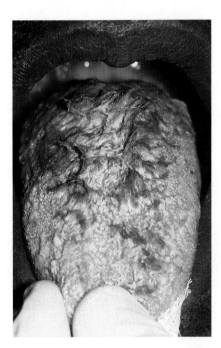

Color Figure 5 (Fig. 1–25). **Hairy tongue**. Marked elongation and brown staining of the filiform papillae resulting in a hair-like appearance. (Courtesy of Dr. Robert Strohaver.)

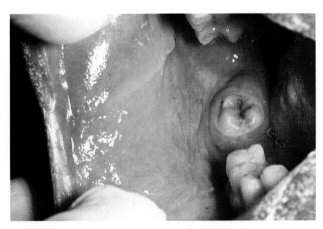

Color Figure 3 (Fig. 1–14). **Leukoedema**. Same lesion as depicted in Color Figure 2 showing disappearance of whiteness when the cheek is stretched.

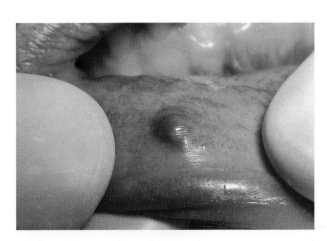

Color Figure 6 (Fig. 1–28). **Varicosity**. Firm, thrombosed varix on the lower lip.

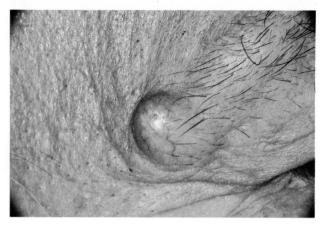

Color Figure 7 (Fig. 1–63). **Epidermoid cyst**. Fluctuant nodule at the lateral edge of the eyebrow.

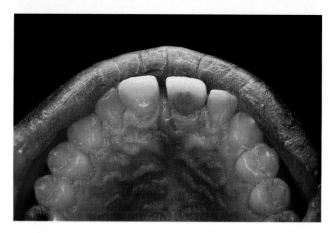

Color Figure 10 (Fig. 2–18). **Internal resorption (pink tooth of Mummery)**. Pink discoloration of the maxillary central incisor.

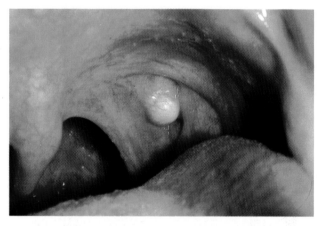

Color Figure 8 (Fig. 1–75). **Oral lymphoepithelial cyst**. Small yellow-white nodule of the tonsillar fossa.

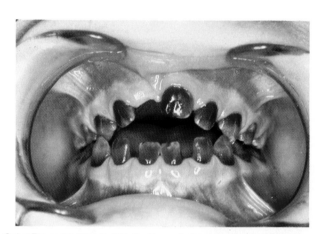

Color Figure 11 (Fig. 2–30). **Erythropoietic porphyria-related discoloration of teeth**. Reddish-brown discoloration of the maxillary dentition.

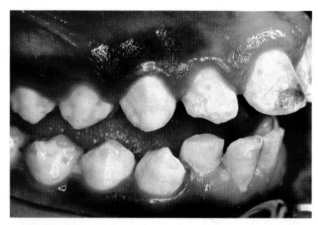

Color Figure 9 (Fig. 2–7). **Dental fluorosis**. Dentition exhibiting lusterless, white, and opaque enamel.

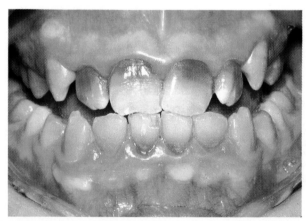

Color Figure 12 (Fig. 2–31). **Hyperbilirubinemia-related tooth discoloration**. Diffuse grayish-blue discoloration of the dentition. Cervical portions are stained most intensely. (Courtesy of Dr. John Giunta.)

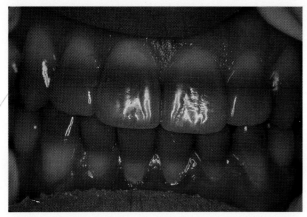

Color Figure 13 (Fig. 2–32). **Tetracycline-related tooth discoloration.** Diffuse brownish discoloration of the permanent dentition. (Courtesy of Dr. John Fantasia.)

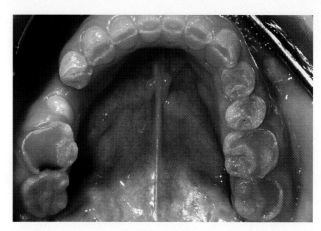

Color Figure 16 (Fig. 2–99). **Dentinogenesis imperfecta.** Dentition exhibiting grayish discoloration with significant enamel loss and attrition.

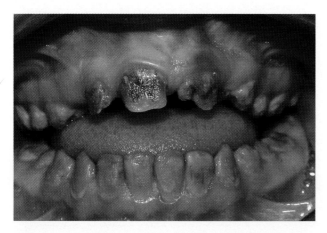

Color Figure 14 (Fig. 2–94). **Hypocalcified amelogenesis imperfecta.** Dentition exhibiting diffuse yellow-brown discoloration. Note numerous teeth with loss of coronal enamel except for the cervical portion.

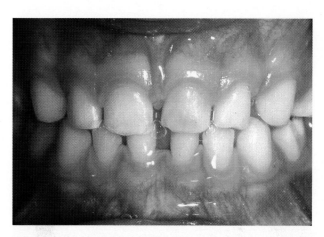

Color Figure 17 (Fig. 3–8). **Calcific metamorphosis.** Left deciduous maxillary central incisor exhibiting yellow discoloration. (Courtesy of Dr. Jackie L. Banahan.)

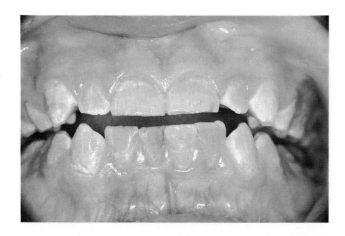

Color Figure 15 (Fig. 2–98). **Dentinogenesis imperfecta.** Dentition exhibiting diffuse brownish discoloration and slight translucence.

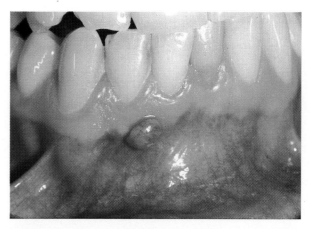

Color Figure 18 (Fig. 3–43). **Parulis.** Asymptomatic yellowish nodule of the anterior mandibular alveolar ridge. Adjacent teeth were clinically normal and also asymptomatic.

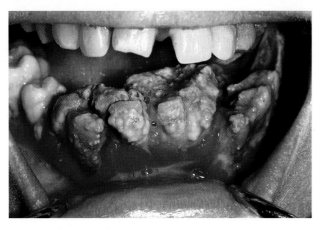

Color Figure 19 (Fig. 4–4). **Chronic gingivitis**. Bright-red gingiva is blunted, receded, and hyperplastic secondary to a total lack of oral hygiene. Note the extensive calculus build-up.

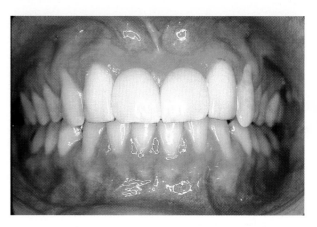

Color Figure 22 (Fig. 4–11). **Plasma cell gingivitis**. Same patient as depicted in Color Figure 21 after elimination of the inciting allergen. Note significant reduction in gingival enlargement and erythema. (Courtesy of Dr. George Blozis.)

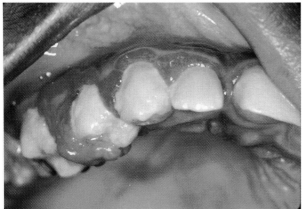

Color Figure 20 (Fig. 4–6). **Hyperplastic gingivitis with pyogenic granuloma**. Diffuse erythematous enlargement of marginal and papillary gingiva with hemorrhagic, tumor-like proliferation (which arose during pregnancy) between the maxillary bicuspid and first molar.

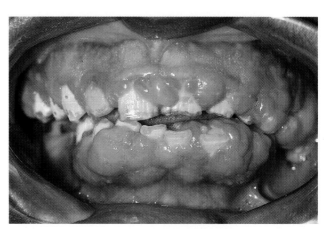

Color Figure 23 (Fig. 4–18). **Cyclosporine and nifedipine-related gingival hyperplasia**. Dramatic gingival hyperplasia in a patient using two drugs associated with gingival enlargement.

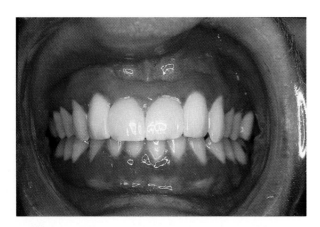

Color Figure 21 (Fig. 4–10). **Plasma cell gingivitis**. Diffuse, bright-red enlargement of the free and attached gingiva. (Courtesy of Dr. George Blozis.)

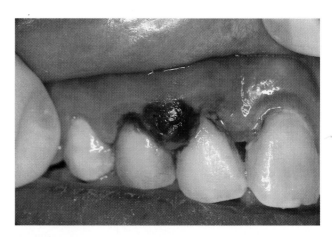

Color Figure 24 (Fig. 4–32). **Periodontal abscess**. Dark-red and hemorrhagic enlargement of the interdental papilla between the maxillary right lateral incisor and cuspid.

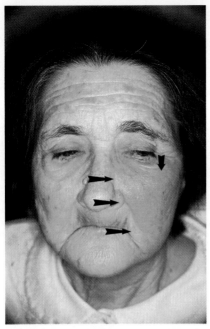

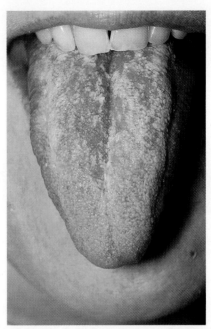

Color Figure 25 (Fig. 5–2). **Erysipelas**. Red, swollen area of the left cheek (*arrows*).

Color Figure 28 (Fig. 6–3). **Erythematous candidiasis**. The patchy, denuded areas (not the white areas) of the dorsal tongue represent erythematous candidiasis. The patient had received broad-spectrum antibiotics.

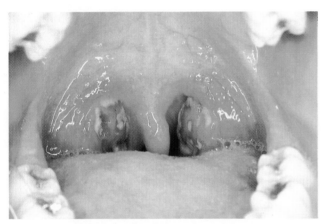

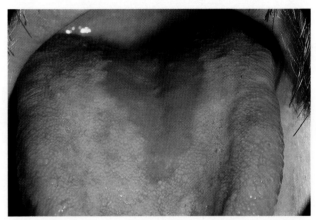

Color Figure 26 (Fig. 5–3). **Tonsillitis**. Hyperplastic pharyngeal tonsils with yellowish exudate of crypts.

Color Figure 29 (Fig. 6–4). **Erythematous candidiasis**. Severe presentation of central papillary atrophy. In this patient, the lesion was asymptomatic.

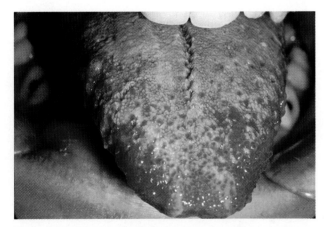

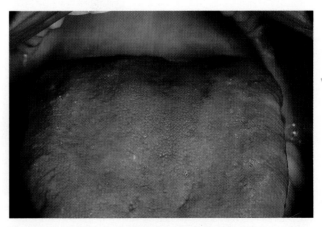

Color Figure 27 (Fig. 5–4). **Scarlet fever**. Dorsal surface of the tongue exhibiting white coating in association with numerous enlarged and erythematous fungiform papillae (white strawberry tongue).

Color Figure 30 (Fig. 6–5). **Erythematous candidiasis**. Same patient as depicted in Color Figure 29. Two weeks after antifungal therapy with fluconazole, there was marked regeneration of the dorsal tongue papillae.

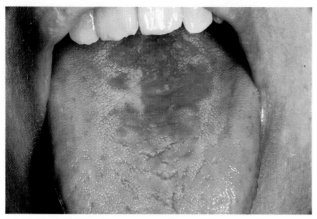

Color Figure 31 (Fig. 6–6). **Candidiasis**. Multifocal oral candidiasis, characterized by central papillary atrophy of the tongue as well as other areas of involvement.

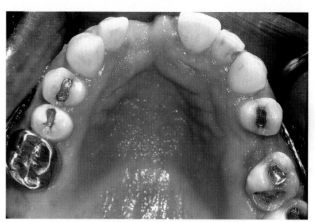

Color Figure 34 (Fig. 6–9). **Denture stomatitis**. Denture stomatitis in association with an interim partial denture. Note that the mucosal alteration is confined to the denture-bearing mucosa.

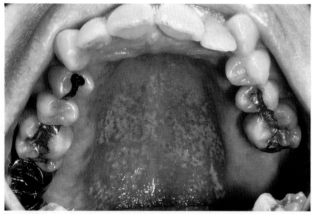

Color Figure 32 (Fig. 6–7). **Candidiasis**. Same patient as in Color Figure 31. A "kissing" lesion of oral candidiasis involves the hard palate.

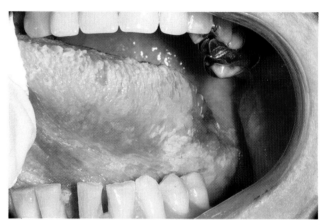

Color Figure 35 (Fig. 6–12A). **Hyperplastic candidiasis**. These diffuse white plaques clinically appear as leukoplakia, but they actually represent an unusual presentation of hyperplastic candidiasis.

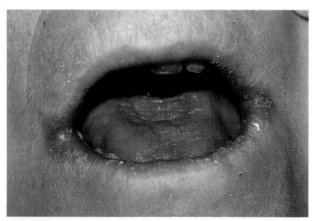

Color Figure 33 (Fig. 6–8). **Angular cheilitis**. Characteristic lesions appear as fissured, erythematous alterations of the skin at the corners of the mouth.

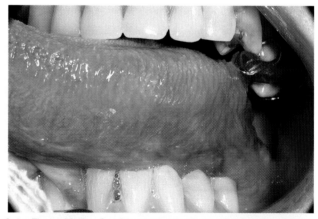

Color Figure 36 (Fig. 6–12B). **Hyperplastic candidiasis**. Treatment of the patient in Color Figure 35 with clotrimazole oral troches shows complete resolution of the white lesions within 2 weeks, essentially confirming the diagnosis of hyperplastic candidiasis. If any white mucosal alteration had persisted, a biopsy of that area would have been mandatory.

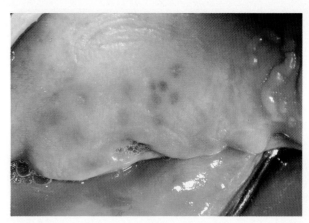

Color Figure 37 (Fig. 7–3). **Acute herpetic gingivostomatitis**. Painful, enlarged, and erythematous palatal gingiva.

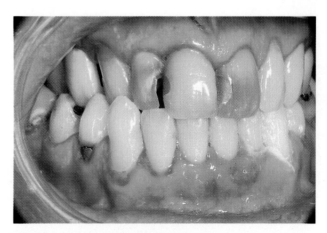

Color Figure 40 (Fig. 7–7). **Intraoral recurrent herpetic infection**. Early lesions presenting as multiple erythematous macules on the hard palate. Lesions had arisen a few days after extraction of a tooth.

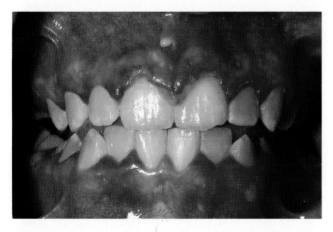

Color Figure 38 (Fig. 7–4). **Acute herpetic gingivostomatitis**. Painful, enlarged, and erythematous facial gingiva. Note erosions of the free gingival margin.

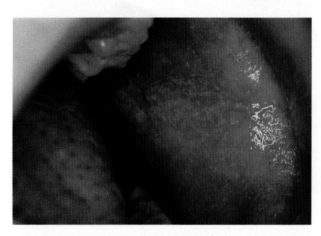

Color Figure 41 (Fig. 7–29). **Rubeola**. Numerous bluish-white Koplik spots of buccal mucosa. (Courtesy of Dr. Robert J. Achterberg.)

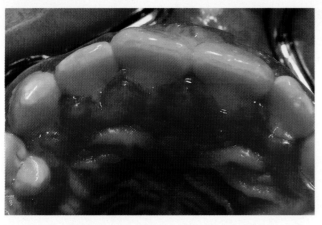

Color Figure 39 (Fig. 7–5). **Herpes labialis**. Multiple fluid-filled vesicles adjacent to the lip vermilion.

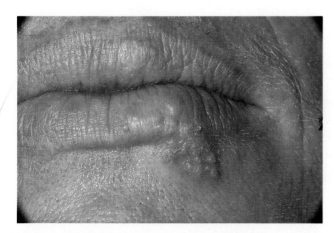

Color Figure 42 (Fig. 7–34). **HIV-associated gingivitis**. Band of erythema involving the free gingival margin.

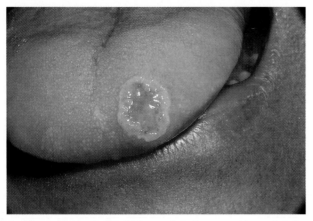

Color Figure 43 (Fig. 7–38). **HIV-associated recurrent herpetic infection**. Mucosal erosion of the anterior dorsal surface of the tongue on the left side. Note the yellowish circinate border.

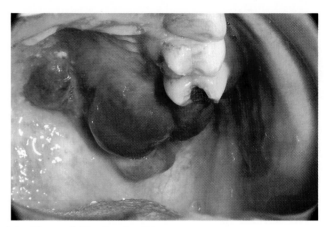

Color Figure 46 (Fig. 7–45). **HIV-associated Kaposi's sarcoma**. Diffuse, reddish-blue nodular enlargement of the left hard palate.

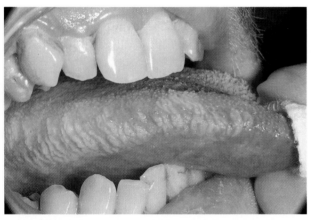

Color Figure 44 (Fig. 7–39). **HIV-associated oral hairy leukoplakia**. Vertical streaks of keratin along the lateral border of the tongue.

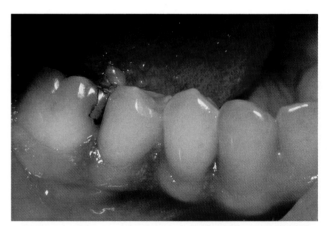

Color Figure 47 (Fig. 8–37). **Floss-related amalgam implantation**. Linear strips of mucosal pigmentation that align with the interdental papillae. The patient used dental floss on the mandibular first molar immediately after the placement of the amalgam restoration. Because the area was still anesthetized, the patient impaled the floss on the gingiva, then continued forward using the amalgam-impregnated floss in the bicuspid area to create additional amalgam tattoos.

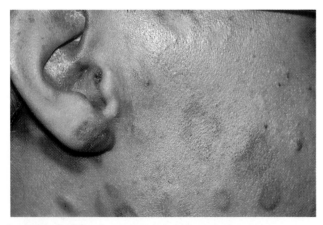

Color Figure 45 (Fig. 7–42). **HIV-associated Kaposi's sarcoma**. Multiple purple macules on the right side of the face.

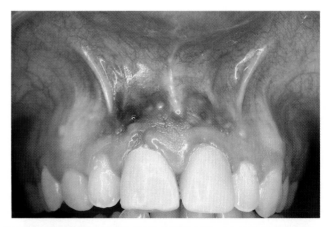

Color Figure 48 (Fig. 8–38). **Endodontic-related amalgam implantation**. Multifocal areas of mucosal discoloration overlying the maxillary anterior incisors, which have been treated with apical retrofill procedures.

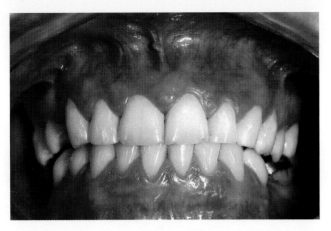

Color Figure 49 (Fig. 8–45). **Smoker's melanosis**. Light, diffuse melanin pigmentation in a white female who is a heavy smoker. Pigmentary changes are limited to the anterior facial gingiva.

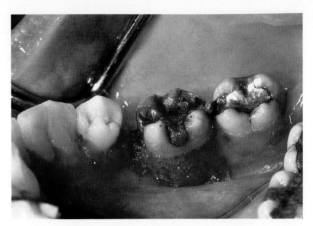

Color Figure 52 (Fig. 9–19). **Wegener's granulomatosis**. Hemorrhagic and friable gingiva (strawberry gingivitis) of the lingual mandible, which demonstrates numerous short bulbous projections. The area developed within 10 days after removal of similar lesions, which affected the entire facial gingiva of the anterior maxilla.

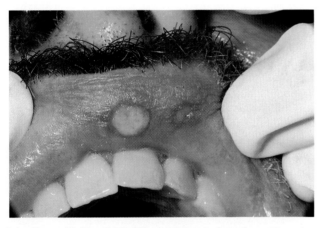

Color Figure 50 (Fig. 9–2). **Minor aphthous ulcerations**. Two ulcerations of different size located on the maxillary labial mucosa.

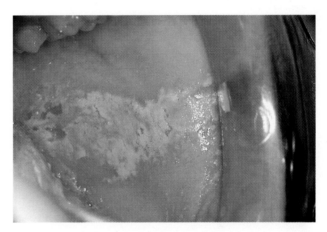

Color Figure 53 (Fig. 9–29). **Contact stomatitis from cinnamon flavoring**. Oblong area of sensitive erythema with overlying shaggy hyperkeratosis.

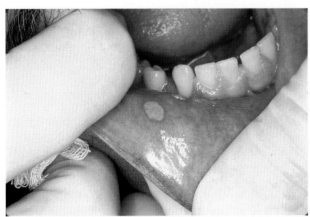

Color Figure 51 (Fig. 9–3). **Minor aphthous ulceration**. Single ulceration of the lower labial mucosa. (Courtesy of Dr. Dean K. White.)

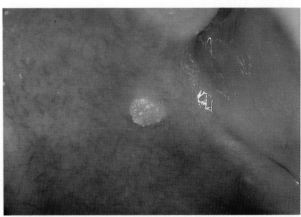

Color Figure 54 (Fig. 10–1). **Squamous papilloma**. An exophytic lesion of the soft palate with multiple short, white surface projections.

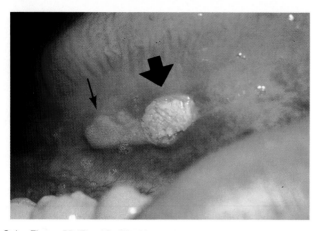

Color Figure 55 (Fig. 10–23). **Verruciform xanthoma**. A lesion of the ventral tongue exhibits a biphasic appearance. The anterior aspect demonstrates elongated white (well-keratinized) projections (*large arrow*). The posterior aspect demonstrates a surface of yellow, blunted projections (*small arrow*).

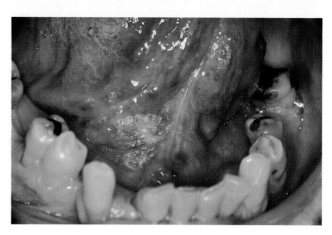

Color Figure 58 (Fig. 10–66). **Erythroleukoplakia**. Rough red and white lesion in the floor of the mouth. Biopsy revealed invasive squamous cell carcinoma.

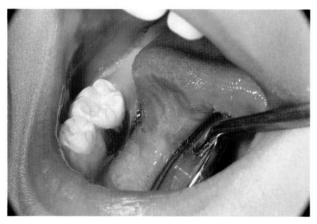

Color Figure 56 (Fig. 10–54). **Congenital melanocytic nevus**. Deeply pigmented lesion of the lingual mandibular gingiva in a 3-year-old child.

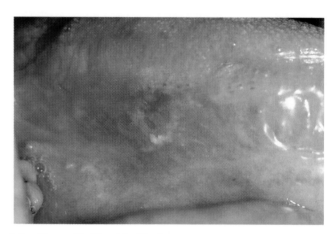

Color Figure 59 (Fig. 10–67). **Erythroleukoplakia**. Mixed red and white lesion of the lateral border of the tongue. Biopsy revealed carcinoma *in situ*.

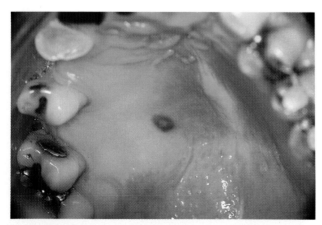

Color Figure 57 (Fig. 10–55). **Blue nevus**. A well-circumscribed, deep-blue macular lesion is seen on palatal mucosa.

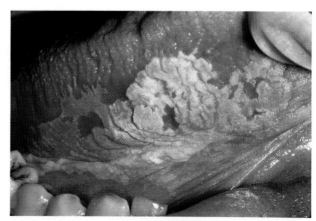

Color Figure 60 (Fig. 10–68). **Leukoplakia**. Extensive ventral and lateral tongue lesion containing multiple areas representing the various possible phases or clinical appearances.

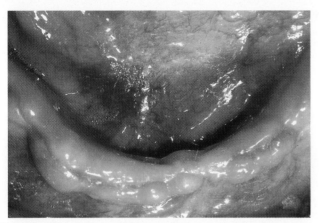

Color Figure 61 (Fig. 10–76). **Erythroplakia**. An erythematous macular lesion is seen on the right floor of the mouth with no associated leukoplakia. Biopsy showed early invasive squamous cell carcinoma.

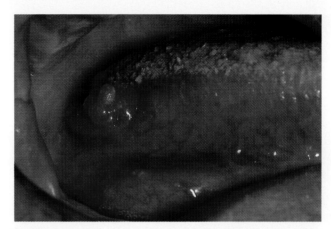

Color Figure 64 (Fig. 10–93). **Squamous cell carcinoma**. An exophytic lesion of the posterior lateral tongue demonstrates surface nodularity and minimal surface keratin production. It is painless and indurated.

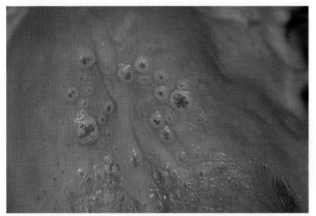

Color Figure 62 (Fig. 10–83). **Nicotine stomatitis**. Closeup of the inflamed ductal openings of involved salivary glands of the hard palate. Note the white keratotic ring at the lip of many of the inflamed ducts.

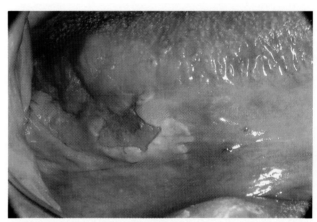

Color Figure 65 (Fig. 10–101). **Squamous cell carcinoma**. Ulcerated lesion with surrounding leukoplakia on the posterior lateral and ventral tongue.

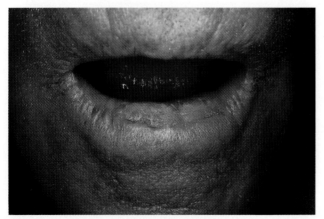

Color Figure 63 (Fig. 10–89). **Actinic cheilosis**. A blurring of the interface between the vermilion mucosa and the skin of the lip is especially noted in this case.

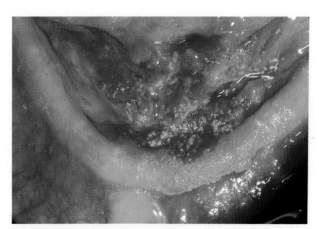

Color Figure 66 (Fig. 10–103). **Squamous cell carcinoma**. Oral floor lesions are typically ulcerated or present as an admixed red and white pebbled surface change, as depicted here.

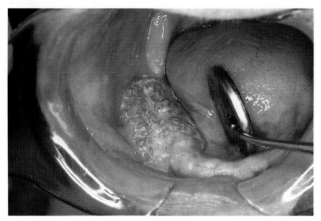

Color Figure 67 (Fig. 10–104). **Squamous cell carcinoma**. An exophytic lesion with an irregular and pebbled surface has a linear indentation along its facial aspect resulting from pressure from the patient's lower denture. Underlying alveolar bone was extensively destroyed.

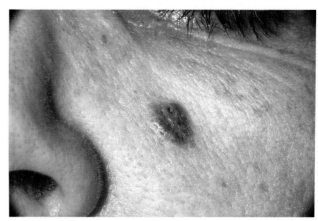

Color Figure 70 (Fig. 10–126). **Basal cell carcinoma**. Pigmented basal cell carcinoma of the cheek.

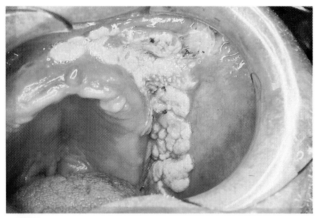

Color Figure 68 (Fig. 10–114). **Verrucous carcinoma**. Extensive papillary, white lesion of the maxillary vestibule.

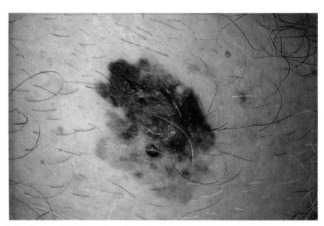

Color Figure 71 (Fig. 10–131). **Superficial spreading melanoma**. This lesion also demonstrates the ABCD warning signs of melanoma: **a**symmetry, **b**order irregularity, **c**olor variegation, and **d**iameter larger than a pencil eraser.

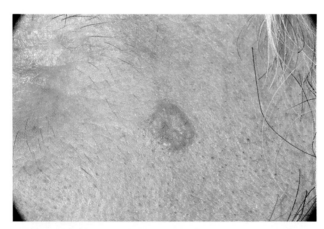

Color Figure 69 (Fig. 10–124). **Basal cell carcinoma**. Early noduloulcerative basal cell carcinoma of the facial skin showing raised, rolled borders and a central depression. Fine, telangiectatic blood vessels can be seen on the surface.

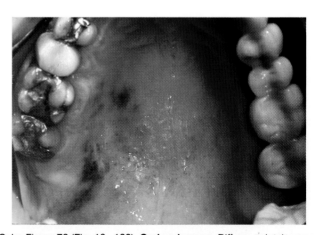

Color Figure 72 (Fig. 10–133). **Oral melanoma**. Diffuse, splotchy area of pigmentation of the lateral hard palate.

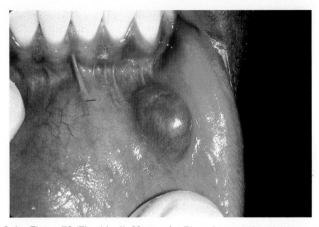

Color Figure 73 (Fig. 11–1). **Mucocele**. Blue-pigmented nodule on the lower lip.

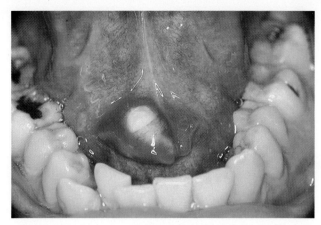

Color Figure 76 (Fig. 11–12). **Sialolithiasis**. Hard mass at the orifice of Wharton's duct.

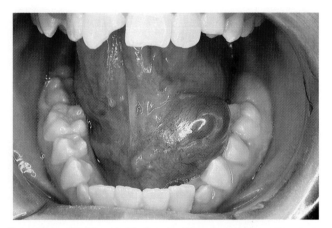

Color Figure 74 (Fig. 11–7). **Ranula**. Blue-pigmented swelling in the left floor of the mouth. (Courtesy of Dr. George Blozis.)

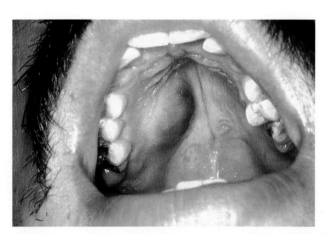

Color Figure 77 (Fig. 11–54). **Mucoepidermoid carcinoma**. Blue-pigmented mass of the posterior lateral hard palate. (Courtesy of Dr. James F. Drummond.)

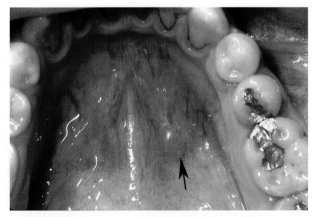

Color Figure 75 (Fig. 11–9). **Salivary duct cyst**. Nodular swelling (*arrow*) overlying Wharton's duct.

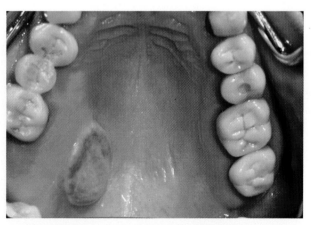

Color Figure 78 (Fig. 11–73). **Polymorphous low-grade adenocarcinoma**. Ulcerated mass of the posterior lateral hard palate.

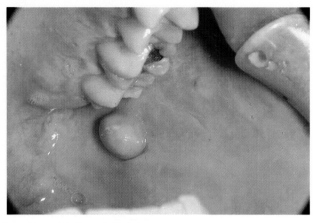

Color Figure 79 (Fig. 12–2). **Irritation fibroma**. Nodule of the posterior buccal mucosa near the level of the occlusal plane.

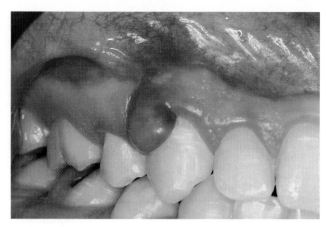

Color Figure 82 (Fig. 12–35). **Peripheral giant cell granuloma**. Nodular reddish-purple mass of the maxillary gingiva. (Courtesy of Dr. Lewis Claman.)

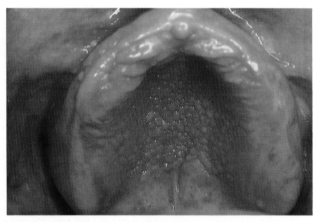

Color Figure 80 (Fig. 12–18). **Inflammatory papillary hyperplasia**. An advanced case exhibiting more pronounced papular lesions of the hard palate.

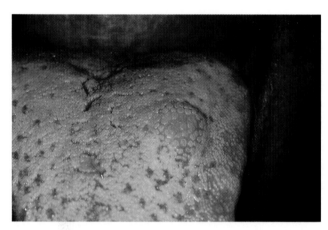

Color Figure 83 (Fig. 12–78). **Granular cell tumor**. Submucosal nodule on the dorsum of the tongue.

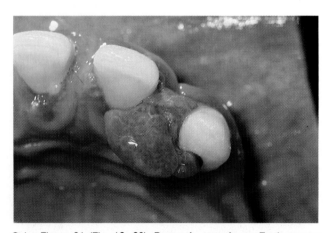

Color Figure 81 (Fig. 12–30). **Pyogenic granuloma**. Erythematous, hemorrhagic mass arising from the maxillary anterior gingiva.

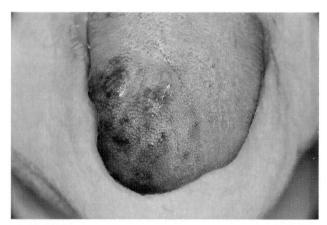

Color Figure 84 (Fig. 12–86). **Hemangioma**. Mass of the anterior tongue.

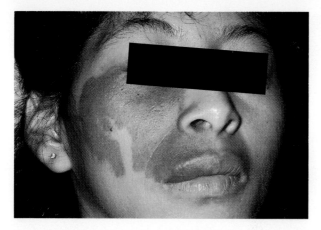

Color Figure 85 (Fig. 12–92). **Port-wine stain**. "Nevus flammeus" of the malar area in a patient without Sturge-Weber angiomatosis. Unless the vascular lesion includes the region innervated by the ophthalmic branch of the trigeminal nerve, the patient usually does not have central nervous system involvement.

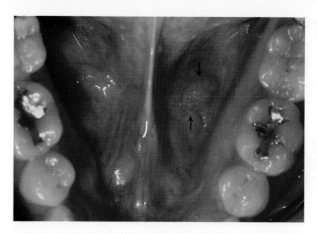

Color Figure 88 (Fig. 13–3). **Lymphoid hyperplasia**. Lymphoid aggregates (*arrows*) are frequently noted in the floor of the mouth, as in this photograph.

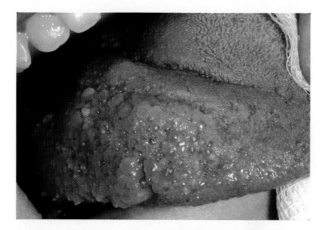

Color Figure 86 (Fig. 12–102). **Lymphangioma**. Pebbly, vesicle-like appearance of a tumor of the right lateral tongue.

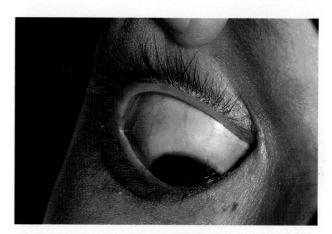

Color Figure 89 (Fig. 14–1). **Osteogenesis imperfecta**. Blue sclera in a patient with osteogenesis imperfecta.

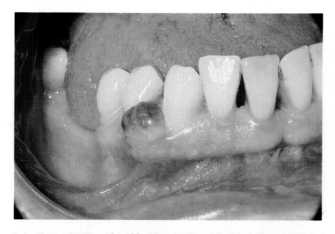

Color Figure 87 (Fig. 12–138). **Metastatic melanoma**. Pigmented nodule of the mandibular gingiva.

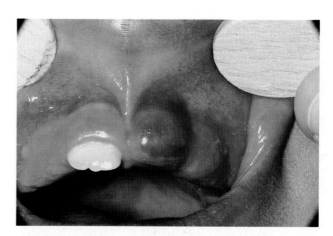

Color Figure 90 (Fig. 15–8). **Eruption cyst**. This soft gingival swelling contains considerable blood and can also be designated as an eruption hematoma.

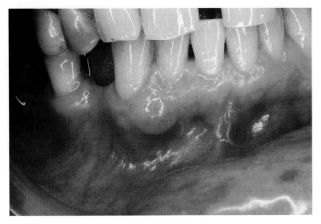

Color Figure 91 (Fig. 15–28). **Gingival cyst of the adult**. Tense, fluid-filled swelling on the facial gingiva.

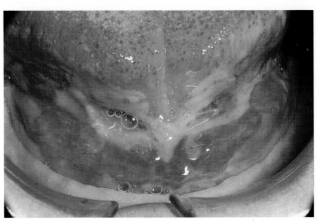

Color Figure 94 (Fig. 16–42). **Pemphigus vulgaris**. Large, irregularly shaped ulcerations involving the floor of the mouth and ventral tongue.

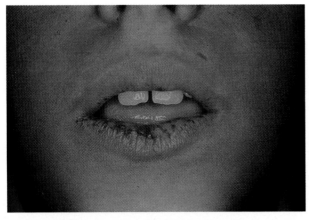

Color Figure 92 (Fig. 16–22). **Peutz-Jeghers syndrome**. Oral manifestations include multiple, dark, freckle-like lesions of the lips. (Courtesy of Dr. Ahmed Uthman.)

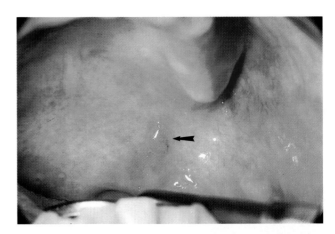

Color Figure 95 (Fig. 16–52). **Cicatricial pemphigoid**. One or more intraoral vesicles, as seen on the soft palate (*arrow*), may be detected in patients with cicatricial pemphigoid. Usually, ulcerations of the oral mucosa are also present.

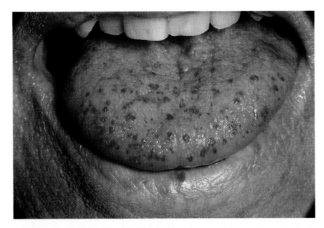

Color Figure 93 (Fig. 16–23). **Hereditary hemorrhagic telangiectasia**. The tongue of this patient shows multiple red papules, which represent superficial collections of dilated capillary spaces.

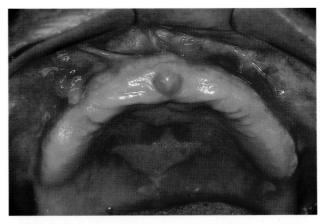

Color Figure 96 (Fig. 16–53). **Cicatricial pemphigoid**. Large, irregular oral ulcerations characterize the lesions after the initial bullae rupture.

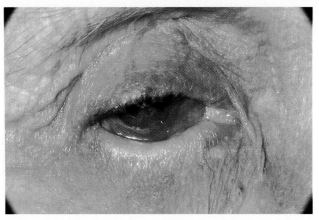

Color Figure 97 (Fig. 16–57). **Cicatricial pemphigoid**. A patient with ocular involvement shows severe conjunctival inflammation. The lower eyelashes were removed by an ophthalmologist because of trichiasis associated with entropion.

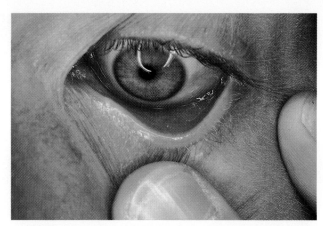

Color Figure 100 (Fig. 16–66). **Stevens-Johnson syndrome**. With erythema multiforme major (Stevens-Johnson syndrome), other mucosal surfaces may show involvement, such as the severe conjunctivitis depicted in this photograph.

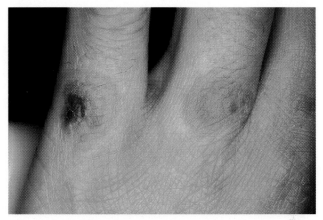

Color Figure 98 (Fig. 16–63). **Erythema multiforme**. The concentric erythematous pattern of the cutaneous lesions on the fingers resembles a target or bull's-eye.

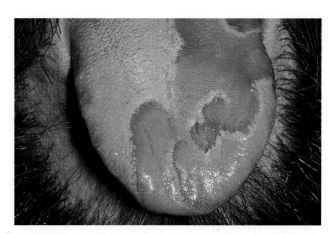

Color Figure 101 (Fig. 16–72). **Erythema migrans**. The erythematous, well-demarcated areas of papillary atrophy are characteristic of erythema migrans affecting the tongue (benign migratory glossitis). Note the asymmetric distribution and the tendency to involve the lateral aspects of the tongue.

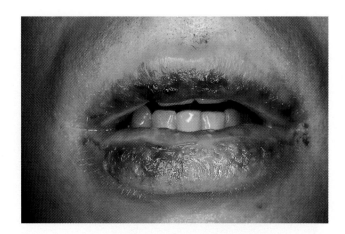

Color Figure 99 (Fig. 16–65). **Erythema multiforme**. Ulceration of the labial mucosa with hemorrhagic crusting of the vermilion zone of the lips.

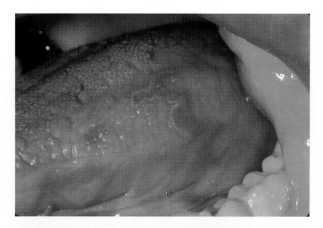

Color Figure 102 (Fig. 16–74). **Erythema migrans**. This photograph illustrates the slightly elevated, yellowish-white, scalloped margin that is characteristically associated with the periphery of the erythematous, atrophic regions.

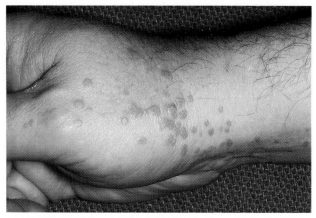

Color Figure 103 (Fig. 16–78). **Lichen planus**. The cutaneous lesions on the wrist appear as purple, polygonal papules. Careful examination shows a network of fine white lines (Wickham's striae) on the surface of the papules.

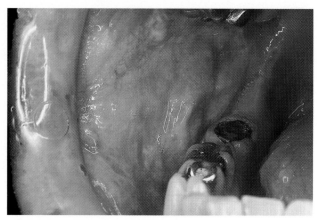

Color Figure 106 (Fig. 16–91). **Lichen planus**. These relatively nondescript white lesions affected the buccal mucosa of a patient who had complained of a burning sensation. Histopathologic evaluation of the lesion showed a lichenoid mucositis with superimposed candidiasis.

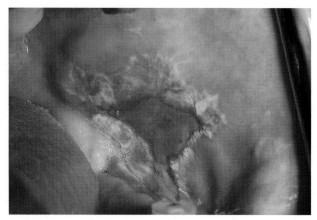

Color Figure 104 (Fig. 16–85). **Lichen planus**. Ulceration of the buccal mucosa shows peripheral radiating keratotic striae, characteristic of oral erosive lichen planus.

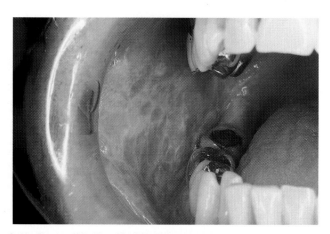

Color Figure 107 (Fig. 16–92). **Lichen planus**. Same patient as depicted in Color Figure 106 two weeks following antifungal therapy. Once the mucosal reaction to the candidal organism has been eliminated, the characteristic white striae of reticular lichen planus can be identified.

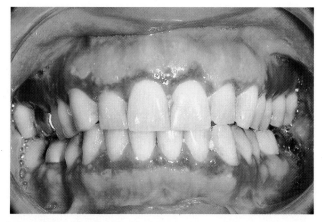

Color Figure 105 (Fig. 16–88). **Lichen planus**. Erosive lichen planus often presents as a desquamative gingivitis, producing gingival erythema and tenderness.

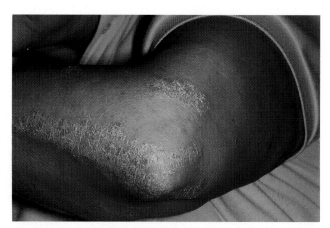

Color Figure 108 (Fig. 16–98). **Psoriasis**. Characteristic cutaneous lesions on the skin of the elbow. Note the erythematous plaques surmounted by silvery keratotic scales.

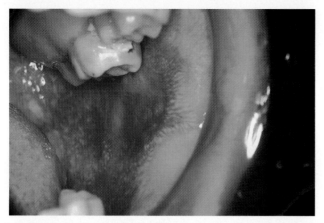

Color Figure 109 (Fig. 16–104). **Chronic cutaneous lupus erythematosus**. Erythematous zones of the buccal mucosa are surrounded by radiating keratotic striae. These features are similar to those of erosive lichen planus.

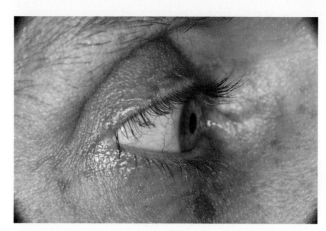

Color Figure 112 (Fig. 17–4). **Jaundice**. The yellow color of the sclera represents a common finding.

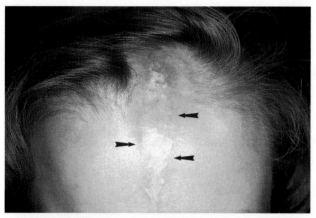

Color Figure 110 (Fig. 16–114). **Localized scleroderma**. The cutaneous alteration on the patient's forehead (*arrows*) represents a limited form of scleroderma called *coup de sabre* because the lesion resembles a scar that might result from a cut with a sword.

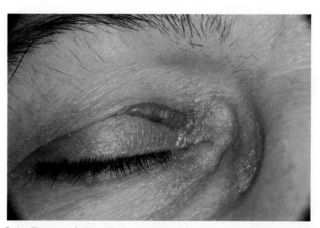

Color Figure 113 (Fig. 17–5). **Amyloidosis**. This patient exhibits a firm, waxy nodular lesion in the periocular region, a finding characteristic for this condition.

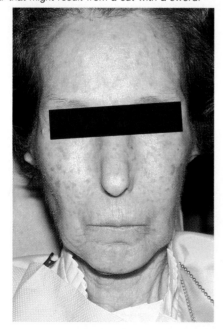

Color Figure 111 (Fig. 16–118). **CREST syndrome**. The patient shows numerous red facial macules representing telangiectatic blood vessels.

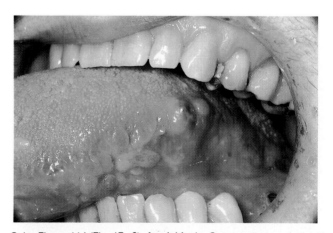

Color Figure 114 (Fig. 17–6). **Amyloidosis**. Same patient as depicted in Color Figure 113. Note amyloid nodules of lateral tongue, some of which are ulcerated. The patient's amyloidosis was due to previously undiagnosed multiple myeloma.

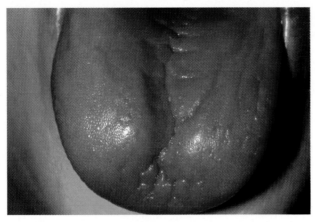

Color Figure 115 (Fig. 17-10). **Plummer-Vinson syndrome**. The diffuse papillary atrophy of the dorsal tongue is characteristic of the oral changes. (From Neville BW, Damm DD, White DK, Waldron CA. Color Atlas of Clinical Oral Pathology. Philadelphia, Lea & Febiger, 1991, p 319.)

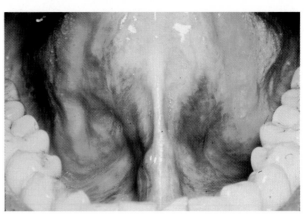

Color Figure 118 (Fig. 17-31). **Addison's disease**. Diffuse pigmentation of the floor of the mouth and ventral tongue in a patient with Addison's disease. (Courtesy of Dr. George Blozis.)

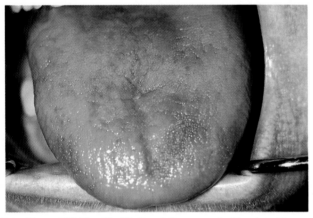

Color Figure 116 (Fig. 17-11). **Pernicious anemia**. The dorsal tongue shows erythema and atrophy.

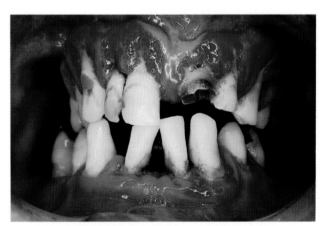

Color Figure 119 (Fig. 17-32). **Diabetes mellitus**. The diffuse, strikingly erythematous enlargement of the gingival tissues is an oral feature that has been identified in diabetic patients.

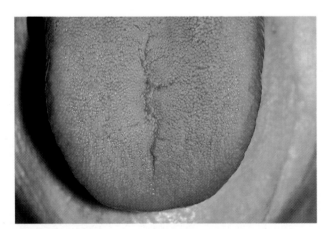

Color Figure 117 (Fig. 17-12). **Pernicious anemia**. Same patient as depicted in Color Figure 116. After therapy with vitamin B$_{12}$, the mucosal alteration resolved.

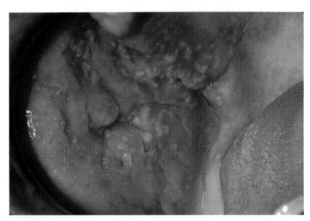

Color Figure 120 (Fig. 17-40). **Pyostomatitis vegetans**. The characteristic lesions are seen on the buccal mucosa, presenting as yellow-white, "snail-track" pustules.

1

Developmental Defects of the Oral and Maxillofacial Region

OROFACIAL CLEFTS

The formation of the face and oral cavity is complex in nature and involves the development of multiple tissue processes that must merge and fuse in a highly orchestrated fashion. Disturbances in the growth of these tissue processes or their fusion may result in the formation of **orofacial clefts.**

Development of the central face begins with the appearance of the nasal placodes on either side of the inferior aspect of the frontonasal process. Proliferation of ectomesenchyme on both sides of each placode results in the formation of the medial and lateral nasal processes. Between each pair of processes is a depression, or nasal pit, that represents the primitive nostril.

During the sixth and seventh weeks of development, the upper lip forms when the medial nasal processes merge with each other and with the maxillary processes of the first branchial arches. Thus, the midportion of the upper lip is derived from the medial nasal processes and the lateral portions are derived from the maxillary processes. The lateral nasal processes are not involved in the formation of the upper lip, but they give rise to the alae of the nose.

The **primary palate** is also formed by the merger of the medial nasal processes to form the intermaxillary segment. This segment gives rise to the premaxilla, a triangular-shaped piece of bone that will include the four incisor teeth. The **secondary palate,** which makes up 90 percent of the hard and soft palates, is formed from the maxillary processes of the first branchial arches.

During the sixth week, bilateral projections emerge from the medial aspects of the maxillary processes to form the palatal shelves. Initially, these shelves are oriented in a vertical position on each side of the developing tongue. As the mandible grows, the tongue drops down, allowing the palatal shelves to rotate to a horizontal position and grow toward one another. By the eighth week, sufficient growth has occurred to allow the anterior aspects of these shelves to begin fusion with one another. The palatal shelves also fuse with the primary palate and the nasal septum. The fusion of the palatal shelves begins in the anterior palate and progresses posteriorly, to be completed by around the 12th week.

Defective fusion of the medial nasal process with the maxillary process leads to **cleft lip** (CL). Likewise, failure of the palatal shelves to fuse results in **cleft palate** (CP). Frequently, CL and CP occur together. Approximately 45 percent of cases present as CL + CP, with 30 percent being isolated CP and 25 percent being isolated CL. Both isolated CL and CL associated with CP are thought to be etiologically related conditions and can be considered as a group: cleft lip, with or without cleft palate (CL ± CP). **Isolated cleft palate** appears to represent a separate entity from CL ± CP.

The etiology of CL ± CP and CP is still being debated. First of all, it is important to distinguish isolated clefts from cases associated with specific syndromes. Although most facial clefts are isolated anomalies, more than 250 developmental syndromes have been identified that may be associated with CL ± CP or CP. Some of these syndromes are single-gene conditions that may

1

follow autosomal dominant, autosomal recessive, or X-linked inheritance patterns. Other syndromes are the result of chromosome anomalies or are idiopathic. The cause of nonsyndromic clefts does not follow any simple mendelian pattern of inheritance but appears to be heterogeneous. Thus, the propensity for cleft development may be related to a number of major genes, minor genes, and environmental factors that can combine to surpass a developmental threshold.

CL ± CP and CP represent the vast majority of orofacial clefts. However, other rare clefts may also occur.

The **lateral facial cleft** is caused by lack of fusion of the maxillary and mandibular processes and represents 0.3 percent of all facial clefts. The lateral facial cleft may occur as an isolated defect or may be associated with other disorders, such as **mandibulofacial dysostosis** (see p. 39). This cleft may be unilateral or bilateral, extending from the commissure toward the ear, resulting in macrostomia.

The **oblique facial cleft** extends from the upper lip to the eye. It is nearly always associated with cleft palate, and severe forms are often incompatible with life. The oblique facial cleft may involve the nostril, as in cleft lip, or it may laterally bypass the nose as it extends to the eye. This cleft is rare, representing only 1 in 1300 facial clefts. Some of these clefts may represent failure of fusion of the lateral nasal process with the maxillary process; others may be caused by amniotic bands.

Median cleft of the upper lip is an extremely rare anomaly that results from failure of fusion of the medial nasal processes. It may be associated with a number of syndromes, including oral-facial-digital syndrome and Ellis–van Creveld syndrome. Most apparent median clefts of the upper lip actually represent agenesis of the primary palate associated with holoprosencephaly.

Median maxillary anterior alveolar clefts have also been reported. Such clefts may cause a bony defect in the midline of the maxilla between the central incisors.

Clinical and Radiographic Features

Clefting is one of the most common major congenital defects in humans. Considerable racial variation in prevalence is seen. In whites, CL ± CP occurs in 1 of every 700 to 1000 births. The frequency of CL ± CP in Oriental (Asian) populations is about 1.5 times higher than in whites. In contrast, the prevalence of CL ± CP in blacks is much lower, occurring in 0.4 per 1000 births. Native Americans appear to have the highest frequency, around 3.6 per 1000 births. Isolated CP is less common than CL ± CP, with a frequency of 0.4 per 1000 births in whites and blacks.

CL ± CP is more common in males than in females. The more severe the defect, the greater the male predilection; the male-to-female ratio for isolated CL is 1.5:1; the ratio for CL + CP is 2:1. In contrast, isolated CP is more common in females. Likewise, the more severe the cleft, the greater the female predilection. Clefts of both the hard and soft palates are twice as common in females, but the ratio is nearly equal for clefts of the soft palate only.

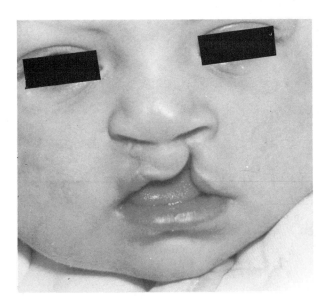

FIGURE 1–1. **Cleft lip.** Infant with bilateral cleft of the upper lip. (Courtesy of Dr. William Bruce.)

About 80 percent of cases of CL will be unilateral, with 20 percent bilateral (Fig. 1–1). Approximately 70 percent of unilateral CLs occur on the left side. A complete CL extends upward into the nostril, but an incomplete CL does not involve the nose. Complete clefts involving the alveolus usually occur between the lateral incisor and cuspid. It is not unusual for teeth, especially the lateral incisor, to be missing in the cleft area. Conversely, supernumerary teeth may be discovered. The bony defect can be observed on radiographs.

A cleft palate shows considerable range in severity (Fig. 1–2). The defect may involve the hard and soft palates or the soft palate alone. The most minimal manifestation of CP is a **cleft** or **bifid uvula** (Fig. 1–3). The prevalence of cleft uvula is much higher than that of cleft palate, with a frequency of 1 in every 80 white individuals. The frequency in Asian and Native American populations is as high as 1 in 10. Cleft uvula is less common in blacks, occurring in 1 out of every 250 persons.

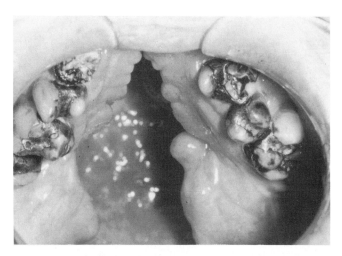

FIGURE 1–2. **Cleft palate.** Palatal defect resulting in communication with the nasal cavity.

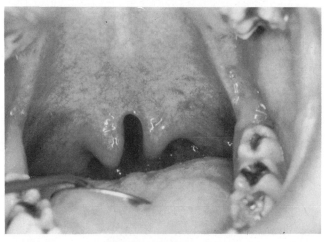

FIGURE 1–3. **Bifid uvula.**

In some instances, a **submucous palatal cleft** develops. The surface mucosa is intact, but there is a defect in the underlying musculature of the soft palate. Frequently, a notch in the bone is present along the posterior margin of the hard palate. This incomplete cleft occasionally appears as a bluish midline discoloration but is best identified by palpation with a blunt instrument. An associated cleft uvula also usually is seen.

The **Pierre Robin sequence** (Pierre Robin anomalad) (Fig. 1–4) is a well-recognized presentation characterized by cleft palate, mandibular micrognathia, and glossoptosis (airway obstruction due to lower, posterior displacement of the tongue). The Pierre Robin sequence may occur as an isolated phenomenon, or it may be associated with a wide variety of syndromes or other anomalies. It has been theorized that constraint of mandibular growth *in utero* results in failure of the tongue to descend, thus preventing fusion of the palatal shelves. The retruded mandible results in the following:

- Posterior displacement of the tongue
- Lack of support of the tongue musculature
- Airway obstruction

Respiratory difficulty, especially when the child is in a supine position, is usually noted from birth and can cause asphyxiation. The palatal cleft is often U-shaped and wider than isolated CP.

The patient with a cleft is burdened with a variety of problems, some obvious and some less so. The most obvious problem is the clinical appearance, which may lead to psychosocial difficulties. Feeding and speech difficulties are inherent, especially with CP. Malocclusion is caused by collapse of the maxillary arch, possibly along with missing teeth, supernumerary teeth, or both.

Treatment and Prognosis

The management of the patient with an orofacial cleft is challenging. Ideally, treatment should involve a multidisciplinary approach, including (but not limited to) a pediatrician, oral and maxillofacial surgeon, otolaryngologist, plastic surgeon, pediatric dentist, orthodontist, prosthodontist, speech pathologist, and geneticist.

Surgical repair often involves multiple primary and secondary procedures throughout childhood. The specific types of surgical procedures and their timing will vary, depending on the severity of the defect and the philosophy of the treatment team. A detailed discussion of these procedures is beyond the scope of this text. However, primary lip closure is usually accomplished during the first few months of life, followed later by repair of the palate. Prosthetic and orthopedic appliances are often used to mold or expand the maxillary segments before closure of the palatal defect. Later in childhood, autogenous bone grafts can be placed in the area of the alveolar bone defect. Secondary soft tissue and orthognathic procedures may be used to improve function and cosmetic appearance.

Genetic counseling is important for the patient and family. In nonsyndromic cases, the risk for cleft development in a sibling or offspring of an affected person is 3 to 5 percent if no other first-degree relatives are also affected. The risk increases to 10 to 20 percent if other first-degree relatives are affected. The risk may be even higher for those with clefts that are associated with syndromes, depending on the possible inheritance pattern.

COMMISSURAL LIP PITS

Commissural lip pits are small mucosal invaginations that occur at the corners of the mouth on the vermilion

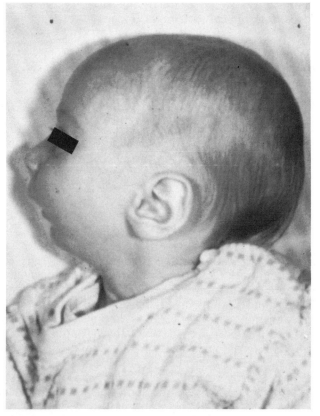

FIGURE 1–4. **Pierre Robin sequence.** Micrognathic mandible in an infant with cleft palate. (Courtesy of Dr. Robert Gorlin.)

border. Their location suggests that they may represent a failure of normal fusion of the embryonal maxillary and mandibular processes.

Commissural lip pits appear to be common in adults, where they have been reported in 12 to 20 percent of the population. Their prevalence in children is considerably lower, ranging from 0.2 to 0.7 percent of those examined.

Although commissural lip pits are generally considered to be congenital lesions, these figures suggest that these invaginations often develop later in life. Commissural pits are seen more often in males than in females. A family history suggestive of autosomal dominant transmission has been noted in some cases.

Clinical Features

Commissural lip pits are usually discovered on routine examination, and the patient is often unaware of their presence. These pits may be unilateral or bilateral. They present as blind fistulas that may extend to a depth of 1 to 4 mm (Fig. 1–5). In some cases, a small amount of fluid may be expressed from the pit when the pit is squeezed, presumably representing saliva from minor salivary glands that drain into the depth of the invagination.

Unlike **paramedian lower lip pits** (described next), commissural lip pits are not associated with facial or palatal clefts. However, there does appear to be a significantly higher incidence of preauricular pits (aural sinuses) in these patients.

Histopathologic Features

Although biopsy is rarely performed for patients with commissural lip pits, microscopic examination reveals a narrow invagination lined by stratified squamous epithelium. Ducts from minor salivary glands may drain into this invagination.

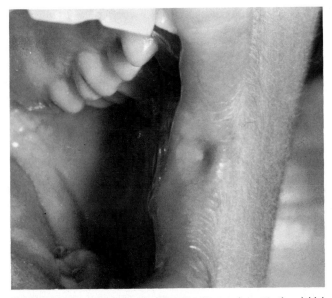

FIGURE 1–5. **Commissural lip pit.** Depression at the labial commissure.

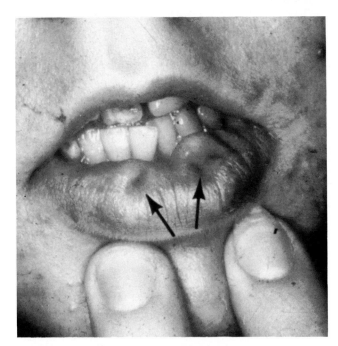

FIGURE 1–6. **Paramedian lip pits.** Bilateral pits (*arrows*) on the lower lip in a patient with van der Woude syndrome.

Treatment and Prognosis

Because commissural lip pits are virtually always asymptomatic and innocuous, no treatment is usually necessary. In extremely rare instances, salivary secretions may be excessive or secondary infection may occur, necessitating surgical excision of the pit.

PARAMEDIAN LIP PITS (Congenital Fistulas of the Lower Lip; Congenital Lip Pits)

Paramedian lip pits are rare congenital invaginations of the lower lip. They are believed to arise from persistence of the lateral sulci on the embryonic mandibular arch. These sulci normally disappear by 6 weeks of embryonic age.

Clinical Features

Paramedian lip pits typically present as bilateral and symmetric fistulas on either side of the midline of the vermilion of the lower lip (Fig. 1–6). Their appearance can range from subtle depressions to prominent humps. These blind sinuses can extend down to a depth of 1.5 cm and may express salivary secretions. Occasionally, only a single pit is present that may be centrally located or lateral to the midline.

The greatest significance of paramedian lip pits is that they are usually inherited as an autosomal dominant trait in combination with cleft lip and/or cleft palate (**van der Woude syndrome**). Some people who carry the trait may not demonstrate clefts or may have a submucous cleft palate; however, they may pass the full syndrome on to their offspring. Paramedian lip pits may also be a feature of the **popliteal pterygium syndrome,** characterized by popliteal webbing *(pterygia),* cleft lip and/or cleft palate, genital abnormalities, and congenital bands connecting the upper and lower jaws *(syngnathia).*

Histopathologic Features

Microscopic examination of a paramedian lip pit shows a tract that is lined by stratified squamous epithelium. Minor salivary glands may communicate with the sinus.

Treatment and Prognosis

If necessary, the labial pits may be excised for cosmetic reasons. The most significant problems are related to associated congenital anomalies, such as cleft lip and/or cleft palate and the potential for transmission of the trait to subsequent generations.

DOUBLE LIP

Double lip is a rare oral anomaly characterized by a redundant fold of tissue on the mucosal side of the lip. It is most often congenital in nature, but it may be acquired later in life. Congenital cases are believed to arise during the second to third month of gestation as a result of the persistence of the sulcus between the pars glabrosa and pars villosa of the lip. Acquired double lip may be a component of **Ascher syndrome,** or it may result from trauma or oral habits, such as sucking on the lip.

Clinical Features

In a patient with double lip, the upper lip is affected much more often than the lower lip, and occasionally both lips are involved. With the lips at rest, the condition is usually unnoticeable, but when the patient smiles or when the lips are tensed, the excess fold of tissue is visible (Fig. 1–7).

Ascher syndrome is characterized by a triad of features:

- Double lip
- Blepharochalasis
- Nontoxic thyroid enlargement

In a person with blepharochalasis, recurring edema of the upper eyelid leads to sagging of the lid at the outer canthus of the eye (Fig. 1–8). This drooping may be severe enough to interfere with vision. Both the double lip and blepharochalasis usually occur abruptly and simultaneously, but in some cases they develop more gradually.

The nontoxic thyroid enlargement occurs in about 50 percent of patients with Ascher syndrome and may be mild in degree. The cause of Ascher syndrome is not certain; autosomal dominant inheritance has been suggested in some cases.

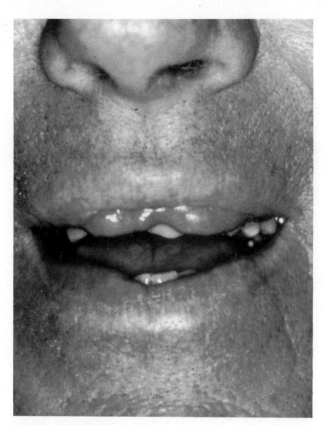

FIGURE 1–7. Double lip. Redundant fold of tissue on the upper lip in a patient with Ascher syndrome. (From Neville BW, Damm DD, White DK, Waldron CA. Color Atlas of Clinical Oral Pathology. Philadelphia, Lea & Febiger, 1991.)

Histopathologic Features

On microscopic examination, double lip shows essentially normal structures. Often there is an abundance of minor salivary glands. The blepharochalasis of Ascher syndrome usually shows hyperplasia of the lacrimal glands or prolapse of orbital fat.

Treatment and Prognosis

In mild cases of double lip, no treatment may be required. In more severe cases, simple surgical excision of the excess tissue can be performed for aesthetic purposes.

FORDYCE GRANULES

Fordyce granules are sebaceous glands that occur on the oral mucosa. Because sebaceous glands are typically considered to be dermal adnexal structures, those found in the oral cavity have often been considered to be "ectopic." However, because Fordyce granules have been reported in more than 80 percent of the population, their presence must be considered a normal anatomic variation.

Clinical Features

Fordyce granules present as multiple yellow or yellow-white papular lesions that are most common on the

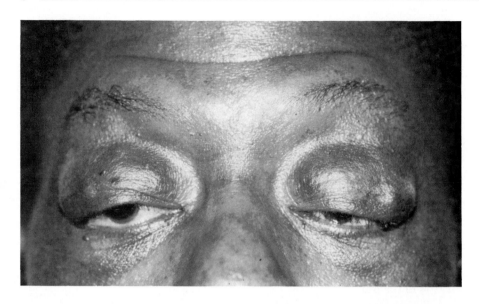

FIGURE 1–8. **Ascher syndrome.** Edema of the upper eyelids (blepharochalasis).

buccal mucosa and vermilion of the lateral upper lip (Figs. 1–9 and 1–10; see Color Figure 1). Occasionally, these glands may also appear in the retromolar area and anterior tonsillar pillar. They are more common in adults than in children, probably as a result of hormonal factors; puberty appears to stimulate their development. The lesions are typically asymptomatic, although patients may be able to feel a slight roughness to the mucosa. There may be considerable clinical variation; some patients may have only a few lesions, whereas others may have literally hundreds of these "granules."

Histopathologic Features

Except for the absence of associated hair follicles, Fordyce granules are closely similar to normal sebaceous glands found in the skin. Acinar lobules can be seen immediately beneath the epithelial surface, often communicating with the surface through a central duct (Fig. 1–11). The sebaceous cells in these lobules are polygonal in shape, containing centrally located nuclei and abundant foamy cytoplasm.

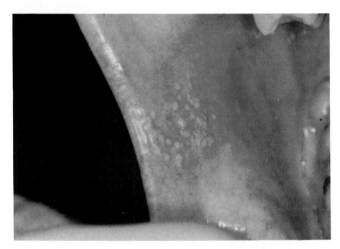

FIGURE 1–10. **Fordyce granules.** Lesions at the commissure. See Color Plates.

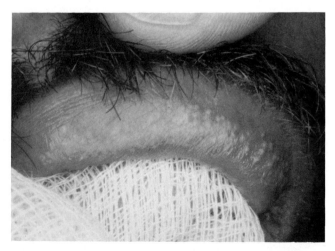

FIGURE 1–9. **Fordyce granules.** Yellow papules on the vermilion of the upper lip.

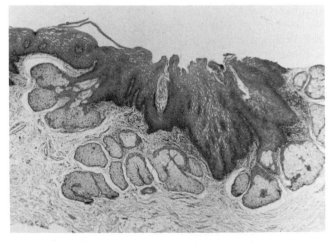

FIGURE 1–11. **Fordyce granules.** Multiple sebaceous glands below the surface epithelium.

Treatment and Prognosis

Because Fordyce granules represent a normal anatomic variation and are asymptomatic, no treatment is indicated. Usually, the clinical appearance is characteristic and biopsy is not necessary for diagnosis.

On occasion, Fordyce granules may become hyperplastic or may form keratin-filled pseudocysts. Tumors arising from these glands are exceedingly rare.

LEUKOEDEMA

Leukoedema is a common oral mucosal condition of unknown cause. It occurs more commonly in blacks than in whites, supporting the likelihood of an ethnic predisposition to its development. Leukoedema has been reported in 90 percent of black adults and in 50 percent of black children. The prevalence in whites is considerably less, although published reports have ranged from less than 10 percent to more than 90 percent. This variation may reflect differing population groups, examination conditions, and stringency of criteria used to make the diagnosis. At any rate, leukoedema shows a much milder presentation in whites, and it is often hardly noticeable. The difference in racial predilection may partially be explained by the presence of background mucosal pigmentation in blacks that makes the edematous changes more noticeable.

Because leukoedema is so common, it can reasonably be argued that it represents a variation of normal rather than a "disease." This argument can be further supported by the finding of similar edematous mucosa in the vagina and larynx. Although leukoedema appears to be developmental in nature, some studies have indicated that it is more common and more severe in smokers and becomes less pronounced with cessation of smoking.

Clinical Features

Leukoedema is characterized by a diffuse, grayishwhite, milky, opalescent appearance of the mucosa (Fig. 1–12). The surface frequently appears folded, resulting

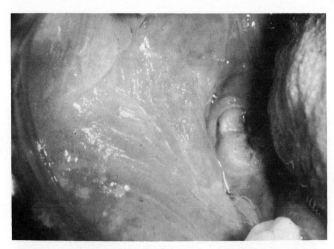

FIGURE 1–13. **Leukoedema.** Diffuse white appearance of the buccal mucosa. See Color Plates.

in wrinkles or whitish streaks. The lesions do not rub off. Leukoedema typically occurs bilaterally on the buccal mucosa and may extend forward onto the labial mucosa. On rare occasions, it can also involve the floor of the mouth and palatopharyngeal tissues. Leukoedema can be easily diagnosed clinically because the white appearance greatly diminishes or disappears when the cheek is everted and stretched (Figs. 1–13 and 1–14; see Color Figures 2 and 3).

Histopathologic Features

Biopsy specimens of leukoedema demonstrate an increase in thickness of the epithelium with striking intracellular edema of the spinous layer (Fig. 1–15). These vacuolated cells appear large and have pyknotic nuclei. The epithelial surface is frequently parakeratinized, and the rete ridges are broad and elongated.

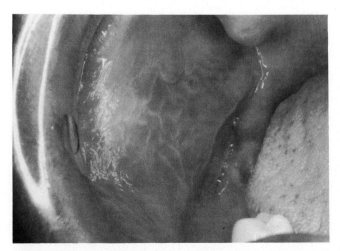

FIGURE 1–12. **Leukoedema.** White wrinkled appearance of the buccal mucosa.

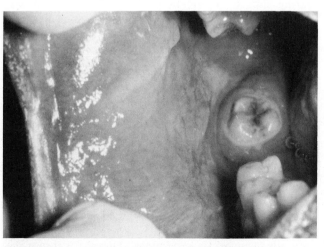

FIGURE 1–14. **Leukoedema.** Same lesion as depicted in Figure 1–13 showing disappearance of whiteness when the cheek is stretched. See Color Plates.

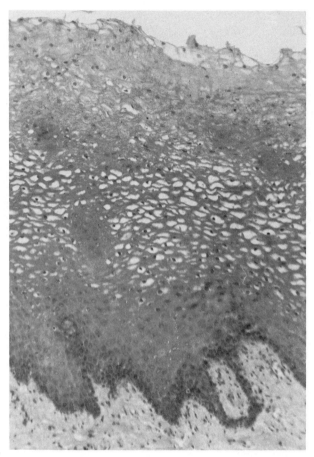

FIGURE 1–15. **Leukoedema.** Parakeratosis and intracellular edema of the spinous layer.

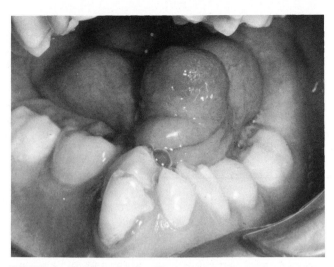

FIGURE 1–16. **Microglossia.** Abnormally small tongue associated with constricted mandibular arch.

Treatment and Prognosis

Leukoedema is a benign condition, and no treatment is required. The characteristic milky-white, opalescent lesions of the buccal mucosa that disappear when stretched help to distinguish it from other common white lesions, such as leukoplakia, candidiasis, and lichen planus. The affected mucosa should always be stretched during clinical examination to rule out any underlying lesions that may be hidden by the edematous change.

MICROGLOSSIA (Hypoglossia)

Clinical Features

Microglossia is an uncommon developmental condition of unknown cause that is characterized by an abnormally small tongue. In rare instances, virtually the entire tongue may be missing **(aglossia)**. Isolated microglossia is known to occur, and mild degrees of microglossia may be difficult to detect and may go unnoticed. However, most reported cases have been associated with one of a group of overlapping conditions known as **oromandibular-limb hypogenesis syndromes**. These syndromes feature associated limb anomalies, such as *hypodactylia* (absence of digits) and *hypomelia* (hypoplasia of part or

all of a limb). Other patients have had coexisting anomalies, such as cleft palate, intraoral bands, and situs inversus. Microglossia is frequently associated with hypoplasia of the mandible, and the lower incisors may be missing (Figs. 1–16 and 1–17).

Treatment and Prognosis

Treatment of the patient with microglossia depends on the nature and severity of the condition. Surgery and orthodontics may improve oral function. Surprisingly, speech development is often quite good but depends on tongue size.

MACROGLOSSIA

Macroglossia is an uncommon condition characterized by enlargement of the tongue. The enlargement may be caused by a wide variety of conditions, including both

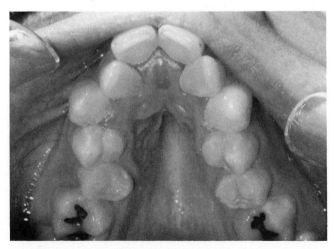

FIGURE 1–17. **Microglossia.** Associated constriction of the maxillary arch in the same patient shown in Figure 1–16.

congenital malformations and acquired diseases. The most frequent causes are vascular malformations and muscular hypertrophy. Table 1–1 lists the most common and important causes of macroglossia. Many of these diseases are discussed in greater detail in subsequent chapters of this book.

Clinical Features

Macroglossia most commonly occurs in children and can range from mild to severe in degree (Fig. 1–18). In infants, macroglossia may be first manifested by noisy breathing, drooling, and difficulty in eating. The tongue

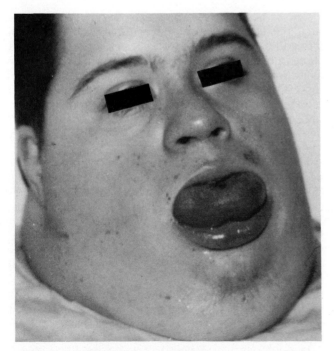

FIGURE 1–18. **Macroglossia.** Large tongue in a patient with Down syndrome. (Courtesy of Dr. Sanford Fenton.)

enlargement may result in a lisping speech. The pressure of the tongue against the mandible and teeth can produce a crenated lateral border to the tongue, open bite, and mandibular prognathism. If the tongue constantly protrudes from the mouth, it may ulcerate and become secondarily infected or may even undergo necrosis. Severe macroglossia can produce airway obstruction.

Macroglossia is a characteristic feature of **Beckwith-Wiedemann syndrome**, a rare hereditary condition that includes many other possible defects, such as:

- Omphalocele (protrusion of part of the intestine through a defect in the abdominal wall at the umbilicus)
- Visceromegaly
- Gigantism
- Neonatal hypoglycemia

Individuals with Beckwith-Wiedemann syndrome have an increased risk for several childhood visceral tumors, including Wilms tumor, adrenal carcinoma, and hepatoblastoma. Facial features may include nevus flammeus of the forehead and eyelids, linear indentations of the earlobes, and maxillary hypoplasia resulting in relative mandibular prognathism. The mode of inheritance of Beckwith-Wiedemann syndrome is uncertain, but autosomal dominant transmission has been suggested, with variable expressivity and incomplete penetrance.

In patients with **hypothyroidism** (see p. 608) or Beckwith-Wiedemann syndrome, the tongue usually shows a diffuse, smooth, generalized enlargement. In those with other forms of macroglossia, the tongue usually has a multinodular appearance. Examples of this nodular type include **amyloidosis** (see p. 509) and neoplastic conditions, such as **neurofibromatosis** (see p. 381) and **multiple endocrine neoplasia, type III** (see p. 384).

In patients with **lymphangiomas** (see p. 395), the tongue surface is characteristically pebbly and exhibits multiple vesicle-like blebs that represent superficial dilated lymphatic channels. The enlarged tongue in those with **Down syndrome** typically demonstrates a papillary, fissured surface.

In patients with **hemifacial hyperplasia** (described later in the chapter), the enlargement will be unilateral. Some patients with neurofibromatosis can also have unilateral lingual enlargement.

In edentulous patients, the tongue often appears elevated and tends to spread out laterally because of loss of the surrounding teeth; as a result, wearing a denture may become difficult.

Histopathologic Features

The histologic appearance of macroglossia depends on the specific cause. In some cases, such as the tongue enlargement seen in Down syndrome or edentulous patients, no histologic abnormality can be detected. When macroglossia is due to tumor, a neoplastic proliferation of a particular tissue can be found (lymphatic vessels, blood vessels, neural tissue). Muscular enlargement occurs in those with hemihypertrophy and Beckwith-

Wiedemann syndrome. In the patient with amyloidosis, an abnormal protein material is deposited in the tongue.

Treatment and Prognosis

The treatment and prognosis of macroglossia depend on the cause and severity of the condition. In mild cases, surgical treatment may not be necessary, although speech therapy may be helpful if speech is affected. In symptomatic patients, reduction glossectomy may be needed.

ANKYLOGLOSSIA (Tongue-Tie)

Ankyloglossia is a developmental anomaly of the tongue characterized by a short, thick lingual frenum resulting in limitation of tongue movement. Although mild forms are probably not unusual, severe ankyloglossia is a relatively uncommon condition that has been estimated to occur in about 2 to 3 of every 10,000 people.

Clinical Features

Ankyloglossia can range in severity from mild cases with little clinical significance to rare examples of complete ankyloglossia in which the tongue is actually fused to the floor of the mouth (Fig. 1–19). Sometimes the frenum extends forward and attaches to the tip of the tongue, and there may be slight clefting of the tip.

Some investigators have speculated that ankyloglossia may contribute to the development of an anterior open bite because the inability to raise the tongue to the roof of the mouth prevents development of the normal adult swallowing pattern. However, others have questioned this theory.

It has also been suggested that tongue-tie may result in speech defects. Usually, however, the shortened frenum results in only minor difficulties because most people can compensate for the limitation in tongue movement. Yet, there are rare examples of patients who have experienced an immediate noticeable improvement in speech after

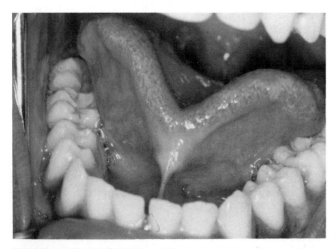

FIGURE 1–19. **Ankyloglossia.** Abnormal attachment of the lingual frenum, limiting tongue mobility.

surgical correction of ankyloglossia. It is also possible that a high mucogingival attachment of the lingual frenum may lead to periodontal problems.

Treatment and Prognosis

Because most cases of ankyloglossia result in few or no clinical problems, treatment is often unnecessary. If there are functional or periodontal difficulties, a frenectomy may allow greater freedom of tongue movement. In young children, it is usually recommended that surgery be postponed until age 4 or 5. Because the tongue is always short at birth, it is difficult in the infant's early life to assess the degree of tongue limitation caused by ankyloglossia. As the infant grows, the tongue becomes longer and thinner at the tip, often decreasing the severity of the tongue-tie. The condition is probably self-correcting in many cases because it is less common in adults.

LINGUAL THYROID

During the third to fourth week of fetal life, the thyroid gland begins as an epithelial proliferation in the floor of the pharyngeal gut. This thyroid bud normally descends into the neck to its final resting position anterior to the trachea and larynx. The site where this descending bud invaginates later becomes the foramen cecum, located at the junction of the anterior two thirds and posterior third of the tongue in the midline. If the primitive gland does not descend normally, ectopic thyroid tissue may be found between the foramen cecum and the epiglottis. Of all ectopic thyroids, 90 percent are found in this region.

Clinical Features

On the basis of autopsy studies, small asymptomatic remnants of thyroid tissue can be discovered on the posterior dorsal tongue in about 10 percent of both men and women. However, clinically evident or symptomatic **lingual thyroids** are much less common and are four times more frequent in females, presumably because of hormonal influences. Symptoms most often develop during puberty, adolescence, pregnancy, or menopause. In 70 percent of cases, this ectopic gland is the patient's only thyroid tissue.

Lingual thyroids may range from small, asymptomatic nodular lesions to large masses that can block the airway (Fig. 1–20; see Color Figure 4). The most common clinical symptoms are dysphagia, dysphonia, and dyspnea. The mass is often vascular, but the physical appearance is variable and there are no reliable features to distinguish it from other masses that might develop in this area. Hypothyroidism has been reported in 15 to 33 percent of patients. Many authors say that lingual thyroid enlargement is a secondary phenomenon, compensating for thyroid hypofunction. Interestingly, as many as 75 percent of patients with infantile hypothyroidism have some ectopic thyroid tissue.

Diagnosis is best established by thyroid scan using iodine isotopes (Fig. 1–21). Biopsy is often avoided be-

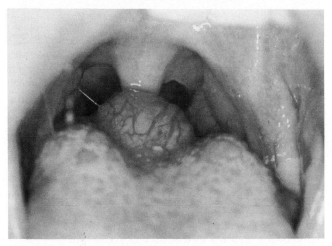

FIGURE 1–20. **Lingual thyroid.** Nodular mass of the posterior dorsal midline of the tongue in a 4-year-old girl. See Color Plates.

cause of the risk of hemorrhage and because the mass may represent the patient's only functioning thyroid tissue. In some cases, incisional biopsy may be needed to confirm the diagnosis or to rule out malignant changes.

Treatment and Prognosis

No treatment except periodic follow-up is required for patients with asymptomatic lingual thyroids. In symptomatic patients, suppressive therapy with supplemental thyroid hormone can often reduce the size of the lesion.

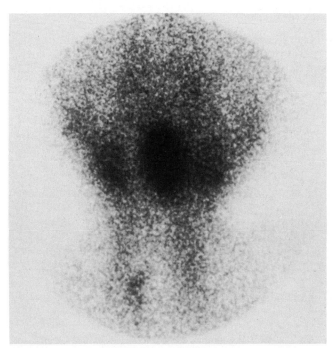

FIGURE 1–21. **Lingual thyroid.** Thyroid scan of the same patient as in Figure 1–20. The scan shows localization (central dark zone) of iodine isotope in the tongue mass and minimal uptake in the neck.

Some authors advise that this treatment should also be tried in asymptomatic patients to prevent possible subsequent enlargement. If hormone therapy does not eliminate symptoms, surgical removal or ablation with radioactive iodine-131 can be performed. If the mass is surgically excised, autotransplantation to another body site can be attempted to maintain functional thyroid tissue and to prevent hypothyroidism.

Rare examples of carcinomas arising in lingual thyroids have been reported; malignancy develops in about 1 percent of identified cases. Although lingual thyroids are decidedly more common in females, this predilection for females is less pronounced in regard to lingual thyroid carcinomas. Because a disproportionate number of these malignancies have been documented in males, some authors have advocated prophylactic excision of lingual thyroids in men older than 30 years of age.

FISSURED TONGUE (Scrotal Tongue)

Fissured tongue is relatively common. Numerous grooves, or fissures, are present on the dorsal tongue surface. The cause is uncertain, but heredity appears to play a significant role. There is evidence that the condition may be either a polygenic trait or an autosomal dominant trait with incomplete penetrance. Aging or local environmental factors may also contribute to its development.

Clinical Features

Patients with fissured tongue exhibit multiple grooves, or furrows, on the surface of the tongue, ranging from 2 to 6 mm in depth (Figs. 1–22 and 1–23). Considerable variation can be seen. In the most severe cases, numerous fissures cover the entire dorsal surface and divide the tongue papillae into multiple separate "islands." Some patients have fissures that are located mostly on the dorsolateral areas of the tongue. Other patients exhibit a large central fissure, with smaller fissures branching outward at right angles. The condition is usually asymptomatic, although some patients may complain of mild burning or soreness.

Most studies have shown that the prevalence of fissured tongue ranges from 2 to 5 percent of the overall population. The condition may be seen in children or adults, but the prevalence and severity appear to increase with age. In some investigations, a male predilection has been noted.

A strong association has been found between fissured tongue and **geographic tongue** (see p. 569), with many patients having both conditions. A hereditary basis has also been suggested for geographic tongue, and the same gene(s) may possibly be linked to both conditions. In fact, it has even been suggested that geographic tongue may cause fissured tongue. Fissured tongue may also be a component of **Melkersson-Rosenthal syndrome** (see p. 243).

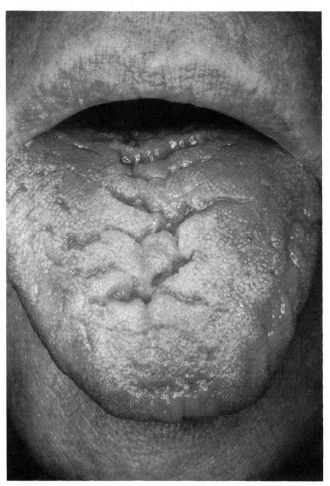

FIGURE 1-22. **Fissured tongue.** Moderate fissuring of the dorsal tongue. (From Allen CM, Camisa C. Diseases of the mouth and lips. _In:_ Principles of Dermatology. Edited by Sams WM, Lynch P. New York, Churchill Livingstone, 1990, pp 913-941.)

Histopathologic Features

Microscopic examination of fissured tongue reveals hyperplasia of the rete ridges and loss of the keratin "hairs" on the surface of the filiform papillae. The papillae vary in size and are often separated by deep grooves. Polymorphonuclear leukocytes can be seen migrating into the epithelium, often forming microabscesses in the upper epithelial layers. A mixed inflammatory cell infiltrate is present in the lamina propria.

Treatment and Prognosis

Fissured tongue is a benign condition, and no specific treatment is indicated. The patient should be encouraged to brush the tongue because food or debris entrapped in the grooves may act as a source of irritation.

HAIRY TONGUE (Black Hairy Tongue)

Hairy tongue is characterized by marked accumulation of keratin on the filiform papillae of the dorsal tongue, resulting in a hair-like appearance. The condition apparently represents an increase in keratin production or a decrease in normal keratin desquamation. Hairy tongue is found in about 0.5 percent of adults.

Although the cause is uncertain, many affected people are heavy smokers. Other possible associated factors include:

- Antibiotic therapy
- Poor oral hygiene
- General debilitation
- Radiation therapy
- Use of oxidizing mouthwashes or antacids
- Overgrowth of fungal or bacterial organisms

Clinical Features

Hairy tongue most commonly affects the midline just anterior to the circumvallate papillae, sparing the lateral and anterior borders (Fig. 1-24). The elongated papillae

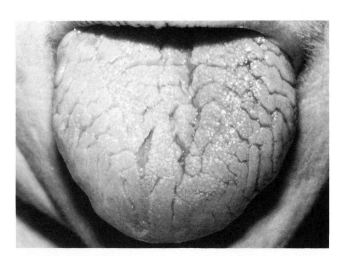

FIGURE 1-23. **Fissured tongue.** Extensive fissuring involving the entire dorsal tongue surface.

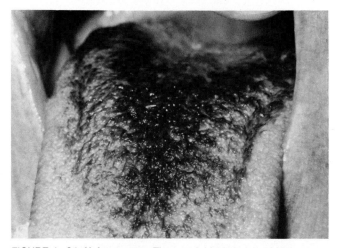

FIGURE 1-24. **Hairy tongue.** Elongated, black-staining filiform papillae on the posterior dorsal tongue.

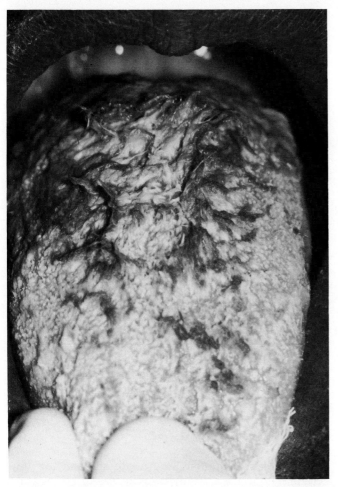

FIGURE 1–25. **Hairy tongue.** Marked elongation and brown staining of the filiform papillae resulting in a hair-like appearance. (Courtesy of Dr. Robert Strohaver.) See Color Plates.

are usually brown, yellow, or black as a result of growth of pigment-producing bacteria or staining from tobacco and food. Sometimes most of the dorsal tongue may be involved, resulting in a thick, matted appearance (Fig. 1–25; see Color Figure 5). Multiple individual elongated filiform papillae may be elevated by using gauze or a dental instrument. The condition is typically asymptomatic, although occasional patients complain of a gagging sensation or a bad taste in the mouth. Because the diagnosis can usually be made from the clinical appearance, biopsy is unnecessary in most instances.

Because of the similarity in names, care should be taken to avoid confusing hairy tongue with **hairy leukoplakia** (see p. 202), which typically occurs on the lateral border of the tongue. Hairy leukoplakia is an Epstein-Barr virus–induced lesion usually associated with human immunodeficiency virus (HIV) infection or other immunosuppressive conditions.

Histopathologic Features

On histopathologic examination, hairy tongue is characterized by marked elongation and hyperparakeratosis

of the filiform papillae (Fig. 1–26). Usually, numerous bacteria can be seen growing on the epithelial surface.

Treatment and Prognosis

Hairy tongue is a benign condition with no serious sequelae. The major concern is often the aesthetic appearance of the tongue along with possible associated bad breath. Any predisposing factors, such as tobacco, antibiotics, or mouthwashes, should be eliminated, and excellent oral hygiene should be encouraged. Desquamation of the hyperkeratotic papillae can be promoted by periodic scraping or brushing with a toothbrush. Keratolytic agents, such as podophyllin, have also been tried with success, but for safety reasons their use should probably not be encouraged.

VARICOSITIES (Varices)

A **varicosity**, or **varix**, is an abnormally dilated and tortuous vein. The exact cause of oral varicosities is uncertain. Age is an important factor because varices are rare in children but common in older adults. Varices have not been associated with systemic hypertension or

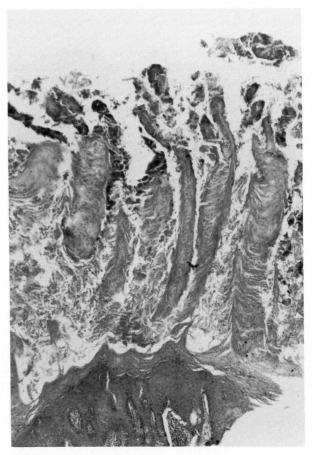

FIGURE 1–26. **Hairy tongue.** Elongation and marked hyperkeratosis of the filiform papillae with bacterial accumulation on the surface.

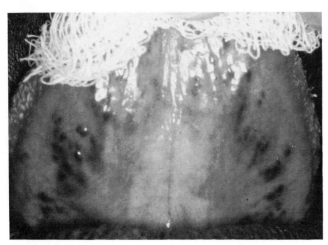

FIGURE 1–27. **Varicosities.** Multiple purple dilated veins on the ventral surface of the tongue.

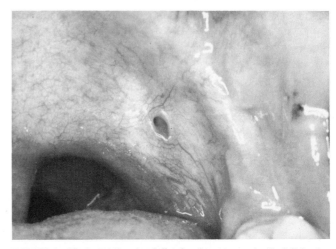

FIGURE 1–28. **Varicosity.** Firm, thrombosed varix on the lower lip. See Color Plates.

other cardiopulmonary diseases, although one study did find that people with varicose veins of the legs were more likely to have varicosities of the tongue.

Clinical Features

The most common type of oral varicosity is the **sublingual varix**, which occurs in two thirds of people older than 60 years of age. Sublingual varicosities classically present as multiple bluish-purple, elevated or papular blebs on the ventral-lateral border of the tongue (Fig. 1–27). The lesions are usually asymptomatic, except in rare instances when secondary thrombosis occurs.

Less frequently, **solitary varices** occur in other areas of the mouth, especially the lips and buccal mucosa. These isolated varicosities are often first noticed after they have become thrombosed (Fig. 1–28; see Color Figure 6). Clinically, a thrombosed varix presents as a firm, nontender, bluish-purple nodule that may feel like a piece of buckshot beneath the mucosal surface.

Histopathologic Features

Microscopic examination of a varix reveals a dilated vein, the wall of which shows little smooth muscle and poorly developed elastic tissue. If secondary thrombosis has occurred, the lumen may contain concentrically layered zones of platelets and erythrocytes (lines of Zahn). The clot can undergo organization via granulation tissue, with subsequent recanalization. Older thrombi may exhibit dystrophic calcification, resulting in formation of a **phlebolith** (*phlebo* = vein; *lith* = stone).

Treatment and Prognosis

Sublingual varicosities are typically asymptomatic, and no treatment is indicated. Solitary varicosities of the lips and buccal mucosa may need to be surgically removed to confirm the diagnosis or because of secondary thrombus formation.

LATERAL SOFT PALATE FISTULAS

Lateral soft palate fistulas are rare anomalies of uncertain pathogenesis. Many cases appear to be congenital, possibly related to a defect in the development of the second pharyngeal pouch. Some fistulas may be the result of infection or surgery of the tonsillar region.

Clinical Features

Lateral soft palate fistulas are usually bilateral, but they may occur only on one side. They are more common on the anterior tonsillar pillar (Figs. 1–29 and 1–

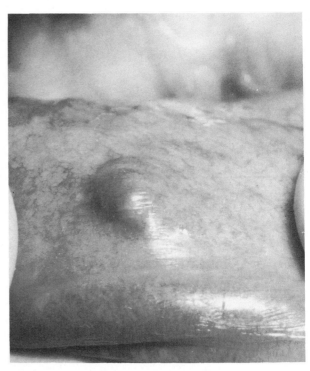

FIGURE 1–29. **Lateral palatal fistula.** Asymptomatic "hole" in the anterior tonsillar pillar.

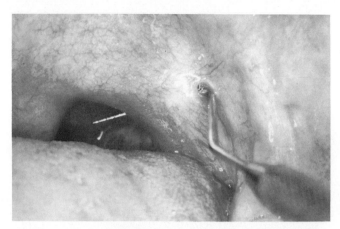

FIGURE 1–30. **Lateral palatal fistula.** A periodontal probe has been used to demonstrate the communication of the lesion (also shown in Figure 1–29) with the tonsillar fossa.

30), but they also may involve the posterior pillar. The perforations are typically asymptomatic, ranging from a few millimeters to more than 1 cm. A few cases have been associated with other anomalies, such as absence or hypoplasia of the palatine tonsils, hearing loss, and preauricular fistulas.

Treatment and Prognosis

The lesions are innocuous, and no treatment is necessary.

CORONOID HYPERPLASIA

Hyperplasia of the coronoid process of the mandible is a rare developmental anomaly that may result in limitation of mandibular movement. The condition may be unilateral or bilateral. **Unilateral coronoid hyperplasia** may be a result of an osteoma or osteochondroma, although some authors believe the enlargement is a hyperplastic process rather than a true neoplasm.

The cause of **bilateral coronoid hyperplasia** is unknown. Because most bilateral cases have been seen in pubertal males, an endocrine influence has been suggested. Heredity may also play a role, as cases have been noted in siblings.

Clinical and Radiographic Features

In a person with **unilateral coronoid hyperplasia**, the enlarged coronoid process impinges on the posterior surface of the zygoma, restricting mandibular opening. In addition, the mandible may deviate toward the affected side. Usually, there is no pain or associated abnormality in occlusion. Radiographs often reveal an irregular, nodular growth of the tip of the coronoid process.

Bilateral coronoid hyperplasia is much more common in males than females and often is first noted at puberty. Limitation of mandibular opening may progressively worsen over several years, reaching maximum severity during the late teens. The radiographic appearance is characterized by regular elongation of both processes.

Because the coronoid process is often superimposed on the zygoma on conventional radiographs, tomograms or computed tomography (CT) scans often better demonstrate the hyperplasia.

Treatment and Prognosis

Treatment of coronoid hyperplasia consists of surgical removal of the elongated coronoid process(es) to allow freedom of mandibular motion. Postoperative physiotherapy is important for re-establishing normal function.

CONDYLAR HYPERPLASIA

Condylar hyperplasia is an uncommon malformation of the mandible created by excessive growth of one of the condyles. The cause of this hyperplasia is unknown, but local circulatory problems, endocrine disturbances, and trauma have been suggested as possible etiologic factors.

Condylar hyperplasia can be difficult to distinguish from **hemifacial hyperplasia** (see p. 34); however, in the latter condition the associated soft tissues and teeth may also be enlarged.

Clinical and Radiographic Features

Condylar hyperplasia may manifest itself in a variety of ways, including facial asymmetry, prognathism, crossbite, and open bite. Sometimes there is compensatory maxillary growth and tilting of the occlusal plane. The condition is most commonly discovered in adolescents and young adults.

The radiographic features are quite variable. Some patients have an irregular enlargement of the condylar head (Fig. 1–31); others show elongation of the condylar neck. Many cases also demonstrate hyperplasia of the entire ramus, suggesting that the condition sometimes affects more than just the condyle.

Histopathologic Features

During active growth, proliferation of the condylar cartilage is noted. Once condylar growth has ceased, the condyle has a normal histologic appearance.

Treatment and Prognosis

Condylar hyperplasia is a self-limiting condition, and treatment is determined by the degree of functional difficulty and aesthetic change. Some patients can be treated with unilateral condylectomy, whereas others require unilateral or bilateral mandibular osteotomies. In patients with compensatory maxillary growth, a maxillary osteotomy may also be needed. Concomitant orthodontic therapy is frequently necessary.

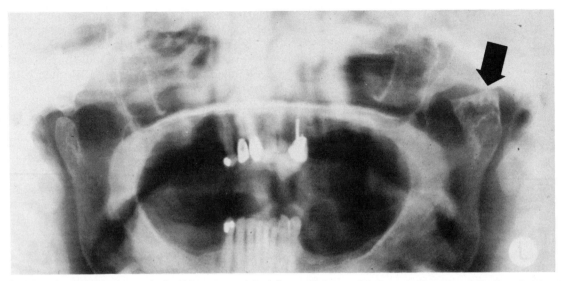

FIGURE 1–31. **Condylar hyperplasia.** Enlargement of the left mandibular condyle (*arrow*). (Courtesy of Dr. Gary Reinhart.)

CONDYLAR HYPOPLASIA

Condylar hypoplasia, or underdevelopment of the mandibular condyle, can be either congenital or acquired. **Congenital condylar hypoplasia** is often associated with head and neck syndromes, including **mandibulofacial dysostosis** (see p. 39), **oculoauriculovertebral syndrome (Goldenhar syndrome),** and **hemifacial microsomia**. In the most severe cases, there is complete agenesis of the condyle or ramus.

Acquired condylar hypoplasia results from disturbances of the growth center of the developing condyle. The most frequent cause is trauma to the condylar region during infancy or childhood. Other causes include infections, radiation therapy, and rheumatoid or degenerative arthritis.

Clinical and Radiographic Features

Condylar hypoplasia can be unilateral or bilateral, producing a small mandible with a Class II malocclusion. Unilateral hypoplasia results in distortion and depression of the face on the affected side. The mandibular midline shifts to the involved side when the mouth is opened, accentuating the deformity. Ankylosis of the temporomandibular joint (TMJ) can develop in cases caused by trauma.

The deformity is easily observed on panoramic films and can range in severity. In severe cases, the condyle or ramus may be totally absent. Milder types demonstrate a short condylar process, shallow sigmoid notch, and poorly formed condylar head. A prominent antegonial notch may be present.

Treatment and Prognosis

Treatment of the patient with condylar hypoplasia depends on the cause and severity of the defect, but surgery is often required. If the condyle is missing, a costochondral rib graft can be placed to help establish an active growth center. Osteotomies sometimes provide a cosmetically acceptable result.

BIFID CONDYLE

A **bifid condyle** is a rare developmental anomaly characterized by a double-headed mandibular condyle. Most bifid condyles have a medial and lateral head divided by an anteroposterior groove. Some condyles may be divided into an anterior and posterior head.

The cause of bifid condyle is uncertain. Anteroposterior bifid condyles may be of traumatic origin, such as a childhood fracture. Mediolaterally divided condyles may result from abnormal muscle attachment, teratogenic agents, or persistence of a fibrous septum within the condylar cartilage.

Clinical and Radiographic Features

A bifid condyle is usually unilateral, but occasionally both sides may be affected. The malformation is often asymptomatic and may be discovered on routine radiographs, although some patients may have a "pop" or "click" of the TMJ when opening their mouths. Rarely does the patient present with TMJ complaints. Radiographs demonstrate a bi-lobed appearance of the condylar head (Fig. 1–32).

Treatment and Prognosis

Because a bifid condyle is usually asymptomatic, most of the time no treatment is necessary. If the patient has joint complaints, the appropriate temporomandibular therapy may be required.

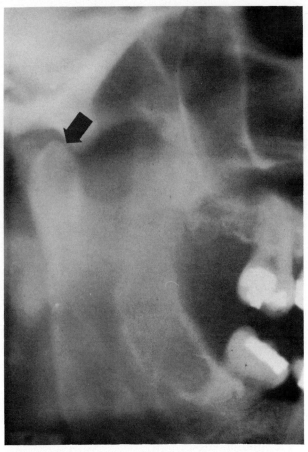

FIGURE 1–32. **Bifid condyle.** Radiograph of the mandibular condyle showing a double head (*arrow*). (Courtesy of Dr. Ed McGaha.)

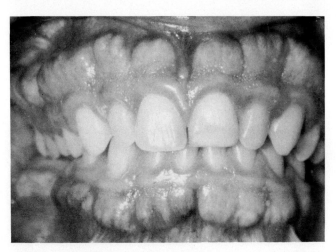

FIGURE 1–33. **Exostoses.** Multiple buccal exostoses of the maxillary and mandibular alveolar ridges.

velop from the alveolar bone beneath free gingival grafts and skin grafts. Presumably, placement of the graft acts as a stimulant to the periosteum to form new bone.

Another rare, interesting variant is the **reactive subpontine exostosis (subpontic osseous proliferation; subpontic osseous hyperplasia)**, which may develop from the alveolar crestal bone beneath the pontic of a posterior mandibular bridge.

If enough excess bone is present, exostoses may exhibit a relative radiopacity on dental radiographs (Fig. 1–35). In rare instances, an exostosis may become so large that it is difficult to distinguish from a tumor such as an osteoma (see p. 472).

EXOSTOSES

Exostoses are localized bony protuberances that arise from the cortical plate. These benign growths frequently affect the jaws. The most common oral exostoses, the **torus palatinus** and the **torus mandibularis**, are described later. Other less common types of exostoses may also affect the jaws and are considered here.

Clinical and Radiographic Features

Exostoses are discovered most often in adults. **Buccal exostoses** occur as a bilateral row of bony hard nodules along the facial aspect of the maxillary and/or mandibular alveolar ridge (Fig. 1–33). They are usually asymptomatic unless the thin overlying mucosa becomes ulcerated from trauma. They occur equally in males and females and in 1 of every 1000 adults.

Palatal exostoses are similar bony protuberances that develop from the lingual aspect of the maxillary tuberosities. These lesions are usually bilateral but may affect only one side (Fig. 1–34). Some patients with buccal and palatal exostoses may also have palatal or mandibular tori.

Less commonly, **solitary exostoses** may occur, possibly in response to local irritation. Such lesions may de-

Histopathologic Features

Microscopic examination reveals a mass of dense, lamellar, cortical bone with a small amount of fibrofatty marrow. In some cases, an inner zone of trabecular bone is also present.

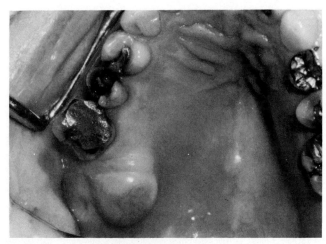

FIGURE 1–34. **Exostosis.** Secondarily ulcerated palatal exostosis.

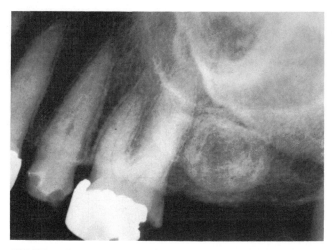

FIGURE 1-35. **Exostosis.** Radiograph of the same lesion shown in Figure 1-34. An ovoid radiopacity is distal to the molar.

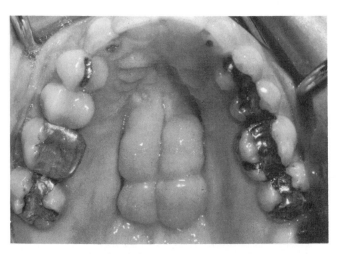

FIGURE 1-37. **Torus palatinus.** Large, lobulated palatal mass.

Treatment and Prognosis

Most exostoses are distinctive enough clinically so that biopsy is unnecessary. If the diagnosis is uncertain, biopsy should be performed to rule out other bony pathosis. Sometimes the exostosis must be removed if it has been exposed to trauma repeatedly or has become ulcerated and painful. In addition, surgical removal may be required to accommodate a dental prosthesis.

TORUS PALATINUS

The **torus palatinus** is a common exostosis that occurs in the midline of the vault of the hard palate. The pathogenesis of these tori has long been debated, with arguments centering around genetic versus environmental factors, such as masticatory stress. The most likely cause is multifactorial, including both genetic and environmental influences. In this model, patients are affected by a variety of hereditary and local environmental factors; if enough of these factors are present, a "threshold" is surpassed and the trait (torus palatinus) will be expressed.

Clinical and Radiographic Features

The torus palatinus presents as a bony hard mass that arises along the midline suture of the hard palate (Figs. 1-36 to 1-38). Tori are sometimes classified according to their morphology:

The **flat torus** has a broad base and a slightly convex, smooth surface. It extends symmetrically onto both sides of the midline raphe.

The **spindle torus** presents as a midline ridge along the palatal raphe. A median groove is sometimes present.

The **nodular torus** arises as multiple protuberances, each with an individual base. These protuberances may coalesce, forming grooves between them.

The **lobular torus** also presents as a lobulated mass, but it rises from a single base. Lobular tori can be either sessile or pedunculated.

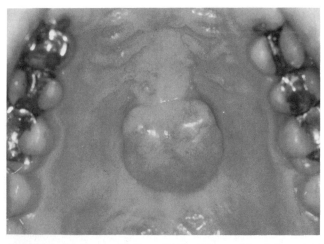

FIGURE 1-36. **Torus palatinus.** Midline bony nodule of the palatal vault.

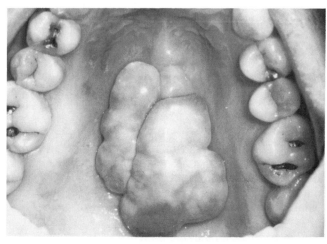

FIGURE 1-38. **Torus palatinus.** Asymmetric, lobulated bony mass.

Most palatal tori are small, measuring less than 2 cm in diameter; however, they can slowly increase in size throughout life, sometimes to the extent that they fill the entire palatal vault. Most tori cause no symptoms, but in some cases, the thin overlying mucosa may become ulcerated secondary to trauma.

The torus palatinus usually does not appear on routine dental radiographs. Rarely, it may be seen as a radiopacity on periapical films if the film is placed behind the torus when the radiograph is taken.

The prevalence of palatal tori has varied widely in a number of population studies, ranging from 9 to 60 percent. Some of this variation may be due to the criteria used to make the diagnosis and also may be based on whether the study was conducted on live patients or skulls. There do appear to be significant racial differences, however, with a higher prevalence in Asian and Eskimo (Inuit) populations. In the United States, most studies have shown a prevalence of 20 to 35 percent, with little difference between whites and blacks. Almost all studies from around the world have shown a pronounced female-to-male ratio of 2:1. The prevalence peaks during early adult life, tapering off in later years. This finding supports the theory that tori are dynamic lesions that are related, in part, to environmental factors; in later life, some may undergo resorption remodeling in response to decreased functional stresses.

Histopathologic Features

Microscopic examination of the torus shows a mass of dense, lamellar, cortical bone. An inner zone of trabecular bone is sometimes seen.

Treatment and Prognosis

Most palatal tori can be diagnosed clinically on the basis of their characteristic appearance; therefore, biopsy is rarely necessary. In edentulous patients, the torus may need to be removed surgically to accommodate a denture base. Surgical removal may also be indicated for palatal tori that become repeatedly ulcerated or that interfere with oral function.

TORUS MANDIBULARIS

The **torus mandibularis** is a common exostosis that develops along the lingual aspect of the mandible. As with torus palatinus, the cause of mandibular tori is probably multifactorial, including both genetic and environmental influences.

Clinical and Radiographic Features

The mandibular torus presents as a bony protuberance along the lingual aspect of the mandible above the mylohyoid line in the region of the premolars (Fig. 1–39). Bilateral involvement occurs in more than 90 percent of cases. Most mandibular tori occur as single nodules, although multiple lobules paralleling the teeth are not unusual. Patients are often unaware of their presence unless

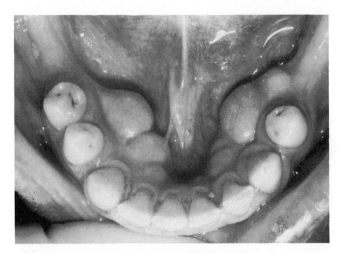

FIGURE 1–39. **Torus mandibularis.** Bilateral lobulated bony protuberances of the mandibular lingual alveolar ridge.

the overlying mucosa becomes ulcerated secondary to trauma. In rare instances, bilateral tori may become so large that they almost meet in the midline (Fig. 1–40). A large mandibular torus may appear on periapical radiographs as a radiopacity superimposed on the roots of the teeth (Fig. 1–41), especially on anterior films.

Studies indicate that the torus mandibularis is not as common as the torus palatinus; the prevalence ranges from 5 to 40 percent. Like the torus palatinus, the mandibular torus appears to be more common in Asians and Inuits. The prevalence in the United States ranges from 7 to 10 percent, with little difference between blacks and whites. A slight male predilection has been noted.

The prevalence of mandibular torus peaks in early adult life, tapering slightly in later years. In addition, the prevalence has been correlated with both bruxism and the number of teeth remaining present. These findings support the theory that the torus mandibularis is multifactorial in development and responds to functional stresses.

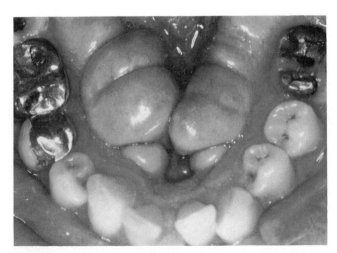

FIGURE 1–40. **Torus mandibularis.** Massive "kissing" tori meet in the midline.

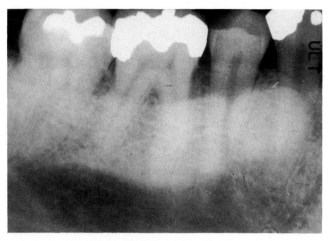

FIGURE 1-41. **Torus mandibularis.** The torus is causing a radiopacity that is superimposed over the roots of the mandibular teeth.

Histopathologic Features

The histopathology of the torus mandibularis is similar to that of other exostoses, consisting primarily of a nodular mass of dense, cortical lamellar bone (Fig. 1-42). An inner zone of trabecular bone with associated fatty marrow is sometimes visible.

Treatment and Prognosis

Most mandibular tori are easily diagnosed clinically, and no treatment is necessary. In edentulous patients, surgical removal of the torus may be required to accommodate a lower denture.

EAGLE SYNDROME (Stylohyoid Syndrome; Carotid Artery Syndrome)

The styloid process is a slender bony projection that originates from the inferior aspect of the temporal bone, anterior and medial to the stylomastoid foramen. It is connected to the lesser cornu of the hyoid bone by the stylohyoid ligament. The external and internal carotid arteries lie on either side. Elongation of the styloid process or mineralization of the stylohyoid ligament complex is not unusual, having been reported in 18 to 40 percent of the population in some radiographic reviews. Such mineralization is usually bilateral, but it may affect only one side. Most cases are asymptomatic; however, a small number of such patients experience symptoms known as **Eagle syndrome,** caused by impingement or compression of adjacent nerves or blood vessels.

Clinical and Radiographic Features

Eagle syndrome most commonly affects adults. The patient experiences vague facial pain, especially while swallowing, turning the head, or opening the mouth. Other symptoms may include dysphagia, dysphonia, otalgia, headache, dizziness, and transient syncope.

Elongation of the styloid process or mineralization of the stylohyoid ligament complex can be seen on panoramic or lateral jaw radiographs (Fig. 1-43). The mineralized stylohyoid complex may be palpated in the tonsillar fossa area, and pain is often elicited.

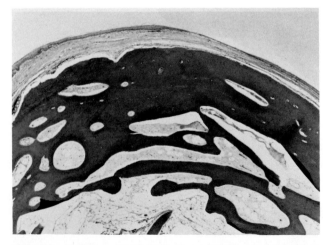

FIGURE 1-42. **Torus mandibularis.** Nodular bony mass with atrophic overlying epithelium. Some fatty marrow is visible at the base of the specimen.

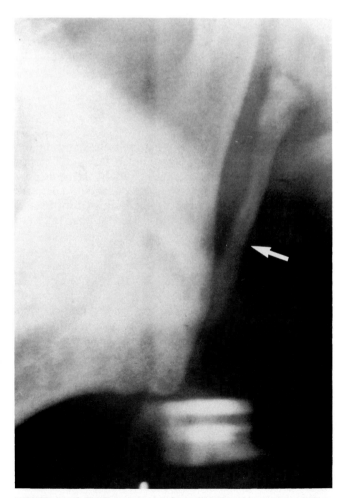

FIGURE 1-43. **Eagle syndrome.** Mineralization of the stylohyoid ligament is visible posterior to the mandibular ramus.

Classic Eagle syndrome occurs after a tonsillectomy. Development of scar tissue in the area of a mineralized stylohyoid complex then results in cervicopharyngeal pain in the region of cranial nerves V, VII, IX, and X, especially during swallowing. Some authors reserve the term "Eagle syndrome" only for those cases in which the ossification of the stylohyoid chain occurs as a result of the tonsillectomy or other neck trauma.

A second form of this condition unrelated to tonsillectomy is sometimes known as **carotid artery syndrome** or **stylohyoid syndrome**. The elongated, mineralized complex is thought to impinge on the internal or external carotid arteries and associated sympathetic nerve fibers. The patient may complain of pain in the neck when turning the head, and this pain may radiate to other sites in the head or neck.

Traumatic Eagle syndrome has also been reported, in which symptoms develop after fracture of a mineralized stylohyoid ligament.

Treatment and Prognosis

Treatment of Eagle syndrome depends on the severity of the symptoms. For mild cases, no treatment may be necessary except reassurance of the patient. Local injection of corticosteroids sometimes provides relief. In more severe cases, partial surgical excision of the elongated styloid process or mineralized stylohyoid ligament is required. This is usually accomplished with an intraoral approach, although an extraoral approach can also be used. The prognosis is good.

STAFNE DEFECT (Stafne Bone Cyst; Lingual Mandibular Salivary Gland Depression; Latent Bone Cyst; Static Bone Cyst; Static Bone Defect; Lingual Cortical Mandibular Defect)

In 1942, Stafne described a series of asymptomatic radiolucent lesions that were located near the angle of the mandible. Subsequent reports of similar lesions have shown that this condition represents a focal concavity of the cortical bone on the lingual surface of the mandible. In most cases, biopsy has revealed histologically normal salivary gland tissue, suggesting that these lesions represent developmental defects containing a portion of the submandibular gland. However, a few of these defects have been reported to be devoid of contents or to contain muscle, fibrous connective tissue, blood vessels, fat, or lymphoid tissue.

Similar lingual cortical defects have also been noted more anteriorly in the mandible, in the area of the incisor, canine, or premolar teeth. These rare defects have been related to the sublingual gland or to aberrant salivary gland tissue. In addition, one report has implicated the parotid gland as the cause of an apparent cortical defect in the upper mandibular ramus. Therefore, all of the major salivary glands appear to be capable of causing such cortical concavities.

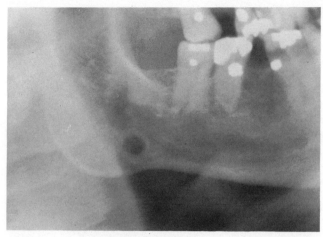

FIGURE 1–44. **Stafne defect.** Radiolucency of the posterior mandible below the mandibular canal.

Clinical and Radiographic Features

The classic **Stafne defect** presents as an asymptomatic radiolucency below the mandibular canal in the posterior mandible, between the molar teeth and the angle of the mandible (Fig. 1–44). The lesion is typically well circumscribed and has a sclerotic border. Sometimes the defect may interrupt the continuity of the inferior border of the mandible, with a palpable notch observed clinically in this area. Most Stafne defects are unilateral, although bilateral cases may be seen. Anterior lingual salivary defects associated with the sublingual gland present as well-defined radiolucencies that may appear superimposed over the apices of the anterior teeth (Figs. 1–45 and 1–46).

Posterior Stafne defects are not rare, having been reported in 0.3 percent of panoramic radiographs. A striking male predilection is observed, with 80 to 90 percent of all cases seen in men.

Although the defect is believed to be developmental in nature, it does not appear to be present from birth. Most

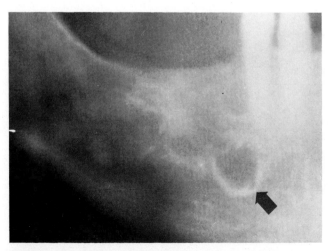

FIGURE 1–45. **Stafne defect.** Anterior radiolucent lesion (arrow) of the body of the mandible associated with the sublingual gland.

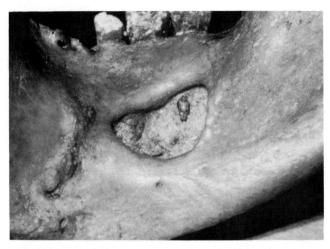

FIGURE 1–46. **Stafne defect.** Lingual surface of the mandible showing an anterior cortical defect caused by the sublingual gland.

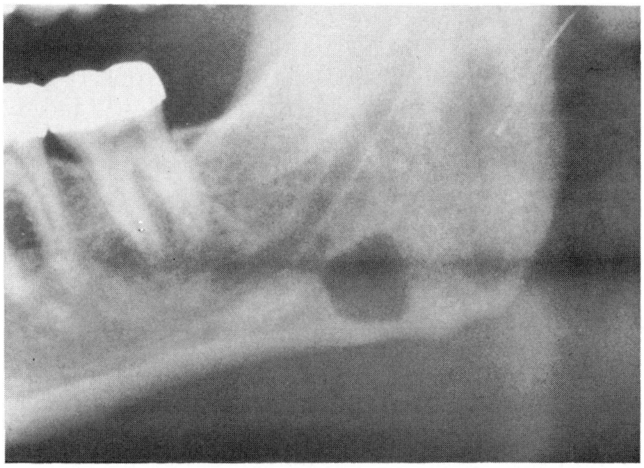

FIGURE 1–48. **Stafne defect.** Radiographic appearance of the same defect depicted in Figure 1–47 several years later. The lesion has enlarged. (Courtesy of Dr. Carroll Gallagher.)

cases have been reported in middle-aged and older adults, with children rarely affected; this implies that the lesion usually "develops" at a later age. Stafne defects typically remain stable in size, hence, the name **static bone cyst**. In a few cases, however, the lesion has increased in size over time (Figs. 1–47 and 1–48). This also indicates that these lesions are not congenital.

The diagnosis can usually be made on a clinical basis by the typical radiographic location and lack of symptoms. If the clinical diagnosis is in doubt, it can be confirmed by CT scans or by sialography. CT scans show a well-defined concavity on the lingual surface of the mandible (Fig. 1–49). Sialograms may be able to demonstrate the presence of salivary gland tissue in the area of the defect.

Histopathologic Features

Because of the typical radiographic appearance, biopsy is usually not necessary to establish the diagnosis of

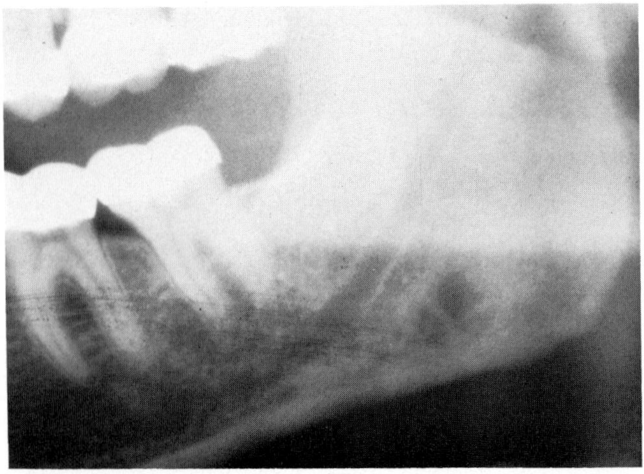

Stafne defects of the posterior mandible. If biopsy is performed, normal submandibular gland tissue is usually seen. However, some defects are devoid of tissue or contain muscle, blood vessels, fat, connective tissue, or lymphoid tissue. In cases reported to be devoid of contents, it is possible that the gland was simply displaced at the time of biopsy.

Treatment and Prognosis

No treatment is necessary for patients with Stafne defects of the posterior mandible, and the prognosis is excellent. Because anterior lingual salivary defects may be difficult to recognize, biopsy may be necessary to rule out other pathologic lesions.

FIGURE 1–47. **Stafne defect.** Ill-defined radiolucency near the angle of the mandible. (Courtesy of Dr. Carroll Gallagher.)

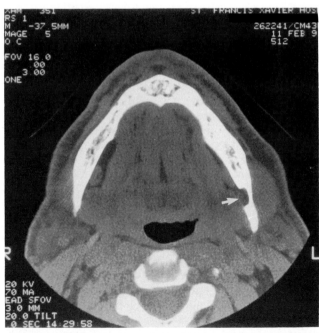

FIGURE 1–49. **Stafne defect.** Computed tomographic (CT) image of the same lesion in Figure 1–48 showing a left lingual cortical defect (*arrow*). (Courtesy of Dr. Carroll Gallagher.)

Developmental Cysts

By definition, a **cyst** is a cavity (often fluid-filled) that is lined by epithelium. A number of different developmental cysts of the head and neck have been described. Some of these have been considered historically as "fissural" cysts because they were thought to arise from epithelium entrapped along embryonal lines of fusion. However, the concept of a fissural origin for many of these cysts has been questioned in more recent years. In many instances, the exact pathogenesis of these lesions is still uncertain. Regardless of their origin, once cysts develop in the oral and maxillofacial region, they tend to slowly increase in size, possibly in response to a slightly elevated hydrostatic luminal pressure.

PALATAL CYSTS OF THE NEWBORN
(Epstein's Pearls; Bohn's Nodules)

Small developmental cysts are a common finding on the palate of newborn infants. It has been theorized that these "inclusion" cysts may arise in one of two ways. First, as the palatal shelves meet and fuse in the midline during embryonic life to form the secondary palate, small islands of epithelium may become entrapped below the surface along the median palatal raphe and form cysts. Second, these cysts may arise from epithelial remnants derived from the development of the minor salivary glands of the palate.

As originally described, **Epstein's pearls** occur along the median palatal raphe and presumably arise from epithelium entrapped along the line of fusion. **Bohn's nodules** are scattered over the hard palate, often near the soft palate junction and are believed to be derived from the minor salivary glands. However, these two terms have been used almost interchangeably in the literature and have often been used to describe gingival cysts of the newborn (see p. 503), similar-appearing lesions of dental lamina origin. Therefore, the term **palatal cysts of the newborn** may be preferable to help distinguish them from gingival cysts of the newborn. Also, because these cysts are most common near the midline at the junction of the hard and soft palates, it is usually difficult to ascertain clinically whether they are arising from epithelium entrapped by fusion of the palate or from the developing minor salivary glands.

Clinical Features

Palatal cysts of the newborn are quite common and have been reported in 65 to 85 percent of neonates. The cysts are small, 1- to 3-mm white or yellowish-white papules that appear most often along the midline near the junction of the hard and soft palates (Fig. 1–50). Occasionally, they may occur in a more anterior location along the raphe or on the posterior palate lateral to the midline. Frequently, a cluster of two to six cysts is observed, although the lesions can also occur singly.

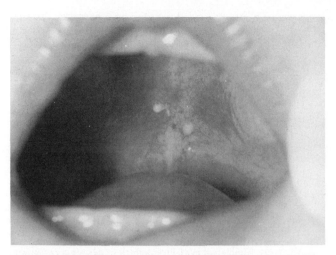

FIGURE 1–50. **Epstein's pearls.** Small keratin-filled cysts at the junction of the hard and soft palates. (From Neville BW, Damm DD, White DK, Waldron CA. Color Atlas of Clinical Oral Pathology. Philadelphia, Lea & Febiger, 1991.)

Histopathologic Features

Microscopic examination reveals keratin-filled cysts that are lined by stratified squamous epithelium. Sometimes these cysts demonstrate a communication with the mucosal surface.

Treatment and Prognosis

Palatal cysts of the newborn are innocuous lesions, and no treatment is required. They are self-healing and rarely observable several weeks after birth. Presumably, the epithelium degenerates, or the cysts rupture onto the mucosal surface and eliminate their keratin contents.

NASOLABIAL CYST (Nasoalveolar Cyst)

The **nasolabial cyst** is a rare developmental cyst that occurs in the upper lip lateral to the midline. Its pathogenesis is uncertain, although there are two major theories. One theory considers the nasolabial cyst to be a "fissural" cyst arising from epithelial remnants entrapped along the line of fusion of the maxillary, medial nasal, and lateral nasal processes. A second theory suggests that these cysts develop from misplaced epithelium of the nasolacrimal duct because of their similar location and histology.

Clinical and Radiographic Features

The nasolabial cyst usually presents as a swelling of the upper lip lateral to the midline, resulting in elevation of the ala of the nose (Fig. 1–51). The enlargement often elevates the mucosa of the nasal vestibule and obliterates the maxillary mucolabial fold (Fig. 1–52). On occasion, this expansion may result in nasal obstruction or may interfere with the wearing of a denture. Pain is uncommon unless the lesion is secondarily infected. The cyst may rupture spontaneously and may drain into the oral cavity or nose.

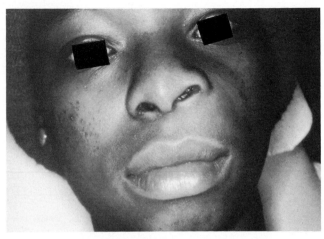

FIGURE 1–51. **Nasolabial cyst.** Enlargement of the left upper lip with elevation of the ala of the nose. (Courtesy of Dr. Jim Weir.)

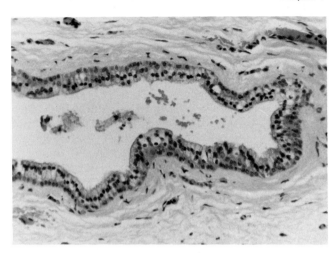

FIGURE 1–53. **Nasolabial cyst.** Pseudostratified columnar epithelial lining.

Nasolabial cysts are most commonly seen in adults, with a peak prevalence in the fourth and fifth decades of life. There is a significant predilection for women, with a female-to-male ratio of 3:1. Approximately 10 percent of the reported cases have been bilateral.

Because the nasolabial cyst arises in soft tissues, in most cases there are no radiographic changes. Occasionally, pressure resorption of the underlying bone may occur.

Histopathologic Features

The nasolabial cyst is characteristically lined by pseudostratified columnar epithelium, often demonstrating goblet cells and cilia (Fig. 1–53). Areas of cuboidal epithelium and squamous metaplasia are not unusual. The cyst wall is composed of fibrous connective tissue with adjacent skeletal muscle. Inflammation may be seen if the lesion is secondarily infected.

Treatment and Prognosis

Complete surgical excision of the cyst via an intraoral approach is the treatment of choice. Because the lesion is often close to the floor of the nose, it is sometimes necessary to sacrifice a portion of the nasal mucosa to ensure total removal. Recurrence is rare.

GLOBULOMAXILLARY CYST

As originally described, the **globulomaxillary cyst** was purported to be a fissural cyst that arose from epithelium entrapped during fusion of the globular portion of the medial nasal process with the maxillary process. This concept has been questioned, however, because the globular portion of the medial nasal process is primarily united with the maxillary process and a fusion does not occur. Therefore, epithelial entrapment should not occur during embryologic development of this area. Current theory holds that most, if not all, cysts that develop in the "globulomaxillary" area are actually of odontogenic origin.

Clinical and Radiographic Features

The "globulomaxillary cyst" classically develops between the maxillary lateral incisor and cuspid teeth, although occasional globulomaxillary lesions have been reported between the central and lateral incisors. Radiographs typically demonstrate a well-circumscribed unilocular radiolucency between and apical to the teeth (Fig. 1–54). Because this radiolucency is often constricted as it extends down between the teeth, it may resemble an inverted pear. As the lesion expands, tipping of the tooth roots may occur.

Histopathologic Features

Virtually all cysts in the globulomaxillary region can be explained on an odontogenic basis. Many are lined by

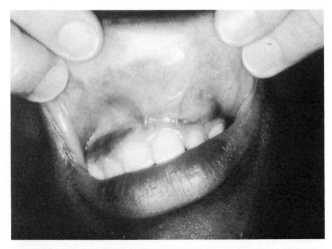

FIGURE 1–52. **Nasolabial cyst.** Same lesion as in Figure 1–51. Intraoral swelling fills the maxillary labial fold. (Courtesy of Dr. Jim Weir.)

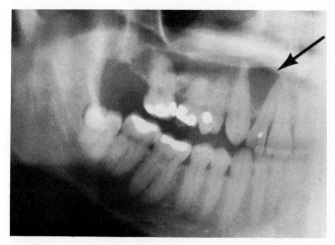

FIGURE 1–54. **"Globulomaxillary cyst."** Inverted pear-shaped radio-lucency (*arrow*) between the maxillary right cuspid and the lateral incisor. Biopsy revealed a periapical cyst.

inflamed stratified squamous epithelium and are consistent with **periapical cysts** (see p. 105). Some exhibit specific histologic features of an **odontogenic keratocyst** (see p. 497) or developmental **lateral periodontal cyst** (see p. 504). It has also been theorized that some of these lesions may arise from inflammation of the reduced enamel epithelium at the time of eruption of the teeth.

On rare occasions, cysts in the globulomaxillary area may be lined by pseudostratified, ciliated columnar epithelium. Such cases may lend credence to the fissural theory of origin. However, this epithelium may be explained by the close proximity of the sinus lining. In addition, respiratory epithelium has also been reported in periapical cysts, dentigerous cysts, and glandular odontogenic cysts found in other locations.

Treatment and Prognosis

Treatment of cysts in the globulomaxillary area usually consists of surgical enucleation. If the lesion can be related to an adjacent nonvital tooth, then endodontic therapy may be appropriate. Prognosis depends on the specific histopathologic type of cyst. Except for the odontogenic keratocyst, the recurrence potential should be low.

NASOPALATINE DUCT CYST (Incisive Canal Cyst)

The **nasopalatine duct cyst** is the most common nonodontogenic cyst of the oral cavity, occurring in about 1 percent of the population. The cyst is believed to arise from remnants of the **nasopalatine duct**, an embryologic structure connecting the oral and nasal cavities in the area of the incisive canal.

In the 7-week-old fetus, the developing palate consists of the **primary palate**, which is formed by the fusion of the medial nasal processes. Behind the primary palate, downgrowth of the nasal septum produces two communications between the oral and nasal cavities, the primitive nasal choanae. Formation of the **secondary palate** begins around the eighth intrauterine week with downward growth of the medial parts of the maxillary processes (the **palatine processes**) to a location on either side of the tongue.

As the mandible develops and the tongue drops down, these palatine processes grow horizontally, fusing with the nasal septum in the midline and with the primary palate along their anterior aspect. Two passageways persist in the midline between the primary and secondary palates (the **incisive canals**). Also formed by this fusion and found within the incisive canals are epithelial structures—the **nasopalatine ducts**. These ducts normally degenerate in humans but may leave epithelial remnants behind in the incisive canals.

The incisive canals begin on the floor of the nasal cavity on either side of the nasal septum, coursing downward and forward to exit the palatal bone via a common foramen in the area of the incisive papilla. In addition to the nasopalatine ducts, these canals contain the nasopalatine nerve plus anastomosing branches of the descending palatine and sphenopalatine arteries. Occasionally, two smaller foramina carrying the nasopalatine nerves—the **canals of Scarpa**—are found within the incisive foramen.

In some mammals, the nasopalatine ducts remain patent and provide communication between the oral and nasal cavities. On rare occasions, patent or partially patent nasopalatine ducts may be encountered in humans. In mammals, the nasopalatine ducts may communicate with the vomer-nasal **organs of Jacobson**, acting as an accessory olfactory organ. However, in humans, Jacobson's organ usually recedes in uterine life to become a vestigial structure.

It has been suggested that the nasopalatine duct cyst may arise from the epithelium of Jacobson's organ, but this appears highly unlikely. Trauma or infection of the duct and mucous retention of adjacent minor salivary glands also have been mentioned as possible etiologic factors, but the role of each has been questioned. Although the pathogenesis of this lesion is still uncertain, the lesion most likely represents a spontaneous cystic degeneration of remnants of the nasopalatine duct.

Clinical and Radiographic Features

The nasopalatine duct cyst may develop at almost any age, but is most common in the fourth to sixth decades of life. In spite of its being a "developmental" cyst, the nasopalatine duct cyst is rarely seen during the first decade. Most studies have shown a male predilection.

The most common presenting symptoms include swelling of the anterior palate, drainage, and pain (Fig. 1–55). Patients sometimes relate a long history of these symptoms, probably because of their intermittent nature. However, many lesions are asymptomatic and are discovered on routine radiographs. Rarely, a large cyst may produce a "through-and-through" fluctuant expansion involving the anterior palate and labial alveolar mucosa.

Radiographs usually demonstrate a well-circumscribed

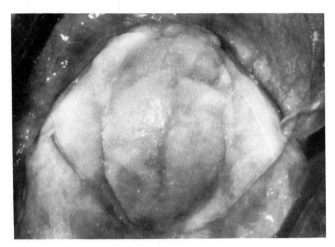

FIGURE 1–55. **Nasopalatine duct cyst.** Fluctuant swelling of the anterior hard palate.

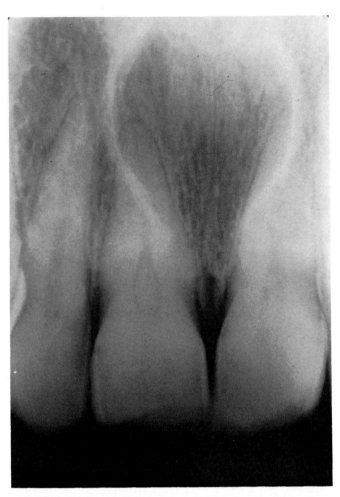

FIGURE 1–57. **Nasopalatine duct cyst.** Well-circumscribed radiolucency between and apical to the roots of the maxillary central incisors.

radiolucency in or near the midline of the anterior maxilla between and apical to the central incisor teeth (Figs. 1–56 and 1–57). Root resorption is rarely noted. The lesion is most often round or oval with a sclerotic border. Some cysts may have an inverted pear shape, presumably because of resistance of adjacent tooth roots. Other examples may show a classic heart shape as a result of superimposition of the nasal spine or because they are notched by the nasal septum.

The radiographic diameter of nasopalatine duct cysts can range from small lesions, less than 6 mm, to destructive lesions as large as 6 cm. However, most cysts are in the range of 1.0 to 2.5 cm, with an average diameter of 1.5 to 1.7 cm. It may be difficult to distinguish a small nasopalatine duct cyst from a large incisive foramen. It is generally accepted that a diameter of 6 mm is the upper limit of normal size for the incisive foramen. Therefore, a radiolucency that is 6 mm or smaller in this area is usually considered a normal foramen unless other clinical signs or symptoms are present.

In rare instances, a nasopalatine duct cyst may develop in the soft tissues of the incisive papilla area without any bony involvement. Such lesions are often called **cysts of the incisive papilla.** These cysts frequently demonstrate bluish discoloration as a result of the fluid contents in the cyst lumen (Fig. 1–58).

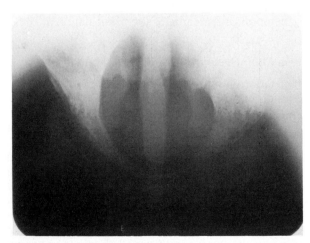

FIGURE 1–56. **Nasopalatine duct cyst.** Radiograph of the same lesion depicted in Figure 1–55. A large, well-circumscribed radiolucency of the anterior hard palate is apparent.

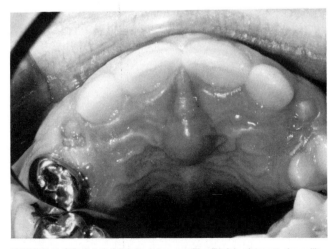

FIGURE 1–58. **Cyst of the incisive papilla.** Bluish-pigmented swelling of the incisive papilla.

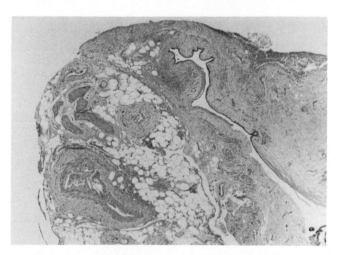

FIGURE 1–59. **Nasopalatine duct cyst.** Low-power view showing a cyst with adjacent blood vessels, nerves, and adipose tissue.

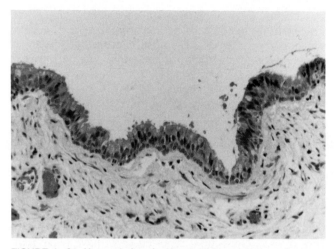

FIGURE 1–61. **Nasopalatine duct cyst.** High-power view of a nasopalatine duct cyst lined by pseudostratified, ciliated columnar epithelium.

Histopathologic Features

The epithelial lining of nasopalatine duct cysts is highly variable (Figs. 1–59 to 1–61). It may be composed of:

- Stratified squamous epithelium
- Pseudostratified columnar epithelium
- Simple columnar epithelium
- Simple cuboidal epithelium

Frequently, more than one epithelial type is found in the same cyst.

Stratified squamous epithelium is most common, present in about three fourths of all cysts. Pseudostratified columnar epithelium has been reported in approximately one third of all cases. Simple columnar and cuboidal epithelium are discovered less frequently.

Cilia and goblet cells may be found in association with columnar linings. The type of epithelium may be related to the vertical position of the cyst within the incisive canal. Cysts developing within the superior aspect of the canal near the nasal cavity are more likely to demonstrate respiratory epithelium; those in an inferior position near the oral cavity are more likely to exhibit squamous epithelium.

The contents of the cyst wall can be a helpful diagnostic aid. Because the nasopalatine duct cyst arises within the incisive canal, moderate-sized nerves and small muscular arteries and veins are usually found in the wall of the cyst. Small mucous glands have been reported in as many as one third of cases. Occasionally, one may see small islands of hyaline cartilage. An inflammatory response is frequently noted in the cyst wall and may range from mild to heavy. This inflammation is usually chronic in nature and is composed of lymphocytes, plasma cells, and histiocytes. Associated acute inflammatory cells (neutrophils) may sometimes be seen.

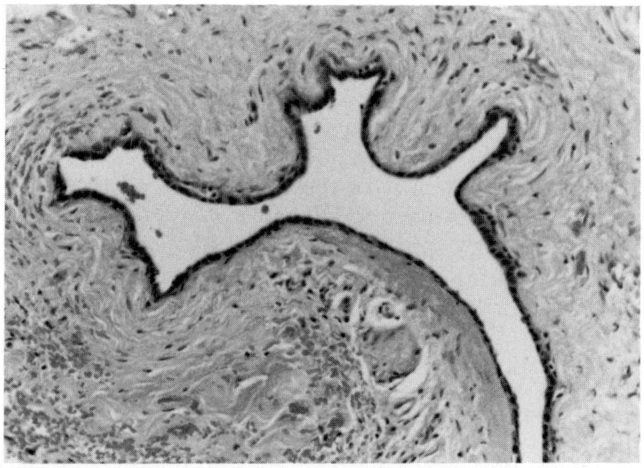

Treatment and Prognosis

Nasopalatine duct cysts are treated by surgical enucleation. Biopsy is recommended because the lesion is not radiographically diagnostic; other benign and malignant lesions have been known to mimic the nasopalatine duct cyst. The lesion is best approached with a palatal flap that is reflected after an incision is made along the lingual gingival margin of the anterior maxillary teeth. Recurrence is rare.

MEDIAN PALATAL (PALATINE) CYST

The **median palatal (palatine) cyst** is a rare fissural cyst that theoretically develops from epithelium entrapped along the embryonic line of fusion of the lateral palatal shelves of the maxilla. This cyst may be difficult to distinguish from a **nasopalatine duct cyst.** In fact, most "median palatal cysts" may represent posteriorly positioned nasopalatine duct cysts. Because the nasopalatine ducts course posteriorly and superiorly as they extend from the incisive canal to the nasal cavity, a nasopalatine duct cyst that arises from posterior remnants of this duct near the

FIGURE 1–60. **Nasopalatine duct cyst.** High-power view of the same cyst in Figure 1–59 showing flattened cuboidal epithelial lining.

nasal cavity might be mistaken for a median palatal cyst. On the other hand, if a true median palatal cyst were to develop toward the anterior portion of the hard palate, it could easily be mistaken for a nasopalatine duct cyst.

Clinical and Radiographic Features

The median palatal cyst presents as a firm or fluctuant swelling of the midline of the hard palate posterior to the palatine papilla. The lesion appears most frequently in young adults. It is often asymptomatic, but some patients complain of pain or expansion. The average size of this cyst is 2 × 2 cm, but it can sometimes become quite large. Occlusal radiographs demonstrate a well-circumscribed radiolucency in the midline of the hard palate (Fig. 1–62). Occasional reported cases have been associated with divergence of the central incisors, although it may be difficult to rule out a nasopalatine duct cyst in these instances.

It must be stressed that a true median palatal cyst should present with clinical enlargement of the palate. A midline radiolucency without clinical evidence of expansion is probably a nasopalatine duct cyst.

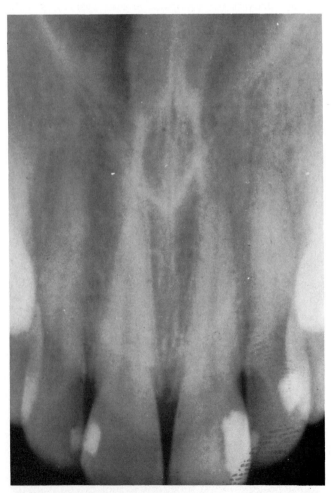

FIGURE 1–62. **Median palatal cyst.** Well-circumscribed radiolucency apical to the maxillary incisors in the midline. At surgery, the lesion was unrelated to the incisive canal. (Courtesy of Dr. Timothy Armanini.)

Histopathologic Features

Microscopic examination shows a cyst that is usually lined by stratified squamous epithelium. Areas of ciliated pseudostratified columnar epithelium have been reported in some cases. Chronic inflammation may be present in the cyst wall.

Treatment and Prognosis

The median palatal cyst is treated by surgical removal. Recurrence should not be expected.

MEDIAN MANDIBULAR CYST

The **median mandibular cyst** is a controversial lesion of questionable existence. Theoretically, it represents a fissural cyst in the anterior midline of the mandible that develops from epithelium entrapped during fusion of the halves of the mandible during embryonic life. However, the mandible actually develops as a single bi-lobed proliferation of mesenchyme with a central isthmus in the midline. As the mandible develops, this isthmus is eliminated. Therefore, because no fusion of epithelium-lined processes occurs, entrapment of epithelium should not be possible. For this reason, it appears likely that most, if not all, of these midline cysts are of odontogenic origin.

Clinical and Radiographic Features

Reported cases of median mandibular cyst have presented as a midline radiolucency found between or apical to the mandibular central incisor teeth. Cortical expansion may be noted. A couple of purported cases have been partially within bone and partially within soft tissue.

Histopathologic Features

The type of epithelial lining varies in reported cases of median mandibular cyst. The most common lining is composed of stratified squamous epithelium, and most of these cases may actually have been periapical or residual cysts. Some cysts in this location may be classified as odontogenic keratocysts or developmental lateral periodontal cysts.

A few reported cysts have been lined with pseudostratified, ciliated columnar epithelium. These findings raise the greatest possibility of the existence of an actual fissural cyst in this location. However, **periapical cysts** exhibit respiratory epithelium in rare instances. Also, these types may now fit into the category of **glandular odontogenic cyst** (see p. 509), a more recently recognized developmental cyst of odontogenic origin.

Treatment and Prognosis

The treatment of choice for median mandibular cysts is surgical enucleation. Recurrence is not expected in most cases.

EPIDERMOID CYST OF THE SKIN

The **epidermoid cyst** is a common cyst of the skin that is lined by epidermis-like epithelium. Most epidermoid cysts are derived from the follicular infundibulum and are also called **infundibular cysts**. These cysts often arise after localized inflammation of the hair follicle and probably represent a non-neoplastic proliferation of the infundibular epithelium resulting from the healing process. The term **sebaceous cyst** is sometimes mistakenly used as a synonym for both the epidermoid cyst and another cyst of the scalp known as a **pilar**, or **trichilemmal, cyst**. However, because both the epidermoid cyst and pilar cyst are derived from the hair follicle rather than the sebaceous gland, the term "sebaceous cyst" should be avoided.

Epidermoid cysts of the skin occasionally may arise after traumatic implantation of epithelium. Rarely, such **epidermal inclusion cysts** can also develop in the mouth. These small inclusion cysts should probably be distinguished from oral epidermoid cysts that occur in the midline floor of mouth region and represent the minimal manifestation of the teratoma/dermoid cyst/epidermoid cyst spectrum (see p. 30).

Clinical Features

Epidermoid cysts of the skin are most common in the acne-prone areas of the head, neck, and back. They are unusual before puberty unless they are associated with **Gardner syndrome** (see p. 473). Young adults are more likely to have cysts on the face, whereas older adults are more likely to have cysts on the back. Males are affected more frequently than females.

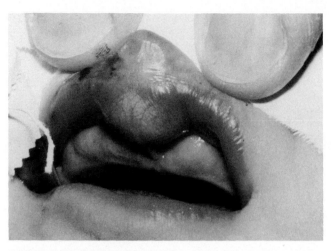

FIGURE 1–64. **Epidermoid cyst.** Infant with a mass in the upper lip.

Epidermoid cysts present as nodular, fluctuant subcutaneous lesions that may or may not be associated with inflammation (Figs. 1–63 and 1–64; see Color Figure 7). If a non-inflamed lesion presents in an area of thin skin, such as the earlobe, it may be white or yellow.

Histopathologic Features

Microscopic examination reveals a cavity that is lined by stratified squamous epithelium resembling epidermis (Fig. 1–65). A well-developed granular cell layer is seen, and the lumen is filled with degenerating orthokeratin (Fig. 1–66). Not infrequently, the epithelial lining will be disrupted. When this occurs, a prominent granulomatous inflammatory reaction, including multinucleated giant cells, can be present in the cyst wall because the exposed keratin is recognized as a foreign material.

Treatment and Prognosis

Epidermoid cysts are usually treated by conservative surgical excision, and recurrence is uncommon. Malig-

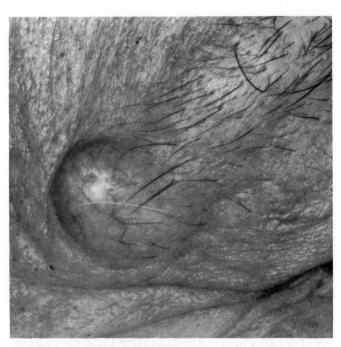

FIGURE 1–63. **Epidermoid cyst.** Fluctuant nodule at the lateral edge of the eyebrow. See Color Plates.

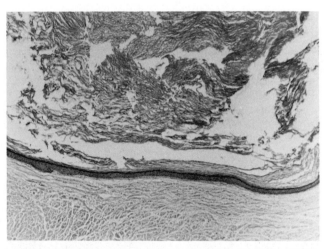

FIGURE 1–65. **Epidermoid cyst.** Low-power view showing a keratin-filled cystic cavity.

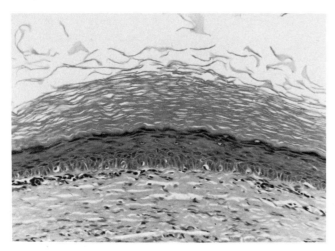

FIGURE 1–66. Epidermoid cyst. Stratified squamous epithelial lining with a prominent granular cell layer and orthokeratin production.

nant transformation has been reported but is exceedingly rare.

DERMOID CYST

The **dermoid cyst** is an uncommon developmental cystic malformation. The cyst is lined by epidermis-like epithelium and contains dermal adnexal structures in the cyst wall. It is generally classified as a benign cystic form of **teratoma.**

By definition, a *true* teratoma is a developmental tumor composed of tissue from all three germ layers: ectoderm, mesoderm, and endoderm. Such tumors are believed to arise from germ cells or entrapped totipotent blastomeres, which can produce derivatives of all three germ layers.

Teratomatous malformations have a spectrum of complexity. In their most complex form, these lesions produce multiple types of tissue that are arranged in a disorganized fashion. These "complex" teratomas are most common in the ovaries or testes and can be benign or malignant. Occasionally, ovarian teratomas (or "dermoids") produce well-formed teeth, or even partially complete jaws. Complex teratomas of the oral cavity are rare and are usually congenital in nature. When they occur, they usually extend through a cleft palate from the pituitary area via Rathke's pouch. Cervical teratomas have also been reported.

The term **teratoid cyst** has been used to describe a cystic form of teratoma that contains a variety of germ layer derivatives:

1. Skin appendages, including hair follicles, sebaceous glands, and sweat glands.
2. Connective tissue elements, such as muscle, blood vessels, and bone.
3. Endodermal structures, such as gastrointestinal lining.

Rarely, oral cysts may be lined entirely by gastrointestinal epithelium. These **heterotopic oral gastrointestinal cysts (enterocystomas; enteric duplication cysts)** are usually considered to be **choristomas,** or histologically normal tissue found in an abnormal location. However, these lesions probably can be included under the broad umbrella of teratomatous lesions, especially since they occasionally are found in combination with dermoid cysts.

Dermoid cysts are simpler in structure than complex teratomas or teratoid cysts. Although they do not contain tissue from all three germ layers, they probably represent a *forme fruste* of a teratoma. Similar cysts of the oral cavity can be seen that are lined by epidermis-like epithelium, but contain no dermal appendages in the cyst wall. These lesions have been called **epidermoid cysts** and represent the simplest expression of the teratoma spectrum. These intraoral epidermoid cysts should not be confused with the more common **epidermoid cyst of the skin** (see p. 29), a non-teratomatous lesion that arises from the hair follicle.

Clinical Features

Dermoid cysts most commonly occur in the midline of the floor of the mouth (Fig. 1–67), although occasionally they are displaced laterally or develop in other locations. If the cyst develops above the geniohyoid muscle, a sublingual swelling may displace the tongue toward the roof of the mouth and create difficulty in eating, speaking, or even breathing. Cysts that occur below the geniohyoid muscle often produce a submental swelling with a "double chin" appearance.

Oral dermoid cysts can vary in size from a few millimeters to 12 cm in diameter. They rarely occur in infants but are most common in young adults. The lesion is usually slow-growing and painless, presenting as a doughy or rubbery mass that frequently retains pitting after application of pressure. Secondary infection can occur, and the lesion may drain intraorally or onto the skin.

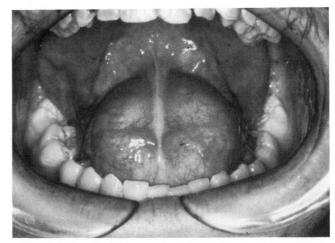

FIGURE 1–67. Dermoid cyst. Fluctuant midline swelling in the floor of the mouth. (From Budnick SD: Handbook of Pediatric Oral Pathology. Chicago, Year Book Medical, 1981, p 240.)

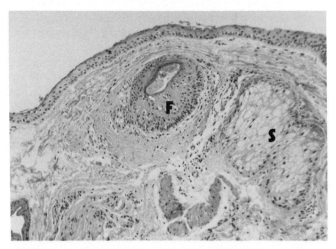

FIGURE 1–68. **Dermoid cyst.** Squamous epithelial lining (*top*) with hair follicle (F) and sebaceous glands (S) in the cyst wall.

Histopathologic Features

Dermoid cysts are lined by orthokeratinized stratified squamous epithelium with a prominent granular cell layer. Abundant keratin is often found within the cyst lumen. On rare occasions, areas of respiratory epithelium can be seen. The cyst wall is composed of fibrous connective tissue that contains one or more skin appendages, such as sebaceous glands, hair follicles, or sweat glands (Fig. 1–68).

Treatment and Prognosis

Dermoid cysts are treated by surgical removal. Those located above the geniohyoid muscle can be removed by an intraoral incision, and those below the geniohyoid muscle may require an extraoral approach. Recurrence is uncommon. Malignant transformation into squamous cell carcinoma has been reported only rarely.

THYROGLOSSAL DUCT CYST
(Thyroglossal Tract Cyst)

The thyroid gland begins its development at the end of the third week of embryonic life as a proliferation of endodermal cells from the ventral floor of the pharynx between the tuberculum impar and copula of the developing tongue—a point that later becomes the foramen cecum. This thyroid anlage descends into the neck as a bi-lobed diverticulum anterior to the developing hyoid bone, and reaches its definitive level below the thyroid cartilage by the seventh embryonic week. Along this path of descent, an epithelial tract or duct is formed, maintaining an attachment to the base of the tongue. This thyroglossal duct becomes intimately associated with the developing hyoid bone. As the hyoid matures and rotates to its adult position, the thyroglossal duct passes in front and beneath the hyoid, looping upward and behind it before curving downward again into the lower neck. The caudal segment of this duct often persists, forming the pyramidal lobe of the thyroid gland.

The thyroglossal duct epithelium normally undergoes atrophy and is obliterated. However, remnants of this epithelium may persist and give rise to cysts along this tract known as **thyroglossal duct cysts**. The impetus for cystic degeneration is uncertain. Inflammation is the most frequently suggested stimulus, especially from adjacent lymphoid tissue that may react to draining infections of the head and neck. Retention of secretions within the duct is another possible factor. In addition, there are several reports of familial occurrence of such cysts.

Clinical Features

Thyroglossal duct cysts classically develop in the midline and may occur anywhere from the foramen cecum area of the tongue to the suprasternal notch. Suprahyoid cysts may be submental in location. In 60 to 80 percent of cases, the cyst develops below the hyoid bone. Intralingual cysts are rare. Cysts that develop in the area of the thyroid cartilage are often deflected lateral to the midline because of the sharp anterior margin of the thyroid cartilage.

Thyroglossal duct cysts may develop at any age, but they are most commonly diagnosed in the first two decades of life; about 50 percent of cases occur before the age of 20. There is no sex predilection. The cyst usually presents as a painless, fluctuant, movable swelling unless it is complicated by secondary infection (Fig. 1–69). Most thyroglossal duct cysts are smaller than 3 cm in diameter, but occasional cysts may reach 10 cm in size. If the cyst maintains an attachment to the hyoid bone or tongue, it will move vertically during swallowing or protrusion of the tongue. Fistulous tracts to the skin or mucosa develop in as many as one third of cases, usually from rupture of an infected cyst or as a sequela of surgery.

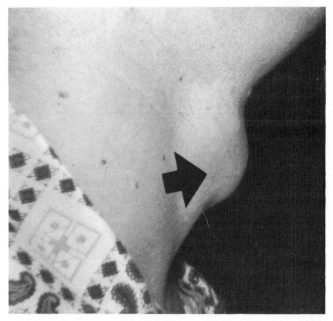

FIGURE 1–69. **Thyroglossal duct cyst.** Swelling (*arrow*) of the anterior midline of the neck. (Courtesy of Dr. Philip Sprinkle.)

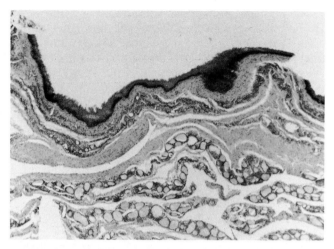

FIGURE 1–70. **Thyroglossal duct cyst.** Cyst (*top*) lined by stratified squamous epithelium. Thyroid follicles can be seen in the cyst wall (*bottom*).

Histopathologic Features

Thyroglossal duct cysts are usually lined by columnar or stratified squamous epithelium, although occasionally cuboidal or even small intestine epithelium may be documented (Fig. 1–70). Sometimes a mixture of epithelial types is present. Thyroid tissue may occur in the cyst wall, but this is not a constant finding.

Treatment and Prognosis

Thyroglossal duct cysts are best treated by a Sistrunk procedure. In this operation, the cyst is removed in addition to the midline segment of the hyoid bone and a generous portion of muscular tissue along the entire thyroglossal tract. The recurrence rate associated with this procedure is less than 10 percent. A much higher recurrence rate can be expected with less aggressive surgery.

Carcinoma arising in a thyroglossal duct cyst is a rare complication that occurs in less than 1 percent of cases. Most of these have been papillary thyroid adenocarcinomas. Fortunately, metastases from thyroglossal carcinoma are rare, and the prognosis for people with these tumors is good.

CERVICAL LYMPHOEPITHELIAL CYST
(Branchial Cleft Cyst)

The **cervical lymphoepithelial cyst,** a developmental cyst of the lateral neck, has a disputed pathogenesis. The classic theory holds that the cyst develops from remnants of the branchial clefts because it occurs in the area of the embryonic gill arch apparatus. A second theory considers that it arises from cystic changes in parotid gland epithelium that becomes entrapped in the upper cervical lymph nodes during embryonic life.

Clinical Features

The cervical lymphoepithelial cyst most commonly occurs in the upper lateral neck along the anterior border of the sternocleidomastoid muscle (Figs. 1–71 and 1–72). It most frequently affects young adults between the ages of 20 and 40. Clinically, the cyst appears as a soft, fluctuant mass that can range from 1 to 10 cm in diameter. Associated tenderness or pain may sometimes occur with secondary infection. Occasionally, the lesion becomes evident after an upper respiratory tract infection or trauma. In rare instances, bilateral cysts may develop.

Although one popular theory suggests that these cysts are derived from parotid epithelium that becomes entrapped within lymph node tissue, lymphoepithelial cysts are uncommon within the parotid gland itself. In recent years, however, increased numbers of parotid lymphoepithelial cysts have been reported in patients with human immunodeficiency virus (HIV) infection. These are probably related to intraparotid lymphadenopathy associated with HIV infection.

Histopathologic Features

More than 90 percent of cervical lymphoepithelial cysts are lined by stratified squamous epithelium that may or may not be keratinized (Fig. 1–73). Some cysts demonstrate respiratory epithelium. The wall of the cyst typically contains lymphoid tissue, often demonstrating germinal center formation (Fig. 1–74). However, occasional cysts have been reported without lymphoid tissue.

Treatment and Prognosis

The cervical lymphoepithelial cyst is treated by surgical removal. The lesion almost never recurs.

Rare examples of malignant transformation in these cysts have been reported. Although such an occurrence is theoretically possible, most of these cases probably represent cystic metastases from previously undetected carci-

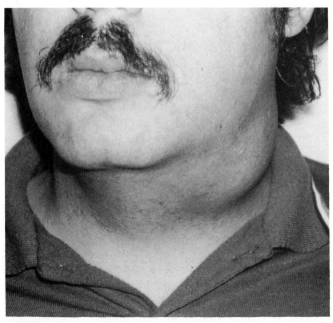

FIGURE 1–71. **Cervical lymphoepithelial cyst.** Fluctuant swelling of the lateral neck.

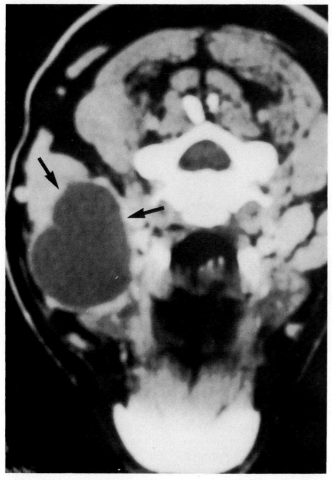

FIGURE 1-72. **Cervical lymphoepithelial cyst.** Imaging study of the same cyst depicted in Figure 1-71 showing a well-circumscribed lesion of the lateral neck (*arrows*).

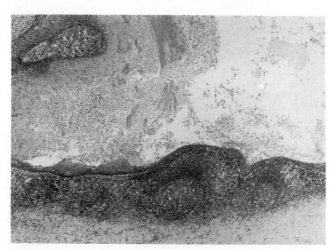

FIGURE 1-73. **Cervical lymphoepithelial cyst.** Low-power view showing the cystic cavity with lymphoid tissue in the cyst wall.

nomas of the head and neck region, especially the nasopharynx.

ORAL LYMPHOEPITHELIAL CYST

The **oral lymphoepithelial cyst** is an uncommon lesion of the mouth that develops within oral lymphoid tissue. It is microscopically similar to the cervical lymphoepithelial cyst but much smaller in size.

Lymphoid tissue is normally found in the oral cavity and pharynx, principally consisting of **Waldeyer's ring**, which includes the palatine tonsils, lingual tonsils, and pharyngeal adenoids. In addition, accessory oral tonsils or lymphoid aggregates may occur in the floor of the mouth, ventral surface of the tongue, and soft palate.

Oral lymphoid tissue has a close relationship with the overlying mucosal epithelium. This epithelium demonstrates invaginations into the tonsillar tissue, resulting in blind pouches or tonsillar crypts that may fill up with keratin debris. The tonsillar crypt may become obstructed or pinched off from the surface, producing a keratin-filled cyst within the lymphoid tissue just below the mucosal surface. It is also possible that oral lympho-

epithelial cysts may develop from salivary or surface mucosal epithelium that becomes enclaved in lymphoid tissue during embryogenesis. It has even been suggested that these cysts may arise from the excretory ducts of the sublingual gland or minor salivary glands and that the associated lymphoid tissue represents a secondary immune response.

Clinical Features

The oral lymphoepithelial cyst presents as a small submucosal mass that is usually less than 1 cm in diameter; rarely will the lesion be greater than 1.5 cm (Figs. 1-75 and 1-76; see Color Figure 8). The cyst may feel firm or soft to palpation, and the overlying mucosa is smooth and non-ulcerated. The lesion is typically white or yellow and often contains creamy or cheesy keratinaceous material in the lumen. The cyst is usually asymptomatic, although occasionally patients may complain of swelling or drainage. Pain is rare but may occur secondary to trauma.

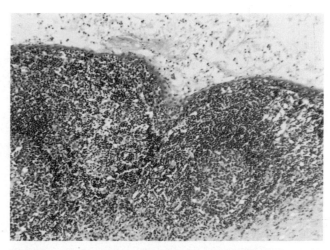

FIGURE 1-74. **Cervical lymphoepithelial cyst.** Lymphoid tissue with germinal centers adjacent to squamous epithelial lining.

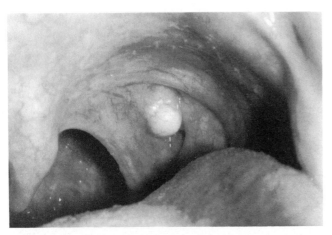

FIGURE 1–75. **Oral lymphoepithelial cyst.** Small yellow-white nodule of the tonsillar fossa. See Color Plates.

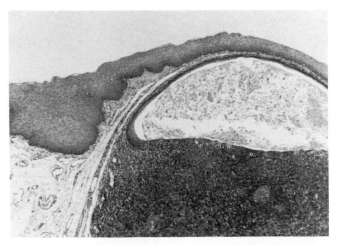

FIGURE 1–77. **Oral lymphoepithelial cyst.** Keratin-filled cyst below the mucosal surface. Lymphoid tissue is present in the cyst wall.

Oral lymphoepithelial cysts may develop in people of almost any age, but they are most common in young adults. The most frequent location is the floor of the mouth, with at least half of all cases found there. The ventral surface and posterior lateral border of the tongue are the next most common sites. Rarely, these cysts develop in the area of the palatine tonsil or soft palate. All of these locations represent sites of normal or accessory oral lymphoid tissue.

Histopathologic Features

Microscopic examination of the oral lymphoepithelial cyst demonstrates a cystic cavity that is lined by stratified squamous epithelium without rete ridges (Fig. 1–77). This epithelium is typically parakeratinized, with desquamated epithelial cells seen filling the cyst lumen. In rare instances, the epithelial lining may also contain mucous cells. Occasional cysts may communicate with the overlying mucosal surface.

The most striking feature is the presence of lymphoid tissue in the cyst wall. In most instances, this lymphoid tissue encircles the cyst but sometimes involves only a portion of the cyst wall. Germinal centers are usually, but not always, present.

Treatment and Prognosis

The oral lymphoepithelial cyst is usually treated with surgical excision and should not recur. Because the lesion is typically asymptomatic and innocuous, biopsy may not always be necessary if the lesion is distinctive enough to make the diagnosis on a clinical basis.

Other Rare Developmental Anomalies

HEMIHYPERPLASIA (Hemihypertrophy)

Hemihyperplasia is a rare developmental anomaly characterized by unilateral enlargement of the body. Although the condition is known more commonly as **hemihypertrophy**, it actually represents a hyperplasia of the tissues rather than a hypertrophy.

Almost all cases are sporadic. A number of possible etiologic factors have been suggested, but the cause remains obscure. Various theories include vascular or lymphatic abnormalities, central nervous system disturbances, endocrine dysfunctions, and aberrant twinning mechanisms. Occasionally, chromosomal anomalies have been documented.

Clinical and Radiographic Features

In a person with hemihyperplasia, one whole side of the body (**complex hyperplasia**) may be affected, or the enlargement may be limited to a single digit (**simple hyperplasia**) or limb (**segmental hyperplasia**). If the en-

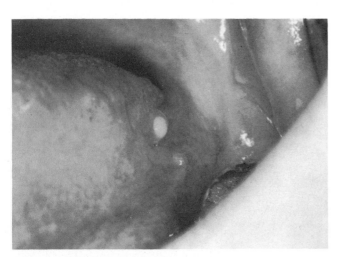

FIGURE 1–76. **Oral lymphoepithelial cyst.** Small white nodule of the posterior lateral border of the tongue.

largement is confined to one side of the face, the term **hemifacial hyperplasia** (or **hemifacial hypertrophy**) may apply. The condition can occasionally be crossed, involving different areas on both sides of the body.

Asymmetry often is noted at birth, although in some cases the condition may not become evident until later in childhood (Fig. 1–78). The enlargement becomes more accentuated with age, especially at puberty. This disproportionate growth continues until the patient's overall growth ceases, resulting in permanent asymmetry.

The changes may involve all the tissues on the affected side, including the underlying bone. The skin is often thickened and may demonstrate increased pigmentation, hypertrichosis, telangiectasias, or nevus flammeus. About 20 percent of those affected are mentally retarded. One of the most significant features is an increased incidence of abdominal tumors, especially Wilms tumor, adrenal cortical carcinoma, and hepatoblastoma. These tumors do not necessarily occur on the same side as the hyperplasia.

Unilateral **macroglossia** featuring prominent tongue papillae is common (Fig. 1–79). Enlargement of other oral soft tissues and bone can occur (Fig. 1–80). The mandibular canal may be increased in size on radiographs. The crowns of the teeth on the affected side, especially the permanent cuspids, premolars, and first molars, can be larger. Premature development of these teeth along with precocious eruption may be obvious.

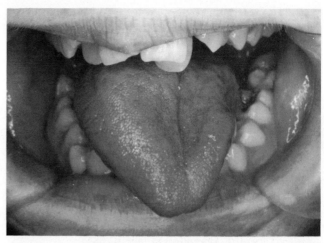

FIGURE 1–79. **Hemihyperplasia.** Same patient as depicted in Figure 1–78 with associated enlargement of the right half of the tongue. (Courtesy of Dr. George Blozis.)

The roots may also be larger, but some reports have described root resorption. Malocclusion with open bite is not unusual.

Histopathologic Features

Microscopic examination shows an increase in thickness of the epithelium with hyperplasia of the underlying connective tissues.

Treatment and Prognosis

A complete workup should be undertaken to rule out other possible causes of unilateral growth, especially neurofibromatosis (see p. 381), which can mimic hemihyperplasia. During childhood, periodic ultrasound examination should be performed to rule out development of abdominal tumors. After the patient's growth has ceased, cosmetic surgery can be performed, including soft tissue debulking, face lifts, and orthognathic surgery. Orthodontic therapy is also frequently needed.

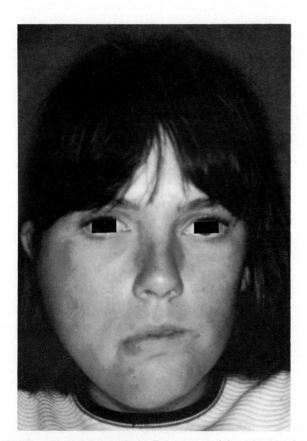

FIGURE 1–78. **Hemihyperplasia.** Enlargement of the right side of the face. (Courtesy of Dr. George Blozis.)

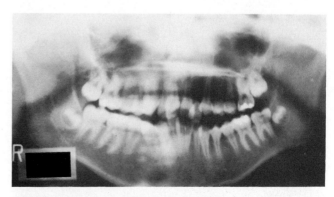

FIGURE 1–80. **Hemihyperplasia.** Radiograph of the same patient in Figures 1–78 and 1–79. The mandible and teeth on the right side are enlarged. (Courtesy of Dr. George Blozis.)

PROGRESSIVE HEMIFACIAL ATROPHY
(Romberg Syndrome; Parry-Romberg Syndrome)

Progressive hemifacial atrophy is an uncommon and poorly understood degenerative condition characterized by atrophic changes affecting one side of the face. The cause of these changes remains obscure. Speculation has considered trophic malfunction of the cervical sympathetic nervous system. A history of prior trauma has been documented in some cases, although other reports have considered a viral or *Borrelia* infection. The condition is usually sporadic, but a few familial cases have been reported, suggesting a possible hereditary influence. Many investigators believe that hemifacial atrophy represents a localized form of **scleroderma** (see p. 585).

Clinical and Radiographic Features

The onset of the syndrome is usually during the first two decades of life. The condition begins as atrophy of the skin and subcutaneous structures in a localized area of the face (Fig. 1–81). This atrophy progresses at a variable rate and affects the dermatome of one or more branches of the trigeminal nerve. Hypoplasia of the underlying bone may also occur. Osseous hypoplasia is more common when the condition begins during the first decade. Occasionally, bilateral facial atrophy may occur, or the condition may affect one side of the entire body. Females are affected more often than males.

The overlying skin often exhibits dark pigmentation. Some patients have a sharp line of demarcation, resembling a large linear scar, between normal and abnormal skin near the midline of the forehead, known as *coup de sabre* ("strike of the sword"). Ocular involvement is common, and the most frequent manifestation is enophthalmos due to loss of periorbital fat. Local alopecia may occur. Occasionally, trigeminal neuralgia, facial paresthesia, migraine, or contralateral jacksonian epilepsy may develop.

The mouth and nose are deviated toward the defective side. Atrophy of the upper lip may expose the maxillary teeth. Unilateral atrophy of the tongue can also occur. Unilateral posterior open bite often develops as a result of mandibular hypoplasia and delayed eruption of the teeth. The teeth on the affected side may exhibit deficient root development.

Histopathologic Features

Microscopic examination of the affected skin reveals atrophy of the epidermis and a variable perivascular infiltrate of lymphocytes and monocytes. Degenerative changes in the vascular endothelium can be identified with electron microscopy.

Treatment and Prognosis

The atrophy typically progresses slowly for several years, and then becomes stable. Plastic surgery may be tried to correct the cosmetic deformity, and orthodontic therapy may be helpful to treat any associated malocclusion.

CROUZON SYNDROME (Craniofacial Dysostosis)

Crouzon syndrome is one of a rare group of syndromes characterized by craniosynostosis, or premature closing of the cranial sutures. The condition occurs in about 1 of every 25,000 births and is inherited as an autosomal dominant trait. A significant number of cases, however, represent new mutations, often apparently related to increased paternal age.

Clinical and Radiographic Features

Crouzon syndrome exhibits a wide variability in expression. The premature sutural closing leads to cranial malformations, such as **brachycephaly** (short head), **scaphocephaly** (boat-shaped head), or **trigonocephaly** (triangle-shaped head). The most severely affected patients can demonstrate a "cloverleaf" skull *(kleeblattschädel)*. The orbits are shallow, resulting in characteristic ocular proptosis (Fig. 1–82). Visual impairment or total blindness as well as a hearing deficit may occur. Some patients report headaches, attributable to increased intracranial pressure. Marked mental deficiency is rarely seen. Skull ra-

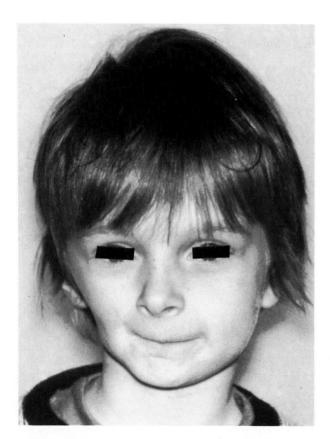

FIGURE 1–81. **Progressive hemifacial atrophy.** Young girl with right-sided facial atrophy.

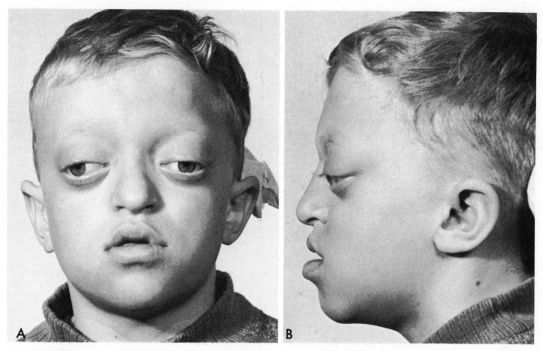

FIGURE 1–82. **Crouzon syndrome.** Ocular proptosis and mid-face hypoplasia. (Courtesy of Dr. Robert Gorlin, with permission of Paparella MM, Shumrick DA. Otolaryngology, 3rd ed. Philadelphia, WB Saunders, 1991.)

diographs typically show increased digital markings ("beaten metal" pattern).

The maxilla is underdeveloped, resulting in mid-face hypoplasia. The maxillary teeth are often crowded, and there is usually occlusal disharmony. Cleft lip and cleft palate are rare, but lateral palatal swellings may produce a midline maxillary pseudocleft.

Treatment and Prognosis

The clinical defects of Crouzon syndrome can be treated surgically, but multiple procedures may be necessary. Early craniectomy is often needed to alleviate the raised intracranial pressure. Fronto-orbital advancement can be performed to correct the ocular defects, with midfacial advancement used to correct the maxillary hypoplasia.

APERT SYNDROME
(Acrocephalosyndactyly)

Like Crouzon syndrome, **Apert syndrome** is a rare condition that is characterized by craniosynostosis. It occurs in about 1 of every 100,000 to 160,000 births. Although it is inherited as an autosomal dominant trait, most cases represent sporadic new mutations, often associated with increased paternal age.

Clinical and Radiographic Features

Craniosynostosis typically produces **acrobrachycephaly** (tower skull); severe cases may demonstrate the

kleeblattschädel deformity (cloverleaf skull). The occiput is flattened, and there is a tall appearance to the forehead. Ocular proptosis is a characteristic finding along with hypertelorism and downward slanting lateral palpebral fissures (Fig. 1–83). Visual loss can result from:

- Chronic exposure of the unprotected eyes
- Increased intracranial pressure
- Compression of the optic nerves

Skull films may demonstrate digital impressions similar to those of Crouzon syndrome (Fig. 1–84).

The middle third of the face is markedly retruded and hypoplastic, resulting in a relative mandibular prognathism. The reduced size of the nasopharynx and narrowing of the posterior choanae can lead to respiratory distress in the young child. To compensate for this, most infants become mouth-breathers, contributing to an "openmouth" appearance. Sleep apnea may develop. Middle ear infections are common, as is conductive hearing loss.

Characteristic limb defects help to distinguish Apert syndrome from other craniosynostosis syndromes. Syndactyly of the second, third, and fourth digits of the hands and feet is always observed (Fig. 1–85). Associated synonychia may also occur. The first and fifth digits may be separate or be joined to the middle digits. Synostosis of adjacent phalanges may be observed on radiographs. The average height of affected patients is below that of the general population.

Mental retardation is common in a large proportion of patients with Apert syndrome. An unusual acne-like eruption develops in most of the patients and involves the forearms.

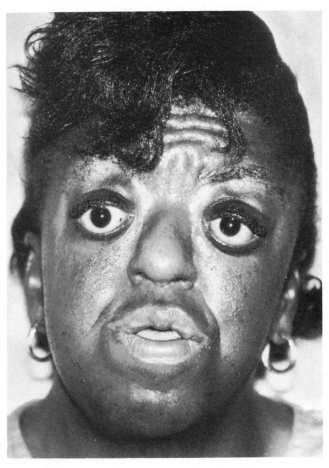

FIGURE 1–83. **Apert syndrome.** Mid-face hypoplasia and ocular proptosis.

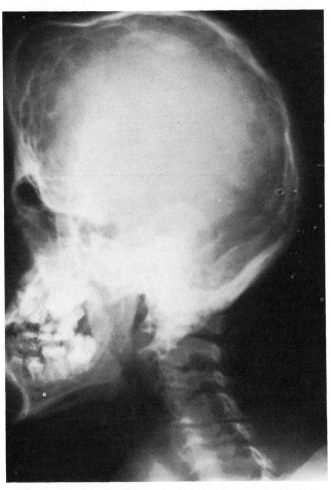

FIGURE 1–84. **Apert syndrome.** Radiograph showing "tower skull," mid-face hypoplasia, and digital markings. Similar digital impressions are apparent in people with Crouzon syndrome. (Courtesy of Dr. Robert Gorlin.)

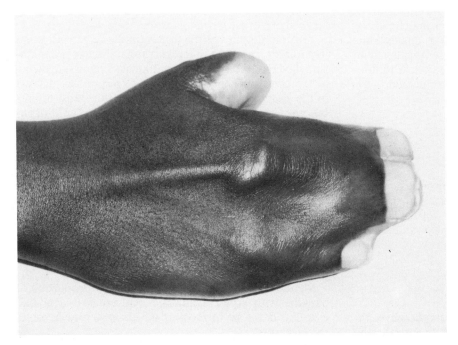

FIGURE 1–85. **Apert syndrome.** Syndactyly of the hand.

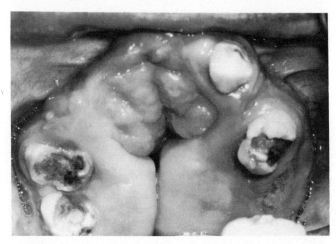

FIGURE 1–86. **Apert syndrome.** Abnormal shape of the maxilla, with swellings of the posterior lateral hard palate resulting in pseudocleft formation.

Specific oral manifestations include a trapezoid-shaped appearance to the lips when they are relaxed, resulting from the mid-face hypoplasia and mouth-breathing. Three fourths of all patients exhibit either a cleft of the soft palate or a bifid uvula. The maxillary hypoplasia leads to a V-shaped arch and crowding of the teeth. Class III malocclusion typically occurs and may be associated with anterior open bite plus anterior and posterior crossbite. Swellings are observed along the lateral hard palate from the accumulation of glycosaminoglycans, especially hyaluronic acid (Fig. 1–86). These swellings often enlarge with age to produce a pseudocleft of the hard palate. Gingival thickening may be associated with delayed eruption of the teeth. Shovel-shaped incisors have been reported in one third of patients.

Treatment and Prognosis

The cosmetic and functional defects of Apert syndrome can be treated by an interdisciplinary approach using multiple surgical procedures. Craniectomy is often performed during the first year of life to treat the craniosynostosis. Frontofacial advancement and mid-face advancement can be done later to correct the proptosis and mid-face hypoplasia. Coordinated orthodontic therapy is often necessary to bring unerupted teeth into place and to improve occlusion. Surgery can also be used to separate the fused fingers.

MANDIBULOFACIAL DYSOSTOSIS
(Treacher Collins Syndrome; Franceschetti-Zwahlen-Klein Syndrome)

Mandibulofacial dysostosis is a rare syndrome that is characterized primarily by defects of structures derived from the first and second branchial arches. It is inherited as an autosomal dominant trait and occurs in around 1

of every 10,000 births. The condition has variable expressivity, and the severity of the clinical features often tends to be greater in subsequent generations of the same family. Approximately 60 percent of cases represent new mutations, and these often are associated with increased paternal age.

Clinical and Radiographic Features

Individuals with mandibulofacial dysostosis exhibit a characteristic facies (Figs. 1–87 and 1–88). The zygomas are hypoplastic, resulting in a narrow face with depressed cheeks and downward-slanting palpebral fissures. In 75 percent of patients, a **coloboma**, or notch, occurs on the outer portion of the lower eyelid. About half of the patients have no eyelashes medial to the coloboma. Often, the sideburns show a tongue-shaped extension toward the cheek.

The ears may demonstrate a number of anomalies. The pinnae are often deformed or misplaced, and extra ear tags may be seen. Ossicle defects or absence of the external auditory canal can cause conductive hearing loss.

The mandible is underdeveloped, resulting in a markedly retruded chin. Radiographs often demonstrate hypoplasia of the condylar and coronoid processes, with prominent antegonial notching. The mouth is downturned, and about 15 percent of patients have lateral facial clefting (see p. 2) that produces macrostomia. Cleft

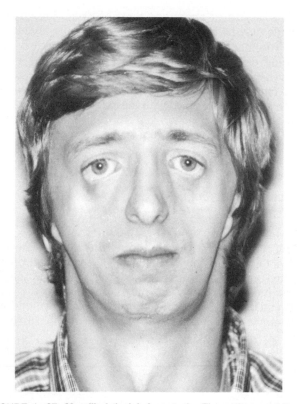

FIGURE 1–87. **Mandibulofacial dysostosis.** The patient exhibits a hypoplastic mandible and downward-slanting palpebral fissures. (Courtesy of Dr. Tom Brock.)

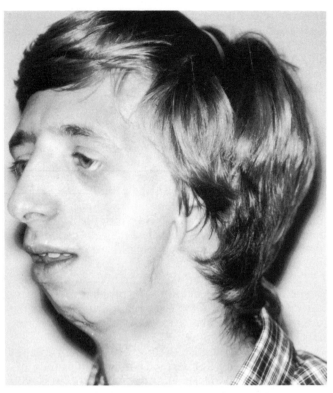

FIGURE 1–88. **Mandibulofacial dysostosis.** Lateral view of the same patient depicted in Figure 1–87 more clearly demonstrates mandibular hypoplasia and ear deformity. (Courtesy of Dr. Tom Brock.)

palate is seen in about one third of cases. The parotid glands may be hypoplastic or may be totally absent.

A number of infants may experience respiratory and feeding difficulties because of hypoplasia of the nasopharynx, oropharynx, and hypopharynx. Choanal atresia is a common finding, and the larynx and trachea are often narrow. Combined with the mandibular hypoplasia and resultant improper tongue position, these defects can lead to the infant's death from respiratory complications.

Treatment and Prognosis

Patients with mild forms of mandibulofacial dysostosis may not require treatment. In more severe cases, the clinical appearance can be improved with cosmetic surgery. Because of the extent of facial reconstruction required, multiple surgical procedures are usually necessary. Individual operations may be needed for the eyes, zygomas, jaws, ears, and nose. Combined orthodontic therapy is needed along with the orthognathic surgery.

REFERENCES

Orofacial Clefts

Gier RE, Fast TB. Median maxillary anterior alveolar cleft: Case reports and discussion. Oral Surg Oral Med Oral Pathol 24:496–502, 1967.

Gorlin RJ, Cohen MM Jr, Levin LS. Orofacial clefting syndromes: General aspects. *In:* Syndromes of the Head and Neck, 3rd ed. New York, Oxford University Press, 1990, pp 693–713.

Hartsfield JK Jr, Bixler D. Bilateral macrostomia in one of monozygotic twins. Oral Surg Oral Med Oral Pathol 57:648–651, 1984.

Kaufman FL. Managing the cleft lip and palate patient. Pediatr Clin North Am 38:1127–1147, 1991.

Kernahan DA, Rosenstein SW. Cleft Lip and Palate: A System of Management. Baltimore, Williams & Wilkins, 1990.

Millard DR Jr, Latham RA. Improved primary surgical and dental treatment of clefts. Plast Reconstr Surg 86:856–871, 1990.

Rintala A, et al. Oblique facial clefts. Scand J Plast Reconstr Surg 14:291–297, 1980.

Shprintzen RJ. Pierre Robin, micrognathia, and airway obstruction: The dependency of treatment on accurate diagnosis. Int Anesthesiol Clin 26:64–71, 1988.

Vanderas AP. Incidence of cleft lip, cleft palate, and cleft lip and palate among races: A review. Cleft Palate J 24:216–225, 1987.

Commissural Lip Pits

Baker BR. Pits of the lip commissures in Caucasoid males. Oral Surg Oral Med Oral Pathol 21:56–60, 1966.

Everett FG, Wescott WB. Commissural lip pits. Oral Surg Oral Med Oral Pathol 14:202–209, 1961.

Gorsky M, Buchner A, Cohen C. Commissural lip pits in Israeli Jews of different ethnic origin. Community Dent Oral Epidemiol 13:195–196, 1985.

Paramedian Lip Pits

Burdick AB, Bixler D, Puckett CL. Genetic analysis in families with van der Woude syndrome. J Craniofac Genet Dev Biol 5:181–208, 1985.

Cervenka J, Gorlin RJ, Anderson VE. The syndrome of pits of the lower lip and cleft lip and/or palate: Genetic considerations. Am J Hum Genet 19:416–432, 1967.

Gorlin RJ, Cohen MM Jr, Levin LS. Popliteal pterygium syndrome (facio-genito-popliteal syndrome). *In:* Syndromes of the Head and Neck, 3rd ed. New York, Oxford University Press, 1990, pp 629–631.

McConnel FMS, Zellweger H, Lawrence RA. Labial pits—cleft lip and/or palate syndrome. Arch Otolaryngol 91:407–411, 1970.

Double Lip

Barnett ML, Bosshardt LL, Morgan AF. Double lip and double lip with blepharochalasis (Ascher's syndrome). Oral Surg Oral Med Oral Pathol 34:727–733, 1972.

Kenny KF, Hreha JP, Dent CD. Bilateral redundant mucosal tissue of the upper lip. J Am Dent Assoc 120:193–194, 1990.

Fordyce Granules

Fordyce JA. A peculiar affection of the mucous membrane of the lips and oral cavity. J Cutan Genito-Urin Dis 14:413, 1896.

Halperin V, et al. The occurrence of Fordyce spots, benign migratory glossitis, median rhomboid glossitis, and fissured tongue in 2,478 dental patients. Oral Surg Oral Med Oral Pathol 6:1072–1077, 1953.

Miles AEW. Sebaceous glands in the lip and cheek mucosa of man. Br Dent J 105:235–248, 1958.

Orlian AI, et al. Sebaceous adenoma of the oral mucosa. J Oral Med 42:38–39, 1987.

Sewerin I. The sebaceous glands in the vermilion border of the lips and in the oral mucosa of man. Acta Odontol Scand 33(Suppl 68):13–226, 1975.

Sewerin I, Prætorius F. Keratin-filled pseudocysts of ducts of sebaceous glands in the vermilion border of the lip. J Oral Pathol 3:279–283, 1974.

Leukoedema

Archard HO, Carlson KP, Stanley HR. Leukoedema of the human oral mucosa. Oral Surg Oral Med Oral Pathol 25:717–728, 1968.

Axéll T, Henricsson V. Leukoedema—an epidemiologic study with special reference to the influence of tobacco habits. Community Dent Oral Epidemiol 9:142–146, 1981.

Durocher RT, Thalman R, Fiore-Donno G. Leukoedema of the oral mucosa. J Am Dent Assoc 85:1105–1109, 1972.

Martin JL, Crump EP. Leukoedema of the buccal mucosa in Negro children and youth. Oral Surg Oral Med Oral Pathol 34:49–58, 1972.

Sandstead HR, Lowe JW. Leukoedema and keratosis in relation to leukoplakia of the buccal mucosa in man. J Natl Cancer Inst 14:423–437, 1953.

Van Wyk CW, Ambrosio SC. Leukoedema: Ultrastructural and histochemical observations. J Oral Pathol 12:319–329, 1983.

Microglossia

Dunham ME, Austin TL. Congenital aglossia and situs inversus. Int J Pediatr Otorhinolaryngol 19:163–168, 1990.

Gorlin RJ, Cohen MM Jr, Levin LS. Oromandibular-limb hypogenesis syndromes. *In:* Syndromes of the Head and Neck, 3rd ed. New York, Oxford University Press, 1990, pp 666–675.

Hall BD. Aglossia-adactylia. Birth Defects 7(7):233–236, 1971.

Shah RM. Palatomandibular and maxillo-mandibular fusion, partial aglossia and cleft palate in a human embryo: Report of a case. Teratology 15:261–272, 1977.

Macroglossia

Engström W, Lindham S, Schofield P. Wiedemann-Beckwith syndrome. Eur J Pediatr 147:450–457, 1988.

Myer CM III, Hotaling AJ, Reilly JS. The diagnosis and treatment of macroglossia in children. Ear Nose Throat J 65:444–448, 1986.

Salman RA. Oral manifestations of Beckwith-Wiedemann syndrome. Special Care in Dentistry 8:23–24, 1988.

Siddiqui A, Pensler JM. The efficacy of tongue resection in treatment of symptomatic macroglossia in the child. Ann Plast Surg 25:14–17, 1990.

Vogel JE, Mulliken JB, Kaban LB. Macroglossia: A review of the condition and a new classification. Plast Reconstr Surg 78:715–723, 1986.

Ankyloglossia

Catlin FI, De Haan V. Tongue-tie. Arch Otolaryngol 94:548–557, 1971.

Ewart NP. A lingual mucogingival problem associated with ankyloglossia: A case report. N Z Dent J 86:16–17, 1990.

Wallace AF. Tongue-tie controversy. Nurs Times 60:527–528, 1964.

Williams WN, Waldron CM. Assessment of lingual function when ankyloglossia (tongue-tie) is suspected. J Am Dent Assoc 110:353–356, 1985.

Lingual Thyroid

Baughman RA. Lingual thyroid and lingual thyroglossal tract remnants. A clinical and histopathologic study with review of the literature. Oral Surg Oral Med Oral Pathol 34:781–799, 1972.

Chanin LR, Greenberg LM. Pediatric upper airway obstruction due to ectopic thyroid: Classification and case reports. Laryngoscope 98:422–427, 1988.

Diaz-Arias AA, et al. Follicular carcinoma with clear cell change arising in lingual thyroid. Oral Surg Oral Med Oral Pathol 74:206–211, 1992.

Kansal P, et al. Lingual thyroid. Diagnosis and treatment. Arch Intern Med 147:2046–2048, 1987.

Montgomery ML. Lingual thyroid: A comprehensive review. West J Surg Obstet Gynecol 43:661–669, 1935; 44:54–62, 122–128, 189–195, 237–247, 303–309, 373–379, 442–446, 1936.

Sauk JJ Jr. Ectopic lingual thyroid. J Pathol 102:239–243, 1970.

Fissured Tongue

Bouquot JE, Gundlach KKH. Odd tongues: The prevalence of common tongue lesions in 23,616 white Americans over 35 years of age. Quintessence Int 17:719–730, 1986.

Eidelman E, Chosack A, Cohen T. Scrotal tongue and geographic tongue: Polygenic and associated traits. Oral Surg Oral Med Oral Pathol 42:591–596, 1976.

Halperin V, et al. The occurrence of Fordyce spots, benign migratory glossitis, median rhomboid glossitis, and fissured tongue in 2,478 dental patients. Oral Surg Oral Med Oral Pathol 6:1072–1077, 1953.

Kullaa-Mikkonen A. Familial study of fissured tongue. Scand J Dent Res 96:366–375, 1988.

Kullaa-Mikkonen A, Sorvari T. Lingua fissurata: A clinical, stereomicroscopic and histopathological study. Int J Oral Maxillofac Surg 15:525–533, 1986.

Hairy Tongue

Bouquot JE, Gundlach KKH. Odd tongues: The prevalence of common tongue lesions in 23,616 white Americans over 35 years of age. Quintessence Int 17:719–730, 1986.

Celis A, Little JW. Clinical study of hairy tongue in hospital patients. J Oral Med 21:139–145, 1966.

Farman AG. Hairy tongue (lingua villosa). J Oral Med 32:85–91, 1977.

Sarti GM, et al. Black hairy tongue. Am Fam Physician 41:1751–1755, 1990.

Standish SM, Moorman WC. Treatment of hairy tongue with podophyllin resin. J Am Dent Assoc 68:535–540, 1964.

Varicosities

Ettinger RL, Manderson RD. A clinical study of sublingual varices. Oral Surg Oral Med Oral Pathol 38:540–545, 1974.

Kleinman HZ. Lingual varicosities. Oral Surg Oral Med Oral Pathol 23:546–548, 1967.

Southam JC, Ettinger RL. A histologic study of sublingual varices. Oral Surg Oral Med Oral Pathol 38:879–886, 1974.

Weathers DR, Fine RM. Thrombosed varix of oral cavity. Arch Dermatol 104:427–430, 1971.

Lateral Soft Palate Fistulas

Gorlin RJ, Cohen MM Jr, Levin LS. Fistulas of lateral soft palate and associated anomalies. *In:* Syndromes of the Head and Neck, 3rd ed. New York, Oxford University Press, 1990, pp 902–903.

Miller AS, Brookreson KR, Brody BA. Lateral soft-palate fistula: Report of a case. Arch Otolaryngol 91:200, 1970.

Coronoid Hyperplasia

Giacomuzzi D. Bilateral enlargement of the mandibular coronoid processes: Review of the literature and report of case. J Oral Maxillofac Surg 44:728–731, 1986.

Hall RE, Orbach S, Landesberg R. Bilateral hyperplasia of the mandibular coronoid processes: A report of two cases. Oral Surg Oral Med Oral Pathol 67:141–145, 1989.

Rowe NL. Bilateral developmental hyperplasia of the mandibular coronoid process: A report of two cases. Br J Oral Surg 1:90–104, 1963.

Tucker MR, Guilford WB, Howard CW. Coronoid process hyperplasia causing restricted opening and facial asymmetry. Oral Surg Oral Med Oral Pathol 58:130–132, 1984.

Condylar Hyperplasia

Bruce RA, Hayward JR. Condylar hyperplasia and mandibular asymmetry: A review. J Oral Surg 26:281–290, 1968.

Iannetti G, et al. Condylar hyperplasia: Cephalometric study, treatment planning, and surgical correction (our experience). Oral Surg Oral Med Oral Pathol 68:673–681, 1989.

Obwegeser HL, Makek MS. Hemimandibular hyperplasia–hemimandibular elongation. J Max-Fac Surg 14:183–208, 1986.

Slootweg PJ, Müller H. Condylar hyperplasia: A clinico-pathological analysis of 22 cases. J Max-Fac Surg 14:209–214, 1986.

Condylar Hypoplasia

Berger SS, Stewart RE. Mandibular hypoplasia secondary to perinatal trauma: Report of case. J Oral Surg 35:578–582, 1977.

Jerrell RG, Fuselier B, Mahan P. Acquired condylar hypoplasia: Report of case. ASDC J Dent Child 58:147–153, 1991.

Sapp JP, Cherrick HM. Pathological aspects of developmental, inflammatory, and neoplastic disease. *In:* The Temporomandibular Joint:

A Biological Basis for Clinical Practice, 4th ed. Edited by Sarnat BG, Laskin DM. Philadelphia, WB Saunders, 1991, pp 150–151.

Bifid Condyle

Gundlach KKH, Fuhrmann A, Beckmann–Van der Ven G. The double-headed mandibular condyle. Oral Surg Oral Med Oral Pathol 64:249–253, 1987.

Loh FC, Yeo JF. Bifid mandibular condyle. Oral Surg Oral Med Oral Pathol 69:24–27, 1990.

McCormick SU, et al. Bilateral bifid mandibular condyles: Report of three cases. Oral Surg Oral Med Oral Pathol 68:555–557, 1989.

Szentpétery A, Kocsis G, Marcsik A. The problem of the bifid mandibular condyle. J Oral Maxillofac Surg 48:1254–1257, 1990.

Exostoses

Blakemore JR, Eller DJ, Tomaro AJ. Maxillary exostoses: Surgical management of an unusual case. Oral Surg Oral Med Oral Pathol 40:200–204, 1975.

Bouquot JE, Gundlach KKH. Oral exophytic lesions in 23,616 white Americans over 35 years of age. Oral Surg Oral Med Oral Pathol 62:284–291, 1986.

Hegtvedt AK, et al. Skin graft vestibuloplasty exostosis: A report of two cases. Oral Surg Oral Med Oral Pathol 69:149–152, 1990.

Morton TH Jr, Natkin E. Hyperostosis and fixed partial denture pontics: Report of 16 patients and review of literature. J Prosthet Dent 64:539–547, 1990.

Pack ARC, Gaudie WM, Jennings AM. Bony exostosis as a sequela to free gingival grafting: Two case reports. J Periodontol 62:269–271, 1991.

Torus Palatinus and Torus Mandibularis

Eggen S. Torus mandibularis: An estimation of the degree of genetic determination. Acta Odontol Scand 47:409–415, 1989.

Eggen S, Natvig B. Relationship between torus mandibularis and number of present teeth. Scand J Dent Res 94:233–240, 1986.

Eggen S, Natvig B. Variation in torus mandibularis prevalence in Norway: A statistical analysis using logistic regression. Community Dent Oral Epidemiol 19:32–35, 1991.

Haugen LK. Palatine and mandibular tori: A morphologic study in the current Norwegian population. Acta Odontol Scand 50:65–77, 1992.

Kolas S, et al. The occurrence of torus palatinus and torus mandibularis in 2,478 dental patients. Oral Surg Oral Med Oral Pathol 6:1134–1141, 1953.

Reichart PA, Neuhaus F, Sookasem M. Prevalence of torus palatinus and torus mandibularis in Germans and Thai. Community Dent Oral Epidemiol 16:61–64, 1988.

Suzuki M, Sakai T. A familial study of torus palatinus and torus mandibularis. Am J Phys Anthropol 18:263–272, 1960.

Eagle Syndrome

Blatchford SJ, Coulthard SW. Eagle's syndrome: An atypical cause of dysphonia. Ear Nose Throat J 68:48–51, 1989.

Camarda AJ, Deschamps C, Forest D. I. Stylohyoid chain ossification: A discussion of etiology. Oral Surg Oral Med Oral Pathol 67:508–514, 1989.

Camarda AJ, Deschamps C, Forest D. II. Stylohyoid chain ossification: A discussion of etiology. Oral Surg Oral Med Oral Pathol 67:515–520, 1989.

Correll RW, et al. Mineralization of the stylohyoid-stylomandibular ligament complex: A radiographic incidence study. Oral Surg Oral Med Oral Pathol 48:286–291, 1979.

Eagle WW. Elongated styloid processes: Report of two cases. Arch Otolaryngol 25:584–587, 1937.

Smith RG, Cherry JE. Traumatic Eagle's syndrome: Report of a case and review of the literature. J Oral Maxillofac Surg 46:606–609, 1988.

Stafne Defect

Ariji E, et al. Stafne's bone cavity: Classification based on outline and content determined by computed tomography. Oral Surg Oral Med Oral Pathol 76:375–380, 1993.

Barker GR. A radiolucency of the ascending ramus of the mandible associated with invested parotid salivary gland material and analogous with a Stafne bone cavity. Br J Oral Maxillofac Surg 26:81–84, 1988.

Correll RW, Jensen JL, Rhyne RR. Lingual cortical mandibular defects: A radiographic incidence study. Oral Surg Oral Med Oral Pathol 50:287–291, 1980.

Miller AS, Winnick M. Salivary gland inclusion in the anterior mandible: Report of a case with a review of the literature on aberrant salivary gland tissue and neoplasms. Oral Surg Oral Med Oral Pathol 31:790–797, 1971.

Oikarinen VJ, Wolf J, Julku M. A stereosialographic study of developmental mandibular bone defects (Stafne's idiopathic bone cavities). Int J Oral Surg 4:51–54, 1975.

Stafne EC. Bone cavities situated near the angle of the mandible. J Am Dent Assoc 29:1969–1972, 1942.

Palatal Cysts of the Newborn

Burke GW Jr, et al. Some aspects of the origin and fate of midpalatal cysts in human fetuses. J Dent Res 45:159–164, 1966.

Cataldo E, Berkman MD. Cysts of the oral mucosa in newborns. Am J Dis Child 116:44–48, 1968.

Fromm A. Epstein's pearls, Bohn's nodules and inclusion-cysts of the oral cavity. J Dent Child 34:275–287, 1967.

Jorgenson RJ, et al. Intraoral findings and anomalies in neonates. Pediatrics 69:577–582, 1982.

Monteleone L, McLellan MS. Epstein's pearls (Bohn's nodules) of the palate. J Oral Surg 22:301–304, 1964.

Nasolabial Cyst

Allard RHB. Nasolabial cyst: Review of the literature and report of 7 cases. Int J Oral Surg 11:351–359, 1982.

Kuriloff DB. The nasolabial cyst—nasal hamartoma. Otolaryngol Head Neck Surg 96:268–272, 1987.

Roed-Petersen B. Nasolabial cysts: A presentation of five patients with a review of the literature. Br J Oral Surg 7:84–95, 1969.

Globulomaxillary Cyst

Christ TF. The globulomaxillary cyst: An embryologic misconception. Oral Surg Oral Med Oral Pathol 30:515–526, 1970.

D'Silva NJ, Anderson L. Globulomaxillary cyst revisited. Oral Surg Oral Med Oral Pathol 76:182–184, 1993.

Ferenczy K. The relationship of globulomaxillary cysts to the fusion of embryonal processes and to cleft palates. Oral Surg Oral Med Oral Pathol 11:1388–1393, 1958.

Little JW, Jakobsen J. Origin of the globulomaxillary cyst. J Oral Surg 31:188–195, 1973.

Vedtofte P, Holmstrup P. Inflammatory paradental cysts in the globulomaxillary region. J Oral Pathol Med 18:125–127, 1989.

Wysocki GP. The differential diagnosis of globulomaxillary radiolucencies. Oral Surg Oral Med Oral Pathol 51:281–286, 1981.

Wysocki GP, Goldblatt LI. The so-called "globulomaxillary cyst" is extinct. Oral Surg Oral Med Oral Pathol 76:185–186, 1993.

Nasopalatine Duct Cyst

Abrams AM, Howell FV, Bullock WK. Nasopalatine cysts. Oral Surg Oral Med Oral Pathol 16:306–332, 1963.

Allard RHB, van der Kwast WAM, van der Waal I. Nasopalatine duct cyst: Review of the literature and report of 22 cases. Int J Oral Surg 10:447–461, 1981.

Anneroth G, Hall G, Stuge U. Nasopalatine duct cyst. Int J Oral Maxillofac Surg 15:572–580, 1986.

Brown FH, et al. Cyst of the incisive (palatine) papilla: Report of a case. J Periodontol 58:274–275, 1987.

Chapple IL, Ord RA. Patent nasopalatine ducts: Four case presentations and review of the literature. Oral Surg Oral Med Oral Pathol 69:554–558, 1990.

Shear M. Nasopalatine duct (incisive canal) cyst. In: Cysts of the Oral Regions. Bristol, England, J Wright & Sons Ltd, 1976, pp 67–79.

Swanson KS, Kaugars GE, Gunsolley JC. Nasopalatine duct cyst: An analysis of 334 cases. J Oral Maxillofac Surg 49:268–271, 1991.

Median Palatal Cyst

Courage GR, North AF, Hansen LS. Median palatine cysts. Oral Surg Oral Med Oral Pathol 37:745–753, 1974.

Gordon NC, Swann NP, Hansen LS. Median palatine cyst and maxillary antral osteoma: Report of an unusual case. J Oral Surg 38:361–365, 1980.

Median Mandibular Cyst

Gardner DG. An evaluation of reported cases of median mandibular cysts. Oral Surg Oral Med Oral Pathol 65:208–213, 1988.

Soskolne WA, Shteyer A. Median mandibular cyst. Oral Surg Oral Med Oral Pathol 44:84–88, 1977.

White DK, Lucas RM, Miller AS. Median mandibular cyst: Review of the literature and report of two cases. J Oral Surg 33:372–375, 1975.

Epidermoid Cyst

Headington JT. Epidermoid and tricholemmal cysts. *In:* Clinical Dermatology. Edited by Demis DJ. Philadelphia, Harper & Row, 1982, chap. 4–57.

Kligman AM. The myth of the sebaceous cyst. Arch Dermatol 89:253–256, 1964.

McGavran MH, Binnington B. Keratinous cysts of the skin. Arch Dermatol 94:499–508, 1966.

Dermoid Cyst

Arcand P, Granger J, Brochu P. Congenital dermoid cyst of the oral cavity with gastric choristoma. J Otolaryngol 17:219–222, 1988.

Lipsett J, Sparnon AL, Byard RW. Embryogenesis of enterocystomas —enteric duplication cysts of the tongue. Oral Surg Oral Med Oral Pathol 75:626–630, 1993.

Meyer I. Dermoid cysts (dermoids) of the floor of the mouth. Oral Surg Oral Med Oral Pathol 8:1149–1164, 1955.

Triantafillidou E, Karakasis D, Laskin J. Swelling of the floor of the mouth. J Oral Maxillofac Surg 47:733–736, 1989.

Tuffin JR, Theaker E. True lateral dermoid cyst of the neck. Int J Oral Maxillofac Surg 20:275–276, 1991.

Thyroglossal Duct Cyst

Allard RHB. The thyroglossal cyst. Head Neck Surg 5:134–146, 1982.

Fernandez JF, et al. Thyroglossal duct carcinoma. Surgery 110:928–935, 1991.

Girard M, DeLuca SA. Thyroglossal duct cyst. Am Fam Physician 42:665–668, 1990.

Hoffman MA, Schuster SR. Thyroglossal duct remnants in infants and children: Reevaluation of histopathology and methods for resection. Ann Otol Rhinol Laryngol 97:483–486, 1988.

Issa MM, deVries P. Familial occurrence of thyroglossal duct cyst. J Pediatr Surg 26:30–31, 1991.

Katz AD, Hachigian M. Thyroglossal duct cysts: A thirty-year experience with emphasis on occurrence in older patients. Am J Surg 155:741–744, 1988.

Cervical Lymphoepithelial Cyst

Bhaskar SN, Bernier JL. Histogenesis of branchial cysts: A report of 468 cases. Am J Pathol 35:407–423, 1959.

Elliott JN, Oertel YC. Lymphoepithelial cysts of the salivary glands. Am J Clin Pathol 93:39–43, 1990.

Foss RD, et al. Malignant cyst of the lateral aspect of the neck: Branchial cleft carcinoma or metastasis? Oral Surg Oral Med Oral Pathol 71:214–217, 1991.

Little JW, Rickles NH. The histogenesis of the branchial cyst. Am J Pathol 50:533–547, 1967.

Mandel L, Reich R. HIV parotid gland lymphoepithelial cysts: Review and case reports. Oral Surg Oral Med Oral Pathol 74:273–278, 1992.

Skouteris CA, Patterson GT, Sotereanos GC. Benign cervical lymphoepithelial cyst: Report of cases. J Oral Maxillofac Surg 47:1106–1112, 1989.

Oral Lymphoepithelial Cyst

Bhaskar SN. Lymphoepithelial cysts of the oral cavity: Report of twenty-four cases. Oral Surg Oral Med Oral Pathol 21:120–128, 1966.

Buchner A, Hansen LS. Lymphoepithelial cysts of the oral cavity. Oral Surg Oral Med Oral Pathol 50:441–449, 1980.

Chaudhry AP, et al. A clinico-pathological study of intraoral lymphoepithelial cysts. J Oral Med 39:79–84, 1984.

Giunta J, Cataldo E. Lymphoepithelial cysts of the oral mucosa. Oral Surg Oral Med Oral Pathol 35:77–84, 1973.

Hemihyperplasia

Bell RA, McTigue DJ. Complex congenital hemihypertrophy: A case report and literature review. J Pedodont 8:300–313, 1984.

Gorlin RJ, Cohen MM Jr, Levin LS. Hemihyperplasia (hemihypertrophy). *In:* Syndromes of the Head and Neck, 3rd ed. New York, Oxford University Press, 1990, pp 329–332.

Horswell BB, et al. Primary hemihypertrophy of the face: Review and report of two cases. J Oral Maxillofac Surg 45:217–222, 1987.

Progressive Hemifacial Atrophy

Abele DC, et al. Progressive facial hemiatrophy (Parry-Romberg syndrome) and borreliosis. J Am Acad Dermatol 22:531–533, 1990.

Foster TD. The effects of hemifacial atrophy on dental growth. Br Dent J 146:148–150, 1979.

Glass D. Hemifacial atrophy. Br J Oral Surg 1:194–199, 1963.

Moore MH, et al. Progressive hemifacial atrophy (Romberg's disease): Skeletal involvement and treatment. Br J Plast Surg 46:39–44, 1993.

Pensler JM, Murphy GF, Mulliken JB. Clinical and ultrastructural studies of Romberg's hemifacial atrophy. Plast Reconstr Surg 85:669–674, 1990.

Crouzon Syndrome

David DJ, Sheen R. Surgical correction of Crouzon syndrome. Plast Reconstr Surg 85:344–354, 1990.

Gorlin RJ, Cohen MM Jr, Levin LS. Crouzon syndrome (craniofacial dysostosis). *In:* Syndromes of the Head and Neck, 3rd ed. New York, Oxford University Press, 1990, pp 524–526.

Kreiborg S. Crouzon syndrome. Scand J Plast Reconstr Surg Suppl 18:1–198, 1981.

Apert Syndrome

Ferraro NF. Dental, orthodontic, and oral/maxillofacial evaluation and treatment in Apert syndrome. Clin Plast Surg 18:291–307, 1991.

Gorlin RJ, Cohen MM Jr, Levin LS. Apert syndrome (acrocephalosyndactyly). *In:* Syndromes of the Head and Neck, 3rd ed. New York, Oxford University Press, 1990, pp 520–524.

Kreiborg S, Cohen MM Jr. The oral manifestations of Apert syndrome. J Craniofac Genet Dev Biol 12:41–48, 1992.

Marsh JL, Galic M, Vannier MW. Surgical correction of the craniofacial dysmorphology of Apert syndrome. Clin Plast Surg 18:251–275, 1991.

Mandibulofacial Dysostosis

Argenta LC, Iacobucci JJ. Treacher Collins syndrome: Present concepts of the disorder and their surgical correction. World J Surg 13:401–409, 1989.

Gorlin RJ, Cohen MM Jr, Levin LS. Mandibulofacial dysostosis (Treacher Collins syndrome, Francheschetti-Zwahlen-Klein syndrome). *In:* Syndromes of the Head and Neck, 3rd ed. New York, Oxford University Press, 1990, pp 649–652.

Environmental Alterations of Teeth

The abnormalities of the teeth can be divided into those that are influenced by environmental forces and those that are idiopathic or appear hereditary in nature. Later parts of this chapter delineate the idiopathic or hereditary alterations of teeth. Table 2–1 lists the major categories of tooth alteration that can be affected by environmental influences. In many cases, the cause and effect are obvious; in others, the primary nature of the problem is less distinct.

ENVIRONMENTAL EFFECTS ON TOOTH STRUCTURE DEVELOPMENT

The ameloblasts in the developing tooth germ are extremely sensitive to external stimuli, and many factors can result in abnormalities in the enamel (Table 2–2). The primary hereditary abnormalities of the enamel that are unrelated to other disorders are termed **amelogenesis imperfecta** (see p. 79).

The enamel develops in two major stages: **secretory** and **maturation**. During the secretory phase, the enamel matrix is laid down and mineralization of the matrix occurs during the subsequent maturation phase, which is divided into early and late stages. In the early stage of maturation, the enamel is dull, white, and relatively soft. During the late stage of maturation, this diffuse opaque enamel is replaced by the final hard translucent enamel.

The timing of the ameloblastic damage has a great impact on the location and appearance of the defect in the enamel. The cause of the damage does not appear to be of major importance because many different local and systemic stimuli can result in defects that have similar clinical appearances. The final enamel represents a record of all significant insults received during tooth development. Deciduous enamel contains a neonatal ring, and the rate of enamel apposition is estimated to be 0.023 mm/day. Using this knowledge, one can estimate the timing of an insult in these teeth to an accuracy of as little as 1 week.

Clinical Features

Almost all visible environmental enamel defects can be classified into one of three patterns:

- Hypoplasia
- Diffuse opacities
- Demarcated opacities

The altered enamel may be localized or present on numerous teeth, and all or part of the surfaces of each affected tooth may be involved. **Enamel hypoplasia** occurs in the form of pits, grooves, or larger areas of missing enamel. **Diffuse opacities of enamel** present as variations in the translucency of the enamel. The affected enamel is of normal thickness but has an increased white opacity with no clear boundary with the adjacent normal enamel. **Demarcated opacities of enamel** show areas of decreased translucence, increased opacity, and a sharp boundary with the adjacent enamel. The enamel is of normal thickness, and the affected opacity may be white, cream, yellow, or brown.

The crowns of the deciduous dentition develop between the 15th week of gestation to the 12th month of age; development of the crowns of the permanent dentition is extended from approximately 6 months to 15 years of age. The site of coronal damage correlates with the area of ameloblastic activity at the time of the injury; the affected enamel is restricted to the areas in which there was secretory activity or active maturation of the enamel matrix.

A common pattern occurs as a result of systemic influences, such as exanthematous fevers, which occur during the first 2 years of life. Horizontal rows of pits or diminished enamel are present on the anterior teeth and first molars (Figs. 2–1 and 2–2). The enamel loss is bilaterally symmetric and correlates well with the developmen-

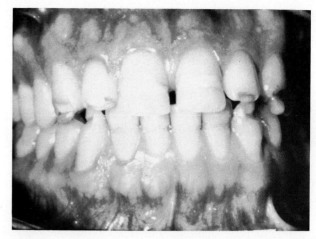

FIGURE 2–1. **Environmental enamel hypoplasia.** Bilaterally symmetric pattern of horizontal enamel hypoplasia of the anterior dentition. Maxillary central incisors previously have been restored. (From Neville BW, Damm DD, White DK, Waldron CA. Color Atlas of Clinical Oral Pathology. Philadelphia, Lea & Febiger, 1991, p 57.)

tal pattern of the affected teeth. A similar pattern of enamel defects can be seen in the cuspids, bicuspids, and second molars when the inciting event occurs around the age of 4 to 5 years (Fig. 2–3).

Turner's Hypoplasia

Another frequent pattern of enamel defects is seen in permanent teeth secondary to periapical inflammatory disease of the overlying deciduous tooth. The altered tooth is called a **Turner's tooth** after the dental clinician whose publications allowed this problem to be widely recognized. The appearance of the affected area varies according to the timing and severity of the insult. The enamel defects vary from focal areas of white, yellow, or brown discoloration to extensive hypoplasia, which can involve the entire crown. The process is noted most frequently in the permanent bicuspids because of their rela-

Table 2–2. FACTORS ASSOCIATED WITH ENAMEL DEFECTS

Systemic
1. *Birth-related trauma*: breech presentations, hypoxia, multiple births, premature birth, prolonged labor.
2. *Chemicals*: fluoride, lead, tetracycline, thalidomide, vitamin D.
3. *Chromosomal abnormalities*: trisomy 21.
4. *Infections*: chicken pox, cytomegalovirus, gastrointestinal infections, measles, pneumonia, respiratory infections, rubella, syphilis, tetanus.
5. *Inherited diseases*: amelo-cerebro-hypohidrotic syndrome, amelo-onycho-hypohidrotic syndrome, epidermolysis bullosa, galactosemia, mucopolysaccharidosis IV, oculo-dento-osseous dysplasia, phenylketonuria, pseudohypoparathyroidism, tricho-dento-osseous syndrome, tuberous sclerosis, vitamin D–dependent rickets.
6. *Malnutrition*: generalized malnutrition, vitamin D deficiency, vitamin A deficiency.
7. *Metabolic disorders*: cardiac disease, gastrointestinal malabsorption, gastrointestinal lymphangiectasia, hepatobiliary disease, hyperbilirubinemia, hypocalcemia, hypothyroidism, hypoparathyroidism, maternal diabetes, renal disease, toxemia of pregnancy.
8. *Neurologic disorders*: cerebral palsy, mental retardation, sensorineural hearing defects.

Local
1. *Local acute mechanical trauma*: falls, gunshots, neonatal mechanical ventilation, ritual mutilation, surgery, vehicular accidents, etc.
2. *Electric burn.*
3. *Irradiation.*
4. *Local infection*: acute neonatal maxillitis, periapical inflammatory disease.

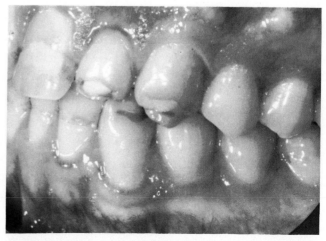

FIGURE 2–2. **Environmental enamel hypoplasia.** Same patient as depicted in Figure 2–1. Note the lack of enamel damage on bicuspids.

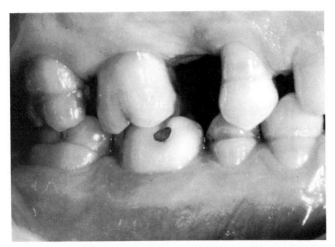

FIGURE 2–3. **Environmental enamel hypoplasia.** Horizontal enamel hypoplasia of the bicuspids and second molars. Note sparing of the first molars. (From Neville BW, Damm DD, White DK, Waldron CA. Color Atlas of Clinical Oral Pathology. Philadelphia, Lea & Febiger, 1991, p 57.)

tionship to the overlying deciduous molars (Figs. 2–4 and 2–5). Anterior teeth are involved less frequently because crown formation is usually complete before the development of any apical inflammatory disease in the relatively caries-resistant anterior deciduous dentition.

In addition to primary inflammatory disorders, traumatic injury to deciduous teeth can also cause significant alterations of the underlying dentition and the formation of Turner's teeth. This is not a rare occurrence; up to 45 percent of all children sustain injuries to their primary teeth. In a prospective study of 114 children with 255 traumatized primary teeth, 23 percent of the correspond-

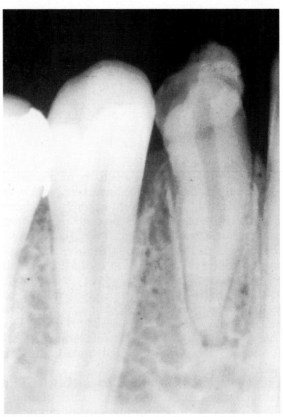

FIGURE 2–5. **Turner's hypoplasia.** Radiograph of the same tooth depicted in Figure 2–4. Note the lack of significant enamel and irregularity of the dentin surface. (From Halstead CL, Blozis GG, Drinnan AJ, Gier RE. Physical Evaluation of the Dental Patient. St. Louis, CV Mosby, 1982, p 350.)

ing permanent teeth demonstrated developmental disturbances. The maxillary central incisors are affected in the majority of the cases; the maxillary lateral incisors are altered less frequently (Fig. 2–6). The prevalence of involvement of the posterior teeth or mandibular incisors was less than 10 percent of all cases in several large reviews.

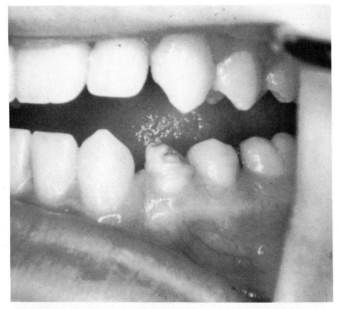

FIGURE 2–4. **Turner's hypoplasia.** Extensive enamel hypoplasia of mandibular first bicuspid secondary to previous inflammatory process associated with overlying first deciduous molar. (From Halstead CL, Blozis GG, Drinnan AJ, Gier RE. Physical Evaluation of the Dental Patient. St. Louis, CV Mosby, 1982, p 350.)

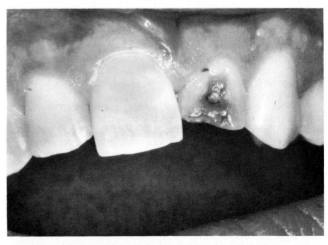

FIGURE 2–6. **Turner's hypoplasia.** Extensive coronal hypoplasia of permanent maxillary left central incisor secondary to previous trauma to deciduous central incisor.

The frequency of traumatic damage of the anterior maxillary dentition is not surprising, considering the common occurrence of trauma to the deciduous dentition of the prominent anterior maxilla and the close anatomic relationship between the developing tooth bud and the apices of the overlying primary incisors. As would be expected, the clinical appearance of the alteration varies according to the timing and severity of the damage.

Because of the position of the primary apices relative to the tooth bud, the facial surface of the maxillary incisors is the location most frequently affected. Typically, the affected area presents as a zone of white or yellowish-brown discoloration with or without an area of horizontal enamel hypoplasia. The trauma also can cause displacement of the already formed hard tooth substance in relation to the soft tissue of the remaining developing tooth. This results in a bend of the tooth known as **dilaceration** and can affect either the crown or the root of a tooth (see Developmental Alterations in the Shape of Teeth, p. 65). Severe trauma early in the development of the tooth can result in such disorganization of the bud that the resultant product may resemble a complex odontoma (see p. 532). Similar levels of damage late in the formative process can lead to partial or total arrest in root formation.

Dental Fluorosis

The ingestion of fluoride also can result in significant enamel defects known as **dental fluorosis**. These alterations consist of permanent hypomaturation of the enamel in which there is an increased surface and subsurface porosity of the enamel. The fluoride-induced enamel alterations occur during the maturation phase of tooth development. Most of the problems associated with dental fluorosis are aesthetic and concern the appearance of the anterior teeth. Therefore, the critical period for clinically significant dental fluorosis is during the 2nd and 3rd years of life, when these teeth are forming, and if fluoride levels greater than 1 part per million are ingested.

During the early studies on dental fluorosis in the 1930s and 1940s, the major source of fluoride was naturally fluoridated water. Since that time, the prevalence of fluorosis appears to be increasing among children and is most likely a result of an accumulation of the element obtained from several sources. Adult-strength fluoride toothpastes, fluoride supplements, infant foods, soft drinks, and fruit juices all represent potential sources of fluoride for children in their formative years. Infant formulas also used to contain significant amounts of fluoride, but more recent efforts have resulted in a dramatic decrease in the fluoride content from this source. When fluoride supplementation is being considered for non-fluoridated areas, all sources of fluoride must be analyzed.

The severity of dental fluorosis is dose-dependent, with higher intakes during critical periods of tooth development associated with more severe fluorosis. The affected teeth are caries-resistant, and the altered tooth structure presents as areas of lusterless white opaque enamel, which may have zones of yellow to dark-brown discolor-

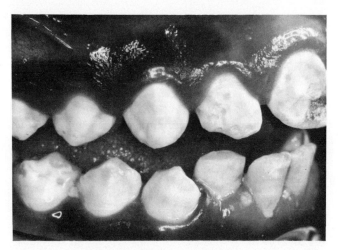

FIGURE 2–7. **Dental fluorosis.** Dentition exhibiting lusterless, white, and opaque enamel. See Color Plates.

ation (Figs. 2–7 and 2–8; see Color Figure 9). True enamel hypoplasia is uncommon but can occur as deep, irregular, and brownish pits. Because other factors can result in a similar pattern of enamel damage, a definitive diagnosis requires that the defects be present in a bilaterally symmetric distribution, and evidence of prior excessive fluoride intake or elevated levels of fluoride in the enamel or other tissues should be found.

Syphilitic Hypoplasia

Congenital syphilis (see p. 148) results in a pattern of enamel hypoplasia that is well known but currently so rare that significant discussion is not warranted. Anterior teeth altered by syphilis are termed *Hutchinson's incisors* and exhibit crowns that are shaped like straight-edge screwdrivers, with the greatest circumference present in the middle one third of the crown and a constricted incisal edge. The middle portion of the incisal edge often demonstrates a central hypoplastic notch. Altered poste-

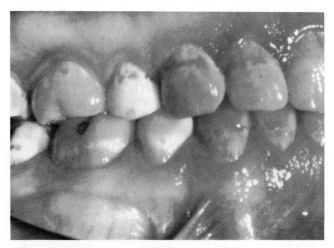

FIGURE 2–8. **Dental fluorosis.** White opaque alteration of the bicuspids and second molars in a patient who also exhibits discoloration of the teeth secondary to tetracycline use. Patient moved to area of endemic fluorosis at 3 years of age.

rior teeth are termed *mulberry molars* and demonstrate constricted occlusal tables with a disorganized surface anatomy that resembles the bumpy surface of a mulberry.

Treatment and Prognosis

Except for rare severe cases, most defects in the enamel are cosmetic rather than functional dental problems. Aesthetically or functionally defective teeth can be restored through a variety of cosmetically pleasing techniques, such as:

- Acid-etched composite resin restorations
- Labial veneers
- Full crowns

POSTDEVELOPMENTAL LOSS OF TOOTH STRUCTURE

Tooth structure can be lost after its formation by a variety of influences beyond the obvious cases related to caries or traumatic fractures. Destruction can begin on the enamel surface of the crown through abrasion, attrition, or erosion; in addition, loss of tooth structure can begin on the dentin or cemental surfaces of the teeth by external or internal resorption.

Attrition, Abrasion, and Erosion

Attrition is the loss of tooth structure caused by tooth-to-tooth contact during occlusion and mastication. Some degree of attrition is physiologic, and the process becomes more noticeable with age. When the amount of tooth loss is extensive and begins to affect the aesthetic appearance and function, the process must be considered pathologic. The destruction can be accelerated by:

- Poor quality or absent enamel (e.g., fluorosis, environmental or hereditary enamel hypoplasia, or dentinogenesis imperfecta)
- Premature contacts (edge-to-edge occlusion)
- Intraoral abrasives, erosion, and grinding habits

Abrasion is the pathologic loss of tooth structure secondary to the action of an external agent. The most common source of abrasion is toothbrushing that combines an abrasive toothpaste with heavy pressure and a horizontal brushing stroke. Other items frequently associated with dental abrasion include pencils, toothpicks, pipe stems, and bobby pins (hair grips). Chewing tobacco, biting thread, and using dental floss inappropriately also can cause clinically significant abrasion.

Erosion is the loss of tooth structure caused by a chemical reaction beyond that associated with bacteria (caries). Typically, the process is secondary to the presence of an acid, but chelating agents occasionally are the primary cause. The source can be dietary (e.g., lemons, soft drinks, or vinegar), internal (e.g., gastric secretions), or external (e.g., acidic industrial atmosphere or poorly

monitored swimming pools). Erosion secondary to gastric secretions is termed *perimolysis*. It may result from a hiatal hernia, esophagitis, regurgitation from inappropriate digestion of certain foods, or chronic vomiting, such as that seen in association with bulimia. Erosion can accelerate attrition and abrasion because acid-etched enamel is more susceptible to the effects of mechanical forces.

Erosion is often used as the "trash-bag" diagnosis for postdevelopmental coronal tooth loss ("if it is not abrasion or attrition, it must be erosion!"). Many cases can be diagnosed easily from the clinical appearance and history, but often no obvious cause can be found. Even after extensive investigation, a definite diagnosis often is not possible. Because the establishment of the specific cause often is necessary to stop the process, the lack of ability to arrive at a definitive diagnosis demonstrates that research still is needed in this area.

Clinical Features

Attrition

Attrition can occur in both the deciduous and permanent dentitions. As would be expected, the surfaces predominantly affected are those that interdigitate with the opposing dentition. Most frequently, the incisal and occlusal surfaces are involved, in addition to the lingual of the anterior maxillary teeth and the labial of the anterior mandibular teeth. Large flat wear facets are found in a relationship that corresponds to the pattern of occlusion. The interproximal contact points also are affected from the vertical movement of the teeth during function. Over time, this interproximal loss can result in a shortening of the arch length. Pulp exposure and dentin sensitivity are rare because of the slow loss of tooth structure and the apposition of reparative secondary dentin within the pulp chamber (Fig. 2–9).

Abrasion

Abrasion has a variety of patterns, depending on the cause. Toothbrush abrasion typically presents as horizontal cervical notches on the buccal surface of exposed radicular cementum and dentin (Figs. 2–10 and 2–11). The degree of loss is greatest on prominent teeth (cuspids, bicuspids, and teeth adjacent to edentulous areas) and on the side of the arch opposite the dominant hand. Thread biting or the use of pipes or bobby pins usually produces rounded or V-shaped notches in the incisal edges of anterior teeth (Figs. 2–12 and 2–13). The inappropriate use of dental floss or toothpicks results in the loss of interproximal radicular cementum and dentin. Pulp exposure and dentin sensitivity are rare.

Erosion

In patients with erosion, the tooth loss does not correlate with functional wear patterns or with those typically associated with known abrasives. In contrast to abrasion, erosion commonly affects the facial surfaces of the maxillary anteriors and appears as shallow spoon-shaped depressions in the cervical portion of the crown. The posterior teeth frequently exhibit extensive loss of the occlusal surface, and the edges of metallic restorations subse-

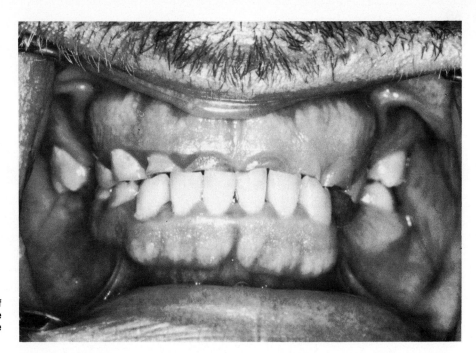

FIGURE 2–9. **Attrition.** Extensive loss of coronal tooth height without pulp exposure in patient with anterior edge-to-edge occlusion.

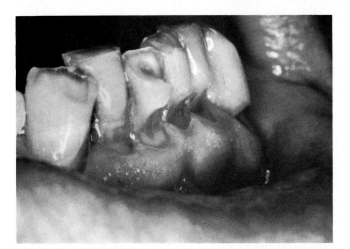

FIGURE 2–10. **Abrasion.** Horizontal cervical notches on the anterior mandibular dentition.

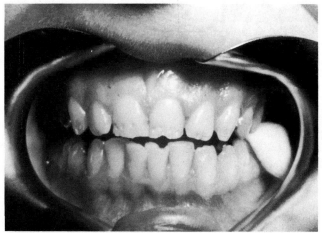

FIGURE 2–12. **Abrasion.** Notching of the right central incisor caused by improper use of bobby pins. The patient also exhibits environmental enamel hypoplasia of the anterior dentition. (Courtesy of Dr. Robert J. Gorlin.)

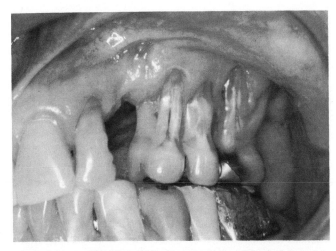

FIGURE 2–11. **Abrasion.** Extensive recession and loss of buccal radicular dentin. Note visible pulp canals, which have been filled with tertiary dentin.

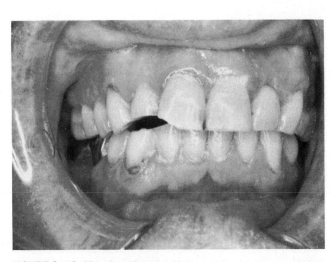

FIGURE 2–13. **Abrasion.** Notching of the anterior dentition on the right side caused by long-term use of tobacco pipe.

49

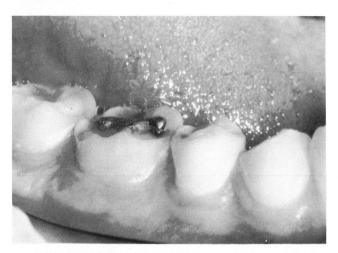

FIGURE 2–14. **Erosion.** Extensive loss of buccal and occlusal tooth structure. Note that the amalgam margins are above the surface of the dentin.

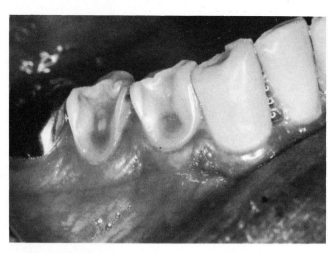

FIGURE 2–16. **Erosion.** Extensive loss of enamel and dentin on the buccal surface of the maxillary bicuspids. The patient had chronically sucked on tamarinds (acidic fruit).

quently may be above the level of the tooth structure (Fig. 2–14). After a portion of the cuspal enamel has been lost, the dentin is destroyed more rapidly than the remaining enamel, often resulting in a concave depression of the dentin surrounded by an elevated rim of enamel (Fig. 2–15). On occasion, entire buccal cusps are lost and replaced by ski slope–like depressions that extend from the lingual cusp to the buccal cemento-enamel junction (Fig. 2–16). When palatal surfaces are affected, the exposed dentin has a concave surface and shows a peripheral white line of enamel (Fig. 2–17).

Erosion limited to the facial surfaces of the maxillary anterior dentition is often associated with dietary sources of acid. When the tooth loss is confined to the incisal portions of the anterior dentition of both arches, an external environmental source is indicated. When erosion is located on the palatal surfaces of the maxillary anterior teeth and the occlusal surfaces of the posterior teeth of both dentitions, regurgitation of gastric secretions is probable. Although not common, erosion can proceed rapidly and result in dentinal sensitivity or pulp exposure.

On occasion, the tooth loss may appear as wedge-shaped defects limited to the cervical area of the teeth. Many of these cases cannot be associated with acid exposure or mechanical abrasion and have been termed **idiopathic cervical erosions**. Investigators have proposed that these defects are created from occlusal stresses that cause the teeth to bend. The bending disrupts the chemical bonds of the enamel and dentin. The damaged area then demonstrates an increased susceptibility to dissolution and abrasion.

Treatment and Prognosis

Attrition, abrasion, and erosion are best treated with early diagnosis and intervention to restrict the severity of tooth loss. Patients should be informed of the potential

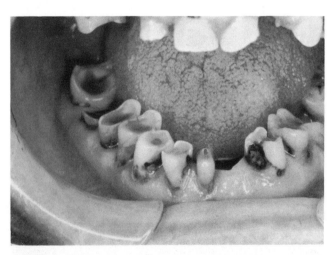

FIGURE 2–15. **Erosion.** Occlusal surface of the mandibular dentition exhibiting concave dentin depressions surrounded by elevated rims of enamel.

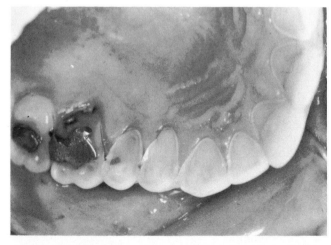

FIGURE 2–17. **Erosion.** Palatal surfaces of the maxillary dentition in which the exposed dentin exhibits a concave surface and a peripheral white line of enamel. The patient suffered from bulimia.

for loss of tooth structure associated with the use of acidic foods and drinks, chronic regurgitation, and improper oral hygiene techniques. Mouth guards can be used to protect the teeth from frequent exposure to acid from regurgitation or industrial sources. Patients with erosion should limit their toothbrushing to once a day in the morning because of the increased vulnerability of acid-etched enamel to abrasion and attrition. Replacement of lost posterior teeth and avoidance of edge-to-edge occlusion limit the effects of attrition. Lost tooth structure can be restored with composite resins, veneers, onlays, or full crowns.

Loss of tooth structure is compensated by continual eruption of the teeth, appositional alveolar bone deposition, and compensatory skeletal growth. If the process of tooth loss is slow, the vertical dimension often is maintained; in patients with rapid destruction, there is a loss of facial length. Restoration of extensive loss of tooth structure is complex and should be performed only after a complete evaluation of the dentoalveolar complex.

Internal/External Resorption

In addition to loss of tooth structure that begins on the exposed coronal surfaces, destruction of teeth also can occur through resorption, which is accomplished by cells located in the dental pulp (**internal resorption**) or in the periodontal ligament (**external resorption**). Internal resorption is a relatively rare occurrence, and most cases follow injury to pulpal tissues, such as physical trauma or caries-related pulpitis. The resorption can continue as long as vital pulp tissue remains. The process often proceeds, resulting in communication with the periodontal ligament.

By contrast, external resorption is extremely common; with close examination, all patients are most likely to have root resorption on one or more teeth. In one radiographic review of 13,263 teeth, all patients showed evidence of root resorption, and 86.4 percent of the examined teeth demonstrated external resorption, with an average of 16 affected teeth per patient. Most areas of resorption are mild and of no clinical significance, but 10 percent of patients exhibit unusual amounts of external resorption.

The given resorption potential is inherent within the periodontal tissue of each patient, and this individual susceptibility to resorption is the most important factor in the degree of resorption that will occur after a stimulus. The factors reported to increase the severity of external resorption are delineated in Table 2–3. Many cases have been termed idiopathic because no factor could be found to explain the accelerated resorption. When pretreatment radiographs of a given patient exhibit a degree of resorption beyond that which is normally seen, the clinician should realize the risks involved in initiating procedures (such as orthodontics) that are known to be associated with an increased risk of external resorption.

Clinical Features

Resorption of dentin or cementum can occur at any site that contacts vital tissue. Internal resorption usually

Table 2–3. FACTORS ASSOCIATED WITH EXTERNAL RESORPTION
1. Cysts
2. Dental trauma
3. Excessive mechanical forces (e.g., orthodontic therapy)
4. Excessive occlusal forces
5. Grafting of alveolar clefts
6. Hormonal imbalances
7. Intracoronal bleaching of pulpless teeth
8. Local involvement by herpes zoster
9. Paget's disease of bone
10. Periodontal treatment
11. Periradicular inflammation
12. Pressure from impacted teeth
13. Reimplantation of teeth
14. Tumors

presents as a uniform, well-circumscribed symmetric radiolucent enlargement of the pulp chamber or canal. When it affects the coronal pulp, the crown can display a pink discoloration (**pink tooth of Mummery**) as the vascular resorptive process approaches the surface (Figs. 2–18 and 2–19; see Color Figure 10). When it occurs in the root, the original outline of the canal is lost and a balloon-like radiographic dilation of the canal is seen (Fig. 2–20).

By contrast, external resorption typically presents with a "moth-eaten" loss of tooth structure in which the radiolucency is less well defined and demonstrates variations in density (Figs. 2–21 to 2–24). If the lesion overlies the pulp canal, close examination demonstrates the retention of the unaltered canal through the area of the defect. Most cases involve the apical or midportions of the root. On occasion, the resorption may begin in the cervical area and extend from a small opening to involve a large area of the dentin between the cementum and the pulp. The resorption can extend apically into the pulp or coronally under the enamel and simulate the pink tooth seen in internal resorption. The cervical pattern of external resorption often is rapid and has been termed **inva-**

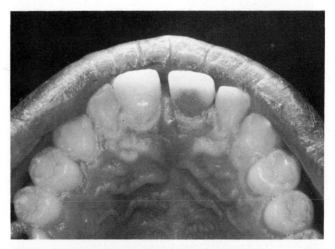

FIGURE 2–18. **Internal resorption (pink tooth of Mummery).** Pink discoloration of the maxillary central incisor. See Color Plates.

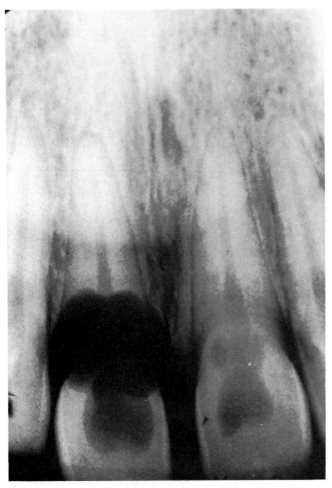

FIGURE 2–19. **Internal resorption.** Same patient as depicted in Figure 2–18. Note extensive resorption of both maxillary central incisors.

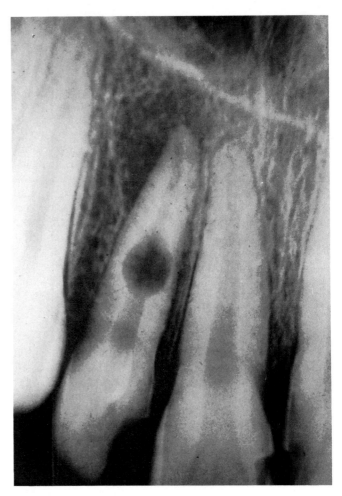

FIGURE 2–20. **Internal resorption.** Balloon-like enlargement of the root canal.

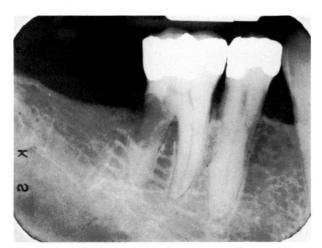

FIGURE 2–21. **External resorption.** Ragged radiolucency of the distal root of the mandibular first molar. (Courtesy of Dr. Michael Strong.)

sive resorption (Figs. 2–25 and 2–26). In some instances, several teeth may be involved, and an underlying cause for the accelerated destruction may not be obvious (**multiple idiopathic root resorption**).

If difficulty arises in separation between external and internal resorption, the mesial-buccal-distal rule can be used through two radiographic exposures: one perpendicular and one mesial (objects closer to the source of radiation will shift distally). With this technique, the sites of external resorption appear to shift away from the pulp canal when the radiographs are compared. In addition, the radiographs can reveal which side of the root is affected in cases of external resorption.

Histopathologic Features

In patients with internal resorption, the pulp tissue in the area of destruction is vascular and exhibits an in-

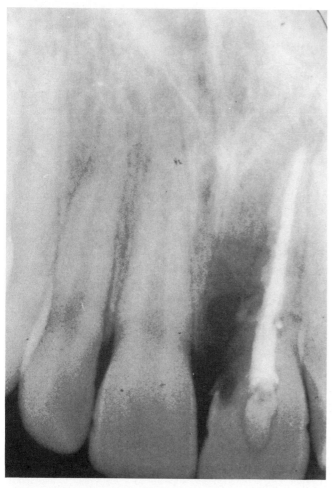

FIGURE 2-22. **External resorption.** "Moth-eaten" radiolucent alteration of the maxillary left central incisor. The tooth had been reimplanted following traumatic avulsion. (Courtesy of Dr. Harry Meyers.)

creased cellularity and collagenization. Immediately adjacent to the dentinal wall are numerous multinucleated dentinoclasts, which are histologically identical to osteoclasts. Inflammation by lymphocytes, histiocytes, and polymorphonuclear leukocytes is not uncommon (Figs. 2-27 and 2-28). External resorption is similar in appearance, with numerous multinucleated dentinoclasts located in the areas of structure loss. Areas of resorption are often repaired through deposition of osteodentin.

Treatment and Prognosis

The treatment of internal and external resorption centers around the removal of all soft tissue from the sites of dental destruction. Internal resorption can be consistently stopped if endodontic therapy successfully removes all vital pulp tissue before perforation into the periodontal ligament. On perforation, therapy becomes more difficult; curettage of the adjacent soft tissue with restoration of the site of perforation is necessary. Apical perforations often limit effective therapy.

The first approach in treating external resorption is to investigate the presence of an accelerating factor and to eliminate this influence. Apically located sites cannot be approached without significant damage created from attempts at access. Those cases located in the cervical areas can be treated by surgical exposure, removal of all soft tissue from the defects, and restoration of the lost structure of the tooth.

ENVIRONMENTAL DISCOLORATION OF TEETH

The color of normal teeth varies and depends on the shade, translucency, and thickness of the enamel. Translucent enamel appears bluish-white; opaque enamel is gray-white. Therefore, teeth with translucent enamel appear yellow at the cervical one third and blue-white at the incisal edge; those with opaque enamel are a more uniform gray-white. Abnormal colorations may be **extrinsic**

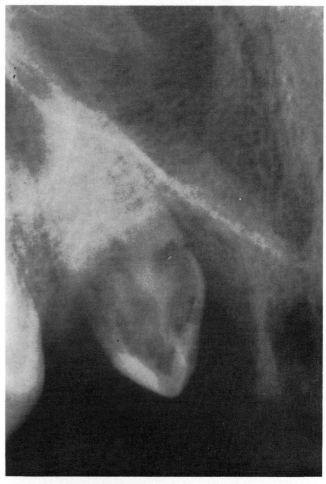

FIGURE 2-23. **External resorption.** Extensive external resorption of the crown of the impacted right maxillary cuspid. Histologic examination revealed resorption without bacterial contamination or caries.

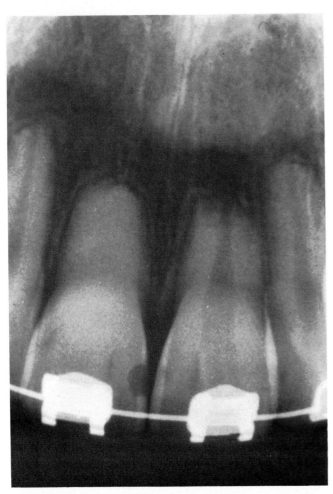

FIGURE 2-24. **External resorption.** Diffuse external resorption of radicular dentin of maxillary dentition. This process arose after initiation of orthodontics.

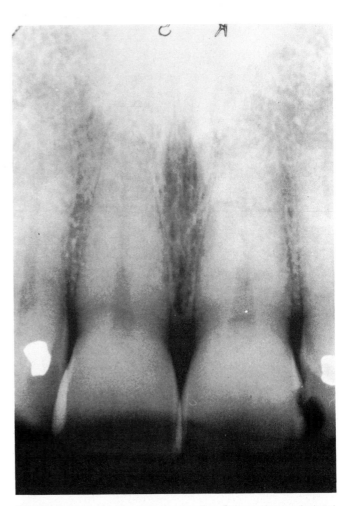

FIGURE 2-26. **Cervical external resorption.** Same patient as depicted in Figure 2-25. Radiographic appearance 3 years prior to alterations noted in Figure 2-25. (Courtesy of Dr. H. Dwaine Blakeman.)

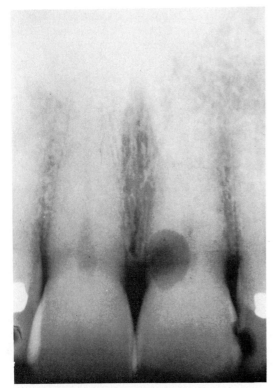

FIGURE 2-25. **Cervical external resorption.** Well-defined radiolucent alteration of the cervical area of the maxillary left central incisor. (Courtesy of Dr. H. Dwaine Blakeman.)

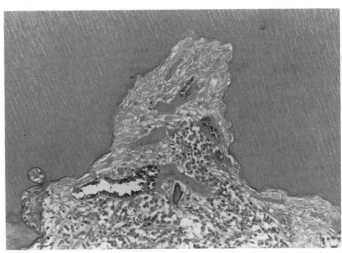

FIGURE 2-27. **Internal resorption.** Resorption of the inner dentinal wall of the pulp. Note cellular and vascular fibrous connective tissue, which exhibits an adjacent inflammatory infiltrate.

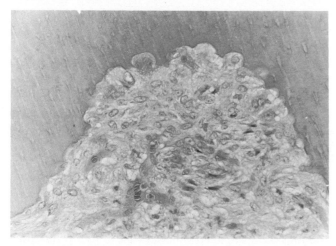

FIGURE 2-28. **Internal resorption.** Higher power of the area of resorption depicted in Figure 2-27. Note dentinoclasts within resorptive lacunae and cellularity of the adjacent connective tissue.

(arising from the surface accumulation of exogenous pigment) or **intrinsic** (secondary to endogenous factors that result in the discoloration of the underlying dentin). Table 2-4 lists the most frequently documented causes of tooth discolorations.

Dental fluorosis is discussed under environmental effects on the structural development of the teeth (see p. 47). The alterations associated with **amelogenesis imperfecta** (see p. 79) and **dentinogenesis imperfecta** (see p. 84) are presented later in this chapter in the text devoted to primary developmental alterations of the teeth.

Clinical Features

Extrinsic Stains

Bacterial stains are not an uncommon cause of surface staining of exposed enamel, dentin, and cementum. Chromogenic bacteria can produce colorations that vary from green or black-brown to orange. The discoloration occurs most frequently in children and usually is seen initially on the labial surface of the maxillary anterior teeth in the gingival one third. In contrast to most plaque-related discolorations, the black-brown stains most likely are not primarily of bacterial origin but are secondary to the formation of ferric sulfide from an interaction between bacterial ferric sulfide and iron in the saliva or gingival crevicular fluid.

Extensive use of **tobacco** products, **tea**, or **coffee** often results in significant brown discoloration of the surface enamel. The tar within the tobacco dissolves in the saliva and easily penetrates the pits and fissures of the enamel. Smokers (tobacco or marijuana) most frequently exhibit involvement of the lingual surface of the mandibular incisors; users of smokeless tobacco often demonstrate involvement of the enamel in the area of tobacco placement. Stains due to beverages also often involve the lingual surface of the anterior teeth, but the stains are usually more widespread and less intense. In addition, **foods** that contain abundant chlorophyll can produce a green discoloration of the enamel surface.

The green discoloration associated with chromogenic bacteria or the frequent consumption of chlorophyll-containing foods can resemble the pattern of green staining seen secondary to **gingival hemorrhage**. As would be expected, this pattern of discoloration occurs most frequently in patients with poor oral hygiene and erythematous, hemorrhagic, and enlarged gingiva. The color results from the breakdown of hemoglobin into green biliverdin.

Dental **restorative materials**, especially amalgam, can result in black-gray discolorations of teeth. This most frequently arises in younger patients, who have more open dentinal tubules. Large Class II proximal restorations of posterior teeth can produce discoloration of the overlying facial surface. In addition, deep lingual metallic restorations on anterior incisors can stain significant underlying dentin and produce visible labial grayish discoloration. To help prevent significant discoloration, one should not restore endodontically treated anterior teeth with amalgam (Fig. 2-29).

Table 2-4. TOOTH DISCOLORATIONS

Extrinsic
1. Bacterial stains
2. Tobacco
3. Foods and beverages
4. Gingival hemorrhage
5. Restorative materials
6. Medications

Intrinsic
1. Amelogenesis imperfecta
2. Dentinogenesis imperfecta
3. Dental fluorosis
4. Erythropoietic porphyria
5. Hyperbilirubinemia
6. Localized red blood cell breakdown
7. Medications

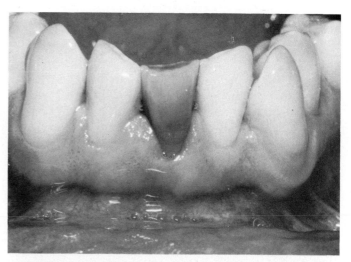

FIGURE 2-29. **Amalgam discoloration.** Greenish-gray discoloration of mandibular central incisor, which had endodontic access preparation restored with amalgam.

A large number of **medications** may result in surface staining of the teeth. In the past, use of products containing high amounts of iron or iodine was associated with significant black pigmentation of the teeth. Exposure to sulfides, silver nitrate, or manganese can cause stains that vary from gray to yellow to brown to black. Copper or nickel may produce a green stain; cadmium may be associated with a yellow to golden-brown discoloration.

More recently, the most frequently reported culprits include **stannous fluoride** and **chlorhexidine**.

Fluoride staining may be associated with the use of 8 percent stannous fluoride and is thought to be secondary to the combination of the stannous (tin) ion with bacterial sulfides. This black stain was seen predominantly in people with poor oral hygiene in areas previously affected by early carious involvement. The labial surfaces of anterior teeth and the occlusal surfaces of posterior teeth are the most frequently affected.

Chlorhexidine is associated with a yellowish-brown stain that predominantly involves the interproximal surfaces near the gingival margins. The degree of staining varies with the concentration of the medication and the patient's susceptibility. Although an increased frequency has been associated with the use of tannin-containing beverages, such as tea and wine, the stain can be minimized by effective brushing and flossing. Chlorhexidine is not alone in its association with tooth staining; many oral antiseptics, such as Listerine and sanguinarine, also may produce similar changes.

Intrinsic Stains

Congenital erythropoietic porphyria (Günther's disease) is an autosomal recessive disorder of porphyrin metabolism that results in the increased synthesis and excretion of porphyrins and their related precursors. Significant diffuse discoloration of the dentition is noted as a result of the deposition of porphyrin in the teeth (Fig. 2–30; see Color Figure 11). Affected teeth demonstrate a marked reddish-brown coloration that exhibits a red fluorescence when exposed to a Wood's ultraviolet (UV) light. The deciduous teeth demonstrate a more intense coloration because porphyrin is present in the enamel and the dentin; in the permanent teeth, only the dentin is affected.

Bilirubin is a breakdown product of red blood cells, and excess levels can be released into the blood in a number of conditions. The increased amount of bilirubin can accumulate in the interstitial fluid, mucosa, serosa, and skin, resulting in a yellow-green discoloration known as **jaundice**. During periods of **hyperbilirubinemia**, developing teeth also may accumulate the pigment and become intrinsically stained. In most cases, the deciduous teeth are affected as a result of hyperbilirubinemia during the neonatal period. The two most common causes are **erythroblastosis fetalis** and **biliary atresia**. Other diseases less frequently involved include:

- Premature birth
- ABO incompatibility
- Neonatal respiratory distress
- Significant internal hemorrhage
- Congenital hypothyroidism
- Biliary hypoplasia
- Metabolic diseases (tyrosinemia, α_1-antitrypsin deficiency)
- Neonatal hepatitis

Erythroblastosis fetalis is a hemolytic anemia of newborns secondary to a blood incompatibility (usually Rh factor) between the mother and the fetus. Currently, this disorder is relatively uncommon because of the use of antiantigen gamma globulin at delivery in mothers who are Rh-negative.

Biliary atresia is a sclerosing process of the biliary tree

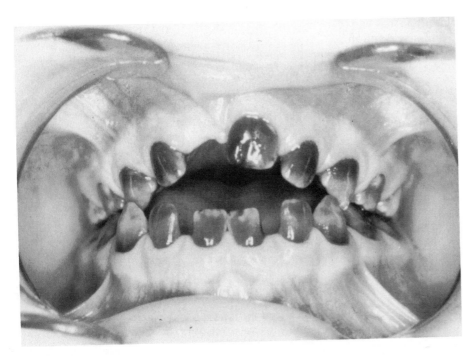

FIGURE 2–30. **Erythropoietic porphyria-related discoloration of teeth.** Reddish-brown discoloration of the maxillary dentition. See Color Plates.

that is the most important cause of death from hepatic failure in children in North America. Many affected children live after successful liver transplantation.

The extent of the dental changes correlates with the period of hyperbilirubinemia, and most patients exhibit involvement limited to the primary dentition. On occasion, the cusps of the permanent first molars may be affected. In addition to enamel hypoplasia, the affected teeth frequently demonstrate a green discoloration (**chlorodontia**). The color is secondary to biliverdin, the breakdown product of bilirubin that causes jaundice, and may vary from yellow to deep shades of green (Fig. 2–31; see Color Figure 12). The color of tooth structure formed after the resolution of the hyperbilirubinemia appears normal. The teeth often demonstrate a sharp dividing line, separating green portions (which formed during hyperbilirubinemia) from normal-colored portions (which formed after normal levels of bilirubin were restored).

A related process secondary to **localized red blood cell destruction** also can result in discoloration of the teeth. On occasion during a postmortem examination, a pink discoloration of teeth is found. The crowns and necks of the teeth are affected most frequently, and the process is thought to arise from hemoglobin breakdown within the necrotic pulp tissue in patients in whom blood has accumulated in the head.

A similar pink or red discoloration of the maxillary incisors has been reported in living patients with **lepromatous leprosy** (see p. 153). These teeth are involved selectively because of the decreased temperature required for the survival of the causative organism. This process is thought to be secondary to infection-related necrosis and the rupture of numerous small blood vessels within the pulp with a secondary release of hemoglobin into the adjacent dentinal tubules.

Several different **medications** can become incorporated into the developing tooth and result in clinically evident discoloration. The severity of the alterations is dependent on the time of administration, the dose, and the duration of the drug's use. The most infamous is **tetracycline**,

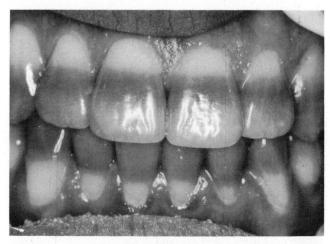

FIGURE 2–32. Tetracycline-related tooth discoloration. Diffuse brownish discoloration of the permanent dentition. See Color Plates. (Courtesy of Dr. John Fantasia.)

producing dental discolorations that vary from bright yellow to dark brown and, in ultraviolet light, show a bright yellow fluorescence (Fig. 2–32; see Color Figure 13). The drug and its homologues can cross the placental barrier; therefore, administration must be avoided during pregnancy and in children up to age 8 years. Homologues of tetracycline also associated with discoloration include chlortetracycline (gray-brown discoloration) and oxytetracycline (yellow). Synthetic tetracyclines, such as minocycline, also cause tooth discoloration, which varies from green to gray to black.

The effects of tetracyclines on developing teeth are well known, but it must be emphasized that the long-term use of these drugs in adults also can result in significant objectionable discoloration. When given over long periods in adults, tetracyclines are incorporated into the continually forming physiologic secondary dentin. Reports have documented the occurrence of patients with clinically obvious discoloration secondary to the involvement of the underlying secondary dentin.

Treatment and Prognosis

Most extrinsic stains on the teeth can be removed by careful polishing with fine pumice; typically, normal prophy paste is insufficient. Stubborn stains often are resolved by mixing 3 percent hydrogen peroxide with the pumice or by using bicarbonated spray solutions. The use of jet prophylactic devices with a mild abrasive is the most effective. Recurrence of the stains is not uncommon unless the associated cause is altered. Improving the level of oral hygiene often minimizes the chance of recurrence.

Intrinsic discoloration is much more difficult to resolve because of the frequent extensive involvement of the dentin. Suggested aesthetic solutions include full crowns, external bleaching of vital teeth, internal bleaching of nonvital teeth, bonded restorations, composite build-ups, and laminate veneer crowns. The treatment must be individualized to fulfill the unique needs of each patient and his or her specific pattern of discoloration.

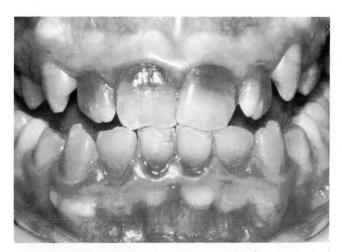

FIGURE 2–31. Hyperbilirubinemia-related tooth discoloration. Diffuse grayish-blue discoloration of the dentition. Cervical portions are stained most intensely. See Color Plates. (Courtesy of Dr. John Giunta.)

LOCALIZED DISTURBANCES IN ERUPTION

Primary Impaction

Eruption is the continuous process of movement of a tooth from its developmental location to its functional location. Teeth that cease to erupt before emergence are **impacted**. Some authors subdivide these nonerupted teeth into those that are obstructed by a physical barrier *(impacted)* and those that appear to exhibit a lack of eruptive force *(embedded)*. In many cases, a tooth may appear to be embedded but, on removal, a previously undetected overlying odontogenic hamartoma or neoplasm is discovered. Therefore, it appears appropriate to classify all these teeth as "impacted."

Clinical Features

Primary impaction of deciduous teeth is extremely rare and, when seen, most commonly involves second molars (Fig. 2–33). Analysis of cases suggests ankylosis plays a major role in the pathogenesis. In permanent teeth, third molars are impacted most frequently, followed by maxillary cuspids. The remaining order of frequency of tooth impaction is mandibular premolars, mandibular canines, maxillary premolars, maxillary central incisors, maxillary lateral incisors, and mandibular second molars. First molars and maxillary second molars are rarely affected.

Lack of eruption most frequently is due to crowding and insufficient maxillofacial development. Impacted teeth are frequently diverted or angulated and eventually lose their potential to erupt (on completion of root development). Other factors known to be associated with impaction include:

- Overlying cysts or tumors
- Trauma
- Reconstructive surgery
- Thickened overlying bone or soft tissue
- A host of systemic disorders, diseases, and syndromes

Impacted teeth may be partially erupted or completely encased within the bone (full bony impaction). In addition, the impaction may be classified according to the angulation of the tooth in relationship to the remaining dentition: mesioangular, distoangular, vertical, horizontal, or inverted.

Treatment and Prognosis

The choices of treatment for impacted teeth include:

- Long-term observation
- Orthodontically assisted eruption
- Transplantation
- Surgical removal

The presence of infection, nonrestorable carious lesions, cysts, tumors, or destruction of adjacent tooth and bone mandate extraction. Surgical removal of impacted teeth is the procedure performed most frequently by oral and maxillofacial surgeons. The choice of therapy in asymptomatic cases is an area of hot debate, and no immediate resolution is obvious.

The risks associated with nonintervention include:

- Crowding of dentition
- Resorption and worsening of the periodontal status of adjacent teeth (Fig. 2–34)
- Development of pathologic conditions, such as infections, cysts, and tumors

The risks of intervention include:

- Transient or permanent sensory loss
- Alveolitis
- Trismus

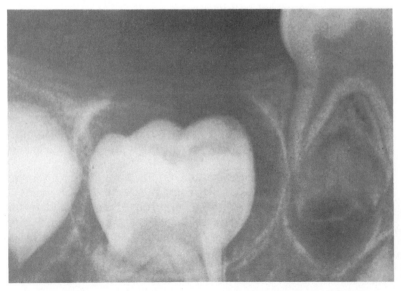

FIGURE 2–33. Primary impaction of deciduous tooth. The right secondary primary molar demonstrates delayed eruption and enlarged pericoronal radiolucency. (Courtesy of Dr. G. Thomas Kluemper.)

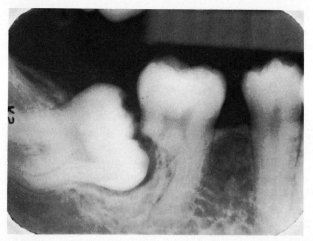

FIGURE 2–34. **Impaction-related tooth resorption.** Mesioangular impaction of the right mandibular third molar associated with significant resorption of the distal root of the second molar. (Courtesy of Dr. Richard Brock.)

- Infection
- Fracture
- Temporomandibular joint injury
- Periodontal injury
- Injury to adjacent teeth

Dental referral patterns provide a variety of perspectives of different dental practitioners. Many specialists, such as oral/maxillofacial surgeons and oral/maxillofacial pathologists, see a large percentage of significant pathologic conditions associated with impacted teeth compared with the experience of other clinicians. One large review of pericoronal tissue submitted to an active oral pathology service revealed that 32.9 percent of cases had pathologically significant lesions. In this 6-year review were six primary squamous cell carcinomas arising from dentigerous cysts in addition to numerous neoplastic odontogenic cysts and tumors. The variable patient pool of specialists leads to an alteration in the therapeutic approach that is based on personal experience, hence the different therapeutic opinions chosen by different areas of dentistry.

Ankylosis

Eruption continues after the emergence of the teeth in order to compensate for masticatory wear and the growth of the jaws. The cessation of eruption after emergence is termed **ankylosis**. Although the areas of union may be too subtle to be detected clinically and radiographically, histologic examination will demonstrate fusion between the affected tooth and the adjacent bone in almost all cases. Other terms for this process within the literature include *infraocclusion, secondary retention, submergence, reimpaction,* and *reinclusion.* "Secondary retention" is an acceptable term but may be confused with "retained primary teeth," which maintain their emergence. "Submergence," "reimpaction," and "reinclu-

sion" connote an active depression, and this is not the case.

The pathogenesis of ankylosis is unknown and may be secondary to one of many factors. Disturbances from changes in local metabolism, trauma, injury, chemical or thermal irritation, local failure of bone growth, and abnormal pressure from the tongue have been suggested. Some propose a genetically decreased periodontal ligament gap; others point to a disturbance between normal root resorption and hard tissue repair.

Clinical and Radiographic Features

Ankylosis may occur at any age, but clinically it is most obvious if the fusion develops during the first two decades of life. Most patients reported in the literature with obvious alterations in occlusion are between the ages of 9 and 18 years. The occlusal plane of the involved tooth is below that of the adjacent dentition (infraocclusion) in a patient with a history of previous full occlusion (Fig. 2–35). A sharp, solid sound may be noted on percussion of the involved tooth but can be detected only when more than 20 percent of the root is fused to the bone. Radiographically, absence of the periodontal ligament space may be noted, but the area of fusion is often in the bifurcation and inter-radicular root surface, making radiographic detection most difficult (Fig. 2–36).

Ankylosed teeth that are allowed to remain in position can lead to a number of dental problems. The adjacent teeth often incline toward the affected tooth, frequently with the development of subsequent occlusal and periodontal problems. In addition, the opposing teeth often exhibit overeruption.

Treatment and Prognosis

Because they are fused to the adjacent bone, ankylosed teeth fail to respond to orthodontic forces. Ankylosis of primary molars is best treated with extraction and space maintenance. Failure to do so results in a high incidence of tilting, carious destruction, and periodontal disease of

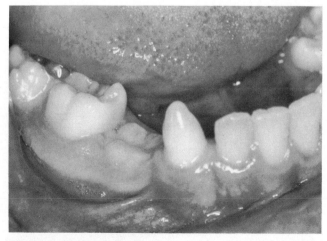

FIGURE 2–35. **Ankylosis.** Deciduous molar well below the occlusal plane of the adjacent teeth.

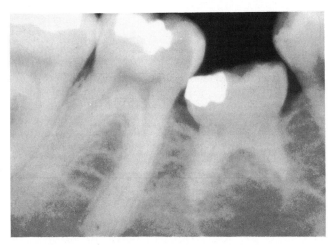

FIGURE 2–36. **Ankylosis.** Radiograph of an ankylosed deciduous molar. Note the lack of periodontal ligament space.

the teeth in the area. Ankylosis in adulthood may be treated with prosthetic build-up if the occlusal discrepancy is limited. Finally, luxation of affected permanent teeth may be attempted with extraction forceps in an effort to break the ankylosis. It is hoped that the subsequent inflammatory reaction may result in the formation of a new fibrous ligament in the area of previous fusion. In these cases, re-evaluation in 6 months is mandatory.

Developmental Alterations of Teeth

Numerous developmental alterations of teeth can occur. Table 2–5 delineates the major reported alterations, and the following text pertains to these entities.

Table 2–5. DEVELOPMENTAL ALTERATIONS OF TEETH

1. **Number**
   a. Hypodontia
   b. Hyperdontia

2. **Size**
   a. Microdontia
   b. Macrodontia

3. **Shape**
   a. Gemination
   b. Fusion
   c. Concrescence
   d. Accessory cusps
   e. Dens invaginatus
   f. Ectopic enamel
   g. Taurodontism
   h. Hypercementosis
   i. Accessory roots
   j. Dilaceration

4. **Structure**
   a. Amelogenesis imperfecta
   b. Dentinogenesis imperfecta
   c. Dentin dysplasia, type I
   d. Dentin dysplasia, type II
   e. Regional odontodysplasia

These alterations may be primary or arise secondary to environmental influences (such as concrescence, hypercementosis, or dilaceration). For the sake of convenience, both the primary and environmental forms will be discussed together.

DEVELOPMENTAL ALTERATIONS IN THE NUMBER OF TEETH

Variations in the number of teeth that develop are common. Several terms are useful in the discussion of the numeric variations of teeth. **Anodontia** refers to a total lack of tooth development. **Hypodontia** denotes the lack of development of one or more teeth; **oligodontia** (subdivision of hypodontia) indicates the lack of development of six or more teeth. **Hyperdontia** is the development of an increased number of teeth, and the additional teeth are termed **supernumerary**. Terms such as "partial anodontia" are oxymorons and should be avoided. In addition, these terms pertain to teeth that failed to develop and should not be applied to teeth that developed but are impacted or have been removed.

Genetic control appears to exert a strong influence on the development of teeth. Numerous hereditary syndromes have been associated with both hypodontia (Table 2–6) and hyperdontia (Table 2–7). In addition,

Table 2–6. SYNDROMES ASSOCIATED WITH HYPODONTIA

1. Ankyloglossia superior
2. Böök
3. Cockayne
4. Coffin-Lowry
5. Cranio-oculo-dental
6. Crouzon
7. Down
8. Ectodermal dysplasia
9. Ectodermal dysplasia, cleft lip, cleft palate
10. Ehlers-Danlos
11. Ellis–van Creveld
12. Focal dermal hypoplasia
13. Freire-Maia
14. Frontometaphyseal dysplasia
15. Goldenhar
16. Gorlin
17. Gorlin-Chaudhry-Moss
18. Hallermann-Streiff
19. Hanhart
20. Hurler
21. Hypoglossia-hypodactylia
22. Incontinentia pigmenti
23. Johanson-Blizzard
24. Lipoid proteinosis
25. Marshall-White
26. Melanoleukoderma
27. Monilethrix-anodontia
28. Oral-facial-digital, type I
29. Otodental dysplasia
30. Palmoplantar keratosis, hypotrichosis, cysts of eyelid
31. Progeria
32. Rieger
33. Robinson
34. Rothmund
35. Sturge-Weber
36. Tooth and nail
37. Turner

Table 2-7. SYNDROMES ASSOCIATED
WITH HYPERDONTIA

1. Angio-osteohypertrophy
2. Cleidocranial dysplasia
3. Curtius
4. Fabry-Anderson
5. Gardner
6. Hallermann-Streiff
7. Oral-facial-digital, type I
8. Sturge-Weber

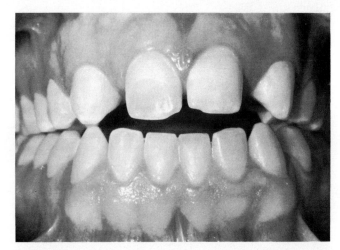

FIGURE 2-37. **Hypodontia.** Developmentally missing maxillary lateral incisors. Radiographs revealed no underlying teeth, and there was no history of trauma or extraction.

many nonsyndromic numeric alterations of teeth demonstrate a strong genetic correlation. Primary hypodontia appears to be autosomal dominant with incomplete penetrance, but the environment is not without its influence. Less information is available on the genetics of hyperdontia, but many cases also suggest an autosomal dominant pattern of inheritance with incomplete penetrance. The variable expression and penetrance of the gene defects may be due to the influence of environmental factors.

Some investigators have implied that hypodontia is a normal variant, suggesting that humans are in an intermediate stage of dentitional evolution. A proposed future dentition would contain one incisor, one canine, one premolar, and two molars per quadrant. Conversely, others have suggested that hyperdontia represents *atavism*, the reappearance of an ancestral condition. The latter hypothesis is difficult to accept because patients have presented with as many as four premolars in one quadrant, a situation that has never been reported in other mammals.

The pathogenesis of hyperdontia has been related to the development of excess dental lamina, which leads to the formation of additional tooth germs. As expected, hypodontia correlates with the absence of appropriate dental lamina. As discussed, the loss of the developing tooth buds in most instances appears to be genetically controlled. In spite of this, the environment most likely influences the final result or, in some cases, may be totally responsible for the lack of tooth formation. The dental lamina is extremely sensitive to external stimuli, and damage before tooth formation can result in hypodontia. Trauma, infection, radiation, chemotherapeutic medications, endocrine disturbances, and severe intrauterine disturbances have been associated with missing teeth.

Clinical Features

Hypodontia

Anodontia is rare, and most cases occur in the presence of hereditary hypohidrotic ectodermal dysplasia (see p. 541). Hypodontia is uncommon in the deciduous dentition (less than 1 percent of the population) and, when present, most frequently involves the mandibular incisors. Missing teeth in the permanent dentition are not rare, with third molars being the most commonly affected (the prevalence varies in different races from 2.5 to 35 percent). After the molars, the second premolars and lateral incisors are absent the most frequently (Fig.

2-37). Hypodontia is associated positively with microdontia (see p. 64) and occurs more frequently in females than males (approximate ratio, 1.5:1) (Figs. 2-38 and 2-39).

Hyperdontia

Single-tooth hyperdontia occurs more frequently in the permanent dentition, and approximately 90 percent present in the maxilla, with a strong predilection for the anterior region. The most common site is the maxillary incisor region, followed by maxillary fourth molars and mandibular fourth molars, premolars, canines, and lateral incisors (Fig. 2-40). Although supernumerary teeth may be bilateral, most occur unilaterally (Figs. 2-41 and 2-42). In contrast to single-tooth hyperdontia, nonsyndromic multiple supernumerary teeth occur most frequently in the mandible. These multiple supernumerary teeth occur most often in the premolar region, followed by the molar and anterior regions, respectively (Fig. 2-43). Although most supernumerary teeth occur in the

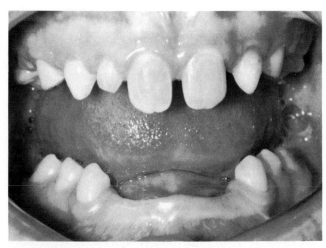

FIGURE 2-38. **Hypodontia.** Multiple developmentally missing permanent teeth and several retained deciduous teeth in a female adult.

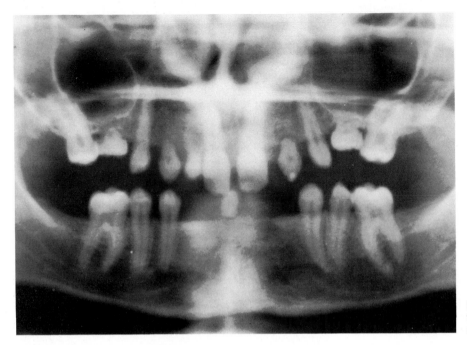

FIGURE 2–39. **Hypodontia.** Radiograph of the same patient depicted in Figure 2–38. No unerupted teeth were noted within the jaws.

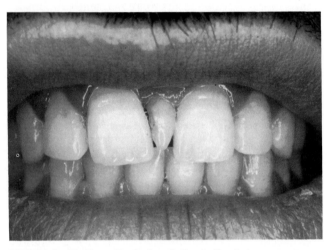

FIGURE 2–40. **Hyperdontia (mesiodens).** Erupted supernumerary, rudimentary tooth of the anterior maxilla.

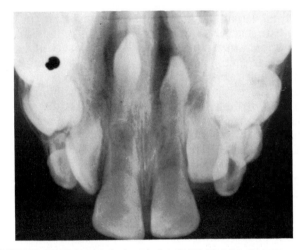

FIGURE 2–42. **Hyperdontia (mesiodens).** Bilateral inverted supernumerary teeth of the anterior maxilla.

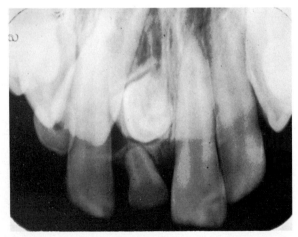

FIGURE 2–41. **Hyperdontia (mesiodens).** Unilateral supernumerary tooth of the anterior maxilla, which has altered the eruption path of the maxillary right permanent central incisor.

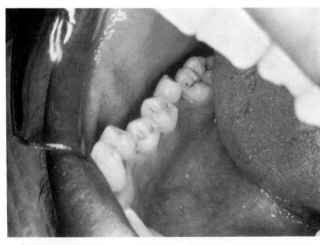

FIGURE 2–43. **Hyperdontia.** Right mandibular dentition exhibiting four erupted bicuspids.

jaws, examples have been reported in the gingiva, maxillary tuberosity, soft palate, sphenomaxillary fissure, and nasal cavity. The eruption of accessory teeth is variable and dependent on the degree of space available; 75 percent of supernumerary teeth in the anterior maxilla fail to erupt. The converse of hypodontia, hyperdontia is positively correlated with macrodontia (see p. 64) and exhibits a 2:1 male predominance. Although late cases do occur, most supernumerary teeth develop during the first two decades of life.

Several terms have been applied to supernumerary teeth, according to the location of their origin. A supernumerary tooth in the maxillary anterior incisor region is termed a **mesiodens** (see Fig. 2–40); an accessory fourth molar is often called a **distomolar** or **distodens**. A posterior supernumerary tooth situated lingually or buccally to a molar tooth is termed a **paramolar** (Figs. 2–44 and 2–45).

On occasion, normal teeth may erupt into an inappropriate position (such as a canine present between two premolars). This pattern of abnormal eruption is called **dental transposition.** Such misplaced teeth have been confused with supernumerary teeth. Crowding or malocclusion of these normal teeth may dictate reshaping, orthodontics, or extraction.

Accessory teeth may be present at or shortly after birth. Historically, teeth present in newborns have been called **natal teeth**; those arising within the first 30 days of life are designated **neonatal teeth.** This is an artificial distinction, and it appears appropriate to call all these teeth "natal teeth" (Fig. 2–46). Although some authors have suggested that these teeth may represent prededuous supernumerary teeth, most of these teeth represent prematurely erupted portions of the deciduous dentition, not supernumerary teeth. Approximately 85 percent of natal teeth are mandibular incisors, 11 percent are maxillary incisors, and 4 percent are posterior teeth.

Treatment and Prognosis

The management of the patient with hypodontia depends on the severity of the case. No treatment may be

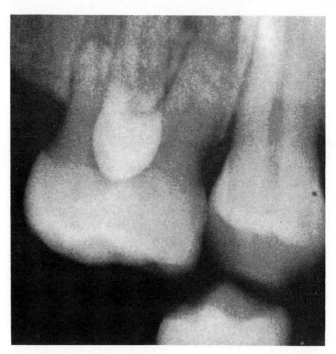

FIGURE 2–45. **Paramolar.** Radiograph of the same patient depicted in Figure 2–44. Note the fully formed tooth overlying the crown of the adjacent molar.

required for individual missing teeth; prosthetic replacement is often needed when multiple teeth are absent.

The presence of supernumerary teeth should be suspected if there is a significant delay in the eruption of a localized portion of the dentition. Early diagnosis and treatment often are crucial in minimizing the aesthetic and functional problems of the adjacent teeth. The standard of care is early removal of the accessory tooth.

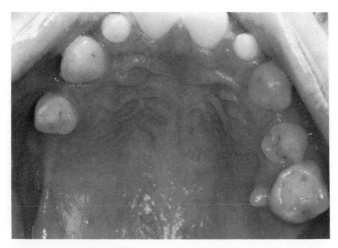

FIGURE 2–44. **Paramolar.** Rudimentary tooth situated palatal to a maxillary molar in a patient who also exhibits hypodontia.

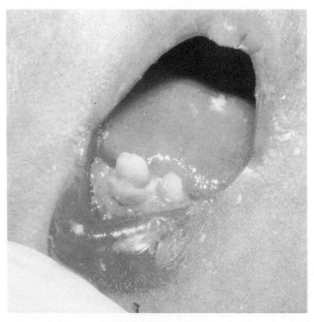

FIGURE 2–46. **Natal teeth.** Mandibular central incisors, which were erupted at birth.

Reports have documented spontaneous eruption of the adjacent dentition in 75 percent of the cases if the supernumerary tooth is removed early.

A consequence of delayed therapy may include the delayed eruption of the adjacent teeth or the displacement of the teeth with associated crowding and malocclusion. Supernumerary teeth also predispose the area to subacute pericoronitis, gingivitis, periodontitis, abscess formation, and the development of any one of a large number of odontogenic cysts and tumors. In selected cases, clinical judgment may not dictate surgical removal or patient resistance to therapy may be present. In these instances, regular monitoring is mandatory.

Natal teeth must be approached individually, with sound clinical judgment guiding appropriate therapy. As stated, the erupted teeth in most cases represent the deciduous dentition and removal should not be performed hastily. If the teeth are mobile and at risk for aspiration, removal is indicated. If mobility is not a problem and the teeth are stable, they should be retained. Traumatic ulcerations of the adjacent soft tissue (**Riga-Fede disease**, see p. 213) may occur during breast-feeding but can be resolved with appropriate measures.

DEVELOPMENTAL ALTERATIONS IN THE SIZE OF TEETH

Tooth size is variable among different races and between the sexes. The presence of unusually small teeth is termed **microdontia**; the presence of teeth larger than average is termed **macrodontia**. Although heredity is the major factor, both genetic and environmental influences affect the size of developing teeth. The deciduous dentition appears to be affected more by maternal intrauterine influences; the permanent teeth seem to be more affected by environment.

Clinical Features

Although the size of teeth is variable, there usually is symmetry of the two sides of the jaws. In spite of this, when significant size variation is present, the entire dentition rarely is affected. Typically, only a few teeth are altered significantly in size. Differences in tooth sizes cannot be considered in isolation. Microdontia is strongly associated with hypodontia (see p. 60); macrodontia often is seen in association with hyperdontia (see p. 60). Females demonstrate a higher frequency of microdontia and hypodontia; males have a greater prevalence of macrodontia and hyperdontia.

Microdontia

The term "microdontia" should be applied only when the teeth are physically smaller than usual. Normal-sized teeth may appear small when widely spaced within jaws that are larger than normal. This appearance historically has been termed **relative microdontia**, but it represents **macrognathia**, not microdontia. Diffuse true microdontia is uncommon but may occur as an isolated finding in Down syndrome, in pituitary dwarfism, and in association with a small number of rare hereditary disorders that

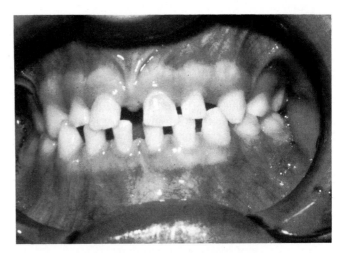

FIGURE 2–47. **Diffuse microdontia.** Dentition in which the teeth are smaller than normal and widely spaced within the arch.

exhibit multiple abnormalities of the dentition (Fig. 2–47).

Isolated microdontia within an otherwise normal dentition is not uncommon. The maxillary lateral incisor is affected most frequently and typically presents as a peg-shaped crown overlying a root that often is of normal length (Fig. 2–48). The mesiodistal diameter is reduced, and the proximal surfaces converge toward the incisal edge. The reported prevalence varies from 0.8 to 8.4 percent of the population, and the alteration appears to be autosomal dominant with incomplete penetrance. In addition, isolated microdontia often affects third molars. Interestingly, both the maxillary lateral incisors and third molars are among the most frequent teeth to be congenitally missing.

Macrodontia

Analogous to microdontia, the term "macrodontia" (**megalodontia**, **megadontia**) should be applied only when teeth are physically larger than usual and should not

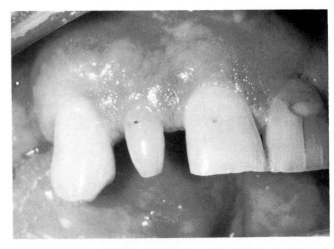

FIGURE 2–48. **Isolated microdontia (peg lateral).** Small, cone-shaped right maxillary lateral incisor.

include normal-sized teeth crowded within a small jaw (previously termed **relative macrodontia**). In addition, the term macrodontia should not be used to describe teeth that have been altered by fusion or gemination. Diffuse involvement is rare, and typically only a few teeth are abnormally large. Diffuse macrodontia has been noted in association with pituitary gigantism (see p. 606) and pineal hyperplasia with hyperinsulinism. Macrodontia with unilateral premature eruption is not infrequently a finding in hemifacial hyperplasia (see p. 34). Authors have postulated that the influence resulting in the unilateral bone growth also affects the developing teeth on the altered side.

Treatment and Prognosis

Treatment of the dentition is not necessary unless desired for aesthetic considerations. Maxillary peg laterals often are restored to full size by porcelain crowns.

DEVELOPMENTAL ALTERATIONS IN THE SHAPE OF TEETH

Gemination, Fusion, and Concrescence

Double teeth are two separate teeth exhibiting union by dentin and maybe their pulps. The union may be the result of fusion of two adjacent tooth buds or the partial splitting of one into two. The development of isolated large or joined (double) teeth is not rare, but the literature is confusing when the appropriate terminology is presented. Historically, "gemination" was defined as an attempt of a single tooth bud to divide, with the resultant formation of a tooth with a bifid crown and, usually, a common root and root canal. Likewise, "fusion" was considered the union of two normally separated tooth buds with the resultant formation of a joined tooth with confluence of dentin. Finally, "concrescence" was the union of two teeth by cementum without confluence of the dentin.

Many investigators have found these definitions confusing and open to debate. A double tooth found in the place of a maxillary permanent central incisor is a good example of the controversy. If the joined tooth is counted as one and the tooth number is correct, the anomaly could result from the division of a single tooth bud or the fusion of the permanent tooth bud with the bud of an adjacent mesiodens. Some have suggested that the terms gemination, fusion, and concrescence should be discontinued, and all of these anomalies should be termed **twinning**. This also is confusing because other investigators use "twinning" to refer to the development of two separate teeth that arose from the complete separation of one tooth bud (this also is arguable).

Secondary to this confusion in terminology, the use of the term "twinning" cannot be recommended. Extra teeth are termed supernumerary, and another name is not necessary. Even though the exact pathogenesis may be questionable in some cases (fusion of adjacent buds or partial split of one bud?), the terms gemination, fusion,

and concrescence serve a useful purpose because they are the most descriptive of the clinical presentation. **Gemination** is defined as a single enlarged tooth or joined (double) tooth in which the tooth count is normal when the anomalous tooth is counted as one. **Fusion** is defined as a single enlarged tooth or joined (double) tooth in which the tooth count reveals a missing tooth when the anomalous tooth is counted as one.

Concrescence is union of two adjacent teeth by cementum alone without confluence of the underlying dentin. Unlike fusion and gemination, concrescence may be developmental or postinflammatory. When two teeth develop in close proximity, developmental union by cementum is possible. In addition, areas of inflammatory damage to the roots of teeth are repaired by cementum once the inciting process resolves. Concrescence of adjacent teeth may arise in initially separated teeth in which cementum deposition extends between two closely approximated roots in a previous area of damage.

Clinical Features

Gemination/Fusion

Double teeth (gemination and fusion) occur in both the primary and permanent dentitions, with a higher frequency in the anterior and maxillary regions (Figs. 2–49 to 2–53). The literature reveals a prevalence of 0.5 percent in the deciduous teeth and 0.1 percent in the permanent dentition. Bilateral cases are seen less frequently, with a prevalence of 0.02 percent in both dentitions (Fig. 2–54). Gemination and fusion appear similar and may be differentiated by assessing the number of teeth in the dentition. Some authors have suggested that gemination demonstrates a single root canal. Separate canals are present in fusion, but this does not hold true in all cases (Fig. 2–55). A variety of appearances are noted with both fusion and gemination. The processes may result in an otherwise anatomically correct tooth that is greatly enlarged. A bifid crown may be seen overlying two completely separated roots, or the joined crowns may blend into one enlarged root with a single canal.

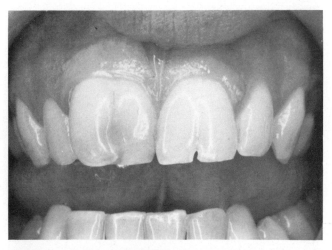

FIGURE 2–49. Bilateral gemination. Two "double teeth." The tooth count was normal when each anomalous tooth was counted as one.

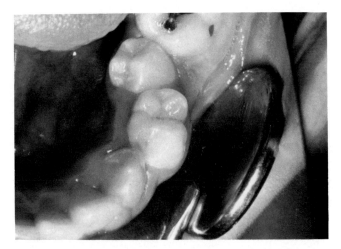

FIGURE 2-50. **Gemination.** Mandibular bicuspid exhibiting bifid crown.

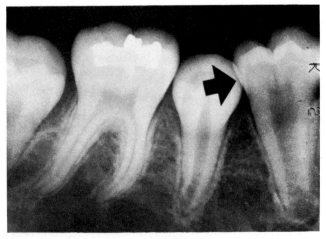

FIGURE 2-51. **Gemination.** Same patient as depicted in Figure 2-50. Note the bifid crown and shared root canal.

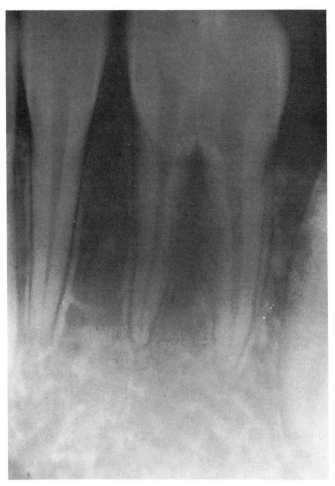

FIGURE 2-53. **Fusion.** Radiographic view of ''double tooth'' in the place of the mandibular central and lateral incisors. Note separate root canals.

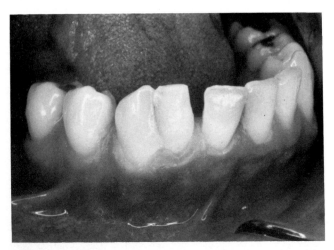

FIGURE 2-52. **Fusion.** ''Double tooth'' in the place of the mandibular right lateral incisor and cuspid.

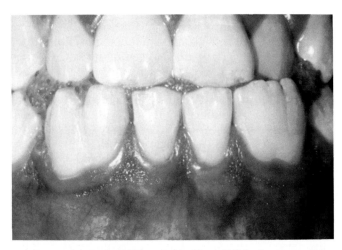

FIGURE 2-54. **Fusion.** Bilateral ''double teeth'' in the place of the mandibular lateral incisors and cuspids.

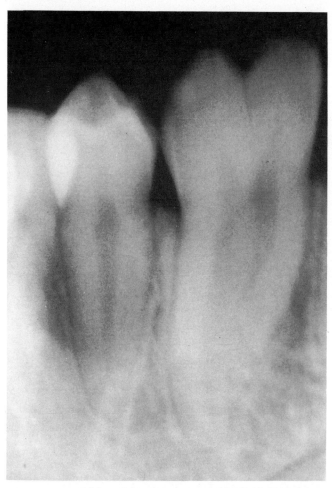

FIGURE 2-55. **Fusion.** Radiograph of the same patient depicted in Figure 2-54. Note the bifid crown overlying the single root canal; the contralateral radiograph revealed a similar pattern.

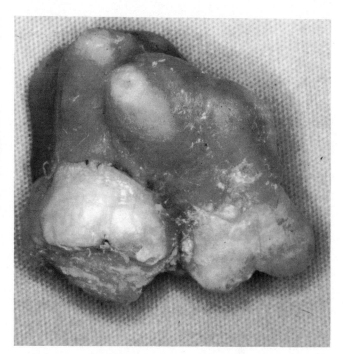

FIGURE 2-56. **Concrescence.** Union by cementum of adjacent maxillary molars.

Concrescence

Concrescence presents with two fully formed teeth, joined along the root surfaces by cementum. The process is noted more frequently in the posterior and maxillary regions. The developmental pattern often involves a second molar tooth in which its roots closely approximate the adjacent impacted third molar (Fig. 2-56). The postinflammatory pattern frequently involves carious molars in which the apices overlie the roots of horizontally or distally angulated third molars. This latter pattern most frequently arises in a carious tooth that exhibits large coronal tooth loss. The resultant large pulpal exposure often permits pulpal drainage, leading to a resolution of a portion of the intrabony pathosis. Cemental repair then occurs (Figs. 2-57 and 2-58).

Treatment and Prognosis

The presence of double teeth (gemination or fusion) in the deciduous dentition can result in delayed or ectopic eruption of the underlying permanent teeth. When detected, the progression of eruption of the permanent teeth should be closely monitored by careful clinical and radiographic observation. When appropriate, extraction may be necessary to prevent an abnormality in eruption.

Several approaches are available for the treatment of joined teeth in the permanent dentition, and the treatment of choice is determined by the patient's particular needs. Rare reports of successful surgical division have been documented. Selected shaping with or without placement of full crowns has been used in many cases. Many patients exhibit pulpal or coronal anatomic features that are resistant to reshaping and require surgical removal with prosthetic replacement.

Patients with concrescence often require no therapy unless the union interferes with eruption; then surgical removal may be warranted. Postinflammatory concrescence must be kept in mind whenever extraction is planned for nonvital teeth with apices that overlie the roots of an adjacent tooth. Significant extraction difficulties can be experienced on attempted removal of a tooth that is unexpectedly joined to its neighbor. Surgical separation often is required to complete the procedure without loss of a significant portion of the surrounding bone.

Accessory Cusps

The cuspal morphology of teeth exhibits minor variations among different populations; of these, three distinctive patterns deserve further discussion: (1) **talon cusps**, (2) **cusps of Carabelli**, and (3) **dens evaginatus**.

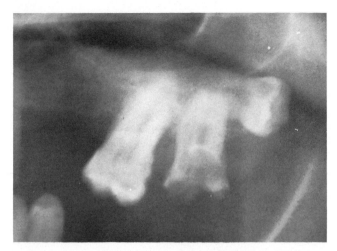

FIGURE 2–57. **Concrescence.** Union by cementum of maxillary second and third molars. Note the large carious defect of the second molar.

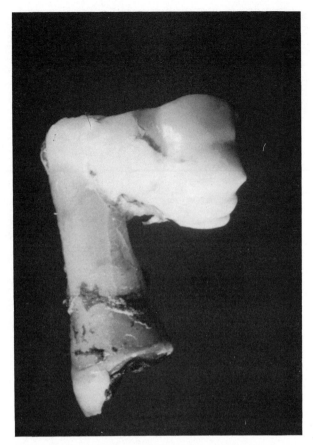

FIGURE 2–58. **Concrescence.** Gross photograph of the same teeth depicted in Figure 2–57. Histologic examination revealed that union occurred in the area of cemental repair previously damaged by a periapical inflammatory lesion.

Clinical and Radiographic Features

Talon Cusp

A talon cusp is a well-delineated additional cusp that is located on the surface of an anterior tooth and extends at least half the distance from the cemento-enamel junction to the incisal edge. The cusps predominantly occur on permanent maxillary incisors but have been seen less frequently on mandibular incisors and maxillary canines (Fig. 2–59). Their occurrence on maxillary deciduous central incisors has been reported but is rare. In almost all cases, the accessory cusp projects from the lingual surface of the affected tooth and forms a three-pronged pattern, which resembles an eagle's talon. On rare occasions, the cusp may project from the facial surface. A deep developmental groove may be present where the cusp fuses with the underlying surface of the affected tooth. Most, but not all, talon cusps contain a pulpal extension. Radiographically, the cusp is seen overlying the central portion of the crown and includes enamel and dentin (Fig. 2–60). Only a few cases demonstrate visible pulpal extensions on dental radiographs.

Extensive prevalence studies have not been performed, but estimates suggest that the frequency of talon cusp in

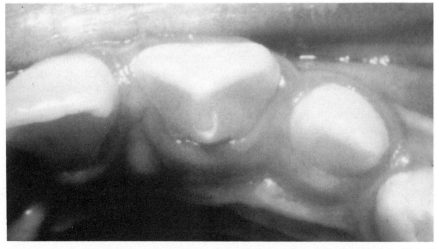

FIGURE 2–59. **Talon cusp.** Accessory cusp present on the palatal surface of the maxillary left central incisor. Note the three-pronged pattern, which resembles an eagle talon.

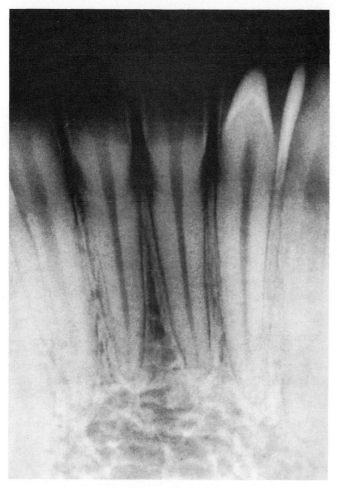

FIGURE 2–60. **Talon cusp.** Radiograph of a talon cusp on a mandibular lateral incisor. Note the enamel and dentin layers within the accessory cusp.

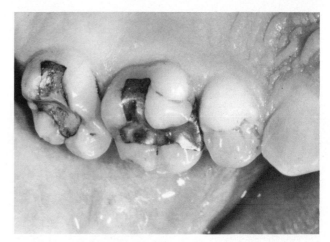

FIGURE 2–61. **Cusp of Carabelli.** Accessory cusp on the mesiolingual surface of the maxillary first molar.

Dens Evaginatus

Dens evaginatus is a cusp-like elevation of enamel located in the central groove or lingual ridge of the buccal cusp of permanent premolar or molar teeth (Fig. 2–62). Although this pattern of accessory cusps has been

the population ranges from 0.17 to 5.2 percent. Variations within different population groups make a definitive calculation difficult. Both sexes may be affected, and the occurrence may be unilateral or bilateral. The accessory cusp has been seen in association with other dental anomalies (e.g., odontomas, impacted teeth, peg-shaped lateral incisors, dens invaginatus). Talon cusps have been seen in patients with Mohr, Rubinstein-Taybi, and Sturge-Weber syndromes.

Cusp of Carabelli

The cusp of Carabelli is an accessory cusp that is located on the palatal surface of the mesiolingual cusp of a maxillary molar (Fig. 2–61). The cusp may be seen in the permanent or deciduous dentitions and varies from a definite cusp to a small indented pit or fissure. When present, the cusp is most pronounced on the first molar and is increasingly less obvious on the second and third molars. There is a significant variation between different populations, with the prevalence reported to be as high as 90 percent in whites and rare in Asians.

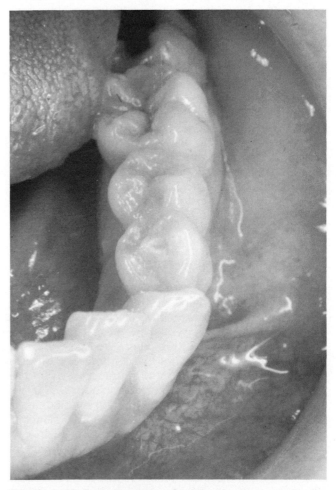

FIGURE 2–62. **Dens evaginatus.** Cusp-like elevation located in the central groove of mandibular first bicuspid.

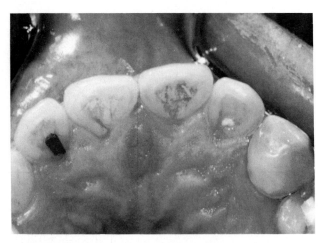

FIGURE 2-63. **Shovel-shaped incisors.** Chinese patient exhibiting maxillary incisors with prominent lateral margins, which create a hollowed lingual surface.

reported on molars, dens evaginatus typically occurs on premolar teeth, usually is bilateral, and demonstrates a marked mandibular predominance. The accessory cusp normally consists of enamel, dentin, and pulp. The process is rare in whites, but the prevalence has been reported to be as high as 15 percent in Asians. Radiographically, the occlusal surface exhibits a tuberculated appearance, and often a pulpal extension is seen in the cusp.

Frequently, dens evaginatus is seen in association with another variation of coronal anatomy, **shovel-shaped incisors.** This alteration also occurs predominantly in Asians, with a prevalence of approximately 15 percent in whites but close to 100 percent in Native Americans and Alaskans. Affected incisors demonstrate prominent lateral margins, creating a hollowed lingual surface that resembles the scoop of a shovel (Fig. 2-63). Typically, the thickened marginal ridges converge at the cingulum; not uncommonly, there is a deep pit, fissure, or dens invaginatus at this junction. Maxillary lateral and central incisors most frequently are affected, with mandibular incisors and canines less commonly reported.

Treatment and Prognosis

Patients with talon cusps on mandibular teeth often require no therapy; talon cusps present on maxillary teeth frequently interfere with occlusion and should be removed. Because many of these cusps contain pulp, rapid removal often results in pulpal exposure. Removal without the loss of vitality may be accomplished through periodic grinding of the cusp, with time allowed for tertiary dentin deposition and pulpal recession. One investigator covered the exposed dentin with fluoride at the end of each grinding session. After successful removal, the exposed dentin is covered with calcium hydroxide and the peripheral enamel is etched, with the placement of an unfilled composite resin.

On eruption, the affected tooth should be inspected for the presence of a deep fissure at the junction between the talon cusp and the surface of the tooth. If a fissure is

present, it should be restored to avoid early carious extension into the nearby dental pulp. Reports also have documented the continuation of this fissure down the surface of the root, with subsequent development of lateral radicular inflammatory lesions secondary to the access provided to oral flora by the deep groove. In these latter cases, further surgery is required to expose the groove for appropriate cleansing.

Patients with cusps of Carabelli require no therapy unless a deep groove is present between the accessory cusp and the surface of the mesiolingual cusp of the molar. These deep grooves should be sealed to prevent carious involvement.

Dens evaginatus often results in occlusal problems and is prone to fracture, frequently resulting in pulpal exposure. Pulpal necrosis results in the cessation of root formation; apexification with calcium hydroxide often is required to achieve closure. The removal of the cusps is often indicated, but attempts to maintain vitality have met with only partial success. The elimination of opposing occlusal interferences, combined with gradual grinding of the tubercle and indirect pulp capping with calcium hydroxide, has been suggested as the best approach when one is considering removal. Other investigators have protected the cusp from fracture by the placement of composite reinforcement around the projection until root formation is complete.

If shovel-shaped incisors are present, the affected teeth should be inspected for surface defects at the point where the marginal ridges converge. Any deep fissures or invaginations should be restored shortly after eruption to prevent carious exposure of the adjacent pulp.

Dens Invaginatus (Dens in Dente)

Dens invaginatus is a deep surface invagination of the crown or root that is lined by enamel. Oehlers described this condition thoroughly in three classic articles published from 1957 to 1958. Two forms—coronal and radicular—are recognized.

Clinical and Radiographic Features

By a great margin, **coronal dens invaginatus** is seen most frequently and the reported prevalence varies from 0.04 to 10 percent of all patients. In order of decreasing frequency, the teeth affected most often include the permanent lateral incisors, central incisors, premolars, canines, and molars (Fig. 2-64). A maxillary predominance is seen. On occasion, the invagination may be rather large and resemble a tooth within a tooth, hence the nickname **dens in dente.** In other cases, the invagination may be dilated and disturb the formation of the tooth, resulting in anomalous tooth development nicknamed **dilated odontome.** Involvement may be singular, multiple, or bilateral.

Radiographically, the invagination is lined by radiopaque enamel and may be small without extension past the level of the cemento-enamel junction or large with extension into the substance of the root (Figs. 2-65 and 2-66). Large invaginations may become dilated and

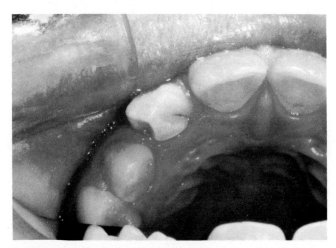

FIGURE 2–64. **Coronal dens invaginatus.** Coronal opening of enamel invagination of the right maxillary lateral incisor.

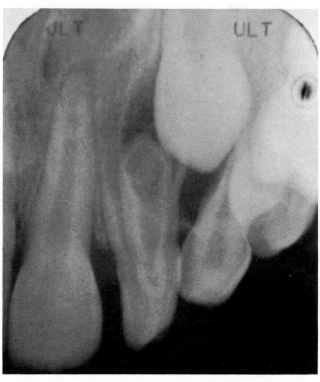

FIGURE 2–66. **Coronal dens invaginatus.** Deep invagination of the surface enamel, which extends to the apical area of the left maxillary lateral incisor. Note the dilatation of the apical portion of the invagination, which contains faintly radiopaque dystrophic enamel.

contain dystrophic enamel in the base of the dilatation (Fig. 2–67). On occasion, the coronal invagination may rupture out the side of the root and result in a lateral inflammatory lesion in the presence of a vital pulp (Figs. 2–68 and 2–69).

Radicular dens invaginatus is rare and thought to arise secondary to a proliferation of Hertwig's root sheath, with the formation of a strip of enamel that extends along the surface of the root. This pattern of enamel deposition is similar to that frequently seen in association with radicular **enamel pearls** (see Ectopic Enamel below). Rather than protrude from the surface, as seen in an enamel pearl, the altered enamel forms a surface in-

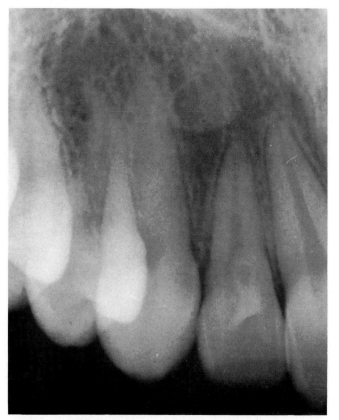

FIGURE 2–65. **Coronal dens invaginatus.** Radiograph of the right maxillary lateral incisor, which exhibits surface enamel invagination originating in the area of the cingulum with extension to just below the level of the cemento-enamel junction. Note the radiopaque enamel lining the invagination.

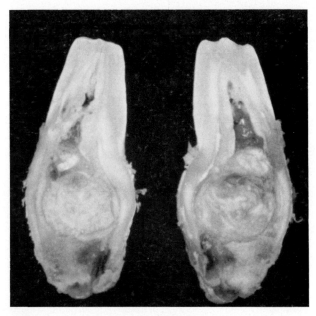

FIGURE 2–67. **Coronal dens invaginatus.** Gross photograph of a sectioned tooth. Note the dilated invagination with apical accumulation of dystrophic enamel.

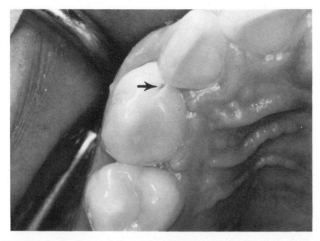

FIGURE 2-68. **Coronal dens invaginatus associated with a lateral inflammatory lesion.** Maxillary cuspid exhibiting opening of surface enamel invagination *(arrow)*. A parulis was present on the alveolar ridge buccal to the altered tooth, which was responsive to electric pulp testing. (Courtesy of Dr. Jill Harris.)

vagination into the dental papilla. Cementum-lined invaginations of the root have been reported, but these represent a simple variation of root morphology and should not be included under the term radicular dens invaginatus.

Radiographically, the affected tooth demonstrates an enlargement of the root. Close examination often reveals a dilated invagination lined by enamel with the opening of the invagination situated along the lateral aspect of the root.

Treatment and Prognosis

Minor cases of coronal dens invaginatus do not sufficiently disrupt formation to require removal of the tooth. The opening of the invagination should be restored on eruption in an attempt to prevent carious involvement of the invagination and subsequent pulpal inflammation. If the invagination is not detected quickly, pulpal necrosis frequently results. Large invaginations often disrupt normal coronal development and necessitate extraction. Invaginations associated with lateral radicular inflammatory lesions in vital teeth require restoration of the opening in conjunction with the surgical removal of the inflammatory lesion and filling of the apical portion of the defect.

If the invagination does not significantly disrupt the tooth's morphology, complications of radicular dens invaginatus are rare unless the radicular opening is exposed to the oral cavity. After exposure occurs, carious involvement often leads to pulpal necrosis. Openings close to the anatomic neck of the tooth should be exposed and restored, if possible, without significant damage to the tooth and surrounding structures.

Ectopic Enamel

Ectopic enamel refers to the presence of enamel in unusual locations, mainly the tooth root. The most widely known are **enamel pearls**. These are hemispherical structures that may consist entirely of enamel or contain underlying dentin and pulp tissue. Most project from the surface of the root and are thought to arise from a localized bulging of the odontoblastic layer. This bulge may provide prolonged contact between Hertwig's root sheath and the developing dentin, triggering induction of enamel formation. Similar internal projections of enamel into the underlying dentin rarely have been reported in the crowns of teeth.

In addition to enamel pearls, **cervical enamel extensions** also occur along the surface of dental roots. These extensions represent a dipping of the enamel from the cemento-enamel junction toward the bifurcation of molar teeth. This pattern of ectopic enamel forms a triangular extension of the coronal enamel, which develops on the buccal surface of molar teeth directly overlying the bifurcation. The base of the triangle is continuous with the inferior portion of the coronal enamel; the leading point of the triangle extends directly toward the bifurcation of the tooth. These areas of ectopic enamel have been called "cervical enamel projections," but this terminology is confusing because no significant exophytic projections are seen.

Clinical and Radiographic Features

Enamel Pearls

Enamel pearls are found most frequently on the roots of maxillary molars, with mandibular molars being the

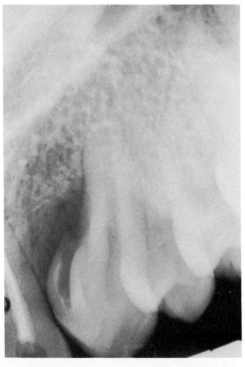

FIGURE 2-69. **Coronal dens invaginatus associated with a lateral inflammatory lesion.** Radiograph of the same tooth depicted in Figure 2-68. Note the enamel-lined coronal invagination that has perforated the lateral aspect of the root, resulting in a lateral inflammatory lesion in association with a vital tooth.

second most frequent site. Maxillary premolars and incisors are reported to be uncommonly affected. Involvement of deciduous molars is not rare. The prevalence of enamel pearls varies (1.1 to 9.7 percent of all patients), according to the population studied and is highest in Asians. In most cases, one pearl is found, but as many as four pearls have been documented on a single tooth. The majority occur on the roots at the furcation area or near the cemento-enamel junction (Fig. 2–70). Radiographically, pearls present as well-defined radiopaque nodules along the root's surface (Fig. 2–71). Mature internal enamel pearls present as well-defined circular areas of radiodensity extending from the enamel-dentin junction into the underlying coronal dentin.

The enamel surface of pearls precludes normal periodontal attachment with connective tissue, and a hemidesmosomal junction probably exists. This junction is less resistant to breakdown, and once separation occurs, rapid loss of attachment is likely (Fig. 2–71). In addition, the exophytic nature of the pearl is conducive to plaque retention and inadequate cleansing.

Cervical Enamel Extensions

As mentioned previously, cervical enamel extensions are located on the buccal surface of the root overlying the bifurcation (Fig. 2–72). Mandibular molars are affected more frequently than are maxillary molars. The prevalence is greater in Asians and varies from 8.6 to 32.6 percent of all patients, depending on the population that is under study. In descending order, the teeth most fre-

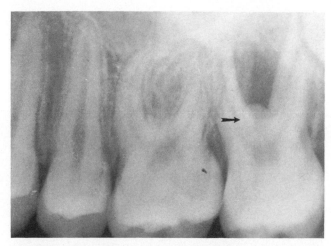

FIGURE 2–71. **Enamel pearl.** Radiopaque nodule in the bifurcation area of the maxillary second molar *(arrow)*. Extensive loss of attachment has occurred at the site of the enamel pearl.

quently affected are the first, second, and third molars, respectively.

These apical extensions of enamel have been correlated positively to localized loss of periodontal attachment with furcation involvement. On review of a large number of dentitions with periodontal furcation involvement, a significantly higher frequency of cervical enamel extensions was found compared with dentitions without furcation involvement. In addition, the greater the degree of cervical extension, the higher the frequency of furcation involvement.

In addition to periodontal furcation involvement, cervical enamel extensions in some cases have been associated with the development of inflammatory cysts,

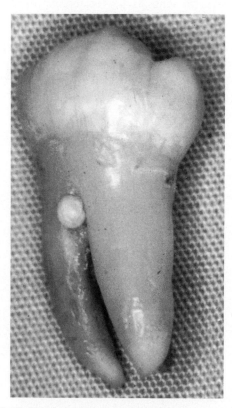

FIGURE 2–70. **Enamel pearl.** Mass of ectopic enamel located in the furcation area of a molar tooth. (Courtesy of Dr. Joseph Beard.)

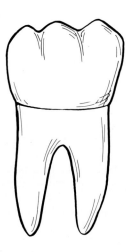
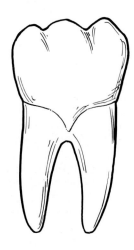

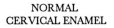
NORMAL   CERVICAL
CERVICAL ENAMEL   ENAMEL EXTENSION

FIGURE 2–72. **Cervical enamel extension.** Illustration of a normal molar adjacent to a molar exhibiting V-shaped elongation of enamel extending toward the bifurcation.

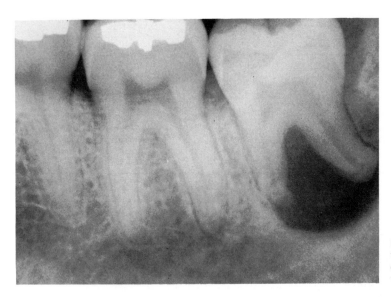

FIGURE 2–73. **Buccal bifurcation cyst.** Radiograph of a vital tooth that developed buccal soft tissue enlargement. The lucency associated with the cyst enveloped the entire root system and extended below the level of the apex.

which are histologically identical to inflammatory periapical cysts. The cysts develop along the buccal surface over the bifurcation, and most appropriately are called **buccal bifurcation cysts.** Several investigators have called these "paradental cysts," but this name should be avoided because of its use for a number of different pathologic disorders (e.g., distally oriented coronal radiolucencies associated with partially erupted third molars).

Radiographically, a buccal bifurcation cyst presents as a well-defined radiolucency overlying the furcation area of the affected tooth. The lucency may involve only the upper third of the roots or extend to envelop the entire root system, with involvement of the bone below the level of the apices (Fig. 2–73). Occlusal radiographs demonstrate a buccally positioned radiolucency with occasional lingual migration of the affected tooth. In cases with significant inflammation, proliferative periostitis (see p. 118) may result in laminar reduplication of the cortex overlying the cyst.

Treatment and Prognosis

When enamel pearls are detected radiographically, the area should be viewed as a weak point of periodontal attachment. Meticulous oral hygiene should be maintained in an effort to prevent localized loss of periodontal support. If removal of the lesion is contemplated, one must remember that enamel pearls occasionally contain vital pulp tissue.

Buccal bifurcation cysts need to be removed surgically and appropriate periodontal therapy instituted to eliminate future loss of attachment. For teeth with cervical enamel extensions and associated periodontal furcation involvement, therapy is directed at achieving a more durable attachment and providing access to the area for appropriate cleaning. Reports have suggested that this may be accomplished by flattening or removing the enamel in combination with an excisional new attachment procedure and furcation plasty.

Taurodontism

Taurodontism is an enlargement of the body and pulp chamber of a multirooted tooth with apical displacement of the pulpal floor and bifurcation of the roots. This pattern of molar formation has been found in ancient Neanderthals and occurs in cud-chewing animals (*tauro* = bull and *dont* = tooth).

Clinical and Radiographic Features

Affected teeth tend to be rectangular in shape and exhibit pulp chambers with a dramatically increased apico-occlusal height and a bifurcation close to the apex (Fig. 2–74). The diagnosis usually is made subjectively from the radiographic appearance. The degree of taurodontism has been classified into mild (**hypotaurodon-**

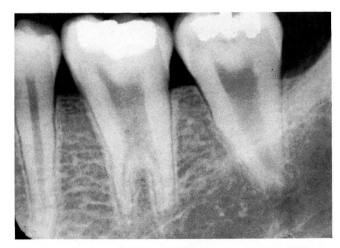

FIGURE 2–74. **Taurodontism.** Mandibular molar teeth exhibiting increased pulpal apico-occlusal height with apically positioned pulpal floor and bifurcation.

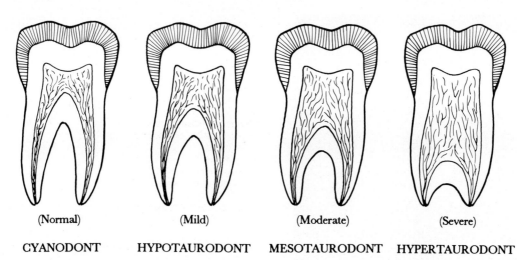

(Normal)   (Mild)   (Moderate)   (Severe)

CYANODONT   HYPOTAURODONT   MESOTAURODONT   HYPERTAURODONT

FIGURE 2–75. **Taurodontism.** Classification of taurodontism according to the degree of apical displacement of the pulpal floor.

tism), moderate (**mesotaurodontism**), and severe (**hypertaurodontism**), according to the degree of apical displacement of the pulpal floor (Fig. 2–75). Useful biometric criteria for the determination of taurodontism were presented by Witkop and colleagues and by Shifman and Chanannel. These reports contain information that is useful in epidemiologic studies of the process.

Some investigators include examples of taurodontism in premolar teeth; others argue that taurodontism is not shown by premolars. This argument is academic because the presence of taurodontism in premolars cannot be documented *in situ*. Investigations of taurodontism in premolar teeth require the examination of extracted teeth because the necessary radiographs depict the tooth in a mesiodistal orientation.

Taurodontism may be unilateral or bilateral and affects permanent teeth more frequently than deciduous teeth. There is no sex predilection. The reported prevalence is variable and is most likely related to different diagnostic criteria and racial variations. In the United States, most reports indicate a prevalence of 2.5 to 3.2 percent of the population. The process often demonstrates a field effect with the involvement of all molars. When this occurs, the first molar usually is least affected, with increasing severity noted in the second and third molars, respectively.

Taurodontism may occur as an isolated trait or as a component of a specific syndrome (Table 2–8). Investigations have shown that taurodontism may develop in the presence of any one of a large number of different genetic alterations. These findings suggest that chromosomal abnormalities may disrupt the development of the tooth's form and that taurodontism is not the result of a specific genetic abnormality.

Treatment and Prognosis

Patients with taurodontism require no specific therapy. Coronal extension of the pulp is not seen; therefore, the process does not interfere with routine restorative procedures. Some investigators have suggested that the taurodontic shape may exhibit decreased stability and strength as an abutment tooth in prosthetic procedures, but this hypothesis has not been verified. If endodontic therapy is required, the shape of the pulp chamber frequently increases the difficulty of locating, instrumenting, and obturating the pulp canals. One bit of good news is that patients have to demonstrate significant periodontal destruction before bifurcation involvement occurs.

Hypercementosis

Hypercementosis is a non-neoplastic deposition of excessive cementum that is continuous with the normal radicular cementum.

Table 2–8. SYNDROMES ASSOCIATED WITH TAURODONTISM
1. Amelogenesis imperfecta, hypoplastic, type IE
2. Amelogenesis imperfecta–taurodontism, type IV
3. Cranioectodermal
4. Ectodermal dysplasia
5. Hyperphosphatasia-oligophrenia-taurodontism
6. Hypophosphatasia
7. Klinefelter
8. Microdontia-taurodontia-dens invaginatus
9. Microcephalic dwarfism–taurodontism
10. Oculo-dento-digital dysplasia
11. Oral-facial-digital, type II
12. Rapp-Hodgkin
13. Scanty hair-oligodontia-taurodontia
14. Sex chromosomal aberrations (XXX, XYY)
15. Down
16. Tricho-dento-osseous, types I, II, and III
17. Tricho-onycho-dental

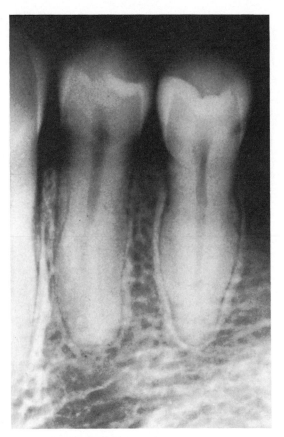

FIGURE 2–76. **Hypercementosis.** Bicuspid teeth exhibiting thickening and blunting of the roots.

Clinical and Radiographic Features

Radiographically, affected teeth demonstrate a thickening or blunting of the root, but the exact amount of increased cementum often is difficult to ascertain because cementum and dentin demonstrate similar radiodensities. The enlarged root is surrounded by the radiolucent periodontal ligament space and the adjacent intact lamina dura. Hypercementosis may be isolated, may involve multiple teeth, or may present as a generalized process. Premolar teeth are involved most frequently (Fig. 2–76).

Hypercementosis occurs predominantly in adulthood, and the frequency increases with age. Its occurrence has been reported in younger patients, and many of these cases demonstrate a familial clustering, suggesting hereditary influence.

Table 2–9 lists several local and systemic factors that have been associated with an increased frequency of the cemental deposition. Of these factors, **Paget's disease of bone** (see p. 449) has received the most attention. Numerous authors have reported significant hypercementosis in patients with Paget's disease, and this disorder should be considered whenever generalized hypercementosis is discovered in a patient of the appropriate age. In spite of the association with a number of disorders, most localized cases of hypercementosis are not related to any systemic disturbance.

Table 2–9. FACTORS ASSOCIATED WITH HYPERCEMENTOSIS

Local Factors
Abnormal occlusal trauma
Adjacent inflammation
Unopposed teeth (impacted, embedded, without antagonist)

Systemic Factors
Acromegaly and pituitary gigantism
Arthritis
Calcinosis
Paget's disease of bone
Rheumatic fever
Thyroid goiter
Vitamin A deficiency (possibly)

Histopathologic Features

The periphery of the root exhibits deposition of an excessive amount of cementum over the original layer of primary cementum. The excessive cementum may be hypocellular or exhibit areas of cellular cementum that resembles bone (osteocementum). Often, the material is arranged in concentric layers and may be applied over the entire root or be limited to the apical portion. On routine light microscopy, the distinction between dentin and cementum often is difficult, but the use of polarized light clearly separates the two different layers (Figs. 2–77 and 2–78).

Treatment and Prognosis

Patients with hypercementosis require no treatment. As a consequence of radicular enlargement, occasional problems have been reported during the extraction of affected teeth. Sectioning of the teeth may be necessary in selected cases to aid in removal.

Dilaceration

Dilaceration is an abnormal angulation or bend in the root or, less frequently, the crown of a tooth (Fig. 2–79).

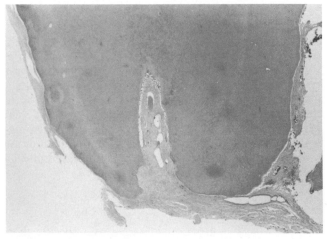

FIGURE 2–77. **Hypercementosis.** Dental root exhibiting excessive deposition of cellular and acellular cementum. The dividing line between dentin and cementum is indistinct.

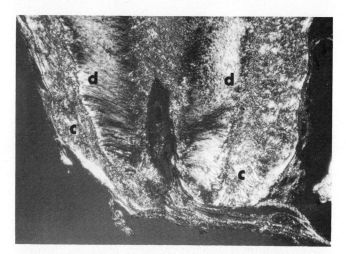

FIGURE 2–78. **Hypercementosis.** Polarized light demonstration of the same tooth depicted in Figure 2–77. Note the sharp dividing line between the tubular dentin (d) and the woven pattern of osteocementum (c).

Although a corroborating history may be absent, the majority appear to arise following an injury that displaces the calcified portion of the tooth germ, and the remainder of the tooth is formed at an abnormal angle. Less frequently, the bend develops secondary to the presence of an adjacent cyst, tumor, or odontogenic hamartoma (e.g., odontoma or supernumerary tooth) (Fig. 2–80). Some cases cannot be related to local injury and appear to be an idiopathic developmental disturbance (Fig. 2–81).

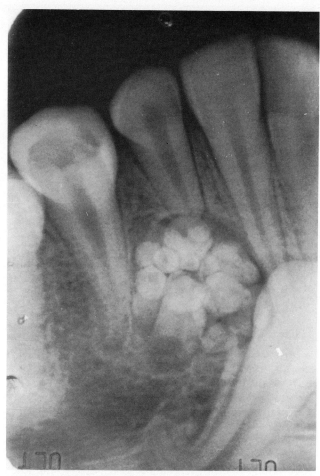

FIGURE 2–80. **Dilaceration.** Root angulation of a mandibular cuspid. Development has been altered by the presence of an adjacent compound odontoma. (Courtesy of Dr. Brent Bernard.)

Clinical and Radiographic Features

Although any tooth may be affected, the most frequently involved teeth are the permanent maxillary incisors, followed by the mandibular anterior dentition (Fig. 2–82). Occasionally, involvement of the deciduous teeth

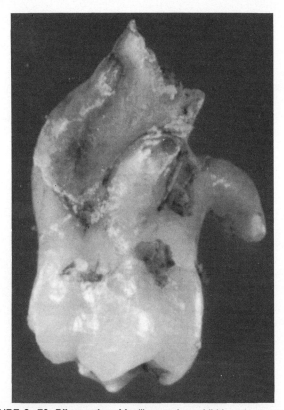

FIGURE 2–79. **Dilaceration.** Maxillary molar exhibiting sharp angulation of the roots. Note the inter-radicular bone.

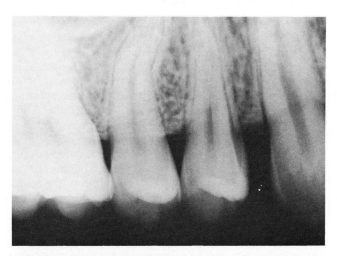

FIGURE 2–81. **Dilaceration.** Maxillary second bicuspid exhibiting mesial inclination of the root. There was no history of local injury to the area.

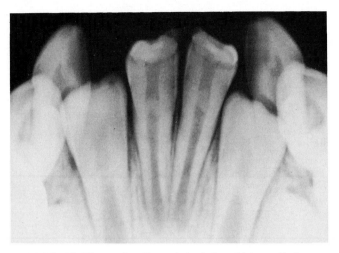

FIGURE 2-82. **Dilaceration.** Coronal angulation of the mandibular central incisors has developed after trauma to the overlying deciduous dentition. (From Neville BW, Damm DD, White DK, Waldron CA. Color Atlas of Clinical Oral Pathology. Philadelphia, Lea & Febiger, 1991, p 55.)

is reported, and some have been associated with prior trauma secondary to neonatal laryngoscopy and endotracheal intubation. The age of the patient and the direction and degree of force appear to determine the extent of the tooth's malformation. The abnormal angulation may be present anywhere along the length of the tooth.

Altered maxillary anterior teeth frequently demonstrate the bend in the crown or the coronal half of the root; failure of eruption often is seen. Affected mandibular incisors also exhibit involvement of the crown or the superficial portion of the root but more frequently erupt into full occlusion. Many of the affected teeth, especially anterior mandibular teeth, are nonvital and associated with periapical inflammatory lesions. Typically, altered posterior teeth demonstrate involvement of the apical half of the root and frequently do not exhibit delayed eruption.

Treatment and Prognosis

The treatment and prognosis vary according to the severity of the deformity. Altered deciduous teeth often demonstrate inappropriate resorption and result in delayed eruption of the permanent teeth. Extraction is indicated when necessary for the normal eruption of the succedaneous teeth. Patients with minor dilaceration of permanent teeth frequently require no therapy. Those teeth that exhibit delayed or abnormal eruption may be exposed and orthodontically moved into position. In some cases, orthodontic therapy is not indicated because of extensive deformation of the affected tooth or the possibility, on repositioning, of perforation of the buccal alveolar ridge by the malpositioned root. Grossly deformed teeth require surgical removal. The extraction of affected teeth may be difficult and result in root fracture on removal. When attempting to perform endodontic procedures, one must use great care to avoid root perforation of teeth with significant dilaceration.

Root dilaceration concentrates stress if the affected

tooth is used as an abutment for a dental prosthetic appliance. This increased stress may affect the stability and longevity of the abutment tooth. Splinting of the dilacerated tooth to an adjacent tooth results in a multirooted abutment and overcomes the stress-related problems.

Supernumerary Roots

The term **supernumerary roots** refers to the development of an increased number of roots on a tooth compared with that classically described in dental anatomy.

Clinical and Radiographic Features

Any tooth may develop accessory roots, and involvement has been reported in both the deciduous and permanent dentitions. Data on the frequency of supernumerary roots are sparse, but the prevalence appears to vary significantly among different races. The most frequently affected teeth are the permanent molars (especially third molars) from either arch and mandibular cuspids and premolars (Figs. 2-83 and 2-84). In some instances, the supernumerary root is divergent and easily seen on radiographs; in other cases, the additional root is small, superimposed over other roots, and difficult to ascertain (Fig. 2-85).

Treatment and Prognosis

No treatment is required for supernumerary roots, but the detection of the accessory root is of critical impor-

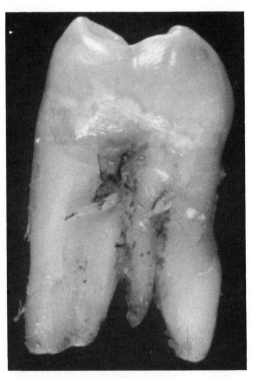

FIGURE 2-83. **Supernumerary root.** Gross photograph exhibiting a maxillary molar with a small supernumerary root.

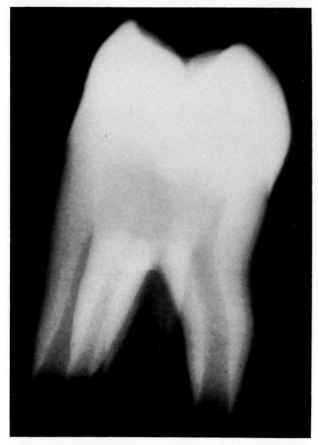

FIGURE 2-84. **Supernumerary root.** Mesial-to-distal radiographic view of the same tooth depicted in Figure 2-83. Note the accessory root with central pulp canal. If a buccal-to-lingual radiographic view had been taken (as would be necessary in patient care), the additional root would not have been evident.

tance when endodontic therapy or exodontia is undertaken. Extracted teeth always should be closely examined to ensure that all roots have been successfully removed because accessory roots may not be obvious on the presurgical radiographs. Just as important is the search for accessory canals during endodontic access procedures

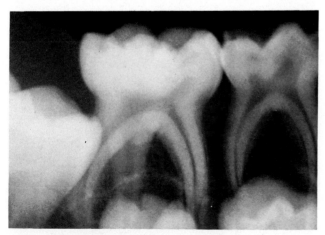

FIGURE 2-85. **Supernumerary root.** Radiograph of a mandibular second deciduous molar, which exhibits divergent and easily discernible accessory root.

because failure to discover these additional openings often results in a lack of resolution of the associated inflammatory process.

DEVELOPMENTAL ALTERATIONS IN THE STRUCTURE OF TEETH

Amelogenesis Imperfecta

Amelogenesis imperfecta encompasses a complicated group of conditions that demonstrate developmental alterations in the structure of the enamel in the absence of a systemic disorder. Table 2-2 (see p. 45) lists several systemic diseases associated with enamel disorders that are not considered isolated amelogenesis imperfecta.

At least 14 different hereditary subtypes of amelogenesis imperfecta exist, with numerous patterns of inheritance and a wide variety of clinical manifestations. As proof of the complicated nature of the process, several different classification systems exist. The most widely accepted is that developed by Witkop (Table 2-10), and this part of the text adheres to this classification. The dissertation by Witkop and Sauk plus Witkop's more recent review are works of art and should be used if more information is desired.

The formation of enamel is a multistep process, and problems may arise in any one of the steps. In general, the development of enamel can be divided into three major stages:

- Elaboration of the organic matrix
- Mineralization of the matrix
- Maturation of the enamel

The hereditary defects of the formation of enamel also are divided along these lines: hypoplastic, hypocalcified, and hypomaturation.

Clinical and Radiographic Features

The estimated frequency of amelogenesis imperfecta in the population varies between 1:8000 and 1:700. As in any hereditary disorder, clustering in certain geographic areas may occur, resulting in a wide range of reported prevalences. In general, both the deciduous and permanent dentitions are diffusely involved.

Hypoplastic Amelogenesis Imperfecta

In patients with **hypoplastic amelogenesis imperfecta**, the basic alteration centers around inadequate deposition of enamel matrix. Any matrix present is appropriately mineralized and radiographically contrasts well with the underlying dentin. In the **generalized pattern**, pinpoint-to-pinhead-sized pits are scattered across the surface of the teeth and do not correlate with a pattern of environmental damage (Figs. 2-86 and 2-87). The buccal surfaces of the teeth are more severely affected, and the pits may be arranged in rows or columns. Staining of the pits may occur. Variable expressivity is seen within groups of affected patients. The enamel between the pits is of normal thickness, hardness, and coloration.

Table 2–10. CLASSIFICATION OF AMELOGENESIS IMPERFECTA

Type	Pattern	Specific Features	Inheritance
I	*Hypoplastic*		
IA	Hypoplastic	Pitted	Autosomal dominant
IB	Hypoplastic	Localized	Autosomal dominant
IC	Hypoplastic	Localized	Autosomal recessive
ID	Hypoplastic	Smooth	Autosomal dominant
IE	Hypoplastic	Smooth	X-linked dominant
IF	Hypoplastic	Rough	Autosomal dominant
IG	Hypoplastic	Enamel agenesis	Autosomal recessive
II	*Hypomaturation*		
IIA	Hypomaturation	Pigmented	Autosomal recessive
IIB	Hypomaturation		X-linked recessive
IIC	Hypomaturation	Snow capped	X-linked
IID	Hypomaturation	Snow capped	Autosomal dominant?
III	*Hypocalcified*		
IIIA	Hypocalcified		Autosomal dominant
IIIB	Hypocalcified		Autosomal recessive
IV	*Hypomaturation/Hypoplastic*	*With Taurodontism*	
IVA	Hypomaturation/hypoplastic	With taurodontism	Autosomal dominant
IVB	Hypoplastic/hypomaturation	With taurodontism	Autosomal dominant

In the **localized pattern**, the affected teeth demonstrate horizontal rows of pits, a linear depression, or one large area of hypoplastic enamel surrounded by a zone of hypocalcification. Typically, the altered area is located in the middle third of the buccal surfaces of the teeth. The incisal edge or occlusal surface usually is not affected. Both dentitions or only the primary teeth may be affected. All the teeth may be altered, or only scattered teeth may be affected. When the involvement is not diffuse, the pattern of affected teeth does not correlate with a specific time in development. The autosomal recessive type (type IC) is more severe and typically demonstrates involvement of all teeth in both dentitions.

In the **autosomal dominant smooth pattern**, the enamel of all teeth exhibits a smooth surface and is thin, hard, and glossy (Fig. 2–88). The absence of appropriate enamel thickness results in teeth that are shaped like crown preparations and demonstrate open contact points. The color of the teeth varies from opaque white to translucent brown. Anterior open bite is not rare. Radiographically, the teeth exhibit a thin peripheral outline of radiopaque enamel (Fig. 2–89). Often, unerupted teeth exhibiting resorption are seen.

The **X-linked dominant smooth pattern** is a lesson in the *lyonization effect*. On approximately the 16th day of embryonic life in all individuals with two X chromo-

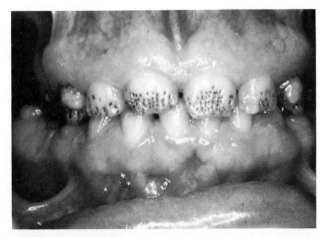

FIGURE 2–86. **Hypoplastic amelogenesis imperfecta, generalized pattern.** Numerous pinpoint pits scattered across the surface of the teeth. The enamel between the pits is of normal thickness, hardness, and coloration. (Courtesy of Stewart RE, Prescott GH. Oral Facial Genetics. St. Louis, CV Mosby, 1976, p 157.)

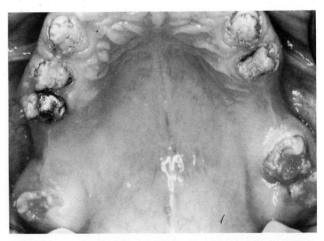

FIGURE 2–87. **Hypoplastic amelogenesis imperfecta, generalized pattern.** Same patient as depicted in Figure 2–86. Note diffuse involvement of all maxillary teeth; this is inconsistent with environmental damage. (Courtesy of Dr. Joseph S. Giansanti.)

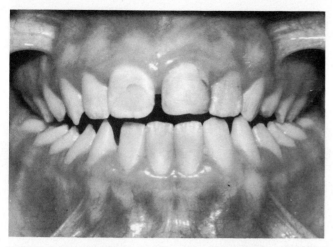

FIGURE 2-88. **Hypoplastic amelogenesis imperfecta, autosomal dominant smooth pattern.** Small, yellowish teeth exhibiting hard, glossy enamel with numerous open contact points and anterior open bite.

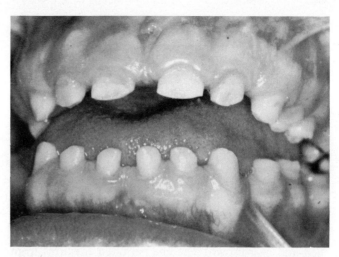

FIGURE 2-90. **Hypoplastic amelogenesis imperfecta, rough pattern.** Small, yellow teeth with rough enamel surface, open contact points, significant attrition, and anterior open bite.

somes, one member of the pair is inactivated in each cell. As a result of this event, females are mosaics, with a mixture of cells, some with active maternal X chromosomes and others with active paternal X chromosomes. Usually, the mix is of approximately equal proportions. If one X were to direct the formation of defective enamel and the other X were to form normal enamel, the teeth would exhibit alternating zones of normal and abnormal enamel.

Males with the X-linked dominant smooth pattern exhibit diffuse thin, smooth, and shiny enamel in both dentitions. The teeth often have the shape of crown preparations, and the contact points are open. The color varies from brown to yellow-brown. Radiographs demonstrate a peripheral outline of radiopaque enamel. Unerupted teeth may undergo resorption. On the other hand, females exhibit vertical furrows of thin hypoplastic enamel, alternating between bands of normal thickness.

The banding often is detectable with dental radiographs. An open bite is seen in almost all males and in a minority of females.

In the **rough pattern**, the enamel is thin, hard, and rough-surfaced. As in the smooth forms, the teeth taper toward the incisal-occlusal surface and demonstrate open contact points (Fig. 2-90). The color varies from white to yellow-white. The enamel is denser than that seen in the smooth patterns, and the teeth are less vulnerable to attrition. Radiographs exhibit a thin peripheral outline of radiodense enamel (Fig. 2-91). Unerupted teeth, often undergoing resorption, may be seen. An anterior open bite is common.

As the name implies, **enamel agenesis** demonstrates a total lack of enamel formation. The teeth are the shape and color of the dentin, with a yellow-brown hue, open contact points, and crowns that taper toward the incisal-occlusal surface. The surface of the dentin is rough, and

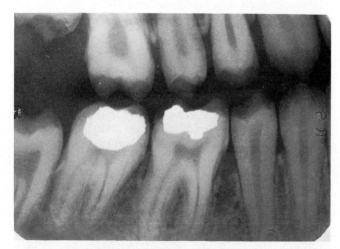

FIGURE 2-89. **Hypoplastic amelogenesis imperfecta, autosomal dominant smooth pattern.** Radiograph of the same patient depicted in Figure 2-88. Note the thin peripheral outline of radiopaque enamel. (Courtesy of Dr. John G. Stephenson.)

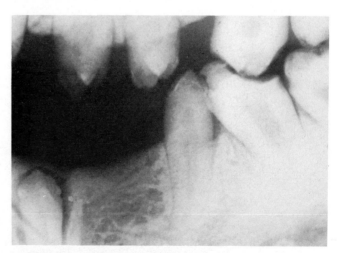

FIGURE 2-91. **Hypoplastic amelogenesis imperfecta, rough pattern.** Radiograph of the same patient as depicted in Figure 2-90. Note the impacted tooth and the thin peripheral outline of radiodense enamel.

an anterior open bite is seen frequently. Radiographs demonstrate no peripheral enamel overlying the dentin. A lack of eruption of many teeth with significant resorption frequently occurs.

Hypomaturation Amelogenesis Imperfecta

In a person with **hypomaturation amelogenesis imperfecta**, the enamel matrix is laid down appropriately and begins to mineralize, but there is a defect in the maturation of the enamel's crystal structure. Affected teeth are normal in shape but exhibit a mottled, opaque white-brown-yellow discoloration (Fig. 2–92). The enamel is softer than normal and tends to chip from the underlying dentin. Radiographically, the affected enamel exhibits a radiodensity that is similar to dentin.

In the **pigmented pattern**, the surface enamel is mottled and agar-brown. The enamel often fractures from the underlying dentin and is soft enough to be punctured by a dental explorer. Anterior open bite and unerupted teeth exhibiting resorption are uncommon. On occasion, the surface enamel may be severely affected and similar in softness to that of hypocalcified patterns. These cases often demonstrate extensive calculus deposition.

The **X-linked pattern** is another lesson in lyonization but one that is not as obvious as the X-linked hypoplastic pattern. Affected males exhibit different patterns in the deciduous and permanent dentitions. The deciduous teeth are opaque white with a translucent mottling; the permanent teeth are opaque yellow-white and may darken with age. The enamel tends to chip and often can be pierced with a dental explorer point. The degree of enamel loss is more rapid than that in normal teeth but does not approach that seen in the hypocalcified forms. Focal areas of brown discoloration may develop within the white opaque enamel. Radiographically, the contrast between enamel and dentin is reduced.

Female patients exhibit a similar pattern in both dentitions. The teeth demonstrate vertical bands of white opaque enamel and normal translucent enamel. The bands are random and asymmetric. The banding is not

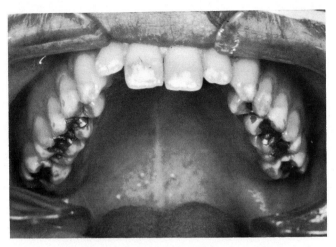

FIGURE 2–93. **Hypomaturation amelogenesis imperfecta, snow-capped pattern.** Dentition exhibiting zone of white opaque enamel in the incisal/occlusal one fourth of the enamel surface. (Courtesy of Dr. Heddie O. Sedano.)

obvious under regular lighting, and transillumination often is required to demonstrate the pattern. Radiographically, the band is not perceptible, and the contrast between enamel and dentin is within normal limits.

The **snow-capped patterns** exhibit a zone of white opaque enamel on the incisal or occlusal one quarter to one third of the crown (Fig. 2–93). The altered areas do not exhibit a distribution that would support an environmental origin, and the surface lacks the iridescent sheen seen with mild fluorosis. The affected teeth often demonstrate an anterior to posterior distribution and have been compared with a denture dipped in white paint (only affected anteriors, the anteriors back to the bicuspids, or the anteriors back to the molars, and so forth). Both the deciduous and permanent dentitions are affected. Most cases demonstrate an X-linked pattern of inheritance, but there possibly is an autosomal dominant form.

Hypocalcified Amelogenesis Imperfecta

In this type, the enamel matrix is laid down appropriately but no significant mineralization occurs. In both patterns of **hypocalcified amelogenesis imperfecta**, the teeth are appropriately shaped on eruption, but the enamel is very soft and easily lost. On eruption, the enamel is yellow-brown or orange but often becomes stained brown to black and exhibits rapid calculus apposition (Fig. 2–94; see Color Figure 14). With years of function, much of the coronal enamel is removed, except for the cervical portion, which occasionally is better calcified. Unerupted teeth and anterior open bite are not rare. Both patterns are similar, but the autosomal recessive examples are generally more severe than are the autosomal dominant cases. Radiographically, the density of the enamel and dentin are similar. Before eruption, the teeth are normal in shape, but after a period of function, much of the cuspal enamel is lost, with the occlusal surface becoming the most irregular (Fig. 2–95).

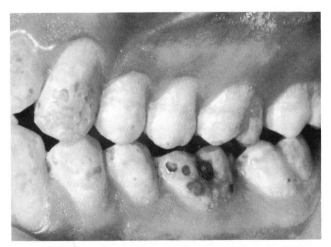

FIGURE 2–92. **Hypomaturation amelogenesis imperfecta.** Dentition exhibiting mottled, opaque white enamel with scattered areas of brown discoloration.

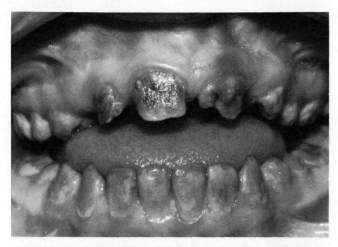

FIGURE 2–94. **Hypocalcified amelogenesis imperfecta.** Dentition exhibiting diffuse yellow-brown discoloration. Note numerous teeth with loss of coronal enamel except for the cervical portion. See Color Plates.

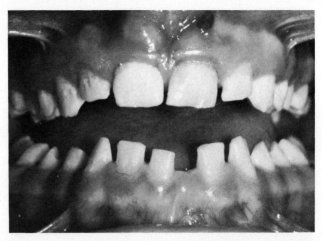

FIGURE 2–96. **Tricho-dento-osseous syndrome.** Dentition exhibiting diffuse enamel hypoplasia and hypomaturation. At birth, the patient exhibited a kinky "steel wool"–like texture to her hair; with time, the hair straightened. A high index of suspicion was required to arrive at the diagnosis.

Hypomaturation/Hypoplastic Amelogenesis Imperfecta

This type of amelogenesis imperfecta exhibits enamel hypoplasia in combination with hypomaturation. Both the deciduous and permanent dentitions are involved diffusely. Two patterns are recognized that are similar but differentiated by the thickness of the enamel and the overall tooth size. Both patterns have been reported in a single kindred, and these may represent a range of the same process.

In the **hypomaturation-hypoplastic pattern**, the predominant defect is one of enamel hypomaturation in which the enamel appears as mottled yellowish-white to yellow-brown. Pits are frequently seen on the buccal surfaces of the teeth. Radiographically, the enamel appears similar to dentin in density, and large pulp chambers may be seen in single-rooted teeth in addition to varying degrees of taurodontism.

In the **hypoplastic-hypomaturation pattern**, the predominant defect is one of enamel hypoplasia in which the enamel is thin; the enamel that is present demonstrates hypomaturation. Except for the decrease in the thickness of the enamel, this pattern is radiographically similar to the hypomaturation-hypoplastic variant.

Both patterns are seen in the systemic disorder, **tricho-dento-osseous syndrome**. This autosomal dominant syndrome is mentioned here because the diagnosis may not be readily apparent without a high index of suspicion (Fig. 2–96). In addition to the dental findings, the predominant systemic changes are present variably and include kinky hair, osteosclerosis, and brittle nails. The kinky hair is present at birth but may straighten with age. The osteosclerosis primarily affects the base of skull and the mastoid process. The mandible often exhibits a shortened ramus and an obtuse angle.

Some authors suggest that hypomaturation-hypoplastic amelogenesis imperfecta may represent partial expression of the tricho-dento-osseous syndrome. If only dental changes are seen in the absence of hair or bone changes, either in the individual or within the family, the diagnosis of amelogenesis imperfecta appears appropriate. One investigator reviewed the controversy and believes the disorders can be distinguished by the degree of taurodontism present in the mandibular first molars. This review indicated that no severe taurodontism of the mandibular first molar was found in cases of hypomaturation-hypoplastic amelogenesis imperfecta; however, all examples of tricho-dento-osseous syndrome demonstrated severe hypertaurodontism of this tooth (Fig. 2–97).

Histopathologic Features

The histopathologic alterations present in amelogenesis imperfecta are not evident in routine preparations. Decalcification of the teeth is necessary before processing to allow sectioning of paraffin-embedded specimens. To

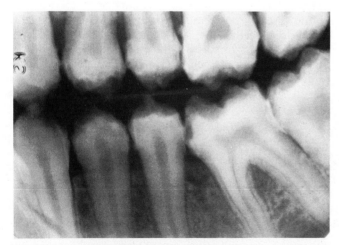

FIGURE 2–95. **Hypocalcified amelogenesis imperfecta.** Radiograph of the same patient depicted in Figure 2–94. Note the extensive loss of coronal enamel and the similar density of enamel and dentin.

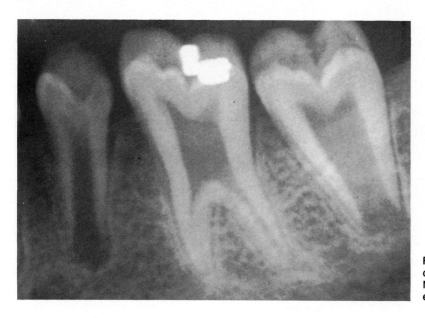

FIGURE 2-97. **Tricho-dento-osseous syndrome.** Radiograph of the same patient depicted in Figure 2-96. Note significant taurodontism of the first molar and the enamel, which is thin and similar in density to the dentin.

examine the enamel structure of altered teeth, ground sections of non-decalcified specimens are prepared. The alterations discovered are highly diverse and vary with each clinical type of amelogenesis imperfecta. Detailed descriptions of such alterations were provided by Witkop and Sauk.

Treatment and Prognosis

The treatment and prognosis are highly variable and relate to the severity of the enamel's involvement. Types ID, IE, IG, IIA, IIIA, IIIB, and IVB demonstrate very thin enamel or highly defective enamel, which leads to rapid attrition. These variants require full coverage as soon as is practical; if the treatment is delayed, a loss of usable crown length occurs. In those patients without sufficient crown lengths, full dentures (overdentures in some cases) often become the only satisfactory approach.

The other types of amelogenesis imperfecta demonstrate less rapid tooth loss, and the aesthetic appearance often is the prime consideration. Many less severe cases can be improved by the placement of full crowns or facial veneers on clinically objectionable teeth. In some cases, a lack of good enamel bonding of veneers occurs and does not result in a durable restoration. The use of glass-ionomer cements with dentinal adhesives often overcomes this weakness.

Dentinogenesis Imperfecta (Hereditary Opalescent Dentin; Capdepont's Teeth)

Dentinogenesis imperfecta is a hereditary developmental disturbance of the dentin that may be seen alone or in conjunction with the systemic hereditary disorder of bone, **osteogenesis imperfecta** (see p. 443). Like amelogenesis imperfecta, the disorders of dentin also involve disagreements in classification. Two systems, one by Witkop and the other by Shields, are well accepted but not totally satisfactory (Table 2-11). This text does not adhere strictly to either. It is evident that the third type of dentinogenesis imperfecta (Shields' type III or Witkop's Brandywine isolate) is not a separate disease and merely represents a variation of expression of Shields' type II.

The best nomenclature system was suggested by Levin. Analogous to amelogenesis imperfecta, the diagnosis of dentinogenesis imperfecta should be reserved for defective dentin formation with opalescent teeth (deciduous and permanent) in the absence of systemic disease. Appropriately, dentin defects associated with the systemic bone disease are termed **osteogenesis imperfecta with opalescent teeth**. Extensive pedigrees of individuals with dentinogenesis imperfecta have been studied, and none has exhibited other changes suggestive of osteogenesis imperfecta. Therefore, dentinogenesis imperfecta is clearly a disorder distinct from osteogenesis imperfecta.

Table 2-11. DENTINOGENESIS IMPERFECTA

Shields	Clinical Presentation	Witkop
Dentinogenesis imperfecta I	Dentinogenesis and osteogenesis imperfecta	Dentinogenesis imperfecta
Dentinogenesis imperfecta II	Isolated dentinogenesis imperfecta	Hereditary opalescent dentin
Dentinogenesis imperfecta III		Brandywine isolate

Arguably, the dentin dysplasias could be included under the heading of isolated dentin defects, but such a confusing disruption of the nomenclature is undesirable.

Clinical and Radiographic Features

The prevalence of dentinogenesis imperfecta is not randomly distributed throughout the United States and Europe. Most cases can be traced to whites (English or French ancestry) from communities close to the English Channel. The disorder is autosomal dominant and occurs in about 1:8000 whites in the United States.

The dental alterations in dentinogenesis imperfecta and osteogenesis imperfecta with opalescent teeth are similar clinically, radiographically, and histopathologically. All teeth in both dentitions are affected. The severity of the dental alterations varies with the age at which the tooth developed. Deciduous teeth are affected most severely, followed by the permanent incisors and first molars, with the second and third molars being least altered.

The dentitions have a blue to brown discoloration, often with a distinctive translucence (Fig. 2–98; see Color Figure 15). The enamel frequently separates easily from the underlying defective dentin. Once exposed, the dentin often demonstrates significantly accelerated attrition (Fig. 2–99; see Color Figure 16). Radiographically, the teeth have bulbous crowns, cervical constriction, thin roots, and early obliteration of the root canals and pulp chambers (Fig. 2–100).

The trait exhibits close to 100 percent penetrance but variable expressivity. Significant clinically obvious enamel hypoplasia is noted in some patients. The enamel abnormality is thought to be a secondary defect and not a direct expression of the dentinogenesis imperfecta gene (Fig. 2–101). Although the pulps usually are obliterated by excess dentin production, some teeth may show normal-sized pulps or pulpal enlargement ("shell teeth").

Shell teeth demonstrate normal-thickness enamel in association with extremely thin dentin and dramatically

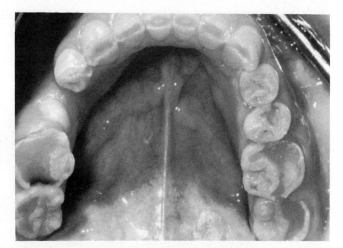

FIGURE 2–99. **Dentinogenesis imperfecta.** Dentition exhibiting grayish discoloration with significant enamel loss and attrition. See Color Plates.

enlarged pulps (Fig. 2–102). The thin dentin may involve the entire tooth or be isolated to the root. This rare abnormality has been seen most frequently in deciduous teeth in the presence of dentinogenesis imperfecta. The alteration may be unassociated with dentinogenesis imperfecta as an isolated finding in both dentitions and demonstrate normal tooth shape and coloration, a negative family history, and diffuse involvement. In the isolated variant, slow but progressive root resorption occurs.

Initially, this pulpal enlargement was discovered in the large Maryland Brandywine isolate and thought to be a new variant of dentinogenesis imperfecta (type III or Brandywine isolate). Current evidence strongly supports the Brandywine isolate representing nothing more than variable expressivity of the gene for dentinogenesis imperfecta. A review of the isolate revealed only 8 percent of the kindred with enlarged pulp chambers. Investiga-

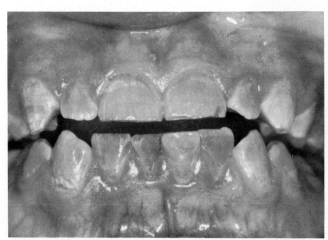

FIGURE 2–98. **Dentinogenesis imperfecta.** Dentition exhibiting diffuse brownish discoloration and slight translucence. See Color Plates.

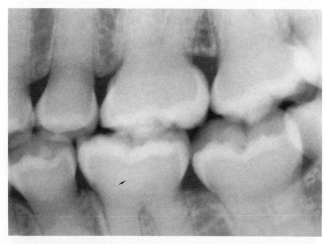

FIGURE 2–100. **Dentinogenesis imperfecta.** Radiograph of dentition exhibiting bulbous crowns, cervical constriction, and obliterated pulp canals and chambers.

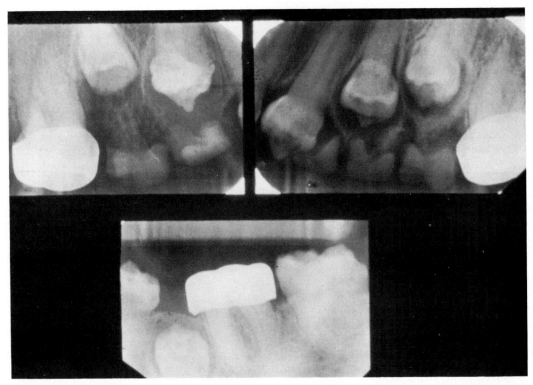

FIGURE 2–101. **Dentinogenesis imperfecta.** Radiograph of dentition exhibiting bulbous crowns, early obliteration of the pulp, and enamel hypoplasia. (Courtesy of Levin LS, Leaf SH, Jelmine RJ, Rose JJ, et al. Dentinogenesis imperfecta in the Brandywine isolate (DI type III): Clinical, radiologic, and scanning electron microscopic studies of the dentition. Oral Surg Oral Med Oral Pathol 56:267–274, 1983.)

tors have documented affected people with enlarged pulps in association with parents and children with classic dentinogenesis imperfecta. Finally, identical patterns of variable expressivity have been seen in other large affected kindreds with no connection to the Brandywine isolate.

Histopathologic Features

As expected, affected teeth demonstrate altered dentin. The dentin adjacent to the enamel junction appears similar to normal dentin, but the remainder is distinctly abnormal. Short misshapen tubules course through an

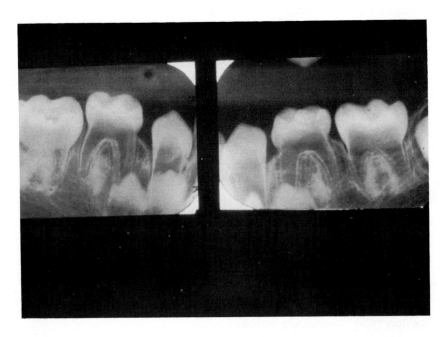

FIGURE 2–102. **Shell teeth.** Dentition exhibiting normal thickness enamel, extremely thin dentin, and dramatically enlarged pulps.

FIGURE 2–103. **Dentinogenesis imperfecta.** Coronal dentin exhibiting short misshapen tubules within atypical granular dentin matrix.

Table 2–12. SYSTEMIC DISEASES CORRELATED WITH DENTIN DYSPLASIA-LIKE ALTERATIONS
1. Calcinosis universalis
2. Rheumatoid arthritis and vitaminosis D
3. Sclerotic bone and skeletal anomalies
4. Tumoral calcinosis

category, there should be no correlation with systemic disease or dentinogenesis imperfecta. Systemic diseases reported to be associated with similar dentin changes are listed in Table 2–12.

Clinical and Radiographic Features

Dentin Dysplasia Type I (Radicular Dentin Dysplasia; Rootless Teeth)

Dentin dysplasia type I has been referred to as **rootless teeth** because the loss of organization of the root dentin often leads to a shortened root length. The process exhibits an autosomal dominant pattern of inheritance. The enamel and coronal dentin are normal clinically and well formed (Fig. 2–104), but the radicular dentin loses all organization and subsequently is shortened dramatically (Fig. 2–105). Wide variation in root formation is produced because dentinal disorganization may occur during different stages of tooth development. If the dentin organization is lost early in tooth development, markedly deficient roots are formed; later disorganization results in minimal root malformation. The variability is most pronounced in permanent teeth and may vary not only from patient to patient but also from tooth to tooth in a single patient.

Radiographically, the deciduous teeth are affected severely, with little or no detectable pulp and roots that are markedly short or absent. The permanent teeth vary according to the proportion of organized versus disor-

atypical granular dentin matrix, which often demonstrates interglobular calcification (Fig. 2–103). Scanty atypical odontoblasts line the pulp surface, and cells can be seen entrapped within the defective dentin. In ground sections, the enamel is normal in most patients but about one third have hypoplastic or hypocalcified defects.

Treatment and Prognosis

The entire dentition is at risk because of numerous problems. The root canals become thread-like and may develop microexposures, resulting in periapical inflammatory lesions. In spite of the risk of enamel loss and significant attrition, the teeth are not good candidates for full crowns because of cervical fracture. The success of full coverage is best in teeth with crowns and roots that exhibit close to a normal shape and size. Overlay dentures placed on teeth that are covered with fluoride-releasing glass-ionomer cement have been used with success in some cases.

Additional therapeutic approaches have been used, but long-term follow-up is incomplete. In patients with extensive attrition, the vertical dimension has been rebuilt by placing nonprecious metal castings with adhesive luting agents on teeth that have received no preparation and are not subject to significant occlusal stress. The newer composites combined with a dentin-bonding agent have been used in areas subject to occlusal wear. When large kindreds have been followed over a long term, most of those affected are candidates for full dentures or implants by age 30 years in spite of the numerous interventions. Newer materials and interventions may alter this outlook.

Dentin Dysplasia

Dentin dysplasia was categorized initially in 1939. There are two major patterns, and to be included in this

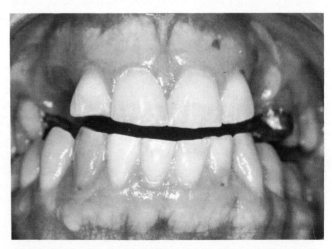

FIGURE 2–104. **Dentin dysplasia, type I.** Dentition exhibiting attrition but otherwise normal coronal coloration and morphology.

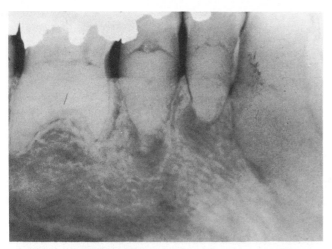

FIGURE 2–105. **Dentin dysplasia, type I.** Dentition exhibiting shortened roots, no pulp canals, and small crescent-shaped pulp chambers. (From Tidwell E, Cunningham CJ. Dentinal dysplasia. Endodontic treatment, with case report. J Endod 5:372–376, 1979. © American Association of Endodontists.)

ganized dentin (Fig. 2–106). With early disorganization, no pulp can be detected and the roots are extremely short or absent. With somewhat later disorganization, crescent or chevron-shaped pulp chambers can be detected overlying shortened roots that exhibit no pulp canals. Late disorganization results in normal pulp chambers overlying roots, each of which exhibits a large pulp stone. The root is flared at the site of the stone, and the canal is constricted distal to the stone. Those teeth without root canals frequently develop periapical inflammatory lesions without obvious cause. The inflammatory lesions appear secondary to caries or spontaneous coronal exposure of microscopic threads of pulpal remnants present within the defective dentin.

A similar but unrelated disorder is **fibrous dysplasia of dentin.** This autosomal dominant disorder presents with teeth that are clinically normal. Radiographically, the teeth are normal in shape but demonstrate a radiodense product filling the pulp chambers and canals. In contrast to dentinogenesis imperfecta, small foci of radiolucency can be seen in the pulp. In contrast to dentin dysplasia type I, no crescent pulp chambers and no decrease in root length are seen. The radiodense intrapulpal material consists of fibrotic dentin.

Dentin Dysplasia Type II
(Coronal Dentin Dysplasia)

Dentin dysplasia type II exhibits numerous features of dentinogenesis imperfecta, and although reclassification was not recommended, Witkop suggested it might be a form of that disease. In contrast to dentin dysplasia type I, the root length is normal in both dentitions. Autosomal dominant inheritance is seen. The deciduous teeth closely resemble those of dentinogenesis imperfecta. Clinically, the teeth demonstrate a blue to amber to brown translucence. Radiographically, the dental changes include bulbous crowns, cervical constriction, thin roots, and early obliteration of the pulp. The permanent teeth demonstrate normal clinical coloration but are enlarged, with apical extension of the pulp chamber radiographically (thistle tube–shaped or flame-shaped) (Figs. 2–107 and 2–108). Pulp stones develop in the enlarged pulp chambers.

A similar but unrelated disorder is **pulpal dysplasia.** This process develops in teeth that are clinically normal. Radiographically, *both* dentitions exhibit thistle tube–shaped pulp chambers and multiple pulp stones.

Histopathologic Features

In patients with dentin dysplasia type I, the coronal enamel and dentin are normal. Apical to the point of disorganization, the central portion of the root forms whorls of tubular dentin and atypical osteodentin. These whorls exhibit a peripheral layer of normal dentin, giving the root the appearance of a "stream flowing around boulders" (Fig. 2–109).

In patients with dentin dysplasia type II, the deciduous teeth demonstrate the pattern described in dentinogenesis imperfecta. The permanent teeth exhibit normal

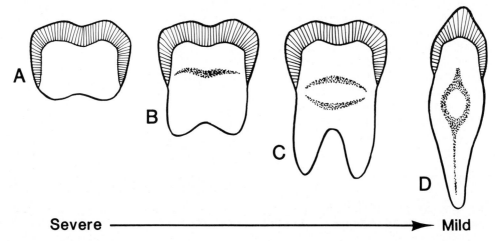

Severe ——————————————————————————▶ Mild

FIGURE 2–106. **Dentin dysplasia, type I.** Variability of the radiograph appearance according to the degree of dentin disorganization within the root.

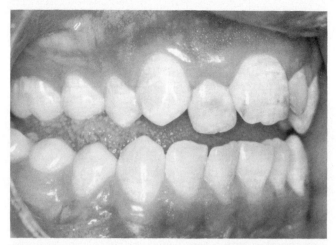

FIGURE 2-107. **Dentin dysplasia, type II.** Permanent dentition that does not exhibit translucence, as noted in the deciduous teeth. The patient also exhibits mild fluorosis of the enamel.

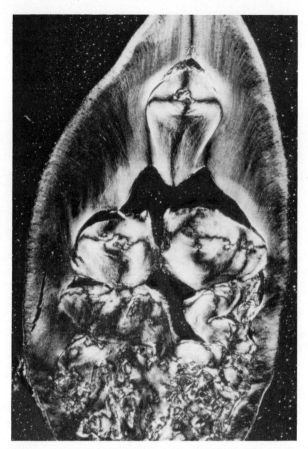

FIGURE 2-109. **Dentin dysplasia, type I.** Polarized light view of affected tooth demonstrating a classic "stream flowing around boulders" appearance.

enamel and coronal dentin. Adjacent to the pulp, numerous areas of interglobular dentin are seen. The radicular dentin is atubular, amorphous, and hypertrophic. Pulp stones develop in any portion of the chamber (Fig. 2-110).

Treatment and Prognosis

In patients with dentin dysplasia type I, preventive care is of foremost importance. Perhaps as a result of

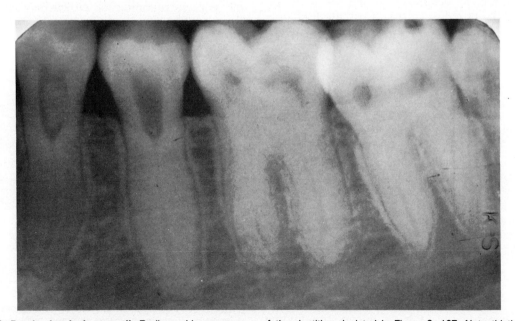

FIGURE 2-108. **Dentin dysplasia, type II.** Radiographic appearance of the dentition depicted in Figure 2-107. Note thistle tube-shaped enlargements of the pulp chambers and numerous pulp stones.

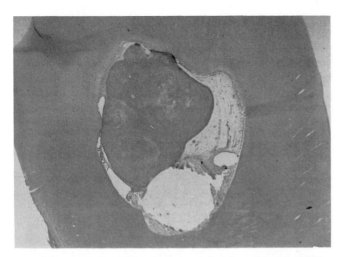

FIGURE 2–110. **Dentin dysplasia, type II.** Affected tooth exhibiting large pulp stone within the pulp chamber.

shortened roots, early loss from periodontitis is frequent. In addition, pulp vascular channels extend close to the dentino-enamel junction; therefore, even shallow occlusal restorations can result in pulpal necrosis. Meticulous oral hygiene must be established and maintained.

If periapical inflammatory lesions develop, the therapeutic choice is guided by the root length. Conventional endodontic therapy requires mechanical creation of canal paths and has been successful in teeth without extremely short roots. Teeth with short roots demonstrate pulpal ramifications that eliminate conventional endodontic treatment as an appropriate therapeutic option. Periapical curettage and retrograde amalgam seals have demonstrated short-term success.

Dentin dysplasia type II demonstrates similar problems, and meticulous oral hygiene must be established. The deciduous teeth can be approached in a manner similar to that used for dentinogenesis imperfecta. In the permanent teeth, an increased risk of periapical inflammatory lesions is also seen. Because the pulp canals usually are not obliterated completely, endodontic therapy is accomplished more readily.

Regional Odontodysplasia (Ghost Teeth)

Regional odontodysplasia is a localized, nonhereditary developmental abnormality of teeth with extensive adverse effects on the formation of enamel, dentin, and pulp. Most cases are idiopathic, but a number have been related to various syndromes, growth abnormalities, neural disorders, and vascular malformations. Several cases have occurred in patients with vascular nevi of the head and neck; in addition, similar changes have been induced in animals through a restriction of the vascular flow.

Clinical and Radiographic Features

Regional odontodysplasia is an uncommon finding that occurs in both dentitions and exhibits no sex or

racial predilection. A review of the age at the time of diagnosis reveals a bimodal peak that correlates with the normal time of eruption of the deciduous (2 to 4 years) and permanent dentitions (7 to 11 years). Typically, the process affects a focal area of the dentition, with involvement of several contiguous teeth. There is a maxillary predominance (2.5:1) and a predilection for the anterior teeth. On occasion, an unaffected tooth may be intermixed within a row of altered teeth. Ipsilateral involvement of both arches and bilateral changes in the same jaw have been reported. Involvement of more than two quadrants is rare. Involvement of the deciduous dentition typically is followed by similarly affected permanent teeth.

Many of the affected teeth fail to erupt. Erupted teeth demonstrate small irregular crowns that are yellow to brown, often with a very rough surface. Caries and associated periapical inflammatory lesions are fairly common. Radiographically, the altered teeth demonstrate extremely thin enamel and dentin surrounding an enlarged radiolucent pulp, resulting in a pale wispy image of a tooth; hence the term, **ghost teeth** (Fig. 2–111). There is a lack of contrast between the dentin and the enamel with an indistinct or "fuzzy" appearance of the coronal silhouette. Short roots and open apices may be seen. The enlarged pulps frequently demonstrate one or more prominent pulp stones.

Histopathologic Features

In ground sections, the thickness of the enamel varies, resulting in an irregular surface. The prism structure of the enamel is irregular or lacking with a laminated appearance. The dentin contains clefts scattered through a mixture of interglobular dentin and amorphous material. Globular areas of poorly organized tubular dentin and scattered cellular inclusions often are seen. The pulp tissue contains free or attached stones, which may exhibit tubules or consist of laminated calcification. The follicular tissue surrounding the crown may be enlarged and

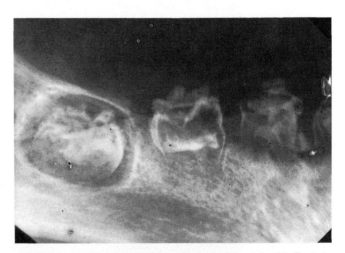

FIGURE 2–111. **Regional odontodysplasia (ghost teeth).** Posterior mandibular dentition exhibiting enlarged pulps and extremely thin enamel and dentin. (Courtesy of Dr. John B. Perry.)

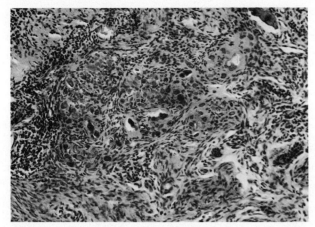

FIGURE 2-112. Regional odontodysplasia. Follicular tissue contains scattered collections of enameloid conglomerates and islands of odontogenic epithelium.

typically exhibit focal collections of basophilic enameloid calcifications called *enameloid conglomerates* (Fig. 2-112). This pattern of calcification is not specific for regional odontodysplasia and has been seen in other processes with disturbed enamel formation, such as amelogenesis imperfecta. Scattered islands of odontogenic epithelium and other patterns of intramural calcification are also seen.

Treatment and Prognosis

The basic approach to therapy of regional odontodysplasia is directed toward retention of the altered teeth, whenever possible, to allow for appropriate development and preservation of the surrounding alveolar ridge. Severely affected and infected teeth often are not salvageable and need to be removed. Endodontic therapy on nonvital teeth that have sufficient hard tissue to allow restoration has been performed successfully. Unerupted teeth are best covered by a removable partial prosthesis until the skeletal growth period has passed. Erupted teeth can be covered with etched-retained restorations or stainless steel crowns until final restorations can be placed after the completion of growth. Because of the fragile nature of the coronal hard tissue and the ease of pulp exposure, tooth preparation is contraindicated.

REFERENCES

General References

Gorlin RJ, Cohen MM, Levin LS. Syndromes of the Head and Neck, 3rd ed. New York, Oxford University Press, 1990.

Stewart RE, Prescott GH. Oral Facial Genetics. St. Louis, CV Mosby, 1976.

Witkop CJ. Clinical aspects of dental anomalies. Int Dent J 26:378–390, 1976.

Witkop CJ, Rao S. Inherited defects in tooth structure. *In*: Birth Defects. Original Article Series. Vol 7, No 7. Edited by Bergsma D. Baltimore, Williams & Wilkins, 1971, pp 153–184.

Environmental Effects on Tooth Structure Development

Andreasen JO, Sundström B, Ravn JJ. The effect of traumatic injuries to primary teeth on their permanent successors. I. A clinical and histologic study of 117 injured permanent teeth. Scand J Dent Res 79:219–283, 1971.

Bhat M, Nelson KB. Developmental enamel defects in primary teeth in children with cerebral palsy, mental retardation, or hearing defects: A review. Adv Dent Res 3:132–142, 1989.

Burt BA. The changing patterns of systemic fluoride intake. J Dent Res 71:1228–1237, 1992.

Cutress TW, Suckling GW. Differential diagnosis of dental fluorosis. J Dent Res 69:714–720, 1990.

Møller IJ. Fluorides and dental fluorosis. Int Dent J 32:135–147, 1982.

Pindborg JJ. Aetiology of developmental enamel defects not related to fluorosis. Int Dent J 32:123–134, 1982.

Seow WK. Enamel hypoplasia in the primary dentition: A review. J Dent Child 58:441–452, 1991.

Small BW, Murray JJ. Enamel opacities: Prevalence, classifications and aetiological considerations. J Dent 6:33–42, 1978.

Suckling GW. Developmental defects of enamel—historical and present day perspective of their pathogenesis. Adv Dent Res 3:87–94, 1989.

Turner JG. Two cases of hypoplasia of enamel. Proc R Soc Med [Odontological Section] 5:73–76, 1912.

von Arx T. Developmental disturbances of permanent teeth following trauma to the primary dentition. Aust Dent J 38:1–10, 1993.

Postdevelopmental Loss of Tooth Structure

Bakland LK. Root resorption. Dent Clin North Am 36:491–507, 1992.

Brezniak N, Wasserstein A. Root resorption after orthodontic treatment: Part 2. Literature review. Am J Orthod Dentofacial Orthop 103:138–146, 1993.

Crothers AJR. Tooth wear and facial morphology. J Dent 20:333–341, 1992.

Eccles JD. Tooth surface loss from abrasion, attrition and erosion. Dent Update 7:373–381, 1982.

Gartner AH, et al. Differential diagnosis of internal and external resorption. J Endod 2:329–334, 1976.

Goultschin J, Nitzan D, Azaz B. Root resorption. Review and discussion. Oral Surg Oral Med Oral Pathol 54:586–590, 1982.

House RC, et al. Perimolysis: Unveiling the surreptitious vomiter. Oral Surg Oral Med Oral Pathol 51:152–155, 1981.

Lee WC, Eakle WS. Possible role of tensile stress in the etiology of cervical erosive lesions of teeth. J Prosthet Dent 52:374–379, 1984.

Mair LH. Wear in dentistry—current terminology. J Dent 20:140–144, 1992.

Massler M, Malone AJ. Root resorption in human permanent teeth: A roentgenographic study. Am J Orthod 40:619–633, 1954.

Moody GH, Muir KF. Multiple idiopathic root resorption. A case report and discussion of pathogenesis. J Clin Periodontol 18:577–580, 1991.

Mummery JH. The pathology of "pink spots" on teeth. Br Dent J 7:301–311, 1920.

Newman WG. Possible etiologic factors in external root resorption. Am J Orthod 67:522–539, 1975.

Rabinowitch BZ. Internal resorption. Oral Surg Oral Med Oral Pathol 33:263–282, 1972.

Smith BGN. Toothwear: Aetiology and diagnosis. Dent Update 16:204–212, 1989.

Smith BGN, Knight JK. A comparison of patterns of tooth wear with aetiological factors. Br Dent J 157:16–19, 1984.

Tronstad L. Root resorption—etiology, terminology and clinical manifestations. Endod Dent Traumatol 4:241–252, 1988.

Wedenberg C, Zetterqvist L. Internal resorption in human teeth—a histological, scanning electron microscopic, and enzyme histochemical study. J Endod 13:255–259, 1987.

Discolorations of Teeth

Chiappinelli JA, Walton RE. Tooth discoloration resulting from long-term tetracycline therapy: A case report. Quintessence Int 23:539–541, 1992.

Cullen CL. Erythroblastosis fetalis produced by Kell immunization: Dental findings. Pediatr Dent 12:393–396, 1990.

Cutbirth ST. Indirect porcelain veneer technique for restoring intrinsically stained teeth. J Esthetic Dent 4:190–196, 1992.

Dayan D, et al. Tooth discoloration—extrinsic and intrinsic factors. Quintessence Int 2:195–199, 1983.

Eisenberg E, Bernick SM. Anomalies of the teeth with stains and discolorations. J Prev Dent 2:7–20, 1975.

Faunce F. Management of discolored teeth. Dent Clin North Am 27:657–670, 1983.

Herbert FL, Delcambre TJ. Unusual case of green teeth resulting from neonatal hyperbilirubinemia. J Dent Child 54:54–56, 1987.

Lang NP, Brecx MC. Chlorhexidine digluconate—an agent for chemical plaque control and prevention of gingival inflammation. J Periodont Res 21(Suppl 16):74–89, 1986.

Merino CC, et al. Stomological manifestations of Günther's disease. J Pedod 14:113–116, 1990.

Morisaki I, et al. Dental findings of children with biliary atresia: Report of seven cases. J Dent Child 57:220–223, 1990.

Parkins FM, Furnish G, Bernstein M. Minocycline use discolors teeth. J Am Dent Assoc 123:87–89, 1992.

Rendall JR, McDougall AC. Reddening of the upper central incisors associated with periapical granuloma in lepromatous leprosy. Br J Oral Surg 13:271–277, 1976.

Sainio P, et al. Postmortem pink teeth phenomenon: An experimental study and a survey of the literature. Proc Finn Dent Soc 86:29–35, 1990.

Seow WK, Shepard RW, Ong TH. Oral changes associated with end-stage liver disease and liver transplantation: Implication for dental management. J Dent Child 58:474–480, 1991.

Localized Disturbances in Eruption

Alling CC III, Catone GA. Management of impacted teeth. J Oral Maxillofac Surg 51(Suppl 1):3–6, 1993.

Ben-Bassat Y, Brin I, Fuks AB. Occlusal disturbances resulting from neglected submerged primary molars. J Dent Child 58:129–133, 1991.

Bianchi SD, Roccuzzo M. Primary impaction of primary teeth: A review and report of three cases. J Clin Pediatr Dent 15:165–168, 1991.

Douglass J, Tinanoff N. The etiology, prevalence, and sequelae of infraocclusion of primary molars. J Dent Child 58:481–483, 1991.

Kokich VG, Mathews DP. Surgical and orthodontic management of impacted teeth. Dent Clin North Am 37:181–204, 1993.

Mercier P, Precious D. Risks and benefits of removal of impacted third molars. J Oral Maxillofac Surg 21:17–27, 1993.

Paleczny G. Treatment of the ankylosed mandibular permanent first molar: A case study. J Can Dent Assoc 57:717–719, 1991.

Peterson LJ. Rationale for removing impacted teeth: When to extract or not to extract. J Am Dent Assoc 123:198–204, 1992.

Raghoebar GM, et al. Secondary retention of permanent molars: A histologic study. J Oral Pathol Med 18:427–431, 1989.

Raghoebar GM, Boering G, Vissink A. Clinical, radiographic and histological characteristics of secondary retention of permanent molars. J Dent 19:164–170, 1991.

Developmental Alterations in Number of Teeth

Bodin I, Julin P, Thomsson M. Hyperdontia. I. Frequency and distribution of supernumerary teeth among 21,609 patients. Dentomaxillofac Radiol 7:15–17, 1978.

Burzynski NJ, Escobar VH. Classification and genetics of numeric anomalies of dentition. In: Birth Defects. Original Article Series. Vol 19. No. 1. Edited by Jorgenson RJ, Paul NW. New York, Alan R. Liss, 1983, pp 95–106.

Grimanis GA, Kyriakides AT, Spyropoulos ND. A survey on supernumerary molars. Quintessence Int 22:989–995, 1991.

Kates GA, Needleman HL, Holmes LB. Natal and neonatal teeth: A clinical study. J Am Dent Assoc 109:441–443, 1984.

King NM, Lee AM, Wan PKC. Multiple supernumerary premolars: Their occurrence in three patients. Aust Dent J 38:11–16, 1993.

Meon R. Hypodontia of the primary and permanent dentition. J Clin Pediatr Dent 16:121–123, 1992.

Schalk-van der Weide Y, Steen WHA, Bosman F. Distribution of missing teeth and tooth morphology in patients with oligodontia. J Dent Child 59:133–140, 1992.

Shapira Y, Kuftinec MM. Tooth transposition—a review of the literature and treatment considerations. Angle Orthod 59:271–276, 1989.

Solares R. The complications of late diagnosis of anterior supernumerary teeth: Case report. J Dent Child 57:209–211, 1990.

Spouge JD, Feasby WH. Erupted teeth in the newborn. Oral Surg Oral Med Oral Pathol 22:198–208, 1966.

To EWH. A study of natal teeth in Hong Kong Chinese. Int J Paediatr Dent 1:73–76, 1991.

Yusof WZ. Non-syndrome multiple supernumerary teeth: Literature review. J Can Dent Assoc 56:147–149, 1990.

Developmental Alterations in Size of Teeth

Bailit HL. Dental variation among populations. An anthropologic view. Dent Clin North Am 19:125–139, 1975.

Bazopoulou-Kyrkanidou E, et al. Microdontia, hypodontia, short bulbous roots and root canals with strabismus, short stature, and border-line mentality. Oral Surg Oral Med Oral Pathol 74:93–95, 1992.

Brook AH. A unifying aetiological explanation for anomalies of human tooth number and size. Arch Oral Biol 29:373–378, 1984.

Holmes J, Tanner MS. Premature eruption and macrodontia associated with insulin resistant diabetes and pineal hyperplasia. Report of two cases. Br Dent J 141:280–284, 1976.

MacMillan ARG, et al. Regional macrodontia and regional bony enlargement associated with congenital infiltrating lipomatosis of the face presenting as unilateral facial hyperplasia. Brief review and case report. Int J Oral Maxillofac Surg 19:283–286, 1990.

Rushton MA. Partial gigantism of face and teeth. Br Dent J 62:572–578, 1937.

Thorburn DN, Ferguson MM. Familial ogee roots, tooth mobility, oligodontia, and microdontia. Oral Surg Oral Med Oral Pathol 74:576–581, 1992.

Townsend GC. Hereditability of deciduous tooth size in Australian aboriginals. Am J Phys Anthropol 53:297–300, 1980.

Townsend GC, Brown T. Hereditability of permanent tooth size. Am J Phys Anthropol 49:497–504, 1978.

Gemination, Fusion, Concrescence

Brook AH, Winter GB. Double teeth. A retrospective study of "geminated" and "fused" teeth in children. Br Dent J 129:123–130, 1970.

Duncan WK, Helpin ML. Bilateral fusion and gemination: A literature analysis and case report. Oral Surg Oral Med Oral Pathol 64:82–87, 1987.

Grover PS, Lorton L. Gemination and twinning in the permanent dentition. Oral Surg Oral Med Oral Pathol 59:313–318, 1985.

Killian CM, Croll TP. Dental twinning anomalies: The nomenclature enigma. Quintessence Int 21:571–576, 1990.

Levitas TC. Gemination, fusion, twinning and concrescence. J Dent Child 32:93–100, 1965.

Ruprecht A, Batniji S, El-Neweihi E. Double teeth: The incidence of gemination and fusion. J Pedod 9:332–337, 1985.

Yuen SWH, Chan JCY, Wei SHY. Double primary teeth and their relationship with the permanent successors: A radiographic study of 376 cases. Pediatr Dent 9:42–48, 1987.

Accessory Cusps

Bailit HL. Dental variation among populations. An anthropologic view. Dent Clin North Am 19:125–139, 1975.

Chen R-J, Chen H-S. Talon cusp in primary dentition. Oral Surg Oral Med Oral Pathol 62:67–72, 1986.

Fabra-Campos H. Failure of endodontic treatment due to a palatal gingival groove in a maxillary lateral incisor with talon cusp and two root canals. J Endod 16:342–345, 1990.

Geist JR. Dens evaginatus. Case report and review of the literature. Oral Surg Oral Med Oral Pathol 67:628–631, 1989.

Jowharji N, Noonan RG, Tylka JA. An unusual case of dental anomaly: A "facial" talon cusp. J Dent Child 59:156–158, 1992.

Mellor JK, Ripa LW. Talon cusp: A clinically significant anomaly. Oral Surg Oral Med Oral Pathol 29:225–228, 1970.

Meon R. Talon cusp in primary dentition. Case report. Singapore Dent J 15:32–34, 1990.

Meon R. Talon cusp in Malaysia. Aust Dent J 36:11–14, 1991.

Meyers CL. Treatment of a talon-cusp incisor: Report of a case. J Dent Child 47:119–121, 1980.

Rusmah M. The cusp of Carabelli in Malaysians. Odonto-Stomatol Trop 15:13–15, 1992.

Saini TS, Kharat DU, Mokeem S. Prevalence of shovel-shaped incisors in Saudi Arabian dental patients. Oral Surg Oral Med Oral Pathol 70:540–544, 1990.

Shey Z, Eytel R. Clinical management of an unusual case of dens evaginatus in a maxillary central incisor. J Am Dent Assoc 106:346–348, 1983.

Wong MT, Augsburger RA. Management of dens evaginatus. Gen Dent 40:300–303, 1992.

Yong SL. Prophylactic treatment of dens evaginatus. J Dent Child 41:289–292, 1974.

Dens Invaginatus

Burton DJ, Saffos RO, Scheffer RB. Multiple bilateral dens in dente as a factor in the etiology of multiple periapical lesions. Oral Surg Oral Med Oral Pathol 49:496–499, 1980.

Karaca İ, Toller MÖ. Multiple bilateral dens in dente involving all the premolars. Case report. Aust Dent J 37:449–452, 1992.

Oehlers FAC. Dens invaginatus (dilated composite odontome). I. Variations of the invagination process and associated anterior crown forms. Oral Surg Oral Med Oral Pathol 10:1204–1218, 1957.

Oehlers FAC. Dens invaginatus (dilated composite odontome). II. Associated posterior crown forms and pathogenesis. Oral Surg Oral Med Oral Pathol 10:1302–1316, 1957.

Oehlers FAC. The radicular variety of dens invaginatus. Oral Surg Oral Med Oral Pathol 11:1251–1260, 1958.

Payne M, Craig GT. A radicular dens invaginatus. Br Dent J 169:94–95, 1990.

Rotstein I, Stabholz A, Friedman S. Endodontic therapy for dens invaginatus in a maxillary second molar. Oral Surg Oral Med Oral Pathol 63:237–240, 1987.

Ectopic Enamel

Bohay RN, Weinberg S, Thorner PS. The paradental cyst of the mandibular first molar: Report of a bilateral case. J Dent Child 59:361–365, 1992.

Cavanha AO. Enamel pearls. Oral Surg Oral Med Oral Pathol 19:373–382, 1965.

Craig GT. The paradental cyst, a specific inflammatory odontogenic cyst. Br Dent J 141:9–14, 1976.

Fowler CB, Brannon RB. The paradental cyst: A clinicopathologic study of six new cases and review of the literature. J Oral Maxillofac Surg 47:243–248, 1989.

Goldstein AR. Enamel pearls as a contributing factor in periodontal breakdown. J Am Dent Assoc 99:210–211, 1979.

Hou G-L, Tsai C-C. Relationship between periodontal furcation involvement and molar cervical enamel projections. J Periodontol 58:715–721, 1987.

Kaugers GE. Internal enamel pearls: Report of case. J Am Dent Assoc 107:941–943, 1983.

Kupietzky A, Rozenfarb N. Enamel pearls in the primary dentition: Report of two cases. J Dent Child 60:63–66, 1993.

Moskow BS, Canut PM. Studies on root enamel. (2) Enamel pearls. A review of their morphology, localization, nomenclature, occurrence, classification, histogenesis and incidence. J Clin Periodontol 17:275–281, 1990.

Packota GV, et al. Paradental cysts on mandibular first molars in children: Report of five cases. Dentomaxillofac Radiol 19:126–132, 1990.

Risnes S. The prevalence, location, and size of enamel pearls on human molars. Scand J Dent Res 82:403–412, 1974.

Wolf J, Hietanen J. The mandibular infected buccal cyst (paradental cyst). A radiographic and histological study. Br J Oral Maxillofac Surg 28:322–325, 1990.

Taurodontism

Durr DP, Campos CA, Ayers CS. Clinical significance of taurodontism. J Am Dent Assoc 100:378–381, 1980.

Llamas R, Jimenez-Planas A. Taurodontism in premolars. Oral Surg Oral Med Oral Pathol 75:501–505, 1993.

Ruprecht A, Batniji S, El-Neweihi E. The incidence of taurodontism in dental patients. Oral Surg Oral Med Oral Pathol 63:743–747, 1987.

Shaw JCM. Taurodont teeth in South African races. J Anat 62:476–498, 1928.

Shifman A, Chanannel I. Prevalence of taurodontism found in radiographic dental examination of 1,200 young adult Israeli patients. Community Dent Oral Epidemiol 6:200–203, 1978.

Witkop CJ, et al. Taurodontism: An anomaly of teeth reflecting disruptive developmental homeostasis. Am J Med Genet 4(Suppl):85–97, 1988.

Hypercementosis

Fox L. Paget's disease (osteitis deformans) and its effect on maxillary bones and teeth. J Am Dent Assoc 20:1823–1829, 1933.

Gardner BS, Goldstein H. The significance of hypercementosis. Dent Cosmos 73:1065–1069, 1931.

Leider AS, Garbarino VE. Generalized hypercementosis. Oral Surg Oral Med Oral Pathol 63:375–380, 1987.

Rao VM, Karasick D. Hypercementosis—An important clue to Paget disease of the maxilla. Skeletal Radiol 9:126–128, 1982.

Weinberger A. The clinical significance of hypercementosis. Oral Surg Oral Med Oral Pathol 7:79–87, 1954.

Dilaceration

Bimstein E. Root dilaceration and stunting in two unerupted primary incisors. J Dent Child 45:223–225, 1978.

Celik E, Aydinlik E. Effect of a dilacerated root in stress distribution to the tooth and supporting tissues. J Prosthet Dent 65:771–777, 1991.

Kilpatrick NM, Hardman PJ, Welbury RR. Dilaceration of a primary tooth. Int J Paediatr Dent 1:151–153, 1991.

Ligh RQ. Coronal dilaceration. Oral Surg Oral Med Oral Pathol 51:567, 1981.

Seow WK, et al. Dilaceration of a primary maxillary incisor associated with neonatal laryngoscopy. Pediatr Dent 12:321–324, 1990.

Smith DMH, Winter GB. Root dilaceration of maxillary incisors. Br Dent J 150:125–127, 1981.

Stewart DJ. Dilacerate unerupted maxillary central incisors. Br Dent J 145:229–233, 1978.

van Gool AV. Injury to the permanent tooth germ after trauma to the deciduous predecessor. Oral Surg Oral Med Oral Pathol 35:2–12, 1973.

Supernumerary Roots

Acs G, Pokala P, Cozzi E. Shovel incisors, three-rooted molars, talon cusp, and supernumerary tooth in one patient. Pediatr Dent 14:263–264, 1992.

Badger GR. Three-rooted mandibular first primary molar. Oral Surg Oral Med Oral Pathol 53:547, 1982.

Krolls SO, Donahue AH. Double-rooted maxillary primary canines. Oral Surg Oral Med Oral Pathol 49:379, 1980.

Oliver RG, Hunter B. An accessory root on a maxillary central incisor. Dent Update 18:306–307, 1991.

Younes SA, Al-Shammery AR, El-Angbawi MF. Three-rooted permanent mandibular first molars of Asian and black groups in the Middle East. Oral Surg Oral Med Oral Pathol 69:102–105, 1990.

Amelogenesis Imperfecta

Crawford PJM, Aldred MJ. X-linked amelogenesis imperfecta. Presentation of two kindreds and a review of the literature. Oral Surg Oral Med Oral Pathol 73:449–455, 1992.

Crawford PJM, Aldred MJ. Amelogenesis imperfecta: Autosomal dominant hypomaturation-hypoplasia type with taurodontism. Br Dent J 164:71–73, 1988.

Crawford PJM, Aldred MJ. Amelogenesis imperfecta with taurodontism and the tricho-dento-osseous syndrome: Separate conditions or a spectrum of disease? Clin Genet 38:44–50, 1990.

McLarty EL, Giansanti JS, Hibbard ED. X-linked hypomaturation type of amelogenesis imperfecta exhibiting lyonization in affected females. Oral Surg Oral Med Oral Pathol 36:678–685, 1973.

Rada RE, Hasiakos PS. Current treatment modalities in the conservative restoration of amelogenesis imperfecta: A case report. Quintessence Int 21:937–942, 1990.

Seow WK. Taurodontism of the mandibular first permanent molar distinguishes between the tricho-dento-osseous (TDO) syndrome and amelogenesis imperfecta. Clin Genet 43:240–246, 1993.

Shields ED. A new classification of heritable human enamel defects and a discussion of dentin defects. *In*: Dentition: Genetic Effects, Birth Defects. Original Article Series. Vol 19. No. 1. Edited by Jorgenson RJ, Paul NW. New York, Alan R. Liss, 1983, pp 107–127.

Sundell S, Koch G. Hereditary amelogenesis imperfecta. I. Epidemiology and clinical classification in a Swedish child population. Swed Dent J 9:157–169, 1985.

Sundell S, Valentin J. Hereditary aspects and classification of hereditary amelogenesis imperfecta. Community Dent Oral Epidemiol 14:211–216, 1986.

Winter GB, Brook AH. Enamel hypoplasia and anomalies of the enamel. Dent Clin North Am 19:3–24, 1975.

Witkop CJ Jr. Partial expression of sex-linked recessive amelogenesis imperfecta in females compatible with the Lyon hypothesis. Oral Surg Oral Med Oral Pathol 23:174–182, 1967.

Witkop CJ Jr. Amelogenesis imperfecta, dentinogenesis imperfecta and dentin dysplasia revisited: Problems in classification. J Oral Pathol 17:547–553, 1988.

Witkop CJ Jr, Sauk JJ Jr. Heritable defects of enamel. *In*: Oral Facial Genetics. Edited by Stewart RE, Prescott GH. St. Louis, CV Mosby, 1976, pp 151–226.

Dentinogenesis Imperfecta

Darendeliler-Kaba A, Maréchaux SC. Hereditary dentinogenesis imperfecta: A treatment program using an overdenture. J Dent Child 59:273–276, 1992.

Harley KE, Ibbetson RJ. Dental anomalies: Are adhesive castings the solution? Br Dent J 174:15–22, 1993.

Harrison R, Kennedy D. Shell teeth: Management from the mixed to the permanent dentition: Case report. Pediatr Dent 14:110–114, 1992.

Heimler A, et al. An unusual presentation of opalescent dentin and Brandywine isolate: Hereditary opalescent dentin in an Ashkenazic Jewish family. Oral Surg Oral Med Oral Pathol 59:608–615, 1985.

Hursey RJ, et al. Dentinogenesis imperfecta in a racial isolate with multiple hereditary defects. Oral Surg Oral Med Oral Pathol 9:641–658, 1956.

Levin LS. The dentition in the osteogenesis imperfecta syndrome. Clin Orthop 159:64–74, 1981.

Levin LS, et al. Dentinogenesis imperfecta in the Brandywine isolate (DI type III): Clinical, radiologic, and scanning electron microscopic studies of the dentition. Oral Surg Oral Med Oral Pathol 56:267–274, 1983.

Mayordomo FG, Estrela F, de Aldecoa EA. Dentinogenesis imperfecta: A case report. Quintessence Int 23:795–802, 1992.

Ranta H, Lukinmaa P-L, Waltimo J. Heritable dentin defects: Nosology, pathology, and treatment. Am J Med Genet 45:193–200, 1993.

Rushton MA. A new form of dentinal dysplasia: Shell teeth. Oral Surg Oral Med Oral Pathol 7:543–549, 1954.

Shields ED, Bixler D, El-Kafrawy AM. A proposed classification for heritable human dentine defects with a description of a new entity. Arch Oral Biol 18:543–553, 1973.

Witkop CJ Jr. Hereditary defects of dentin. Dent Clin North Am 19:25–45, 1975.

Witkop CJ Jr. Amelogenesis imperfecta, dentinogenesis imperfecta and dentin dysplasia revisited: Problems in classification. J Oral Pathol 17:547–553, 1988.

Witkop CJ Jr, et al. Medical and dental findings in the Brandywine isolate. Ala J Med Sci 3:382–403, 1966.

Dentin Dysplasia

Bixler D. Heritable disorders affecting dentin. *In*: Oral Facial Genetics. Edited by Stewart RE, Prescott GH. St. Louis, CV Mosby, 1976, pp 227–262.

Ciola B, Bahn SL, Goviea GL. Radiographic manifestations of an unusual combination of type I and type II dentin dysplasia. Oral Surg Oral Med Oral Pathol 45:317–322, 1978.

Coke JM, et al. Dentinal dysplasia, type I. Report of a case with endodontic therapy. Oral Surg Oral Med Oral Pathol 48:262–268, 1979.

Diamond O. Dentin dysplasia type II: Report of a case. J Dent Child 56:310–312, 1989.

Duncan WK, Perkins TM, O'Carroll MK. Type I dentin dysplasia: Report of two cases. Ann Dent 50:18–21, 1991.

Jasmin JR, Clergeau-Guerithault S. A scanning electron microscopic study of dentin dysplasia type II in primary dentition. Oral Surg Oral Med Oral Pathol 58:57–63, 1984.

Melnick M, et al. Dentin dysplasia, type II: A rare autosomal dominant disorder. Oral Surg Oral Med Oral Pathol 44:592–599, 1977.

O'Carroll MK, Duncan WK, Perkins TM. Dentin dysplasia: Review of the literature and a proposed subclassification based on radiographic findings. Oral Surg Oral Med Oral Pathol 72:119–125, 1991.

Ranta H, Lukinmaa P-L, Waltimo J. Heritable dentin defects: Nosology, pathology, and treatment. Am J Med Genet 45:193–200, 1993.

Rao SR, Witkop CJ Jr, Yamane GM. Pulpal dysplasia. Oral Surg Oral Med Oral Pathol 30:682–689, 1970.

Rosenberg LR, Phelan JA. Dentin dysplasia type II: Review of the literature and report of a family. J Dent Child 50:372–375, 1983.

Rushton MA. A case of dentinal dysplasia. Guy's Hosp Rep 89:369–373, 1939.

Scola SM, Watts PG. Dentinal dysplasia type I. A subclassification. Br J Orthod 14:175–179, 1987.

Shields ED, Bixler D, El-Kafrawy AM. A proposed classification for heritable human dentine defects with a description of a new entity. Arch Oral Biol 18:543–553, 1973.

Steidler NE, Radden BG, Reade PC. Dentinal dysplasia: A clinicopathologic study of eight cases and review of the literature. Br J Oral Maxillofac Surg 22:274–286, 1984.

Tidwell E, Cunningham CJ. Dentinal dysplasia: Endodontic treatment, with case report. J Endod 5:372–376, 1979.

Van Dis ML, Allen CM. Dentinal dysplasia type I: A report of four cases. Dentomaxillofac Radiol 18:128–131, 1989.

Waltimo J, Ranta H, Lukinmaa P-L. Transmission electron microscopic appearance of dentin matrix in type II dentin dysplasia. Scand J Dent Res 99:349–356, 1991.

Wesley RK, et al. Dentin dysplasia type I. Clinical, morphologic, and genetic studies of a case. Oral Surg Oral Med Oral Pathol 41:516–524, 1976.

Witkop CJ Jr. Hereditary defects of dentin. Dent Clin North Am 19:25–45, 1975.

Witkop CJ Jr. Manifestations of genetic diseases in the human pulp. Oral Surg Oral Med Oral Pathol 32:278–316, 1971.

Witkop CJ Jr. Amelogenesis imperfecta, dentinogenesis imperfecta and dentin dysplasia revisited: Problems in classification. J Oral Pathol 17:547–553, 1988.

Regional Odontodysplasia

Crawford PJM, Aldred MJ. Regional odontodysplasia: A bibliography. J Oral Pathol Med 18:251–263, 1989.

Dahllöf G, et al. Concomitant regional odontodysplasia and hydrocephalus. Oral Surg Oral Med Oral Pathol 63:354–357, 1987.

Gardner DG. The dentinal changes in regional odontodysplasia. Oral Surg Oral Med Oral Pathol 38:887–897, 1974.

Guzman R, Elliot MA, Rossie KM. Odontodysplasia in a pediatric patient: Literature review and case report. Pediatr Dent 12:45–48, 1990.

Kahn MA, Hinson RL. Regional odontodysplasia. Case report with etiologic and treatment considerations. Oral Surg Oral Med Oral Pathol 72:462–467, 1991.

Kerebel L-M, Kerebel B. Soft-tissue calcifications of the dental follicle in regional odontodysplasia: A structural and ultrastructural study. Oral Surg Oral Med Oral Pathol 56:396–404, 1983.

Kinirons MJ, O'Brien FV, Gregg TA. Regional odontodysplasia: An evaluation of three cases based on clinical, microradiographic and histopathological findings. Br Dent J 165:136–139, 1988.

Lowery L, Welbury RR, Soames JV. An unusual case of regional odontodysplasia. Int J Paediatr Dent 2:171–176, 1992.

Lustmann J, Klein H, Ulmansky M. Odontodysplasia. Report of two cases and review of the literature. Oral Surg Oral Med Oral Pathol 39:781–793, 1975.

Sadeghi EM, Ashrafi MH. Regional odontodysplasia: Clinical, pathologic and therapeutic considerations. J Am Dent Assoc 102:336–339, 1981.

Steiman HR, Cullen CL, Geist JR. Bilateral mandibular regional odontodysplasia with vascular nevus. Pediatr Dent 13:303–306, 1991.

Walton JL, Witkop CJ Jr, Walker PO. Odontodysplasia. Report of three cases with vascular nevi overlying the adjacent skin of the face. Oral Surg Oral Med Oral Pathol 46:676–684, 1978.

Zegarelli EV, et al. Odontodysplasia. Oral Surg Oral Med Oral Pathol 16:187–193, 1963.

3

Pulpal and Periapical Disease

PULPITIS

The initial response of the dental pulp to injury is not significantly different from that seen in other tissues, but the final result can be dramatically different because of the rigid dentinal walls of the pulp chamber. When external stimuli reach a noxious level, degranulation of mast cells, decreased nutrient flow, and cellular damage occur. Numerous inflammatory mediators (e.g., histamine, bradykinin, neurokinins, neuropeptides, prostaglandins) are released. These mediators cause vasodilation, increased blood inflow, and vascular leakage with edema. In normal tissue, increased blood flow promotes healing through removal of inflammatory mediators, and usually swelling of the injured tissue occurs. However, the dental pulp exists in a very confined area. The active dilation of the arterioles leads to increased pulpal pressure and secondary compression of the venous return, which can lead to strangulation of the arterial inflow. The increased pressure appears to be confined to the area of the pulp receiving the noxious stimulus. The increased pulpal pressures, combined with the accumulation of mediators, can lead to vessel damage, pulpal inflammation, and tissue necrosis. Severe localized pulpal damage can progressively spread to involve the more apical portion of the pulp.

Four main types of noxious stimuli are common causes of pulpal inflammation:

1. *Mechanical damage.* Mechanical sources of injury include traumatic accidents, iatrogenic damage from dental procedures, attrition, abrasion, and barometric changes.
2. *Thermal injury.* Severe thermal stimuli can be transmitted through large uninsulated metallic restorations or may occur from such dental procedures as cavity preparation, polishing, and exothermic chemical reactions of dental materials.
3. *Chemical irritation.* Chemical-related damage can arise from erosion or from the inappropriate use of acidic dental materials.
4. *Bacterial effects.* Bacteria can damage the pulp through toxins or directly after extension from caries or transportation via the vasculature.

Pulpitis can be classified as:

- Acute or chronic
- Subtotal or generalized
- Infected or sterile

The best classification system is one that guides the appropriate treatment. **Reversible pulpitis** denotes a level of pulpal inflammation in which the tissue is capable of returning to a normal state of health if the noxious stimuli are removed. **Irreversible pulpitis** implies that a higher level of inflammation has developed, in which the dental pulp has been damaged beyond the point of recovery. Frank invasion by bacteria is often the cross-over point from reversible to irreversible pulpitis.

Clinical Features

Reversible Pulpitis

When exposed to temperature extremes, patients with reversible pulpitis experience a sudden mild to moderate pain of short duration. Although heat may initiate pain, the affected tooth responds most to cold stimuli, such as ice, beverages, and cold air. Contact with sweet or sour foods and beverages also may cause pain. The pain does not occur without stimulation, and it subsides within seconds after the stimulus is removed. Typically, the tooth responds to electric pulp testing at lower levels of current than an appropriate control tooth. Mobility and sensitivity to percussion are absent. If the pulpitis is allowed to progress, the duration of the pain upon stimulation can become longer and the pulp may become irreversibly affected.

Irreversible Pulpitis

Patients with early irreversible pulpitis generally have sharp, severe pain upon thermal stimulation, and the pain continues after the stimulus is removed. Cold is especially uncomfortable, although heat or sweet and acid foods also can elicit pain. In addition, the pain may be spontaneous or continuous and may be exacerbated when one lies down. The tooth responds to electric pulp testing at lower levels of current.

In the early stages of irreversible pulpitis, the pain often can be easily localized to the individual offending tooth; with increasing discomfort, however, the patient is unable to identify the offending tooth within a quadrant.

In the later stages of irreversible pulpitis, the pain increases in intensity and is experienced as a throbbing pressure that can keep patients awake at night. At this point, heat increases the pain but cold may sometimes produce relief. The tooth responds to electric pulp testing at higher levels of current or demonstrates no response. Mobility and sensitivity to percussion are usually absent because significant inflammation has not yet spread to the apical area. If pulpal drainage occurs (e.g., crown fracture, fistula formation), the symptoms may resolve, only to return if the drainage ceases.

The dramatic and painful cases of acute pulpitis are the ones that are most easily recalled by both patients and clinicians. In spite of this, the process may take years, the pattern of symptomatology is highly variable, and often the patient may have no symptoms.

Chronic Hyperplastic Pulpitis

One unique pattern of pulpal inflammation is **chronic hyperplastic pulpitis (pulp polyp)**. This condition occurs in children and young adults who have large exposures of the pulp in which the entire dentinal roof often is missing. The most frequently involved teeth are the deciduous or succedaneous molars, which have large pulp chambers in these age groups. Mechanical irritation and bacterial invasion result in a level of chronic inflammation that produces hyperplastic granulation tissue that extrudes from the chamber and often fills the associated dentinal defect (Figs. 3–1 to 3–3). The apex may be

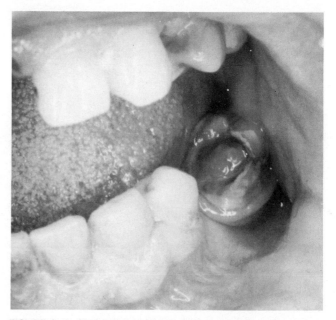

FIGURE 3–1. **Chronic hyperplastic pulpitis.** Erythematous granulation tissue extruding from the pulp chamber of the mandibular first molar.

open and reduces the chance of pulpal necrosis secondary to venous compression. The tooth is asymptomatic except for a possible feeling of pressure when it is placed into masticatory function.

Histopathologic Features

Basically, the histopathology is primarily of academic interest and does not usually affect treatment significantly. Numerous investigations have shown a surprising

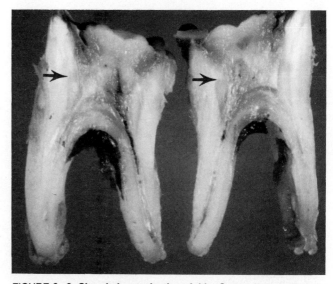

FIGURE 3–2. **Chronic hyperplastic pulpitis.** Gross photograph demonstrating hyperplastic pulp tissue filling a large coronal carious defect. Arrows delineate the previous roof of the pulp chamber.

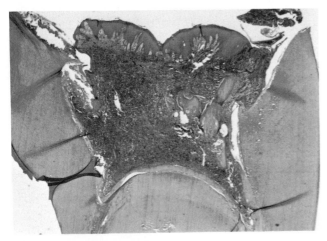

FIGURE 3-3. **Chronic hyperplastic pulpitis.** Same tooth as depicted in Figure 3-2. Chronically inflamed granulation tissue fills the coronal defect. Note surface stratified squamous epithelium.

seen in a pyogenic granuloma. The surface of the polyp may or may not be covered with stratified squamous epithelium, which migrates from the adjacent gingiva or arises from sloughed epithelium within the oral fluids (see Fig. 3-3). The deeper pulp tissue demonstrates a chronic inflammatory infiltrate.

The diagnosis is made from the combination of the clinical presentation and the response to percussion, thermal stimuli, and electric pulp testing. The predictive value of these tests is less than desired. When the procedures demonstrate that the pulp is disease-free, results are highly reliable. However, when a pulp tests positive for irreversible pulpitis, histopathologic examination frequently demonstrates a disease-free state. The practitioner should utilize all available tests, clinical information, and personal judgment in an attempt to arrive at an appropriate diagnosis. Future improvements in diagnostic methods, such as laser Doppler flowmetry, may help to increase accuracy.

Treatment and Prognosis

Reversible pulpitis is treated by removal of the local irritant. The prognosis is good if action is taken early enough. The tooth should be tested for vitality after the symptoms have subsided to ensure that irreversible damage has not occurred.

Irreversible and chronic hyperplastic pulpitis are treated by extraction or by removal of the affected pulp by endodontic procedures.

SECONDARY DENTIN

Formation of dentin proceeds throughout life. The dentin formed before completion of the crown is called **primary dentin.** This process is followed by the formation

lack of correlation between histopathologic findings and the clinical symptoms in the majority of pulps examined.

In patients with reversible pulpitis, the pulp usually shows hyperemia, edema, and a chronic inflammatory cellular infiltrate underlying the area of affected dentinal tubules (Fig. 3-4). Reparative secondary dentin may be noted in the adjacent dentinal wall and scattered acute inflammatory cells are found occasionally.

Irreversible pulpitis often demonstrates congestion of the venules that results in focal necrosis. This necrotic zone contains polymorphonuclear leukocytes and histiocytes (Fig. 3-5). The surrounding pulp tissue usually exhibits fibrosis and a mixture of plasma cells, lymphocytes, and histiocytes (Fig. 3-6).

Chronic hyperplastic pulpitis demonstrates a cap of subacutely inflamed granulation tissue resembling that

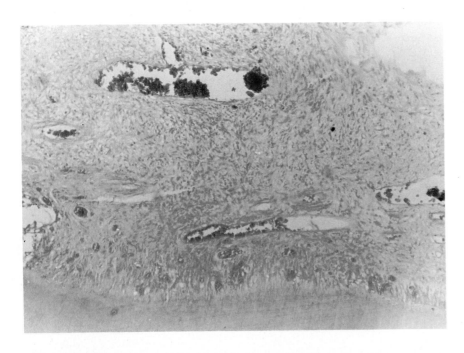

FIGURE 3-4. **Reversible pulpitis.** Dental pulp demonstrating hyperemia and chronic inflammatory infiltrate underlying dentinal tubules. The tooth had recently been prepared for placement of a dental restoration.

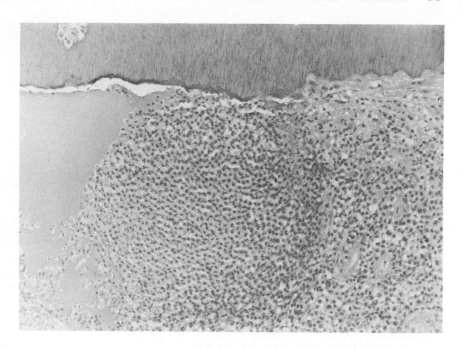

FIGURE 3-5. **Irreversible pulpitis.** Dental pulp exhibiting acute inflammatory infiltrate consisting predominantly of polymorphonuclear leukocytes.

of **secondary dentin**. The same odontoblasts that formed the primary dentin remain functional and produce secondary dentin. With advancing age, deposition of secondary dentin leads to smaller pulp chambers and canal systems. The deposition of dentin is slow and gradual but does increase after the age of 35 to 40. Early widespread formation of secondary dentin has been seen in association with **progeria,** a condition associated with accelerated aging. On occasion, significant traumatic injury can lead to early obliteration of the pulp chamber and canal (**calcific metamorphosis**) in the affected tooth.

In functioning teeth, deposition begins in the coronal portions of the tooth and proceeds to the apical areas.

This type of dentin is thought by many investigators to occur as a result of aging and has been termed **physiologic secondary dentin**. Other authors have noted a significantly decreased amount in impacted teeth and say that the deposition is promoted by environmental functional forces of occlusion. Interestingly, the deposition in impacted teeth appears to begin in the apical areas and spreads coronally.

Localized secondary dentin also is laid down in areas of focal injury. This dentin is more haphazardly organized and is termed **reparative secondary (irregular, tertiary) dentin**. This localized dentin formation may occur in response to:

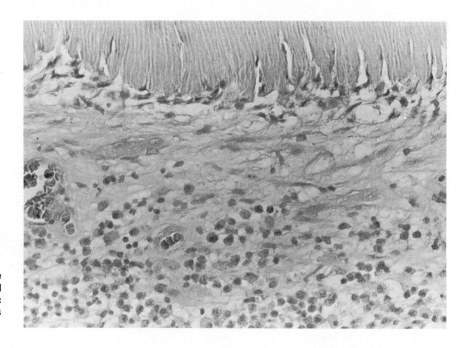

FIGURE 3-6. **Irreversible pulpitis.** Same tooth as depicted in Figure 3-5. The dental pulp exhibits an area of fibrosis and chronic inflammation peripheral to the zone of abscess formation.

- Attrition
- Fracture
- Erosion
- Abrasion
- Caries
- Periodontal disease
- Mechanical injury from dental procedures
- Irritation from dental materials

Injury of the peripheral odontoblastic processes is all that is required to initiate reparative secondary dentin formation. If the damage is severe, the odontoblasts may die, resulting in dentinal tubules filled with degenerated odontoblastic processes known as *dead tracts*. These tubules are usually sealed off by formation of reparative dentin along the pulpal wall of these tracts.

Clinical and Radiographic Features

As noted on periapical radiographs, the deposition of secondary dentin results in diminishing size of pulp chambers and canals. In addition to being used as an estimate of age, secondary dentin appears to reduce sensitivity of the affected teeth, susceptibility to dentinal caries, and the danger of dental procedures. On occasion, large inflammatory lesions may involve more than one

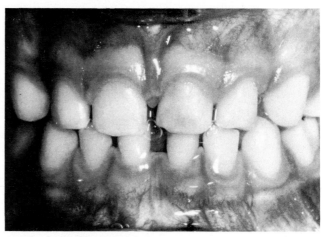

FIGURE 3–8. **Calcific metamorphosis.** Left deciduous maxillary central incisor exhibiting yellow discoloration. See Color Plates. (Courtesy of Dr. Jackie L. Banahan.)

apex and the size of the canals can be used to help determine the original focus of infection because the canal may be larger in the tooth that became nonvital earlier (Fig. 3–7). Teeth affected by calcific metamorphosis are often discovered by a yellow clinical discoloration of the crown; radiographically, the affected teeth exhibit calcification of the pulp chamber and canal (Figs. 3–8 [see Color Figure 17] and 3–9).

Histopathologic Features

Physiologic secondary dentin consists of regular tubular dentin that is applied onto the primary dentin. These two layers of dentin can be separated by a line of demarcation often noted by a bending of the tubules (Fig. 3–10). With advancing age, as the odontoblasts undergo degenerative changes, the physiologic secondary dentin becomes more irregular with fewer tubules.

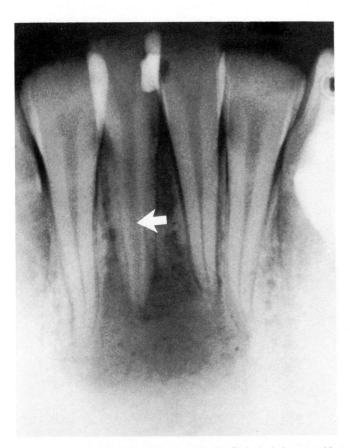

FIGURE 3–7. **Physiologic secondary dentin.** Periapical abscess with all four teeth nonresponsive to electric pulp testing. Increased deposition of physiologic secondary dentin on the right central incisor *(arrow)* delineated the origin of the infection; endodontic treatment of this tooth resolved the lesion.

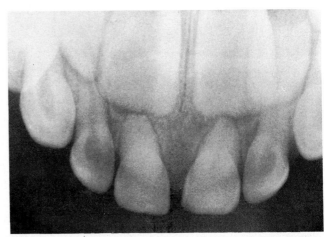

FIGURE 3–9. **Calcific metamorphosis.** Same patient as depicted in Figure 3–8. Deciduous maxillary incisors exhibit total calcification of the pulp chambers and canals. (Courtesy of Dr. Jackie L. Banahan.)

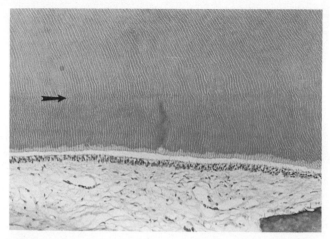

FIGURE 3–10. **Physiologic secondary dentin.** Primary dentin and physiologic secondary dentin are separated by a distinct line of demarcation *(arrow)*.

The quality and appearance of reparative secondary dentin depend on the severity of the noxious stimulus that promoted its formation. This dentin is localized to the pulpal end of the odontoblastic processes that were affected (Fig. 3–11). With a mild stimulus, such as abrasion or attrition, the deposition is slow and demonstrates only slightly irregular tubules. With more severe damage, such as a rapidly progressing carious lesion, the formation is rapid and consists of very irregular dentin with widely scattered, disorganized tubules.

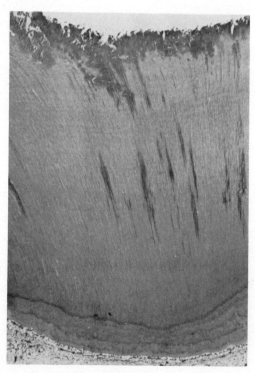

FIGURE 3–11. **Reparative secondary dentin.** Localized deposition of secondary dentin *(bottom)* at the pulpal end of the dentinal tubules affected by the carious process.

PULPAL CALCIFICATIONS

Calcifications within the dental pulp are not rare, but the frequency is difficult to determine. Reported rates vary from 8 to 90 percent. Increased numbers of calcifications are seen in older teeth and those that have been exposed to trauma or caries. There are three types of pulpal calcifications:

- Denticles
- Pulp stones
- Diffuse linear calcifications

All pulpal calcifications start out as free bodies within the pulp tissue but many may become attached or embedded in the dentinal walls of the pulp.

Denticles are believed to form as a result of an epitheliomesenchymal interaction within the developing pulp. Epithelial strands originating from the root sheath or cervical extensions into the pulp chamber adjacent to furcations induce odontoblastic differentiation of the surrounding papilla mesenchyme, forming the core of the denticle. Odontoblasts deposit tubular dentin as they move away from the central epithelium and produce thimble-shaped structures surrounding the epithelium. Denticles form during the period of root development and occur in the root canal and the pulp chamber adjacent to the furcation areas of multirooted teeth. Because denticle development typically precedes completion of the primary dentin, most denticles become attached to or embedded in the dentin.

Pulp stones are thought to develop around a central nidus of pulp tissue, such as a collagen fibril, ground substance, or necrotic cell remnants. Initial calcification begins around the central nidus and extends outward in a concentric or radial pattern of regular calcified material. Pulp stones are formed within the coronal portions of the pulp and may arise as a part of age-related or local pathologic changes. Most pulp stones develop after tooth formation is completed and usually are free or attached. In rare instances, stones may become embedded.

Diffuse linear calcifications do not demonstrate the lamellar organization of pulp stones. They present as areas of fine, fibrillar, irregular calcification that often parallel the vasculature. These calcifications may be present in the pulp chamber or canals, and the frequency increases with age.

Clinical and Radiographic Features

Denticles and pulp stones can reach sufficient size to be detected on intraoral radiographs as radiopaque enlargements within the pulp chamber or canal (Fig. 3–12). Diffuse calcifications are not detectable radiographically.

Other than rare difficulties during endodontic procedures, pulpal calcifications typically are of little clinical significance. Some investigators associate the calcifications with dental neuralgias, but the high frequency of these lesions in the absence of clinical symptoms argues against this relationship. On occasion, the pulpal calcifications may become very large and may interfere with

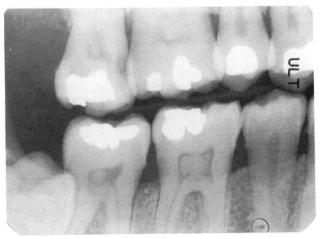

FIGURE 3–12. **Pulp stones.** Multiple teeth demonstrating radiographically obvious calcifications within the pulp chambers.

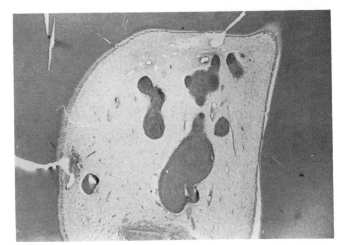

FIGURE 3–13. **Pulp stones.** Multiple stones within the pulp chamber.

root formation, possibly leading to early periodontal destruction and tooth loss. Prominent pulpal calcifications have been noted in association with certain disease processes, such as:

- Dentin dysplasia, type II (see p. 88)
- Pulpal dysplasia (see p. 88)
- Tumoral calcinosis
- Calcinosis universalis
- Ehlers-Danlos syndrome, type I (see p. 552)

Histopathologic Features

Denticles consist of tubular dentin surrounding a central nest of epithelium. With time, the central epithelium degenerates and the tubules undergo sclerosis, making their detection difficult. Most denticles are attached or embedded. Those that remain free in the pulp occasionally develop outer layers of irregular fibrillar calcification or lamellated layers of calcification similar to that seen in pulp stones.

Pulp stones demonstrate a central amorphous mass of irregular calcification surrounded by concentric lamellar rings of regular calcified material (Figs. 3–13 and 3–14). Occasionally, a peripheral layer of tubular dentin may be applied by odontoblasts, which arise from the surrounding pulp tissue in response to the presence of the pulp stone. In addition, fibrillar irregular calcified material also may be evident on the periphery of pulp stones.

Diffuse linear calcifications consist entirely of fine, fibrillar, and irregular calcifications that develop in the pulp chambers and canals (Fig. 3–15). This material often is deposited in a linear fashion along the course of a blood vessel or nerve.

Treatment and Prognosis

No treatment is required. Most pulpal calcifications are not associated with any significant clinical alterations.

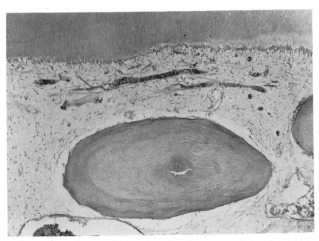

FIGURE 3–14. **Pulp stone.** Pulp stone demonstrating concentric lamellar rings.

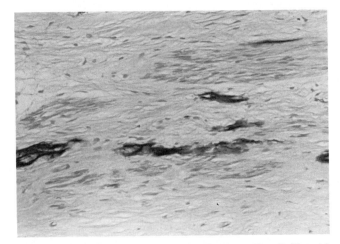

FIGURE 3–15. **Diffuse linear pulpal calcifications.** Fine, fibrillar calcifications parallel the course of the neurovascular channels within the pulp canal.

PERIAPICAL GRANULOMA (Chronic Apical Periodontitis)

The term **periapical granuloma** refers to a mass of chronically inflamed granulation tissue at the apex of a nonvital tooth. This commonly used name is not totally accurate because the lesion does not show true granulomatous inflammation microscopically. Although the term **apical periodontitis** may be more appropriate, it may prove confusing to the clinician. Formation of apical inflammatory lesions represents a defensive reaction secondary to the presence of bacteria in the root canal with spread of related toxic products into the apical zone. Initially, the defense reaction eliminates noxious substances that exit the canals. With time, however, the host reaction becomes less effective with microbial invasion or spread of toxins into the apical area.

Periapical granulomas may arise following quiescence of a **periapical abscess,** or they may develop as the initial periapical pathosis. These lesions are not static and may transform into **periapical cysts** or may demonstrate acute exacerbations with abscess formation.

Clinical and Radiographic Features

Most periapical granulomas are asymptomatic, but pain and sensitivity can develop if acute exacerbation occurs. Typically, the involved tooth does not demonstrate mobility or significant sensitivity to percussion. The soft tissue overlying the apex may or may not be tender. The tooth does not respond to thermal or electric pulp tests unless the pulpal necrosis is limited to a single canal in a multirooted tooth. Periapical granulomas represent approximately 75 percent of apical inflammatory lesions and 50 percent of those that have failed to respond to conservative endodontic measures.

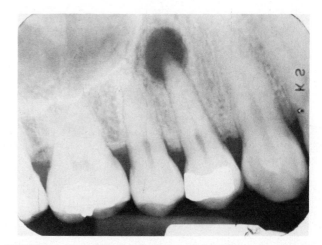

FIGURE 3–17. **Periapical granuloma.** Well-defined radiolucency associated with the apex of the maxillary first bicuspid. (Courtesy of Dr. Frank Beylotte.)

Most lesions are discovered on routine radiographic examination. A radiolucency of variable size is present, and the affected tooth shows loss of the apical lamina dura. The lesion may be circumscribed or ill defined. The size is variable, ranging from small barely perceptible lesions to lucencies exceeding 2 cm in diameter (Figs. 3–16 to 3–18). Root resorption is not uncommon (Fig. 3–19). Although lesions greater than 200 mm^2 often represent periapical cysts, numerous investigators have been unable to distinguish periapical granulomas from periapical cysts on the basis of only size and radiographic appearance.

Histopathologic Features

Periapical granulomas consist of inflamed granulation tissue surrounded by a fibrous connective wall. The

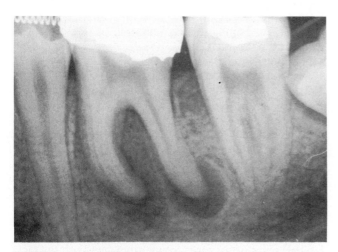

FIGURE 3–16. **Periapical granulomas.** Discrete periapical radiolucencies associated with the apices of the mandibular first molar. (Courtesy of Dr. Garth Bobrowski.)

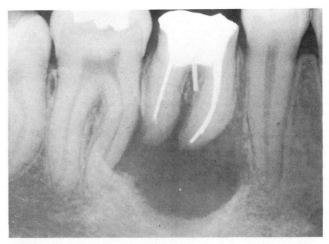

FIGURE 3–18. **Periapical granuloma.** Large, well-defined radiolucency associated with the apices of the mandibular first molar. (Courtesy of Dr. Robert E. Loy.)

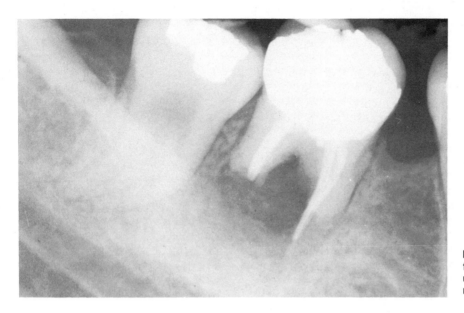

FIGURE 3-19. **Periapical granuloma.** Ill-defined radiolucency associated with the mandibular first molar, which exhibits significant root resorption.

granulation tissue demonstrates a variably dense lymphocytic infiltrate that is frequently intermixed with neutrophils, plasma cells, histiocytes, and, less frequently, mast cells and eosinophils (Fig. 3-20). When numerous plasma cells are present, scattered eosinophilic globules of gamma globulin *(Russell bodies)* may be seen. In addition, clusters of lightly basophilic particles *(pyronine bodies)* also may be present in association with the plasmacytic infiltrate. Both of these plasma cell products are not specific for the periapical granuloma and may be found within any accumulation of plasma cells. Epithelial rests of Malassez may be identified within the granulation tissue. Collections of cholesterol clefts with associated multinucleated giant cells and areas of red blood cell extravasation with hemosiderin pigmentation may be present.

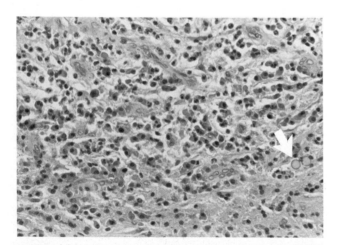

FIGURE 3-20. **Periapical granuloma.** Granulation tissue exhibits mixed inflammatory infiltrate consisting of lymphocytes, plasma cells, histiocytes, and polymorphonuclear leukocytes. Note two adjacent round Russell bodies on the right side of the field of view *(arrow).*

Treatment and Prognosis

Apical inflammatory lesions result from the presence of bacteria or their toxic products in the root canal, the apical tissues, or both. Successful treatment centers on the reduction and elimination of the offending organisms. If the tooth can be maintained, root canal therapy can be performed. Nonrestorable teeth must be extracted, followed by curettage of all apical soft tissue.

Unless they are symptomatic, teeth treated endodontically should be evaluated at 1- and 2-year intervals at a minimum to rule out possible lesional enlargement and to ensure appropriate healing. In addition, many clinicians believe that evaluations at 1, 3, and 6 months are appropriate. Strong emphasis should be placed on the importance of the recall appointments. Lesions may fail to heal for several reasons:

- Cyst formation
- Inadequate endodontics (missed canals, perforated canals, inadequate instrumentation or fill)
- Vertical root fractures
- Periapical foreign material
- Associated periodontal disease
- Penetration of the adjacent maxillary sinus

Following conventional adequate endodontic measures, lesions that do not resolve or that enlarge should be treated with periapical surgery, biopsy, and retrofill of the apices. Standard of care dictates that any tissue warranting removal during apical surgery also warrants a microscopic diagnosis.

On occasion, the defect created by periapical inflammatory lesions may fill with dense collagenous tissue rather than normal bone (Fig. 3-21). These **fibrous (periapical) scars** occur most frequently when both the facial and lingual cortical plates have been lost, but in rare instances they may result from loss of only one plate (Fig. 3-22). If during surgery both plates are discovered to be

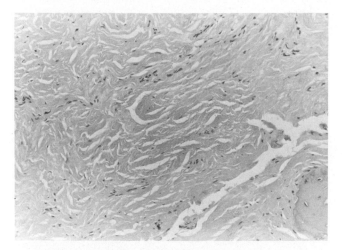

FIGURE 3–21. **Periapical fibrous scar.** Dense, fibrous connective tissue with vital bone and no significant inflammatory infiltrate.

and cellular debris. As the epithelium desquamates into the lumen, the protein content is increased. Fluid enters the lumen in an attempt to equalize the osmotic pressure, and slow enlargement occurs. Most periapical cysts grow slowly and do not attain a large size.

On occasion, a similar cyst, best termed a **lateral radicular cyst,** may appear along the lateral aspect of the root. Like the periapical cyst, this lesion also usually arises from rests of Malassez, and the source of inflammation may be periodontal disease or pulpal necrosis with spread through a lateral foramen. Radiographically, these cysts mimic developmental **lateral periodontal cysts** (see p. 504); histopathologically, however, they are consistent with cysts of inflammatory origin.

Periapical inflammatory tissue that is not curetted at the time of tooth removal may give rise to an inflammatory cyst, called a **residual periapical cyst**. With time, many of these cysts exhibit an overall reduction in size, and spontaneous resolution can occur from a lack of continued inflammatory stimulus.

missing, the patient should be informed of the possibility of scar formation. The development of a periapical scar is not an indication for future surgery.

PERIAPICAL CYST (Radicular Cyst; Apical Periodontal Cyst)

Epithelium at the apex of a nonvital tooth presumably can be stimulated by inflammation to form a true epithelium-lined cyst, or **periapical cyst**. The source of the epithelium is usually rests of Malassez but also may be traced to crevicular epithelium, sinus lining, or epithelial lining of fistulous tracts. Cyst development is common; the reported frequency varies from 7 to 54 percent of periapical radiolucencies. In large reviews of tissue retrieved from lesions that have not responded to conventional endodontics, the prevalence of periapical cysts is approximately 35 percent, with the frequency of occurrence greater in the maxilla.

Periapical cysts represent a fibrous connective tissue wall lined by epithelium with a lumen containing fluid

Clinical and Radiographic Features

Periapical Cysts

Typically, patients with periapical cysts have no symptoms unless there is an acute inflammatory exacerbation. In addition, if the cyst reaches a large size, swelling and mild sensitivity may be noted. Movement and mobility of adjacent teeth are possible as the cyst enlarges. The tooth of origin does not respond to thermal and electric pulp testing.

The radiographic pattern is identical to that of a **periapical granuloma**. Cysts may develop even in small periapical radiolucencies, and the radiographic size cannot be used for the definitive diagnosis (Figs. 3–23 and 3–24). There is a loss of the lamina dura along the adjacent root, and a rounded radiolucency encircles the affected tooth apex (Fig. 3–25). Root resorption is common (Fig. 3–26). With enlargement, the radiolucency often flattens out as it approaches adjacent teeth. Significant growth is possible, and lesions occupying an entire quadrant have

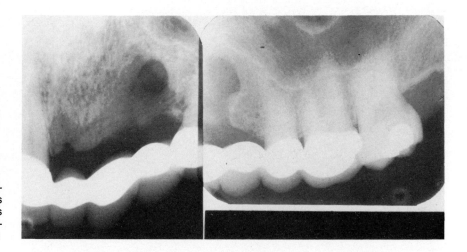

FIGURE 3–22. **Periapical fibrous scar.** Periapical radiolucency of maxilla at the previous site of extraction in which both cortical plates were lost. The site was filled with dense collagenous tissue. (Courtesy of Dr. Brent Klinger.)

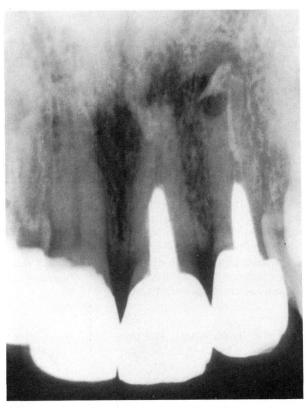

FIGURE 3–23. **Periapical cyst.** Discrete, ill-defined radiolucency associated with the maxillary left central incisor.

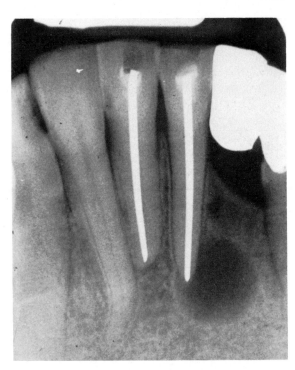

FIGURE 3–25. **Periapical cyst.** Well-circumscribed radiolucency intimately associated with the apex of the mandibular central incisor. Note the loss of lamina dura in the area of the lesion.

been noted (Fig. 3–27). Although periapical cysts more frequently achieve greater size than periapical granulomas, neither the size nor the shape of the lesion can be considered a definitive diagnostic criterion.

Lateral Radicular Cysts

Lateral radicular cysts present as discrete radiolucencies along the lateral aspect of the root (Figs. 3–28 and 3–29). Loss of lamina dura and an obvious source of

inflammation may not be detected without a high index of suspicion. Before surgical exploration of laterally positioned radiolucencies, a thorough evaluation of the periodontal status and vitality of adjacent teeth should be performed.

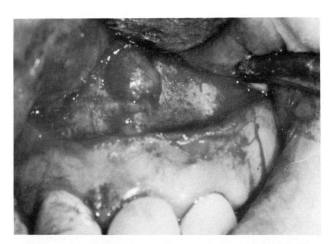

FIGURE 3–24. **Periapical cyst.** Same patient as depicted in Figure 3–23. Note the clinically significant cyst, which was not fully appreciated on the radiograph. (Courtesy of Dr. Brian Blocher.)

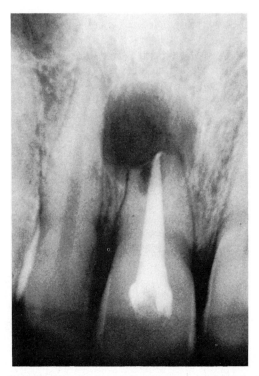

FIGURE 3–26. **Periapical cyst.** Radiolucency associated with the maxillary central incisor, which exhibits significant root resorption.

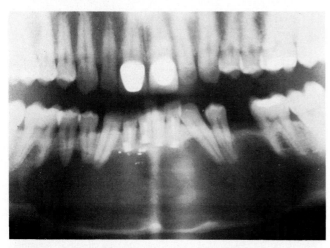

FIGURE 3–27. **Periapical cyst.** Large unilocular radiolucency extending from the mandibular first molar to the contralateral first molar. (Courtesy of Dr. John R. Cramer.)

Residual Periapical Cysts

The residual periapical cyst presents as a round to oval radiolucency of variable size within the alveolar ridge at the site of a previous tooth extraction (Figs. 3–30 to

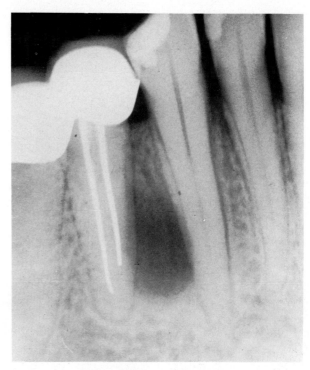

FIGURE 3–29. **Lateral radicular cyst.** Inter-radicular radiolucency associated with the nonvital mandibular first bicuspid. The lesion was a cyst that resulted from the spread of pulpal inflammation from a lateral foramen. (Courtesy of Dr. William Fournier.)

3–32). As the cyst ages, degeneration of the cellular contents within the lumen occasionally leads to dystrophic calcification and central luminal radiopacity (Fig. 3–33).

Histopathologic Features

The histopathologic features of all three types of inflammatory cysts are similar. The cyst is lined by stratified squamous epithelium, which may demonstrate exocytosis, spongiosis, and/or hyperplasia (Fig. 3–34). The lumen will be filled with fluid and cellular debris. On

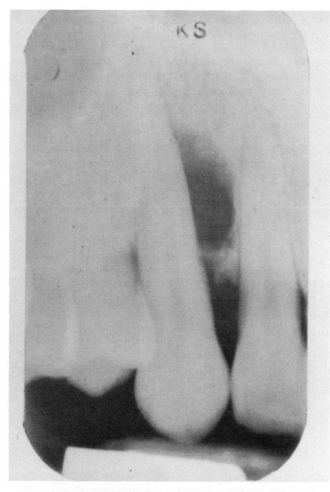

FIGURE 3–28. **Lateral radicular cyst.** An inter-radicular radiolucency has developed as a result of periodontal inflammation along the mesial surface of the right maxillary cuspid. (Courtesy of Dr. Richard Young.)

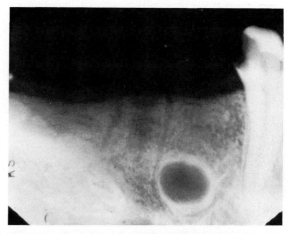

FIGURE 3–30. **Residual periapical cyst.** Persistent radiolucency of the mandibular body at site of previous tooth extraction.

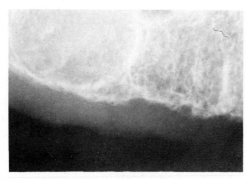

FIGURE 3–31. **Residual periapical cyst.** Well-defined radiolucency of the posterior maxilla.

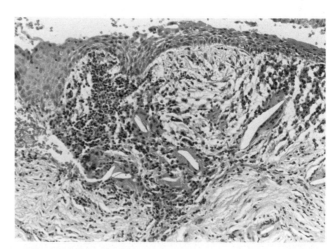

FIGURE 3–34. **Periapical cyst.** Cyst lined by stratified squamous epithelium. Note connective tissue wall, which contains a chronic inflammatory infiltrate and scattered cholesterol clefts with associated multinucleated giant cells.

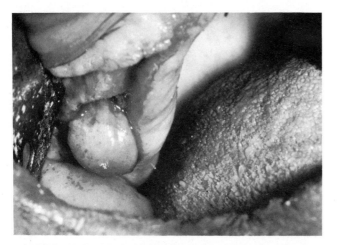

FIGURE 3–32. **Residual periapical cyst.** Same patient as depicted in Figure 3–31. A soft tissue cyst extrudes from the maxillary alveolar ridge after surgical exposure of the site. (Courtesy of Dr. Denise E. Clarke.)

occasion, the lining epithelium may demonstrate linear or arch-shaped calcifications known as *Rushton bodies* (Fig. 3–35). Dystrophic calcification, cholesterol clefts with multinucleated giant cells, red blood cells, and areas of hemosiderin pigmentation may be present in the lumen, wall, or both (see Fig. 3–34). The wall of the cyst consists of dense fibrous connective tissue, often with an inflammatory infiltrate containing lymphocytes variably intermixed with neutrophils, plasma cells, histiocytes and, rarely, mast cells and eosinophils (see Fig. 3–34).

Treatment and Prognosis

A periapical cyst is treated in the same manner as a periapical granuloma. When clinical and radiographic features point to a periapical inflammatory lesion, ex-

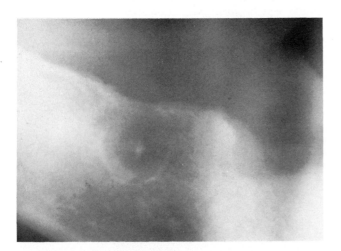

FIGURE 3–33. **Residual periapical cyst.** Radiolucency with central radiopacity of the right mandibular body.

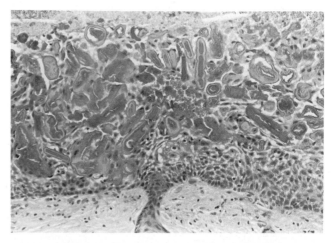

FIGURE 3–35. **Periapical cyst.** Squamous epithelial cyst lining exhibits numerous linear and arch-shaped Rushton bodies.

traction or conservative nonsurgical endodontic therapy is performed. Larger lesions associated with restorable teeth have been treated successfully with conservative endodontic therapy when combined with biopsy and marsupialization, decompression, or fenestration. As with any suspected periapical inflammatory lesion, minimal follow-up at 1 and 2 years is strongly advised.

If the radiolucency fails to resolve and the initial endodontic therapy appears to be of less than optimal quality, the lesion often can be successfully managed by nonsurgical endodontic retreatment. However, if the initial endodontic therapy appears adequate and the lesion has not healed, periapical surgery and biopsy are indicated to rule out other possible pathologic processes. Biopsy also is required if lesions associated with endodontically treated teeth demonstrate enlargement on follow-up.

Because any number of odontogenic and non-odontogenic cysts and tumors can mimic the appearance of a residual periapical cyst, all of these cysts should be surgically excised. All inflammatory foci in the area of a lateral radicular cyst should be eliminated and the patient observed in a manner similar to that described for the periapical cyst. In some instances, lateral radicular cysts are removed before thorough evaluation for the source of the inflammation. If this diagnosis is made, a thorough evaluation for an inflammatory source is mandatory.

Cysts of inflammatory origin do not recur after appropriate management. Fibrous scars are possible, especially when both cortical plates have been lost. In rare instances, development of squamous cell carcinoma has been reported within periapical cysts; therefore, even in the absence of symptoms, treatment is required for all persistent intrabony pathosis.

PERIAPICAL ABSCESS

The accumulation of acute inflammatory cells at the apex of a nonvital tooth is termed a **periapical abscess.** Acute inflammatory lesions with abscess formation may arise as the initial periapical pathosis or from an acute exacerbation (**phoenix abscess**) of a chronic periapical inflammatory lesion. Frequently, the source of the infection is obvious; on occasion, however, pulpal death may be trauma-related and the tooth may contain neither a cavity nor a restoration.

In the very earliest stage, the periapical periodontal ligament fibers may exhibit acute inflammation but no frank abscess formation. This localized alteration, best termed **acute apical periodontitis,** may or may not proceed to abscess formation. Although this process often occurs in association with a nonvital tooth, acute apical periodontitis may present in vital teeth secondary to trauma, high occlusal contacts, or wedging by a foreign object. The clinical presentation often closely resembles that of a periapical abscess and must be considered in the differential diagnosis.

Clinical and Radiographic Features

Many investigators subdivide periapical abscesses into **acute** and **chronic** types, but these are misnomers because both types represent acute inflammatory reactions. Periapical abscesses should be designated as **symptomatic** or **asymptomatic** on the basis of their clinical presentations.

Periapical abscesses become symptomatic as the purulent material accumulates within the alveolus. The initial stages produce tenderness of the affected tooth that is often relieved by direct application of pressure. With progression, the pain becomes more intense, often with extreme sensitivity to percussion, extrusion of the tooth, and swelling of the tissues. The offending tooth does not respond to cold or electric pulp testing. Headache, malaise, fever, and chills may be present.

Radiographically, abscesses may demonstrate a thickening of the apical periodontal ligament, an ill-defined radiolucency, or both, but often no appreciable alterations can be detected because there has been insufficient time for significant bone destruction. Phoenix abscesses demonstrate the outline of the original chronic lesion with or without an associated ill-defined bone loss.

With progression, the abscess spreads along the path of least resistance. The purulence may extend through the medullary spaces away from the apical area, resulting in **osteomyelitis,** or it may perforate the cortex and spread diffusely through the overlying soft tissue as **cellulitis.** Each of these occurrences is described later in the chapter.

Once an abscess is in soft tissue, it can cause cellulitis or it may channelize through the overlying soft tissue. The cortical plate may be perforated in a location that permits entrance into the oral cavity. The purulent material can accumulate in the connective tissue overlying the bone and can create a sessile swelling or perforate through the surface epithelium and drain through an intraoral sinus (Fig. 3–36 and 3–37). At the distal opening of an intraoral sinus tract, there is often a mass of subacutely inflamed granulation tissue known as a **parulis (gum boil)** (Figs. 3–38 and 3–39). On occasion, the

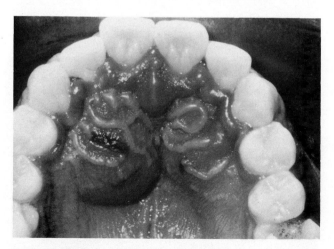

FIGURE 3–36. **Periapical abscess.** Bilateral soft tissue swelling of the anterior palate.

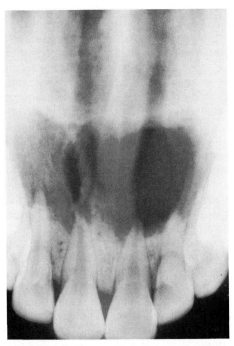

FIGURE 3–37. **Periapical abscess.** Same patient as depicted in Figure 3–36. Multiple, overlapping radiolucencies of the anterior maxilla are present. All four maxillary incisors exhibit pulpal necrosis.

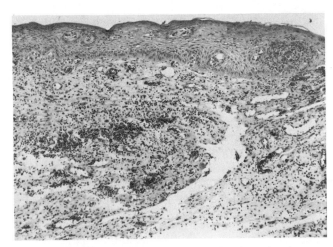

FIGURE 3–39. **Parulis.** The normal connective tissue has been replaced by acutely inflamed granulation tissue, which exhibits focal areas of neutrophilic abscess formation. Note the central sinus tract, which courses from the base of the specimen toward the surface epithelium.

nonvital tooth associated with the parulis may be difficult to determine, and insertion of a gutta-percha point into the tract can aid in detection of the offending tooth during radiographic examination (Figs. 3–40 and 3–41). Dental abscesses also may channelize through the overlying skin and drain via a **cutaneous sinus** (Fig. 3–42).

Most dental-related abscesses perforate buccally because the bone is thinner on the buccal surface. In contrast, infections associated with maxillary lateral incisors, the palatal roots of maxillary molars, and mandibular second and third molars typically drain through the lingual cortical plate.

If a chronic path of drainage is achieved, a periapical abscess typically becomes asymptomatic because of a

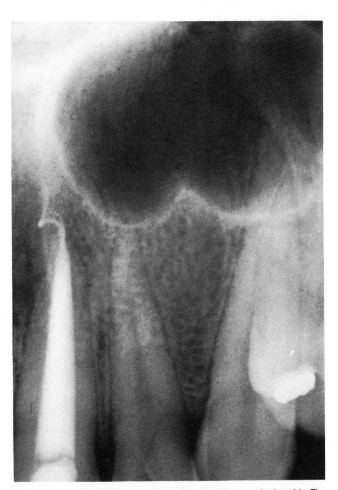

FIGURE 3–40. **Periapical abscess.** Same patient as depicted in Figure 3–38. None of the incisors demonstrates an obvious periapical radiolucency. (The large radiolucency at the top is the anterior portion of the maxillary sinus.)

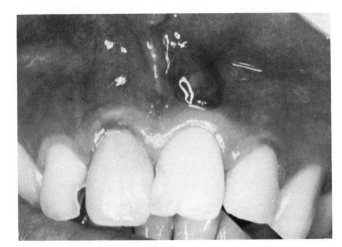

FIGURE 3–38. **Parulis.** Erythematous mass of granulation tissue overlying the left maxillary central incisor. Note discoloration of the maxillary right central incisor.

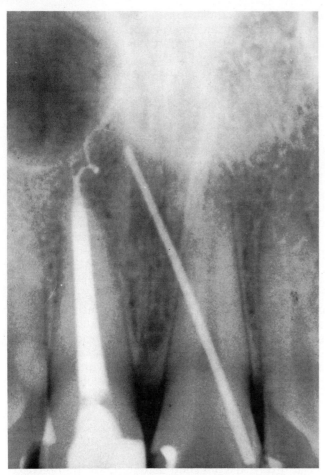

FIGURE 3–41. **Periapical abscess.** Same patient as depicted in Figures 3–38 and 3–40. Gutta-percha point revealed that the right maxillary incisor was the source of the infection.

lack of accumulation of purulent material within the alveolus. Not infrequently, such infections are discovered during a routine oral examination after detection of a parulis or drainage through a large carious defect (Figs. 3–43 [see Color Figure 18] and 3–44). If the drainage

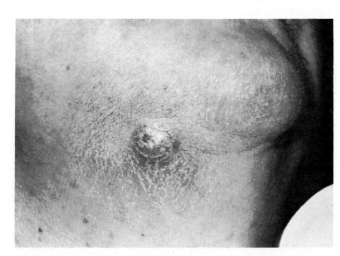

FIGURE 3–42. **Cutaneous sinus.** Erythematous, firm, and sensitive enlargement of the skin inferior to the right body of the mandible.

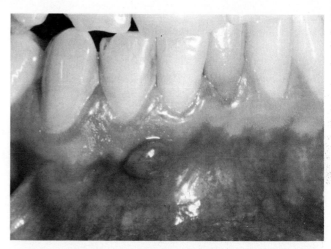

FIGURE 3–43. **Parulis.** Asymptomatic yellowish nodule of the anterior mandibular alveolar ridge. Adjacent teeth were clinically normal and also asymptomatic. See Color Plates.

site becomes blocked, signs and symptoms of the abscess frequently become evident in a short period of time.

The insertion of muscles along the buccal surface of the jaws and the local fasciae help to determine whether a buccally oriented abscess will extend to the surface of the

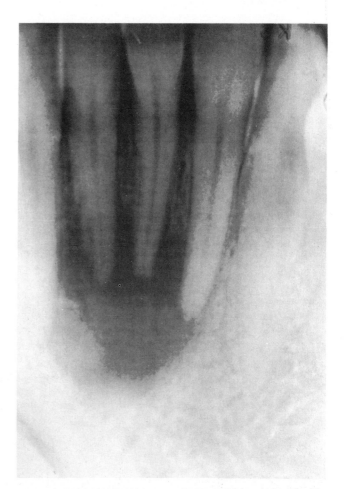

FIGURE 3–44. **Periapical abscess.** Same patient as depicted in Figure 3–43. Periapical radiolucency associated with the nonvital mandibular lateral incisor.

skin, penetrate into the oral cavity, or spread into deeper tissues. The buccinator muscle blocks the spread of infections that are directed buccally from posterior teeth from the oral cavity. These abscesses typically perforate the skin or spread posteriorly, whereas abscesses from the bicuspids can gain access to the oral cavity.

Because of unobstructed access, most buccally oriented infections from anterior teeth achieve intraoral drainage, but infections from teeth with apices located beyond the insertion of the muscles of facial expression typically are blocked from the oral cavity. Abscesses from maxillary canines and mandibular incisors and canines frequently are forced exteriorly because of the insertion of the overlying musculature.

Histopathologic Features

Biopsy specimens from pure abscesses are uncommon because the material is in liquid form. Abscesses consist of a sea of polymorphonuclear leukocytes often intermixed with inflammatory exudate, cellular debris, necrotic material, bacterial colonies, or histiocytes (Fig. 3–45).

Phoenix abscesses can maintain a soft tissue component; they present as subacutely inflamed periapical granulomas or cysts intermixed with areas of significant abscess formation.

Treatment and Prognosis

Treatment of the patient with a periapical abscess consists of drainage and elimination of the focus of infection. Those abscesses associated with a patent sinus tract may be asymptomatic but, nevertheless, should be treated. With localized periapical abscesses, the signs and symptoms typically diminish significantly within 48 hours of initiation of appropriate drainage. If the affected tooth is extruded, reduction of the occlusion is recommended. Analgesics and antibiotics are administered in more severe cases. Once the infection has been resolved by extraction or appropriate endodontic therapy, the affected bone typically heals.

Usually, a parulis resolves spontaneously after the of-

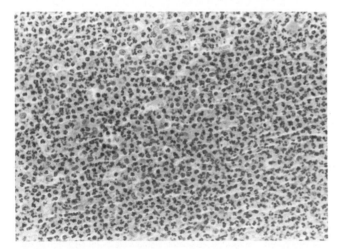

FIGURE 3–45. **Periapical abscess.** Sheet of polymorphonuclear leukocytes intermixed with scattered histiocytes.

fending tooth is extracted or endodontically treated. Parulides that persist are thought to contain sufficient infectious material along the fistulous tract to maintain the surface granulation tissue, and surgical removal with curettage of the tract is required for resolution.

CELLULITIS

If an abscess is not able to establish drainage through the surface of the skin or into the oral cavity, it may spread diffusely through fascial planes of the soft tissue. This acute and edematous spread of an acute inflammatory process is termed **cellulitis**. Although numerous patterns of cellulitis can be seen from the spread of dental infections, two especially dangerous forms warrant further discussion: **Ludwig's angina** and **cavernous sinus thrombosis**.

Ludwig's angina, named after the German physician who described the seriousness of the disorder in 1836, refers to cellulitis of the submandibular region. Angina comes from the Latin word *angere,* which means "to strangle"—an apt term for the clinical features described next. Ludwig's angina develops from spread of an acute infection from the lower molar teeth in about 70 percent of cases. Other situations associated with this clinical presentation are compound fractures of the mandible, traumatic lacerations of the floor of the mouth, and peritonsillar abscesses.

The submandibular space is divided into the sublingual space above the mylohyoid muscle and the submaxillary space below the muscle. These two spaces communicate freely and function as one. Once the infection enters the submandibular space, it may extend to the lateral pharyngeal space and then to the retropharyngeal space. This extension may result in spread to the mediastinum with several serious consequences.

Another serious pattern can occur when infection from maxillary premolar or molar teeth perforates the buccal cortical plate and extends into the maxillary sinus, the pterygopalatine space, or the infratemporal fossa, reaching the orbit via the inferior orbital fissure. In addition to affecting periorbital structures, the infection can then spread into the cavernous sinus at the cranial vault and cause the extremely serious condition known as cavernous sinus thrombosis. Similar involvement can also occur from maxillary anterior teeth by retrograde spread through the valveless anterior facial, angular, and ophthalmic veins to the orbit. Cavernous sinus thrombosis is relatively uncommon, and orodental infections are responsible in approximately 10 percent of the cases.

Clinical Features

Ludwig's Angina

Ludwig's angina presents as a swelling of the floor of mouth, tongue, and submandibular region (Fig. 3–46). Involvement of the sublingual space results in elevation, posterior enlargement, and protrusion of the tongue *(woody tongue).* Submandibular space spread causes enlargement and tenderness of the neck above the level of the hyoid bone *(bull neck).* Although initially unilateral, spread to the contralateral neck typically occurs. Pain in

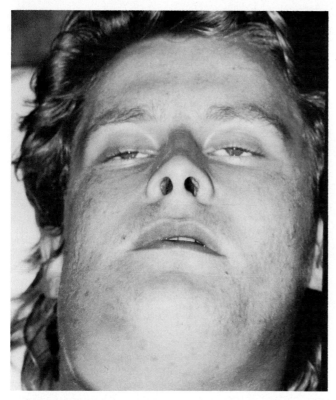

FIGURE 3–46. **Ludwig's angina.** Soft tissue swelling of the right submandibular region. (Courtesy of Dr. Brian Blocher.)

the neck and floor of mouth may be seen in addition to restricted neck movement, dysphagia, dysphonia, dysarthria, drooling, and sore throat. Involvement of the lateral pharyngeal space can cause respiratory obstruction secondary to laryngeal edema. Tachypnea, dyspnea, tachycardia, stridor, restlessness, and the patient's need to maintain an erect position suggest airway obstruction. Fever, chills, leukocytosis, and an elevated sedimentation rate may be seen. Classically, obvious collections of pus are not present.

Cavernous Sinus Thrombosis

Cavernous sinus thrombosis presents as edematous periorbital enlargement with involvement of the eyelids and conjunctiva (Fig. 3–47). Protrusion and fixation of the eyeball are often evident in addition to induration and swelling of the adjacent forehead and nose. Pupil dilation, lacrimation, photophobia, and loss of vision may occur. Pain over the eye and along the distribution of the ophthalmic and maxillary branches of the trigeminal nerve often are present.

Fever, chills, sweating, tachycardia, nausea, and vomiting can occur. With progression, signs of central nervous system involvement develop. Meningitis, tachycardia, tachypnea, irregular breathing, stiffening of the neck, and deepening stupor with or without delirium indicate advanced toxemia and meningeal involvement. Occasionally, brain abscesses may result.

Treatment and Prognosis

Modern interventions and antibiotics have altered the course of these dangerous forms of cellulitis and have dramatically reduced the mortality and morbidity. With appropriate therapy, the incidence of mortality associated with Ludwig's angina has diminished from 60 percent to approximately 8 percent.

Treatment of cavernous sinus thrombosis has met with similar success, but if it is not diagnosed and treated early, morbidity such as blindness can occur.

Ludwig's Angina

Treatment of Ludwig's angina centers around three activities:

1. Maintenance of the airway.
2. Antibiotic therapy.
3. Surgical drainage.

If signs or symptoms of impending airway obstruction develop, endotracheal intubation or tracheostomy is performed. Because intubation may cause laryngospasm or discharge of pus into the bronchial tree, tracheostomy is preferred if there is any chance of significant intubation complications.

High-dose penicillin is the antibiotic of choice. Aminoglycosides are given for resistant organisms, and clindamycin or chloramphenicol is used in penicillin-sensitive

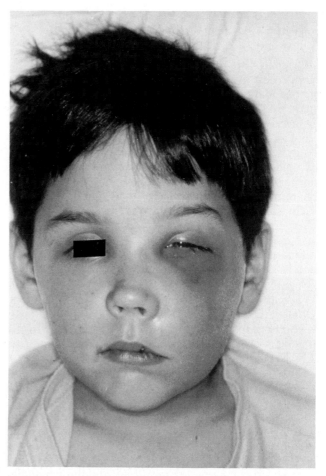

FIGURE 3–47. **Cavernous sinus thrombosis.** Erythematous and edematous enlargement of the left side of the face with involvement of the eyelids and conjunctiva. (Courtesy of Dr. Richard Ziegler.)

patients. The antibiotic therapy is adjusted according to the patient's response and culture results from aspirates of fluid from the enlargements. Some authors recommend the addition of corticosteroids in patients who do not respond to appropriate antibiotic therapy and surgical intervention, but the effectiveness of this addition has not been thoroughly investigated.

Significant accumulation of purulent material is rare. When fluctuance is present, however, surgical drainage is required. If the infection remains diffuse, indurated, and brawny, surgical intervention is at the discretion of the clinician and is often governed by the patient's response to noninvasive therapy.

Cavernous Sinus Thrombosis

The therapeutic cornerstone of cavernous sinus thrombosis secondary to dental infections is high-dose antibiotics similar to those administered for patients with Ludwig's angina. The offending tooth should be extracted, and drainage is required if fluctuance is present. Corticosteroids also are given to decrease inflammation and prevent vascular collapse from pituitary dysfunction. Some investigators also prescribe anticoagulants to prevent thrombosis and septic emboli; others believe that thrombosis limits the infection and that the use of anticoagulants may promote hemorrhagic lesions in the orbit and brain.

OSTEOMYELITIS

Osteomyelitis can be an acute or chronic inflammatory process in the medullary spaces or cortical surfaces of bone that extends away from the initial site of involvement, usually a bacterial infection. **Osteoradionecrosis** is excluded from this discussion because this is primarily a problem of hypoxia, hypocellularity, and hypovascularity, in which the presence of bacteria represents a secondary colonization of non-healing bone rather than a primary bacterial infection (see p. 220). Several patterns of inflammatory bone disease (e.g., **focal** and **diffuse sclerosing osteomyelitis**, **proliferative periostitis**, **alveolar osteitis**) are unique and are covered separately later in the chapter.

True progressive osteomyelitis of the jaws is uncommon in developed countries but continues to be a source of significant difficulties in developing nations. In Europe and North America, most cases arise following odontogenic infections or traumatic fracture of the jaws. In addition, many cases reported in Africa occur in the presence of acute necrotizing ulcerative gingivitis (ANUG) or noma.

Chronic systemic diseases, immunocompromised status, and disorders associated with decreased vascularity of bone appear to predispose people to osteomyelitis. Tobacco use, alcohol abuse, intravenous drug abuse, diabetes mellitus, exanthematous fevers, malaria, anemia, malnutrition, malignancy, and acquired immunodeficiency syndrome (AIDS) have been associated with an increased frequency of osteomyelitis. In addition to radiation, several diseases (e.g., osteopetrosis, dysosteosclerosis, late Paget's disease, end-stage cemento-osseous dysplasia) may result in hypovascularized bone that is predisposed to necrosis and inflammation.

Acute osteomyelitis exists when an acute inflammatory process spreads through the medullary spaces of the bone and there has been insufficient time for the body to react to the presence of the inflammatory infiltrate. **Chronic osteomyelitis** exists when the defensive response leads to the production of granulation tissue, which subsequently forms dense scar in an attempt to wall off the infected area. The encircled dead space acts as a reservoir for bacteria, and antibiotics have great difficulty reaching the site. A smoldering process results that is difficult to manage unless the problem is approached aggressively.

Clinical and Radiographic Features

Patients of all ages can be affected by osteomyelitis. There is a strong male predominance, approaching 75 percent in some reviews. Most cases involve the mandible. Maxillary disease becomes important primarily in pediatric patients and in cases that arise from ANUG or noma (i.e., in African populations).

Acute Osteomyelitis

Patients with acute osteomyelitis have signs and symptoms of an acute inflammatory process that typically has been less than 1 month in duration. Fever, leukocytosis, lymphadenopathy, significant sensitivity, and soft tissue swelling of the affected area may be present. The radiographs may be unremarkable or may demonstrate an ill-defined radiolucency (Fig. 3–48). On occasion, paresthesia of the lower lip, drainage, or exfoliation of fragments of necrotic bone may be discovered. A fragment of necrotic bone that has separated from the adjacent vital bone is termed a *sequestrum*. Sequestra often exhibit spontaneous exfoliation (Fig. 3–49). On occasion, fragments of necrotic bone may become surrounded by vital bone, and the mass of encased nonvital bone is called an *involucrum*.

Chronic Osteomyelitis

If acute osteomyelitis is not resolved expeditiously, the entrenchment of chronic osteomyelitis occurs, or the pro-

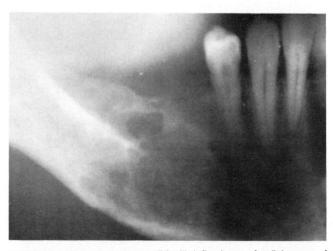

FIGURE 3–48. **Acute osteomyelitis.** Ill-defined area of radiolucency of the right body of the mandible.

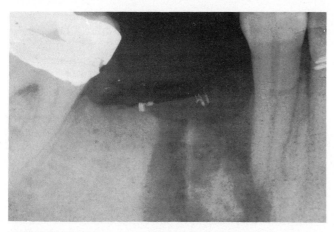

FIGURE 3–49. **Acute osteomyelitis with sequestrum.** Radiolucency of the right body of the mandible with central radiopaque mass of necrotic bone. (Courtesy of Dr. Michael Meyrowitz.)

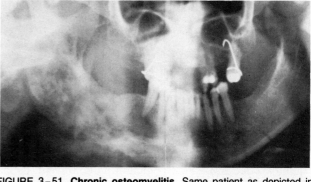

FIGURE 3–51. **Chronic osteomyelitis.** Same patient as depicted in Figure 3–50. After the initial intervention, the patient failed to return for follow-up because of lack of significant pain. An enlarged, ill-defined radiolucency of the right body of the mandible was discovered 2 years after the initial surgery. (Courtesy of Dr. Charles Waldron.)

cess may arise primarily without a previous acute episode. There may be swelling, pain, sinus formation, purulent discharge, sequestrum formation, tooth loss, or pathologic fracture. Patients may experience acute exacerbations or periods of decreased pain associated with chronic smoldering progression (Figs. 3–50 and 3–51).

Radiographs reveal a patchy, ragged, and ill-defined radiolucency that often contains central radiopaque sequestra. On occasion, the surrounding bone may exhibit an increased radiodensity, and the cortical surface can demonstrate significant osteogenic periosteal hyperplasia.

Because of an anatomic peculiarity, large portions of each bone receive their blood supply through multiple arterial loops originating from a single vessel. Involvement of this single feeder vessel can lead to necrosis of a large portion of the affected bone. Sequestration that has involved an entire quadrant of the jaw has been reported in longstanding cases of chronic osteomyelitis.

Histopathologic Features

Acute Osteomyelitis

Generation of biopsy material from patients with acute osteomyelitis is not common because of the predominantly liquid content and lack of a soft tissue component. When submitted, the material consists predominantly of necrotic bone. The bone shows a loss of the osteocytes from their lacunae, peripheral resorption, and bacterial colonization (Fig. 3–52). The periphery of the bone and the haversian canals contain necrotic debris and an acute inflammatory infiltrate consisting of polymorphonuclear leukocytes. The submitted material will be diagnosed as a sequestrum unless a good clinicopathologic correlation points to the appropriate diagnosis of acute osteomyelitis.

Chronic Osteomyelitis

Biopsy material from patients with chronic osteomyelitis demonstrates a significant soft tissue component that consists of chronically or subacutely inflamed fibrous connective tissue filling the intertrabecular areas of the

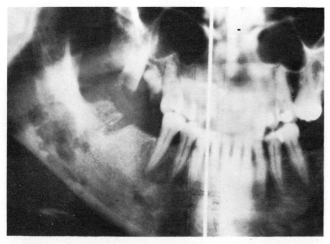

FIGURE 3–50. **Chronic osteomyelitis.** Ill-defined area of radiolucency of the right body of the mandible adjacent to a recent extraction site. (Courtesy of Dr. Charles Waldron.)

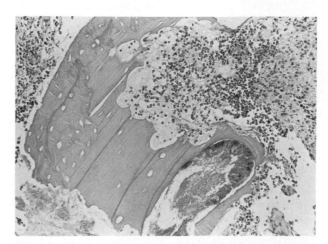

FIGURE 3–52. **Acute osteomyelitis.** Nonvital bone exhibits loss of the osteocytes from the lacunae. Peripheral resorption, bacterial colonization, and surrounding inflammatory response also can be seen.

bone. Scattered sequestra and pockets of abscess formation are common.

Treatment and Prognosis

Acute Osteomyelitis

If obvious abscess formation is noted, the treatment of acute osteomyelitis consists of antibiotics and drainage. Microbiologic study of the infectious material typically reveals a polymicrobial infection of organisms normally present in the oral cavity. The antibiotics most frequently selected include penicillin, clindamycin, cephalexin, cefotaxime, tobramycin, and gentamicin.

In most patients, a sufficient and appropriate antibiotic regimen aborts the infection and averts the need for surgical intervention. Several investigators have suggested that antibiotic therapy can bring about sterilization of the sequestra; therefore, these nonvital bone fragments should be allowed to remain in place as a scaffolding for the future development of new bone.

Chronic Osteomyelitis

Chronic osteomyelitis is difficult to manage medically because pockets of dead bone and organisms are protected from antibiotics by the surrounding wall of fibrous connective tissue. Surgical intervention is mandatory. The antibiotics are similar to those used in the acute form but must be given intravenously in high dosages.

The extent of the surgical intervention depends on the spread of the process. Removal of all infected material down to good bleeding bone is mandatory in all cases. For small lesions, curettage, removal of necrotic bone, and saucerization are sufficient. In patients with more extensive osteomyelitis, decortication or saucerization is often combined with transplantation of cancellous bone chips. In cases of persisting osteomyelitis, resection of the diseased bone, followed by immediate reconstruction with an autologous graft, is required. Weakened jawbones must be immobilized.

Several promising advances have been made in the management of persistent cases of chronic osteomyelitis.

Scintigraphic techniques with technetium-99m (^{99m}Tc-labeled phosphorus compounds) can be used to evaluate the therapeutic response and progress of treatment. Hyperbaric oxygen has been beneficial, but it is recommended primarily for patients who are resistant to the standard therapeutic approach or for disease arising in hypovascularized bone (e.g., osteoradionecrosis, osteopetrosis, Paget's disease, cemento-osseous dysplasia). Finally, direct delivery of antibiotics has been achieved through the use of antibiotic-impregnated polymethylmethacrylate beads implanted into areas of chronic osteomyelitis that have been resistant to other therapeutic approaches.

DIFFUSE SCLEROSING OSTEOMYELITIS AND CHRONIC TENDOPERIOSTITIS

Numerous disease entities have been included under the category of **diffuse sclerosing osteomyelitis**, but this term should be used only when an infectious process is directly responsible for sclerosis of bone. Diseases in which altered bone is secondarily affected by inflammation, such as **florid cemento-osseous dysplasia** (see p. 467) and **chronic tendoperiostitis**, do not represent true primary sclerosing osteomyelitis.

If a direct correlation with a primary infection is required for the diagnosis, diffuse sclerosing osteomyelitis is an extremely rare process. Most cases reported as "diffuse sclerosing osteomyelitis" most likely represent a process that is better termed chronic tendoperiostitis.

Clinical and Radiographic Features

Diffuse Sclerosing Osteomyelitis

Diffuse sclerosing osteomyelitis is similar to the localized variant (**condensing osteitis** [see p. 117]) but is also very different. The disorder arises almost exclusively in adulthood and does not exhibit a sex predominance. It presents primarily in the mandible. An increased radiodensity develops around sites of chronic infection (periodontitis, pericoronitis, apical inflammatory disease) in a manner very similar to the increased radiodensity that may be seen surrounding areas of chronic suppurative osteomyelitis. Typically, the altered area is restricted to a single site, but it may be multifocal or extend to fill an entire quadrant.

The sclerosis centers around the crestal portions of the tooth-bearing alveolar ridge and does not appear to originate in the areas of attachment of the masseter or digastric muscle (Fig. 3–53). The radiodensities do not develop from previously radiolucent fibro-osseous lesions and do not exhibit the predilection for black females, as is found in those patients with florid cemento-osseous dysplasia. Pain and swelling are not typical.

Chronic Tendoperiostitis

Although initially thought to be an obscure infectious process, chronic tendoperiostitis may represent a reactive hyperplasia of bone that is initiated and exacerbated by

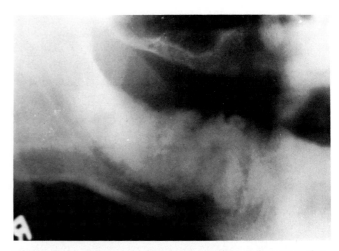

FIGURE 3–53. **Diffuse sclerosing osteomyelitis.** Diffuse area of increased radiodensity of the right body of the mandible in the tooth-bearing area. No other quadrants were involved. (Courtesy of Dr. Louis M. Beto.)

chronic overuse of the masticatory muscles, predominantly the masseter and digastric. In a large series of patients, parafunctional muscle habits, such as bruxism, clenching, nail-biting, co-contraction, or inability to relax jaw musculature, were known or became evident during follow-up. In neurophysiologic studies, masseter inhibitory reflexes were abnormal in the vast majority.

Although the mean age of occurrence is 40, the process may occur in people of all ages. There is no sex predilection. Recurrent pain, swelling of the cheek, and trismus are classic symptoms. Suppuration and an associated infectious cause are not found. Uncommon spontaneous resolution with development of radiographic normalcy has been noted.

In most instances, the sclerosis is limited to a single quadrant and centers around the anterior region of the mandibular angle and posterior portion of the mandibular body (attachment of the masseter muscle). Occasionally, there may be involvement in the cuspid-premolar region and the anterior mandible (attachment of the digastric muscle). Relatively radiolucent zones are apparent within the areas of radiodensity, but histopathologic examination reveals only dense bone, formation of reactive bone, and relatively few signs of inflammation. The inferior border of the mandibular body is typically affected, and significant erosion of the inferior border appears just anterior to the angle of the mandible.

Histopathologic Features

Diffuse Sclerosing Osteomyelitis

Diffuse sclerosing osteomyelitis presents with sclerosis and remodeling of bone. The haversian canals are widely scattered, and little marrow tissue can be found. Although the sclerosis occurs adjacent to areas of inflammation, the bone typically is not intermixed with a significant inflammatory soft tissue component. If the adjacent inflammatory process extends into the sclerotic bone, necrosis often occurs. The necrotic bone separates from the adjacent vital tissue and becomes surrounded by subacutely inflamed granulation tissue. Secondary bacterial colonization often is visible.

Chronic Tendoperiostitis

Chronic tendoperiostitis demonstrates sclerosis and remodeling of the cortical and subcortical bone with a resultant increase in bone volume. If chronic inflammatory cells are present, they are located in cortical resorption defects and the subcortical bone adjacent to sites of muscle insertion.

Treatment and Prognosis

Diffuse Sclerosing Osteomyelitis

Diffuse sclerosing osteomyelitis is best treated through resolution of the adjacent foci of chronic infection. After resolution of the inflammatory causation, the sclerosis remodels in some patients but remains as an area of significant radiodensity in others. The resultant sclerotic bone is hypovascular, does not exhibit typical remodeling, and is very sensitive to inflammation. The patient and the clinician should work together to avoid future

problems with periodontitis or apical inflammatory disease. With long-term alveolar resorption following denture placement, the altered bone does not exhibit typical resorption, and exposure with secondary osteomyelitis can develop. These secondary lesions can be treated in the same fashion as a primary acute or chronic osteomyelitis (see p. 116).

Chronic Tendoperiostitis

Treatment of chronic tendoperiostitis as a form of osteomyelitis has been most unsatisfactory. Large series of patients have been treated with antibiotics, explorations, intraoral decortication, implantation of gentamicin beads, hyperbaric oxygen, and corticosteroids with no significant effect. Treatment directed toward resolution of muscle overuse has resulted in significantly decreased symptoms in most patients and total resolution in a minority. Therapeutic approaches include:

- Muscular relaxation instructions (soft diet, avoidance of parafunctional habits)
- Rotation exercises
- Occlusal splint therapy
- Myofeedback
- Muscle relaxant drugs (diazepam, mefenoxalon).

CONDENSING OSTEITIS (Focal Sclerosing Osteomyelitis)

Localized areas of bone sclerosis associated with the apices of teeth with pulpitis (from large carious lesions or deep coronal restorations) or pulpal necrosis are termed **condensing osteitis**. The association with an area of inflammation is critical because these lesions can resemble several other intrabony processes that produce a somewhat similar pattern.

Clinical and Radiographic Features

This secondary sclerosis of bone is seen most frequently in children and young adults but also can occur in older people. The classic alteration consists of a localized, usually uniform, zone of increased radiodensity adjacent to the apex of a tooth that exhibits a thickened periodontal ligament space or an apical inflammatory lesion (Fig. 3–54). Clinical expansion should not be present. Most cases occur in the premolar and molar areas of the mandible, and the dental pulp of the involved tooth demonstrates pulpitis or necrosis. The lesion does not exhibit a radiolucent border, as is seen in cases of **focal cemento-osseous dysplasia** (see p. 465), although an adjacent radiolucent inflammatory lesion may be present. In addition, the radiopacity is not separated from the apex as would be seen in **idiopathic osteosclerosis** (see p. 447).

Treatment and Prognosis

Treatment of the patient with condensing osteitis consists of resolution of the odontogenic focus of infection.

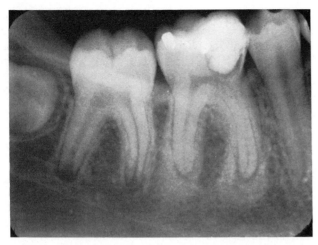

FIGURE 3–54. Condensing osteitis. Increased areas of radiodensity surrounding the apices of the nonvital mandibular first molar.

Following extraction or appropriate endodontic therapy of the involved tooth, approximately 85 percent of cases of condensing osteitis will regress, either partially or totally. Typically, resolution of the lesion is associated with normalization of the associated periodontal membrane. If the lesion persists and the periodontal membrane remains wide, re-evaluation of the endodontic therapy should be considered. A residual area of condensing osteitis which remains after resolution of the inflammatory focus is termed a **bone scar** (Fig. 3–55).

PROLIFERATIVE PERIOSTITIS
(Periostitis Ossificans)

In 1893, a German physician, C. Garrè, reported on patterns of acute osteomyelitis. Since that time, numerous articles have been written that associate Garrè's report with a form of inflammatory periosteal hyperplasia demonstrating an onion skin–like reduplication of the

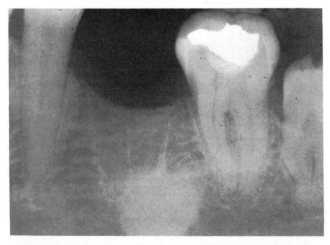

FIGURE 3–55. Bone scar. Residual area of increased radiodensity in the area of extraction of the mandibular first molar. (Courtesy of Dr. Walter Blevins.)

cortical plate. (In these subsequent articles, Garrè's name was consistently misspelled as Garré with an improper accent.) However, Garrè did not have any pathologic specimens for microscopic examination, and Röntgen did not discover x-rays until 2 years after Garrè's publication. Nowhere in the original publication is there any mention of periostitis, periosteal duplication, or "onion skinning." Therefore, although the term "Garrè's osteomyelitis" is often used synonymously for this condition, it is an improper designation for the process, which is described below and should be disassociated with the entity.

Clinical and Radiographic Features

Proliferative periostitis represents a periosteal reaction to the presence of inflammation. The affected periosteum forms several rows of reactive vital bone that parallel each other and expand the surface of the altered bone. This reactive pattern occurs primarily in children and young adults, with a mean age of 13 years. No sex predominance is noted.

As expected, the most frequent cause is dental caries with associated periapical inflammatory disease, although lesions have been reported secondary to periodontal infections, fractures, buccal bifurcation cysts, and non-odontogenic infections. Most cases arise in the premolar-molar area of the mandible. The hyperplasia is located most frequently along the lower border of the mandible, but buccal cortical involvement also is common. Isolated lingual cortical enlargement is infrequent. Most cases are unifocal, although multiple quadrants may be affected.

Appropriate radiographs demonstrate radiopaque laminations of bone that roughly parallel each other and the underlying cortical surface (Fig. 3–56). The laminations vary from 1 to 12 in number, and radiolucent separations often are present between the new bone and the original cortex. Within the new bone, areas of small sequestra or osteolytic radiolucencies may be found. Typically, the alterations are best seen on a panoramic or lateral oblique radiograph. The latter type is often favored because of finer detail of the final image. If lateral oblique radiographs fail to demonstrate the lesion, occlusal views and, less frequently, posteroanterior radiographs may be successful. The radiographic examination should reveal preservation of the underlying cortical surface; if bone destruction is seen in association with the cortical surface or the periosteal new bone, this suggests the possibility of a neoplastic process rather than an inflammatory condition.

Histopathologic Features

Usually, biopsy is not required unless the clinical diagnosis is in question. Specimens often reveal parallel rows of highly cellular and reactive woven bone in which the individual trabeculae frequently are oriented perpendicular to the surface (Fig. 3–57). The trabeculae sometimes form an interconnecting meshwork of bone or are more widely scattered, resembling the pattern seen in immature fibrous dysplasia. Between the cellular trabeculae,

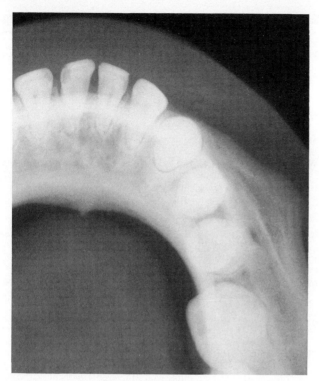

FIGURE 3–56. **Proliferative periostitis.** Radiopaque laminations of cortical bone parallel the cortex adjacent to inflammatory process of the mandibular bicuspid. (Courtesy of Dr. William Bechtold.)

relatively uninflamed fibrous connective tissue is evident. Sequestra, if included, demonstrate the typical features of bone necrosis (see **osteomyelitis,** p. 114).

Treatment and Prognosis

Most cases of proliferative periostitis of the jaws are associated with periapical inflammatory lesions, and treatment in these cases is directed toward eliminating the source of the infection—either extraction of the offending tooth or appropriate endodontic therapy. After

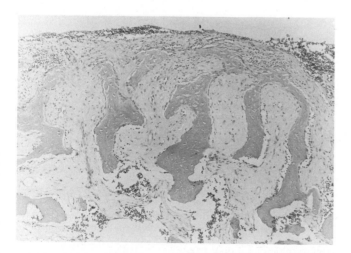

FIGURE 3–57. **Proliferative periostitis.** Cellular and reactive vital bone with individual trabeculae oriented perpendicular to the surface.

the focus of infection has been eliminated and inflammation has resolved, the layers of bone will consolidate in 6 to 12 months as the overlying muscle action helps to remodel the bone to its original state. If a unifocal periosteal reaction similar to proliferative periostitis appears in the absence of an obvious source of inflammation, biopsy is recommended because several neoplastic conditions can result in a similar pattern.

ALVEOLAR OSTEITIS (Dry Socket; Fibrinolytic Alveolitis)

Following extraction of a tooth, a blood clot is formed at the site, with eventual organization of the clot by granulation tissue, and gradual replacement by coarse fibrillar bone and, finally, mature bone. Destruction of the initial clot prevents appropriate healing and causes the clinical syndrome known as **alveolar osteitis.**

Extensive investigations have shown that the clot is lost secondary to transformation of plasminogen to plasmin with subsequent lysis of fibrin and formation of kinins, which are potent pain mediators (**fibrinolytic alveolitis**). Local trauma, estrogens, and bacterial pyrogens are known to stimulate fibrinolysins. This knowledge correlates well with the increased frequency of alveolar osteitis in association with inexperienced surgeons, traumatic extractions, oral contraceptive use, and presurgical infections. In addition, inadequate irrigation at surgery and patient use of tobacco products have been positively related to the development of the problem.

Clinical Features

The frequency of alveolar osteitis is higher in the mandible and the posterior areas. After oral contraceptive use is taken into account, there does not appear to be a significant sex predilection. The prevalence is between 1 and 3 percent of all extractions but increases to 25 to 30 percent for impacted mandibular third molars. The frequency appears to be decreased when impacted teeth are removed prophylactically, rather than for therapeutic reasons, after development of chronic inflammation of pericoronal tissues. The overall prevalence is highest between 20 and 40 years of age (when the majority of teeth are extracted), although the likelihood of developing alveolar osteitis appears greatest for extractions in the 40- to 45-year-old age group.

The affected extraction site is initially filled with a dirty gray clot that is lost and leaves a bare bony socket (**dry socket**). The detection of the bare socket may be hindered by partial retention of the clot or by overlying inflamed tissue that covers the site. The diagnosis is confirmed by probing of the socket, which reveals exposed and extremely sensitive bone. Typically, severe pain, foul odor, and, less frequently, swelling and lymphadenopathy develop 3 to 4 days following extraction of the tooth. The signs and symptoms may last from 10 to 40 days.

Treatment and Prognosis

Upon evaluation of the patient complaining of post-extraction pain, a radiograph should be taken of the affected area to rule out the possibility of a retained root tip or a foreign body. The socket is irrigated with warm saline, followed by thorough clinical inspection of the socket for any unexpected pathosis. Finally, the socket is packed with an obtundent and antiseptic dressing, such as iodoform gauze containing eugenol. Typically, the dressing is changed every 24 hours for the first 3 days, then every 2 to 3 days until granulation tissue covers the exposed bone.

Many investigators have studied preventive measures for alveolar osteitis and have found several that offer promise. Intraoperative irrigation, topical antibiotics, systemic antibiotics, systemic or topical antifibrinolytics, and antimicrobial rinses have been used. The best results have been obtained with intraoperative irrigation, combined with placement of antibiotics into the socket, or chlorhexidine rinsing both before and after the surgical procedure. Tetracycline is the most frequently chosen antibiotic, but lincomycin, clindamycin, and metronidazole also show favorable results.

Many surgeons are hesitant to place a medicament into an extraction socket. Those who do often restrict its use to those patients who are considered "high risk," such as:

- Females on oral contraceptives
- Smokers
- Those with existing signs of pericoronitis
- Those with traumatic extractions
- Those with a previous history of alveolar osteitis

REFERENCES

General References

Cohen S, Burns RC. Pathways of the Pulp, 4th ed. St. Louis, CV Mosby, 1987.
Grossman LI, Oliet S, Del Rio CE. Endodontic Practice, 11th ed. Philadelphia, Lea & Febiger, 1988.
Ingle JI, Taintor JF. Endodontics, 3rd ed. Philadelphia, Lea & Febiger, 1985.

Pulpitis

Baume LJ. Diagnosis of diseases of the pulp. Oral Surg Oral Med Oral Pathol 29:102–116, 1970.
Cecic PA, Hartwell GR, Bellizzi R. Cold as a diagnostic aid in cases of irreversible pulpitis: Report of two cases. Oral Surg Oral Med Oral Pathol 56:647–650, 1983.
Garfunkel A, Sela J, Ulmansky M. Dental pulp pathosis: Clinicopathologic correlations based on 109 cases. Oral Surg Oral Med Oral Pathol 35:110–117, 1973.
Hyman JL, Cohn ME. The predictive value of endodontic diagnostic tests. Oral Surg Oral Med Oral Pathol 58:343–346, 1984.
Johnson RH, Dachi SF, Haley JV. Pulpal hyperemia—a correlation of clinical and histologic data from 706 teeth. J Am Dent Assoc 81:108–124, 1970.
Kim S. Neurovascular interactions in the dental pulp in health and inflammation. J Endod 16:48–53, 1990.
Tønder KJH. Vascular reactions in the dental pulp during inflammation. Acta Odontol Scand 41:247–256, 1983.
Tronstad L. Recent development in endodontic research. Scand J Dent Res 100:52–59, 1992.

Secondary Dentin

Cox CF, et al. Reparative dentin: Factors affecting its deposition. Quintessence Int 23:257–270, 1992.
Gardner DG, Majka M. The early formation of irregular secondary dentine in progeria. Oral Surg Oral Med Oral Pathol 28:877–884, 1969.

Holcomb JB, Gregory WB. Calcific metamorphosis of the pulp: Its incidence and treatment. Oral Surg Oral Med Oral Pathol 24:825–830, 1967.
Ketterl W. Age-induced changes in the teeth and their attachment apparatus. Int Dent J 33:262–271, 1983.
Morse DR. Age-related changes of the dental pulp complex and their relationship to systemic aging. Oral Surg Oral Med Oral Pathol 72:721–745, 1991.
Nitzan DW, et al. The effect of aging on tooth morphology: A study on impacted teeth. Oral Surg Oral Med Oral Pathol 61:54–60, 1986.
Solheim T. Amount of secondary dentin as an indicator of age. Scand J Dent Res 100:193–199, 1992.
Woods MA, Robinson QC, Harris EF. Age-progressive changes in pulp widths and root lengths during adulthood: A study of American blacks and whites. Gerodontology 9:41–50, 1990.

Pulpal Calcifications

Burkes EJ Jr, et al. Dental lesions in tumoral calcinosis. J Oral Pathol Med 20:222–227, 1991.
Kumar S, et al. Pulp calcifications in primary teeth. J Pedod 14:93–96, 1990.
Morse DR. Age-related changes of the dental pulp complex and their relationship to systemic aging. Oral Surg Oral Med Oral Pathol 72:721–745, 1991.
Moss-Salentijn L, Hendricks-Klyvert M. Epithelially induced denticles in the pulps of recently erupted, noncarious human premolars. J Endod 9:554–560, 1983.
Moss-Salentijn L, Hendricks-Klyvert M. Calcified structures in human dental pulps. J Endod 14:184–189, 1988.
Pope FM, et al. Ehlers Danlos syndrome type I with novel dental features. J Oral Pathol Med 21:418–421, 1992.
Rao SR, Witkop CJ, Yamane GM. Pulpal dysplasia. Oral Surg Oral Med Oral Pathol 30:682–689, 1970.
Sayegh FS, Reed AJ. Calcification in the dental pulp. Oral Surg Oral Med Oral Pathol 25:873–882, 1968.
Selden HS. Radiographic pulpal calcifications: Normal or abnormal—a paradox. J Endod 17:34–37, 1991.
Sundell JR, Stanley HR, White CL. The relationship of coronal pulp stone formation to experimental operative procedures. Oral Surg Oral Med Oral Pathol 25:579–589, 1968.

Periapical Inflammatory Disease (Granuloma; Cyst; Abscess)

Azma NEA, el Razzak MYA, el Saaid HY. Correlation between histological and radiographic appearance of periapical radiolucencies. Egypt Dent J 36:245–259, 1990.
Bhaskar SN. Periapical lesions—types, incidence, and clinical features. Oral Surg Oral Med Oral Pathol 21:657–671, 1966.
Dahl EC. Diagnosing inflammatory and non-inflammatory periapical disease. J Indiana Dent Assoc 70(6):22–26, 1991.
High AS, Hirschmann PN. Age changes in residual radicular cysts. J Oral Pathol 15:524–528, 1986.
Iwu C, et al. The microbiology of periapical granulomas. Oral Surg Oral Med Oral Pathol 69:502–505, 1990.
Kontiainen S, Ranta H, Lautenschlager I. Cells infiltrating human periapical inflammatory lesions. J Oral Pathol 15:544–546, 1986.
Morse DR, Bhambhani SM. A dentist's dilemma: Nonsurgical endodontic therapy or periapical surgery for teeth with apparent pulpal pathosis and an associated periapical radiolucent lesion. Oral Surg Oral Med Oral Pathol 70:333–340, 1990.
Piattelli A, et al. Immune cells in periapical granuloma: Morphological and immunohistochemical characterization. J Endod 17:26–29, 1991.
Spatafore CM, et al. Periapical biopsy report: An analysis over a 10-year period. J Endod 16:239–241, 1990.
Stockdale CR, Chandler NP. The nature of the periapical lesion—a review of 1108 cases. J Dent 16:123–129, 1988.
Tronstad L. Recent development in endodontic research. Scand J Dent Res 100:52–59, 1992.
Trowbridge HO, Stevens BH. Microbiologic and pathologic aspects of pulpal and periapical disease. Curr Opin Dent 2:85–92, 1992.
Wayman BE, et al. A bacteriological and histological evaluation of 58 periapical lesions. J Endod 18:152–155, 1992.
Winstock D. Apical disease: An analysis of diagnosis and management with special reference to root lesion resection and pathology. Ann R Coll Surg Engl 62:171–179, 1980.

Wong M. Surgical fenestration of large periapical lesions. J Endod 17:516–521, 1991.

Cellulitis

Allan BP, Egbert MA, Myall RWT. Orbital abscess of odontogenic origin: Case report and review of the literature. J Oral Maxillofac Surg 20:268–270, 1991.

Birn H. Spread of dental infections. Dent Pract Dent Rec 22:347–356, 1972.

Childs HG, Courville CB. Thrombosis of the cavernous sinus secondary to dental infections. Am J Orthodont Oral Surg (Oral Surgery Section) 28:367–373, 402–413, 458–468, 515–521, 1942.

Fritsch DE, Klein DG. Ludwig's angina. Heart Lung 21:39–46, 1992.

Hought RT, et al. Ludwig's angina: Report of two cases and review of the literature from 1945 to January 1979. J Oral Surg 38:849–855, 1980.

Hutchinson IL, James DR. New treatment for Ludwig's angina. Br J Oral Maxillofac Surg 27:83–84, 1989.

Iwu CO. Ludwig's angina: Report of seven cases and review of the current concepts in management. Br J Oral Maxillofac Surg 28:189–193, 1990.

Moreland LW, Corey J, McKenzie R. Ludwig's angina: Report of a case and review of the literature. Arch Intern Med 148:461–466, 1988.

Ogundiya DA, Keith DA, Mirowski J. Cavernous sinus thrombosis and blindness as complication of an odontogenic infection. J Oral Maxillofac Surg 47:1317–1321, 1989.

Osteomyelitis

Adekeye EO, Cornah J. Osteomyelitis of the jaws: A review of 141 cases. Br J Oral Maxillofac Surg 23:24–35, 1985.

Calhoun KH, Shapiro RD, Stiernberg CM. Osteomyelitis of the mandible. Arch Otolaryngol Head Neck Surg 114:1157–1162, 1988.

Chisholm BB, Lew D, Sadasivan K. The use of tobramycin-impregnated polymethylmethacrylate beads in the treatment of osteomyelitis of the mandible. J Oral Maxillofac Surg 51:444–449, 1993.

Daramola JO, Ajagbe HA. Chronic osteomyelitis of the mandible in adults: A clinical study of 34 cases. Br J Oral Surg 20:58–62, 1982.

Davies HT, Carr RJ. Osteomyelitis of the mandible: A complication of routine dental extractions in alcoholics. Br J Oral Maxillofac Surg 28:185–188, 1990.

Khosla VM. Current concepts in the treatment of acute and chronic osteomyelitis: Review and report of four cases. J Oral Surg 28:209–214, 1970.

Kinnman JEG, Lee HS. Chronic osteomyelitis of the mandible: Clinical study of thirteen cases. Oral Surg Oral Med Oral Pathol 25:6–11, 1968.

Koorbusch GF, Fotos P, Terhark K. Retrospective assessment of osteomyelitis: Etiology, demographics, risk factors, and management in 35 cases. Oral Surg Oral Med Oral Pathol 74:149–154, 1992.

Marx RE. Chronic osteomyelitis of the jaws. Oral Maxillofac Clin North Am 3:367–381, 1991.

Rohlin M. Diagnostic value of bone scintigraphy in osteomyelitis of the mandible. Oral Surg Oral Med Oral Pathol 75:650–657, 1993.

van Merkesteyn JPR, et al. Hyperbaric oxygen treatment of chronic osteomyelitis of the jaws. Int J Oral Surg 13:386–395, 1984.

Diffuse Sclerosing Osteomyelitis and Chronic Tendoperiostitis

Groot RH, et al. Diffuse sclerosing osteomyelitis (chronic tendoperiostitis) of the mandible: An 11-year follow-up report. Oral Surg Oral Med Oral Pathol 74:557–560, 1992.

Groot RH, et al. Changes in masseter inhibitory reflex responses in patients with diffuse sclerosing osteomyelitis of the mandible. Oral Surg Oral Med Oral Pathol 74:727–732, 1992.

Jacobsson S. Diffuse sclerosing osteomyelitis of the mandible. Int J Oral Surg 13:363–385, 1984.

Jacobsson S, Dahlén G, Möller ÅJR. Bacteriologic and serologic investigation in diffuse sclerosing osteomyelitis (DSO) of the mandible. Oral Surg Oral Med Oral Pathol 54:506–512, 1984.

Jacobsson S, Hollender L. Treatment and prognosis of diffuse sclerosing osteomyelitis (DSO) of the mandible. Oral Surg Oral Med Oral Pathol 49:7–14, 1980.

Schneider LC, Mesa ML. Differences between florid osseous dysplasia and chronic diffuse sclerosing osteomyelitis. Oral Surg Oral Med Oral Pathol 70:308–312, 1990.

van Merkesteyn JPR, et al. Diffuse sclerosing osteomyelitis of the mandible: A new concept of its etiology. Oral Surg Oral Med Oral Pathol 70:414–419, 1990.

Condensing Osteitis

Boyne PJ. Incidence of osteosclerotic areas in the mandible and maxilla. J Oral Surg Anes Hosp Dent Serv 18:486–491, 1960.

Eliasson S, Halvarsson C, Ljungheimer C. Periapical condensing osteitis and endodontic treatment. Oral Surg Oral Med Oral Pathol 57:195–199, 1984.

Eversole LR, Stone CE, Strub D. Focal sclerosing osteomyelitis/focal periapical osteopetrosis: Radiographic patterns. Oral Surg Oral Med Oral Pathol 58:456–460, 1984.

Farman AG, de V Joubert JJ, Nortjé C. Focal osteosclerosis and apical periodontal pathoses in "European" and Cape Coloured dental outpatients. Int J Oral Surg 7:549–557, 1978.

Hedin M, Polhagen L. Follow-up study of periradicular bone condensation. Scand J Dent Res 79:436–440, 1979.

Proliferative Periostitis

Eisenbud L, Miller J, Roberts IL. Garré's proliferative periostitis occurring simultaneously in four quadrants of the jaws. Oral Surg Oral Med Oral Pathol 51:172–178, 1981.

Eversole LR, et al. Proliferative periostitis of Garré: Its differentiation from other neoperiostoses. J Oral Surg 37:725–731, 1979.

Felsberg GJ, Gore RL, Schweitzer ME. Sclerosing osteomyelitis of Garrè (periostitis ossificans). Oral Surg Oral Med Oral Pathol 70:117–120, 1990.

Lichty G, Langlais RP, Aufdemorte T. Garré's osteomyelitis: Literature review and case report. Oral Surg Oral Med Oral Pathol 50:309–313, 1980.

Nortjé CJ, Wood RE, Grotepass F: Periostitis ossificans versus Garré's osteomyelitis: Part II. Radiologic analysis of 93 cases in the jaws. Oral Surg Oral Med Oral Pathol 66:249–260, 1988.

Smith SN, Farman AG: Osteomyelitis with proliferative periostitis (Garré's osteomyelitis): Report of a case affecting the mandible. Oral Surg Oral Med Oral Pathol 43:315–318, 1977.

van den Bossche LH, Demeulemeester JDA. Periodontal infection leading to periostitis ossificans ("Garré's osteomyelitis") of the mandible: Report of a case. J Periodontol 64:60–62, 1993.

Wood RE, et al. Periostitis ossificans versus Garré's osteomyelitis: Part I. What did Garré really say? Oral Surg Oral Med Oral Pathol 65:773–777, 1988.

Alveolar Osteitis

Al-Khateeb TL, El-Marsafi AI, Butler NP. The relationship between the indications for the surgical removal of impacted third molars and the incidence of alveolar osteitis. J Oral Maxillofac Surg 49:141–145, 1991.

Awang MN. The aetiology of dry socket: A review. Int Dent J 39:236–240, 1989.

Birn H. Etiology and pathogenesis of fibrinolytic alveolitis ("dry socket"). Int J Oral Surg 2:211–263, 1973.

Calhoun NR. Dry socket and other postoperative complications. Dent Clin North Am 15:337–348, 1971.

Catellani JE. Review of factors contributing to dry socket through enhanced fibrinolysis. J Oral Surg 37:42–46, 1979.

Chapnick P, Diamond LH. A review of dry socket: A double-blind study on the effectiveness of clindamycin in reducing the incidence of dry socket. J Can Dent Assoc 58:43–52, 1992.

Fazakerley M, Field EA. Dry socket: A painful post-extraction complication (a review). Dent Update 18(1):31–34, 1991.

Fridrich KL, Olson AJ. Alveolar osteitis following surgical removal of mandibular third molars. Anesth Prog 37:32–41, 1990.

Larsen PE. Alveolar osteitis after surgical removal of impacted mandibular third molars: Identification of the patient at risk. Oral Surg Oral Med Oral Pathol 73:393–397, 1992.

Ragno JR, Szkutnik AJ. Evaluation of .12% chlorhexidine rinse on the prevention of alveolar osteitis. Oral Surg Oral Med Oral Pathol 72:524–526, 1992.

Swanson AE. A double-blind study on the effectiveness of tetracycline in reducing the incidence of fibrinolytic alveolitis. J Oral Maxillofac Surg 47:165–167, 1989.

Swanson AE. Prevention of dry socket: An overview. Oral Surg Oral Med Oral Pathol 70:131–136, 1990.

4

Periodontal Diseases

In this textbook of oral and maxillofacial pathology, the discussion of periodontal diseases is appropriately limited in scope. For greater detail on the background, microbiology, clinical presentations, diagnostic procedures, and current therapies of these diseases, one of several fine textbooks on periodontology can be consulted.

GINGIVITIS

Gingivitis refers to inflammation limited to the soft tissues that surround the teeth. It does not include the inflammatory processes that may extend into the underlying alveolar ridge, periodontal ligament, or cementum. The primary types of gingivitis are listed in Table 4–1. This part of the text concentrates on the plaque-related types. **Acute necrotizing ulcerative gingivitis** (ANUG), **medication-influenced**, and a specific type of allergic gingivitis (**plasma cell gingivitis**) are presented later in this chapter. Additional forms of allergic gingivitis can be found in Chapter 9. The gingivitis that is associated with specific infections (i.e., herpes simplex, human immunodeficiency virus [HIV], etc.) is discussed in Chapters 5 and 7. The gingiva is a frequent site of involvement in several of the dermatologic vesiculoerosive diseases, and these are well described in Chapter 16.

Clinical Features

Most cases of gingivitis occur from lack of proper oral hygiene, which leads to the accumulation of dental plaque and calculus, but many other factors can affect the gingiva's susceptibility to the oral flora. The frequency of gingivitis is high in all age groups, but the true prevalence is difficult to determine because of the lack of a standardized method of measurement. Clinically detectable inflammatory changes of the gingiva begin in childhood and increase with age. Around the time of puberty, there is a period of increased susceptibility to gingivitis, with the peak incidence of involvement occurring around the age of 11 years (**puberty gingivitis**) (Fig. 4–1). Between the ages of 11 and 17 years, the frequency declines, then a slow increase is seen until the prevalence approaches 100 percent in the sixth decade of life.

In most age groups, females demonstrate a lower frequency of gingivitis than do males, even though they have periods of increased susceptibility. This may be due more to better oral hygiene in females rather than a physiologic difference. In addition to the years of puberty, females exhibit a greater susceptibility to gingivitis when they are exposed to the high levels of progesterone associated with pregnancy or some forms of oral contraceptives. Progesterone appears to increase the permeability of gingival blood vessels, thereby rendering the area more sensitive to bacterial, physical, and chemical irritants.

Other factors shown to relate directly to the frequency of gingivitis are diabetes mellitus (see p. 615), metal poisoning (see p. 227), trauma, mouth-breathing, smoking, and nutrition. Injury to the gingiva from mastication, oral hygiene techniques, or other habits may result in a

Table 4-1. TYPES OF GINGIVITIS
1. Plaque-related
2. Acute necrotizing ulcerative gingivitis (ANUG)
3. Medication-influenced
4. Allergic
5. Specific infection-related
6. Dermatosis-related

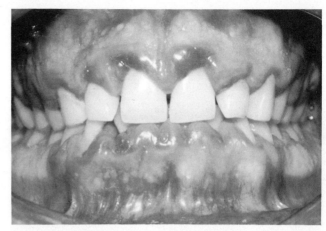

FIGURE 4-2. **Mouth-breathing-related gingivitis.** Slick, swollen, and red gingivitis of the anterior facial gingiva secondary to chronic mouth breathing.

breach of the oral mucosa, with secondary infection from the local flora. Most such injuries result in transient areas of erythema; if the trauma follows a chronic pattern, however, areas of persistently swollen, erythematous gingiva may result. Patients who are mouth-breathers or demonstrate incomplete lip closure can have a unique pattern of gingivitis in which the anterior facial gingiva is slick, swollen, and red (Fig. 4-2).

After such factors as age, sex, family income, education, and race are considered, numerous studies have shown that smoking correlates with a higher frequency of gingivitis and related periodontal diseases in every age group. Inflammation of the gingiva also can be enhanced by a poor nutritional status. Although the lack of vitamin C and its relationship to scorbutic gingivitis is well known (see p. 601), indirect evidence also demonstrates a correlation between gingival health and the intake of protein, folic acid, and zinc.

Inflammation of the gingiva may be localized or generalized. The involved area may be diffuse or confined to the free gingival margins (**marginal gingivitis**) (Fig. 4-3) or the interdental papillae (**papillary gingivitis**). The earliest signs of gingivitis include a loss of stippling plus bleeding on gentle probing. Healthy gingiva is coral pink; with inflammation, the involved gingiva becomes light red. With progression, the area becomes redder and edematous. As the process becomes entrenched, the involved gingiva becomes brighter red or magenta; the gingiva often demonstrates margins that may be blunted, receded, or hyperplastic (Fig. 4-4; see Color Figure 19). When the chronic inflammatory process leads to gingiva

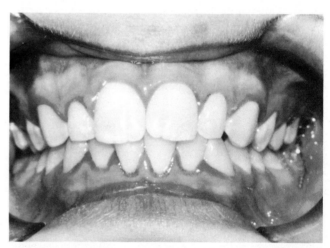

FIGURE 4-3. **Marginal gingivitis.** Diffuse erythematous alteration of the free gingival margins.

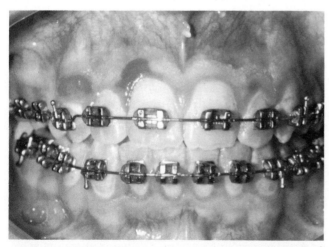

FIGURE 4-1. **Puberty gingivitis.** Erythematous gingivitis that arose at time of initial menses and was slow to respond to local therapy.

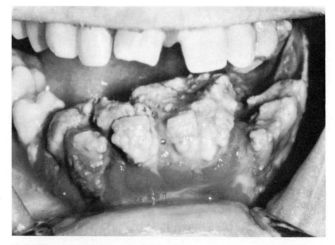

FIGURE 4-4. **Chronic gingivitis.** Bright-red gingiva is blunted, receded, and hyperplastic secondary to a total lack of oral hygiene. Note the extensive calculus build-up. See Color Plates.

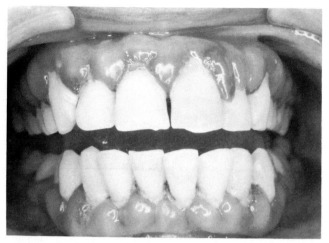

FIGURE 4–5. **Chronic hyperplastic gingivitis.** Diffuse erythema and enlargement of marginal and papillary gingiva.

that is significantly increased in size from edema or fibrosis, the pattern is termed **chronic hyperplastic gingivitis** (Fig. 4–5). Bleeding occurs easily, and exudate can be seen in the gingival sulcus. A localized tumor-like proliferation of subacutely inflamed granulation tissue, known as a **pyogenic granuloma** (see p. 371), can develop on the gingiva in patients with severe gingivitis (Fig. 4–6; see Color Figure 20).

Histopathologic Features

Incipient gingivitis demonstrates a light inflammatory infiltrate consisting of polymorphonuclear leukocytes, which accumulate in the connective tissue adjacent to the sulcular epithelium. With progression, the infiltrate becomes more intense and demonstrates a mixture of lymphocytes, plasma cells, and acute inflammatory cells (Fig. 4–7). Areas of fibrosis, hyperemia, edema, and hemorrhage may be present.

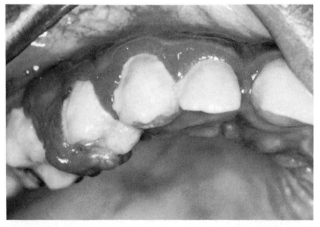

FIGURE 4–6. **Hyperplastic gingivitis with pyogenic granuloma.** Diffuse erythematous enlargement of marginal and papillary gingiva with hemorrhagic, tumor-like proliferation (which arose during pregnancy) between the maxillary bicuspid and first molar. See Color Plates.

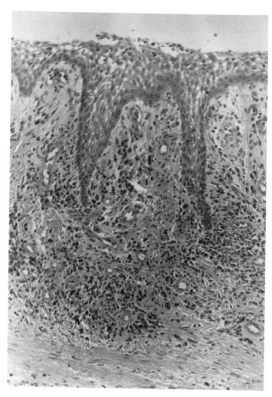

FIGURE 4–7. **Chronic gingivitis.** Sulcular epithelium with exocytosis overlying connective tissue, which contains inflammatory infiltrate consisting of lymphocytes, plasma cells, and polymorphonuclear leukocytes.

Treatment and Prognosis

Treatment of gingivitis consists of elimination (if possible) of any known cause of increased susceptibility and improvement in oral hygiene to decrease the dental plaque responsible for the inflammatory alterations. A further discussion of dental plaque and its relationship to gingival inflammation is presented in the discussion of periodontitis (see p. 133). Mechanical removal of dental plaque can be aided by the use of numerous chemical agents, such as chlorhexidine, essential oils (such as those contained in Listerine), or triclosan-containing products. On occasion, hyperplastic and fibrotic gingiva may have to be surgically recontoured to allow total resolution of the pathosis after improvements in hygiene have been made.

ACUTE NECROTIZING ULCERATIVE GINGIVITIS (ANUG; Vincent's Infection; Trench Mouth)

Acute necrotizing ulcerative gingivitis (ANUG) presents with a distinctive pattern of gingival pathologic changes that have been recognized for hundreds of years. In the 1890s, the French physician Jean Hyacinthe Vincent identified a fusiform bacterium, *Bacillus fusiformis* (currently *Fusobacterium nucleatum*), and a spirochete, *Borrelia vincentii*, after microscopic examination of plaque samples from affected sites. Vincent believed that the fusiform bacteria were principally responsible and the spirochetes were mainly saprophytic opportunists. The spirochete and fusiform bacterium association still remains true today, but more sophisticated techniques have implicated *Prevotella intermedia* and pathogen-related oral spirochetes (PROS), which may represent a new species closely related to *Treponema pallidum*.

The infection frequently occurs in the presence of psychologic stress. People in military service exhibit an increased frequency of ANUG, and the disorder was so common in the battlefield trenches during World War I that the nickname, **trench mouth**, was coined. Stress-related corticosteroids are thought to alter T4/T8 lymphocyte ratios and may cause the decreased neutrophilic chemotaxis and phagocytic response seen in patients with ANUG. Stress-related epinephrine may result in localized ischemia, which predisposes the gingiva to ANUG.

In addition to stress, other factors have been related to an increased frequency of ANUG:

- Smoking
- Local trauma
- Poor nutritional status
- Poor oral hygiene

In addition, immunocompromised status, especially that seen in association with acquired immunodeficiency syndrome (AIDS) (see p. 200) and infectious mononucleosis (see p. 190), has been related to the development of ANUG. The list of predisposing factors clearly supports the association between a depressed systemic immunity and the appearance of the disorder.

Clinical Features

ANUG may occur at any age but is most frequently seen in young and middle-aged adults. The prevalence in the normal population is less than 0.1 percent, but in stressed populations, such as military recruits, the frequency increases up to 7 percent. In a classic case of ANUG, the interdental papillae are highly inflamed and edematous. Typically, the affected papillae are blunted and demonstrate areas of "punched-out," crater-like necrosis, which are covered with a gray pseudomembrane (Fig. 4-8). Early cases may be missed easily because the ulceration initially involves only the tip of the interdental papilla. A fetid odor, exquisite pain, spontaneous hemorrhage, and accumulations of necrotic debris usually are noted. Occasional ancillary clinical features include lymphadenopathy, fever, and malaise. The process sometimes can lead to a loss of attachment and the development of associated periodontitis (**necrotizing ulcerative periodontitis**) or spread to adjacent soft tissue (**acute necrotizing ulcerative mucositis**) (Fig. 4-9).

Histopathologic Features

The histopathologic features of ANUG are not specific. Typically, affected gingival papillae demonstrate

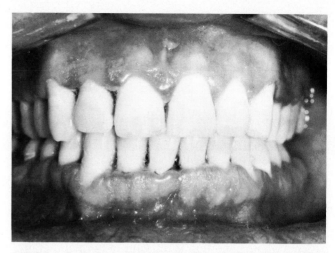

FIGURE 4-8. **Acute necrotizing ulcerative gingivitis.** Gingiva demonstrates blunted interdental papillae, which exhibit early mucosal necrosis.

surface ulceration, which is covered by a thickened fibrinopurulent membrane. The underlying lamina propria demonstrates an intense acute or mixed inflammatory infiltrate and extensive hyperemia. In non-ulcerated affected epithelium, there is often a loss of the typical surface keratinization. Necrotic material and extensive bacterial colonization often are included in the material submitted for microscopic examination.

Treatment and Prognosis

The affected area is best treated with debridement by scaling, curettage, or ultrasonic instrumentation. Topical or local anesthetic often is required before one can debride the tissues adequately. Frequent rinses with chlorhexidine, warm salt water, or diluted hydrogen peroxide are beneficial in increasing the therapeutic response. Antibiotics, such as metronidazole, tetracycline, penicillin,

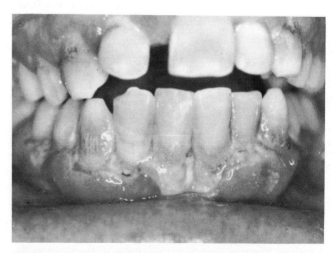

FIGURE 4-9. **Acute necrotizing ulcerative mucositis.** Gingiva exhibits epithelial necrosis that has extended between the adjacent interdental papillae and apically to the alveolar mucosa junction.

or erythromycin, often are necessary, especially in the presence of fever or lymphadenopathy.

The therapeutic interventions should be accompanied with instructions on oral hygiene and patient motivation. Follow-up appointments are necessary to reinforce the home care instructions and to rule out a recurrence of the process.

One must be ever vigilant in the search for other signs and symptoms of immunosuppression. Subtle palatal candidiasis or HIV-related oral hairy leukoplakia (see p. 202) can be easily missed in a patient with ANUG. Appropriate attention must be directed toward the oral soft tissue examination, especially in patients with infections such as ANUG that are related to immunosuppression. In addition, a thorough investigation of underlying causes of immunosuppression should be performed on patients whose condition is resistant to normal therapy.

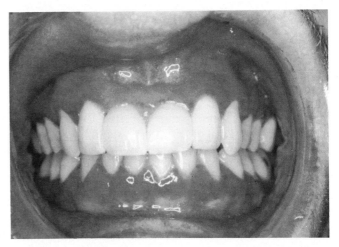

FIGURE 4–10. **Plasma cell gingivitis.** Diffuse, bright-red enlargement of the free and attached gingiva. See Color Plates. (Courtesy of Dr. George Blozis.)

PLASMA CELL GINGIVITIS (Atypical Gingivostomatitis)

A distinctive pattern of gingival alteration, **plasma cell gingivitis**, was brought to the attention of health care practitioners during the late 1960s and early 1970s. A rash of cases occurred during that time, and most appear to have been related to a hypersensitivity to a component of chewing gum. Since that time, the number of cases has dwindled, but similar gingival alterations occasionally are reported.

Plasma cell enlargements of the gingiva can be grouped under three categories:

■ Allergic
■ Neoplastic
■ Idiopathic

Although the association with chewing gum has decreased, allergy still is responsible for many reported cases. One herbal toothpaste, a specific type of mint candy, and peppers used for cooking have been implicated in more recent reports. The list of allergens appears to be variable, and a thorough evaluation is often required to rule out an allergic cause.

Clinical Features

Patients with plasma cell gingivitis present with a rapid onset of sore mouth, which is often intensified by dentifrices and hot or spicy foods. The entire free and attached gingiva demonstrates a diffuse enlargement with bright erythema and loss of normal stippling (Figs. 4–10 and 4–11; see Color Figures 21 and 22). Extension onto the palate can occur, and edentulous areas typically exhibit less intense changes.

Additional sites of involvement may be seen, or the changes may be localized to the gingiva. In the chewing gum–related cases of the early 1970s, involvement of the lips and tongue was typical. The lips presented with dry, atrophic mucosa, which occasionally demonstrated fissuring, and involvement of the lower lip often was more pronounced. A dark-blue hue of the lips and angular

cheilitis were frequent. Tongue involvement resulted in erythematous enlargement with furrows, mild crenation, and loss of the typical dorsal coating.

More recent reports have described lesions often isolated to the gingiva without the classic lip and tongue involvement, as was seen in the past. A larger percentage of these cases are idiopathic, and occasional extraoral involvement of sites such as the supraglottic region occurs.

Histopathologic Features

A review of the tissue specimens from the cases of classic plasma cell gingivitis of the 1970s reveals surface epithelium that demonstrates psoriasiform hyperplasia and spongiosis with intense exocytosis and the formation of microabscesses by polymorphonuclear leukocytes.

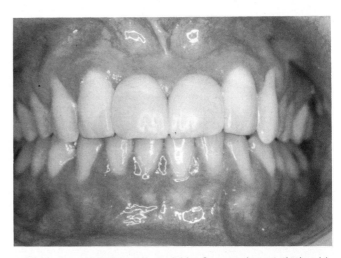

FIGURE 4–11. **Plasma cell gingivitis.** Same patient as depicted in Figure 4–10 after elimination of the inciting allergen. Note significant reduction in gingival enlargement and erythema. See Color Plates. (Courtesy of Dr. George Blozis.)

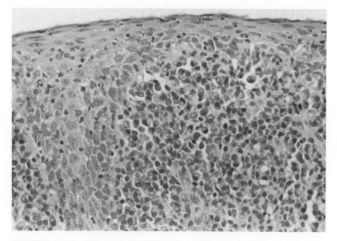

FIGURE 4-12. **Plasma cell gingivitis.** Hyperplastic squamous epithelium exhibiting exocytosis and dense plasmacytic infiltrate of the underlying lamina propria.

The underlying lamina propria contains numerous dilated vascular channels and an extremely dense chronic inflammatory infiltrate, which is composed predominantly of plasma cells (Fig. 4-12). The current cases are frequently similar, but many often demonstrate less involvement of the surface epithelium and a less dense underlying plasmacytic infiltrate.

Investigation of the clonality of the plasma cell infiltrate may be necessary to rule out the possibility of a monoclonal plasma cell neoplasm. All allergic and idiopathic cases of plasma cell gingivitis demonstrate a polyclonal mixture of plasma cells and a normal profile on plasma immunoelectrophoresis.

Treatment and Prognosis

All patients with plasma cell gingivitis should be instructed to keep a complete dietary history with records of everything taken into the mouth (e.g., foods, dentifrice, mouthwash, tobacco, alcohol, chewing gum, candy, medications). Possible allergens should be eliminated in an attempt to discover the underlying causation. If an easy answer is not apparent, extensive allergy testing and an elimination diet can be undertaken.

Many patients in whom no underlying causation could be discovered have been treated with topical or systemic corticosteroids, with variable results. Betamethasone rinses, fluocinonide gel, and topical triamcinolone are several of the reported choices. In spite of all the evaluations and therapeutic interventions, in some patients no cause can be identified, and the patients do not respond to any treatment.

GRANULOMATOUS GINGIVITIS

The discovery of unexplained granulomatous inflammation in an intraoral biopsy specimen is a diagnostic challenge for the pathologist, referring clinician, and patient. The pathologist must rule out histologically distinctive granulomatous diseases and specific granulomatous infectious processes (e.g., deep fungal infections, acid-fast bacteria [see Chapters 5 and 6]); the clini-

cian must search for signs and symptoms of local and systemic granulomatous diseases (e.g., orofacial granulomatosis, Crohn's disease, sarcoidosis, chronic granulomatous disease, Wegener's granulomatosis [see Chapters 9 and 17]); and the patient must endure and pay for these evaluations. Even after a costly workup, some patients who have localized areas of granulomatous inflammation of the gingiva have no signs or symptoms of any of the previously mentioned disorders.

One group investigated a series of non-diagnostic gingival lesions and demonstrated that many were the result of the introduction of dental materials into the connective tissue deep to the sulcular epithelium. When the material is obvious on light microscopy, the areas can be diagnosed easily as foreign-body reactions. In many instances, the material was so fine that it could be overlooked easily and would be missed by many pathologists who were not experienced in searching for this subtle foreign material. Energy-dispersive x-ray microanalysis demonstrated that the material often consisted of elements that are contained in prophylaxis paste. Less frequently, dental metals, such as gold and nickel, were seen. Rarely, nondental foreign material was detected. This investigation suggests the possibility of damage to the sulcular epithelium during dental or oral hygiene procedures, thereby providing avenues for the introduction of foreign material into the gingival tissues. This material can be present even when no microscopically obvious foreign material is detected.

Clinical Features

Granulomatous gingivitis may occur at any age but most frequently is encountered in adulthood. The lesions may be solitary or multifocal, typically with a diameter less than 2 cm. The affected areas appear as red or red-and-white macules, which most frequently involve the interdental papillae. Extension may occur along the marginal gingiva or onto the attached gingiva (Fig. 4-13). Pain or sensitivity is a common finding, and the

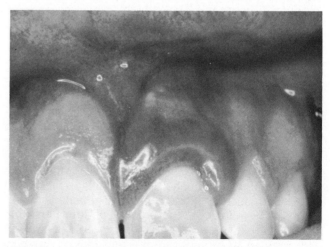

FIGURE 4-13. **Granulomatous gingivitis.** Localized enlarged and erythematous gingiva associated with the maxillary left central incisor. The alterations developed shortly after placement of a porcelain-fused-to-metal full crown and were not responsive to conservative local therapy. (Courtesy of Dr. Timothy L. Gutierrez.)

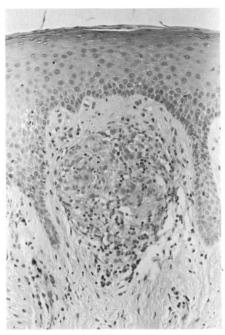

FIGURE 4–14. **Granulomatous gingivitis.** Focal collection of histiocytes, lymphocytes, and multinucleated giant cells within the superficial lamina propria of the gingiva.

lesions persist despite conventional therapy and rigorous oral hygiene. The process can be seen adjacent to clinically normal teeth or next to teeth with restorations.

Histopathologic Features

A biopsy specimen of the affected gingiva demonstrates focal collections of histiocytes intermixed with an intense lymphocytic infiltrate (Fig. 4–14). On occasion, well-formed histiocytic granulomas with multinucleated giant cells are seen. Special stains for organisms should be negative. If foreign material is detected, one can render a diagnosis of a foreign-body granuloma. In some cases, however, the foreign material may be too fine to be detected.

Treatment and Prognosis

When all the histopathologic and clinical investigations have been performed, the final differential diagnosis of granulomatous gingivitis is usually narrowed down to a localized form of orofacial granulomatosis (see p. 243) or a foreign-body reaction. Surgical excision of the affected tissue is the therapy of choice for those cases related to foreign material. In an attempt to prevent future introduction of iatrogenic foreign material, it appears appropriate to postpone dental polishing and prophylaxis for at least 2 days after scaling. Patients who do not respond to surgical removal and have recurrences despite cautious dental care should be classified as having orofacial granulomatosis and managed accordingly.

DESQUAMATIVE GINGIVITIS

Most clinicians use the term **desquamative gingivitis** to describe a clinical presentation in which the patient has a chronic vesiculoerosive process whereby the gingiva spontaneously sloughs or can be removed with minor manipulation. The process most likely represents a manifestation of one of several different vesiculoerosive diseases. Histopathologic and immunologic investigations of this condition reveal that most patients exhibit features that are diagnostic of cicatricial pemphigoid or lichen planus. Other diagnoses that are made less frequently include linear IgA disease, pemphigus vulgaris, epidermolysis bullosa acquisita, systemic lupus erythematosus, and chronic ulcerative stomatitis. (For a complete discussion of these entities, consult Chapter 16.)

In a review of more than 453 patients presenting to a dermatology hospital with manifestations of pemphigoid, pemphigus, or lichen planus, 24.5 percent had involvement of the gingiva. In this group, 63.6 percent had pemphigoid, 25 percent had lichen planus, and 18.4 percent presented with pemphigus.

In another study, 41 patients with desquamative gingivitis were evaluated with the following diagnoses:

	No. of patients
Pemphigus	2
Lichen planus	1
Contact stomatitis	1
Epidermolysis bullosa acquisita	1
Pemphigoid	36

Of the patients with pemphigoid, 18 were diagnosed as having cicatricial pemphigoid because of the presence of extragingival lesions. The remaining 18 patients exhibited lesions localized to the gingiva.

Several investigators have suggested that the form of pemphigoid limited to the gingiva is a separate disease from both bullous and cicatricial pemphigoid. The names suggested for this localized erosive process include **desquamative gingivitis** and **oral non-dystrophic mechanobullous eruption**, but no terminology for this presentation has been uniformly accepted. These patients do not appear to have bullous pemphigoid because extraoral lesions and circulating antibodies to basement membrane material are not present. The diagnosis of cicatricial pemphigoid also does not appear totally appropriate because scarring is minimal and involvement of the eyes and posterior pharynx is not noted.

In some cases, the process demonstrates a subepithelial separation, but the immunofluorescence assay gives negative results and does not support any of the dermatologic disorders previously discussed. Several investigators believe that this process may represent a hormone-mediated desquamative gingivitis. Interestingly, human gingiva has been shown to metabolize estrogens and to contain specific high-affinity estrogen receptors.

Another group has suggested that desquamative lesions localized to the gingiva may represent an abnormal local immunoresponse to certain plaque substances. Frequently, the lesions are topographically related to plaque, and this group's investigations reveal a statistically significant improvement when affected patients are treated with doxycycline monohydrate. Whether this is due to the antibacterial or anti-inflammatory activity of tetracyclines has not been determined.

In conclusion, there is a form of chronic mucosal desquamation that is limited to the gingiva. Whether this represents a separate entity, a *forme fruste* variation of one of the chronic dermatologic vesiculoerosive processes, or a mixture of several different diseases, has yet to be definitively determined. Until the controversy has been resolved, the term **desquamative gingivitis** should be used as a clinical description and not as a definitive diagnosis.

Clinical Features

Most people who are affected with desquamative gingivitis are older than age 40, and there is a significant female predominance (up to 80 percent in those with negative immunofluorescence findings). The process demonstrates a chronic onset in which the involvement is initially limited but, with time, spreads to affect large portions of the gingiva. By definition, the process is limited to the gingiva. The facial surface is involved more frequently than the lingual gingiva. Involvement may be multifocal or may demonstrate a generalized pattern.

Affected sites present as areas of smooth erythema in which there is a loss of normal stippling (Fig. 4–15). With progression, blister formation, spontaneous desquamation, or zones of erosion can be found. The blisters are filled with clear fluid or can be contaminated with blood. Manipulation of the affected erythematous surface epithelium with a cotton swab, gauze pad, or compressed air often can cause desquamation. Areas of frank erosion are covered by yellowish fibrinopurulent membranes, and significant pain usually is present.

Histopathologic Features

The histopathologic findings of desquamative gingivitis are variable, although most patients present with features diagnostic of lichen planus or cicatricial pemphigoid (see Chapter 16). In those cases with immunofluorescence findings that are incompatible with the dermatologic disorders, there is a subepithelial separation with vacuolization of the epithelial-connective tissue junction.

Treatment and Prognosis

An incisional biopsy specimen should be submitted for routine histopathologic examination, typically followed by direct and/or indirect immunofluorescence. The biopsy incision should extend from the adjacent normal epithelium into the area of separation. The type of immunofluorescent investigation necessary for definitive diagnosis is guided by the light microscopic findings. A thorough evaluation of all dermatologic and mucosal surfaces should be performed to rule out the possibility of other occult sites of involvement. Before definitive therapy, the dentition should be cleaned thoroughly and the patient should be taught to maintain excellent oral hygiene. A course of doxycycline monohydrate can be prescribed in an attempt to reduce the degree of mucosal inflammation before immunosuppressive therapy.

Currently, definitive therapy is guided by the histopathologic and immunologic diagnoses. As described in Chapter 16, many patients respond well to topical corticosteroids. Patients whose conditions are resistant to corticosteroids often respond to dapsone or sulfapyridine. In cases that demonstrate negative immunofluorescence findings and are not diagnostic for any of the specific dermatologic erosive disorders, therapy with estrogens has been attempted with equivocal results.

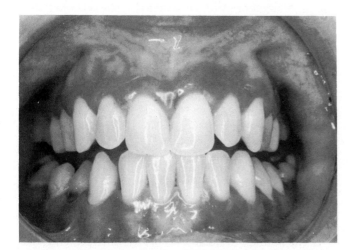

FIGURE 4–15. **Desquamative gingivitis.** Diffuse, slick, red, and painful gingiva.

DRUG-RELATED GINGIVAL HYPERPLASIA

Drug-related gingival hyperplasia associated with the use of phenytoin has been well known for more than 50 years, but the list of offending medications has been lengthening. Numerous calcium channel blockers and the immunosuppressant drug cyclosporine have demonstrated a similar ability (Fig. 4–16). Of the calcium channel blockers, nifedipine produces gingival enlargement with the greatest frequency (Fig. 4–17); diltiazem, felodipine, nitrendipine, and verapamil occasionally cause gingival hyperplasia. Calcium channel blockers belong to a class of drugs known as dihydropyridines; others within the same class that can cause gingival overgrowth include amlodipine, bepridil, bleomycin, isradipine, nicardipine, nimodipine, nisoldipine, and oxidipine.

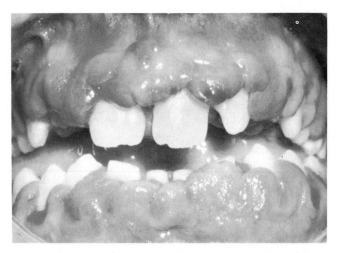

FIGURE 4–16. **Cyclosporine-related gingival hyperplasia.** Diffuse, erythematous, and fibrotic gingival hyperplasia.

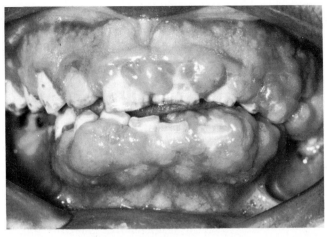

FIGURE 4–18. **Cyclosporine- and nifedipine-related gingival hyperplasia.** Dramatic gingival hyperplasia in a patient using two drugs associated with gingival enlargement. See Color Plates.

The use of sodium valproate, an antiepileptic agent, rarely has been related to gingival hyperplasia. When two drugs known to cause gingival hyperplasia are used concurrently, the severity of the hyperplasia often is increased (Fig. 4–18; see Color Figure 24).

The prevalence of these hyperplasias varies widely; as reported in a critical review of the literature, however, the prevalence related to use of phenytoin is approximately 50 percent. Cyclosporine and the dihydropyridines produce significant changes in about 25 percent of the patients. Whether there is a relationship between the dose and the risk or severity of the hyperplasia is controversial, with reports on both sides.

The degree of gingival enlargement appears to be related to the patient's susceptibility and the level of oral hygiene. The correlation between gingival hyperplasia and oral hygiene inadequacy is positive and significant. In observations of patients with excellent oral hygiene, gingival overgrowth, as ascertained by pseudopocket for-

mation, is dramatically reduced or not present. Even with good oral hygiene, however, some degree of gingival enlargement can be discovered in susceptible individuals, although in many cases the changes are difficult to detect. Rigorous oral hygiene often can limit the severity to clinically insignificant levels. Of the medications discussed, cyclosporine appears to be the least responsive to the institution of a rigorous program of oral hygiene; even with this medication, however, the elimination of gingival inflammation results in noticeable clinical improvement.

Clinical Features

Because phenytoin is most often used by young patients, the gingival hyperplasia it induces is primarily a problem in people younger than age 25; cases related to the dihydropyridines occur mainly in middle-aged or elderly adults. Cyclosporine is used over a broad age range, and this correlates with the age of reported hyperplasia. A greater risk for gingival hyperplasia occurs when the drug is used in children, especially adolescents. No sex or race predilection is present.

After 1 to 3 months of drug use, the enlargements originate in the interdental papillae and spread across the tooth surfaces (Fig. 4–19). The anterior and facial segments are the most frequently involved areas. In extensive cases, the hyperplastic gingiva can cover a portion or all of the crowns of many of the involved teeth (Figs. 4–20 and 4–21). Extension lingually and occlusally can interfere with speech and mastication. In one report, significant lingual expansion of the gingiva resulted in tongue displacement and respiratory distress. Edentulous areas generally are not affected, but significant hyperplasia under poorly maintained dentures has been noted (Fig. 4–22).

In the absence of inflammation, the enlarged gingiva is normal in color and firm with a surface that may be smooth, stippled, or granular. With inflammation, the affected gingiva often becomes dark-red and edematous, with a surface that is friable, bleeds easily, and is occa-

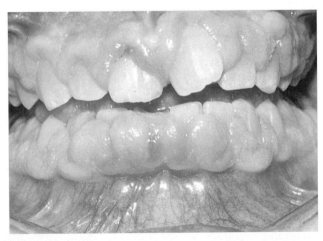

FIGURE 4–17. **Nifedipine-related gingivitis hyperplasia.** Diffuse, fibrotic gingival hyperplasia after 1 month of intensive oral hygiene. Significant erythema, edema, and increased enlargement were present prior to intervention.

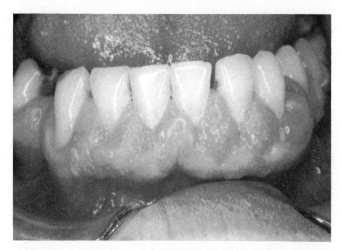

FIGURE 4-19. **Mild phenytoin-related gingival hyperplasia.** Gingival enlargement present predominantly in the interdental papillae.

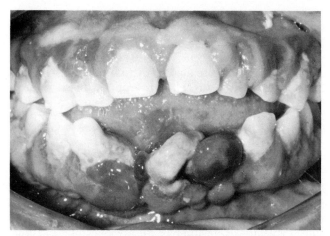

FIGURE 4-20. **Phenytoin-related gingival hyperplasia.** Significant erythematous gingival hyperplasia is covering portions of the crowns of numerous teeth.

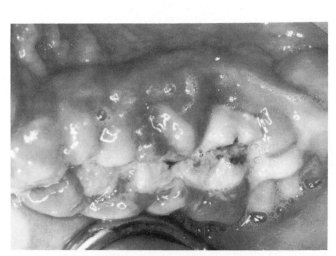

FIGURE 4-21. **Phenytoin-related gingival hyperplasia.** Significant gingival hyperplasia almost totally covers the crowns of the posterior maxillary dentition. (Courtesy of Drs. Ann Drummond and Timothy Johnson.)

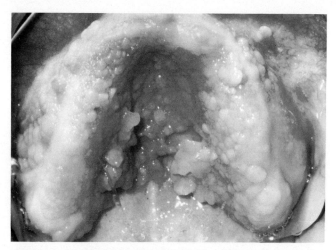

FIGURE 4-22. **Phenytoin-related palatal hyperplasia.** Extensive hyperplasia of palatal mucosa in an edentulous patient with poor denture hygiene.

sionally ulcerated. Pyogenic granuloma-like enlargements are occasionally seen in the presence of heavy inflammation.

Histopathologic Features

The exact histopathologic changes that occur in people with drug-induced gingival hyperplasia are difficult to ascertain because of variations in the techniques of investigation. In spite of this, most controlled microscopic examinations of hyperplastic gingival tissues removed from lesions caused by phenytoin or the dihydropyridines reveal redundant tissue of apparent normal composition. Those cases related to cyclosporine use demonstrate an increased amount of collagen per unit volume, with an increased number of fibroblasts.

The overlying surface epithelium may demonstrate elongation of the rete ridges with long extensions into the underlying lamina propria. In patients with secondary inflammation, there is increased vascularity and a chronic inflammatory cellular infiltrate, which most frequently consists of lymphocytes and plasma cells.

Treatment and Prognosis

Discontinuation of the offending medication often results in cessation, and possibly some regression, of the gingival enlargement; even substitution of one dihydropyridine for another may be beneficial. If the drug use is mandatory, plaque control, scaling, and gingivectomy are used. Antiplaque agents, such as chlorhexidine, have been beneficial in the prevention of plaque build-up and the associated gingival hyperplasia. With subsequent rigorous oral hygiene, recurrence typically is not a problem.

The impact of drug-related gingival hyperplasia on periodontal health in the future is a concern. Until recently, drugs that cause gingival hyperplasia were not prescribed frequently to middle-aged and elderly adults. With the advent of the highly successful dihydropyridines, a rapid increase in the frequency of gingival hyperplasia in adults is expected. When one considers the frequency of periodontitis in this population, the combination may result in increased disease activity in many patients. Clinicians must be ever vigilant and should try to minimize these combined effects through early preventive efforts.

GINGIVAL FIBROMATOSIS (Fibromatosis Gingivae; Elephantiasis Gingivae)

Gingival fibromatosis is a slowly progressive gingival enlargement caused by a collagenous overgrowth of the gingival fibrous connective tissue. In spite of the name, this disorder bears no relationship to the hypercellular and neoplastic fibromatoses that can occur in soft tissue and bone (see pp. 369 and 480).

Clinical Features

Gingival fibromatosis may be familial or idiopathic. The familial variations may occur as an isolated finding or in association with one of several hereditary syndromes (e.g., **Zimmermann-Laband, Murray-Puretic-Drescher, Rutherfurd, multiple hamartoma** [see p. 555], and **Cross** syndromes). Other findings sometimes seen in relationship to gingival fibromatosis include hypertrichosis (Fig. 4–23), epilepsy, mental retardation, sensorineural deafness, hypothyroidism, chondrodystrophia, and growth hormone deficiency. The isolated familial types exhibit both autosomal dominant and autosomal recessive patterns of inheritance.

In most instances, the enlargement begins before age 20 and is often correlated with the eruption of the decid-

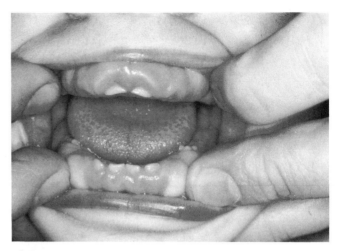

FIGURE 4–24. **Gingival fibromatosis.** A young child with cheeks retracted by the parent. Note erythematous gingival hyperplasia arising in association with erupting deciduous dentition. (Courtesy of Dr. George Blozis.)

uous or permanent teeth (Fig. 4–24). Most investigators believe that the presence of teeth probably is necessary for the condition to occur. After the process has begun, it can overgrow the associated teeth and even interfere with lip closure. Failure or delay in eruption of subsequent teeth may be evident (Fig. 4–25). In some instances, a tooth may have erupted into a normal position but the fibrous connective tissue continues to cover the crown and prevent visualization.

The gingival changes may be generalized or localized to one or more quadrants. Either jaw may be involved, but the maxilla is more frequently affected and demonstrates a greater degree of enlargement. Palatal surfaces typically are increased in thickness more than the buccal side. Typically, extension past the alveolar mucosal junction into the mucobuccal fold is not seen, but palatal extensions can cause significant distortion of the contour of the palate and, at times, can almost meet in the midline.

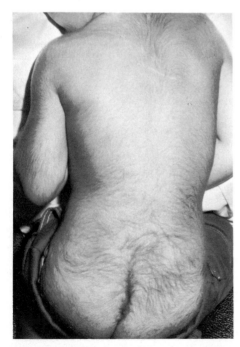

FIGURE 4–23. **Hypertrichosis in association with gingival fibromatosis.** Dramatically increased body hair of the back and buttocks in a patient with gingival fibromatosis. (Courtesy of Dr. George Blozis.)

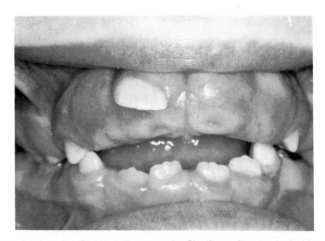

FIGURE 4–25. **Gingival fibromatosis.** Significant fibrotic gingival hyperplasia with resultant delayed eruption of numerous teeth. (From Neville BW, Damm DD, White DK, Waldron CA. Color Atlas of Clinical Oral Pathology. Philadelphia, Lea & Febiger, 1991.)

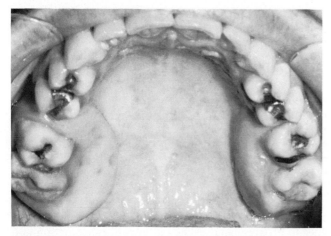

FIGURE 4-26. **Localized gingival fibromatosis.** Bilateral and symmetric fibrotic enlargements of the palatal surfaces of the posterior maxillary alveolar ridges.

In localized cases, the hyperplasia may involve a group of teeth and remain stable, or, at a later date, may extend to other segments of one or both jaws. One distinctive and not uncommon pattern involves the posterior maxillary alveolar ridge. In this pattern, the hyperplastic tissue forms bilaterally symmetric enlargements that extend posteriorly and palatally from the posterior alveolar ridges (Fig. 4-26).

The gingiva is firm, normal in color, and covered by a surface that is smooth or finely stippled. In older patients, the surface may develop numerous papillary projections. The frenular attachments may appear to divide the gingival tissues of the alveolar ridge into lobules.

Histopathologic Features

The enlargements of gingival fibromatosis consist of dense hypocellular, hypovascular collagenous tissue that forms numerous interlacing bundles that appear to be running in all directions. The surface epithelium often exhibits long, thin rete ridges that extend deeply into the

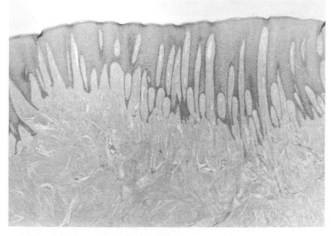

FIGURE 4-27. **Gingival fibromatosis.** Surface stratified squamous epithelium exhibiting long, thin rete ridges and underlying dense, fibrous connective tissue.

underlying fibrous connective tissue (Fig. 4-27). Inflammation is absent to mild, and dystrophic calcification sometimes is seen. Electron microscopic examination demonstrates a mixture of both fibroblasts and myofibroblast-like cells.

Treatment and Prognosis

Conservative treatment consists of gingivectomy in conjunction with a rigorous program of oral hygiene. Follow-up is recommended because there is a tendency for recurrence within a few years. In severe cases, selective extraction of teeth combined with gingivectomy often is required to achieve a normal gingival morphology.

PERIODONTITIS

Periodontitis is an inflammatory disease process that affects the supporting structures of the teeth: periodontal ligament, alveolar bone, and cementum. With progression, the process can lead to the loss of attachment, with destruction of the periodontal ligament and alveolar bone. Apical migration of the crevicular epithelium along the root surface results in the formation of periodontal pockets. Loosening and eventual loss of teeth are possible.

For more than a century, the presence of the disease has been correlated with the accumulation of dental plaque on the tooth and under the gingiva. In spite of this, current evidence suggests that dental plaque is part of the natural human microflora. In some patients with extensive dental plaque, destructive lesions of the periodontium do not develop. Many investigators now believe that periodontitis occurs not from the mere presence of dental plaque but as a result of shifts in the proportions of bacterial species in the plaque, possibly related to changes in the dentogingival environment (e.g., soft diet or a high fermentable carbohydrate content of diet).

Dramatic differences exist in the content of dental plaque in areas of healthy and diseased periodontium. Healthy sites are colonized primarily by facultative gram-positive organisms, such as actinomycetes and streptococci; plaque within areas of active periodontitis contains anaerobic and microaerophilic gram-negative flora. Of the more than 300 types of bacteria that may reside in the oral cavity, only a few have been related to periodontitis, and the specific types often correlate with the clinical patterns of periodontitis. Adult periodontitis is associated predominantly with *Actinobacillus actinomycetemcomitans*, *Porphyromonas gingivalis*, and *Prevotella intermedia*, in addition to a handful of other organisms that occasionally can be involved in active periodontitis.

The cause of periodontitis has not been completely delineated, but three plausible hypotheses exist:

1. Direct tissue destruction by the bacteria or their products.
2. Immune hyperresponsiveness.
3. Immune deficiency.

Table 4-2. CLASSIFICATION OF PERIODONTITIS

1. Adult periodontitis
2. Early-onset periodontitis
   a. Prepubertal periodontitis
   b. Juvenile periodontitis
   c. Rapidly progressive periodontitis
3. Periodontitis associated with systemic disease
4. Necrotizing ulcerative periodontitis
5. Refractory periodontitis

In reality, different forms of periodontitis may be the result of variations in the pathogenesis of the disease.

The classification of periodontitis, as delineated by the American Academy of Periodontology, is listed in Table 4-2. The following text concentrates on the adult form of periodontitis. A later section discusses early-onset periodontitis. From this list, it should be clear that periodontitis represents a heterogeneous group of disorders.

Periodontitis associated with systemic disease is not rare, and Table 4-3 lists many of the disorders that may be associated with a premature loss of periodontal attachment.

Necrotizing ulcerative periodontitis represents the loss of attachment that occurs in association with **acute necrotizing ulcerative gingivitis** (see p. 124). This form has been correlated with aggressive invasion by a number of spirochetes and *P. intermedia*.

Refractory periodontitis refers to the presence of disease in multifocal sites that continues to demonstrate a loss of attachment after appropriate comprehensive periodontal therapy. Various specific periodontopathic organisms have been identified from active sites of refractory periodontitis.

Clinical and Radiographic Features

Periodontitis

With the decline in caries, **adult periodontitis** has become the primary cause of tooth loss in patients older than 35 years of age. A national survey found that 44 percent of adults in the United States had attachment loss of 3 mm or more in at least one site. The disorder demonstrates no sex predilection, and an increased prevalence is seen in association with:

- Advancing age
- An increased quantity of plaque and calculus
- Smoking
- Diabetes mellitus
- A lower socioeconomic level
- Decreased use of professional dental care

In the adult form, no abnormalities of the immune system are found. Periodontitis often takes years to decades to progress, and cyclic patterns of exacerbation and remission are typical.

In patients with periodontitis, gingivitis is present and precedes the development of significant periodontal lesions. Blunting and apical positioning of the gingival margins typically are present (Fig. 4-28). Periodontal disease is present when a loss of attachment can be demonstrated through the use of a periodontal probe. In the absence of significant gingival hyperplasia, a measurement of pockets greater than 3 to 4 mm indicates destruction of the periodontal ligament and resorption of adjacent alveolar bone. High-quality dental radiographs exhibit a decreased vertical height of the bone surrounding the affected teeth. With advanced bone loss, tooth mobility is present (Fig. 4-29).

Periodontal Abscess

On occasion, the entrance into a periodontal pocket can close, resulting in a secondary localized accumulation of pus within the pocket—a **periodontal abscess** (Figs. 4-30 and 4-31). The area presents as a zone of gingival enlargement along the lateral aspect of a tooth. The involved gingiva may be erythematous and edematous with a slick, red surface or hemorrhagic with a dark-red coloration (Fig. 4-32; see Color Figure 24). Common symptoms include:

Table 4-3. SYSTEMIC DISORDERS WITH PREMATURE ATTACHMENT LOSS

1. Acatalasia
2. Acrodynia
3. Acquired immunodeficiency syndrome (AIDS)
4. Blood dyscrasias
   a. Leukemia
   b. Agranulocytosis
   c. Cyclic neutropenia
5. Crohn's disease
6. Diabetes mellitus
7. Dyskeratosis congenita
8. Ehlers-Danlos syndrome, type VIII
9. Hemochromatosis
10. Hypophosphatasia
11. Langerhans cell disease
12. Leukocyte dysfunctions with associated extraoral infections
13. Oxalosis
14. Papillon-Lefèvre syndrome
15. Sarcoidosis
16. Trisomy 21

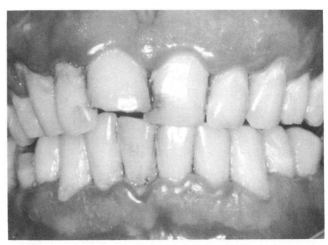

FIGURE 4-28. **Adult periodontitis.** Diffuse gingival erythema with blunting and apical positioning of the gingival margins. (Courtesy of Dr. Dorene Sabulski.)

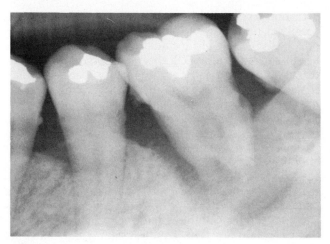

FIGURE 4–29. **Advanced adult periodontitis.** Extensive loss of bone support of the posterior mandibular dentition. Significant mobility of the first molar was noted.

- Throbbing pain
- Extreme sensitivity to palpation of the affected gingiva
- Sensitivity and mobility of the adjacent tooth
- A foul taste
- Lymphadenopathy
- Occasionally, fever, leukocytosis, and malaise.

Probing or gentle pressure on the affected gingiva often results in the expression of pus from the sulcus. The abscess may drain through an overlying sinus tract. With drainage, the abscess becomes asymptomatic but can demonstrate acute exacerbations if the mucosa heals over and the pressure builds again.

Pericoronitis

A similar inflammatory lesion known as **pericoronitis** can develop around impacted or partially erupted teeth when food debris and bacteria are present beneath the gingival flap overlying the crown. These gingival flaps can exhibit long-term periods of chronic inflammation

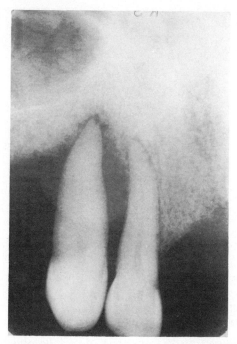

FIGURE 4–31. **Periodontal abscess.** Same patient as depicted in Figure 4–30. Note extensive loss of bone support associated with the maxillary cuspid.

without symptoms. If the debris and bacteria become entrapped deep within the gingival flap, abscess formation develops. Abscess development is most frequently seen in association with the mandibular third molars, and the predominant symptoms are extreme pain in the area, a foul taste, and inability to close the jaws. The pain may radiate to the throat, ear, or floor of the mouth. The affected area is erythematous and edematous, and the patient often has lymphadenopathy, fever, leukocytosis, and malaise (Fig. 4–33). ANUG-like necrosis may develop in areas of persistent pericoronitis.

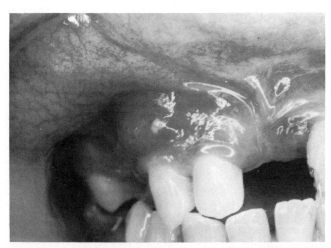

FIGURE 4–30. **Periodontal abscess.** Localized erythematous gingival enlargement with central purulent drainage.

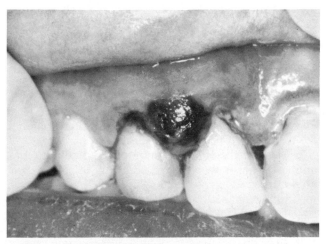

FIGURE 4–32. **Periodontal abscess.** Dark-red and hemorrhagic enlargement of the interdental papilla between the maxillary right lateral incisor and cuspid. See Color Plates.

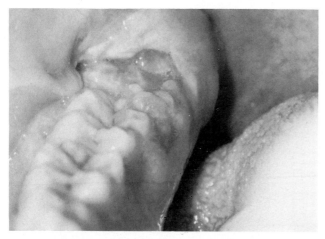

FIGURE 4–33. **Pericoronitis.** Painful erythematous enlargement of the soft tissues overlying the crown of the partially erupted right mandibular third molar.

Histopathologic Features

When soft tissue from areas of periodontitis is examined microscopically, gingivitis is present and the crevicular epithelium lining the pocket is hyperplastic, with extensive exocytosis of acute inflammatory cells. The adjacent connective tissue exhibits an increased vascularity and contains an inflammatory cellular infiltrate consisting predominantly of lymphocytes and plasma cells, but with a variable number of polymorphonuclear leukocytes. Frequently, large colonies of microorganisms, representing plaque and calculus, are noted.

Treatment and Prognosis

Periodontitis

The treatment of periodontitis is directed toward cessation of the destruction of attachment. The foremost goal is the elimination of the presence of the pathogenic bacterial plaque. Early periodontal lesions can be treated by scaling, root planing, and curettage. In deeper pockets, a surgical flap may be required to gain access to the tooth for necessary debridement. At this time, the underlying bone may be recontoured, if necessary, to aid in the resolution of the periodontal pocket.

In some bony defects, regeneration of the attachment can be attempted through interdental denudation or the placement of autogenous bone grafts, allografts, or alloplastic materials. Often, these grafts are used in conjunction with materials such as polytetrafluorethylene in an attempt to achieve guided tissue regeneration in moderate to advanced periodontal defects.

Because of the chronic nature of adult periodontitis, antibiotics generally are not used except in patients who do not respond to conventional therapy. When required, tetracycline or metronidazole are the most common antibiotics used. In addition, several studies suggest that nonsteroidal anti-inflammatory drugs (NSAIDs) may help slow the progression of bone loss in some cases of destructive periodontitis.

In many cases, the prognosis for adult periodontitis correlates directly with the patient's desire to maintain oral health. Long-term studies show that periodontal health can be maintained after appropriate periodontal therapy if a program of rigorous oral hygiene and professional care is established. Professional scaling and root planing modify the composition of the plaque microflora such that pathogenic plaques are converted to those with bacterial types normally found in healthy mouths. Bacterial morphotypes return to pretreatment levels in 42 days after professional prophylaxis, but pathogenic complexes capable of inducing attachment loss require approximately 3 months to be functionally re-established. In patients with less than optimal oral hygiene or with isolated defects that cannot be self-cleaned, a loss of attachment can be prevented if professional scaling and root planing are performed at 3-month intervals.

Periodontal Abscess

A periodontal abscess is treated by drainage through the sulcus or by an incision through the overlying mucosa. Penicillin or other antibiotics are prescribed when a fever is present. Analgesics are prescribed and the patient receives a soft diet, is told to use warm salt water rinses, and is instructed to return each day until the symptoms have resolved. After the acute phase has passed, the patient is treated for the underlying chronic pathologic periodontal condition.

Pericoronitis

Acute pericoronitis is treated with gentle antiseptic lavage under the gingival flap to remove gross food debris and bacteria. Systemic antibiotics are used if a fever or general symptoms are noted. The patient is instructed to use warm salt water rinses and to return in 24 hours. Once the acute phase has subsided, the tooth can be extracted if long-term maintenance is contraindicated. If tooth retention is desirable, the overlying gingival flap is removed surgically, followed by elimination of all food debris and bacterial colonies by thorough curettage.

EARLY-ONSET PERIODONTITIS

Although periodontitis is much more frequent in older adults, it can also be a significant problem in children and young adults. Three forms of **early-onset periodontitis** are seen:

- Prepubertal
- Juvenile
- Rapidly progressive

By definition, these disorders occur in otherwise healthy people and there should be no association with a systemic disease process. In keeping with this definition, these diagnoses are ones of exclusion, and all systemic disorders known to be related to premature loss of attachment (see Table 4–3) should be ruled out before the definitive diagnosis is made. Too many clinicians inappropriately jump to the diagnosis of early-onset periodontitis before undertaking a sufficient evaluation for systemic disease.

In contrast to adult disease, early-onset periodontitis appears to be correlated with one or more deficiencies in the immune response rather than with inappropriate accumulations of plaque and calculus. In addition, a genetic predisposition is suggested in many cases. A review of numerous investigations into the immunology and genetics of these diseases has produced conflicting results, which may be due to the multifactorial nature of early-onset periodontitis. Suspected pathogens that are commonly found in these diseases include *Actinobacillus actinomycetemcomitans*, *Prevotella intermedia*, *Porphyromonas gingivalis*, and a variety of other less common organisms. The response to therapy often hinges on the successful elimination of these organisms.

Clinical and Radiographic Features

Prepubertal Periodontitis

Prepubertal periodontitis develops around the age of 4, with a female predominance reported by several investigators. In the past, the disease was divided into generalized and localized forms, but the generalized variant has been discovered to represent an oral manifestation of a systemic disease known as **leukocyte adhesion deficiency**. In the localized pattern, minimal plaque and gingivitis often are present. Only some of the primary teeth are affected, and there is no localization to specific areas of the jaws. Localized prepubertal periodontitis may lead to juvenile periodontitis.

Localized Juvenile Periodontitis

Juvenile periodontitis can be localized or generalized. One large study of children aged 5 to 17 years in the United States demonstrated a prevalence of 0.53 percent for the localized form and 0.13 percent for the generalized variant. **Localized juvenile periodontitis** most likely represents a specific disease process that begins around the ages of 11 to 13 years with a strong familial tendency. This form appears to localize around the first molars and the incisors, possibly because these teeth have been erupted for the longest duration of time (Figs. 4–34 and 4–35). Typically, there is a lack of gingival inflammation with minimal plaque and calculus; however, subgingival plaque is present on every affected root. The rate of bone destruction is 3 to 5 times faster than that seen in adult periodontitis.

Radiographs reveal vertical bone resorption of the first molars, which is often bilateral and symmetric. In classic cases, an arc-shaped zone of bone loss extends from the distal portion of the second bicuspid to the mesial part of the second molar. Similar involvement is apparent around the anterior teeth. Tooth migration and mobility are common. If untreated, the process continues until the teeth are exfoliated. Progression to more generalized disease may occur.

Of all the pathogens in dental plaque, *A. actinomycetemcomitans* appears to be predominant in localized juvenile periodontitis. This bacterium is present in disease

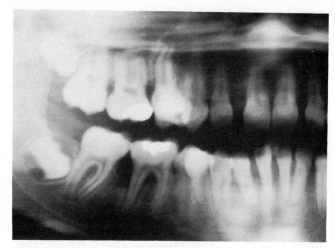

FIGURE 4–34. **Localized juvenile periodontitis.** Loss of bone support in the area of the first molars and incisors of both maxillary and mandibular right quadrants in a 14-year-old patient.

sites in more than 90 percent of the cases. Its ability to invade gingival tissue has created difficulties in mechanical eradication. A knowledge of its importance to the disease process has led to remarkable advances in therapy.

Generalized Juvenile Periodontitis

Generalized juvenile periodontitis may not represent a distinct disease entity but, rather, may be a collection of young adults with advanced periodontal disease. Many cases may represent localized juvenile periodontitis that has become more generalized with time; other cases initially demonstrate generalized disease. Most affected patients are between the ages of 12 and 32. Once again, minimal plaque and calculus are present. Compared with the localized variant, more teeth are affected and the bone loss is not restricted to specific areas of the jaws.

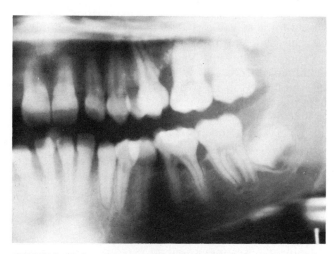

FIGURE 4–35. **Localized juvenile periodontitis.** Left quadrants of the same patient depicted in Figure 4–34. Note the similar pattern of bone loss in the area of the first molars and incisors.

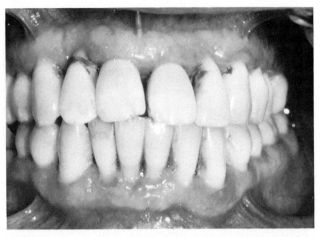

FIGURE 4–36. **Rapidly progressive periodontitis, quiescent phase.** Gingiva exhibiting mild erythema and close adaptation to the dentition. Note blunting and recession of the gingiva margins from prior loss of attachment.

Rapidly Progressive Periodontitis

Rapidly progressive periodontitis is a highly destructive form of periodontitis that occurs primarily in young adults between the ages of 20 and 35. Most patients demonstrate defective leukocyte function and a relationship to pathogenic organisms within the plaque that is similar to that seen in adult periodontitis. The destruction of attachment is widespread and rapid, with loss of much of the alveolar bone within a few weeks to months. Progression may proceed to tooth loss or may be interrupted by periods of quiescence. During the active phase, the gingiva is extremely inflamed, hyperplastic, and hemorrhagic; malaise, weight loss, and depression also may be noted. During the quiescent phase, the gingiva is clinically normal and closely adapted to the teeth (Fig. 4–36).

Histopathologic Features

The microscopic examination of granulation tissue removed from sites of early-onset periodontitis is not dramatically different from that seen in adult periodontitis. In spite of this, histopathologic examination of the material removed from active sites of disease is mandatory to rule out the possibility of other disease processes, such as Langerhans cell disease (see p. 451). Even when the attachment loss presents in a classic localized pattern of juvenile periodontitis, systemic disease cannot be eliminated without an examination of tissue. The definitive diagnosis centers around the clinical, radiographic, histopathologic, and microbiologic findings combined with the family history and leukocyte function tests.

Treatment and Prognosis

Unlike the treatment used for patients with adult periodontitis, scaling and root planing alone do not stop progression of early-onset periodontitis. The defects in leukocyte function along with the invasive capabilities of the involved pathogenic organisms mandate the use of antibiotics in combination with mechanical removal of subgingival plaque and inflamed periodontal tissues. Tetracycline, amoxicillin/clavulanate potassium, and a combination of amoxicillin and metronidazole are the medications of choice, although minocycline and erythromycin also are used.

Antibiotics are prescribed, and surgery is performed 2 days after the initiation of the antimicrobial therapy. Surgery is approached in a manner similar to that described for adult periodontitis. Chlorhexidine rinses are used for 2 weeks after surgery. A re-evaluation with professional prophylaxis is performed once a month for 6 months and then every 3 months thereafter.

Specimens for anaerobic cultures are obtained at each 3-month recall. Patients with refractory disease or significant colonization by pathogenic organisms receive additional courses of appropriate antibiotics. Long-term follow-up is mandatory because of the possibility of reinfection or incomplete elimination of the organisms. Dental practitioners should alert proband patients with early-onset periodontitis of the possible genetic transmission of the disease process.

PAPILLON-LEFÈVRE SYNDROME

Papillon and Lefèvre initially described the syndrome that bears their names in 1924. This autosomal recessive disorder predominantly demonstrates oral and dermatologic manifestations; similar dermatologic changes can be seen in the absence of oral findings (**Meleda's disease**). The predominant oral finding is accelerated periodontitis that appears to be due to multiple leukocyte dysfunctions:

- Impaired T- and B-lymphocyte reactivity
- A chemotactic defect
- Reduced intracellular killing of both bacterial and fungal organisms

Clinical and Radiographic Features

Papillon-Lefèvre syndrome exhibits a prevalence of 1 to 4 per million people in the population, and carriers are thought to be present in 2 to 4 per thousand persons. In most cases, the dermatologic manifestations become clinically evident in the first 3 years of life. Diffuse transgredient (first occurs on the palms and soles and then spreads to the dorsa of the hands and feet) palmar-plantar keratosis develops, with occasional reports of diffuse follicular hyperkeratosis and keratosis on the elbows and knees (Fig. 4–37). Some patients describe worsening in the winter, and others describe keratotic desquamation, which may be confused with psoriasis.

The oral manifestations consist of dramatically advanced periodontitis, which is seen in both the deciduous and permanent dentitions and develops soon after the eruption of the teeth. Extensive hyperplastic and hemorrhagic gingivitis is seen (Fig. 4–38). A rapid loss of attachment occurs, with the teeth soon lacking osseous support and appearing radiographically to float in the soft tissue (Fig. 4–39). The loss of the dentition is inevi-

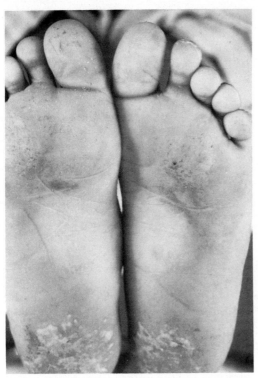

FIGURE 4-37. **Papillon-Lefèvre syndrome.** Plantar keratosis of the soles of both feet. (Courtesy of Dr. James L. Dickson.)

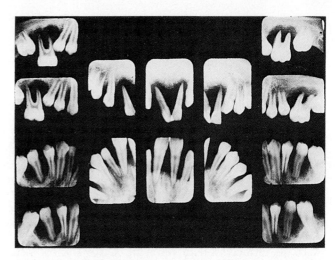

FIGURE 4-39. **Papillon-Lefèvre syndrome.** Multifocal sites of bone loss in all four quadrants. (From Giansanti JS, Hrabak, RP, Waldron CA. Palmar-plantar hyperkeratosis and concomitant periodontal destruction (Papillon-Lefèvre syndrome). Oral Surg Oral Med Oral Pathol 36:40–48, 1973.)

table without aggressive therapy. Mobility and migration of the teeth is observed consistently, and mastication often is painful because of the lack of support. The teeth spontaneously exfoliate or are removed because of sensitivity during function. This process prematurely eliminates the deciduous dentition; with eruption of the permanent teeth, the destructive pattern is duplicated. When the teeth are absent, the alveolar mucosa is normal in appearance.

Although other pathogenic bacteria have been isolated from sites of active disease, *Actinobacillus actinomyce-*

temcomitans has been directly related to the periodontal destruction. Although there is a hereditary component and leukocyte dysfunctions can be demonstrated, it appears that there must be an infection with a specific, potent bacterium, such as *A. actinomycetemcomitans*, for the periodontal component to develop. Interestingly, one investigation documented the development of appropriate peripheral leukocyte function following successful resolution of the pathogenic organisms responsible for the periodontitis. This indicates that the leukocyte dysfunction may be induced by infection with *A. actinomycetemcomitans* (possibly secondary to generated leukotoxins).

In addition to the dermatologic and oral manifestations, less frequent findings have been documented by numerous investigators. Ectopic calcifications of the falx cerebri and choroid plexus have been reported in addition to an increased susceptibility to infections beyond the oral cavity. Pyoderma, furunculosis, pneumonia, hepatic abscesses, and other infections have been documented.

Histopathologic Features

Once again, the histopathologic features of Papillon-Lefèvre resemble those seen in adult periodontitis and are not specific. Submitted tissue often contains hyperplastic crevicular epithelium with exocytosis. The underlying connective tissue exhibits increased vascularity and a mixed inflammatory cellular infiltrate consisting predominantly of polymorphonuclear leukocytes, lymphocytes, histiocytes, and plasma cells. Initially, histopathologic examination is recommended to rule out other pathologic causation for the periodontal destruction.

Treatment and Prognosis

Attempts at resolution of the periodontal disease have often been frustrating. In spite of extensive periodontal

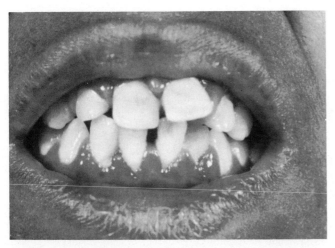

FIGURE 4-38. **Papillon-Lefèvre syndrome.** Diffuse erythematous and hyperplastic gingivitis. (Courtesy of Dr. James L. Dickson.)

therapy and antibiotics, in many patients the disease progresses until all teeth are lost. However, a cessation of attachment loss has been reported by several investigators, and two different treatment approaches have been used.

Despite the use of numerous antibiotics, several reports document a difficulty in resolution of the infection associated with teeth that already exhibit attachment loss. In some of the cases, all of the periodontally involved deciduous teeth were extracted, and treatment with antibiotics was performed in an attempt to remove the causative pathogens. Tetracycline was successful in preventing the redevelopment of periodontitis in the permanent teeth following extraction and the resolution of the infection in the deciduous dentition. However, penicillin, erythromycin, metronidazole, and tetracycline were all unsuccessful in resolving active sites of periodontitis.

The second approach revolves around direct attack against *A. actinomycetemcomitans*. In one investigation, culture and sensitivity testing revealed that the most effective antibiotic regimen was amoxicillin/clavulanate potassium. Ceftriaxone and erythromycin were moderately effective; penicillin, tetracycline, and chloramphenicol were less effective. Metronidazole and ornidazole were ineffective.

Through the use of mechanical plaque control and amoxicillin/clavulanate potassium, the course of the disease may be altered. The progression of attachment loss is slowed dramatically, and the teeth that erupt after the initiation of therapy do not develop periodontal destruction. Rigorous oral hygiene, chlorhexidine mouth rinses, frequent professional prophylaxis, and periodic appropriate antibiotic therapy are necessary for long-term maintenance.

REFERENCES

General References

Carranza FA. Glickman's Clinical Periodontology, 7th ed. Philadelphia, WB Saunders, 1990.

Grant DA, Stern IB, Listgarten MA. Periodontics in the Tradition of Gottlieb and Orban, 6th ed. St. Louis, CV Mosby, 1988.

Schluger S, et al. Periodontal Diseases: Basic Phenomena, Clinical Management, and Occlusal and Restorative Interrelationships, 2nd ed. Philadelphia, Lea & Febiger, 1990.

Gingivitis

Ciancio SG. Agents for the management of plaque and gingivitis. J Dent Res 71:1450–1454, 1992.

Moskow BS, Polson AM. Histologic studies on the extension of the inflammatory infiltrate in human periodontitis. J Clin Periodontol 18:534–542, 1991.

Serio FG, Siegel MA. Periodontal diseases: A review. Cutis 47:55–62, 1991.

Stamm JW. Epidemiology of gingivitis. J Clin Periodontol 13:360–366, 1986.

Suzuki JB. Diagnosis and classification of the periodontal diseases. Dent Clin North Am 32:195–216, 1988.

Acute Necrotizing Ulcerative Gingivitis

Chung CP, et al. Bacterial IgG and IgM antibody titers in acute necrotizing ulcerative gingivitis. J Periodontol 54:557–562, 1983.

Dennison DK, Smith B, Newland JR. Immune responsiveness and ANUG (1985 IADR/AADR abstract). J Dent Res 64:197, 1985.

Haroian A, Vissichelli VP. A patient instruction guide used in treating ANUG. Gen Dent 39:40, 1991.

Hartnett AC, Shiloah J. The treatment of acute necrotizing ulcerative gingivitis. Quintessence Int 22:95–100, 1991.

Johnson BD, Engel D. Acute necrotizing ulcerative gingivitis: A review of diagnosis, etiology and treatment. J Periodontol 57:141–150, 1986.

Loesche WJ, et al. The bacteriology of acute necrotizing ulcerative gingivitis. J Periodontol 53:223–230, 1982.

MacCarthy D, Claffey N. Acute necrotizing ulcerative gingivitis is associated with attachment loss. J Clin Periodontol 18:776–779, 1991.

Riviere GR, et al. Identification of spirochetes related to *Treponema pallidum* in necrotizing ulcerative gingivitis and chronic periodontitis. N Engl J Med 325:539–543, 1991.

Riviere GR, et al. Pathogen-related spirochetes identified within gingival tissue from patients with acute necrotizing ulcerative gingivitis. Infect Immun 59:2653–2657, 1991.

Rowland RW, et al. Serum IgG and IgM levels to bacterial antigens in necrotizing ulcerative gingivitis. J Periodontol 64:195–201, 1992.

Plasma Cell Gingivitis

Kerr DA, McClatchey KD, Regezi JA. Idiopathic gingivostomatitis: Cheilitis, glossitis, gingivitis syndrome: Atypical gingivostomatitis, plasma-cell gingivitis, plasmacytosis of gingiva. Oral Surg Oral Med Oral Pathol 32:402–423, 1971.

Kerr DA, McClatchey KD, Regezi JA. Allergic gingivostomatitis (due to gum chewing). J Periodontol 42:709–712, 1971.

Lubow RM et al. Plasma-cell gingivostomatitis: Report of a case. J Periodontol 55:235–241, 1984.

MacLeod RI, Ellis JE. Plasma cell gingivitis related to the use of herbal toothpaste. Br Dent J 166:375–376, 1989.

Owings JR. An atypical gingivostomatitis: Report of four cases. J Periodontol 40:538–542, 1969.

Perry HO, Deffner NF, Sheridan PJ. Atypical gingivostomatitis: Nineteen cases. Arch Dermatol 107:872–878, 1973.

Serio FG, Siegel MA. Plasma cell gingivitis of unusual origin: Report of a case. J Periodontol 62:390–393, 1991.

Silverman S Jr, Lozada F. An epilogue to plasma-cell gingivostomatitis (allergic gingivostomatitis). Oral Surg Oral Med Oral Pathol 43:211–217, 1977.

Sollecito TP, Greenberg MS. Plasma cell gingivitis: Report of two cases. Oral Surg Oral Med Oral Pathol 73:690–693, 1992.

Timms MS, Sloan P. Association of supraglottic and gingival idiopathic plasmacytosis. Oral Surg Oral Med Oral Pathol 71:451–453, 1991.

Granulomatous Gingivitis

Daley TD, Wysocki GP. Foreign body gingivitis: An iatrogenic disease? Oral Surg Oral Med Oral Pathol 69:708–712, 1990.

Desquamative Gingivitis

Fine RM, Weathers DR. Desquamative gingivitis: A form of cicatricial pemphigoid? Br J Dermatol 102:393–399, 1980.

Forman L, Nally FF. Oral non-dystrophic bullous eruption mainly limited to the gingivae: A mechano bullous response: A variant of cicatricial mucous membrane pemphigoid? Br J Dermatol 96:111–117, 1977.

Laskaris G, Demetriou N, Angelopoulos A. Immunofluorescent studies in desquamative gingivitis. J Oral Pathol 10:398–407, 1981.

Lind PO, Hurlen B. Desquamative gingivitis responding to treatment with tetracycline: A pilot study. Scand J Dent Res 96:232–234, 1988.

Mariotti A. Desquamative gingivitis: Revisited. Today's FDA 3:1C–3C, 1991.

Rogers RS III, Sheridan PJ. Desquamative gingivitis: Clinical, histopathologic, immunopathologic, and therapeutic observations. J Am Acad Dermatol 7:729–735, 1982.

Rønbeck BA, Lind PO, Thrane PS. Desquamative gingivitis: Preliminary observations with tetracycline treatment. Oral Surg Oral Med Oral Pathol 69:694–697, 1990.

Sklavounou A, Laskaris G. Frequency of desquamative gingivitis in skin diseases. Oral Surg Oral Med Oral Pathol 56:141–144, 1983.

Drug-Related Gingival Hyperplasia

Barclay S, Thomason JM, Seymour RA. The incidence and severity of nifedipine-induced gingival overgrowth. J Clin Periodontol 19:311–314, 1992.

Behari M. Gingival hyperplasia due to sodium valproate. J Neurol Neurosurg Psychiatry 54:279–283, 1991.

Butler RT, Kalkwarf KL, Kaldahl WB. Drug-induced gingival hyperplasia: Phenytoin, cyclosporine, and nifedipine. J Am Dent Assoc 114:56–60, 1987.

Dongari A, McDonnell HT, Langlais RP. Drug-induced gingival overgrowth. Oral Surg Oral Med Oral Pathol 76:543–548, 1993.

Hassell TM, Hefti AF. Drug-induced gingival overgrowth: Old problem, new problem. Crit Rev Oral Biol Med 2:103–137, 1991.

Lundergan WP. Drug-induced gingival enlargements. Dilantin® hyperplasia and beyond. Calif Dent Assoc J 17(6):48–52, 1989.

Miller CS, Damm DD. Incidence of verapamil-induced gingival hyperplasia in a dental population. J Periodontol 63:453–456, 1992.

Peñarrocha-Diago M, Bagán-Sebastián JV, Vera-Sempere F. Diphenylhydantoin-induced gingival overgrowths in man: A clinico-pathologic study. J Periodontol 61:571–574, 1990.

Seymour RA. Calcium channel blockers and gingival overgrowth. Br Dent J 170:376–379, 1991.

Seymour RA, Jacobs DJ. Cyclosporin and the gingival tissues. J Clin Periodontol 19:1–11, 1992.

Thomason JM, Seymour RA, Rice N. The prevalence and severity of cyclosporin and nifedipine-induced gingival overgrowth. J Clin Periodontol 20:37–40, 1993.

Gingival Fibromatosis

Bakaeen G, Scully C. Hereditary gingival fibromatosis in a family with the Zimmerman-Laband syndrome. J Oral Pathol Med 20:457–459, 1991.

Jorgenson RJ, Cocker ME. Variation in the inheritance and expression of gingival fibromatosis. J Periodontol 45:472–477, 1974.

Oikarinen K, et al. Hereditary gingival fibromatosis associated with growth hormone deficiency. Br J Oral Maxillofac Surg 28:335–339, 1990.

Rushton MA. Hereditary or idiopathic hyperplasia of the gums. Dent Pract Dent Rec 7:136–146, 1957.

Sciubba JJ, Neibloom T. Juvenile hyaline fibromatosis (Murray-Puretic-Drescher syndrome): Oral and systemic findings in siblings. Oral Surg Oral Med Oral Pathol 62:397–409, 1986.

Takagi M, et al. Heterogeneity in the gingival fibromatoses. Cancer 68:2202–2212, 1991.

Witkop CJ. Heterogeneity in gingival fibromatosis. *In* Birth Defects. Original Article Series. Vol 7. No. 7. Edited by Bergsma D. Baltimore, Williams & Wilkins, 1971, pp 210–221.

Adult Periodontitis

Beck JD, et al. Risk factors for various levels of periodontal disease and treatment needs in Iowa. Community Dent Oral Epidemiol 12:17–22, 1984.

Becker W, Becker BE. Periodontal regeneration updated. J Am Dent Assoc 124 (7):37–43, 1993.

Clemons GP, et al. Current concepts in the diagnosis and classification of periodontitis. Calif Dent Assoc J 18:(5):33–38, 1990.

Fox CH. New considerations in the prevalence of periodontal disease. Curr Opin Dent 2:5–11, 1992.

Greenstein G. The role of metronidazole in the treatment of periodontal diseases. J Periodontol 64:1–15, 1993.

Greenstein G. Supragingival and subgingival irrigation: Practical application in the treatment of periodontal diseases. Compend Contin Educ Dent 13:1098–1125, 1992.

Greenstein G. Periodontal response to mechanical non-surgical therapy: A review. J Periodontol 63:118–130, 1992.

Greenwell H, Bissada NF, Wittwer JW. Periodontics in general practice: Professional plaque control. J Am Dent Assoc 121:642–646, 1990.

Ismail AI, et al. Natural history of periodontal disease in adults: Findings from the Tecumseh periodontal disease study, 1959–87. J Dent Res 69:430–435, 1990.

Lindhe J, Nyman S. Long-term maintenance of patients treated for advanced periodontal disease. J Clin Periodontol 11:504–514, 1984.

Low SB, Ciancio SG. Reviewing nonsurgical periodontal therapy. J Am Dent Assoc 121:467–470, 1990.

Moskow BS, Polson AM. Histologic studies on the extension of the inflammatory infiltrate in human periodontitis. J Clin Periodontol 18:534–542, 1991.

Newman HN. Plaque and chronic inflammatory periodontal disease: A question of ecology. J Clin Periodontol 17:533–541, 1990.

Paquette DW. Potential role of nonsteroidal anti-inflammatory drugs in the treatment of periodontitis. Compend Contin Educ Dent 13:1174–1179, 1992.

Rams TE, NIH Consultant Staff (Periodontics), Slots J. Antibiotics in periodontal therapy: An update. Compend Contin Educ Dent 13:1130–1145, 1992.

Rees JS, Midda M. Update on periodontology: 1. Current concepts in the histopathology of periodontal disease. Dent Update 18:418–422, 1991.

Serio FG, Siegel MA. Periodontal disease: A review. Cutis 47:55–62, 1991.

Tanner A. Microbial etiology of periodontal disease: Where are we? Where are we going? Curr Opin Dent 2:12–24, 1992.

Williams RC. Periodontal disease. N Engl J Med 322:373–382, 1990.

Wilson TG Jr. Supportive periodontal treatment: Maintenance. Curr Opin Dent 1:111–117, 1991.

Early-Onset Periodontitis

Clemons GP, et al. Current concepts in the diagnosis and classification of periodontitis. Calif Dent Assoc J 18:33–38, 1990.

Donly KJ, Ashkenazi M. Juvenile periodontitis: A review of pathogenesis, diagnosis and treatment. J Clin Pediatr Dent 16:73–78, 1992.

Dougherty MA, Slots J. Periodontal disease in young individuals. Calif Dent Assoc J 21:55–69, 1993.

Goené RJ, et al. Microbiology in diagnosis of severe periodontitis: A report of four cases. J Periodontol 61:61–64, 1990.

Lindhe J, Liljenberg B. Treatment of localized juvenile periodontitis: Results after 5 years. J Clin Periodontol 11:399–410, 1984.

Löe H, Brown LJ. Early onset periodontitis in the United States of America. J Periodontol 62:608–616, 1991.

Page RC, et al. Prepubertal periodontitis: I. Definition of a clinical disease entity. J Periodontol 54:257–271, 1983.

Page RC, et al. Rapidly progressive periodontitis: A distinct clinical condition. J Periodontol 54:197–209, 1983.

Pruthi VK. Treatment of rapidly progressive periodontitis: A review and case report. J Can Dent Assoc 56:949–953, 1990.

Pruthi VK, Angier JE, Gelskey SC. Localized juvenile periodontitis: A case analysis and rational approach to treatment. J Can Dent Assoc 56:427–431, 1990.

Watanabe K. Prepubertal periodontitis: A review of diagnostic criteria, pathogenesis, and differential diagnosis. J Periodont Res 25:31–48, 1990.

Papillon-Lefèvre Syndrome

Bimstein E, et al. Periodontitis associated with Papillon-Lefèvre syndrome. J Periodontol 61:373–377, 1990.

Eronat N, Ucar F, Kiline G. Papillon Lefèvre syndrome: Treatment of two cases with a clinical microbiological and histopathological investigation. J Clin Pediatr Dent 17:99–104, 1993.

Glenwright HD, Rock WP. Papillon-Lefèvre syndrome: A discussion of aetiology and a case report. Br Dent J 168:27–29, 1990.

Gorlin RJ, Sedano H, Anderson VE. The syndrome of palmar-plantar hyperkeratosis and premature destruction of the teeth: A clinical and genetic analysis of the Papillon-Lefèvre syndrome. J Pediatr 65:895–908, 1964.

Haneke E. The Papillon-Lefèvre syndrome: Keratosis palmoplantaris with periodontopathy: Report of a case and review of the cases in the literature. Hum Genet 51:1–35, 1979.

Preus HR. Treatment of rapidly destructive periodontitis in Papillon-Lefèvre syndrome: Laboratory and clinical observations. J Clin Periodontol 15:639–643, 1988.

Preus H, Gjermo P. Clinical management of prepubertal periodontitis in 2 siblings with Papillon-Lefèvre syndrome. J Clin Periodontol 14:156–160, 1987.

Tinanoff N, et al. Treatment of periodontal component of Papillon-Lefèvre syndrome. J Clin Periodontol 13:6–10, 1986.

5

Bacterial Infections

IMPETIGO

Impetigo is a superficial infection of the skin that is caused by *Streptococcus pyogenes* and *Staphylococcus aureus*, either separately or together. This infection is endemic in young children and can occur in epidemics. Intact epithelium is normally protective against infection; therefore, most cases arise in areas of dermatitis or previous trauma, such as cuts, abrasions, or insect bites. Individuals harboring the organisms can transmit them through skin contact, and outbreaks are associated with poor hygiene, crowded living conditions, and hot, humid climates.

Clinical Features

Impetigo most commonly occurs on the skin of the face or the extremities. Two clinical patterns are seen. The infection may produce fragile vesicles, which quickly rupture and are replaced by thick, adherent, amber crusts; in other instances, longer-lasting flaccid bullous lesions develop (Fig. 5–1). After the bullae rupture, thin, light-brown crusts develop. Pruritus and regional lymphadenopathy may be seen, but systemic manifestations, such as fever, are not present normally. Some cases have presented as exfoliative cheilitis (see p. 222) or may resemble recurrent herpes simplex (see p. 181).

Diagnosis

A strong presumptive diagnosis can normally be made from the clinical presentation. When the diagnosis is not clinically obvious, the definitive diagnosis requires isolation of *S. pyogenes* or *S. aureus* from cultures of involved skin.

Treatment and Prognosis

Although topical antibiotics may be beneficial in nonbullous forms of impetigo, they are ineffective for the bullous forms, and a 1-week course of a systemic oral antibiotic is the treatment of choice. The best antibiotic is one that is effective against both *S. pyogenes* and penicillin-resistant *S. aureus*. Clindamycin, cephalexin, and dicloxacillin represent good current choices. If left untreated, the lesions often enlarge slowly and spread. Serious complications, such as acute glomerulonephritis, are rare but possible in prolonged cases. Inappropriate diagnosis and treatment with topical corticosteroids may produce resolution of the surface crusts, but infectious, red, raw lesions remain.

ERYSIPELAS

Erysipelas is an infection of the dermis caused by streptococcal organisms, usually *S. pyogenes*. The infection rapidly spreads through the lymphatic channels which become filled with fibrin, leukocytes, and streptococci. Before the use of antibiotics, erysipelas was known as "Saint Anthony's fire" and was associated with a high mortality rate. Today, it is rare and often a forgotten

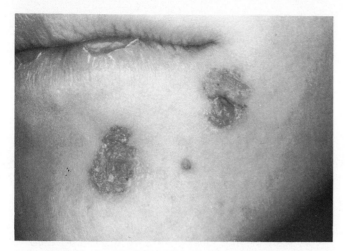

FIGURE 5–1. **Impetigo.** Amber crusts of skin of the chin.

diagnosis. At times, the appropriate diagnosis has been delayed because of confusion with facial cellulitis from dental infections.

Clinical Features

Erysipelas tends to occur primarily in young and elderly patients or in those who are debilitated or diabetic. The infection may occur anywhere on the skin, but the favored sites are the legs and face, often in areas of previous trauma. When lesions occur on the face, they normally present on the cheeks, eyelids, and bridge of the nose, at times producing a butterfly-shaped lesion that may resemble lupus erythematosus (see p. 580). If the eyelids are involved, they may become edematous and shut, thereby resembling angioedema (see p. 253). The affected area is bright-red, well-circumscribed, swollen, indurated, and warm to the touch (Fig. 5–2; see Color Figure 25). Fever and an elevated white blood cell count may be present. The diagnosis is made by the clinical presentation because cultures usually are not beneficial.

Treatment and Prognosis

The treatment of choice is penicillin or erythromycin. On the initiation of therapy, the area of skin involvement often enlarges, probably secondary to the release of toxins from the dying streptococci. A rapid resolution is noted within 48 hours. Recurrences may develop in the same area, most likely in a previous zone of damaged lymphatics. With repeated recurrences, permanent and disfiguring enlargements may result.

STREPTOCOCCAL TONSILLITIS AND PHARYNGITIS

Pharyngeal infections are extremely common and may be caused by many different organisms. The most common causes are group A β-hemolytic streptococci, adenoviruses, enteroviruses, influenza, parainfluenza, and Epstein-Barr virus. The streptococcal variety is one of the most common bacterial infections in humans and represents as many as 25 percent of the cases of pharyngitis. The clinical features of the bacterial and viral varieties are similar.

Clinical Features

The signs and symptoms of **tonsillitis** and **pharyngitis** vary from mild to intense. Common findings include sore throat, dysphagia, tonsillar hyperplasia, redness of the oropharynx and tonsils, palatal petechiae, cervical lymphadenopathy, and a yellowish tonsillar exudate, which may be patchy or confluent (Fig. 5–3; see Color Figure 26). Systemic symptoms, such as fever, headache, malaise, anorexia, abdominal pain, and vomiting, may be noted, especially in younger children. Rhinitis, laryngitis, and bronchitis are typically associated with the viral infections and normally are not present in streptococcal pharyngotonsillitis.

Diagnosis

The diagnosis of streptococcal pharyngotonsillitis can be made by throat culture or much more rapidly by the detection of group A streptococcal antigens on throat swabs.

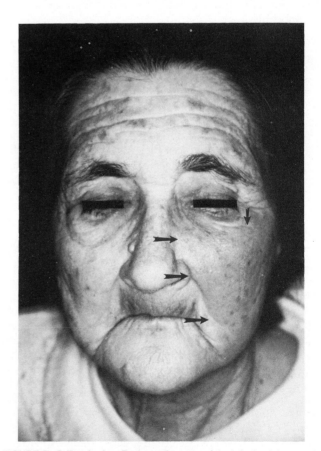

FIGURE 5–2. **Erysipelas.** Red, swollen area of the left cheek (*arrows*). See Color Plates.

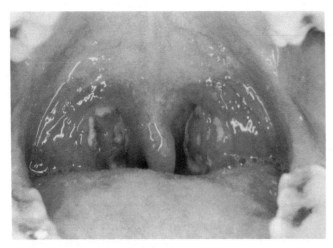

FIGURE 5–3. **Tonsillitis.** Hyperplastic pharyngeal tonsils with yellowish exudate of crypts. See Color Plates.

Treatment and Prognosis

Group A streptococci are uniformly sensitive to penicillin. Erythromycin is used only in patients who have a known sensitivity to penicillin. Streptococcal pharyngitis is a potentially serious infection because of its possible complications, such as rheumatic fever and acute glomerulonephritis. Prompt, appropriate treatment reduces not only the spread and duration of the local infection but also the patient's risk for these significant complications.

SCARLET FEVER

Scarlet fever is a systemic infection produced by group A β-hemolytic streptococci. The disease begins as a streptococcal tonsillitis with pharyngitis in which the organisms elaborate an erythrogenic toxin that attacks the blood vessels and produces the characteristic skin rash. The incubation period ranges from 1 to 7 days, and the significant clinical findings include fever, enanthem, and exanthem.

Clinical Features

Scarlet fever is most common in children from the ages of 3 to 12 years. The enanthem of the oral mucosa involves the tonsils, pharynx, soft palate, and tongue. The tonsils, soft palate, and pharynx become erythematous and edematous, and the tonsillar crypts may be filled with a yellowish exudate. In severe cases, the exudates may become confluent and can resemble diphtheria (see p. 145). Scattered petechiae may be seen on the soft palate. During the first 2 days, the dorsal surface of the tongue demonstrates a white coating through which only the fungiform papillae can be seen; this has been called *white strawberry tongue* (Fig. 5–4; see Color Figure 27). By the fourth or fifth day, *red strawberry tongue* develops when the white coating desquamates to reveal an erythematous dorsal surface with hyperplastic fungiform papillae.

Classically, in untreated cases, fever develops abruptly around the second day, peaks around 103°F, and returns to normal within 6 days. The exanthematous rash develops within the first 2 days and becomes widespread within 24 hours. The classic rash of scarlet fever is distinctive and is often referred to as a "sunburn with goose pimples." Pinhead punctate areas that are normal in color project through the erythema, giving the skin of the trunk and extremities a sandpaper texture. In contrast, the face exhibits a diffuse erythema without punctate zones. The rash is more intense in areas of pressure and skin folds. There are often transverse red streaks, known as *Pastia's lines*, which occur in the skin folds secondary to the capillary fragility in these zones of stress. The mouth demonstrates circumoral pallor.

The rash usually clears within 1 week, and then a period of desquamation of the skin occurs. This scaling begins on the face at the end of the first week and spreads to the rest of the skin by the third week, with the extremities being the last affected. The desquamation of the face produces small flakes; the skin of the trunk comes off in thicker, larger flakes. This period of desquamation may last from 3 to 8 weeks.

Diagnosis

A culture of throat secretions may be used to confirm the diagnosis of streptococcal infection, but this has been replaced by several methods of rapid detection of antigens that are specific for group A β-hemolytic streptococci. Failure to respond to appropriate antibiotics should alert the clinician that the detected streptococci may represent an intercurrent carrier state and other causes of infection should be investigated.

Treatment and Prognosis

Therapy for scarlet fever is indicated to prevent the possibility of complications, such as rheumatic fever or glomerulonephritis. The treatment of choice is oral penicillin, with erythromycin reserved for patients who are

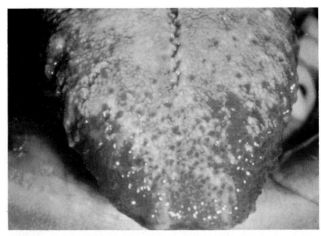

FIGURE 5–4. **Scarlet fever.** Dorsal surface of the tongue exhibiting white coating in association with numerous enlarged and erythematous fungiform papillae (white strawberry tongue). See Color Plates.

allergic to penicillin. The fever and symptoms show dramatic improvement within 48 hours after the initiation of treatment. With appropriate therapy, the prognosis is excellent.

TONSILLOLITHIASIS

Tonsilloliths are calcified structures that grossly resemble sialoliths but develop within tonsillar tissue. Most tonsilloliths develop in tonsillar crypts in which closure of the surface opening leads to the entrapment of organic debris. The calcifications develop within a mass of desquamated epithelium, serum, food debris, and bacterial colonies. Recurrent tonsillar inflammation may promote the development of these tonsillar concretions.

Clinical and Radiographic Features

Tonsillolithiasis can develop over a wide age range, from childhood to old age, with a mean patient age in the early 40s. Males and females are equally affected. These calcifications may vary from small clinically insignificant lesions to massive calcifications more than 14 cm in length. Tonsilloliths may be single or multiple, and bilateral cases have been reported. Many tonsilloliths, especially the smaller examples, are asymptomatic. However, these calcifications can promote recurrent tonsillar infections and may lead to pain, abscess formation, ulceration, dysphagia, and halitosis. In patients with large stones, clinical examination often reveals a hard, yellow submucosal mass of the affected tonsil. In elderly patients, large tonsilloliths can be aspirated and produce significant secondary pulmonary complications. On occasion, tonsilloliths may be discovered on panoramic radiographs as radiopaque objects superimposed on the midportion of the ascending mandibular ramus (Fig. 5–5).

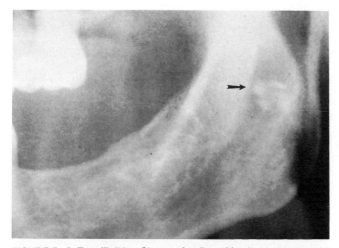

FIGURE 5–5. **Tonsilloliths.** Cluster of radiopacities (*arrow*) in the midportion of the ascending ramus. (Courtesy of Dr. J. R. Cramer.)

Diagnosis

A strong presumptive diagnosis can be made through a combination of the clinical and radiographic features. The definitive diagnosis can be confirmed by the demonstration of the calculi on removal of the affected tonsil.

Treatment and Prognosis

Superficial calculi can be enucleated; deeper tonsilloliths require excision of the affected tonsil.

DIPHTHERIA

Diphtheria is a life-threatening infection produced by *Corynebacterium diphtheriae*. The disease was first described in 1826, and *C. diphtheriae* (also termed Klebs-Löffler bacillus) was initially discovered by Klebs in 1883 and isolated in pure culture by Löffler in 1884. Humans are the sole reservoir, and the infection is acquired through contact with an infected person or carrier. The bacterium produces a lethal exotoxin that causes tissue necrosis, thereby providing nutrients for further growth and leading to peripheral spread. However, an effective antitoxin has been available since 1913, and immunization has been widespread in North America since 1922. Its inclusion in this text is mainly for historical interest, but the infection may still be encountered in developing countries. In addition, infections may occur in people who are immunosuppressed or who have failed to receive booster injections as required. Isolated outbreaks are still reported in the urban poor and Native American populations of North America.

Clinical Features

The signs and symptoms of diphtheria arise 1 to 5 days after exposure to the organism. The initial systemic symptoms, which include a low-grade fever, headache, malaise, anorexia, sore throat, and vomiting, arise gradually and may be mild. Although skin wounds may be involved, the infection predominantly affects mucosal surfaces and may produce exudates of the nasal, tonsillar, pharyngeal, laryngotracheal, conjunctival, or genital areas. Involvement of the nasal cavity often presents with prolonged mucoid or hemorrhagic discharge. The oropharyngeal exudate begins on one or both tonsils as a patchy, yellowish-white, thin film, which thickens to form an adherent gray covering. The superficial epithelium is an integral portion of this exudate, and attempts at removal are difficult and may result in bleeding. The covering may continue to involve the entire soft palate, uvula, larynx, or trachea, resulting in stridor and respiratory difficulties. Palatal perforation rarely has been reported.

The severity of the infection correlates with the spread of the membrane. Local obstruction of the airway can be lethal. Involvement of the tonsils leads to significant cervical lymphadenopathy, which is often associated with an edematous neck enlargement known as "bull neck." Toxin-related paralysis may affect oculomotor, facial, pharyngeal, diaphragmatic, and intercostal muscles. The soft palatal paralysis can lead to nasal regurgitation during swallowing. Oral or nasal involvement has been reported to spread to the adjacent skin of the face and lips.

Although bacteremia is rare, circulating toxin can result in systemic complications. Myocarditis and neurologic difficulties are the most frequently seen and are usually discovered in patients with severe nasopharyngeal diphtheria. Myocarditis may present as progressive weakness and dyspnea or lead to acute congestive heart failure. Neuropathy is not uncommon in patients with severe diphtheria, and palatal paralysis is the most commonly seen manifestation. A peripheral polyneuritis resembling Guillain-Barré syndrome may also occur.

Diagnosis

Although the clinical presentation can be distinctive in severe cases, laboratory confirmation should be sought in all instances. The specimen for culture should be obtained from underneath the diphtheric membrane, if possible, or from the surface of the membrane. Culture material should also be obtained from the nose of each patient.

Treatment and Prognosis

Treatment of the patient with diphtheria should be initiated at the time of the clinical diagnosis and should not be delayed until the results of the culture are received. Antitoxin should be administered in combination with antibiotics to prevent further toxin production, to stop the local infection, and to prevent transmission. Erythromycin, procaine penicillin, or intravenous (IV) penicillin may be used. Most patients are no longer infectious after 4 days of antibiotic therapy, but some may retain vital organisms. The patient is not considered as cured until 3 consecutive negative culture specimens are obtained.

Before the development of the antitoxin, the mortality rate approached 50 percent, usually from cardiac or neurologic complications. The current mortality rate is less than 5 percent, but the outcome is unpredictable.

SYPHILIS (Lues)

Syphilis is a worldwide chronic infection produced by *Treponema pallidum*. The organism is extremely vulnerable to drying; therefore, the primary modes of transmission are venereal or from mother to fetus. In general, the incidence of the infection has been declining in Western nations since the 1860s, but there was a sharp increase during World War II and a smaller peak occurred between 1971 and 1980, primarily in the male homosexual community. Primary infection is concentrated in young adults and is more frequently diagnosed in males. If left untreated, the infection typically progresses through stages.

The first stage is known as **primary syphilis** and becomes clinically evident 2 to 3 weeks after the initial inoculation. At this time, the organism is spreading systemically through the lymphatic channels, setting the stage for future progression. If untreated, the initial lesion heals within 3 to 8 weeks.

The next stage is known as **secondary (disseminated) syphilis** and is discovered clinically 4 to 10 weeks after the initial infection. The lesions of secondary syphilis may arise before the primary lesion has resolved completely. Spontaneous resolution usually occurs within 3 to 12 weeks; however, relapses may occur during the next year.

After the second stage, patients enter a period in which they are free of lesions and symptoms, known as **latent syphilis**. This period of latency may last from 1 to 30 years, and then in approximately 30 percent of patients the third stage, which is known as **tertiary syphilis**, develops.

A syphilitic patient is highly infectious only during the first two stages, but pregnant women may also transmit the infection during the latent stage. Maternal transmission during the first two stages of infection almost always results in miscarriage, stillbirth, or an infant with congenital malformations. The longer the mother has had the infection, the less the chance of fetal infection. Infection of the fetus may occur at any time during pregnancy, but the stigmata do not begin to develop until after the fourth month of gestation. The clinical changes secondary to the fetal infection are known as **congenital syphilis**.

Oral syphilitic lesions are rare but may occur in any stage. Many of the changes are secondary to obliterative endarteritis, which occurs in areas of infection.

Clinical Features

Primary Syphilis

Primary syphilis is characterized by the *chancre* that develops at the site of inoculation. The external genitalia and anus are the most common sites, and the affected area begins as a papular lesion, which develops a central ulceration. Oral lesions are most commonly seen on the lip, but other sites include the tongue, palate, gingiva, and tonsils (Fig. 5–6). The oral lesion presents as a painless, clean-based ulceration or, rarely, as a vascular proliferation resembling a pyogenic granuloma. Regional lymphadenopathy, which may be bilateral, is seen in most patients.

Secondary Syphilis

During secondary syphilis, systemic symptoms often arise. The most common are sore throat, malaise, headache, weight loss, fever, and musculoskeletal pain. A consistent sign is a diffuse, painless, maculopapular cutaneous rash, which is widespread and can even affect the palmar-plantar areas (Fig. 5–7). The rash may also involve the oral cavity and present as red, maculopapular areas. In addition, roughly 30 percent of patients present with superficial areas of irregular, grayish mucosal necrosis known as *mucous patches* (Fig. 5–8). The superficial membrane can be removed to reveal underlying raw connective tissue. These may present on any mucosal

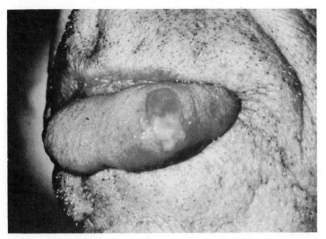

FIGURE 5–6. **Chancre of primary syphilis.** Ulceration of the dorsal surface of the tongue on the left side. (From Neville BW, Damm DD, White DK, Waldron CA. Color Atlas of Clinical Oral Pathology. Philadelphia, Lea & Febiger, 1991.)

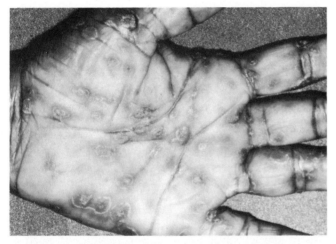

FIGURE 5–7. **Secondary syphilis.** Erythematous rash of secondary syphilis affecting the palms of the hands. (Courtesy of Dr. John Maize.)

surface but are commonly found on the tongue, lip, buccal mucosa, and palate. Occasionally, papillary lesions that resemble viral papillomas may arise during this time and are known as *condylomata lata*.

On occasion, especially in the presence of a compromised immune system, secondary syphilis can exhibit an explosive and widespread form known as **lues maligna.** This form has prodromal symptoms of fever, headache, and myalgia, followed by the formation of necrotic ulcerations, which commonly involve the face and scalp. Oral lesions are present in more than 30 percent of affected patients. Malaise, pain, and arthralgia are occasionally seen. Several cases of lues maligna have been reported in patients with acquired immunodeficiency syndrome (AIDS) (see p. 198), and this possibility should be kept in mind whenever human immunodeficiency virus (HIV)-infected patients present with atypical ulcerations of the skin or oral mucosa.

Tertiary Syphilis

The third stage of syphilis includes the most serious of all complications. The vascular system can be affected significantly through the effects of the earlier arteritis. Aneurysm of the ascending aorta, left ventricular hypertrophy, and congestive heart failure may occur. Effects in the central nervous system may result in tabes dorsalis, psychosis, dementia, paresis, and death. Less significant, but more characteristic, are scattered foci of granulomatous inflammation, which may affect the skin, mucosa, soft tissue, bones, and internal organs. This zone of granulomatous inflammation, known as a *gumma*, presents as an indurated, nodular, or ulcerated lesion which on occasion may be associated with a large amount of tissue destruction. Intraoral involvement most frequently affects the palate or tongue. When the palate is involved, the ulceration frequently perforates through to the nasal cavity (Fig. 5–9). The tongue may be diffusely involved with gummata and appear large, lobulated, and irregularly shaped. Diffuse atrophy and loss of the dorsal tongue papillae produce a condition called *luetic glossitis* (Fig. 5–10). In the past, this atrophic glossitis was

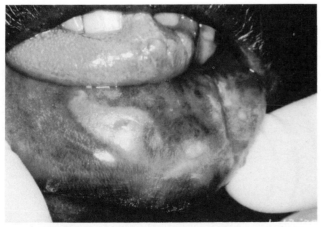

FIGURE 5–8. **Mucous patch of secondary syphilis.** Irregular, grayish area of epithelial necrosis of the lower labial mucosa. (Courtesy of Dr. Michael Kahn.)

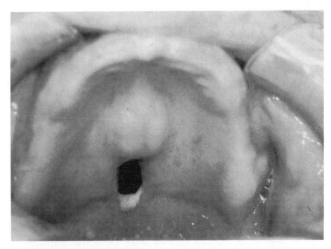

FIGURE 5–9. **Tertiary syphilis.** Perforation of the hard palate. (Courtesy of Dr. George Blozis.)

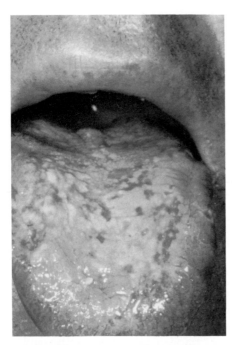

FIGURE 5–10. **Atrophic glossitis of tertiary syphilis.** Dorsal surface of the tongue exhibiting loss of filiform papillae and areas of epithelial atrophy and hyperkeratosis. (Courtesy of Dr. Robert J. Gorlin.)

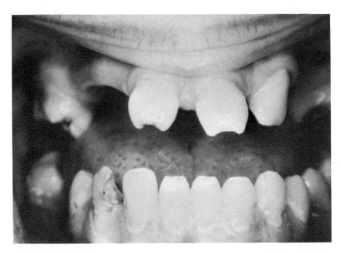

FIGURE 5–11. **Hutchinson's incisors of congenital syphilis.** Dentition exhibiting crowns tapering toward the incisal edges. (From Halstead CL, Blozis GG, Drinnan AJ, Gier RE. Physical Evaluation of the Dental Patient. St. Louis, CV Mosby, 1982.)

thought to be precancerous, but several more recent publications do not support this concept.

Congenital Syphilis

In 1858, Sir Jonathan Hutchinson described the changes found in congenital syphilis and defined three pathognomonic diagnostic features, known as *Hutchinson's triad*:

- Hutchinson's teeth
- Interstitial keratitis
- Eighth nerve deafness

Like many diagnostic triads, few patients exhibit all three features.

The infection alters the formation of both the anterior teeth (*Hutchinson's incisors*) and the posterior dentition (*mulberry molars*). Hutchinson's incisors exhibit their greatest mesiodistal width in the middle third of the crown. The incisal third tapers to the incisal edge, and the resulting tooth resembles a straight-edge screwdriver (Fig. 5–11). The incisal edge often exhibits a central hypoplastic notch. Mulberry molars taper toward the occlusal surface with a constricted grinding surface. The occlusal anatomy is abnormal, with numerous disorganized globular projections that resemble the surface of a mulberry, thus the name (Fig. 5–12).

Interstitial keratitis of the eyes is not present at birth but usually develops between the ages of 5 and 25 years. The affected eye has an opacified corneal surface, with a resultant loss of vision. In addition to Hutchinson's triad, a number of other alterations may be seen. Table 5–1 delineates the prevalence rates of the stigmata of congenital syphilis in a cohort of affected patients.

Histopathologic Features

The histopathologic picture of the oral lesions in the syphilitic patient is not specific. During the first two stages, the pattern is similar. The surface epithelium is ulcerated in primary lesions and may be ulcerated or hyperplastic in the secondary stage. The underlying lamina propria may demonstrate an increase in the number of vascular channels, and an intense chronic inflammatory reaction is present. The infiltrate is predominantly composed of lymphocytes and plasma cells and often demonstrates a perivascular pattern (Fig. 5–13). Although the presence of plasma cells within the infiltrate may suggest the diagnosis of syphilis on the skin, their presence in areas of oral ulceration is commonplace and, therefore, not necessarily of diagnostic significance. The use of special silver impregnation techniques, such as Warthin-Starry or Steiner stains, often shows scattered "corkscrew-like" spirochetal organisms (Fig. 5–14).

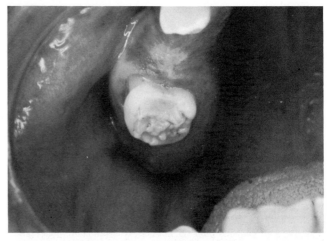

FIGURE 5–12. **Mulberry molar of congenital syphilis.** Maxillary molar demonstrating occlusal surface with numerous globular projections.

Table 5-1. STIGMATA OF CONGENITAL SYPHILIS

Stigmata of Congenital Syphilis in a Cohort of 271 Patients	No. of Patients	% Affected
Frontal bossing	235	86.7
Short maxilla	227	83.8
High-arched palate	207	76.4
Saddle nose	199	73.4
Mulberry molars	176	64.9
Hutchinson's incisors	171	63.1
Higouménaki's sign*	107	39.4
Relative prognathism of mandible	70	25.8
Interstitial keratitis	24	8.8
Rhagades†	19	7.0
Saber shin‡	11	4.1
Eighth nerve deafness	9	3.3
Scaphoid scapulae§	2	0.7
Clutton's joint¶	1	0.3

Modified from Fiumara NJ, Lessel S. Manifestations of late congenital syphilis: An analysis of 271 patients. Arch Dermatol 102:78–83, 1970. Copyright 1970, American Medical Association.

*Enlargement of clavicle adjacent to the sternum.
†Premature perioral fissuring.
‡Anterior bowing of tibia as a result of periostitis.
§Concavity of vertebral border of the scapulae.
¶Painless synovitis and enlargement of joints, usually the knee.

Oral tertiary lesions typically exhibit surface ulceration, with peripheral pseudoepitheliomatous hyperplasia. The underlying inflammatory infiltrate usually demonstrates foci of granulomatous inflammation with well-circumscribed collections of histiocytes and multinucleated giant cells. Even with special stains, the organisms are hard to demonstrate in the third stage, and the inflammatory response is thought to be an immune reaction rather than a direct response to *T. pallidum*.

Diagnosis

The diagnosis of syphilis is best confirmed by demonstrating the spiral organism by dark-field examination of a smear of the exudate of an active lesion. False-positive results are possible in the oral cavity because of the morphologically similar oral inhabitants, such as *T. micro-*

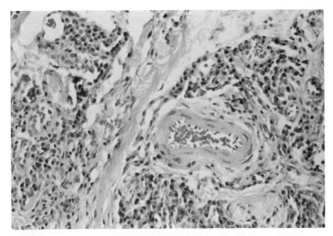

FIGURE 5-13. **Primary syphilis.** A chronic perivascular inflammatory infiltrate of plasma cells and lymphocytes. (Courtesy of Dr. John Metcalf.)

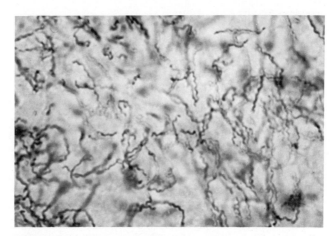

FIGURE 5-14. **Primary syphilis.** Silver stain exhibiting numerous "corkscrew-like" organisms.

dentium, T. macrodentium, and *T. mucosum.* Demonstration of the organism on a smear or in biopsy material should be confirmed through the use of specific immunofluorescent antibody or serologic tests.

Several nonspecific and not highly sensitive serologic screening tests for syphilis are available. These include the Venereal Disease Research Laboratory (VDRL) and the rapid plasma reagin (RPR). After the first 3 weeks of infection, the screening tests are strongly positive throughout the first two stages. After the development of latency, the positivity generally subsides with time.

Specific and highly sensitive serologic tests for syphilis are also available. These include the fluorescent treponemal antibody absorption (FTA-ABS) and *T. pallidum* hemagglutination assays (TPHA). These tests become positive at the time of the development of the first lesion of primary syphilis and remain positive for life. This lifelong persistence of positivity limits their usefulness in the diagnosis of a second incidence of infection. In cases of suspected reinfection, therefore, the organisms should be demonstrated within the tissue or exudates.

Treatment and Prognosis

The treatment for syphilis necessitates an individual evaluation and a customized therapeutic approach. The treatment of choice is penicillin. The dose and administration schedules vary according to the stage, neurologic involvement, and immune status. Most patients obtain a clinical cure with penicillin, but it must be remembered that *T. pallidum* can escape the lethal effects of the antibiotic when the organism is located within the confines of lymph nodes or the central nervous system. Therefore, antibiotic therapy may not always result in a total cure in patients with neurologic involvement but it may arrest only the clinical presentations of the infection. Patients with immunosuppression, such as those with AIDS, may not respond appropriately to standard antibiotic regimens, and numerous reports have documented a continuation to neurosyphilis despite seemingly appropriate single-dose therapy. Tetracycline is given to patients who are allergic to penicillin.

GONORRHEA

Gonorrhea, a sexually transmitted disease that is produced by *Neisseria gonorrhoeae*, represents the most common reportable bacterial infection in the United States. Indirect infection is rare because the organism is sensitive to drying and cannot penetrate intact, stratified squamous epithelium. The disease is epidemic, especially in urban areas, and millions of people are infected each year.

Clinical Features

Most cases of gonorrhea are reported in patients between the ages of 20 and 24 years, although people of any age may be affected. The infection is spread through sexual contact, and most lesions occur in the genital areas. The incubation period is typically 2 to 5 days. Affected areas often demonstrate significant purulent discharge, but approximately 10 percent of men and up to 50 percent of women who contract gonorrhea are asymptomatic.

In men, purulent urethral discharge and dysuria are the most common symptoms. The cervix is the primary site of involvement in women, and the chief complaints are increased vaginal discharge, genital itching, and dysuria. The organism may ascend to involve the uterus and ovarian tubes, leading to the most important female complication of gonorrhea—**pelvic inflammatory disease (PID)**. The symptoms of PID include cramps and abnormal bleeding, and they may be severe or mild. The long-term complications of PID include ectopic pregnancies or infertility from tubal obstruction.

Less than 2 percent of untreated patients with gonorrhea will have disseminated gonococcal infections from systemic bacteremia. The most common signs of dissemination are myalgia, arthralgia, polyarthritis, and dermatitis. Primary involvement of the anorectal areas and oropharyngeal region is not unusual.

Although kissing and cunnilingus have also been implicated as possible modes of transmission, most cases of oral gonorrhea arise as a result of fellatio; therefore, most cases have been reported in females or homosexuals. Because the organism cannot penetrate intact, stratified squamous epithelium, the most common site of oral involvement is the pharyngeal area along with the tonsils and uvula. Involved tonsils typically demonstrate edema and erythema, often with scattered, small yellowish vesicles. Rarely, lesions have been reported in the anterior portion of the oral cavity, with areas of infection appearing erythematous, pustular, erosive, or ulcerated.

During birth, infection of an infant's eyes can occur from an infected mother who may be asymptomatic. This infection is called **gonococcal ophthalmia neonatorum**, and it can rapidly cause blindness.

Diagnosis

To confirm the diagnosis, a Gram stain of the purulent material can be used to demonstrate gram-negative diplococci within the neutrophils. Confirmation of the diagnosis is made through culture and sugar fermentation tests or by a positive fluorescent antibody test.

Treatment and Prognosis

Patients with gonorrhea are at risk for additional sexually transmitted diseases, most commonly *Chlamydia trachomatis*. Isolation of *Chlamydia* is costly and tends to delay therapy. The most cost-effective approach is to co-treat all cases of gonorrhea for possible associated chlamydial infection; the preferred regimen is ceftriaxone and doxycycline. Rescreening is recommended 1 to 2 months after therapy. The most common cause for treatment failure is re-exposure to infected partners, who are often asymptomatic; therefore, the treatment of all recent sexual partners is recommended. Prophylactic ophthalmic erythromycin, tetracycline, or silver nitrate is applied to the newborn's eyes to prevent the occurrence of gonococcal ophthalmia neonatorum.

TUBERCULOSIS

Tuberculosis is a chronic infectious disease caused by *Mycobacterium tuberculosis*. Worldwide, more than 1 billion people are infected, with 8 million new cases and 3 million deaths per year. In the United States, the disease has been declining since the 1800s, especially since the introduction of effective antimicrobials in the 1940s. The decline ceased abruptly in the early 1980s as a result of the AIDS epidemic and increased numbers of the urban poor. Most infections are the result of direct person-to-person spread through airborne droplets from a patient with active disease. Before the tuberculin testing of dairy herds, many cases arose from the consumption of milk infected with *M. bovis*.

Infection must be distinguished from active disease. **Primary tuberculosis** occurs in previously unexposed people and almost always involves the lungs unless it is contracted through consumption of infected milk. The organism initially elicits a nonspecific, chronic inflammatory reaction. In most individuals, the primary infection results only in a localized, fibrocalcified nodule at the initial site of involvement. However, vital organisms may be present in these nodules and remain dormant for years to life.

Less than 5 percent of patients with tuberculosis progress from infection to active disease, and an existing state of immunosuppression is often responsible. In rare instances, active tuberculosis may directly ensue from the primary infection. However, active disease usually develops later in life from a reactivation of organisms in a previously infected person. This reactivation is typically associated with compromised host defenses and is called **secondary tuberculosis**. Diffuse dissemination through the vascular system may occur and has been termed **miliary tuberculosis**. Secondary tuberculosis is often associated with old age, poverty, and crowded living conditions. The immunosuppression of AIDS provides a high risk for progression to active disease.

Clinical and Radiographic Features

Primary tuberculosis is usually asymptomatic. Occasionally, fever and pleural effusion may occur.

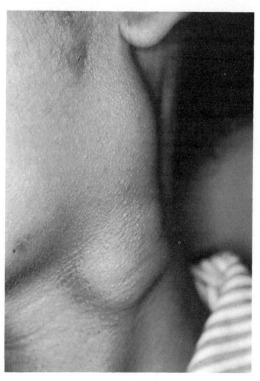

FIGURE 5–15. **Tuberculosis.** Enlargement of numerous cervical lymph nodes. (Courtesy of Dr. George Blozis.)

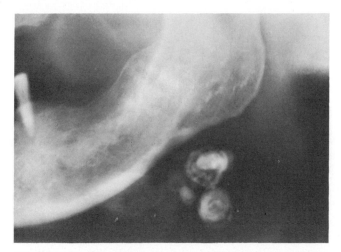

FIGURE 5–17. **Tuberculosis.** Multiple calcified cervical lymph nodes.

Classically, the lesions of secondary tuberculosis are located in the apex of the lungs, but they may spread to many different sites through expectorated infected material or through the lymphatic or vascular channels. Patients typically present with a low-grade fever, malaise, anorexia, weight loss, and night sweats. With pulmonary progression, a productive cough develops and is often combined with hemoptysis or chest pain. In the past, progressive tuberculosis could lead to a cachectic-like wasting termed **consumption.** Involvement of the skin may develop and has been called **lupus vulgaris.**

Drinking of contaminated infected milk can result in a form of tuberculosis known as **scrofula,** but this is rare in North America. Scrofula presents with enlargement of the oropharyngeal lymphoid tissues with involvement of

the cervical lymph nodes (Fig. 5–15). On occasion, the involved nodes may develop significant caseous necrosis and form numerous fistulas through the overlying skin (Fig. 5–16). In addition, areas of nodal involvement may present radiographically as calcified lymph nodes (Fig. 5–17). Pulmonary involvement is unusual in patients with scrofula.

Oral lesions of tuberculosis are uncommon but can occur as nodular, granular, ulcerated, or, rarely, firm leukoplakic areas. Most of the lesions represent secondary infection from the initial pulmonary lesions. It is unclear whether these develop from hematogenous spread or from exposure to infected sputum. The reported prevalence of clinically evident oral lesions varies from 0.5 to 1.5 percent. However, one autopsy study revealed a prevalence of close to 20 percent when the tongues of those infected were examined microscopically. The discovery of pulmonary tuberculosis as a result of the investigation of oral lesions is unusual but not rare. Primary oral tuberculosis without pulmonary involvement is rare.

When present, the oral involvement of primary tuberculosis usually involves the gingiva, mucobuccal fold, and areas of inflammation adjacent to teeth or in extrac-

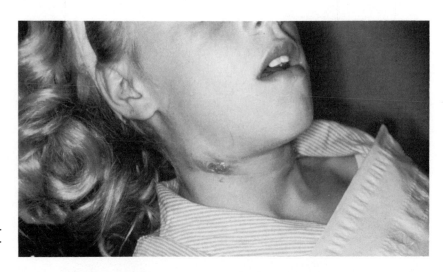

FIGURE 5–16. **Tuberculosis.** Submandibular fistula secondary to involvement of underlying cervical lymph nodes.

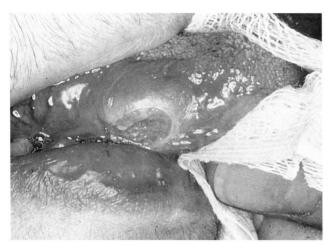

FIGURE 5–18. **Tuberculosis.** Chronic mucosal ulceration of the ventral surface of the tongue on the right side. (Copyright by the American Dental Association. Reprinted by permission.)

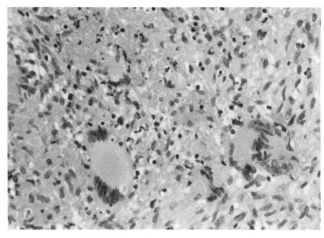

FIGURE 5–20. **Tuberculosis.** Histopathologic presentation of the same lesion depicted in Figure 5–19. Sheets of histiocytes are intermixed with multinucleated giant cells and areas of necrosis.

tion sites; secondary oral lesions mostly present on the tongue, palate, and lip (Figs. 5–18 and 5–19). Primary oral lesions are usually associated with enlarged regional lymph nodes. Tuberculous osteomyelitis has been reported in the jaws and appears as ill-defined areas of radiolucency.

Histopathologic Features

The cell-mediated hypersensitivity reaction is responsible for the classic histopathologic presentation of tuberculosis. Areas of infection demonstrate the formation of granulomas, which are circumscribed collections of epithelioid histiocytes, lymphocytes, and multinucleated giant cells, often with central caseous necrosis (Fig. 5–20). In a person with tuberculosis, one of these granulomas is called a *tubercle*. Special stains, such as the Ziehl-Neelsen or other acid-fast stains, are required to demonstrate the mycobacteria (Fig. 5–21). Special stains sometimes fail to demonstrate the bacteria because of their relative scarcity in the tissue, and a negative result

does not completely rule out the possibility of tuberculosis.

Diagnosis

About 2 to 4 weeks after initial exposure, a cell-mediated hypersensitivity reaction to tubercular antigens develops. This reaction is the basis for the tuberculin (Mantoux or PPD) skin test. Positivity runs as high as 80 percent in developing nations; only 5 to 10 percent of the population in the United States is positive. A positive tuberculin skin test indicates exposure to the organism and does not distinguish infection from active disease. The diagnosis of active disease must be confirmed by special mycobacterial stains or culture of infected sputum or tissue.

Treatment and Prognosis

M. tuberculosis can mutate and develop resistance to single-agent medications. To combat this ability, multi-

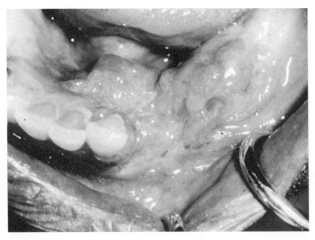

FIGURE 5–19. **Tuberculosis.** Area of granularity and ulceration of the lower alveolar ridge and floor of mouth. (Courtesy of Dr. Brian Blocher.)

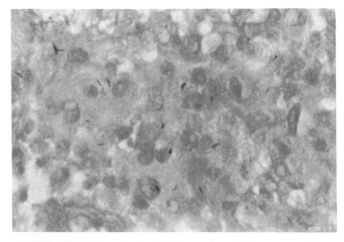

FIGURE 5–21. **Tuberculosis.** Acid-fast stain exhibiting scattered clusters of small mycobacterial organisms.

agent therapy is the treatment of choice. Two multiagent protocols are recommended as first-line therapy against drug-susceptible tuberculosis. The choice is between (1) isoniazid (INH) plus rifampin for 9 months or (2) INH, rifampin, and pyrazinamide for 2 months, followed by INH and rifampin for 4 months. Other first-line medications include ethambutol and streptomycin. Relapse rates of approximately 1.5 percent are seen. With an alteration of doses and the administration schedule, the response to therapy in patients with AIDS has been good, but relapses and progression of infection have been seen.

LEPROSY (Hansen's Disease)

Leprosy is a chronic infectious disease produced by *Mycobacterium leprae*. Worldwide, 10 to 12 million people are affected. The organism has a low infectivity, and exposure rarely results in clinical disease. Small endemic areas of infection are present in Louisiana and Texas, but most patients in the United States have been infected abroad. The organism requires cool host body temperatures for survival. The nine-banded armadillo is unique because of its low core temperature, and it is naturally susceptible to the infection. Naturally infected armadillos have been discovered in Louisiana.

Two main clinical presentations are noted, and these are related to the immune reaction to the organism. The first, called **tuberculoid leprosy**, develops in patients with a high immune reaction. The organisms are typically not found in skin biopsy specimens, skin tests to heat-killed organisms (lepromin) are positive, and the disease is usually localized. The second form, **lepromatous leprosy**, is seen in patients who demonstrate an absence of the cell-mediated immune response. These patients exhibit numerous organisms in the tissue, do not respond to lepromin skin tests, and exhibit diffuse disease. Borderline and less common variations exist. Active disease progresses through stages of invasion, proliferation, ulceration, and resolution with fibrosis. The incubation period is prolonged, with an average of 2 to 5 years for the tuberculoid type and 8 to 12 years for the lepromatous variant.

Clinical Features

M. leprae prefers peripheral nerves and temperatures lower than 37°C. In addition to its neurotropism, the primary sites of involvement are the skin and areas cooled by passing air, such as the nasal cavity.

Tuberculoid leprosy presents with a small number of well-circumscribed, hypopigmented skin lesions. Nerve involvement usually results in anesthesia of the affected skin, often accompanied by a loss of sweating. Oral lesions are rare in the tuberculoid variant.

Lepromatous leprosy begins slowly with numerous, ill-defined, hypopigmented macules or papules on skin that, with time, become thickened (Fig. 5–22). The face is a common site of involvement, and the skin enlargements can lead to a distorted facial appearance *(leonine facies)*. Hair, including the eyebrows and lashes, is often lost (Fig. 5–23). Nerve involvement leads to a loss of sweating and decreased light touch, pain, and tempera-

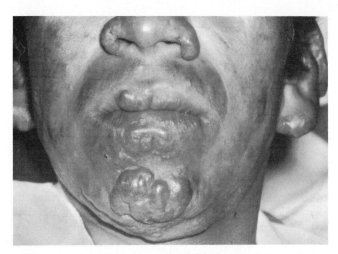

FIGURE 5–22. Lepromatous leprosy. Numerous thickened facial nodules.

ture sensors. This sensory loss begins in the extremities and spreads to most of the body. Nasal involvement presents with nosebleeds, stuffiness, and a loss of the sense of smell. The hard tissue of the floor, septum, and bridge of the nose may be affected. Collapse of the bridge of the nose is considered pathognomonic.

Oral lesions are not rare in lepromatous leprosy, and reports on their incidence vary from 19 to 60 percent. In an excellent review by Prabhu and Daftary of 700 patients with leprosy, the prevalance of facial skin involvement was 28 percent, and oral lesions were noted in 11.5 percent. The lesions tended to be more frequent during the first 5 years of the disease. The sites that are cooled by the passage of air are most frequently affected. The anterior maxillary area, hard and soft palate, uvula, and tongue are the most common sites involved. Affected soft tissue initially presents as yellowish to red, sessile, firm, enlarging papules that develop ulceration and necrosis, followed by attempted healing by secondary intention. Continuous infection of an area can lead to

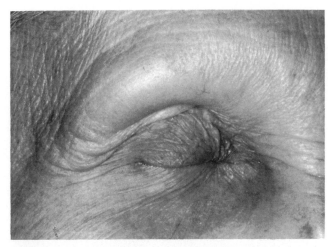

FIGURE 5–23. Lepromatous leprosy. Loss of eyebrows and eyelashes.

significant scarring and loss of tissue. Complete loss of the uvula and fixation of the soft palate may occur. The lingual lesions appear primarily in the anterior third and often begin as areas of erosion, which may develop into large nodules. Infection of the lip can result in significant macrocheilia.

Direct infiltration of lepromatous granulation tissue can destroy the bone underlying the areas of soft tissue involvement. Involvement of the anterior maxilla can result in significant bone erosion, with the loss of the teeth in this area. This classic destruction of the anterior maxilla is responsible for the changes in appearance called *facies leprosa*. Maxillary involvement in children can affect the developing teeth and produce enamel hypoplasia and short tapering roots. Dental pulp infection can lead to internal resorption or pulpal necrosis. Teeth with pulpal involvement may demonstrate a clinically obvious red discoloration of the crown. The cause of the discoloration is unknown but appears to be related to intrapulpal vascular damage secondary to the infection. Granulomatous involvement of the nasal cavity can erode through the palatal tissues and result in perforation.

The facial and trigeminal nerves can be involved with the infectious process. Facial paralysis may be unilateral or bilateral. Sensory deficits may affect any branch of the trigeminal nerve, but the maxillary division is the most commonly affected.

Histopathologic Features

Biopsy specimens of tuberculoid leprosy demonstrate well-formed granulomatous inflammation, with clusters of epithelioid histiocytes, lymphocytes, and multinucleated giant cells (Fig. 5–24). There is a paucity of

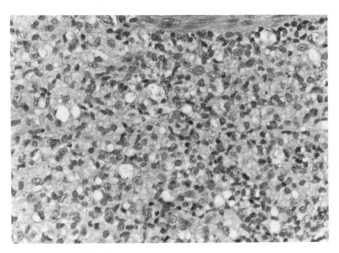

FIGURE 5–25. **Lepromatous leprosy.** Sheets of lymphocytes and histiocytes exhibiting scattered vacuolated lepra cells.

organisms; when present, they can be demonstrated only when stained with acid-fast stains, such as the Fite method. Lepromatous leprosy demonstrates no well-formed granulomas; the typical finding is sheets of lymphocytes intermixed with vacuolated histiocytes known as *lepra cells* (Fig. 5–25). Unlike tuberculoid leprosy, an abundance of organisms can be demonstrated with acid-fast stains in the lepromatous variant (Fig. 5–26).

Diagnosis

The definitive diagnosis is based on the clinical presentation and supported by the demonstration of acid-fast organisms on a smear or in the tissue. The organism cannot be cultivated on artificial media. There is no reliable test to determine whether a person has been exposed to *M. leprae* without developing the disease; this creates difficulties in establishing the diagnosis and determining the prevalence of the infection.

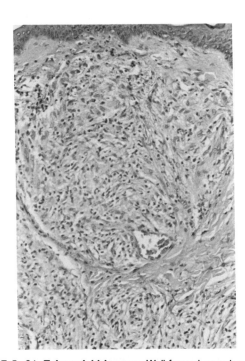

FIGURE 5–24. **Tuberculoid leprosy.** Well-formed granulomatous inflammation demonstrating clusters of lymphocytes and histiocytes.

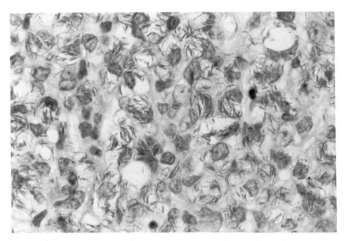

FIGURE 5–26. **Lepromatous leprosy.** Acid-fast stain exhibiting numerous small mycobacterial organisms seen individually and in clusters.

Treatment and Prognosis

The recommended therapy for a person with tuberculoid leprosy is 6 months of rifampin and dapsone, followed by 2 years of observation. The lepromatous variant is best treated with a minimum 2-year course of rifampin, clofazimine, and dapsone followed by 5 years of observation. After resolution of the infection, the therapy must be directed toward reconstruction of the damage in addition to physiotherapy and education of the patients who must live not only with their physical damage but also with the psychological stigmata.

NOMA (Cancrum Oris; Gangrenous Stomatitis; Necrotizing Stomatitis)

Noma is a rapidly progressive, opportunistic infection caused by components of the normal oral flora, which become pathogenic during periods of compromised immune status. *Fusobacterium nucleatum* forms a symbiotic relationship with one or more bacterial organisms, of which the most commonly implicated are *Borrelia vincentii, Staphylococcus aureus, Prevotella intermedia,* and nonhemolytic *Streptococcus* species. The most common predisposing factors include:

- Malnutrition
- Dehydration
- Poor oral hygiene
- Recent illness
- Malignancy
- An immunodeficiency disorder, including AIDS

Commonly associated illnesses include measles, scarlet fever, and tuberculosis; leukemia is one of the more frequently associated malignancies. In many instances, the infection begins as **acute necrotizing ulcerative gingivitis (ANUG)** (see p. 124), and several investigators believe that noma is merely an extension of the same process.

Clinical Features

Noma typically arises in children aged 2 to 10 years and is rare in the United States. The process often begins on the gingiva as ANUG, which may extend either facially or lingually to involve the adjacent soft tissue and form areas called **acute necrotizing ulcerative mucositis**. Zones of necrosis may also develop in soft tissue not continuous with the gingiva, particularly in areas of trauma (Figs. 5–27 and 5–28). The necrosis can extend into deeper tissues; over the next few days, zones of bluish-black discoloration of the overlying skin surface may develop (Fig. 5–29). These discolored zones break down into areas of yellowish necrosis, which also frequently spreads into adjacent bone, with large areas of osteomyelitis possible. Additional lesions may also occur in distant sites, such as the scalp, neck, shoulders, perineum, and vulva. Fetid odor, significant pain, fever, malaise, and regional lymphadenopathy are typical.

A related disorder, **noma neonatorum**, arises in the first month of life in low-birth-weight infants who also dem-

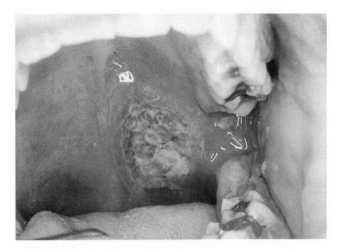

FIGURE 5–27. **Acute necrotizing ulcerative mucositis.** Large area of soft tissue necrosis of the posterior soft palate on the left side.

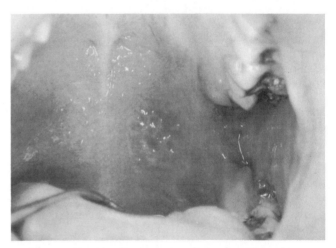

FIGURE 5–28. **Acute necrotizing ulcerative mucositis.** Healing site of necrotizing mucositis (also depicted in Figure 5–27) 6 days after initiation of tetracycline therapy.

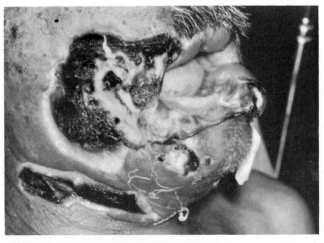

FIGURE 5–29. **Noma.** Extensive blackish orofacial necrosis of the right cheek in an immunocompromised patient.

onstrate malnutrition and frequently a debilitating illness. These patients almost always have infection with *Pseudomonas aeruginosa*, often combined with *Escherichia coli*, *Klebsiella* species, or *Staphylococcus* species. The affected infants frequently have lesions on the lips, nose, mouth, and anal area and less commonly on the scrotum and eyelids. Devastating *Pseudomonas*-related septicemia is often present.

Treatment and Prognosis

In addition to using appropriate antibiotics to treat noma, the clinician must direct therapeutic attention not only to local wound care but also toward correcting the inadequate nutrition, hydration, and electrolyte imbalances. Penicillin and metronidazole are the first-line therapeutic antibiotics in necrotizing stomatitis. The therapy of noma neonatorum is directed against the *Pseudomonas* organisms and often consists of piperacillin, gentamicin, or clindamycin. Conservative debridement of gross necrotic areas is recommended, but aggressive removal is contraindicated because it does not stop the extension of the process and it compounds the reconstruction problems. Necrotic bone is left in place to help hold the facial form, but it is removed as it sequestrates. Reconstruction should be delayed for 1 year to ensure complete recovery.

Prior to the discovery of antibiotics, the mortality rate approached 95 percent, but today less than 10 percent of these patients die. Noma infection can cause significant morbidity when it is not fatal. Facial disfigurement with effects on future growth and development are not rare. Reconstruction is often extremely challenging. Trismus from significant scarring associated with mandibular involvement can occur. Noma neonatorum is much more dangerous because the septicemia that is related to *Pseudomonas* infection is usually fatal.

ACTINOMYCOSIS

Although the term **actinomycosis** seems to imply a fungal infection, it is an infection of filamentous, branching, gram-positive anaerobic bacteria. Actinomycetes are normal saprophytic components of the oral flora. Documented sites of colonization in healthy patients include the tonsillar crypts, dental plaque and calculus, carious dentin, gingival sulci, and periodontal pockets. The colonies within the tonsillar crypts may form concretions and become large enough for the patient to feel the firm plugs within the crypts. Although *Actinomyces israelii* is the most common culprit in clinical infections, *A. naeslundii*, *A. viscosus*, *A. odontolyticus*, *A. meyeri*, and *A. bovis* along with *Arachnia propionica* may produce cases of actinomycosis. In most such cases, the primary organism is synergistically combined with streptococci and staphylococci.

Clinical Features

Actinomycosis may present as either an acute, rapidly progressing infection or as a chronic, slowly spreading lesion that is associated with fibrosis. The most common sites of involvement in actinomycosis are the cervicofacial, abdominal, thoracic, cutaneous, and genital regions. More than 50 percent of cases arise in the cervicofacial region.

The suppurative reaction of the infection may discharge large yellowish flecks that represent colonies of the bacteria called *sulfur granules*. Although common, sulfur granules are not invariably present. In addition, another infection that can also produce sulfur granules and mimic actinomycosis is **botryomycosis**, an unrelated process that represents an unusual host reaction to *Staphylococcus aureus* and other bacteria.

In the cervicofacial region, the organism typically enters tissue through an area of prior trauma, such as a soft tissue injury, periodontal pocket, nonvital tooth, extraction socket, or infected tonsil. The infection does not spread along the typical fascial planes and usually disregards the normal lymphatic and vascular routes. Direct extension through soft tissue is seen, and lymph nodes become involved only if they are in the path of the process. The classic description is of a "wooden" indurated area of fibrosis, which ultimately forms a central, softer area of abscess. The infection may extend to the surface, forming a fistula (Fig. 5–30). Pain is often minimal. The soft tissues of the submandibular, submental, and cheek areas are common sites of involvement, with the area overlying the angle of the mandible being the most frequently affected site.

Localized abscesses without the associated chronic fibrosing reaction have been reported in soft tissue that has received minor trauma. The tongue is the most frequently mentioned site, but any oral mucosal location is possible. Involvement of the tonsils may produce infectious symptoms; in many cases, however, the primary change is one of significant hyperplasia. Investigators have suggested that trial courses of antibiotics be directed against actinomycosis in patients who have obstructive symptoms related to tonsillar hyperplasia.

Salivary gland involvement also is not unusual. Intraductal colonization by the organism may lead to infec-

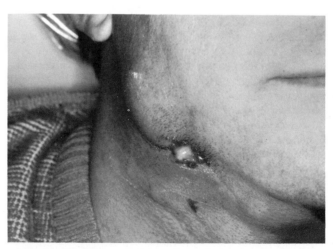

FIGURE 5–30. **Actinomycosis.** Draining fistula of the right submandibular area.

tions in both the submandibular and parotid glands, resulting in abscess formation in the submandibular and masseter spaces, respectively.

Actinomycotic osteomyelitis of the mandible and maxilla has been reported. Trauma, periodontal infections, nonvital teeth, and extraction sites have all provided access. Ill-defined areas of radiolucency, often surrounded by radiopacity, may be found with or without involvement of the overlying soft tissue. Intrabony colonization of dentigerous cysts without other significant clinical or radiographic spread has been reported.

Periapical inflammatory lesions involved by the bacteria can result in lesions that are difficult to resolve with standard endodontic treatment. The anterior maxillary teeth, followed by the mandibular first molars, are the most common areas to be involved. Draining sinuses, pain, and swelling are frequently reported.

Histopathologic Features

The tissue removed from areas of active infection demonstrates chronically inflamed granulation tissue surrounding large collections of polymorphonuclear leukocytes and, with luck, colonies of organisms (Fig. 5–31). The colonies consist of club-shaped filaments that form a radiating rosette pattern (Fig. 5–32). With hematoxylin and eosin stains, the central core stains basophilic, and the peripheral portion is eosinophilic. Methenamine silver stains demonstrate the organisms well. If the colonies of actinomycetes become displaced from the exudate, a rim of neutrophils typically clings to the periphery of the organisms.

Diagnosis

The diagnosis of actinomycosis is ideally achieved by culture, but less than 50 percent of cases are positive because of the overgrowth of associated bacteria, prior antibiotic therapy, or improper anaerobic media conditions. Lacking positive culture results, a strong presumptive diagnosis can be obtained through a demonstration

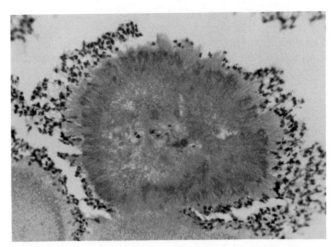

FIGURE 5–32. **Actinomycosis.** Actinomycotic colony exhibiting club-shaped filaments arranged in a radiating rosette pattern.

of the typical colonies in lesional biopsy material. Sulfur granules in infections other than actinomycosis are so rare that their demonstration strongly supports the diagnosis. Finally, fluorescein-conjugated antiserum can be used on the granules to specifically identify the *Actinomyces* species.

Treatment and Prognosis

The treatment of choice for actinomycosis in chronic fibrosing cases is prolonged high doses of antibiotics in association with abscess drainage and excision of the sinus tracts. A high antibiotic concentration is required to penetrate larger areas of suppuration and fibrosis. Penicillin remains the standard of care, and no *in vivo* resistance has been documented. In spite of this, some investigators have demonstrated *in vitro* resistance and recommend tetracycline, which is as effective as penicillin and is the drug of choice for patients with a known allergy to penicillin. Early cervicofacial actinomycosis typically responds to a 5- to 6-week course of penicillin; patients with deep-seated infections may require up to 12 months.

Several authors have indicated that the localized acute infections associated with a dental focus of contamination may be treated more conservatively than the deep, chronic cases of actinomycosis. Localized tongue abscesses, periapical actinomycosis, and pericoronal infections frequently respond well to removal of infected tissue and a shorter 2- to 3-week course of penicillin.

CAT-SCRATCH DISEASE

Cat-scratch disease is an infectious disorder that begins in the skin but classically spreads to the adjacent lymph nodes. Almost all cases arise after contact with a cat, usually a kitten. The organism typically enters the skin through a scratch, bite, or previous site of injury. Infection from other sources is highly unlikely. This disease has been recognized since 1931, but the definitive

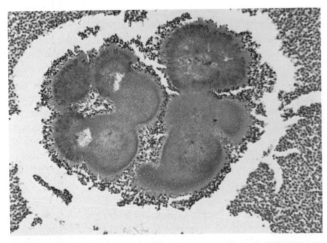

FIGURE 5–31. **Actinomycosis.** Numerous colonies of actinomycotic organisms surrounded by a collection of polymorphonuclear leukocytes.

cause was not determined until the 1980s. Isolation and culture of the organism were finally achieved in 1988. The organism has still not been definitively classified, but findings suggest that *Rochalimaea henselae* or a closely related organism may play an etiologic role.

Clinical Features

Cat-scratch disease begins as a papule or pustule that develops in 3 to 14 days along the initial scratch line (Fig. 5–33). The lymph node changes develop in approximately 3 weeks and often may be accompanied by fever or malaise (Fig. 5–34). Scratches on the face typically lead to submandibular lymphadenopathy and the patient may be referred to dental practitioners to rule out an odontogenic infection. Often, the primary site of trauma may have resolved when the patient presents with the symptomatic lymphadenopathy. Therefore, cat-scratch disease must be strongly considered in the differential diagnosis of patients with unexplained symptomatic lymphadenopathy.

A few patients with cat-scratch disease demonstrate unusual presentations. The infection can present as an intraoral mass in the buccal mucosa when lymphoid aggregates become involved from an adjacent cutaneous primary site. Scratches in the preauricular area may localize in parotid lymphoid tissue and can cause significant parotid pain or even temporary facial paralysis. Primary lesions adjacent to the eye can result in a

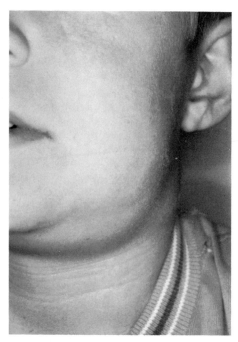

FIGURE 5–34. **Cat-scratch disease.** Submandibular lymphadenopathy has developed after initial trivial injury to skin. (Courtesy of Dr. George Blozis.)

conjunctival granuloma that is associated with preauricular lymphadenopathy (**oculoglandular syndrome of Parinaud**). Other less common presentations include encephalopathy, erythematous and maculopapular rashes, splenomegaly, hepatic lesions, thrombocytopenia, pneumonia, anemia, pleural effusions, and recurrent bacterial infections.

During the past decade, an unusual subcutaneous vascular proliferation, histopathologically similar to histiocytoid hemangioma, has been recognized in patients with AIDS. Because cat-scratch bacilli have been demonstrated microscopically in these lesions and they respond to erythromycin therapy, this disorder is believed to represent a reaction to the cat-scratch bacillus and has been called **bacillary angiomatosis**. The affected areas can resemble Kaposi's sarcoma (see p. 203) and present as variable numbers of red to purple skin lesions. These may be macular, papular, or pedunculated and exhibit a widespread distribution on the skin. Pain and tenderness are common. The larger lesions are friable and bleed easily.

Oral lesions have been seen in bacillary angiomatosis and may also resemble Kaposi's sarcoma. The affected areas may present as zones of alveolar bone loss or may be within the soft tissue and appear as a proliferative vascular lesion.

Histopathologic Features

The involved lymph nodes are enlarged as a result of significant cortical hyperplasia, which classically contains areas of stellate suppurative necrosis surrounded by a band of histiocytes and neutrophils (Fig. 5–35). In some cases, significant necrosis is absent but areas of

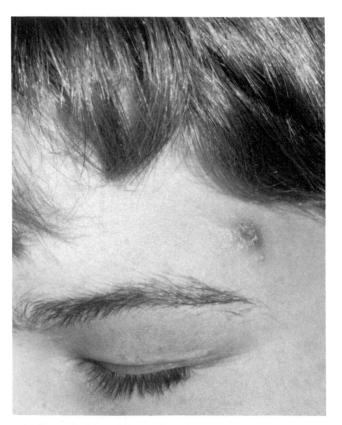

FIGURE 5–33. **Cat-scratch disease.** Papule that developed at initial site of injury.

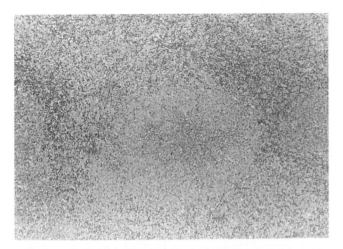

FIGURE 5–35. **Cat-scratch disease.** Intranodal area of abscess formation surrounded by band of histiocytes and neutrophils.

karyorrhexis are present around proliferations of plump vascular channels that often exhibit thickened eosinophilic walls. On staining with the Warthin-Starry method, cat-scratch bacilli are usually found in areas without significant necrosis. As the disease progresses and necrosis increases, the organisms become more difficult to identify. Also, the Brown-Hopps method of Gram staining may be used to highlight the bacilli.

Diagnosis

The clinical diagnosis of cat-scratch disease requires that three of the four following criteria are met.

1. Contact with a cat, presence of a scratch, or a primary dermal or ocular lesion.
2. Positive cat-scratch disease skin test finding (Hanger-Rose skin test).
3. Negative results for other causes of lymphadenopathy.
4. Characteristic histopathologic findings of infected tissue, especially if pleomorphic bacilli can be found on staining with the Warthin-Starry method.

An indirect fluorescent-antibody test for the detection of humoral response to *R. henselae* has been developed. This test has a sensitivity of 88 percent and a specificity of 94 percent for cat-scratch disease. Many clinicians prefer this test to the older Hanger-Rose procedure.

Treatment and Prognosis

Cat-scratch disease is a self-limiting condition and normally resolves within 4 months. The use of local heat, analgesics, and aspiration of the node on suppuration is the typical pattern of therapy. Although the organism has demonstrated sensitivity to a number of antibiotics in culture, the results in immunocompetent patients have been inconsistent. Currently, no controlled therapeutic studies have been performed. Healthy children do not require antibiotics. Acutely ill children have been treated with intravenous gentamicin, oral trimethoprim-sulfamethoxazole, or rifampin. A good response to ciprofloxacin has been reported in adult patients. Antibiotics in patients with AIDS and bacillary angiomatosis have produced dramatic resolution within 2 days. In these patients, erythromycin, doxycycline, or the combination of isoniazid, rifampin, and ethambutol has been efficacious.

SINUSITIS

Sinusitis is one of the most common health care complaints in the United States, with more than 31 million people currently affected. To understand the problem, one must first have at least an elementary knowledge of the sinus anatomy. Adults have bilateral maxillary, frontal, and sphenoid sinuses. These large cavities drain into the nose through openings called ostia. All three of the major sinuses must drain through the middle meatus. Also located bilaterally in this area of the nose is a labyrinth of 3 to 15 small ethmoid sinuses, which drain through smaller ostia. The ostiomeatal complex, with its numerous narrow openings, is the key to sinus disease because it is the primary nasal site for the deposition of foreign matter from inspired air.

Normal sinuses are lined by pseudostratified columnar epithelium with cilia. The cilia are necessary to move the sinus secretions toward the ostia. Gravity also is beneficial in removing the secretions except in the maxillary sinus, where there is a superior location of the ostial opening and, therefore, the ciliary apparatus becomes even more important. Normal function of the paranasal sinuses depends on:

- The patency of the ostial openings
- Proper function of the ciliary apparatus
- The quality of the nasal secretions

Disruption of this balance leads to sinusitis.

Primary inflammation of the lining of the maxillary antrum was long thought to be the major cause of sinusitis, but advances have demonstrated that most sinus disease begins from a blockage of the ostiomeatal complex, which disrupts normal drainage, decreases ventilation, and precipitates disease. Less common localized sinus infections can occur from focal areas of inflammation within a single sinus, such as a dental infection affecting the maxillary sinus.

All of the sinuses contain bacteria. In a person with sinusitis, infection is present initially or as the disease evolves. With bacteria already present in the sinuses, changes as minor as a slight mucosal thickening in the ostiomeatal complex can lead to improper sinus drainage and infection. The most common predisposing factors are a recent upper respiratory viral infection or allergic rhinitis. Other less common causes include cystic fibrosis, immotile cilia syndrome, bronchiectasis, developmental abnormalities, and immunodeficiency, including AIDS.

In otherwise healthy patients, the most common organisms responsible for acute sinusitis are *Streptococcus pneumoniae*, *Haemophilus influenzae*, and *Moraxella catarrhalis*.

If not corrected, some cases of acute sinusitis may become chronic. Chronic sinusitis is defined as recurring episodes of acute sinusitis or symptomatic sinus disease lasting longer than 3 months. In these cases, the bacteria tend to be anaerobes and are most frequently *Streptococcus*, *Bacteroides*, or *Veillonella* species.

Clinical and Radiographic Features

Acute sinusitis in adults presents with headache, fever, and facial pain over the affected sinus. Anorexia, photophobia, and malaise may also be seen. Anterior nasal or posterior pharyngeal discharge is present; it may be thick or thin in consistency and appear clear, mucoid, or purulent. Children, with their less complex sinuses, typically present with only persistent cough, fever, and purulent rhinorrhea. Localized involvement of the maxillary sinus can present as pain over the cheekbone, toothache, periorbital pain, or temporal headache. Maxillary sinusitis is associated with increased pain when the head is held upright and less discomfort when the patient is supine.

Chronic sinusitis is less diagnostic, and radiographic imaging becomes more important. Frequent complaints include facial pressure, pain, or a sensation of obstruction. In some cases, nonspecific symptoms, such as headache, sore throat, lightheadedness, or generalized fatigue, may also be present or even dominate. Radiographically, the involved sinus has a cloudy, increased density (Fig. 5–36).

In addition to the patient's symptoms, the diagnosis in the past was often made by procedures such as transillumination and by plain radiographs, such as the Waters, Caldwell-Luc, lateral, and submental vertex views. Today, when the diagnosis is in question, many clinicians use nasal endoscopy and computed tomography. Areas of infection and sites of improper drainage will be found. These techniques not only confirm the diagnosis but also pinpoint the primary pathologic alteration that led to the obstructive sinusitis.

Treatment and Prognosis

First-line therapy for acute sinusitis in otherwise healthy patients is amoxicillin. Because of drug resistance, additional medications are used if the patient does not respond to the initial antibiotic. Amoxicillin-clavulanate, trimethoprim-sulfamethoxazole, or cefaclor are good antibiotics for resistant cases. Although topical decongestants shrink nasal membranes and improve ostial drainage, they are not recommended because of the resultant decreased ciliary function and decreased mucosal blood flow, which leads to impaired antibiotic delivery. The effect of systemic antihistamines and decongestants on sinusitis has not been studied adequately.

In otherwise healthy adult patients, chronic sinusitis that is not responsive to typical medical management is often corrected surgically. In the past, radical stripping of the diseased sinus mucosa was the therapy of choice. Today, nasal endoscopy has shown that sinusitis is a disease of obstruction and that mucosal inflammation is usually a secondary development. Functional endoscopic sinus surgery enlarges the ostial openings and corrects blockages in the ostiomeatal complex, often with a rapid resolution of the signs and symptoms. The surgery is delicate because it extends close to the orbit and the central nervous system. Each patient's unique anatomy should be carefully evaluated by computed tomography (CT) and nasal endoscopy before surgery.

In children, continued medical management is the therapy of choice for uncomplicated acute or recurrent acute sinusitis. The anatomy in the child, with the increased closeness of the orbit and brain, increases the difficulty of any surgical procedure. Surgical management is indicated in only a small number of childhood sinusitis cases. Suppurative sinusitis extending into surrounding tissues or true chronic sinusitis caused by serious underlying systemic disease are examples of indications for the surgical management of sinus disease in a child.

REFERENCES

General References

Farrar WE, et al. Infectious Diseases, Text and Color Atlas, 2nd ed. New York, Gower Medical, 1992.

Gorbach SL, Bartlett JG, Blacklow NR. Infectious Diseases, 8th ed. Philadelphia, WB Saunders, 1992.

Holmes KK, et al. Sexually Transmitted Diseases, 2nd ed. New York, McGraw-Hill, 1990.

Krugman S, et al. Infectious Diseases of Children, 9th ed. St. Louis, CV Mosby, 1992.

Schuster GS. Oral Microbiology and Infectious Disease. Philadelphia, BC Decker, 1990.

Streptococcal Infections (Impetigo; Erysipelas; Scarlet Fever; Streptococcal Pharyngitis/Tonsillitis)

Bialecki C, Feder HM, Grant-Kels JM. The six classic childhood exanthems: A review and update. J Am Acad Dermatol 21:891–903, 1989.

Demidovich, CW, et al. Impetigo: Current etiology and comparison of penicillin, erythromycin and cephalexin therapies. Am J Dis Child 144:1313–1315, 1990.

Giunta JL. Comparison of erysipelas and odontogenic cellulitis. J Endod 13:291–294, 1987.

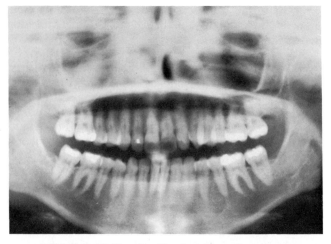

FIGURE 5–36. **Sinusitis.** Cloudy right maxillary antrum.

Macko D, Krutchkoff D, Poole A. Oral manifestations of impetigo: Report of two cases. J Pedod 1:318–326, 1977.

Ochs MW, Dolwick MF. Facial erysipelas: Report of a case and review of the literature. J Oral Maxillofac Surg 49:1116–1120, 1991.

Parnell AG. Facial erysipelas. Oral Surg Oral Med Oral Pathol 27:166–168, 1969.

Peter G, Smith AL. Group A streptococcal infections of the skin and pharynx (first of two parts). N Engl J Med 297:311–317, 1977.

Popowich LD, Brooke RI. Postinjection infection—two unusual cases. J Oral Maxillofac Surg 37:494–495, 1979.

Wannamaker LW, Ferrieri P. Streptococcal infections updated. Dis Mon Oct.:1–40, 1975.

Tonsillolithiasis

Černý R, Bekárek V. Tonsillolith. Acta Univ Palacki Olomuc Fac Med 126:267–273, 1990.

Cooper MM, et al. Tonsillar calculi: Report of a case and review of the literature. Oral Surg Oral Med Oral Pathol 55:239–243, 1983.

Espe BJ, Newmark H. A tonsillolith seen on CT. Comput Med Imaging Graph 16:59–61, 1992.

Hoffman H. Tonsillolith. Oral Surg Oral Med Oral Pathol 45:657–658, 1978.

Marshall WG, Irwin ND. Tonsilloliths. Oral Surg Oral Med Oral Pathol 51:113, 1981.

Diphtheria

Dixon JMS. Diphtheria in North America. J Hyg (Camb) 93:419–432, 1984.

Harnisch JP, et al. Diphtheria among alcoholic urban adults: A decade of experience in Seattle. Ann Intern Med 111:71–82, 1989.

Wyatt GB. Diphtheria. Trop Doct 4:110–114, 1974.

Zizmor J. Diphtherial stomatitis: A complication of immunosuppressive therapy. Arch Dermatol 114:1771, 1978.

Syphilis

Altini M, Peters E, Hill JJ. The causation of oral precancer and cancer. S Afr Med J 18(Suppl):6–10, 1989.

de Swaan B, et al. Solitary oral condylomata lata in a patient with secondary syphilis. Sex Transm Dis 12:238–241, 1985.

Felman YM, Nikitas JA. Sexually transmitted diseases of the oral cavity: Part 1. Cutis 29:552, 560, 562, 564, 634, 635, 650, 1982.

Ficarra G, et al. Early oral presentation of lues maligna in a patient with HIV infection: A case report. Oral Surg Oral Med Oral Pathol 75:728–732, 1993.

Fiumara NJ. Oral lesions of gonorrhea and syphilis. Cutis 17:689–692, 1976.

Fiumara NJ. Venereal diseases of the oral cavity. J Oral Med 31:36–40, 55, 1976.

Fiumara NJ, Lessel S. Manifestations of late congenital syphilis: An analysis of 271 patients. Arch Dermatol 102:78–83, 1970.

Mani NJ. Secondary syphilis initially diagnosed from oral lesions: Report of three cases. Oral Surg Oral Med Oral Pathol 58:47–50, 1984.

Meyer I, Abbey LM. The relationship of syphilis to primary carcinoma of the tongue. Oral Surg Oral Med Oral Pathol 30:678–681, 1970.

Meyer I, Shklar G. The oral manifestations of acquired syphilis: A study of eighty-one cases. Oral Surg Oral Med Oral Pathol 23:45–61, 1967.

Steiner M, Alexander WN. Primary syphilis of the gingiva: Report of two cases. Oral Surg Oral Med Oral Pathol 21:530–535, 1966.

Terezhalmy GT, Cottone JA, Baker BR. Sexual diseases important to dentistry: Clinical diagnoses and treatment. Dentistry 6(2):7–18, 1986.

Viers WA. Primary syphilis of the tonsil: Presentation of four cases. Laryngoscope 91:1507–1511, 1981.

Wong PNC. Secondary syphilis with extensive oral manifestations. Aust Dent J 30:22–24, 1985.

Gonorrhea

Bro-jørgensen A, Jensen T. Gonococcal tonsillar infections. Br Med J 4:660–661, 1971.

Chue PWY. Gonorrhea—its natural history, oral manifestations, diag-nosis, treatment and prevention. J Am Dent Assoc 90:1297–1301, 1975.

Cowan L. Gonococcal ulceration of the tongue in the gonococcal dermatitis syndrome. Br J Vener Dis 45:228–231, 1969.

Felman YM, Nikitas JA. Sexually transmitted diseases of the oral cavity: Part I. Cutis 29:552, 560, 562, 564, 634, 635, 650, 1982.

Guinta JL, Fiumara NJ. Facts about gonorrhea and dentistry. Oral Surg Oral Med Oral Pathol 62:529–531, 1986.

Lightfoot RW, Gotschlich EC. Gonococcal disease. Am J Med 56:347–356, 1974.

Marina D, Veraldi S, Innocenti M. Oral cavity abscess due to *Neisseria gonorrhoeae*. Cutis 40:363–364, 1987.

Merchant HW, Schuster GS. Oral gonococcal infection. J Am Dent Assoc 95:807–809, 1977.

Tuberculosis

Brennan TF, Vrabec DP. Tuberculosis of the oral mucosa. Report of a case. Ann Otol Rhinol Laryngol 79:601–605, 1970.

Cawson RA. Tuberculosis of the mouth and throat with special reference to the incidence and management since the introduction of chemotherapy. Br J Dis Chest 54:40–53, 1960.

Darlington CC, Salman I. Oral tuberculous lesions. Am Rev Tuberc 35:147–179, 1937.

Fujibayashi T, et al. Tuberculosis of the tongue: A case report with immunologic study. Oral Surg Oral Med Oral Pathol 47:427–435, 1979.

Laws IM. Oral tuberculosis: Case reports. Br Dent J 134:146–148, 1973.

Mani NJ. Tuberculosis initially diagnosed by asymptomatic oral lesions: Report of three cases. J Oral Med 40:39–42, 1985.

Rauch DM, Freidman E. Systemic tuberculosis initially seen as an oral ulceration: Report of case. J Oral Surg 36:387–389, 1978.

Sachs SA, Eisenbud L. Tuberculous osteomyelitis of the mandible. Oral Surg Oral Med Oral Pathol 44:425–429, 1977.

Siar CH, et al. Secondary oral tuberculosis ulcerations. Dent J Malaysia 9:29–32, 1986.

Leprosy

Bucci F, et al. Oral lesions in lepromatous leprosy. J Oral Med 42:4–6, 1987.

Epker BN, Via WF. Oral and perioral manifestations of leprosy. Oral Surg Oral Med Oral Pathol 28:342–347, 1969.

Girdhar BK, Desikan KV. A clinical study of the mouth in untreated lepromatous patients. Lepr Rev 50:25–35, 1979.

Lighterman I, Watanabe T, Hidaka T. Leprosy of the oral cavity and adnexa. Oral Surg Oral Med Oral Pathol 15:1178–1194, 1962.

Prabhu SR, Daftary DK. Clinical evaluation of oro-facial lesions of leprosy. Odonto-Stomatol Trop 4:83–95, 1981.

Reichart P. Facial and oral manifestations in leprosy: An evaluation of seventy cases. Oral Surg Oral Med Oral Pathol 41:385–399, 1976.

Reichart P. Pathological changes in the soft palate in lepromatous leprosy: An evaluation of ten patients. Oral Surg Oral Med Oral Pathol 38:898–904, 1974.

Rendall JR, McDougall AC. Reddening of the upper central incisors associated with periapical granuloma in lepromatous leprosy. Br J Oral Surg 13:271–277, 1976.

Scheepers A, Lemmer J, Lownie JF. Oral manifestations of leprosy. Lepr Rev 64:37–43, 1993.

Noma

Adekeye EO, Ord RA. Cancrum oris: Principles of management and reconstructive surgery. J Maxillofac Surg 11:160–170, 1983.

Eisele DW, Inglis AF, Richardson MA. Noma and noma neonatorum. Ear Nose Throat J 69:119–123, 1990.

Goshal SP, Gupta PCS, Mukherjee AK. Noma neonatorum: Its ætiopathogenesis. Lancet 2:289–291, 1969.

Griffin JM, et al. Noma: Report of two cases. Oral Surg Oral Med Oral Pathol 56:605–607, 1983.

Limongelli WA, Clark MS, Williams AC. Nomalike lesion in a patient with chronic lymphocytic leukemia: Review of the literature and report of a case. Oral Surg Oral Med Oral Pathol 41:40–51, 1976.

Nash ES, Cheng HH. Cancrum oris-like lesions. Br J Oral Maxillofac Surg 29:51–53, 1991.

Reinhardt RA, Cohen DM, Lewis JES. Unusual sequelae to necrotizing ulcerative gingivitis (NUG)-like lesions. J Oral Med 37:109–112, 1982.

Sawyer DR, Nwoku AL. Cancrum oris (noma): Past and present. J Dent Child 48:138–141, 1981.

Uohara GI, Knapp MJ. Oral fusospirochetosis and associated lesions. Oral Surg Oral Med Oral Pathol 24:113–123, 1967.

Actinomycosis

Bennhoff DF. Actinomycosis: Diagnostic and therapeutic considerations and a review of 32 cases. Laryngoscope 94:1198–1217, 1984.

Benoliel R, Asquith J. Actinomycosis of the jaws. Int J Oral Surg 14:195–199, 1985.

Brignall ID, Gilhooly M. Actinomycosis of the tongue: A diagnostic dilemma. Br J Oral Maxillofac Surg 27:249–253, 1989.

Neuhauser EBD. Actinomycosis and botryomycosis. Postgrad Med 48(5):59–61, 1970.

O'Grady JF. Periapical actinomycosis involving *Actinomyces israelii.* J Endod 14:147–149, 1988.

Pransky SM, et al. Actinomycosis in obstructive tonsillar hypertrophy and recurrent tonsillitis. Arch Otolaryngol Head Neck Surg 117:883–885, 1991.

Richtsmeier WJ, Johns ME. Actinomycosis of the head and neck. CRC Crit Rev Clin Lab Sci 11:175–202, 1979.

Ruprecht A, Ulstadt H. Actinomycotic osteomyelitis. J Can Dent Assoc 54:837–839, 1988.

Sprague WG, Shafer WG. Presence of actinomyces in dentigerous cyst: Report of two cases. J Oral Surg 21:243–245, 1963.

Stenhouse D, MacDonald DG, MacFarlane TW. Cervico-facial and intra-oral actinomycosis: A 5-year retrospective study. Br J Oral Surg 13:172–182, 1975.

Weir JC, Buck WH: Periapical actinomycosis: Report of a case and review of the literature. Oral Surg Oral Med Oral Pathol 54:336–340, 1982.

Cat-Scratch Disease

Cockerell CJ, et al. Epithelioid angiomatosis: A distinct vascular disorder in patients with the acquired immunodeficiency syndrome or AIDS-related complex. Lancet 2:654–656, 1987.

Donlon WC, Jacobsen PL. An unusual submandibular mass—cat scratch disease: Report of a case. J Am Dent Assoc 109:581–583, 1984.

English CK, et al. Cat-scratch disease: Isolation and culture of the bacterial agent. JAMA 259:1347–1352, 1988.

Glick M, Cleveland DB. Oral mucosal bacillary epithelioid angiomatosis in a patient with AIDS associated with rapid alveolar bone loss: Case report. J Oral Pathol Med 22:235–239, 1993.

Hughes JJ. Cat scratch disease: Report of a case presenting as an intra-oral mass. Ohio State Med J 67:139–140, 1971.

LeBoit PE, et al. Epithelioid haemangioma-like vascular proliferation in AIDS: Manifestation of cat scratch disease bacillus infection? Lancet 1:960–963, 1988.

Margileth AM, Wear DJ, English CK. Systemic cat scratch disease: Report of 23 patients with prolonged or recurrent severe bacterial infection. J Infect Dis 155:390–402, 1987.

Premachandra DJ, Milton CM. Cat scratch disease in the parotid gland presenting with facial paralysis. Br J Oral Maxillofac Surg 28:413–415, 1990.

Roberge RJ. Cat-scratch disease. Emerg Med Clin North Am 9:327–334, 1991.

Walsh LJ, Tuffley M, Young WG. An unusual dental presentation of cat scratch disease. Aust Dent J 30:29–32, 1985.

Wear DJ, et al. Cat scratch disease: A bacterial infection. Science 221:1403–1405, 1983.

Zachariades N, Xypolyta A. Cat scratch disease (report of a case). J Oral Med 41:207–208, 1986.

Zangwill KM, et al. Cat scratch disease in Connecticut: Epidemiology, risk factors, and evaluation of a new diagnostic test. N Engl J Med 329:8–13, 1993.

Sinusitis

Herr RD. Acute sinusitis: Diagnosis and treatment update. Am Fam Physician 44:2055–2062, 1991.

Kennedy DW. First-line management of sinusitis: A national problem? Overview. Otolaryngol Head Neck Surg 103(Suppl):847–854, 1990.

Kennedy DW. First-line management of sinusitis: A national problem? Surgical update. Otolaryngol Head Neck Surg 103(Suppl):884–886, 1990.

Manning SC. Surgical management of sinus disease in children. Ann Otol Rhinol Laryngol 101(Suppl 155):42–45, 1992.

Reilly JS. First-line management of sinusitis: A national problem? The sinusitis cycle. Otolaryngol Head Neck Surg 103(Suppl):856–862, 1990.

Richtsmeier WJ. Medical and surgical management of sinusitis in adults. Ann Otol Rhinol Laryngol 101(Suppl 155):46–50, 1992.

Wald ER. Sinusitis in infants and children. Ann Otol Rhinol Laryngol 101(Suppl 155):37–41, 1992.

Winstead W. An update on chronic sinusitis. J Ky Med Assoc 88:177–183, 1990.

Zinreich SJ. First-line management of sinusitis: A national problem? Paranasal sinus imaging. Otolaryngol Head Neck Surg 103(Suppl):863–869, 1990.

6

Fungal and Protozoal Diseases

CANDIDIASIS

Infection with the yeast-like fungal organism *Candida albicans* is termed **candidiasis** or, as the British prefer, **candidosis**. An older name for this disease is **moniliasis**; this term should be eliminated from use because it is derived from the archaic designation *Monilia albicans*. Other members of the *Candida* genus, such as *C. tropicalis, C. krusei, C. parapsilosis,* and *C. guilliermondi,* may also be found intraorally, but they rarely cause disease.

Like many other pathogenic fungi, *C. albicans* may exist in two forms, a trait known as *dimorphism*. The yeast form of the organism is believed to be relatively innocuous, but the hyphal form is usually associated with invasion of host tissue.

Candidiasis is by far the most common oral fungal infection in humans, and it can be manifested in a variety of clinical presentations, making the diagnosis difficult at times. In fact, *C. albicans* may be a component of the normal oral microflora, with as many as 30 to 50 percent of people simply carrying the organism in their mouths without clinical evidence of infection. Whether or not there is clinical evidence of infection probably depends on at least three general factors:

1. The immune status of the host.
2. The oral mucosal environment.
3. The strain of *C. albicans.*

In the past, candidiasis was considered to be only an opportunistic infection, affecting individuals who were debilitated by another disease. Certainly, such patients make up a large percentage of those with candidal infections today, but we now recognize that oral candidiasis may develop in people who are otherwise healthy. As a result of this complex host/organism interaction, candidal infection may range from mild, superficial mucosal involvement seen in most patients to fatal, disseminated disease in severely immunocompromised patients. Our discussion focuses on those clinical presentations of candidiasis that affect the oral mucosa.

Clinical Features

Candidiasis of the oral mucosa may exhibit a variety of clinical patterns, which are summarized in Table 6–1. Many patients will present with a single pattern, although some individuals will exhibit more than one clinical form of oral candidiasis.

Pseudomembranous Candidiasis

The best recognized form of candidal infection is **pseudomembranous candidiasis**. Also known as "thrush," pseudomembranous candidiasis is characterized by the development of adherent white plaques that resemble cottage cheese or curdled milk on the oral mucosa (Figs. 6–1 and 6–2). The white plaques are composed of tangled masses of hyphae, yeasts, desquamated epithelial cells, and debris. These plaques can be removed by scraping them with a tongue blade or rubbing them with a dry gauze sponge. The underlying mucosa may appear normal or erythematous. If bleeding occurs,

Table 6–1. CLINICAL FORMS OF ORAL CANDIDIASIS

Clinical Type	Appearance and Symptoms	Common Sites	Associated Factors and Comments
Pseudomembranous (thrush)	Creamy-white plaques, removable; burning sensation, foul taste	Buccal mucosa, tongue, palate	Antibiotic therapy, immunosuppression
Erythematous	Red macules; burning sensation	Posterior hard palate, buccal mucosa, dorsal tongue	Antibiotic therapy, xerostomia, immunosuppression, idiopathic
Central papillary atrophy (median rhomboid glossitis)	Red, atrophic mucosal areas; asymptomatic	Midline posterior dorsal tongue	Idiopathic, immunosuppression
Chronic multifocal	Red areas, often with removable white plaques; burning sensation, asymptomatic	Posterior palate, posterior dorsal tongue, angles of mouth	Immunosuppression, idiopathic
Angular cheilitis	Red, fissured lesions; irritated, raw feeling	Angles of mouth	Idiopathic, immunosuppression, loss of vertical dimension
Denture stomatitis (chronic atrophic candidiasis; denture sore mouth)	Red; asymptomatic	Confined to palatal denture-bearing mucosa	Probably not true infection; denture often is positive on culture, but mucosa is not
Hyperplastic (candidal leukoplakia)	White plaques which are not removable; asymptomatic	Anterior buccal mucosa	Idiopathic, immunosuppression; care must be taken not to confuse this with other keratotic lesions with superimposed candidiasis
Mucocutaneous	White plaques, some of which may be removable; red areas	Tongue, buccal mucosa, palate	Rare; inherited or sporadic idiopathic immune dysfunction
Endocrine-candidiasis syndromes	White plaques, most of which are not removable	Tongue, buccal mucosa, palate	Rare; endocrine disorder develops after candidiasis

the mucosa has probably also been affected by another process, such as lichen planus or cancer chemotherapy.

Pseudomembranous candidiasis may be initiated by exposure of the patient to broad-spectrum antibiotics (thus eliminating competing bacteria) or by impairment of the patient's immune system. The immune dysfunctions seen in leukemic patients (see p. 427) or those infected with human immunodeficiency virus (HIV) (see p. 200) are often associated with pseudomembranous

candidiasis. Infants may also be affected, ostensibly because of their underdeveloped immune system. Antibiotic exposure is typically responsible for an acute (rapid) expression of the condition; immunologic problems usually produce a chronic (slow-onset, longstanding) form of pseudomembranous candidiasis.

Symptoms, if present at all, are usually relatively mild, consisting of a burning sensation of the oral mucosa or an unpleasant taste in the mouth. Sometimes patients complain of "blisters," when in fact they feel the elevated plaques rather than true vesicles. The plaques are characteristically distributed on the buccal mucosa, palate, and dorsal tongue.

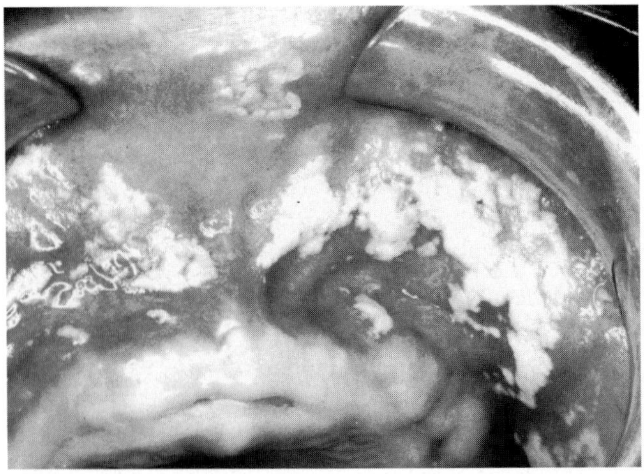

FIGURE 6–1. **Pseudomembranous candidiasis.** Classic "curdled milk" appearance of the oral lesions of pseudomembranous candidiasis. This patient had no apparent risk factors for candidiasis development. (From Allen CM, Blozis GG. Oral mucosal lesions. *In*: Otolaryngology: Head and Neck Surgery, 2nd ed. Edited by Cummings CW, Fredrickson JM, Harker LA, Krause CJ, Schuller DE. St. Louis, CV Mosby, 1993.)

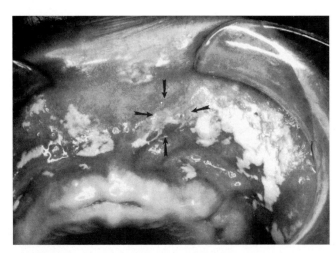

FIGURE 6–2. **Pseudomembranous candidiasis.** Removal of one of the pseudomembranous plaques (*arrows*), shown in Figure 6–1, reveals a mildly erythematous mucosal surface.

Erythematous Candidiasis

In contrast to the pseudomembranous form, patients with **erythematous candidiasis** do not show white flecks. Several clinical presentations may be seen. The first, known as **acute atrophic candidiasis** or "antibiotic sore mouth," typically follows a course of broad-spectrum antibiotics. Patients often complain that their mouth feels as if it had been scalded by a hot beverage. This burning sensation may be accompanied by a diffuse loss of the filiform papillae of the dorsal tongue, resulting in a reddened, "bald" appearance of the tongue (Fig. 6–3; see Color Figure 28).

Other forms of erythematous candidiasis are usually asymptomatic and chronic. Included in this category is the condition known as **central papillary atrophy** of the tongue, or **median rhomboid glossitis**. In the past, this was thought to be a developmental defect of the tongue, occurring in 0.01 to 1.0 percent of adults. The lesion was supposed to have resulted from a failure of the embryologic tuberculum impar to be covered by the lateral processes of the tongue. Theoretically, the prevalence of central papillary atrophy in children should be identical to that seen in adults; however, in one study in which 10,000 children were examined, not a single lesion was detected. Other investigators have noted a consistent re-

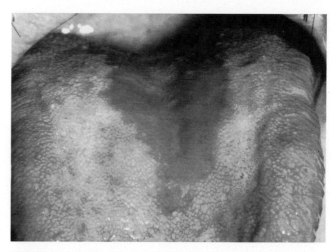

FIGURE 6–4. **Erythematous candidiasis.** Severe presentation of central papillary atrophy. In this patient, the lesion was asymptomatic. See Color Plates.

lationship between the lesion and *C. albicans*, and similar lesions have been induced on the dorsal tongues of rats.

Clinically, central papillary atrophy presents as a well-demarcated erythematous zone that affects the midline posterior dorsal tongue and often is asymptomatic (Figs. 6–4 and 6–5; see Color Figures 29 and 30). The erythema is due in part to the loss of the filiform papillae in this area. The lesion is usually symmetric, and its surface may range from smooth to lobulated. Often the mucosal alteration resolves with antifungal therapy, although occasionally only partial resolution can be achieved.

Some patients with central papillary atrophy may also exhibit signs of oral mucosal candidal infection at other sites. This presentation of erythematous candidiasis has been termed **chronic multifocal candidiasis**. In addition to the dorsal tongue, the sites that show involvement include the junction of the hard and soft palate and the

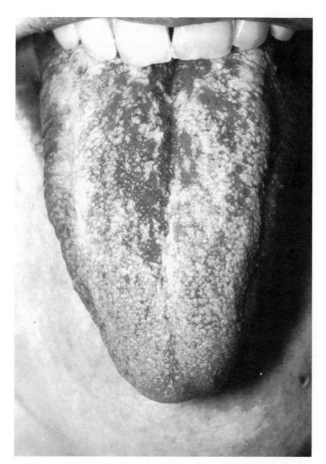

FIGURE 6–3. **Erythematous candidiasis.** The patchy, denuded areas (not the white areas) of the dorsal tongue represent erythematous candidiasis. The patient had received broad-spectrum antibiotics. See Color Plates.

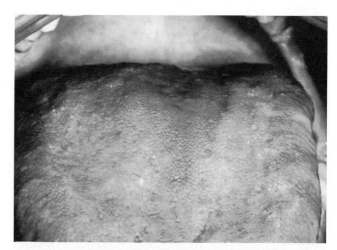

FIGURE 6–5. **Erythematous candidiasis.** Same patient as depicted in Figure 6–4. Two weeks after antifungal therapy with fluconazole, there was marked regeneration of the dorsal tongue papillae. See Color Plates.

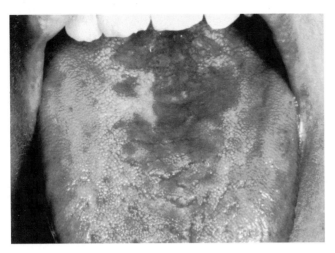

FIGURE 6-6. **Candidiasis.** Multifocal oral candidiasis, characterized by central papillary atrophy of the tongue as well as other areas of involvement. See Color Plates.

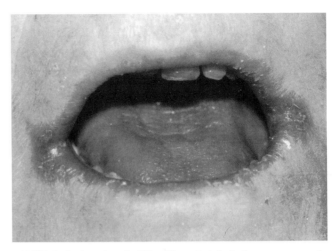

FIGURE 6-8. **Angular cheilitis.** Characteristic lesions appear as fissured, erythematous alterations of the skin at the corners of the mouth. See Color Plates.

angles of the mouth. The palatal lesion appears as an erythematous area that, when the tongue is at rest, contacts the dorsal tongue lesion, resulting in what is called a "kissing lesion" because of their intimate proximity (Figs. 6-6 and 6-7; see Color Figures 31 and 32).

The involvement of the angles of the mouth (**angular cheilitis,** or *perlèche*) is characterized by erythema, fissuring, and scaling (Fig. 6-8; see Color Figure 33). Sometimes this condition is seen as a component of chronic multifocal candidiasis, but it often occurs alone, typically in an older person with reduced vertical dimension and accentuated folds at the corners of the mouth. Saliva tends to pool in these areas, keeping them moist and thus favoring a yeast infection. Patients often indicate that the severity of the lesions waxes and wanes. Microbiologic studies have indicated that 20 percent of these cases are caused by *C. albicans* alone, 60 percent are due to a combined infection with *C. albicans* and *Staphylococcus aureus*, and 20 percent are associated with *S. aureus* alone.

Denture stomatitis should be mentioned at this point because it is often classified as a form of erythematous candidiasis, and the term **chronic atrophic candidiasis** may be used synonymously by some authors. This condition is characterized by varying degrees of erythema, sometimes accompanied by petechial hemorrhage, localized to the denture-bearing areas of a maxillary removable dental prosthesis (Figs. 6-9 [see Color Figure 34] and 6-10). Even though the clinical appearance can be striking, the process is rarely symptomatic. Usually, the patient admits to wearing the denture continuously, removing it only periodically in order to clean it. Whether this represents actual infection by *C. albicans* or is simply a tissue response by the host to the various microorganisms living beneath the denture remains controversial. The clinician should also rule out the possibility that this reaction could be due to improper design of the denture, allergy to the denture base, or inadequate curing of the denture acrylic.

Even though *C. albicans* is often associated with this

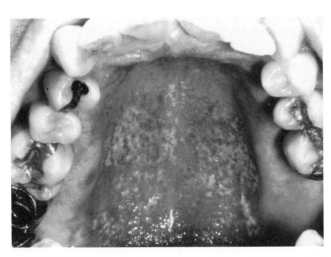

FIGURE 6-7. **Candidiasis.** Same patient as in Figure 6-6. A "kissing" lesion of oral candidiasis involves the hard palate. See Color Plates.

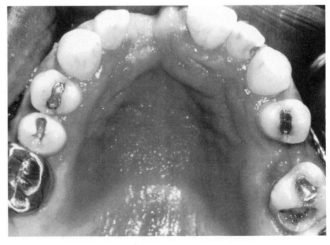

FIGURE 6-9. **Denture stomatitis.** Denture stomatitis in association with an interim partial denture. Note that the mucosal alteration is confined to the denture-bearing mucosa. See Color Plates.

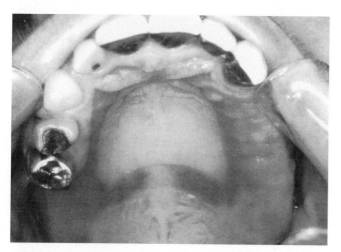

FIGURE 6-10. **Denture stomatitis.** Denture stomatitis, not associated with *Candida albicans*, confined to the denture-bearing mucosa of a maxillary partial denture framework.

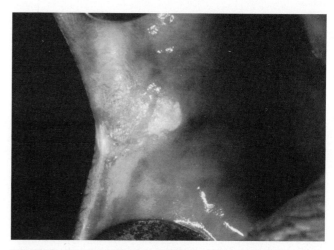

FIGURE 6-11. **Hyperplastic candidiasis.** This lesion of the anterior buccal mucosa clinically resembles a leukoplakia because it is a white plaque that cannot be removed by rubbing. With antifungal therapy, such a lesion should resolve completely.

condition, biopsy specimens of denture stomatitis seldom show candidal hyphae actually penetrating the keratin layer of the host epithelium. Therefore, one of the main defining criteria for the diagnosis of infection — host tissue invasion by the organism — is not met by this lesion.

Chronic Hyperplastic Candidiasis (Candidal Leukoplakia)

In some patients with oral candidiasis, there may be a white patch that cannot be removed by scraping, in which case the term **chronic hyperplastic candidiasis** is appropriate. This form of candidiasis, also known as **candidal leukoplakia**, is the least common and is also somewhat controversial. Some investigators believe that this condition simply represents candidiasis that is superimposed on a pre-existing leukoplakic lesion, a situation that may certainly exist at times. In some instances,

however, the candidal organism alone may be capable of inducing a hyperkeratotic lesion. Such lesions are usually located on the anterior buccal mucosa and cannot clinically be distinguished from a routine leukoplakia (Fig. 6-11). Often the leukoplakic lesion associated with candidal infection has a fine intermingling of red and white areas, resulting in a "**speckled**" **leukoplakia** (see p. 284). Such lesions may have an increased frequency of epithelial dysplasia histopathologically.

The diagnosis is confirmed by the presence of candidal hyphae associated with the lesion as well as by complete resolution of the lesion after antifungal therapy (Fig. 6-12; see Color Figures 35 and 36).

Mucocutaneous Candidiasis

Severe oral candidiasis may also be seen as a component of a relatively rare group of immunologic disorders known as **mucocutaneous candidiasis**. Several distinct

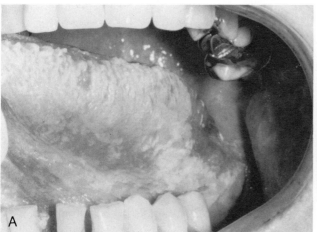 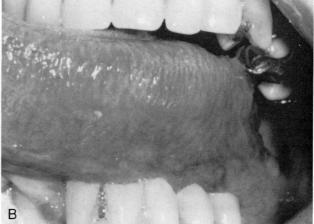

FIGURE 6-12. **Hyperplastic candidiasis.** *A,* These diffuse white plaques clinically appear as leukoplakia, but they actually represent an unusual presentation of hyperplastic candidiasis. *B,* Treatment with clotrimazole oral troches shows complete resolution of the white lesions within 2 weeks, essentially confirming the diagnosis of hyperplastic candidiasis. If any white mucosal alteration had persisted, a biopsy of that area would have been mandatory.

immunologic dysfunctions have been identified, and the severity of the candidal infection correlates with the severity of the immunologic defect. Most cases are sporadic, although an autosomal recessive pattern of inheritance has been identified in some families. The immune problem usually becomes evident during the first few years of life, when the patient begins to have candidal infections of the mouth, nails, skin, and other mucosal surfaces. The oral lesions appear as thick white plaques that typically do not rub off—essentially chronic hyperplastic candidiasis.

Patients should be evaluated periodically because any one of a variety of endocrine abnormalities (**endocrine-candidiasis syndrome**) as well as iron-deficiency anemia may develop in addition to the candidiasis. These endocrine disturbances include hypothyroidism, hypoparathyroidism, hypoadrenocorticism (Addison's disease), and diabetes mellitus. Typically, the endocrine abnormality develops months or even years after the onset of the candidal infection. Interestingly, the candidal infection remains relatively superficial rather than disseminating throughout the body. Both the oral lesions and the rather grotesque, roughened, foul-smelling cutaneous plaques and nodules can be controlled with continuous use of relatively safe systemic antifungal drugs.

Histopathologic Features

The candidal organism can be seen microscopically in either an exfoliative cytologic preparation or in tissue sections obtained from a biopsy specimen. On staining with the periodic acid–Schiff (PAS) method, the candidal hyphae and yeasts can be readily identified (Fig. 6–13). The PAS method stains carbohydrates, contained in abundance by fungal cell walls. The organisms are thus easily identified by the bright magenta color imparted by the stain. To make a diagnosis of candidiasis, one must be able to see hyphae or pseudohyphae (which are essentially elongated yeast cells). These hyphae are approximately 2 μm in diameter, vary in their length, and may show branching. Often the hyphae are accompa-

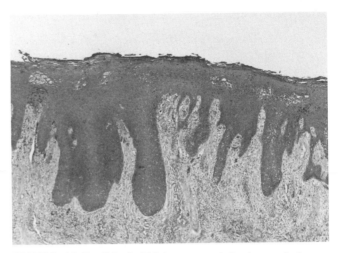

FIGURE 6–14. **Candidiasis.** This low-power photomicrograph shows a characteristic pattern of thickening of the spinous layer, elongation of the rete ridges, and chronic inflammation of the underlying connective tissue associated with longstanding candidal infection of the oral mucosa.

nied by variable numbers of yeasts as well as squamous epithelial cells and inflammatory cells.

A 10 to 20 percent potassium hydroxide (KOH) preparation may also be used to rapidly evaluate specimens for the presence of fungal organisms. With this technique, the KOH lyses the background of epithelial cells, allowing the more resistant hyphae to be visualized.

The disadvantages of the KOH preparation include:

- The lack of a permanent record
- The greater difficulty in identifying the fungal organisms compared with PAS staining
- The inability to assess the nature of the epithelial cell population with respect to epithelial dysplasia or pemphigus vulgaris

The histopathologic pattern of oral candidiasis may vary slightly, depending on which clinical form of the infection has been submitted for biopsy. The features that are found in common include an increased thickness of parakeratin on the surface of the lesion in conjunction with elongation of the epithelial rete ridges (Fig. 6–14). Typically, a chronic inflammatory cell infiltrate can be seen in the connective tissue immediately subjacent to the infected epithelium, and small collections of neutrophils (microabscesses) are often identified in the parakeratin layer and the superficial spinous cell layer near the organisms (Fig. 6–15). The candidal hyphae are embedded in the parakeratin layer and rarely penetrate into the viable cell layers of the epithelium unless the patient is extremely immunocompromised.

Diagnosis

The diagnosis of candidiasis in clinical practice is usually established by the clinical signs in conjunction with exfoliative cytologic examination. Although a culture can definitively identify the organism as *C. albicans*, this process may not be practical in most office settings. The cytologic findings should demonstrate the hyphal phase

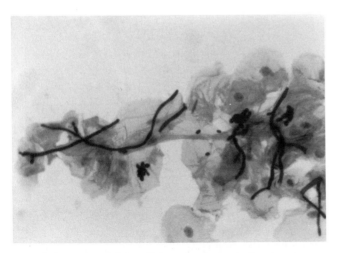

FIGURE 6–13. **Candidiasis.** This cytologic preparation demonstrates tubular-appearing fungal hyphae and ovoid yeasts of *Candida albicans*. (Periodic acid–Schiff stain.)

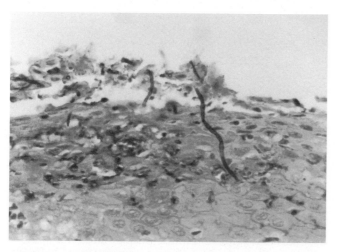

FIGURE 6–15. **Candidiasis.** This high-power photomicrograph shows the tubular hyphae of *Candida albicans* embedded in the parakeratin layer. Neutrophilic microabscesses are visible adjacent to the organism in response to the invasion. (Periodic acid–Schiff stain.)

of the organism, and antifungal therapy can then be instituted. If the lesion is clinically suggestive of chronic hyperplastic candidiasis but does not respond to antifungal therapy, a biopsy should be performed to rule out the possibility of *C. albicans* superimposed on epithelial dysplasia, squamous cell carcinoma, or lichen planus.

The definitive identification of the organism can be made by means of culture. A specimen for culture is obtained by rubbing a sterile cotton swab over the lesion and then streaking the swab on the surface of a Sabouraud's agar slant. *C. albicans* will grow as creamy, smooth-surfaced colonies after 2 to 3 days of incubation at room temperature.

Treatment

Several antifungal medications have been developed for managing oral candidiasis, each with its advantages and disadvantages.

Nystatin

In the 1950s, the polyene antibiotic nystatin was the first effective treatment. Nystatin is formulated for oral use as a suspension or pastille (lozenge). This drug is safe because it is not absorbed across the gastrointestinal tract; unfortunately, however, this means that to be of benefit the medication must remain in direct contact with the organism, thus necessitating multiple daily doses. In addition, many patients report that nystatin has a very bitter taste; the taste has to be disguised with sucrose and flavoring agents, and this problem may reduce patient compliance. If the candidiasis is due to xerostomia, the sucrose content of the nystatin preparation may contribute to xerostomia-related caries in these patients. Nystatin combined with triamcinolone acetonide cream or ointment can be applied topically and is effective for conditions such as angular cheilitis.

Imidazole Agents

The imidazole-derived antifungal agents were developed during the 1970s and represented a major step

forward in the management of candidiasis. The two drugs of this group that are used most frequently are clotrimazole and ketoconazole.

Clotrimazole. Like nystatin, clotrimazole is not well absorbed and must be administered several times each day. It is formulated as a pleasant-tasting troche and produces few side effects. The efficacy of this agent in treating oral candidiasis can be seen in Figure 6–12.

Ketoconazole. Ketoconazole was the first antifungal drug that could be absorbed across the gastrointestinal tract, thereby providing systemic therapy by an oral route of administration. The single daily dose was much easier for the patient to use; however, several disadvantages have been noted. Patients must not take antacids or H_2 blocking agents because an acidic environment is required for proper absorption. If a patient is to take ketoconazole for more than 2 weeks, liver function studies are recommended because approximately 1 in 12,000 individuals will experience idiosyncratic liver toxicity from the agent. For this reason, the U.S. Food and Drug Administration has stated that ketoconazole should not be used as initial therapy for routine oral candidiasis. Furthermore, ketoconazole has been implicated in drug interactions with the macrolide antibiotics (e.g. erythromycin) and with the antihistamine terfenadine, producing potentially life-threatening cardiac arrhythmias.

Triazole Agents

The triazoles are the newest group of antifungal drugs. Fluconazole has been approved for use against candidiasis in the United States, and itraconazole is under consideration.

Fluconazole appears to be more effective than ketoconazole; it is well absorbed systemically, and an acidic environment is not required for absorption. A relatively long half-life allows for once-daily dosing, and liver toxicity is rare at the doses used to treat oral candidiasis. Some reports have suggested that fluconazole may not be appropriate for long-term preventive therapy because resistance to the drug seems to develop in some instances. Known drug interactions include a potentiation of the effects of phenytoin (Dilantin), an antiseizure medication; warfarin compounds (anticoagulants); and sulfonylureas (oral hypoglycemic agents).

HISTOPLASMOSIS

Histoplasmosis, the most common systemic fungal infection in the United States, is caused by the organism *Histoplasma capsulatum.* Like several other pathogenic fungi, *H. capsulatum* is dimorphic, growing as a yeast at body temperature in the human host and as a mold in its natural environment. Humid areas with soil enriched by bird or bat excrement are especially suited to the growth of this organism. This habitat preference explains why histoplasmosis is seen endemically in fertile river valleys, such as the region drained by the Ohio and Mississippi Rivers in the United States. Airborne spores of the organism are inhaled, pass into the terminal passages of the lungs, and germinate.

Approximately 500,000 new cases of histoplasmosis are thought to develop annually in the United States, and other parts of the world, such as Central and South America, Europe, and Asia, also report numerous cases. Epidemiologic studies in endemic areas of the United States suggest that 80 to 90 percent of the population in these regions has been infected.

Clinical and Radiographic Features

Most cases of histoplasmosis either produce no symptoms or such mild symptoms that the patient does not seek medical treatment. The expression of disease depends on the quantity of spores inhaled, the immune status of the host, and perhaps the strain of *H. capsulatum.* Most individuals who become exposed to the organism are relatively healthy and do not inhale a large number of spores; therefore, they have either no symptoms or they have a mild, flu-like illness for 1 to 2 weeks. The inhaled spores are ingested by macrophages within 24 to 48 hours, and specific T-lymphocyte immunity develops in 2 to 3 weeks. Antibodies directed against the organism usually appear several weeks later. With these defense mechanisms, the host is usually able to destroy the invading organism, although sometimes the macrophages simply surround and confine the fungus so that viable organisms can be recovered years later. Thus, patients who formerly lived in an endemic area may have acquired the organism and later express the disease at some other geographic site if they become immunocompromised.

Acute histoplasmosis is a self-limited pulmonary infection that probably develops in only about 1 percent of people who are exposed to a low number of spores. With a high concentration of spores, as many as 50 to 100 percent of individuals may experience acute symptoms. These symptoms (e.g., fever, headache, myalgia, nonproductive cough, anorexia) result in a clinical picture similar to that of influenza. Patients are usually ill for 2 weeks, although calcification of the hilar lymph nodes may be detected as an incidental finding on chest radiographs years later.

Chronic histoplasmosis also primarily affects the lungs, although it is much less common than acute histoplasmosis. The chronic form usually affects elderly, emphysematous, white males or immunosuppressed patients. Clinically, it appears similar to tuberculosis. Patients typically exhibit cough, weight loss, fever, dyspnea, chest pain, hemoptysis, weakness, and fatigue. Chest roentgenograms show upper lobe infiltrates and cavitation.

Disseminated histoplasmosis is even less common than the acute and chronic types. It occurs in 1 of 2000 to 5000 patients who have acute symptoms. This condition is characterized by the progressive spread of the infection to extrapulmonary sites. It usually occurs in either elderly, debilitated, or immunosuppressed patients. In some areas of the United States, from 2 to 10 percent of patients with **acquired immunodeficiency syndrome (AIDS)** (see p. 205) develop disseminated histoplasmosis. Tissues that may be affected include the spleen, adrenal glands, liver, lymph nodes, gastrointestinal tract, central nervous system (CNS), kidneys, and oral mucosa. Adrenal involvement may produce hypoadrenocorticism (**Addison's disease**; see p. 615).

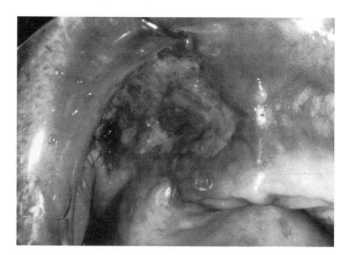

FIGURE 6–16. Histoplasmosis. This ulcerated granular lesion involves the maxillary buccal vestibule and is easily mistaken clinically for carcinoma. Biopsy established the diagnosis. (From Allen CM, Blozis GG. Oral mucosal lesions. *In:* Otolaryngology—Head and Neck Surgery, 2nd ed. Edited by Cummings CW, Fredrickson JM, Harker LA, Krause CJ, Schuller DE. St. Louis, CV Mosby, 1993.)

Most oral lesions of histoplasmosis occur with the disseminated form of the disease. The most commonly affected sites are the tongue, palate, and buccal mucosa. The condition usually presents as a solitary, painful ulceration of several weeks' duration, although some lesions may appear erythematous or white with an irregular surface (Fig. 6–16). The ulcerated lesions have firm, rolled margins, and they may be indistinguishable clinically from a malignancy (Fig. 6–17).

Histopathologic Features

Microscopic examination of lesional tissue shows either a diffuse infiltrate of macrophages or, more commonly, collections of macrophages organized into granulomas (Fig. 6–18). Multinucleated giant cells are usually seen in association with the granulomatous inflammation. The causative organism can be identified with some difficulty in the routine hematoxylin and eosin (H&E)–

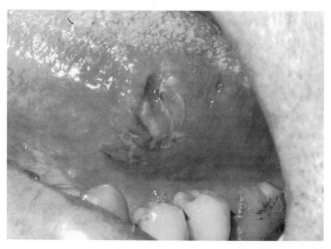

FIGURE 6–17. Histoplasmosis. This chronic ulceration of the ventral/lateral tongue represents an oral lesion of histoplasmosis that had disseminated from the lungs. The lesion clinically resembles carcinoma, and because of this high-risk site, biopsy is mandatory.

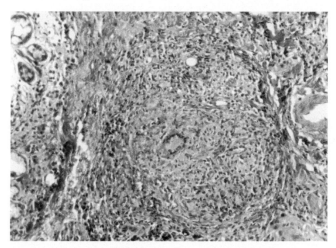

FIGURE 6-18. **Histoplasmosis.** This low-power photomicrograph shows a collection of epithelioid macrophages organized into a granuloma in response to infection by *Histoplasma capsulatum*.

stained section; however, special stains, such as the PAS and Grocott-Gomori methenamine silver methods, readily demonstrate the characteristic 1- to 2-μm yeasts of *H. capsulatum* (Fig. 6-19).

Diagnosis

The diagnosis of histoplasmosis can be made by histopathologic identification of the organism in tissue sections or by culture. Other helpful diagnostic studies include serologic testing, in which antibodies directed against *H. capsulatum* are identified, and detection of antigen produced by the yeast.

Treatment and Prognosis

Acute histoplasmosis, because it is a self-limited process, generally warrants no specific treatment other than supportive care with analgesics and antipyretics.

Patients with chronic histoplasmosis usually require treatment, despite the fact that up to half of them may recover spontaneously. Often the pulmonary damage is

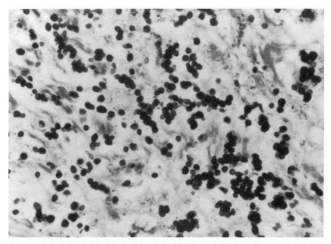

FIGURE 6-19. **Histoplasmosis.** This high-power photomicrograph of a tissue section readily demonstrates the small yeasts of *Histoplasma capsulatum*. (Grocott-Gomori methenamine silver stain.)

progressive if it remains untreated, and death may result in up to 20 percent of these cases. The treatment of choice is intravenous amphotericin B, although significant kidney damage can result from this therapy. For that reason, ketoconazole may be used in non-immunosuppressed patients because it is associated with fewer side effects. The new triazole compound itraconazole has been approved for treatment of histoplasmosis. This agent appears to be more effective than ketoconazole and has less potential to produce toxicity.

Disseminated histoplasmosis is a very serious condition that results in death in 90 percent of the patients if they remain untreated. Amphotericin B is usually indicated for such patients. Despite therapy, however, a mortality rate of 7 to 23 percent is observed. Itraconazole or ketoconazole may also be used if the patient is non-immunocompromised, but the response rate is slower than for patients receiving amphotericin B and the relapse rate may be higher.

BLASTOMYCOSIS

Blastomycosis is a relatively uncommon disease caused by the dimorphic fungus known as *Blastomyces dermatitidis*. Although the organism is rarely isolated from its natural habitat, it seems to prefer rich, moist soil, where it grows as a mold. Much of the region in which it grows overlaps the territory associated with *H. capsulatum*, basically affecting the eastern half of the United States. Sporadic cases have also been reported in Africa, India, Europe, and South America. By way of comparison, histoplasmosis appears to be at least ten times more common than blastomycosis. In several series of cases, a prominent adult male predilection has been noted, often with a male-to-female ratio as high as 9:1. This has been attributed to the greater degree of outdoor activity, such as hunting and fishing, by men in areas where the organism grows. Blastomycosis occurring in immunocompromised patients is relatively rare.

Clinical and Radiographic Features

Blastomycosis infection is almost always acquired by inhalation of spores, particularly after a rain. The spores reach the alveoli of the lungs, where they begin to grow as yeasts at body temperature. In most patients, the infection is probably halted and contained in the lungs, but it may become hematogenously disseminated in a few instances. In order of decreasing frequency, the sites of dissemination include skin, bone, prostate, meninges, oropharyngeal mucosa, and abdominal organs.

Although most cases of blastomycosis are either asymptomatic or produce only very mild symptoms, patients who do experience symptoms usually have pulmonary complaints. **Acute blastomycosis** resembles pneumonia, characterized by high fever, chest pain, malaise, night sweats, and productive cough with mucopurulent sputum. Rarely, the infection may precipitate life-threatening adult respiratory distress syndrome.

Chronic blastomycosis is more common than the acute form, and it may mimic tuberculosis; both conditions are often characterized by low-grade fever, night sweats, weight loss, and productive cough. Chest radio-

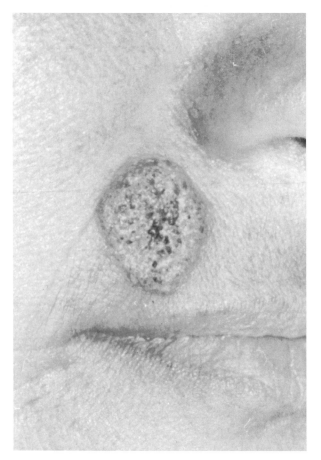

FIGURE 6–20. **Blastomycosis.** This granular erythematous plaque of cutaneous blastomycosis has affected the facial skin. (Courtesy of Dr. William Welton.)

graphs may appear normal, or they may demonstrate diffuse infiltrates or one or more pulmonary or hilar masses. Unlike the situation with tuberculosis and histoplasmosis, calcification is not typically present. Cutaneous lesions usually represent the spread of infection from the lungs, although occasionally they are the only sign of disease. Such lesions begin as erythematous nodules that enlarge and ulcerate (Figs. 6–20 and 6–21).

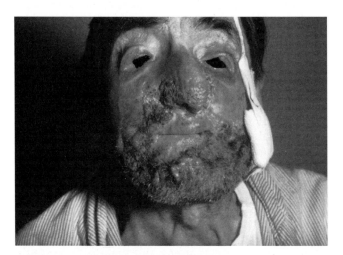

FIGURE 6–21. **Blastomycosis.** Severe cutaneous infection by *Blastomyces dermatitidis*. (Courtesy of Dr. Emmitt Costich.)

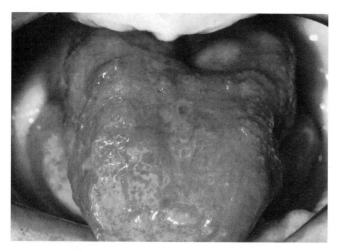

FIGURE 6–22. **Blastomycosis.** These irregular ulcerations of the tongue represent blastomycosis. Direct inoculation was thought to have occurred from the patient's habit of chewing dried horse manure ("Kentucky field candy"), in which the organism was probably growing.

Oral lesions of blastomycosis may result from either extrapulmonary dissemination or local inoculation with the organism. These lesions may have an irregular, pink or white intact surface, or they may appear as ulcerations with irregular rolled borders and varying degrees of pain (Fig. 6–22). Clinically, because the lesions resemble squamous cell carcinoma, biopsy and histopathologic examination are required.

Histopathologic Features

Histopathologic examination of lesional tissue typically shows a mixture of acute inflammation and granulomatous inflammation surrounding variable numbers of yeasts. These organisms are 8 to 20 μ in diameter. They are characterized by a doubly refractile cell wall and a broad attachment between the budding daughter cell and the parent cell. Like many other fungal organisms, *B. dermatitidis* can be detected more easily using special stains, such as the Grocott-Gomori methenamine silver and PAS methods (Fig. 6–23). Identification of

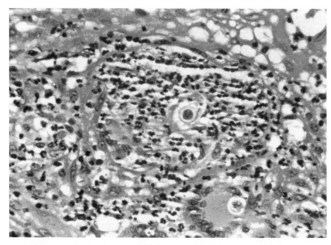

FIGURE 6–23. **Blastomycosis.** This high-power photomicrograph shows the large yeasts of *Blastomyces dermatitidis* and a pronounced host inflammatory response to the organism. (Periodic acid–Schiff stain.)

these organisms is especially important because this infection often induces a benign reaction of the overlying epithelium in mucosal or skin lesions called *pseudoepitheliomatous (pseudocarcinomatous) hyperplasia*. Because this benign elongation of the epithelial rete ridges may look like squamous cell carcinoma at first glance under the microscope, careful inspection of the underlying inflamed lesional tissue is mandatory.

Diagnosis

Rapid diagnosis of blastomycosis can be performed by microscopic examination of either histopathologic sections or an alcohol-fixed cytologic preparation. The most rapid means of diagnosis, however, is the KOH preparation, which may be used for examining scrapings from a suspected lesion. The most accurate method of identifying *B. dermatitidis* is by obtaining a culture specimen from sputum or fresh biopsy material and growing the organism on Sabouraud's agar; however, this is also the slowest technique, sometimes taking as long as 4 weeks. Serologic studies are usually not helpful.

Treatment and Prognosis

As stated earlier, most patients with blastomycosis require no treatment. Even in the case of symptomatic acute blastomycosis, administration of systemic amphotericin B is indicated only if the patient:

- Is seriously ill
- Is not improving clinically
- Is ill for more than 2 or 3 weeks

Patients with chronic blastomycosis or extrapulmonary lesions need treatment. Itraconazole or ketoconazole is generally recommended, particularly if infection is mild or moderate. Amphotericin B is reserved for patients who are severely ill or show no response to ketoconazole.

Most investigators believe that disseminated blastomycosis occurs in a small percentage of infected patients and with proper treatment the outlook for the patient is reasonably good.

PARACOCCIDIOIDOMYCOSIS (South American Blastomycosis)

Paracoccidioidomycosis is a deep fungal infection that is caused by *Paracoccidioides brasiliensis*. The condition is seen most frequently in patients who live in either South America (primarily Brazil, Colombia, Venezuela, Uruguay, and Argentina) or Central America, but immigrants from those regions and visitors to those areas have the potential for acquiring the infection. There is a distinct predilection for males, with a 25:1 male-to-female ratio typically reported. This striking difference is thought to be due to a protective effect of female hormones because beta-estradiol inhibits the transformation of the hyphal form of the organism to the pathogenic yeast form. This theory is supported by the finding of an equal number of men and women who have antibodies directed against the yeast.

Clinical Features

Patients with paracoccidioidomycosis are typically middle-aged at the time of diagnosis, and most are employed in agriculture. Most cases of paracoccidioidomycosis are thought to present initially as pulmonary infections following exposure to the spores of the organism. Although infections are generally self-limiting, *P. brasiliensis* may spread by a hematogenous or lymphatic route to a variety of tissues, including lymph nodes, skin, and adrenal glands. Adrenal involvement often results in hypoadrenocorticism (**Addison's disease**; see p. 615).

Oral lesions appear as mulberry-like ulcerations that most commonly affect the alveolar mucosa, gingiva, and palate. The lip and buccal mucosa are also involved in a significant percentage of cases. In most patients with oral lesions, more than one oral mucosal site is affected.

Histopathologic Features

Microscopic evaluation of tissue obtained from an oral lesion may reveal pseudoepitheliomatous hyperplasia in addition to ulceration of the overlying surface epithelium. *P. brasiliensis* elicits a granulomatous inflammatory host response that is characterized by collections of epithelioid macrophages and multinucleated giant cells. Scattered, large (up to 30μ in diameter) yeasts are readily identified following staining of the tissue sections with the Grocott-Gomori methenamine silver or PAS method. The organisms often show multiple daughter buds on the parent cell, resulting in an appearance that has been described as resembling "Mickey Mouse ears" or the spokes of a ship's steering wheel ("mariner's wheel").

Diagnosis

Demonstration of the characteristic multiple budding yeasts in the appropriate clinical setting is usually adequate to establish a diagnosis of paracoccidioidomycosis. Specimens for culture can be obtained, but *P. brasiliensis* grows quite slowly.

Treatment and Prognosis

The method of management of patients with paracoccidioidomycosis depends on the severity of the disease presentation. Sulfonamide derivatives have been used since the 1940s to treat this infection, and these drugs are still used in many instances today. For severe involvement, intravenous amphotericin B is usually indicated. Cases that are not life-threatening are best managed by oral itraconazole, although therapy may be needed for several months. Ketoconazole can also be used, although the side effects are typically greater than those associated with itraconazole.

COCCIDIOIDOMYCOSIS (San Joaquin Valley Fever; Valley Fever; Cocci)

Coccidioides immitis is the fungal organism responsible for development of **coccidioidomycosis**. *C. immitis* grows saprophytically in the alkaline, semiarid, desert soil of the southwestern United States and Mexico, with isolated regions also noted in Central and South America. As with several other pathogenic fungi, *C. immitis* is a dimorphic organism, appearing as a mold in its natural environment of the soil and as a yeast in tissues of the infected host. Arthrospores produced by the mold become airborne and can be inhaled into the lungs of the human host, producing infection.

Coccidioidomycosis is confined to the Western Hemisphere and is endemic throughout the desert regions of southwestern United States and Mexico; however, with modern travel taking many visitors to and from the "Sun Belt," this disease can be encountered virtually anywhere in the world. An estimated 100,000 people are believed to be newly infected annually, although 60 percent of this group are asymptomatic.

Clinical Features

Most infections with *C. immitis* are asymptomatic, although approximately 40 percent of infected patients experience a flu-like illness and pulmonary symptoms within 1 to 3 weeks after inhaling the arthrospores. Fatigue, cough, chest pain, myalgias, and headache are commonly reported, lasting several weeks with spontaneous resolution in most cases. Occasionally, the immune response may trigger a hypersensitivity reaction that causes the development of erythema multiforme (see p. 567) or erythema nodosum. Erythema nodosum is characterized by the appearance of multiple painful erythematous inflammatory nodules in the subcutaneous connective tissue. This hypersensitivity reaction occurring in conjunction with coccidioidomycosis is termed **Valley fever**, and it resolves as the host cell-mediated immune response controls the pulmonary infection.

Chronic progressive pulmonary coccidioidomycosis is relatively rare. It mimics tuberculosis, with its clinical presentation of persistent cough, hemoptysis, chest pain, low-grade fever, and weight loss.

Disseminated coccidioidomycosis occurs when the organism spreads hematogenously to extrapulmonary sites. This occurs in less than 1 percent of the cases, but it is a more serious problem. The most commonly involved areas include skin, lymph nodes, bone and joints, and the meninges. Immunosuppression greatly increases the risk of dissemination. The following groups are particularly susceptible:

- Patients taking large doses of systemic corticosteroids (such as organ transplant recipients)
- Patients being treated with cancer chemotherapy
- Patients in the end stages of HIV infection

Infants and elderly patients, both of whom may have suboptimally functioning immune systems, also may be at increased risk for disseminated disease. Persons of color (blacks, Filipinos, Native Americans) also seem to have an increased risk, but it is unclear whether their susceptibility is due to genetic causes or socioeconomic factors, such as poor nutrition.

The cutaneous lesions may appear as papules, subcuta-

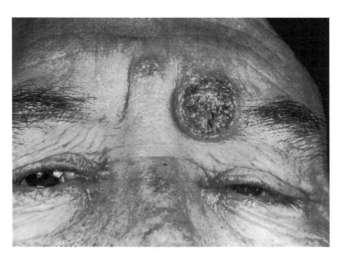

FIGURE 6–24. **Coccidioidomycosis.** This fungating ulceration of the facial skin represents a lesion of disseminated coccidioidomycosis. (Courtesy of Boni E. Elewski, MD, from the book *Cutaneous Fungal Infections*, Igaku-Shoin Medical Publishers, New York, New York, 1992.)

neous abscesses, verrucous plaques, and granulomatous nodules. Of prime significance to the clinician is the predilection for these lesions to develop in the area of the central face, especially the nasolabial fold (Fig. 6–24). Oral lesions are distinctly uncommon.

Histopathologic Features

Biopsy material shows large (20 to 60 μ), round spherules that may contain numerous endospores. The host response may be variable, ranging from a suppurative, neutrophilic infiltrate to a granulomatous inflammatory response. In some cases, the two patterns of inflammation are seen concurrently. Special stains, such as the PAS and Grocott-Gomori methenamine silver methods, enable the pathologist to identify the organism more readily.

Diagnosis

The diagnosis of coccidioidomycosis can be confirmed by culture or identification of characteristic organisms in biopsy material. Cytologic preparations from bronchial swabbings or sputum samples may also reveal the organisms.

Serologic studies are helpful in supporting the diagnosis, and they may be performed at the same time as skin testing. Skin testing by itself may be of limited value in determining the diagnosis because many patients in endemic areas have already been exposed to the organism and have positive test findings.

Treatment

The decision whether or not to treat a particular patient affected by coccidioidomycosis depends on the severity and extent of the infection as well as the patient's immune status. Relatively mild symptoms in an immunocompetent person do not warrant treatment. Amphotericin B is administered for:

- Immunosuppressed patients
- Patients with severe pulmonary infection
- Patients who have disseminated disease
- Patients who appear to be in a life-threatening situation in regard to the infection

For less severe cases of coccidioidomycosis, ketoconazole and fluconazole have been used. The response of the disease to these drugs is slower, but the side effects and complications are fewer compared with those associated with amphotericin B.

CRYPTOCOCCOSIS

Cryptococcosis is a relatively uncommon fungal disease caused by the yeast *Cryptococcus neoformans*. This organism normally causes no problem in immunocompetent people, but it can be devastating to the immunocompromised patient. The incidence of cryptococcosis has increased dramatically during the past decade primarily because of the AIDS epidemic, and it is the most common life-threatening fungal infection in these patients. The disease has a worldwide distribution because of its association with the pigeon, with the organism living in the bird's gut without harming the animal. Unlike many other pathogenic fungi, *C. neoformans* grows as a yeast both in the soil and in infected tissue. The organism usually produces a prominent mucopolysaccharide capsule that appears to protect it from host immune defenses.

The disease is acquired by inhalation of *C. neoformans* spores into the lungs, resulting in an immediate influx of neutrophils that destroy most of the yeasts. Macrophages soon follow, although resolution of infection in the immunocompetent host ultimately depends on an intact cell-mediated immune system.

Clinical Features

Primary cryptococcal infection of the lungs is often asymptomatic; however, a mild flu-like illness may develop. Patients complain of productive cough, chest pain, fever, and malaise. Most patients with a diagnosis of cryptococcosis have a significant underlying medical problem related to immune suppression (e.g., systemic corticosteroid therapy, cancer chemotherapy, malignancy, AIDS). It is estimated that 5 to 8 percent of AIDS patients acquire this infection (see p. 198).

Dissemination of the infection is common in these immunocompromised patients, and the most frequent site of involvement is the meninges, followed by skin, bone, and the prostate gland.

Cryptococcal meningitis is characterized by headache, fever, vomiting, and neck stiffness. In many instances, this is the initial sign of the disease.

Cutaneous lesions develop in 10 to 20 percent of patients with disseminated disease. These are of particular importance to the clinician because the skin of the head and neck is often involved. The lesions present as erythematous papules or pustules that may ulcerate, discharging a pus-like material rich in cryptococcal organisms.

Although oral lesions are relatively rare, they have been described as crater-like, non-healing ulcers that are tender on palpation.

Histopathologic Features

Microscopic sections of a cryptococcal lesion generally show a granulomatous inflammatory response to the organism. The extent of the response may vary, however, depending on the host's immune status and the strain of the organism. The yeasts appear as round to ovoid structures, 4 to 6 μ in diameter, surrounded by a clear halo that represents the capsule. Staining with the PAS or Grocott-Gomori methenamine silver method can readily identify the fungus; moreover, a mucicarmine stain uniquely demonstrates its mucopolysaccharide capsule.

Diagnosis

The diagnosis of cryptococcosis can be made by several methods, including biopsy and culture. Detection of cryptococcal antigen in the serum or cerebrospinal fluid is also useful as a diagnostic procedure.

Treatment and Prognosis

Management of cryptococcal infections can be very difficult because most of the affected patients have an underlying medical problem. Before amphotericin B was developed, cryptococcosis was almost uniformly fatal. A combination of systemic amphotericin B and another antifungal drug (flucytosine) is usually used to treat this disease. The triazoles fluconazole and itraconazole have been effective in controlling cryptococcosis, and fluconazole has been approved for this purpose. These drugs produce far fewer side effects than do amphotericin B and flucytosine and should prove useful in the future.

ZYGOMYCOSIS (Mucormycosis; Phycomycosis)

Zygomycosis is an opportunistic, frequently fulminant, fungal infection that is caused by normally saprobic organisms of the class Zygomycetes, including such genera as *Absidia*, *Mucor*, and *Rhizopus*. These organisms are found throughout the world, growing in their natural state on a variety of decaying organic materials. Numerous spores may be liberated into the air and inhaled by the human host.

Zygomycosis may involve any one of several areas of the body, but the rhinocerebral form is most relevant to the oral health care provider. Zygomycosis is noted especially in insulin-dependent diabetics who have uncontrolled diabetes and are ketoacidotic; however, as with many other fungal diseases, this infection affects immunocompromised patients as well. Only rarely has zygomycosis been reported in apparently healthy individuals.

Clinical and Radiographic Features

Rhinocerebral zygomycosis may present in several ways. Patients experience such signs and symptoms as nasal obstruction, bloody nasal discharge, facial pain or headache, facial swelling or cellulitis, and visual disturbances with concurrent proptosis. Symptoms related to cranial nerve involvement (e.g., facial paralysis) are often present. With progression of disease into the cranial vault, blindness, lethargy, and seizures may develop, followed by death.

If the maxillary sinus is involved, the initial presentation may be seen as intraoral swelling of the maxillary alveolar process, the palate, or both. If the condition remains untreated, palatal ulceration may evolve, with the surface of the ulcer typically appearing black and necrotic. Massive tissue destruction may result if the condition is not treated (Fig. 6–25).

Radiographically, opacification of the sinuses may be observed in conjunction with patchy effacement of the bony walls of the sinuses (Fig. 6–26). Such a picture may be difficult to distinguish from that of a malignancy affecting the sinus area.

Histopathologic Features

Histopathologic examination of lesional tissue shows extensive necrosis with numerous large (6 to 50 μ in diameter), branching, nonseptate hyphae at the periphery (Fig. 6–27). The extensive tissue destruction and necrosis associated with this disease are undoubtedly due to the preference of the fungi for invasion of small blood vessels. This disrupts normal blood flow to the tissue, resulting in infarction and necrosis.

Diagnosis

Diagnosis of zygomycosis is usually based on the histopathologic findings. Because of the grave nature of this infection, appropriate therapy must be instituted in a timely manner, often without the benefit of definitive culture results.

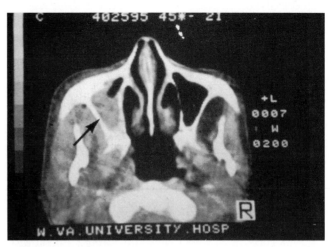

FIGURE 6–26. **Zygomycosis.** This CT scan demonstrates the opacification of the left maxillary sinus (*arrow*).

Treatment and Prognosis

Treatment of zygomycosis consists of radical surgical debridement of the infected, necrotic tissue and systemic administration of high doses of amphotericin B. In addition, control of the patient's underlying disease must be attempted. Despite such therapy, the prognosis is usually poor.

ASPERGILLOSIS

Aspergillosis is a fungal disease that may present as an allergy in the normal host, as a localized infection of damaged tissue, or as an invasive infection in the immunocompromised patient. The various species of the *Aspergillus* genus normally reside worldwide as saprobic organisms in soil, water, or decaying organic debris. The resistant spores that are produced are released into the air and are inhaled by the human host, resulting in opportunistic fungal infection second in frequency only to candidiasis.

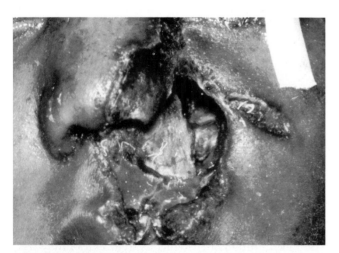

FIGURE 6–25. **Zygomycosis.** Diffuse tissue destruction involving the nasal and maxillary structures caused by a *Mucor* species. (Courtesy of Dr. Sadru Kabani.)

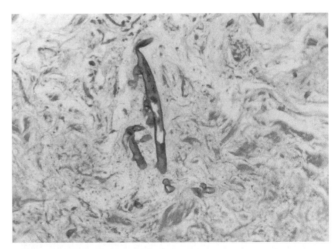

FIGURE 6–27. **Zygomycosis.** This high-power photomicrograph shows the large, nonseptate fungal hyphae characteristic of the zygomycotic organisms.

The two most commonly encountered species of *Aspergillus* in the medical setting are *A. flavus* and *A. fumigatus*. Interestingly, such infections may be acquired by the patient in the hospital, especially if remodeling or building construction is being performed in the immediate area. Such activity often stirs up the spores, which are then inhaled by the patient.

Clinical Features

The clinical manifestations of aspergillosis vary, depending on the host immune status and the presence or absence of tissue damage. In the normal host, the disease may present as an allergy affecting either the sinuses or the bronchopulmonary tract. An asthma attack may be triggered by inhalation of spores by a susceptible person. Sometimes a low-grade infection becomes established in the maxillary sinus, resulting in a mass of fungal hyphae called an *aspergilloma*.

Another presentation that may be encountered by the oral health care provider is aspergillosis following tooth extraction or endodontic treatment, particularly in the maxillary posterior segments. Apparently, the tissue damage predisposes the sinus to infection, resulting in symptoms of localized pain and tenderness accompanied by nasal discharge. If this problem is not treated, it may lead to necrotic palatal perforation, seen clinically as a yellow or black ulcer, and facial swelling. Such lesions occur much more commonly in the immunocompromised host.

Disseminated aspergillosis occurs primarily in immunocompromised patients, particularly in those who have leukemia or who are taking high daily doses of corticosteroids. Such patients usually present with symptoms related to the primary site of inoculation: the lungs. The patient typically has chest pain, cough, and fever, but such symptoms are vague; thus, obtaining an early, accurate diagnosis may be difficult. Once the fungal organism obtains access to the blood stream, infection can spread to such sites as the central nervous system (CNS), eye, skin, liver, gastrointestinal tract, bone, and thyroid gland.

Histopathologic Features

Tissue sections of *Aspergillus* lesions show varying numbers of branching, septate hyphae, 3 to 4 μ in diameter (Fig. 6–28). These hyphae show a tendency to invade adjacent small blood vessels. Occlusion of the vessels often results in the characteristic pattern of necrosis that is associated with this disease. In the immunocompetent host, a granulomatous inflammatory response in addition to necrosis can be expected. In the immunocompromised patient, however, the inflammatory response is often weak or absent, leading to extensive tissue destruction.

Diagnosis

The diagnosis of aspergillosis can be established by identification of the organism in tissue sections. This finding should be supported by cultures of the organism from the lesion. Culture specimens of sputum and blood

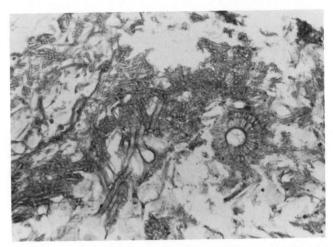

FIGURE 6–28. **Aspergillosis.** This photomicrograph reveals fungal hyphae and a fruiting body of an *Aspergillus* species.

are of limited value because they are often negative despite disseminated disease.

Treatment and Prognosis

Immunocompetent patients with aspergillosis usually respond to systemic amphotericin B therapy, with or without debridement of the lesional area. The prognosis for immunocompromised patients, however, is much worse, particularly if the infection is disseminated. Even with amphotericin B therapy, fewer than one third of these patients survive. Because aspergillosis in the immunocompromised patient usually develops while the individual is hospitalized, particular attention should be given to the ventilation system in the hospital in order to prevent patient exposure to the airborne spores of *Aspergillus*.

TOXOPLASMOSIS

Toxoplasmosis is a relatively common disease caused by the obligate intracellular protozoal organism *Toxoplasma gondii*. For normal, healthy adults, the organism poses no problems, and 30 to 50 percent of adults in the United States may have had asymptomatic infection. Unfortunately, the disease can be devastating for the developing fetus or the immunocompromised patient. Other mammals, particularly members of the cat family, are vulnerable to infection, and cats are considered to be the definitive host. *T. gondii* multiplies in the intestinal tract of the cat by means of a sexual life cycle, discharging numerous oocysts in the cat feces. These oocysts can then be ingested by another animal or human, resulting in the production of disease.

Clinical Features

In the normal, immunocompetent individual, infection with *T. gondii* is often asymptomatic. If symptoms develop, they are usually mild; patients may have a low-grade fever, cervical lymphadenopathy, fatigue, and muscle or joint pain. These symptoms may last from a few weeks up to a few months, although the host typically recovers without therapy. Sometimes the lymphadenopathy may involve one or more of the lymph nodes in the paraoral region, such as the buccal lymph node; in such instances, the disease may be discovered by the oral health care provider.

In immunosuppressed patients, toxoplasmosis may represent a new, primary infection or reactivation of previously encysted organisms. The principal groups at risk include:

- AIDS patients
- Transplant recipients
- Cancer patients

Manifestations of infection can include necrotizing encephalitis, pneumonia, and myositis or myocarditis. In the United States, it is estimated that from 3 to 10 percent of AIDS patients (see p. 198) will experience central nervous system (CNS) involvement. CNS infection is very serious. Clinically, the patient may present with headache, lethargy, disorientation, and hemiparesis.

Congenital toxoplasmosis occurs when a non-immune mother contracts the disease during her pregnancy and the organism crosses the placental barrier, infecting the developing fetus. The potential effects of blindness, mental retardation, and delayed psychomotor development are most severe if the infection occurs during the first trimester of pregnancy.

Histopathologic Features

Histopathologic examination of a lymph node obtained from a patient with active toxoplasmosis shows characteristic reactive germinal centers exhibiting an accumulation of eosinophilic macrophages. The macrophages encroach on the germinal centers and accumulate within the subcapsular and sinusoidal regions of the node (Fig. 6–29).

Diagnosis

The diagnosis of toxoplasmosis is usually established by identification of rising serum antibody titers to *T. gondii* within 10 to 14 days after infection. Immunocompromised patients, however, may not be able to generate an antibody response; therefore, the diagnosis may rest on the clinical findings and the response of the patient to therapy.

Biopsy of an involved lymph node may suggest the diagnosis; however, the diagnosis should be confirmed by serologic studies if possible.

Treatment and Prognosis

Most healthy adults with toxoplasmosis require no specific treatment because of the mild symptoms and self-limiting course. Perhaps more importantly, pregnant

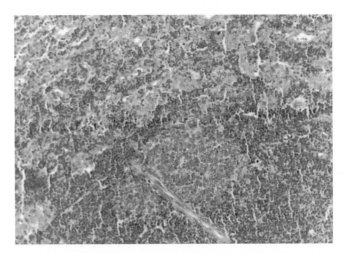

FIGURE 6–29. **Toxoplasmosis.** This medium-power photomicrograph shows the characteristic pattern of disruption of the lymph node architecture by toxoplasmosis. Infiltrates of eosinophilic macrophages accumulate beneath the capsule and encroach on the germinal centers.

women should avoid situations that place them at risk for the disease. Handling or eating raw meat or cleaning a cat litter box should be avoided until after delivery. If exposure during pregnancy is suspected, treatment with a combination of sulfadiazine and pyrimethamine often prevents transmission of *T. gondii* to the fetus. A similar drug regimen is used to treat immunosuppressed individuals with toxoplasmosis, although one study has shown that clindamycin may be substituted for sulfadiazine in managing patients who are allergic to sulfa drugs.

REFERENCES

Candidiasis

Allen CM. Diagnosing and managing oral candidiasis. J Am Dent Assoc 123:77–82, 1992.

Arendorf TM, Walker DM. The prevalence and intra-oral distribution of *Candida albicans* in man. Arch Oral Biol 25:1–10, 1980.

Baughman RA. Median rhomboid glossitis: A developmental anomaly? Oral Surg Oral Med Oral Pathol 31:56–65, 1971.

Bergendal T, Isacsson G. A combined clinical, mycological and histological study of denture stomatitis. Acta Odontol Scand 41:33–44, 1983.

Budtz-Jörgensen E. Etiology, pathogenesis, therapy, and prophylaxis of oral yeast infections. Acta Odontol Scand 48:61–69, 1990.

Field EA, Field JK, Martin MV. Does *Candida* have a role in oral epithelial neoplasia? J Med Vet Mycol 27:277–294, 1989.

Fotos PG, Vincent SD, Hellstein JW. Oral candidosis: Clinical, historical and therapeutic features of 100 cases. Oral Surg Oral Med Oral Pathol 74:41–49, 1992

Heimdahl A, Nord CE. Oral yeast infections in immunocompromised and seriously diseased patients. Acta Odontol Scand 48:77–84, 1990.

Holmstrup P, Axéll T. Classification and clinical manifestations of oral yeast infections. Acta Odontol Scand 48:57–59, 1990.

Lehner T. Oral thrush, or acute pseudomembranous candidiasis: A clinicopathologic study of forty-four cases. Oral Surg Oral Med Oral Pathol 18:27–37, 1964.

Lewis MAO, Samaranayake LP, Lamey P-J. Diagnosis and treatment of oral candidosis. J Oral Maxillofac Surg 49:996–1002, 1991.

Monaco JG, Pickett AB. The role of *Candida* in inflammatory papillary hyperplasia. J Prosthet Dent 45:470–471, 1981.

Morimoto K, Kihara A, Suetsugu T. Clinico-pathological study on denture stomatitis. J Oral Rehabil 14:513–522, 1987.

Odds FC, et al. Nomenclature of fungal diseases: A report and recommendations from a sub-committee of the International Society for Human and Animal Mycology (ISHAM). J Med Vet Mycol 30:1–10, 1992.

Öhman S-C, et al. Angular cheilitis: A clinical and microbial study. J Oral Pathol 15:213–217, 1986.

Rodu B, Griffin IL, Gockerman JP. Oral candidiasis in cancer patients. South Med J 77:312–314, 1984.

Samaranayake LP. Superficial oral fungal infections. Curr Opin Dent 1:415–422, 1991.

Samaranayake LP, Holmstrup P. Oral candidiasis and human immunodeficiency virus. J Oral Pathol Med 18:554–564, 1989.

Sanguineti A, Carmichael JK, Campbell K. Fluconazole-resistant *Candida albicans* after long-term suppressive therapy. Arch Intern Med 153:1122–1124, 1993.

Histoplasmosis

Dijkstra JWE. Histoplasmosis. Dermatol Clin 7:251–258, 1989.

Nightingale SD, et al. Disseminated histoplasmosis in patients with AIDS. South Med J 83:624–630, 1990.

Samaranayake LP. Oral mycoses in HIV infection. Oral Surg Oral Med Oral Pathol 73:171–180, 1992.

Sarosi GA, Johnson PC. Disseminated histoplasmosis in patients infected with human immunodeficiency virus. Clin Infect Dis 14(Suppl 1):S60–S67, 1992.

Sharma OP. Histoplasmosis: A masquerader of sarcoidosis. Sarcoidosis 8:10–13, 1991.

Wheat LJ. Diagnosis and management of histoplasmosis. Eur J Clin Microbiol Infect Dis 8:480–490, 1989.

Wheat LJ. Histoplasmosis in Indianapolis. Clin Infect Dis 14(Suppl 1):S91–S99, 1992.

Blastomycosis

Bradsher RW. Blastomycosis. Clin Infect Dis 14(Suppl 1):S82–S90, 1992.

Davies SF, Sarosi GA. Blastomycosis. Eur J Clin Microbiol Infect Dis 8:474–479, 1989.

Dismukes WE, et al. Itraconazole therapy for blastomycosis and histoplasmosis. Am J Med 93:489–497, 1992.

Klein BS, et al. Isolation of *Blastomyces dermatitidis* in soil associated with a large outbreak of blastomycosis in Wisconsin. N Engl J Med 314:529–534, 1986.

Maxson S, et al. Perinatal blastomycosis: A review. Pediatr Infect Dis J 11:760–763, 1992.

Meyer KC, McManus EJ, Maki DG. Overwhelming pulmonary blastomycosis associated with the adult respiratory distress syndrome. N Engl J Med 329:1231–1236, 1993.

Reder PA, Neel B. Blastomycosis in otolaryngology: Review of a large series. Laryngoscope 103:53–58, 1993.

Rose HD, Gingrass DJ. Localized oral blastomycosis mimicking actinomycosis. Oral Surg Oral Med Oral Pathol 54:12–14, 1982.

Serody JS, et al. Blastomycosis in transplant recipients: Report of a case and review. Clin Infect Dis 16:54–58, 1993.

Steck WD. Blastomycosis. Dermatol Clin 7:241–250, 1989.

Weingardt J, Li Y-P. North American blastomycosis. Am Fam Physician 43:1245–1248, 1991.

Winer-Muram HT, Rubin SA. Pulmonary blastomycosis. J Thorac Imaging 7:23–28, 1992.

Paracoccidioidomycosis

Brummer E, Castaneda E, Restrepo A. Paracoccidioidomycosis: An update. Clin Microbiol Rev 6:89–117, 1993.

Paes de Almeida O, et al. Oral manifestations of paracoccidioidomycosis (South American blastomycosis). Oral Surg Oral Med Oral Pathol 72:430–435,1991.

San-Blas G, et al. Paracoccidioidomycosis. J Med Vet Mycol 30(Suppl 1):59–71, 1992.

San-Blas G. Paracoccidioidomycosis and its etiologic agent *Paracoccidioides brasiliensis*. J Med Vet Mycol 31:99–113, 1993.

Sposto MR, et al. Oral paracoccidioidomycosis: A study of 36 South American patients. Oral Surg Oral Med Oral Pathol 75:461–465, 1993.

Coccidioidomycosis

Ampel NM, Dols CL, Galgiani JN. Coccidioidomycosis during human immunodeficiency virus infection: Results of a prospective study in a coccidioidal endemic area. Am J Med 94:235–240, 1993.

Bronnimann DA, Galgiani JN. Coccidioidomycosis. Eur J Clin Microbiol Infect Dis 8:466–473, 1989.

Einstein HE, Johnson RH. Coccidioidomycosis: New aspects of epidemiology and therapy. Clin Infect Dis 16:349–356, 1993.

Galgiani JN. Coccidioidomycosis: Changes in clinical expression, serological diagnosis, and therapeutic options. Clin Infect Dis 14(Suppl 1):S100–S105, 1992.

Galgiani JN. Coccidioidomycosis. West J Med 159:153–171, 1993.

Hedges E, Miller S. Coccidioidomycosis: Office diagnosis and treatment. Am Fam Physician 41:1499–1506, 1990.

Hobbs ER. Coccidioidomycosis. Dermatol Clin 7:227–239, 1989.

Pappagianis D, et al. Coccidioidomycosis—United States, 1991–1992. MMWR Morb Mortal Wkly Rep 42:21–24, 1993.

Cryptococcosis

Glick M, et al. Oral manifestations of disseminated *Cryptococcus neoformans* in a patient with acquired immunodeficiency syndrome. Oral Surg Oral Med Oral Pathol 64:454–459, 1987.

Hernandez AD. Cutaneous cryptococcosis. Dermatol Clin 7:269–274, 1989.

Kwon-Chung KJ, et al. Recent advances in biology and immunology of *Cryptococcus neoformans*. J Med Vet Mycol 30(Suppl 1):133–142, 1992.

Leggiadro RJ, Barrett FF, Hughes WT. Extrapulmonary cryptococcosis in immunocompromised infants and children. Pediatr Infect Dis J 11:43–47, 1992.

Levitz SM. The ecology of *Cryptococcus neoformans* and the epidemiology of cryptococcosis. Rev Infect Dis 13:1163–1169, 1991.

Patterson TF, Andriole VT. Current concepts in cryptococcosis. Eur J Clin Microbiol Infect Dis 8:457–465, 1989.

Patz EF, Goodman PC. Pulmonary cryptococcosis. J Thorac Imaging 7:51–55, 1992.

Saag MS, et al. Comparison of amphotericin B with fluconazole in the treatment of acute AIDS-associated cryptococcal meningitis. N Engl J Med 326:83–89, 1992.

Scully C, Paes De Almeida O. Orofacial manifestations of the systemic mycoses. J Oral Pathol Med 21:289–294, 1992.

Sugar AM. Overview: Cryptococcosis in the patient with AIDS. Mycopathologia 114:153–157, 1991.

Zygomycosis

de Biscop J, et al. Mucormycosis in an apparently normal host: Case study and literature review. J Craniomaxillofac Surg 19:275–278, 1991.

Hauman CHJ, Raubenheimer EJ. Orofacial mucormycosis. Oral Surg Oral Med Oral Pathol 68:624–627, 1989.

Jones AC, Bentsen TY, Freedman PD. Mucormycosis of the oral cavity. Oral Surg Oral Med Oral Pathol 75:455–460, 1993.

Radentz WH. Opportunistic fungal infections in immunocompromised hosts. J Am Acad Dermatol 20:989–1003, 1989.

Rinaldi MG. Zygomycosis. Infect Dis Clin North Am 3:19–41, 1989.

Rosenberg SW, Lepley JB. Mucormycosis in leukemia. Oral Surg Oral Med Oral Pathol 54:26–32, 1982.

Sugar AM. Mucormycosis. Clin Infect Dis 14(Suppl 1):S126–S129, 1992.

Van der Westhuijzen AJ, et al. A rapidly fatal palatal ulcer: Rhinocerebral mucormycosis. Oral Surg Oral Med Oral Pathol 68:32–36, 1989.

Aspergillosis

Bodey GP, Vartivarian S. Aspergillosis. Eur J Clin Microbiol Infect Dis 8:413–437, 1989.

Dixon DM, Walsh TJ. Human pathogenesis. In: *Aspergillus*: Biology and Industrial Applications. Edited by Bennett JW, Klich MA. Boston, Butterworth-Heinemann, Biotechnology 23:249–267, 1992.

Rhodes JC, et al. *Aspergillus* and aspergillosis. J Med Vet Mycol 30(Suppl 1):51–57, 1992.

Shannon MT, Sclaroff A, Cohen SJ. Invasive aspergillosis of the maxilla in an immunocompromised patient. Oral Surg Oral Med Oral Pathol 70:425–427, 1990.

Burchard KW. Fungal sepsis. Infect Dis Clin North Am 6:677–692, 1992.

Toxoplasmosis

Appel BN, Mendelow H, Pasqual HN. Acquired toxoplasma lymphadenitis. Oral Surg Oral Med Oral Pathol 47:529–532, 1979.

Buxton D. Toxoplasmosis. Practitioner 234:42–44, 1990.

Decker CF, Tuazon CU. Toxoplasmosis: An update on clinical and therapeutic aspects. Prog Clin Parasitol 3:21–41, 1993.

Luft BJ, et al: Toxoplasmic encephalitis in patients with the acquired immunodeficiency syndrome. N Engl J Med 329:995–1000, 1993.

McCabe R, Remington JS. Toxoplasmosis: The time has come. N Engl J Med 318:313–315, 1988.

Moran WJ, et al. Toxoplasmosis lymphadenitis occurring in a parotid gland. Otolaryngol Head Neck Surg 94:237–240, 1986.

7

Viral Infections

HERPES SIMPLEX VIRUS

Herpes simplex virus (HSV) is a DNA virus and a member of the human herpesvirus (HHV) family, officially known as Herpetoviridae. Two HSVs are known to exist: type 1 (HSV-1 or HHV-1) and type 2 (HSV-2 or HHV-2). Other members of the HHV family include varicella-zoster virus (VZV or HHV-3), Epstein-Barr virus (EBV or HHV-4), cytomegalovirus (CMV or HHV-5), and two more recently discovered members, HHV-6 and HHV-7. Humans are the only natural reservoir, and all HHVs have the ability to reside for life within the infected host. After the initial infection, variable periods of latency and reactivation with viral shedding are seen. Because each affected individual remains a reservoir of infection for life, the virus is endemic worldwide.

The two types of HSV are structurally similar but antigenically different. In addition, the two exhibit epidemiologic variations.

HSV-1 is spread predominantly through infected saliva or active perioral lesions. HSV-1 is adapted best and performs more efficiently in the oral, facial, and ocular areas. The pharynx, intraoral sites, lips, eyes, and skin above the waist are the most commonly involved locations.

HSV-2 is adapted best to the genital zones, is transmitted predominantly through sexual contact, and typically involves the genitalia and skin below the waist. Exceptions to these rules do occur, and HSV-1 can be seen in a pattern similar to that of HSV-2 and vice versa. The clinical lesions produced by both types are identical, and both produce the same changes in tissue. The viruses are so similar that antibodies directed against one cross-react against the other. Antibodies to one of the types decrease the chance of infection with the other type; if infection does occur, the manifestations are less severe.

Clinically evident infections with HSV-1 present in two patterns. The initial exposure to an individual without antibodies to the virus is called the **primary infection**. This typically occurs at a young age, is often asymptomatic, and usually does not cause significant morbidity. At this point, the virus is taken up by the sensory nerves and transported to the associated sensory or, less frequently, the autonomic ganglia. With oral HSV-1 infection, the trigeminal ganglion is colonized, and the virus remains at this site in a latent state. The virus uses the axons of the sensory neurons to travel back and forth to the peripheral skin or mucosa.

Secondary or **recurrent HSV-1 infection** occurs with reactivation of the virus, although many patients may show only asymptomatic viral shedding in the saliva. Symptomatic recurrences are fairly common and affect the epithelium supplied by the sensory ganglion. Spread to an uninfected host can easily occur during periods of asymptomatic viral shedding or from symptomatic active lesions. When repeatedly tested, approximately one third of individuals with HSV-1 antibodies occasionally shed infectious viral particles, even without active lesions being present. In addition, the virus may spread to other sites in the same host to establish residency at the sensory ganglion of the new location. Numerous conditions, such

181

as old age, ultraviolet light, emotional stress, pregnancy, allergy, trauma, respiratory illnesses, menstruation, systemic diseases, or malignancy, have been associated with reactivation of the virus, but only ultraviolet light exposure has been unequivocally demonstrated experimentally to induce lesions. More than 80 percent of the primary infections are purported to be asymptomatic, and reactivation with asymptomatic viral shedding greatly exceeds clinically evident recurrences.

HSV does not survive long in the external environment, and almost all primary infections occur from contact with an infected person who is releasing the virus. The usual incubation period is 3 to 9 days. Because HSV-1 is usually acquired from contact with contaminated saliva or active perioral lesions, crowding and poor hygiene promote exposure. Lower socioeconomic status correlates with earlier exposure. In poor, developing countries, more than 50 percent of the population is exposed by age 5 years, 95 percent by age 15 years, and almost universal exposure by age 30 years. On the other hand, upper socioeconomic groups in developed nations exhibit less than 20 percent exposure at age 5 years and only 50 to 60 percent in adults. The low exposure during childhood in the privileged groups is followed by a second peak during the college years of life. The age of initial infection also affects the clinical presentation of the symptomatic primary infections. People exposed to HSV-1 at an early age tend to exhibit gingivostomatitis; those initially exposed later in life often demonstrate pharyngotonsillitis.

As mentioned earlier, antibodies to HSV-1 decrease the chance of infection with HSV-2 or lessen the severity of the clinical manifestations. The dramatic increase recently seen in HSV-2 is partly due to lack of prior exposure to HSV-1 as well as to increased sexual activity and lack of barrier contraception. HSV-2 exposure correlates directly with sexual activity. Exposure of those younger than age 14 is close to zero, and most initial infections occur between the ages of 15 and 35. The prevalence varies from near zero in celibate adults to more than 80 percent in prostitutes.

In addition to clinically evident infections, HSV has been implicated in a number of noninfectious processes. More than 15 percent of cases of **erythema multiforme** are preceded by a symptomatic recurrence of HSV 3 to 10 days earlier (see p. 567). In some instances, the attacks of erythema multiforme are chronic enough to warrant antiviral prophylaxis. An association with cluster headaches and a number of cranial neuropathies has been proposed, but definitive proof is lacking.

On rare occasions, asymptomatic release of HSV will coincide with attacks of aphthous ulcerations. The ulcerations are not infected with the virus. In these rare cases, the virus may be responsible for the initiation of the autoimmune destruction; conversely, the immunodysregulation that produces aphthae may have allowed the release of the virions. In support of the lack of association between HSV and aphthae in the general population of patients with aphthous ulcerations, prophylactic oral acyclovir does not decrease the recurrence rate of the aphthous ulcerations. Although the association between

HSV and recurrent aphthous ulcerations is weak, it may be important in small subsets of patients (see p. 236).

HSV also has been associated with oral carcinomas, but much of the evidence is circumstantial. The DNA from HSV has been extracted from the tissues of some tumors but not from others. HSV may aid carcinogenesis through the promotion of mutations, but the oncogenic role, if any, is uncertain.

Clinical Features

Acute herpetic gingivostomatitis is the most common pattern of symptomatic primary HSV infection, and more than 90 percent are the result of HSV-1. In a study of more than 4000 children with antibodies to HSV-1, Juretić found that only 12 percent of those infected had clinical symptoms and signs severe enough to be remembered by the affected patients.

In spite of this study, some health care practitioners suspect that the percentage of primary infections that exhibit clinical symptoms is much higher. Further studies are needed to fully answer this question.

Most cases of acute herpetic gingivostomatitis arise between the ages of 6 months and 5 years. The onset is abrupt and accompanied by anterior cervical lymphadenopathy, fever (103 to 105°F), anorexia, irritability, and sore mouth lesions. The manifestations vary from mild to severely debilitating. Initially, the affected mucosa develops numerous pinhead vesicles, which rapidly collapse to form numerous small, red lesions. These initial lesions enlarge slightly and develop central areas of ulceration, which are covered by yellow fibrin (Fig. 7–1). Adjacent ulcerations may coalesce to form larger, shallow, irregular ulcerations (Fig. 7–2). Both the movable and attached oral mucosa can be affected, and the number of lesions is highly variable. In all cases, the gingiva is enlarged, painful, and extremely erythematous (Fig. 7–3; see Color Figure 37). In addition, the affected gingiva often exhibits distinctive punched-out erosions along the mid-facial free gingival margins (Fig. 7–4; see Color Figure 38). It is not unusual for the involvement of the labial

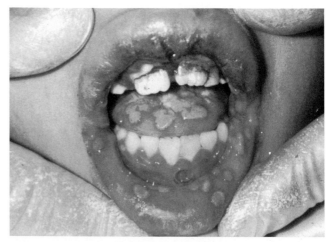

FIGURE 7–1. **Acute herpetic gingivostomatitis**. Widespread yellowish mucosal ulcerations. (Courtesy of Dr. David Johnsen.)

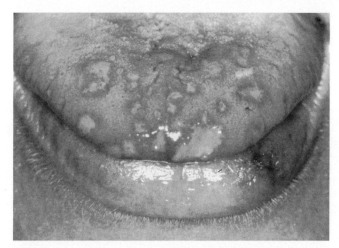

FIGURE 7-2. **Acute herpetic gingivostomatitis**. Numerous coalescing, irregular, and yellowish ulcerations of the dorsal surface of the tongue.

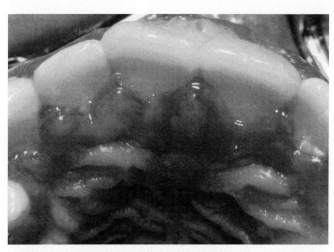

FIGURE 7-3. **Acute herpetic gingivostomatitis**. Painful, enlarged, and erythematous palatal gingiva. See Color Plates.

mucosa to extend past the wet line to include the adjacent vermilion border of the lips. Satellite vesicles of the perioral skin are fairly common. Self-inoculation of the fingers, eyes, and genital areas can occur. Mild cases usually resolve within 5 to 7 days; severe cases may extend to 2 weeks.

As mentioned earlier, when the primary infection occurs in adults, some symptomatic cases present as **pharyngotonsillitis**. Sore throat, fever, malaise, and headache are the initial symptoms. Numerous small vesicles develop on the tonsils and posterior pharynx. The vesicles rapidly rupture to form numerous shallow ulcerations, which often coalesce with one another. A diffuse, grayish-yellow exudate forms over the ulcers in many cases. Involvement of the oral mucosa anterior to Waldeyer's ring occurs in less than 10 percent of these cases. HSV appears to be a significant cause of pharyngotonsillitis in young adults who are from the higher socioeconomic groups with previously negative test findings for HSV antibodies. Most of these infections are HSV-1, but an increasing proportion are HSV-2. The clinical presen-

tation closely resembles pharyngitis secondary to streptococci or infectious mononucleosis, making the true frequency difficult to determine.

Recurrent infections may occur either at the site of primary inoculation or in adjacent areas of surface epithelium supplied by the involved ganglion. The most common site of recurrence for HSV-1 is the vermilion border and adjacent skin of the lips. This is known as **herpes labialis** ("cold sore" or "fever blister"). Prevalence studies suggest that from 15 to 45 percent of the United States population have a history of herpes labialis. In some patients, ultraviolet light or trauma can trigger recurrences. Six to 24 hours before the lesions develop, prodromal signs and symptoms arise, such as pain, burning, itching, tingling, a localized warmth, or erythema of the involved epithelium. Multiple small, erythematous papules develop and form clusters of fluid-filled vesicles (Fig. 7-5; see Color Figure 39). The vesicles rupture and crust within 2 days. Healing usually occurs within 7 to 10 days. Mechanical rupture of intact vesicles and the release of the virus-filled fluid may result

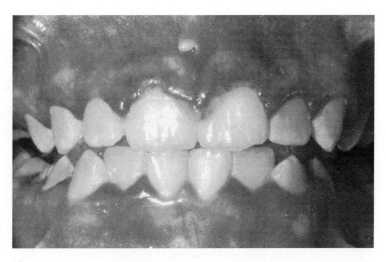

FIGURE 7-4. **Acute herpetic gingivostomatitis**. Painful, enlarged, and erythematous facial gingiva. Note erosions of the free gingival margin. See Color Plates.

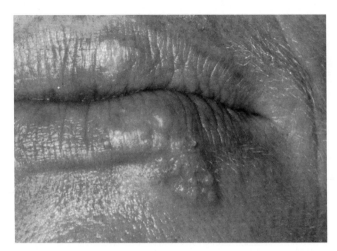

FIGURE 7–5. **Herpes labialis**. Multiple fluid-filled vesicles adjacent to the lip vermilion. See Color Plates.

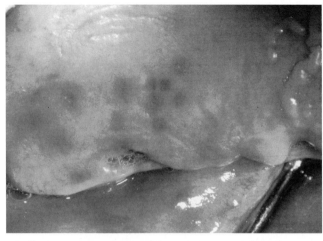

FIGURE 7–7. **Intraoral recurrent herpetic infection.** Early lesions presenting as multiple erythematous macules on the hard palate. Lesions had arisen a few days after extraction of a tooth. See Color Plates.

in the spreading of the lesions on lips previously cracked from sun exposure (Fig. 7–6). Recurrences are less commonly observed on the skin of the nose, chin, or cheek.

Recurrences can also affect the oral mucosa. In the immunocompetent patient, involvement is almost always limited to the keratinized mucosa, which is bound to bone (attached gingiva and hard palate). These sites often exhibit subtle changes, and the symptoms are less intense. The lesions begin as 1- to 3-mm vesicles, which rapidly collapse to form a cluster of erythematous macules, which may coalesce or slightly enlarge (Figs. 7–7 [see Color Figure 40] and 7–8). The damaged epithelium is lost, and a central yellowish area of ulceration develops. Healing takes place within 7 to 10 days.

Less common presentations of HSV-1 do occur. Infection of the thumbs or fingers is known as **herpetic whitlow (herpetic paronychia)**, which may occur as a result of self-inoculation in children with orofacial herpes (Fig. 7–9). Before the uniform use of gloves, medical and dental personnel could infect their digits from contact with infected patients, and they were the most likely

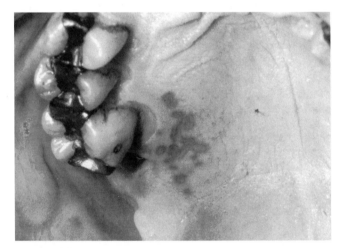

FIGURE 7–8. **Intraoral recurrent herpetic infection.** Multiple coalescing ulcerations on the hard palate.

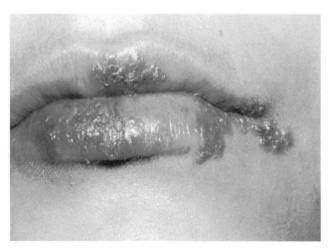

FIGURE 7–6. **Herpes labialis**. Multiple sites of recurrent herpetic infection secondary to spread of viral fluid over cracked lips.

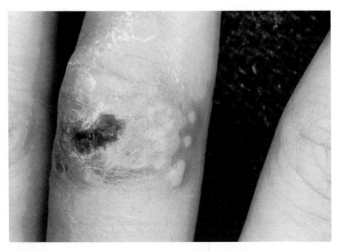

FIGURE 7–9. **Herpetic whitlow**. Recurrent herpetic infection of the finger.

group affected by this form of HSV-1 infection. Recurrences on the digits are not unusual and may result in paresthesia and permanent scarring.

Primary cutaneous herpetic infections can also arise in areas of previous epithelial damage. Parents kissing areas of dermatologic injury in children represent one vector. Wrestlers and rugby players also may contaminate areas of abrasion, a lesion called **herpes gladiatorum** or **scrumpox**. Ocular involvement may occur in children, often resulting from self-inoculation. Patients with diffuse chronic skin diseases, such as eczema, pemphigus, and Darier's disease, may develop diffuse life-threatening HSV infection, known as **eczema herpeticum (Kaposi's varicelliform eruption)**. Newborns may become infected after delivery through a birth canal contaminated with HSV, usually HSV-2. Without treatment, there is greater than a 50 percent mortality rate.

HSV recurrence in immunocompromised hosts can be significant. Without proper immune function, recurrent herpes can persist and spread until the infection is treated with antivirals, until immune status returns, or until the patient dies. On the skin, the lesions continue to enlarge peripherally, with the formation of an increasing zone of superficial cutaneous erosion. Oral mucosa can also be affected and is usually present in conjunction with herpes labialis. Although most oral mucosal involvement begins on the bound mucosa, it often is not confined to these areas. The involved sites often begin as areas of necrotic epithelium, which is brownish and raised above the surface of the adjacent intact epithelium. These areas are typically much larger than the usual pinhead lesions found in immunocompetent patients. With time, the area of involvement spreads laterally. The enlarging lesion presents as a zone of superficial necrosis or erosion, often with a distinctive circinate, raised, yellow border (Figs. 7–10 and 7–11). This border represents the advancing margin of active viral destruction. Microscopic demonstration of HSV infection in a chronic ulceration on the movable oral mucosa is ominous, and all such patients should be evaluated thoroughly for possible immune dysfunction or underlying occult disease processes.

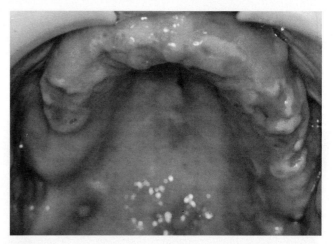

FIGURE 7–11. **Chronic herpetic infection**. Numerous shallow herpetic erosions with raised, yellow, and circinate borders on the maxillary alveolar ridge in an immunocompromised patient.

Histopathologic Features

The virus exerts its main effects on the epithelial cells. Infected epithelial cells exhibit acantholysis, nuclear clearing, and nuclear enlargement, which has been termed "ballooning degeneration" (Fig. 7–12). The acantholytic epithelial cells are termed "Tzanck cells." Nucleolar fragmentation occurs with a condensation of chromatin around the periphery of the nucleus. Multinucleated, infected epithelial cells are formed when fusion occurs between adjacent cells (see Fig. 7–12). Intercellular edema develops and leads to the formation of an intraepithelial vesicle. Mucosal vesicles rapidly rupture; those on the skin persist and develop secondary infiltration by inflammatory cells (Fig. 7–13). Once they have ruptured, the mucosal lesions demonstrate a surface fibrinopurulent membrane. Often at the edge of the ulceration, or mixed within the fibrinous exudate, are the scattered Tzanck or multinucleated epithelial cells.

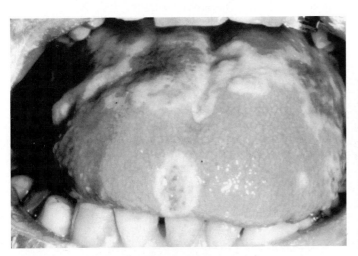

FIGURE 7–10. **Chronic herpetic infection**. Numerous mucosal erosions, each of which is surrounded by a slightly raised, yellowish-white border, in a patient with acute myelogenous leukemia.

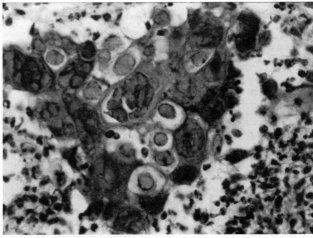

FIGURE 7–12. **Herpes simplex**. Altered epithelial cells exhibiting ballooning degeneration, margination of chromatin, and multinucleation.

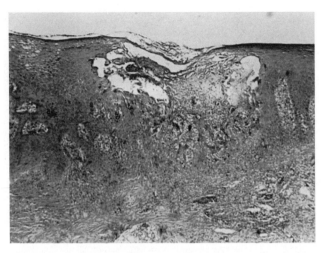

FIGURE 7-13. **Herpes simplex**. Superficial ruptured vesicle. Changes correlate with early erythematous macule of an intraoral recurrent lesion.

Diagnosis

With a thorough knowledge of the clinical presentations, one can make a strong presumptive diagnosis of HSV infection. On occasion, HSV infections can be confused with other diseases, and laboratory confirmation is desirable. Viral isolation from tissue culture inoculated with the fluid of fresh vesicles is the most definitive diagnostic procedure. The problem with this technique in primary infections is that up to 2 weeks can be required for a definitive result. Clinical tests for HSV antigens or nucleic acids in specimens of active lesions are also available. Serologic tests for HSV antibodies are positive 4 to 8 days after the initial exposure. These antibody titers are useful in documenting past exposure and are used primarily in epidemiologic studies.

Two of the most commonly used diagnostic procedures are the cytologic smear and tissue biopsy, with cytologic study being the least invasive and most cost-effective. The virus produces distinctive histologic alterations within the infected epithelium. Only varicella-zoster virus produces similar changes, but these two infections can usually be differentiated on a clinical basis. Fluorescent monoclonal antibody typing can be performed on the direct smears or on infected cells obtained from tissue culture.

Treatment and Prognosis

At this time, primary herpetic gingivostomatitis is best treated symptomatically. Patients should be instructed to restrict contact with active lesions to prevent the spread to other sites and people. As mentioned previously, autoinoculation of the eyes can result in ocular involvement with the possibility of recurrence. Repeated ocular reinfection can produce permanent damage and blindness. HSV is the leading infectious cause of blindness in the United States.

Topical rinsing with 0.5 or 1 percent dyclonine hydrochloride dramatically, but temporarily, decreases the mucosal discomfort. Viscous lidocaine should be avoided in pediatric patients because of reports of lidocaine-induced seizures in children. Nonsteroidal anti-inflammatory medications, such as ibuprofen, also help alleviate the discomfort. Most patients present at too late a stage for systemic antiviral medications to exert a significant effect. Acyclovir suspension is available and can be used with a rinse-and-swallow technique. This formulation provides immediate delivery to the infected area; with time, systemic absorption also occurs. Good placebo-controlled studies need to be performed in this area.

Recurrent herpes labialis has been treated with everything from ether to voodoo. Nothing has solved the problem. Some minor successes have been achieved with the current brand of antivirals. In 1989, Scully wrote an excellent review on the numerous medications that were then in use. Of all these, only acyclovir exhibited significant promise. Oral acyclovir can suppress recurrences prophylactically; if begun early in the prodrome, it may reduce the number of lesions and the length of time to crusting. Pain and the length of time to healing are not significantly affected if the medication is not initiated during the prodrome.

Acyclovir ointment in polyethylene glycol has been of limited benefit for herpes labialis in immunocompetent patients. It was thought that the base might prevent significant absorption; therefore, new trials evaluated acyclovir in a modified aqueous cream. It appears that the initiation of topical acyclovir during the prodrome may be too late, and significant success may be possible only in patients who associate recurrences with a known trigger and are able to begin prophylactic treatment before the first symptoms. Additional studies need to be performed on the aqueous base and on stronger formulations of acyclovir with other bases.

The pain associated with intraoral secondary herpes is usually not intense, and many patients do not require treatment. Some studies have shown chlorhexidine to exert antiviral effects in vivo and in vitro. In addition, acyclovir appears to function synergistically with chlorhexidine. Extensive clinical trials have not been performed, but chlorhexidine alone or in combination with acyclovir suspension may be beneficial in patients who desire or require therapy of intraoral lesions.

Immunocompromised hosts with HSV infections often require intravenous acyclovir to control the problem. Furthermore, severely immunosuppressed individuals, such as bone marrow transplant patients and those with acquired immunodeficiency syndrome (AIDS) often need prophylactic doses of oral acyclovir. On occasion, viral resistance develops, resulting in the onset of significant herpetic lesions. These resistant strains have been successfully treated with trisodium phosphonoformate hexahydrate (foscarnet), but this medication is reserved as a second-line therapy because of its significant side effects. In these cases, it appears that only the peripheral virus mutates, because future recurrences are once again sensitive to acyclovir.

VARICELLA (Chickenpox)

The varicella-zoster virus (VZV; HHV-3) is similar to herpes simplex virus (HSV) in many respects. **Chicken-**

pox represents the primary infection with the VZV; latency ensues, and recurrence is possible as **herpes zoster**, often after many decades. The virus is presumed to be spread through air droplets or direct contact with active lesions. Most cases of chickenpox arise between the ages of 5 and 9, with greater than 90 percent of the United States population being infected by age 15 years. In contrast to infection with HSV, most cases are symptomatic. The incubation period is 10 to 21 days, with an average of 15 days.

Clinical Features

The symptomatic phase of VZV infection usually begins with malaise, pharyngitis, and rhinitis. This is followed by a characteristic, intensely pruritic exanthem. The rash begins on the face and trunk, followed by involvement of the extremities. Each lesion rapidly progresses through stages of erythema, vesicle, pustule, and hardened crust (Figs. 7–14 and 7–15). The early vesicular stage is the most classic presentation. The centrally located vesicle is surrounded by a zone of erythema and has been described as "a dewdrop on a rose petal." The lesions come forth in successive crops over 3 to 4 days, and often lesions in various stages are present at the same time. Affected individuals are contagious from 2 days before the exanthem until all the lesions crust, usually 4 days after the arrival of the initial lesions. Fever is usually present during the active phase of the exanthem. The severity of the cutaneous involvement is variable and often more severe in adults and in household members secondarily infected by the initial patient.

Oral lesions are fairly common and may precede the skin lesions. The palate and the buccal mucosa are the most frequently involved sites. Occasionally, there are gingival lesions that resemble those noted in primary herpes simplex virus (HSV) infections, but distinguishing between the two is not difficult because the lesions of varicella tend to be relatively painless. The lesions begin as 3- to 4-mm white opaque vesicles that rupture to form 1- to 3-mm ulcerations (Fig. 7–16).

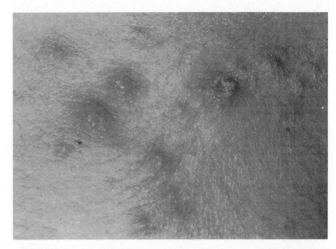

FIGURE 7–15. **Varicella**. Numerous vesicles with surrounding erythema and early crusting.

Complications can occur and are more frequent in adult patients. Before the discovery of antibiotics, secondary bacterial infections were a serious problem. In children, the most significant problems are **encephalitis** and **Reye's syndrome**. With enhanced public education and decreased use of aspirin in children, the incidence of Reye's syndrome is decreasing. Encephalitis and clinically significant pneumonia present in 1 in 375 affected adults older than 20 years of age. The central nervous system involvement typically produces ataxia but may result in headaches, drowsiness, convulsions, or coma. The pneumonia presents as dry cough and chest pain. Chest radiographs typically reveal large areas of patchy pneumonitis.

Infection during pregnancy can produce congenital or neonatal chickenpox. Involvement early in the pregnancy can result in spontaneous abortion or congenital defects. Although complications can occur in newborns, the effects of maternal varicella infection appear minimal. A recent multi-center prospective study of live births associated with maternal varicella infection revealed only a 1.2 percent prevalence of embryopathy.

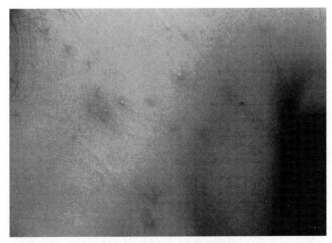

FIGURE 7–14. **Varicella**. Numerous erythematous vesicles on the right side of the neck.

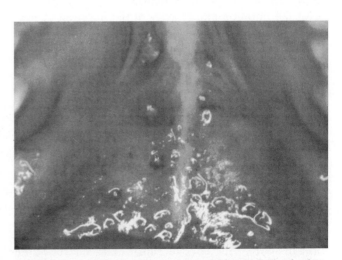

FIGURE 7–16. **Varicella**. White opaque vesicles on the hard palate.

Infection close to delivery can result in a severe fetal infection caused by a lack of maternal antibodies.

Infection in immunocompromised patients can also be most severe. The cutaneous involvement is typically extensive and may be associated with high fever, hepatitis, pneumonitis, pancreatitis, gastrointestinal obstruction, and encephalitis. Before effective antiviral therapy, the mortality rate in immunocompromised individuals was approximately 7 percent. Secondary bacterial infections often complicate the process.

Histopathologic Features

The cytologic alterations are virtually identical to those described for HSV. The virus causes acantholysis, with formation of numerous free-floating Tzanck cells, which exhibit nuclear margination of chromatin and occasional multinucleation.

Diagnosis

The diagnosis of chickenpox can usually be made from a history of exposure to VZV within the last 3 weeks and the presence of the typical exanthem. Confirmation can be obtained through a demonstration of viral cytopathologic effects present within the epithelial cells harvested from the vesicular fluid. These cytologic changes are identical to those found in herpes simplex, and further confirmation is sometimes desired. Viral isolation in cell culture or rapid diagnosis from fluorescein-conjugated VZV monoclonal antibodies can be performed. Finally, serum samples can be obtained during the acute stage and 14 to 28 days later. The later sample should demonstrate a significant (fourfold) increase in antibody titers to VZV.

Treatment and Prognosis

Before the current antiviral medications became available, the treatment of varicella was primarily symptomatic. Warm baths with baking soda, application of calamine lotion, and systemic or topical diphenhydramine are still used to relieve pruritus. Antipyretics other than aspirin should be given to reduce fever. Acyclovir reduces the duration and severity of the infection in normal children if it is administered within the first 24 hours of the rash; however, the drug is not widely used in immunocompetent children. Many clinicians reserve this approach for adults, neonates, immunosuppressed patients, or patients exhibiting progression of their illness. The intravenous form of acyclovir should be used for patients with a high risk for severe infection.

In immunocompromised patients who become exposed to VZV, varicella-zoster immune globulin (VZIG) can be given to significantly modify the clinical manifestations of the infection. VZIG is available commercially and prevents severe varicella infections in immunocompromised patients.

A live attenuated VZV vaccine has been available since 1974 and has been used extensively outside the United States, especially in Japan. The vaccine is 98 percent effective, with a 1 percent prevalence of rash and fever. Currently, the vaccine is being given in the United States on a limited basis and has been combined into one vaccine with measles, mumps, and rubella. Booster vaccines may be required to maintain lifelong immunity. Some clinicians have expressed concern that the vaccine may only delay the infection until adulthood when the clinical manifestations are more severe. In spite of this, the complication rate from varicella supports the wider use of the vaccine. Each year, slightly fewer than 100 deaths are reported secondary to VZV in the United States. However, the number of deaths is decreasing as a result of the use of antiviral medications.

HERPES ZOSTER (Shingles)

After the initial infection with VZV (chickenpox), the virus is transported up the sensory nerves and presumed to establish latency in the dorsal spinal ganglia. Clinically evident **herpes zoster** occurs after reactivation of the virus, with the involvement of the distribution of the affected sensory nerve. Zoster occurs during the lifetime of 10 to 20 percent of individuals, and the prevalence of attacks increases with age. With the increasing average age of the population, an increased prevalence of herpes zoster is expected. Unlike herpes simplex virus (HSV), single rather than multiple recurrences are the rule. Immunosuppression, treatment with cytotoxic drugs, radiation, presence of malignancies, old age, alcohol abuse, and dental manipulation are predisposing factors for reactivation.

Clinical Features

The recurrence begins with pain in the area of epithelium innervated by the affected sensory nerve (dermatome). Typically, one dermatome is affected, but involvement of two or more can occur. This prodromal pain, which may be accompanied by fever, malaise, and headache, is normally present 1 to 4 days before the development of the cutaneous or oral lesions. During this period, before the exanthem, the pain may masquerade as sensitive teeth, otitis media, migraine headache, myocardial infarction, or appendicitis, depending on which dermatome is affected.

The involved skin shows a cluster of vesicles set on an erythematous base (Fig. 7–17). Within 3 to 4 days, the vesicles become pustular and ulcerate, with crusts developing after 7 to 10 days. Scarring is not unusual. The lesions tend to follow the path of the affected nerve and terminate at the midline (Fig. 7–18). The exanthem typically resolves within 2 to 3 weeks in otherwise healthy individuals.

On occasion, there may be recurrence in the absence of vesiculation of the skin or mucosa. This pattern is called **zoster sine herpete**, and affected patients have severe pain of abrupt onset and hyperesthesia over a specific dermatome. Fever, headache, myalgia, and lymphadenopathy may or may not accompany the recurrence.

Pain lasting longer than 1 month after an episode of zoster is called **postherpetic neuralgia** and occurs in up to

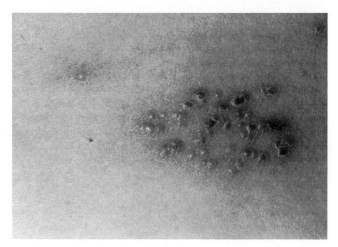

FIGURE 7–17. **Herpes zoster**. Cluster of vesicles with surrounding erythema of the skin.

14 percent of affected patients, especially those older than 60 years of age. Most of these neuralgias resolve within 1 year, with one half of the patients experiencing resolution after 2 months. Rare cases may last up to 20 years, and patients have been known to commit suicide as a result of the severe, lancinating quality of the pain.

Facial paralysis has been seen in association with herpes zoster of the face or external auditory canal. **Ramsay Hunt syndrome** is the combination of cutaneous lesions of the external auditory canal combined with involvement of the ipsilateral facial and auditory nerves. The syndrome causes facial paralysis, hearing deficits, vertigo, and a number of other auditory and vestibular symptoms.

Ocular involvement is not unusual and can be the source of significant morbidity, including permanent blindness. The ocular manifestations are highly variable and may arise from direct viral-mediated epithelial damage, neuropathy, immune-mediated damage, or secondary vasculopathy. If the tip of the nose is involved, this is a sign that the nasociliary branch of the fifth cranial nerve is involved, suggesting the potential for ocular infection. In these cases, referral to an ophthalmologist is mandatory.

Oral lesions occur with trigeminal nerve involvement and may be present on the movable or bound mucosa. The lesions often extend to the midline and are frequently present in conjunction with involvement of the skin overlying the affected quadrant. Like varicella, the individual lesions present as 1- to 4-mm white opaque vesicles, which rupture to form shallow ulcerations (Fig. 7–19). Involvement of the maxilla may be associated with devitalization of the teeth in the affected area. In addition, numerous reports have documented significant bone necrosis with loss of teeth in areas involved with herpes zoster.

Histopathologic Features

The active vesicles of herpes zoster are microscopically identical to those seen in the primary infection, varicella. For more information, refer to the earlier portions of the chapter on the histopathologic presentation of varicella and herpes simplex.

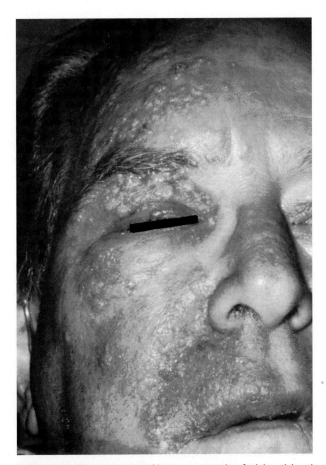

FIGURE 7–18. **Herpes zoster**. Numerous crusting facial vesicles that extend to the midline.

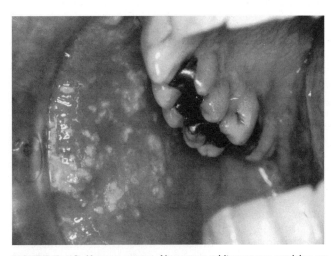

FIGURE 7–19. **Herpes zoster**. Numerous white opaque vesicles on the right buccal mucosa of the same patient depicted in Figure 7–18.

Diagnosis

The diagnosis of herpes zoster often can be made from the clinical presentation, but other procedures may be necessary in atypical cases. Viral culture can confirm the clinical impression but takes at least 24 hours. Cytologic smears demonstrate viral cytopathologic effects, as seen in varicella and HSV. In most cases, the clinical presentation allows the clinician to differentiate zoster from HSV, but cases of zosteriform recurrent HSV infection, although uncommon, do exist. A rapid diagnosis can be obtained through the use of direct staining of cytologic smears with fluorescent monoclonal antibodies for VZV. This technique gives positive results in almost 80 percent of the cases.

Treatment and Prognosis

Therapy for herpes zoster is directed toward supportive and symptomatic measures. Fever should be treated with antipyretics that do not contain aspirin. Topical or systemic antipruritics, such as diphenhydramine, can be administered to decrease itching. Skin lesions should be kept dry and clean to prevent secondary infection; antibiotics may be administered to treat such secondary infections. Once the skin lesions have healed, the pain associated with the neuralgia may be lessened through the use of topical analgesics, such as capsaicin. Corticosteroids have been used to minimize the associated neuralgia that may arise, but studies on the effectiveness of this technique are inconclusive. High doses of acyclovir can decrease the duration of the exanthem and the severity of the pain. This medication is given primarily to:

- Immunocompromised patients
- Patients who have severe disease
- Patients who have disseminated lesions
- Patients in whom the course has become chronic

Preliminary studies of the use of a live attenuated varicella vaccine have shown an improved immune response to the virus in elderly patients. Larger studies may lead to the use of this vaccine in an attempt to decrease the frequency of disease in this vulnerable population.

INFECTIOUS MONONUCLEOSIS (Mono; Glandular Fever; "Kissing Disease")

Infectious mononucleosis is a symptomatic disease resulting from exposure to Epstein-Barr virus (EBV, HHV-4). The infection usually occurs by intimate contact. Intrafamilial spread is common, and once a person is exposed, EBV remains in the host for life. Children usually become infected through contaminated saliva on fingers, toys, or other objects. Adults usually contract the virus through direct salivary transfer, such as shared straws or kissing, hence, the nickname "kissing disease." Exposure during childhood is usually asymptomatic, and most symptomatic infections arise in young adults. In developing nations, exposure usually occurs by age 3 and is universal by adolescence. In the United States, intro-

duction to the virus is often delayed, with close to 50 percent of college students lacking previous exposure. These unexposed adults become infected at a rate of 10 to 15 percent per year while in college. Infection in adulthood is associated with a higher risk (30 to 50 percent) for symptomatic disease.

Besides infectious mononucleosis, EBV has been demonstrated in the lesions of hairy leukoplakia (HL) (see p. 202) and has been associated with a number of cancers, such as African Burkitt's lymphoma (see p. 436), nasopharyngeal carcinoma (see p. 308), and several other types of lymphoma. However, direct proof of a cause-and-effect relationship is lacking.

Clinical Features

Most EBV infections in children are asymptomatic. In children younger than 4 years of age with symptoms, most have fever, lymphadenopathy, pharyngitis, hepatosplenomegaly, and rhinitis or cough. Children older than 4 years of age are similarly affected but exhibit a much lower prevalence of hepatosplenomegaly, rhinitis, and cough.

Most young adults present with fever, lymphadenopathy, pharyngitis, and tonsillitis. Hepatosplenomegaly and rash are seen less frequently. In adults older than 40 years of age, fever and pharyngitis are the predominant findings, with less than 30 percent demonstrating lymphadenopathy. Less frequent signs and symptoms in this group include hepatosplenomegaly, rash, and rhinitis or cough. Possible significant complications include thrombocytopenia and neurologic problems with seizures. These complications are uncommon at any age but more frequently develop in children.

In classic infectious mononucleosis in a young adult, prodromal fatigue, malaise, and anorexia occur up to 2 weeks before the development of pyrexia. The fever usually lasts from 2 to 14 days. Prominent lymphadenopathy is noted in more than 90 percent of the cases and typically presents as enlarged, symmetric, and tender nodes, frequently with involvement of the posterior and anterior cervical chains. Enlargement of parotid lymphoid tissue rarely has been reported and can be associated with facial nerve palsy. More than 80 percent of affected young adults have oropharyngeal tonsillar enlargement, sometimes with diffuse surface exudates and secondary tonsillar abscesses (Fig. 7–20). In rare instances, this enlargement may increase to the point of airway obstruction and even death.

Oral lesions other than lymphoid enlargement may also be seen. Petechiae on the hard or soft palate are present in about 25 percent of patients (Fig. 7–21). The petechiae are transient and usually disappear within 24 to 48 hours. Acute necrotizing ulcerative gingivitis (ANUG) (see p. 124) is also fairly common. ANUG-like pericoronitis (see p. 135) and acute necrotizing ulcerative mucositis (see p. 125) occur less frequently. Cases of ANUG that are refractory to normal therapy should be evaluated to rule out the possibility of EBV.

A controversial symptom complex called **chronic fatigue syndrome** has been described, and several investigators have tried to associate EBV with this problem.

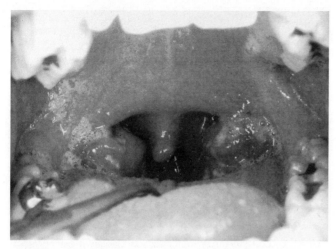

FIGURE 7–20. **Infectious mononucleosis.** Hyperplastic pharyngeal tonsils with yellowish crypt exudates. (Courtesy of Dr. George Blozis.)

Patients present with rather nonspecific findings of chronic fatigue, fever, pharyngitis, myalgias, headaches, arthralgias, paresthesias, depression, and cognitive defects. These patients often demonstrate elevations in EBV antibody titers, but this finding alone is insufficient to prove a definite cause-and-effect relationship.

Diagnosis

The diagnosis of EBV is suggested by the clinical presentation and should be confirmed through laboratory procedures. The white blood cell (WBC) count is increased, with the differential count showing relative lymphocytosis that can become as high as 70 to 90 percent during the second week. Atypical lymphocytes usually are present in the peripheral blood. The classic serologic finding in EBV is the presence of the Paul-Bunnell heterophil antibody; a rapid test for these antibodies (Monospot, Mono-Test) is available and inexpensive. More than 90 percent of infected young adults have positive

findings for the heterophil antibody, but infected children younger than age 4 frequently have negative results. Indirect immunofluorescence testing to detect EBV-specific antibodies should be used in those suspected of having an EBV infection but whose findings were negative on the Paul-Bunnell test. Enzyme-linked immunosorbent assays (ELISA) and recombinant DNA–derived antigens may soon replace the indirect immunofluorescence test.

Treatment and Prognosis

In most cases, infectious mononucleosis resolves within 4 to 6 weeks. Non–aspirin-containing antipyretics and nonsteroidal anti-inflammatory medications can be used to minimize the most common symptoms. On occasion, the fatigue may become chronic. In immunocompromised patients, a polyclonal B-lymphocyte proliferation may occur and possibly lead to death.

Because hairy leukoplakia of AIDS is associated with EBV and responds well to acyclovir, infectious mononucleosis should be responsive also. However, well-controlled studies using acyclovir in infectious mononucleosis have shown no significant effect on clinical outcome. *In vitro* inhibition of EBV by acyclovir suggests that future studies should manipulate the dose to try to improve the clinical response. Reports of ganciclovir use have provided similar results.

The tonsillar involvement may, on occasion, resemble streptococcal pharyngitis or tonsillitis (see p. 143). However, treatment with ampicillin and penicillin should be avoided because the use of these antibiotics in infectious mononucleosis has been associated with a higher than normal prevalence of allergic morbilliform skin rashes.

Corticosteroid use is the recommended therapy in many textbooks. Such drugs, however, should not be used indiscriminately because the person's immune response appears to be the most important factor in fighting the infection and preventing the possibly fatal polyclonal B-lymphocyte proliferation. Corticosteroid use produces a shortened duration of fever and a shrinkage of enlarged lymphoid tissues, but its use should be restricted to life-threatening cases.

CYTOMEGALOVIRUS

Cytomegalovirus (CMV, HHV-5) is similar to the other human herpes viruses (HHVs), in that, after the initial infection, latency is established and reactivation is possible under conditions favorable to the virus. CMV can reside latently in salivary gland cells, endothelium, macrophages, and lymphocytes. Most clinically evident disease is found in neonates or in immunosuppressed adults. In infants, the virus is contracted through the placenta, during delivery, or during breast-feeding. The next peak of transmission occurs during adolescence, predominantly from the exchange of bodily fluids as this group begins sexual activity. Transmission has also been documented from blood transfusion and organ transplantation. The prevalence of neonatal CMV infection varies from 0.5 to 2.5 percent. By the age of 30, almost

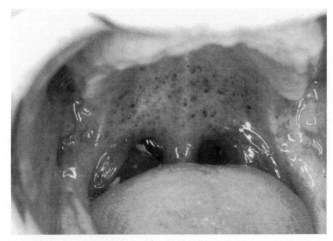

FIGURE 7–21. **Infectious mononucleosis.** Numerous petechiae of the soft palate. (Courtesy of Dr. George Blozis.)

40 percent of the population is infected; by age 60, 80 to 100 percent are infected. Screening of healthy middle-aged adult blood donors reveals that approximately 50 percent have been exposed to CMV.

Clinical Features

At any age, almost 90 percent of CMV infections are asymptomatic. In clinically evident neonatal infection, the infant appears ill within a few days. Typical features include hepatosplenomegaly, extramedullary cutaneous erythropoiesis, and thrombocytopenia, often with associated petechial hemorrhages. Significant encephalitis frequently leads to severe mental and motor retardation.

Acute adult infection presents with a clinical pattern that is similar to that of infectious mononucleosis. Most patients have fever, malaise, myalgia, abnormal liver function tests, and atypical peripheral lymphocytes. In contrast to patients with infectious mononucleosis, only about one third of patients with CMV demonstrate pharyngitis and lymphadenopathy.

Evident CMV involvement is not unusual in immunocompromised transplant patients. In some cases, a temporary mild fever is the only evidence; in others, the infection becomes aggressive and is characterized by significant hepatitis, leukopenia, pneumonitis, and, more rarely, a progressive wasting syndrome.

CMV disease is common in patients with AIDS (see p. 198). CMV chorioretinitis affects almost one third of patients with AIDS and tends to progress rapidly, often resulting in blindness. Bloody diarrhea from CMV colitis is fairly common but may respond to appropriate antiviral medications.

Although oral lesions from CMV infection have been documented in a number of immunosuppressive conditions, reports of oral involvement by CMV have been increasing since the advent of the AIDS epidemic. Most patients present with chronic mucosal ulcerations, in which CMV changes are found on biopsy, or with intraoral Kaposi's sarcoma, which some investigators believe may be associated with CMV infection.

Neonatal CMV can also produce developmental tooth defects, which can be discovered in later years. Examination of 118 people with a history of neonatal CMV infection revealed tooth defects in 40 percent of those with symptomatic infections and slightly more than 5 percent of those with asymptomatic infections. The teeth exhibited diffuse enamel hypoplasia, significant attrition, areas of enamel hypomaturation, and yellow coloration from the underlying dentin.

Histopathologic Features

Biopsy specimens of intraoral CMV lesions usually demonstrate changes within the vascular endothelial cells. Scattered infected cells are extremely swollen, showing both intracytoplasmic and intranuclear inclusions and prominent nucleoli. This enlarged cell has been called an "owl eye" cell. Gomori's methenamine silver and periodic acid–Schiff stains demonstrate the cytoplasmic inclusions but not the intranuclear changes. Sali-

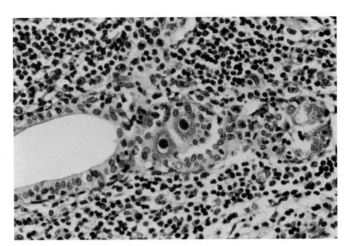

FIGURE 7–22. **Cytomegalovirus infection.** Salivary ductal epithelium exhibiting distinctive "owl eye" alterations.

vary ductal epithelium may also be affected and form "owl eye" cells (Fig. 7–22).

Electron microscopy can be used to differentiate CMV from the other herpes viruses. Paranuclear dense material is found in the round to oval cytoplasmic bodies that surround the individual particles of CMV. These complexes may fuse to form larger dense bodies.

Diagnosis

The diagnosis of CMV is made from a combination of the clinical features as well as from other examinations. Biopsy material can demonstrate cellular changes that suggest infection, and electron microscopic examination demonstrates the viral particles within the infected tissue. Because effective therapies exist for CMV infections in immunocompromised patients, biopsies are recommended for chronic ulcerations that are not responsive to conservative therapy. More specific verification can be made from viral cultures, detection of viral antigens by immunohistochemistry, in situ hybridization, polymerase chain reaction, or a demonstration of rising viral antibody titers.

Treatment and Prognosis

Although most CMV infections resolve spontaneously, therapy is often required in the immunosuppressed patient. Ganciclovir has resolved clinical symptoms in more than 75 percent of treated immunocompromised patients. However, the medication must be continued to prevent a relapse if the immune dysfunction persists. The development of resistance to ganciclovir has been reported, but successful resolution of these resistant infections has been achieved with foscarnet.

ENTEROVIRUSES

More than 30 **enteroviruses** exist that can result in symptomatic infections associated with rashes. Few are clinically distinctive enough to allow differentiation from one another. Most are asymptomatic or subclinical. These infections may arise at any age, but most occur in infants or young children. Neonatal cases have also been reported. Only **herpangina; hand-foot-and-mouth disease**; and **acute lymphonodular pharyngitis** deserve discussion.

Herpangina is usually produced by any 1 of 10 strains of coxsackievirus A and less commonly by coxsackievirus B or echoviruses. Hand-foot-and-mouth disease is usually caused by coxsackievirus A16 but may also arise from a number of other coxsackievirus A or B strains. Acute lymphonodular pharyngitis is less recognized, and coxsackievirus A10 has been found in the few reported cases. The incubation period for these viruses is 4 to 7 days. Most cases arise in the summer or early fall in nontropical areas, with crowding and poor hygiene aiding their spread. Infection confers immunity against reinfection to that one strain. In spite of the developed immunity, people may become infected numerous times with different enterovirus types over several years while still remaining susceptible to other different strains.

Clinical Features

Herpangina

Herpangina begins with an acute onset of significant sore throat, dysphagia, and fever, occasionally accompanied by vomiting, myalgia, and headache. Most cases, however, are mild or subclinical. A small number of oral lesions (usually two to six) develop in the posterior areas of the mouth, usually the soft palate or tonsillar pillars (Fig. 7–23). The affected areas begin as red macules, which form fragile vesicles that rapidly ulcerate. The ulcerations average 2 to 4 mm in diameter. The systemic symptoms resolve within a few days; as would be expected, the ulcerations usually take 7 to 10 days to heal.

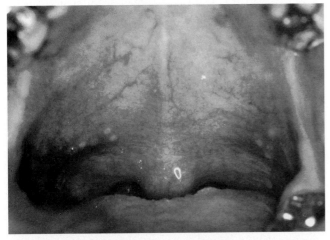

FIGURE 7–23. **Herpangina**. Numerous aphthous-like ulcerations of the soft palate. (From Allen CM, Camisa C. Diseases of the mouth and lips. *In:* Principles of Dermatology. Edited by Sams WM, Lynch P. New York, Churchill Livingstone, 1990, p 918.)

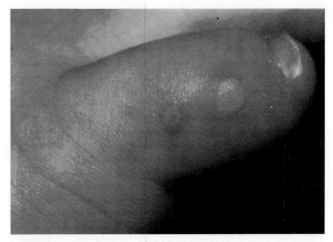

FIGURE 7–24. **Hand-foot-and-mouth disease**. Multiple vesicles of the skin of the toe. (Courtesy of Dr. Samuel J. Jasper.)

Hand-Foot-and-Mouth Disease

Hand-foot-and-mouth disease is the most well-known enterovirus infection. The name fairly well describes the location of the lesions. The oral lesions are almost always present; the presence of cutaneous lesions is more variable. The oral lesions arise without prodromal symptoms and precede the development of the cutaneous lesions. Sore throat and mild fever are present. The cutaneous lesions number from 1 to 100 and affect primarily the borders of the palms and soles and the ventral surfaces and sides of the fingers and toes (Fig. 7–24). Rarely, other sites, especially the buttocks, may be involved. The individual cutaneous lesions begin as erythematous macules that develop central vesicles and heal without crusting (Fig. 7–25).

The oral lesions resemble those of herpangina but may be more numerous and are not confined to the posterior areas of the mouth. The lesions may number from 1 to 30. The buccal mucosa, labial mucosa, and tongue are the most common sites to be affected, but any area of the oral mucosa may be involved (Fig. 7–26). The individual vesicular lesions rapidly ulcerate, are typically 2 to 7 mm in diameter, but may be larger than 1 cm. Most of these ulcerations resolve within 1 week.

Acute Lymphonodular Pharyngitis

Acute lymphonodular pharyngitis is characterized by sore throat, fever, and mild headache, which may last from 4 to 14 days. Low numbers (one to five) of yellow to dark pink nodules develop on the soft palate or tonsillar pillars (Fig. 7–27). The nodules represent hyperplastic lymphoid aggregates and resolve within 10 days without vesiculation or ulceration. Few cases have been described, and whether this represents a distinct clinical entity is as yet unresolved. The possibility that the sore throat and palatal lymphoid hyperplasia represent features of herpangina or some other infection cannot be excluded without further documentation of additional cases.

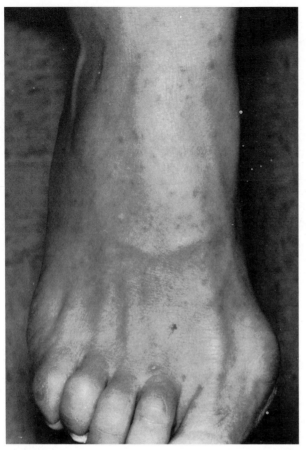

FIGURE 7–25. **Hand-foot-and-mouth disease**. Numerous erythematous macules of the foot.

Histopathologic Features

In patients with herpangina and hand-foot-and-mouth disease, the areas of affected epithelium exhibit intracellular and intercellular edema, which leads to extensive spongiosis and the formation of an intraepithelial vesicle.

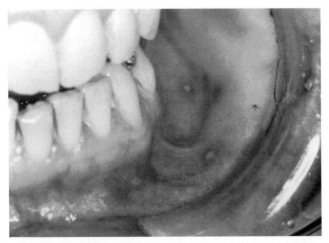

FIGURE 7–26. **Hand-foot-and-mouth disease**. Multiple aphthous-like ulcerations of the mucobuccal fold.

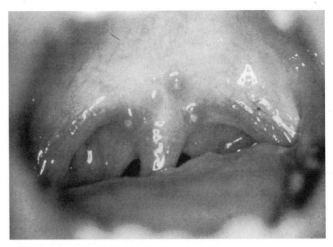

FIGURE 7–27. **Acute lymphonodular pharyngitis**. Numerous dark-pink and yellow lymphoid aggregates. (Courtesy of Dr. George Blozis.)

The vesicle enlarges and ruptures through the epithelial basal cell layer, with the resultant formation of a sub-epithelial vesicle. Epithelial necrosis and ulceration soon follow. Inclusion bodies and multinucleated epithelial cells are absent.

Diagnosis

The diagnoses of herpangina, hand-foot-and-mouth disease, and acute lymphonodular pharyngitis are usually made from the distinctive clinical manifestations. In patients with atypical presentations, laboratory confirmation appears prudent. Viral isolation from culture can be performed, and analysis of stool specimens is the best technique in patients with only mucosal lesions. Throat culture findings tend to be positive, predominantly during the early acute stage. The culture of cutaneous lesions is best for the diagnosis of hand-foot-and-mouth disease. A serologic demonstration of rising enteroviral antibody titers between the acute and convalescent stages can be used to confirm the diagnosis in questionable cases.

Treatment and Prognosis

Therapy for patients with an enterovirus infection is directed toward symptomatic relief. Non-aspirin antipyretics and topical anesthetics, such as dyclonine hydrochloride, are often beneficial.

RUBEOLA (Measles)

Rubeola is produced by a paramyxovirus and would have been included in this text mainly for historical purposes if it had not exhibited a dramatic resurgence in the late 1980s. Measles vaccine has been in wide use since 1963 and is 95 percent effective, resulting in a 98 percent reduction in the incidence of this infection. During 1989 and 1990, isolated outbreaks developed, predominantly in children younger than 5 years of age. The cases occurred primarily in blacks and Hispanics who resided in densely populated areas of several large metropolitan areas and who were not vaccinated. In addition, a smaller number occurred in the 5- to 19-year-old age group as a result of vaccine failure. The infection demonstrated an 800 percent increase in incidence during 1989 to 1990 in contrast to the rest of the 1980s.

Clinical Features

Most cases of measles arise in the spring and are spread through respiratory droplets. After an incubation period of 10 to 12 days, the infection begins with prodromal symptoms of fever, malaise, coryza (runny nose), conjunctivitis, and cough. The well-known exanthematous rash follows after a few days and lasts from 4 to 7 days. The face is involved first, with eventual downward spread to the trunk and extremities. Ultimately, a diffuse erythematous maculopapular eruption is formed (Fig. 7–28). The rash clears in a similar downward progression and is replaced by a brown pigmentary staining. The infected person is contagious from the day before the prodrome to 4 days after the rash develops.

In the most recent resurgence, 21 percent of infected patients had secondary complications, the most common of which were diarrhea, otitis media, pneumonia, and encephalitis. The mortality rate in the 1989 to 1990 infections was close to 3 per 1000 cases. Of the patients who died, 92 percent had not been previously vaccinated and only 12 percent had a serious underlying illness.

Measles in immunocompromised patients can be serious, with a high risk of complications and death. Most of these patients exhibit either an atypical rash or no exanthem. Pneumonitis is the primary complication. The fatality rate of measles in patients with a malignancy is greater than 50 percent; AIDS-associated measles results in death of more than one third of the affected patients.

The most distinctive oral manifestation of measles are lesions known as *Koplik's spots*, which develop early in the course of the infection. Multiple areas of mucosal erythema are visible on the buccal and labial mucosa,

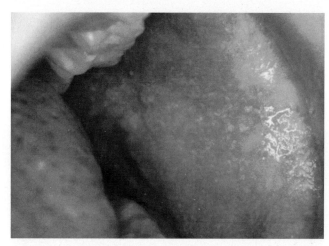

FIGURE 7–29. **Rubeola**. Numerous bluish-white Koplik spots of buccal mucosa. See Color Plates. (Courtesy of Dr. Robert J. Achterberg.)

and within these areas there are numerous small bluish-white macules (Fig. 7–29; see Color Figure 41). These pathognomonic spots represent foci of epithelial necrosis and have been described as "grains of salt" on a red background. The height of the mucosal eruption occurs just as the exanthem begins to develop and spread.

Koplik's spots are not the only oral manifestation that may be associated with measles. Candidiasis, acute necrotizing ulcerative mucositis, and necrotizing stomatitis may occur if significant malnutrition is also present. Severe measles in early childhood can affect odontogenesis and result in pitted enamel hypoplasia of the developing permanent teeth.

Diagnosis

The diagnosis of typical measles in an epidemic setting is usually straightforward and based on the clinical features and history. Laboratory confirmation can be of value in isolated or atypical cases. Viral isolation or rapid detection of viral antigens is possible, but confirmation is usually established through a demonstration of rising serologic antibody titers. The antibodies appear within 1 to 3 days after the beginning of the exanthem and peak in about 3 to 4 weeks.

Treatment and Prognosis

With a complication rate of 21 percent, the best treatment for measles is a good vaccination program; rubeola is part of the widely used measles-mumps-rubella (MMR) vaccine. Renewed emphasis in the noncompliant sections of society must be stressed. In addition, a new two-dose vaccination schedule has been adopted in an attempt to decrease the vaccine failures.

In otherwise healthy patients with measles, fluids and non-aspirin antipyretics are recommended for symptomatic relief. Immunocompromised patients also may be treated with one of a number of medications that have shown promise but that have not yet definitively proved to be efficacious. The most promising is ribavirin, but

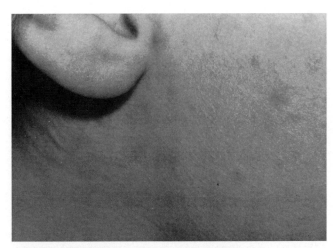

FIGURE 7–28. **Rubeola**. Erythematous maculopapular rash of the face. (Courtesy of Dr. Robert J. Achterberg.)

immunoglobulin, interferon, and vitamin A are also being used.

RUBELLA (German Measles)

Rubella is a mild viral illness that is produced by a togavirus. The greatest importance of this infection lies not in its effects on those who contract the acute illness but in its capacity to induce birth defects in the developing fetus. The virus is contracted through respiratory droplets and is transmitted to nearly 100 percent of individuals in close living conditions. The incubation time is from 14 to 21 days, and infected patients are contagious from 1 week before the exanthem to about 5 days after the development of the rash. Infants with a congenital infection may release virus for up to 1 year.

In the past, this infection occurred in cycles, with localized epidemics every 6 to 9 years and pandemics every 10 to 30 years. The last pandemic occurred from 1962 to 1964. In 1964 and 1965, the United States alone had more than 12.5 million cases, which resulted in more than 10,000 fetal deaths (direct effects or secondary to therapeutic abortions) and 20,000 infants born with **congenital rubella syndrome.**

First released in 1969, an effective vaccine is widely used and has dramatically affected the epidemiology of the infection and broken the cycle of occurrences. The inoculation is given at the age of 15 months as part of the MMR vaccine, with a booster given at ages 4 to 6. The vaccine is contraindicated in:

- Pregnant women
- Immunodeficient patients
- Patients with acute febrile illnesses
- Patients with a known allergy to components of the vaccine

It was postulated that the protection of children would also eliminate the risk of exposure to women in the childbearing years. A 99 percent decrease in the infection was seen between 1969 and 1988, but young adults remain susceptible. A low of 225 cases was reported to the Centers for Disease Control and Prevention (CDC) during 1988. Like rubeola, 1989 and 1990 demonstrated a slight resurgence of rubella, which was caused by a lack of vaccination diligence. More than 70 percent of the current cases occur in patients older than 15 years of age, and 10 to 25 percent of young adults remain susceptible. Of course, this should change when the previously vaccinated children grow into adults. For the present, the vaccination of postpubertal females must be stressed.

Clinical Features

A large percentage of infections are asymptomatic; the frequency of symptoms is greater in adolescents and adults. Prodromal symptoms may be seen 1 to 5 days before the exanthem and include fever, headache, malaise, anorexia, myalgia, mild conjunctivitis, coryza, pharyngitis, cough, and lymphadenopathy. The lymphadenopathy may persist for weeks and is noted primarily in the suboccipital, postauricular, and cervical chains. The most common complication is arthritis, which increases in frequency with age and usually arises subsequent to the rash. Rare complications include encephalitis and thrombocytopenia.

The exanthematous rash is often the first sign of the infection and begins on the face and neck, with spread to the entire body within 1 to 3 days. The rash forms discrete pink macules, then papules, and finally fades with flaky desquamation. The rash fades as it spreads and often exhibits facial clearing before the completion of its spread into the lower body areas.

Oral lesions, known as *Forchheimer's sign*, are present in about 20 percent of the cases. These consist of small, discrete, dark-red papules that develop on the soft palate and may extend onto the hard palate. This characteristic enanthem arises simultaneously with the rash, becoming evident in about 6 hours after the first symptoms and not lasting longer than 12 to 14 hours. Palatal petechiae may also occur.

The risk of congenital rubella syndrome correlates with the time of infection. The frequency of transmission from an infected mother is greater than 80 percent during the first 12 weeks of pregnancy, with the risk of fetal damage decreasing dramatically at 8 weeks and becoming rare after 20 weeks of gestation. The classic triad of congenital rubella syndrome consists of deafness, heart disease, and cataracts. Deafness is the most common manifestation, affecting more than 80 percent of the patients. This hearing loss may not become evident until 2 years of age and is usually bilateral. Less common, late-emerging complications include encephalopathy, mental retardation, diabetes mellitus, and thyroid disorders.

Diagnosis

The diagnosis of rubella is contingent on laboratory tests because the clinical presentation of the acquired infection is typically subclinical, mild, or nonspecific. Although viral culture is possible, serologic analysis is the mainstay of diagnosis.

Treatment and Prognosis

Rubella is mild, and therapy is not usually required. Non-aspirin antipyretics and antipruritic medications may be useful in patients with significant fever or symptomatic cutaneous involvement. Passive immunity may be provided by the administration of human rubella immunoglobulin. If immunoglobulin is given within a few days of exposure, it decreases the severity of the infection. This therapy is typically reserved for pregnant patients who decline abortion.

MUMPS (Epidemic Parotitis)

Mumps is a paramyxovirus infection that primarily affects the salivary glands. As with measles and rubella, the epidemiology has been dramatically affected by the MMR vaccine. Before the advent of widespread vaccination, epidemics were seen every 2 to 5 years. The vaccine directed against mumps was released in 1967, but its use was not nationally accepted until 1977. At that time, vaccination became the norm for children 12 to 15 months of age. The vaccine has a success rate of 75 to 95 percent. Most individuals born before 1957 are thought to have immunity from exposure to naturally occurring mumps virus. What has been created is a population born between 1967 and 1977 who have not been uniformly vaccinated but whose natural exposure to mumps virus in childhood has been dramatically decreased.

The incidence of mumps decreased by 98 percent and reached an all-time low in 1985. In 1986, a resurgence developed. In the past, most cases occurred in children aged 5 to 9 years; during the resurgence, the disease was more prevalent in 10- to 19-year-old patients. Outbreaks have been reported in high schools, on college campuses, and in the workplace. This increased incidence has been attributed to lack of vaccination, not vaccine failure. Immunization continues as part of the MMR vaccine, which is recommended for all 15-month-old children, with a booster at 4 to 6 years of age. In an attempt to decrease the incidence in the older age groups, it is recommended that individuals lacking a history of mumps or MMR vaccination be immunized. This primarily affects those born between 1967 and 1977 and, to a lesser extent, those born between 1957 and 1967.

The mumps virus can be transmitted through urine, saliva, or respiratory droplets. The incubation period is usually 16 to 18 days, with a range of 12 to 25 days. Patients are contagious from 1 day before the clinical appearance of infection to 14 days after its clinical resolution.

Clinical Features

Approximately 30 percent of mumps infections are subclinical. In symptomatic cases, prodromal symptoms of low-grade fever, headache, malaise, anorexia, and myalgia arrive first. These nonspecific findings are most frequently followed within a day by significant salivary gland changes. The parotid gland is involved most frequently, but the sublingual and submandibular glands can also be affected. Discomfort and swelling develop in the tissues surrounding the lower half of the external ear and extending down along the posterior inferior border of the adjacent mandible (Fig. 7–30). The enlargement typically peaks within 2 to 3 days, and the pain is most intense during this period of maximal enlargement. Chewing movements of the jaw or eating saliva-stimulating foods tends to increase the pain. Enlargement of the glands usually begins on one side and is followed by contralateral glandular changes within a few days. Unilateral involvement is seen in about 25 percent of patients.

The second most common finding is epididymoorchitis, which occurs in 14 to 35 percent of postpubertal males. Less commonly, oophoritis can be seen in females. In affected males, the testicle exhibits rapid swelling with significant pain and tenderness. The enlargement can range from a minimal swelling to a fourfold increase in size. Unilateral involvement is most common. On resolution of the swelling, atrophy occurs in

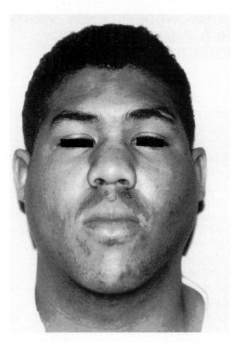

FIGURE 7–30. **Mumps**. Bilateral parotid enlargement. (From Neville BW, Damm DD, White DK, Waldron CA. Color Atlas of Clinical Oral Pathology. Philadelphia, Lea & Febiger, 1991.)

the affected testicle. Permanent sterility from testicular changes is rare.

Less commonly, meningoencephalitis, hearing loss, pancreatitis, arthritis, carditis, and decreased renal function may occur. Isolated changes such as orchitis or meningitis, may occur in the absence of salivary gland involvement, thereby making diagnosis difficult in nonepidemic settings.

The most frequently reported oral manifestation is redness and enlargement of Wharton's and Stensen's salivary gland duct openings. In addition, involvement of the sublingual gland may produce bilateral enlargements of the floor of the mouth.

Diagnosis

The diagnosis of mumps can be made easily from the clinical presentation when the infection is occurring in an epidemic fashion; however, isolated cases must be differentiated from other causes. Saliva, urine, or cerebrospinal fluid specimens can be obtained for culture. The most frequently used confirmatory measures are acute and convalescent mumps-specific antibody measurements.

Treatment and Prognosis

The treatment of mumps is palliative in nature. Nonaspirin analgesics and antipyretics are frequently administered. In an attempt to minimize orchitis, bed rest is recommended for males until the fever breaks. Avoidance of sour foods and drinks helps to decrease the salivary gland discomfort. As with measles and rubella, the best results come from prior vaccination, thereby preventing the infection.

HUMAN IMMUNODEFICIENCY VIRUS/ ACQUIRED IMMUNODEFICIENCY SYNDROME (HIV; AIDS)

During the last decade, more articles have been written on **human immunodeficiency virus** (HIV) and its related disease states than any other infectious process. A complete bibliography alone would easily be thicker than the entire infectious disease portion of this text. Entire texts dedicated to HIV infection and **acquired immunodeficiency syndrome** (AIDS) are available and should be consulted for more detailed information.

AIDS came into the limelight in 1981. By 1992, 8 million people worldwide were thought to have been infected by HIV, with more than 5 million progressing to AIDS. Estimations at that time suggested the United States had between 1 and 1.5 million inhabitants infected with HIV. Without a more effective therapy or vaccine, by the year 2000 it is estimated that more than 18 million people worldwide will be infected with HIV and 6 million will have developed AIDS. The infection is thought to be nearly 100 percent fatal, although the rate of progression is highly variable.

In infected individuals, the virus can be found in most bodily fluids. HIV has been recovered from serum, blood, saliva, semen, tears, urine, breast milk, ear secretions, and vaginal secretions. The most frequent routes of transmission are sexual contact, parenteral exposure to blood, or transmission from mother to fetus during the perinatal period. Infection has also been documented to be caused by artificial insemination, breast-feeding from infected mothers, and organ transplantation. Although heterosexual transmission is increasing, most of the adults infected in the United States have been homosexual or bisexual males, intravenous drug abusers, hemophiliac patients receiving factor VIII before 1985, recipients of blood products, or heterosexual contacts with one of the other high-risk groups.

Researchers have debated the infectiousness of oral fluids. HIV has been found to be present in oral fluids, but saliva appears to reduce the ability of HIV to infect its target cells, lymphocytes. Reports of transmission by oral fluids are rare, and it appears this is not a significant source for the transmission of AIDS. In spite of this, anecdotal reports have documented the transmission of AIDS during breast-feeding from the oral fluids of postpartum infected infants to their previously noninfected mothers. In addition, rare examples have been documented reporting the transmission of HIV infection by contamination of the oral fluids during cunnilingus or repeated passionate kissing. Although rare, these anecdotal reports point out that oral fluids can be infectious and are not totally protective against oral introduction of HIV. In summary, the best safety against infection is avoidance of all body fluids of infected patients.

The primary target cell of HIV is the CD4+ helper T lymphocyte. The DNA of HIV is incorporated into the DNA of the lymphocyte and is thus present for the life of the cell. In most viral infections, host antibodies are usually formed that are protective against the organism. In people with HIV infection, antibodies are developed but are not protective. The virus may remain silent, cause cell death, or produce fusion of the cells into syncytia, which may not function properly. A subsequent decrease in T-helper cell numbers occurs, with a resultant loss in immune function. The normal response to viruses, fungi, and encapsulated bacteria is diminished.

On introduction of the HIV, an indefinite percentage of those infected will have an acute self-limited viral syndrome. This is followed by an asymptomatic stage, which averages 8 to 10 years. The length of the asymptomatic period is variable and may be affected by the nature of the virus, the host immune reaction or external factors that may delay or accelerate the process. Almost inevitably, the final symptomatic stage develops.

A new clinical syndrome complex has been described called **idiopathic CD4+ T lymphocytopenia.** Those affected may resemble patients with AIDS, but there is no evidence of HIV infection. The cases are rare and probably represent various disorders that all share the common finding of a low CD4+ T-lymphocyte count. The absence of immunodeficiency in the contacts of affected patients and the absence of significant clustering of the cases provide no evidence of a new infectious agent or environmental cause of the disease.

Clinical Features

HIV infection may be asymptomatic initially, or an acute response may be seen. The acute viral syndrome that occurs typically develops within 1 to 6 weeks after exposure. The symptoms bear some resemblance to those of infectious mononucleosis (e.g., generalized lymphadenopathy, sore throat, fever, a maculopapular rash, headache, myalgia, arthralgia, diarrhea, photophobia, peripheral neuropathies). Oral changes may include mucosal erythema and focal ulcerations.

The acute viral syndrome clears within a few weeks; during this period, HIV infection is usually not considered or investigated. A variable asymptomatic period follows. Some patients have persistent generalized lymphadenopathy, which may later resolve. In some patients before overt AIDS develops, a period of chronic fever, weight loss, diarrhea, oral candidiasis, herpes zoster, and/or hairy leukoplakia (HL) develops. This has been termed **AIDS-related complex** (ARC).

The presentation of symptomatic overt AIDS is highly variable and is often affected by a person's prior exposure to a number of chronic infections. The signs and symptoms described under ARC are often present along with an increasing number of opportunistic infections or neoplastic processes. In 50 percent of the cases, pneumonia caused by the protozoan, *Pneumocystis carinii*, is the presenting feature leading to the diagnosis. Other infections of diagnostic significance include disseminated cytomegalovirus (CMV) infection, severe herpes simplex virus (HSV) infection, atypical mycobacterial infection, cryptococcal meningitis, and central nervous system (CNS) toxoplasmosis. Persistent diarrhea is commonplace and may be bacterial or protozoal in origin. Clinically significant neurologic dysfunction is present in 30 to 50 percent of patients, and the most common manifestation is a progressive encephalopathy known as **AIDS-dementia complex.**

Certain neoplastic processes are also associated with AIDS. Clinical descriptions of these cancers are presented in the portion of this text dealing with the oral manifestations of HIV infection. A vascular malignancy, **Kaposi's sarcoma** (KS), which is otherwise rare in the United States, has been reported in about 15 to 20 percent of patients with AIDS. This cancer may be secondary to a sexually transmitted agent other than HIV. AIDS-associated KS occurs primarily in homosexuals, and KS has been reported in homosexuals without HIV infection. The prevalence of KS in HIV-infected patients has been decreasing, and this may be due to the use of condoms, which may be decreasing the unknown second agent. This should remind clinicians that homosexuals with KS should not be labeled "HIV-infected" until there is serologic proof.

Non-Hodgkin's lymphoma is the second most common malignancy. It frequently presents in non-nodal sites, especially the CNS. Other cancers, including squamous cell carcinoma, have been implicated, but the association is not as strong.

A list of oral manifestations of AIDS is presented in Table 7–1. The discussion here concentrates primarily on the clinical presentations. (For detailed information on the histopathology, diagnosis, and treatment of each condition, see the text covering the individual disease.) When the infections are treated differently in HIV-infected patients, these variations are presented here. The most common manifestations are presented first, followed by a selection of the less frequently encountered disorders.

Common Oral and Maxillofacial Manifestations of HIV Infection

Persistent Generalized Lymphadenopathy. After seroconversion, HIV disease often remains silent except for persistent generalized lymphadenopathy (PGL). The prevalence of this early clinical sign varies but, in several studies, approaches 70 percent. PGL consists of lymphadenopathy that has been present for longer than 3 months and involves two or more extrainguinal sites.

Table 7–1. ORAL MANIFESTATIONS OF ACQUIRED IMMUNODEFICIENCY SYNDROME

	More Common	Less Common
Infections		
Fungal	Candidiasis	Aspergillosis
		Histoplasmosis
		Cryptococcosis
		Geotrichosis
Bacterial	HIV-related gingivitis	*Mycobacterium avium-intracellulare*
	HIV-associated periodontitis	*Klebsiella pneumoniae*
	Acute necrotizing ulcerative gingivitis (ANUG)	*Enterobacter cloacae*
		Escherichia coli
		Salmonella enteritidis
		Cat-scratch disease
		Sinusitis
		Exacerbation of periapical inflammatory disease
		Submandibular cellulitis
Viral	Herpes simplex virus (HSV)	Human papillomavirus (HPV)
	Varicella-zoster virus (VZV)	Cytomegalovirus (CMV)
	Epstein-Barr virus (EBV)	
Neoplasms	Kaposi's sarcoma	Non-Hodgkin's lymphoma
		Squamous cell carcinoma
Lymphadenopathy	Cervical	
Neurologic		Trigeminal neuropathy
		Facial palsy
Miscellaneous		Aphthous ulcerations
		Necrotizing stomatitis
		Toxic epidermolysis
		Delayed wound healing
		Thrombocytopenia
		Xerostomia or sicca-like syndrome
		HIV-related embryopathy
		Hyperpigmentation
		Granuloma annulare
		Exfoliative cheilitis
		Lichenoid reactions

Modified from Scully C, et al. Oral manifestations of HIV infection and their management: I. More common lesions. Oral Surg Oral Med Oral Pathol 71:158–166, 1991.
HIV, human immunodeficiency virus.

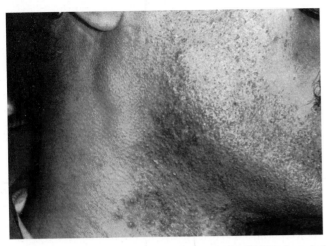

FIGURE 7–31. **HIV-associated lymphadenopathy.** Enlarged cervical lymph nodes in a patient with persistent generalized lymphadenopathy.

Although any site may be involved, the head and neck area is the initial location in most patients. Nodal enlargement fluctuates, is usually larger than 1 cm, and varies from 0.5 to 5 cm (Fig. 7–31). Almost all patients have axillary involvement, and this is closely followed by posterior cervical enlargement. The submandibular and submental chains are affected in more than one third of the cases.

Because lymphoma is known to occur in this population, a lymph node biopsy may be indicated for localized or bulky adenopathy, when cytopenia or an elevated erythrocyte sedimentation rate is present, or when requested for patient reassurance. Histopathologic examination reveals florid follicular hyperplasia. Although not as predictive as oral candidiasis or hairy leukoplakia, PGL does warn of progression to AIDS, and almost one-third of affected patients have diagnostic features of AIDS within 5 years.

Candidiasis. Oral candidiasis is the most common intraoral manifestation of HIV infection and is often the presenting sign that leads to the initial diagnosis (Fig. 7–32). Its presence in a patient infected with HIV is not diagnostic of AIDS but appears to be predictive for the subsequent development of full-blown AIDS within 2 years. Prevalence studies vary widely, but most patients with AIDS exhibit candidal involvement in 45 to 90 percent of the cases. Four clinical patterns are seen:

- Pseudomembranous
- Erythematous
- Hyperplastic
- Angular cheilitis

The first two variants constitute most of the cases (see p. 163). Although infrequently seen in immunocompetent patients, chronic multifocal oral involvement is common in patients who are infected with HIV.

Biopsy specimens of involved mucosa demonstrate the candidal organisms embedded in the superficial keratin, but the typical inflammatory reaction is often deficient (Fig. 7–33). The response to therapy also is altered. The antifungal medications (e.g., nystatin, clotrimazole, amphotericin B) produce transient responses with rapid recurrence. Much better control has been obtained with the systemic medications, such as ketoconazole, fluconazole, and itraconazole.

HIV-Associated Periodontal Disease. HIV-associated periodontal disease is not rare or unexpected. Four patterns are seen:

- Gingivitis
- Periodontitis
- Necrotizing stomatitis of periodontal origin
- Acute necrotizing ulcerative gingivitis

HIV-related gingivitis (linear gingival erythema) presents with a distinctive linear band of erythema involving the free gingival margin and extending 2 to 3 mm apically (Fig. 7–34; see Color Figure 42). Although not responsive to improved plaque control, this unique pattern of gingivitis has been associated with the presence of *Candida.* Systemic fluconazole appears highly effective

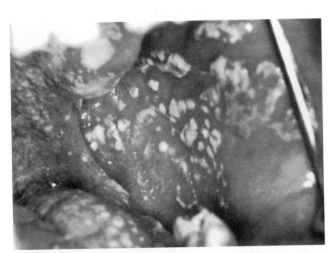

FIGURE 7–32. **HIV-associated candidiasis.** Extensive removable white plaques of the left buccal mucosa.

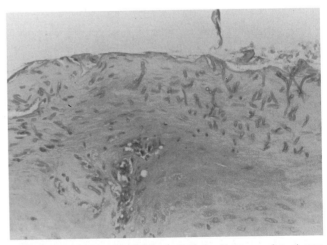

FIGURE 7–33. **HIV-associated candidiasis.** Numerous fungal organisms embedded in superficial keratin.

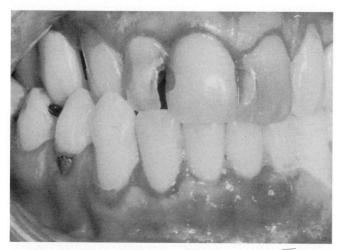

FIGURE 7-34. **HIV-associated gingivitis.** Band of erythema involving the free gingival margin. See Color Plates.

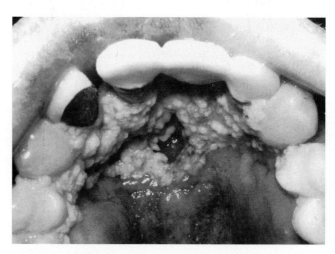

FIGURE 7-36. **HIV-associated necrotizing stomatitis.** Massive necrosis of soft tissue and bone of the anterior maxilla.

in resolving the changes. In addition, the alveolar mucosa and gingiva demonstrate punctate or diffuse erythema in more than 75 percent of cases.

Many patients also have **HIV-associated periodontitis (necrotizing periodontitis).** As periodontitis emerges, severe deep pain, gingival hemorrhage, soft tissue necrosis, and rapid loss of periodontal support occur. Most patients seek care because of significant discomfort. Deep pocketing is not typical because gingival necrosis reduces the height of the soft tissue as the bone is lost (Fig. 7-35). More than 90 percent of the tooth support may be lost in a few weeks. The defects are usually localized and not in the diffuse pattern of routine periodontitis. HIV-associated periodontitis does not respond to conventional periodontal therapy.

HIV periodontitis may be complicated by massively destructive necrotizing lesions known as **HIV-associated necrotizing stomatitis.** Extensive bone sequestration and soft tissue loss can occur (Fig. 7-36).

Acute necrotizing ulcerative gingivitis (ANUG) (see p. 124) is relatively frequent but presents in a different distribution and appears to be microbiologically different from HIV-associated periodontitis and necrotizing stomatitis. Patients with ANUG present with interproximal gingival necrosis, bleeding, pain, and halitosis (Fig. 7-37).

The treatment of HIV-associated periodontal disease revolves around debridement, antimicrobial therapy, immediate follow-up care, and long-term maintenance. The initial removal of necrotic tissue is necessary, combined with povidone-iodine irrigation. The use of systemic antibiotics is usually not necessary, but metronidazole has been administered to patients with extensive involvement that is associated with severe acute pain. All patients should use chlorhexidine mouth rinses initially and for long-term maintenance. After initial debridement, follow-up removal of additional diseased tissue should be performed within 24 hours and again every 7 to 10 days for two to three appointments, depending on the patient's response. At this point, monthly recalls are necessary until the process stabilizes; evaluations are then performed every 3 months.

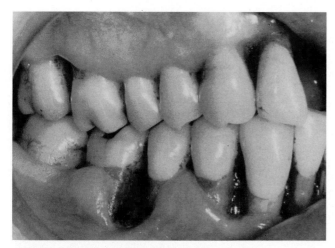

FIGURE 7-35. **HIV-associated periodontitis.** Extensive loss of periodontal support without deep pocketing.

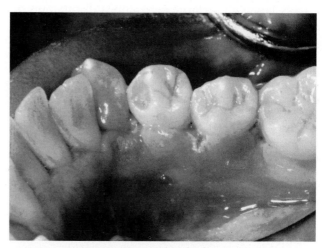

FIGURE 7-37. **HIV-associated necrotizing ulcerative gingivitis.** Necrotic interdental papillae of the lingual mandibular gingiva.

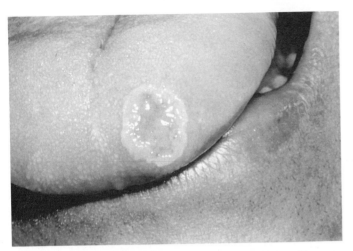

FIGURE 7–38. **HIV-associated recurrent herpetic infection**. Mucosal erosion of the anterior dorsal surface of the tongue on the left side. Note the yellowish circinate border. See Color Plates.

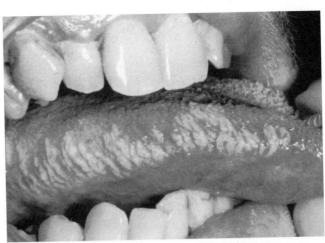

FIGURE 7–39. **HIV-associated oral hairy leukoplakia**. Vertical streaks of keratin along the lateral border of the tongue. See Color Plates.

Herpes Simplex Virus (HSV). Recurrent HSV infections occur in about the same percentage of HIV-infected patients as they do in the immunocompetent population (10 to 15 percent); however, the lesions are more widespread, occur in an atypical pattern, and may persist for months (Fig. 7–38; see Color Figure 43). Herpes labialis may extend to the facial skin and may exhibit extensive lateral spread. Persistence of active sites of HSV infection for more than 1 month in a patient infected with HIV is one accepted definition of AIDS. The clinical presentations of recurrences in immunocompromised patients and appropriate therapy and maintenance have been discussed in the text on herpesvirus (see p. 185).

Varicella-Zoster Virus (VZV). Recurrent VZV infection (herpes zoster) is fairly common in HIV-infected patients, and the course is more severe, with increased morbidity and mortality rates. Many of these patients are younger than age 40, in contrast to cases in immunocompetent patients which usually arise later in life. In the early stages of HIV-related immunosuppression, herpes zoster usually is confined to a dermatome but persists longer than usual. In full-blown AIDS, herpes zoster usually begins in a classic dermatomal distribution but subsequent cutaneous dissemination is not unusual.

Epstein-Barr Virus (EBV). EBV is thought to cause the lesion known as **hairy leukoplakia** (HL). This lesion presents a somewhat distinctive, but not diagnostic, pattern of hyperkeratosis and epithelial hyperplasia that is characterized by white mucosal lesions that do not rub off.

Most cases of HL occur on the lateral border of the tongue and range in appearance from faint white vertical streaks to thickened and furrowed areas of leukoplakia, exhibiting a shaggy keratotic surface (Fig. 7–39; see Color Figure 44). The lesions may become extensive and cover the entire dorsal and lateral surfaces of the tongue. Occasionally, the involvement of other mucosal sites occurs.

Histopathologically, HL exhibits thickened parakeratin, which demonstrates surface corrugations or thin projections (Fig. 7–40). The epithelium is hyperplastic and contains a patchy band of lightly stained "balloon cells" in the upper spinous layer (Fig. 7–41). Dysplasia is not noted. Heavy candidal infestation of the parakeratin layer is typical, and the normal inflammatory reaction to the fungus usually is absent. This pattern of epithelial alteration is not specific, however, and documentation of EBV within the lesion is a diagnostic requirement.

Treatment of HL is usually not needed, although slight discomfort or esthetic concerns may necessitate therapy. Acyclovir or desciclovir produces rapid resolution, but recurrence is expected with a discontinuation of therapy. Topical treatment with podophyllum resin has resulted in temporary remissions for as long as 28 weeks.

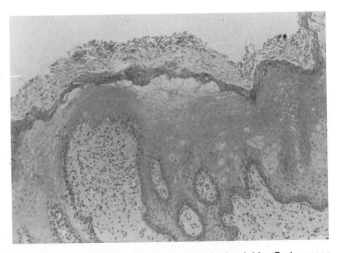

FIGURE 7–40. **HIV-associated oral hairy leukoplakia**. Oral mucosa exhibiting hyperparakeratosis with surface corrugations.

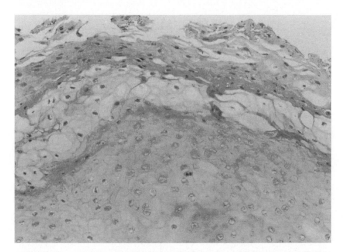

FIGURE 7–41. **HIV-associated oral hairy leukoplakia**. Oral epithelium exhibiting hyperparakeratosis and layer of "balloon cells" in the upper spinous layer.

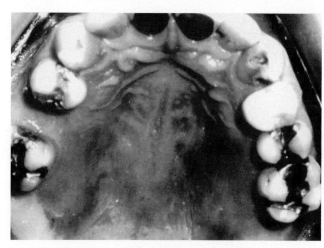

FIGURE 7–43. **HIV-associated Kaposi's sarcoma**. Large zones of Kaposi's sarcoma presenting as a flat, brownish discoloration of the hard palate.

Although rare instances of HL have been reported in immunocompetent individuals, most cases arise in immunocompromised persons. HL also has been reported in heart, kidney, liver, and bone marrow transplant recipients, but its presence in the absence of a known cause of immunosuppression strongly suggests HIV infection. HL documentation in HIV-infected patients is a strong harbinger of the development of AIDS within 2 years.

Kaposi's Sarcoma (KS). KS is a multifocal neoplasm of vascular endothelial cell origin. Before AIDS, KS was rare in North America and was classically found in patients over the age of 60 (see p. 404). Since the beginning of the HIV epidemic, however, most cases have been seen in association with AIDS.

KS begins with single or, more frequently, multiple lesions of the skin or oral mucosa. The trunk, arms, head, and neck are the most commonly involved anatomic sites (Fig. 7–42; see Color Figure 45). Oral lesions

are seen in 50 percent of affected patients, with the hard palate and gingiva involved most frequently (Figs. 7–43 and 7–44). The lesions begin as flat, brown or reddish-purple zones of discoloration that do not blanch with pressure. With time, the involved areas may develop into plaques or nodules (Fig. 7–45; see Color Figure 46). Pain and bleeding may become a problem and necessitate therapy.

A biopsy is required to make the definitive diagnosis, although a presumptive diagnosis is sometimes made from the clinical presentation and history. It must be remembered that similar clinical lesions can occur in HIV-infected patients who exhibit bacillary angiomatosis, the multifocal vascular proliferation associated with the cat-scratch bacillus (see pp. 157 and 158).

Microscopically, the tumor often presents in the superficial connective tissue, and this location allows discoloration to occur while the tumor's size is limited (Fig.

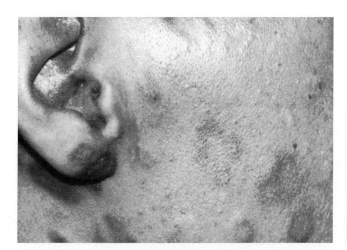

FIGURE 7–42. **HIV-associated Kaposi's sarcoma**. Multiple purple macules on the right side of the face. See Color Plates.

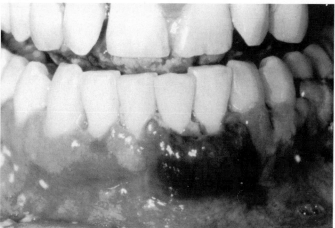

FIGURE 7–44. **HIV-associated Kaposi's sarcoma**. Raised, dark-red enlargement of the mandibular anterior facial gingiva on the left side.

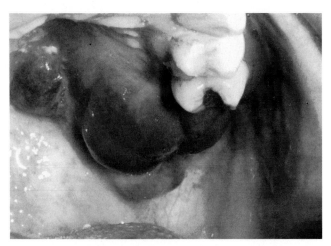

FIGURE 7–45. **HIV-associated Kaposi's sarcoma**. Diffuse, reddish-blue nodular enlargement of the left hard palate. See Color Plates.

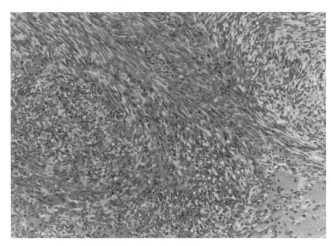

FIGURE 7–47. **HIV-associated Kaposi's sarcoma**. Interweaving bundles of spindle cells associated with numerous small vascular slits.

7–46). The malignancy forms interweaving bundles of spindle-shaped cells, which are associated with numerous vascular slits and large areas of red blood cell extravasation (Fig. 7–47). Numerous atypical vascular channels (often lined by plump endothelial cells) are noted. Scattered collections of eosinophilic globules are present, intermixed with the cellular tumor. An overlying chronic inflammatory cellular infiltrate typically is seen.

KS is a progressive malignancy that may disseminate widely to lymph nodes and various organ systems. Treatment objectives are usually palliative. Extensive systemic therapy often further depresses the immune system, thereby increasing the susceptibility of the patient to infection and other cancers. KS responds to radiation or single-agent systemic chemotherapy, such as vinblastine, vincristine, or etoposide. Oral lesions frequently are a cause of major morbidity, as a result of pain, bleeding, and functional interferences. Intralesional injection of oral lesions with vinblastine is effective and may be repeated if required. Intralesional injection of a sclerosing agent, sodium tetradecyl sulfate, has been effective for problematic intraoral lesions less than 2.5 cm in diameter.

Less Common Oral and Maxillofacial Manifestations of HIV Infection

Aphthous Ulcerations. Lesions that are clinically similar to aphthous ulcerations occur with increased frequency in patients infected with HIV. Although these lesions have not been definitively accepted as aphthous ulcerations, they are considered to be such until proven otherwise. All three forms (minor, major, and herpetiform) are seen; surprisingly, however, almost two thirds of the patients have the usually uncommon herpetiform and major variants (Fig. 7–48). As immunosuppression becomes more profound, major aphthous ulcerations demonstrate an increased prevalence. In most cases, all three lesions respond well to potent topical corticosteroids. Secondary candidiasis may be a complication of therapy. Biopsy should be considered if the lesion is

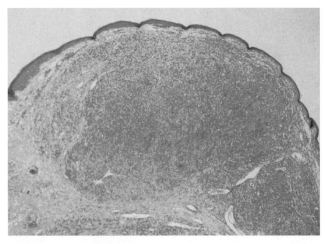

FIGURE 7–46. **HIV-associated Kaposi's sarcoma**. Cellular spindle cell neoplasm present immediately below the atrophic surface epithelium.

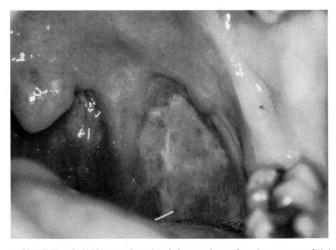

FIGURE 7–48. **HIV-associated aphthous ulceration**. Large superficial ulceration of the posterior soft palate.

clinically atypical or does not respond to therapy. (For further information on aphthous ulcerations and the pathogenesis of these lesions in patients infected with HIV, see p. 236.)

Human Papillomavirus (HPV). HPV is responsible for several facial and oral lesions in immunocompetent patients, the most frequent of which is the **verruca vulgaris (common wart)** (see p. 262). HPV-related lesions are not uncommon in HIV-infected patients, and most are located in the anogenital areas. Oral involvement also may be seen. In addition to the usual types of HPV, oral lesions in HIV-infected individuals are also frequently caused by HPV-7, a strain that is usually associated with **butcher's warts** and is most uncommon in the mouth. The oral lesions are usually multiple and may be located on any mucosal surface. The labial mucosa, tongue, buccal mucosa, and gingiva are frequent sites. The lesions may present as papules or papillary areas, which are sessile or pedunculated (Fig. 7–49).

Histopathologically, the lesions may be sessile or papillary and covered by acanthotic or even hyperplastic stratified squamous epithelium (Fig. 7–50). The affected epithelium often demonstrates vacuolization of numerous epithelial cells (koilocytosis) and may occasionally exhibit mild variation in nuclear size (Fig. 7–51).

Histoplasmosis. Histoplasmosis, the most common endemic respiratory fungal infection in the United States, is produced by *Histoplasma capsulatum* (see p. 169). In healthy patients, the infection typically is subclinical and self-limiting, but clinically evident infections do occur in immunocompromised individuals. Disseminated disease develops in approximately 5 percent of AIDS patients residing in areas where the fungus is endemic.

The signs and symptoms associated with dissemination are nonspecific and include fever, weight loss, splenomegaly, and pulmonary infiltrates. Oral lesions are not uncommon and are usually due to blood-borne organisms. On occasion, the initial diagnosis is made from the oral changes. Although intrabony infection in the jaws has been reported, the most common oral lesion is a

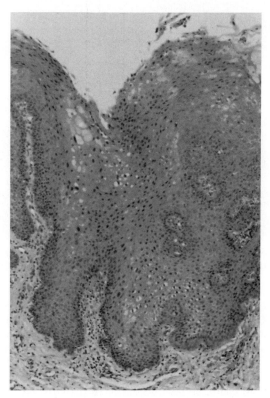

FIGURE 7–50. **HIV-associated human papillomavirus infection**. Oral mucosa exhibiting acanthosis and mild nuclear pleomorphism.

chronic, indurated mucosal ulceration with a raised border (Fig. 7–52). The oral lesions may be singular or multiple, and any area of the oral mucosa may be involved.

Microscopically, the small fungal organisms are visible within the cytoplasm of histiocytes and multinucleated giant cells. These phagocytic cells may be present in sheets or in organized granulomas (Fig. 7–53). Disseminated histoplasmosis is treated with amphotericin B, and ketoconazole is used as the first alternative therapy.

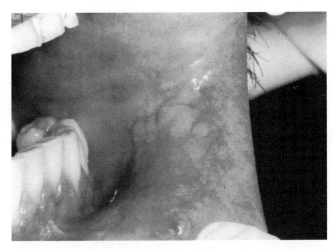

FIGURE 7–49. **HIV-associated human papillomavirus infection**. Multiple elevated and sessile papules of labial mucosa.

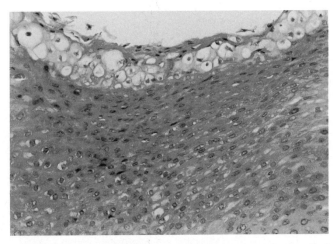

FIGURE 7–51. **HIV-associated human papillomavirus infection**. Oral mucosa exhibiting extensive koilocytosis in the superficial spinous cell layer.

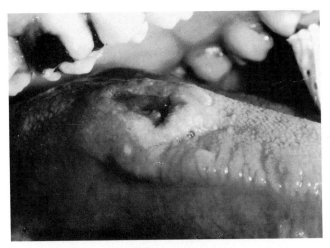

FIGURE 7-52. **HIV-associated histoplasmosis.** Indurated ulceration with a rolled border on the dorsal surface of the tongue on the right side.

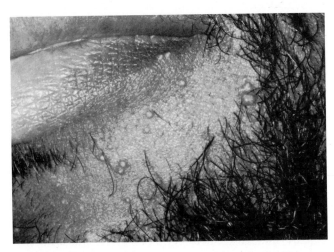

FIGURE 7-54. **HIV-associated molluscum contagiosum.** Numerous perioral papules.

Molluscum Contagiosum. Molluscum contagiosum is an infection of the skin caused by a poxvirus (see p. 266). The lesions present as small, waxy, dome-shaped papules that often demonstrate a central depressed crater. In immunocompetent individuals, the lesions typically demonstrate spontaneous resolution. In patients with AIDS, hundreds of lesions may be present and exhibit little tendency to undergo spontaneous resolution. The facial skin is commonly involved (Fig. 7-54).

Histopathologically, the surface epithelium forms numerous hyperplastic downgrowths. This involuting epithelium contains numerous large, intracytoplasmic inclusions known as *molluscum bodies* (Fig. 7-55). In the center of the lesion, the keratin layer often disintegrates and releases the adjacent molluscum bodies, hence the central crater.

Thrombocytopenia. Thrombocytopenia has been reported in nearly 10 percent of patients with HIV infection and may occur at any time during the course of the disease. Some reports show that megakaryocytes have

CD4 molecules and may be an additional target for the HIV virus. Cutaneous lesions are present in most cases, but oral lesions do occur, presenting as petechiae, ecchymosis, or spontaneous gingival hemorrhage.

HIV-Associated Salivary Gland Disease. HIV-associated salivary gland disease also can arise anytime during infection. In children, it is a common phenomenon; the prevalence is low in adults. The main clinical sign is one of salivary gland enlargement, particularly affecting the parotid. Bilateral involvement is seen in about 60

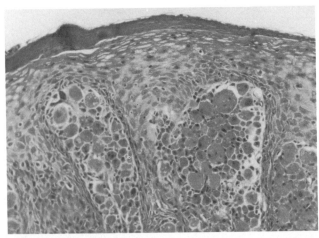

FIGURE 7-53. **HIV-associated histoplasmosis.** Mucosal biopsy in which the connective tissue is filled with numerous enlarged histiocytes. Numerous small, clear-appearing fungal organisms are located within the cytoplasm of the histiocytes.

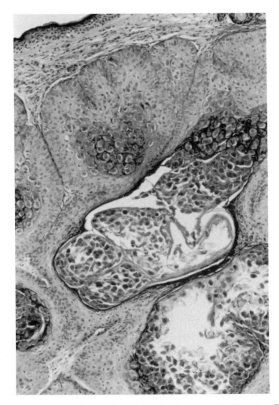

FIGURE 7-55. **HIV-associated molluscum contagiosum.** Downgrowth of surface epithelium exhibiting numerous "molluscum bodies."

percent of the patients with glandular changes. The swellings may fluctuate or progress in size, but most are chronic and stable. Cysts may develop, resulting in objectionable enlargements that need to be removed. Xerostomia is variable and is treated in a similar manner to that of cases associated with non-HIV disease (i.e., maintenance of good oral health and the use of sialogogues and saliva substitutes).

Hyperpigmentation. Hyperpigmentation of the skin, nails, and mucosa has been reported in HIV-infected patients. The changes are microscopically similar to focal melanosis, with increased melanin pigmentation observed in the basal cell layer of the affected epithelium. Several medications taken by AIDS patients (ketoconazole, clofazimine, pyrimethamine, zidovudine) may cause the increased melanin pigmentation. Adrenocortical destruction has been reported from several of the infections associated with AIDS, resulting in an addisonian pattern of pigmentation. Finally, pigmentation with no apparent cause has arisen in HIV-infected patients, and some investigators have theorized that this may be a direct result of the HIV infection.

Lymphoma. Lymphoma is the second most common malignancy in HIV-infected individuals, occurring primarily in intravenous drug abusers. Most are non-Hodgkin's B-cell lymphomas, but reports of T-cell and Hodgkin's lymphomas exist. A relationship between EBV and non-Hodgkin's lymphomas has been documented, and many investigators believe that these tumors arise from a combination of EBV, antigenic stimulation, and immunodysfunction. Lymphoma in patients with AIDS typically presents in non-nodal locations, with the CNS being the most common site. Oral lesions may occur and most often present as a soft tissue enlargement of the palate or gingiva (Fig. 7–56).

The treatment is usually combination chemotherapy, and radiation is reserved for local control of the disease. These malignancies are aggressive, and survival is usually measured in months from the date of discovery.

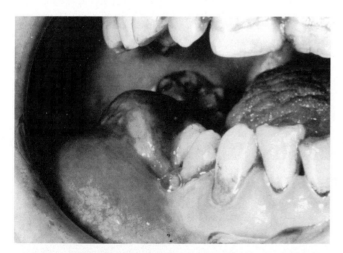

FIGURE 7–56. **HIV-associated lymphoma.** Erythematous and ulcerated soft tissue enlargement of the posterior mandibular gingiva and mucobuccal fold on the right side.

Oral Squamous Cell Carcinoma. Oral squamous cell carcinoma occasionally has been reported in patients with AIDS. A correlation between this malignancy and HIV infection has been suggested because the few cases of oral squamous cell carcinoma have arisen in a much younger age group and often are not associated with the typical risk factors.

Diagnosis

Confirmation of HIV infection can be made by viral culture or by detection of HIV antibodies or antigens. The most frequently used method is the enzyme-linked immunosorbent assay (ELISA) for HIV-related antibodies. This test can have false-positive results or cross-reactions; therefore, it should be repeated and followed by the more accurate Western blot antibody assay.

Two methods of viral antigen detection—the *sandwich assay* and the *competition assay*—can be used to discover HIV infection before antibody development. In these assays, anti-HIV antibodies are exposed to the test specimen and the viral antigen will attach to the antibodies. A third method, the *polymerase chain reaction* (PCR), has also been developed. This method is a molecular biologic technique that can detect small fragments of HIV DNA that may be integrated into the host DNA. Thus, this method may be used to identify HIV carriers who otherwise have negative antigen or antibody findings.

The diagnosis of AIDS is indicated if the patient has laboratory evidence of HIV infection combined with documentation of less than 200 CD4+ T lymphocytes per microliter or a CD4+ T-lymphocyte percentage of total lymphocytes of less than 14. In addition, the diagnosis of AIDS can be made in an HIV-infected person if one of the indicator diseases listed in Table 7–2 has been documented.

Treatment and Prognosis

Even though the progression of HIV infection is variable, the disease is considered fatal. In a study of a San Francisco cohort, the average time from seroconversion to full-blown AIDS was 10.1 years, and the subsequent average survival time from the date of the AIDS diagnosis was 1.4 years. In spite of this, rare HIV-infected patients have been observed for more than 10 years and have demonstrated no signs of immune deficits, which suggests a small percentage of patients may not progress to AIDS. Although no cure exists, survival times are increasing as a result of earlier diagnosis, improved therapy of infections and malignancies, and therapy with zidovudine (AZT). Many other anti-HIV agents are being investigated and may be beneficial. Work is also proceeding toward the development of a safe and effective vaccine against the HIV infection, but complex issues slow the progress. Advances in the therapy and prevention of HIV infection occur daily; however, the best defense against the disease is prevention of the initial infection.

Table 7-2. INDICATOR DISEASES USED IN THE DIAGNOSIS OF ACQUIRED IMMUNODEFICIENCY SYNDROME (AIDS)

1. Candidiasis of bronchi, trachea, or lungs
2. Candidiasis, esophageal
3. Cervical cancer, invasive
4. Coccidioidomycosis, disseminated or extrapulmonary
5. Cryptococcosis, extrapulmonary
6. Cryptosporidiosis, chronic intestinal (>1 month's duration)
7. Cytomegalovirus disease (other than liver, spleen, or nodes)
8. Cytomegalovirus-induced retinitis (with loss of vision)
9. Encephalopathy, HIV-related
10. Herpes simplex: chronic ulcer(s) (>1 month's duration) or bronchitis, pneumonitis, or esophagitis
11. Histoplasmosis, disseminated or extrapulmonary
12. Isosporiasis, chronic intestinal (>1 month's duration)
13. Kaposi's sarcoma
14. Lymphoma, Burkitt's (or equivalent term)
15. Lymphoma, immunoblastic (or equivalent term)
16. Lymphoma, primary, of brain
17. *Mycobacterium avium* complex or *M. kansasii*, disseminated or extrapulmonary
18. *Mycobacterium tuberculosis*, any site (pulmonary or extrapulmonary)
19. *Mycobacterium*, other species or unidentified species, disseminated or extrapulmonary
20. *Pneumocystis carinii* pneumonia
21. Pneumonia, recurrent
22. Progressive multifocal leukoencephalopathy
23. *Salmonella* septicemia, recurrent
24. Toxoplasmosis of brain
25. Wasting syndrome due to AIDS

REFERENCES

General References

Bialecki C, Feder HM, Grant-Kels JM. The six classic childhood exanthems: A review and update. J Am Acad Dermatol 21:891–903, 1989.

Boodley CA, Jaquis JL. Measles, mumps, rubella and chickenpox in the adult population. Nurse Pract 14:12–22, 1989.

Gorbach SL, Bartlett JG, Blacklow NR. Infectious Diseases, 8th ed. Philadelphia, WB Saunders, 1992.

Krugman S et al. Infectious Diseases of Children, 8th ed. St. Louis, CV Mosby, 1985.

Nahmias AJ, Dowdle WR, Schinazi RF. The Human Herpesviruses: An Interdisciplinary Perspective. New York, Elsevier, 1981.

Schuster GS. Oral Microbiology and Infectious Disease. Philadelphia, BC Decker, 1990.

Herpes Simplex Virus

Axéll T, Liedholm R. Occurrence of recurrent herpes labialis in an adult Swedish population. Acta Odontol Scand 48:119–123, 1990.

Barrett AP. Chronic indolent orofacial herpes simplex virus infection in chronic leukemia: A report of three cases. Oral Surg Oral Med Oral Pathol 66:387–390, 1988.

Cohen SG, Greenberg MS. Chronic oral herpes simplex virus infection in immunocompromised patients. Oral Surg Oral Med Oral Pathol 59:465–471, 1985.

Epstein JB, et al. Clinical study of herpes simplex virus infection in leukemia. Oral Surg Oral Med Oral Pathol 70:38–43, 1990.

Gibson JR, et al. Prophylaxis against herpes labialis with acyclovir cream—a placebo-controlled study. Dermatology 172:104–107, 1986.

Hess GP, Walson PD. Seizures secondary to oral viscous lidocaine. Ann Emerg Med 17:725–727, 1988.

Juretić M. Natural history of herpetic infection. Helv Pediatr Acta 21:356–368, 1966.

Kinghorn GR. Long-term suppression with oral acyclovir of recurrent herpes simplex virus infections in otherwise healthy patients. Am J Med 85(Suppl 2A):26–29, 1988.

Lafferty WE, et al. Recurrences after oral and genital herpes simplex virus infection: Influence of site of infection and viral type. N Engl J Med 316:1444–1449, 1987.

Leigh IM. Management of non-genital herpes simplex virus infections in immunocompetent patients. Am J Med 85(Suppl 2A):34–38, 1988.

MacPhail LA, et al. Acyclovir-resistant, foscarnet-sensitive oral herpes simplex type 2 lesion in a patient with AIDS. Oral Surg Oral Med Oral Pathol 67:427–432, 1989.

Main DMG. Acute herpetic stomatitis: Referrals to Leeds Dental Hospital 1978–1987. Br Dent J 166:14–16, 1989.

Merchant VA, Molinari JA, Sabes WR. Herpetic whitlow: Report of a case with multiple recurrences. Oral Surg Oral Med Oral Pathol 55:568–571, 1983.

Nesbit SP, Gobetti JP. Multiple recurrence of oral erythema multiforme after secondary herpes simplex: Report of case and review of literature. J Am Dent Assoc 112:348–352, 1986.

Overall JC. Oral herpes simplex: Pathogenesis, clinical and virologic course, approach to treatment. *In:* Viral Infections in Oral Medicine. Edited by Hooks JJ, Jordan G. New York, Elsevier, 1982, pp 53–78.

Park JB, Park N. Effect of chlorhexidine on the in vitro and in vivo herpes simplex virus infection. Oral Surg Oral Med Oral Pathol 67:149–153, 1989.

Park N, et al. Combined synergistic antiherpetic effect of acyclovir and chlorhexidine in vitro. Oral Surg Oral Med Oral Pathol 71:193–196, 1991.

Pedersen A. Are recurrent oral aphthous ulcers of viral etiology? Med Hypotheses 36:206–210, 1991.

Perna JJ, Eskinazi DP. Treatment of oro-facial herpes simplex infections with acyclovir: A review. Oral Surg Oral Med Oral Pathol 65:689–692, 1988.

Raborn GW, et al. Treatment of herpes labialis with acyclovir. Review of three clinical trials. Am J Med 85(Suppl 2A):39–42, 1988.

Raborn GW, et al. Herpes labialis treatment with acyclovir 5% modified aqueous cream: A double-blind randomized trial. Oral Surg Oral Med Oral Pathol 67:676–679, 1989.

Redding SW, Montgomery MT. Acyclovir prophylaxis for oral herpes simplex virus infection in patients with bone marrow transplant. Oral Surg Oral Med Oral Pathol 67:680–683, 1989.

Saral R. Management of mucocutaneous herpes simplex virus infections in immunocompromised patients. Am J Med 85(Suppl 2A):57–60, 1988.

Schmitt DL, Johnson DW, Henderson FW. Herpes simplex type 1 infections in group day care. Pediatr Infect Dis J 10:729–734, 1991.

Scully C. Orofacial herpes simplex virus infections: Current concepts in the epidemiology, pathogenesis, and treatment, and disorders in which the virus may be implicated. Oral Surg Oral Med Oral Pathol 68:701–710, 1989.

Spruance SL, et al. The natural history of ultraviolet radiation-induced herpes simplex labialis and response to therapy with peroral and topical formulations of acyclovir. J Infect Dis 163:728–734, 1991.

Spruance SL, et al. Acyclovir prevents reactivation of herpes simplex labialis in skiers. JAMA 260:1597–1598, 1988.

Spruance SL, et al. Treatment of recurrent herpes simplex labialis with oral acyclovir. J Infect Dis 161:185–190, 1990.

Taieb A, et al. Clinical epidemiology of symptomatic primary herpetic infection in children. A study of 50 cases. Acta Paediatr Scand 76:128–132, 1987.

Weathers DR, Griffin JW. Intraoral ulcerations of recurrent herpes simplex and recurrent aphthae: Two distinct clinical entities. J Am Dent Assoc 81:81–88, 1970.

Wheeler CE. The herpes simplex problem. J Am Acad Dermatol 18:163–168, 1988.

Wheeler CE. Pathogenesis of recurrent herpes simplex infections. J Invest Dermatol 65:341–346, 1975.

Wormser GP, et al. Lack of effect of oral acyclovir on prevention of aphthous stomatitis. Otolaryngol Head Neck Surg 98:14–17, 1988.

Varicella-Zoster Virus

Adelstein AM, Donovan JW. Malignant disease in children whose mothers had chickenpox, mumps, or rubella in pregnancy. Br Med J 4:629–631, 1972.

Arbeter AM, et al. Combination measles, mumps, rubella, and varicella vaccine. Pediatrics 78(Suppl):742–747, 1986.

Badger GR. Oral signs of chickenpox (varicella): Report of two cases. J Dent Child 47:349–351, 1980.

Bagg J, et al. Rapid diagnosis of oral herpes simplex or zoster virus infections by immunofluorescence: Comparison with Tzanck cell preparations and viral culture. Br Dent J 167:235–238, 1989.

Balfour HH, et al. Acyclovir halts progression of herpes zoster in immunocompromised patients. N Engl J Med 308:1448–1453, 1983.

Barrett AP, et al. Zoster sine herpete of the trigeminal nerve. Oral Surg Oral Med Oral Pathol 75:173–175, 1993.

Dunkle LM, et al. A controlled trial of acyclovir for chickenpox in normal children. N Engl J Med 325:1539–1544, 1991.

Feldman SR, Ford MJ, Briggaman RA. Herpes zoster and facial paralysis. Cutis 42:523–524, 1988.

Gordon JE. Chickenpox: An epidemiological review. Am J Med Sci 244:362–389, 1962.

Guess HA, Melton LJ, Kurland LT. Population-based studies of varicella complications. Pediatrics 78(Suppl):723–727, 1986.

Levin MJ, et al. Immune response of elderly individuals to a live attenuated varicella vaccine. J Infect Dis 166:253–259, 1992.

McKendrick MW, et al. Oral acyclovir in acute herpes zoster. Br Med J 293:1529–1532, 1986.

McKenzie CD, Gobetti JP. Diagnosis and treatment of orofacial herpes zoster: Report of cases. J Am Dent Assoc 120:679–681, 1990.

Mintz SM, Anavi K. Maxillary osteomyelitis and spontaneous tooth exfoliation after herpes zoster. Oral Surg Oral Med Oral Pathol 73:664–666, 1992.

Mostofi R, Marchmont-Robinson H, Freije S. Spontaneous tooth exfoliation and osteonecrosis following a herpes zoster infection of the fifth cranial nerve. J Oral Maxillofac Surg 45:264–266, 1987.

Pastuszak AL, et al. Outcome after maternal varicella infection in the first 20 weeks of pregnancy. N Engl J Med 330:901–905, 1994.

Ross AH. Modification of chicken pox in family contacts by administration of gamma globulin. N Engl J Med 267:369–376, 1962.

Strauss SE, et al. Varicella-zoster virus infections. Biology, natural history, treatment and prevention. Ann Intern Med 108:221–237, 1988.

Takahashi M. Clinical overview of varicella vaccine: Development and early studies. Pediatrics 78(Suppl):736–741, 1986.

Infectious Mononucleosis

Burton JA. The management of severe tonsillitis in infectious mononucleosis. Practitioner 231:1085, 1987.

Carrington P, Hall JI. Fatal airway obstruction in infectious mononucleosis. Br Med J 292:195, 1986.

Courant P, Sobkov T. Oral manifestations of infectious mononucleosis. J Periodontol 40:279–283, 1979.

Englund JA. The many faces of Epstein-Barr virus. Postgrad Med 83(2):167–179, 1988.

Evans AS: The transmission of EB viral infections. *In:* Viral Infections in Oral Medicine. Edited by Hooks J, Jordan G. New York, Elsevier North Holland, 1982, pp 211–225.

Fraser-Moodie W. Oral lesions in infectious mononucleosis. Oral Surg Oral Med Oral Pathol 12:685–691, 1959.

Har-El G, Josephsen JS. Infectious mononucleosis complicated by lingual tonsillitis. J Laryngol Otol 104:651–653, 1990.

Johnson PA, Avery C. Infectious mononucleosis presenting as a parotid mass with associated facial nerve palsy. Int J Oral Maxillofac Surg 20:193–195, 1991.

Portman M, et al. Peritonsillar abscess complicating infectious mononucleosis. J Pediatr 104:742–744, 1984.

Purtilo DT, et al. Epstein-Barr as an etiological agent in the pathogenesis of lymphoproliferative and aproliferative diseases in immune deficient patients. Int Rev Exp Pathol 27:113–183, 1985.

van der Horst C, et al. Lack of effect of peroral acyclovir for the treatment of acute infectious mononucleosis. J Infect Dis 164:788–791, 1991.

Cytomegalovirus

Berman S, Jensen J. Cytomegalovirus-induced osteomyelitis in a patient with the acquired immunodeficiency syndrome. South Med J 83:1231–1232, 1990.

Deibel R, et al. Cytomegalovirus infections in New York State: Laboratory studies of patients and healthy individuals. N Y State J Med 74:785–791, 1974.

Epstein JB, Scully C. Cytomegalovirus: A virus of increasing relevance to oral medicine and pathology. J Oral Pathol Med 22:348–353, 1993.

Epstein JB, Sherlock CH, Wolber RA. Oral manifestations of cytomegalovirus infection. Oral Surg Oral Med Oral Pathol 75:443–451, 1993.

French PD, Birchall MA, Harris JRW. Cytomegalovirus ulceration of the oropharynx. J Laryngol Otol 105:739–742, 1991.

Jones AC, et al. Cytomegalovirus infections of the oral cavity. A report of six cases and review of the literature. Oral Surg Oral Med Oral Pathol 75:76–85, 1993.

Kanas RJ, et al. Oral mucosal cytomegalovirus as a manifestation of the acquired immune deficiency syndrome. Oral Surg Oral Med Oral Pathol 64:183–189, 1987.

Langford A, et al. Cytomegalovirus associated oral ulcerations in HIV-infected patients. J Oral Pathol Med 19:71–76, 1990.

Newland JR, Adler-Storthz K. Cytomegalovirus in intraoral Kaposi's sarcoma. Oral Surg Oral Med Oral Pathol 67:296–300, 1989.

Schubert MM, Epstein JB, Lloid ME. Oral infections due to cytomegalovirus in immunocompromised patients. J Oral Pathol Med 22:268–273, 1993.

Stagno S, et al. Defects of tooth structure in congenital cytomegalovirus infection. Pediatrics 69:646–648, 1982.

Enteroviruses

Alsop J, Flewett TH, Foster JR. "Hand-foot-and-mouth disease" in Birmingham in 1959. Br Med J 2:1708–1711, 1960.

Buchner A. Hand, foot, and mouth disease. Oral Surg Oral Med Oral Pathol 41:333–337, 1976.

Chawareewong S, et al. Neonatal herpangina caused by Coxsackie A-5 virus. J Pediatr 93:492–494, 1978.

Cherry JD, Nelson DB. Enterovirus infections: Their epidemiology and pathogenesis. Clin Pediatr (Phila) 5:659–664, 1966.

Cooper DJ, et al. Fatal rhabdomyolysis and renal failure associated with hand, foot and mouth disease. Med J Aust 151:232–234, 1989.

Higgins PG, Warin RP. Hand, foot, and mouth disease: A clinically recognizable virus infection seen mainly in children. Clin Pediatr (Phila) 6:373–376, 1967.

Steigman AJ, Lipton MM, Braspennickx H. Acute lymphonodular pharyngitis: A newly described condition due to coxsackie virus. J Pediatr 61:331–336, 1962.

Tindall JP, Callaway JL. Hand-foot-mouth disease—it's more common than you think. Am J Dis Child 124:372–375, 1972.

Yamadera S, et al. Herpangina surveillance in Japan, 1982–1989. Jpn J Med Sci Biol 44:29–39, 1991.

Rubeola

Atkinson WL, Orenstein WA, Krugman S. The resurgence of measles in the United States, 1989–1990. Annu Rev Med 43:451–463, 1992.

Campos-Outcalt D. Measles update. Am Fam Physician 42:1274–1283, 1990.

Kaplan LJ, et al. Severe measles in immunocompromised patients. JAMA 267:1237–1241, 1992.

Koplik H. The diagnosis of the invasion of measles from a study of the exanthema as it appears on the buccal mucosa membrane. Arch Pediatr 13:918–922, 1896.

Martinson FD. Otolaryngological complications of measles in West Africa. J Laryngol Otol 89:631–640, 1975.

Scully C, Williams G. Oral manifestations of communicable diseases. Dent Update 5:295–311, 1978.

Rubella

Best JM. Rubella vaccines: Past, present and future. Epidemiol Infect 107:17–30, 1991.

Bligard CA, Millikan LE. Acute exanthems in children. Clues to differential diagnosis of viral disease. Postgrad Med 79(5):150–167, 1986.

Forchheimer F. German measles (Rubella). *In:* Twentieth Century Practice; An International Encyclopedia of Modern Medical Science by Leading Authorities of Europe and America. Edited by Stedman TL. New York, W. Wood, 1898, pp 175–188.

Herrmann KL. Rubella in the United States: Toward a strategy for disease control and elimination. Epidemiol Infect 107:55–61, 1991.

Lindergren ML, et al. Update: Rubella and congenital rubella syndrome, 1980–1990. Epidemiol Rev 13:341–348, 1991.

Miller E. Rubella reinfection. Arch Dis Child 65:820–821, 1990.

Mumps

Cochi SL, Preblud SR, Orenstein WA. Perspectives on the relative resurgence of mumps in the United States. Am J Dis Child 142:499–507, 1988.

Kaplan KM, et al. Mumps in the workplace. Further evidence of the changing epidemiology of a childhood vaccine-preventable disease. JAMA 260:1434–1438, 1988.

Manson AL. Mumps orchitis. Urology 36:355–358, 1990.

Scully C, Williams G. Oral manifestations of communicable diseases. Dent Update 5:295–311, 1978.

Wharton M, et al. A large outbreak of mumps in the postvaccine era. J Infect Dis 158:1253–1260, 1988.

Human Immunodeficiency Virus

Castro KG, et al. 1993 Revised classification system for HIV infection and expanded surveillance case definition for AIDS among adolescents and adults. MMWR Morb Mortal Wkly Rep 41(RR-17):1–19, 1993.

Cohen PT, Sande MA, Volberding PA. The AIDS Knowledge Base: A Textbook on HIV Disease from the University of California, San Francisco, and the San Francisco General Hospital. Waltham, Mass, The Medical Publishing Group, 1990.

Davey RT. Current issues in the development of a vaccine against HIV infection. Ear Nose Throat J 69:497–505, 1990.

Davidson BJ, et al. Lymphadenopathy in the HIV-seropositive patient. Ear Nose Throat J 69:478–485, 1990.

Eisenberg E, Krutchkoff D, Yamase H. Incidental oral hairy leukoplakia in immunocompetent persons: A report of two cases. Oral Surg Oral Med Oral Pathol 74:332–333, 1992.

Epstein JB, Sherlock CH, Wolber RA. Hairy leukoplakia after bone marrow transplantation. Oral Surg Oral Med Oral Pathol 75:690–695, 1993.

Epstein JB, Silverman S, Jr. Head and neck malignancies associated with HIV infection. Oral Surg Oral Med Oral Pathol 73:193–200, 1992.

Eversole LR. Viral infections of the head and neck among HIV-seropositive patients. Oral Surg Oral Med Oral Pathol 73:155–163, 1992.

Fallon J. Current treatment for human immunodeficiency virus infection. Ear Nose Throat J 69:487–496, 1990.

Felix DH, et al. Detection of Epstein-Barr virus and human papillomavirus type 16 in hairy leukoplakia by *in situ* hybridisation and the polymerase chain reaction. J Oral Pathol Med 22:277–281, 1993.

Ficarra G. Oral lesions of iatrogenic and undefined etiology and neurologic disorders associated with HIV infection. Oral Surg Oral Med Oral Pathol 73:201–211, 1992.

Ficarra G, Shillitoe EJ. HIV-related infection of the oral cavity. Crit Rev Oral Biol Med 3:207–231, 1992.

Gilmore N. HIV disease: Present status and future directions. Oral Surg Oral Med Oral Pathol 73:236–243, 1992.

Greenspan D, et al. AIDS and the Mouth. Diagnosis and Management of Oral Lesions. Copenhagen, Munksgaard, 1990.

Greenspan D, Greenspan JS. Significance of oral hairy leukoplakia. Oral Surg Oral Med Oral Pathol 73:151–154, 1992.

Greenspan JS, et al. Oral manifestations of HIV infection: Definitions, diagnostic criteria, and principles of therapy. Oral Surg Oral Med Oral Pathol 73:142–144, 1992.

Heinic GS, et al. Oral *Histoplasma capsulatum* infection in association with HIV infection: A case report. J Oral Pathol Med 21:85–89, 1992.

Hicks MJ, et al. Intraoral presentation of anaplastic large-cell Ki-1 lymphoma in association with HIV infection. Oral Surg Oral Med Oral Pathol 76:73–81, 1993.

Lucatorto FM, Sapp JP. Treatment of oral Kaposi's sarcoma with a sclerosing agent in AIDS patients: A preliminary study. Oral Surg Oral Med Oral Pathol 75:192–198, 1993.

MacPhail LA, et al. Recurrent aphthous ulcerations in association with HIV infection: Description of ulcer types and analysis of T-lymphocyte subsets. Oral Surg Oral Med Oral Pathol 71:678–683, 1991.

MacPhail LA, Greenspan D, Greenspan JS. Recurrent aphthous ulcerations in association with HIV infection: Diagnosis and treatment. Oral Surg Oral Med Oral Pathol 73:283–288, 1992.

Phelan JA, et al. Oral findings in patients with acquired immunodeficiency syndrome. Oral Surg Oral Med Oral Pathol 64:50–56, 1987.

Regezi JA, et al. Human immunodeficiency virus-associated oral Kaposi's sarcoma: A heterogeneous cell population dominated by spindle-shaped endothelial cells. Am J Pathol 143:240–249, 1993.

Robertson PB, Greenspan JS. Perspectives on Oral Manifestations of AIDS: Diagnosis and Management of HIV-Associated Infections. Littleton, Mass, PSG Publishing, 1988.

Samaranayake LP. Oral mycoses in HIV infection. Oral Surg Oral Med Oral Pathol 73:171–180, 1992.

Schiødt M. HIV-associated salivary gland disease: A review. Oral Surg Oral Med Oral Pathol 73:164–167, 1992.

Schmidt-Westhausen A, et al. Epstein-Barr virus in lingual epithelium of liver transplant patients. J Oral Pathol Med 22:274–276, 1993.

Scully C, et al. Oral manifestations of HIV infection and their management: I. More common lesions. Oral Surg Oral Med Oral Pathol 71:158–166, 1991.

Scully C, et al. Oral manifestations of HIV infection and their management: II. Less common lesions. Oral Surg Oral Med Oral Pathol 71:167–171, 1991.

Smith DK, et al. Unexplained opportunistic infections and CD4+ T-lymphocytopenia without HIV infection. An investigation of cases in the United States. N Engl J Med 328:373–379, 1993.

Smith GLF, Felix DH. Current classifications of HIV-associated periodontal diseases. Br Dent J 174:102–105, 1993.

8

Physical and Chemical Injuries

LINEA ALBA

Linea alba ("white line") is a common alteration of the buccal mucosa that is most likely associated with pressure, frictional irritation, or sucking trauma from the facial surfaces of the teeth. In one study of 256 young males, the alteration was present in 13 percent. No other associated problem, such as insufficient horizontal overlap or rough restorations of the teeth, is necessary for the development of linea alba.

Clinical Features

As the name implies, the alteration consists of a white line that is usually bilateral. It may be scalloped and is located on the buccal mucosa at the level of the occlusal plane of the adjacent teeth (Fig. 8–1). The line varies in prominence and is restricted to dentulous areas. It is often more pronounced adjacent to the posterior teeth.

Histopathologic Features

Biopsy is rarely indicated. If a biopsy is performed, hyperorthokeratosis is seen overlying otherwise normal oral mucosa. On occasion, intracellular edema of the epithelium and mild chronic inflammation of the underlying connective tissue may be noted.

Treatment and Prognosis

No treatment is required for patients with linea alba, and no difficulties are documented as a result of its development. Spontaneous regression may occur.

MORSICATIO BUCCARUM ("Chronic Cheek Chewing")

Morsicatio buccarum is a classic example of medical terminology gone astray; it is the scientific term for chronic cheek chewing. *Morsicatio* comes from the Latin word *morsus,* or bite. Chronic nibbling produces lesions that are located most frequently on the buccal mucosa; however, the labial mucosa (**morsicatio labiorum**) and the lateral border of the tongue (**morsicatio linguarum**) may also be involved. Similar changes have been seen as a result of suction and in glass blowers whose technique produces chronic irritation of the buccal mucosa. A higher prevalence has been found in people who are under stress or who exhibit psychologic conditions. Most patients are aware of their habit, although many deny the self-inflicted injury or perform the act subconsciously. The occurrence is twice as prevalent in females and three times more prevalent after age 35. At any given time, one in every 800 adults has active lesions.

Clinical Features

The lesions in patients with morsicatio are most frequently found bilaterally on the buccal mucosa. They may also be unilateral, combined with lesions of the lips or the tongue, or isolated to the lips or tongue. Thick-

211

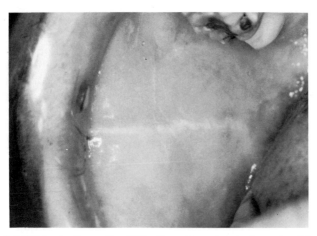

FIGURE 8-1. **Linea alba.** White line of hyperkeratosis on the right buccal mucosa at the level of the occlusal plane.

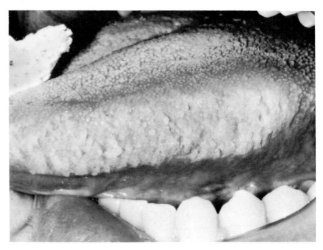

FIGURE 8-3. **Morsicatio linguarum.** Thickened, rough areas of white hyperkeratosis of the lateral border of the tongue on the left side.

ened, shredded white areas infrequently are combined with intervening zones of erythema, erosion, or focal traumatic ulceration (Figs. 8-2 and 8-3). The areas of white mucosa demonstrate an irregular ragged surface, and the patient may describe being able to remove shreds of white material from the involved area.

The altered mucosa is located typically in the midportion of the anterior buccal mucosa along the occlusal plane. Large lesions may extend some distance above or below the occlusal plane in patients whose habit involves pushing the cheek between the teeth with a finger.

Histopathologic Features

Biopsy reveals extensive hyperparakeratosis that often results in an extremely ragged surface with numerous projections of keratin. Surface bacterial colonization is typical (Fig. 8-4). On occasion, clusters of vacuolated cells are present in the superficial portion of the prickle cell layer. This histopathologic pattern is not pathogno-

monic of morsicatio and may bear a striking resemblance to oral hairy leukoplakia, a lesion that most often occurs in people who are infected with the human immunodeficiency virus (HIV) (see p. 202). Similarities with linea alba and leukoedema may also be seen.

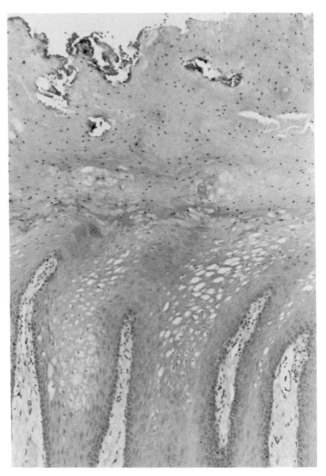

FIGURE 8-4. **Morsicatio buccarum.** Oral mucosa exhibiting greatly thickened layer of parakeratin with ragged surface colonized by bacteria.

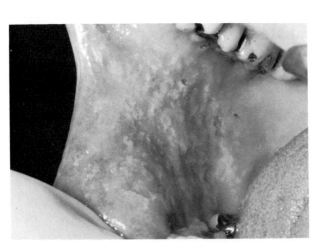

FIGURE 8-2. **Morsicatio buccarum.** Thickened, shredded areas of white hyperkeratosis of the right buccal mucosa.

Diagnosis

The clinical presentation of morsicatio buccarum normally is sufficient for a strong presumptive diagnosis, and biopsy is rarely performed by clinicians familiar with these alterations. Some cases of morsicatio may not be completely diagnostic from the clinical presentation, and biopsy may be necessary. In patients at high risk for HIV infection with isolated involvement of the lateral border of the tongue, further investigation is desirable to rule out HIV-associated hairy leukoplakia.

Treatment and Prognosis

No treatment of the oral lesions is required, and no long-term difficulties arise from the presence of the mucosal changes. For patients who desire treatment, an oral acrylic shield that covers the facial surfaces of the teeth may be constructed to eliminate the lesions by restricting access to the buccal and labial mucosa. Several authors also have suggested psychotherapy as the treatment of choice, but no extensive well-controlled studies have indicated benefits from this approach.

TRAUMATIC ULCERATIONS/ TRAUMATIC GRANULOMA

Acute injuries of the oral mucosa are frequently observed. Injury can result from mechanical damage, such as contact with sharp foodstuffs or accidental biting during mastication, talking, or even sleeping. Damage may also result from thermal, electrical, or chemical burns. (Oral mucosal manifestations of such burns are discussed later in the chapter.)

Acute or chronic trauma to the oral mucosa may result in surface ulcerations. The ulcerations may remain for extended periods of time, but most usually heal within days. A histopathologically unique type of chronic traumatic ulceration is the **traumatic granuloma (traumatic ulcerative granuloma with stromal eosinophilia),** which exhibits a deep "pseudoinvasive" inflammatory reaction and typically is slow to resolve. Lesions microscopically similar to traumatic granuloma have been reproduced in rat tongues following repeated crushing trauma. In addition, similar sublingual ulcerations may occur in infants as a result of chronic mucosal trauma from adjacent anterior primary teeth, often associated with nursing. These distinctive ulcerations have been termed **Riga-Fede disease** and should be considered a variation of traumatic granuloma. In rare instances, the inflammatory infiltrate is very extensive and histopathologically atypical, creating a pseudolymphomatous pattern. This pattern has been termed **atypical histiocytic granuloma** and occasionally has been misdiagnosed as lymphoma.

In most cases of traumatic ulceration, there is an adjacent source of irritation, although this is not invariably present. The clinical presentation often suggests the cause, but many cases resemble early ulcerative squamous cell carcinoma; biopsy is performed to rule out that possibility.

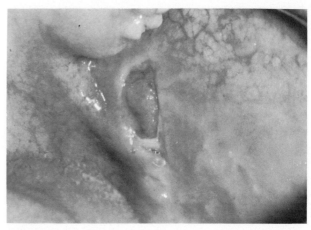

FIGURE 8–5. Traumatic ulceration. Well-circumscribed ulceration of the posterior buccal mucosa on the left side.

Clinical Features

As would be expected, simple chronic traumatic ulcerations occur most often on the tongue, lips, and buccal mucosa—sites that may be injured by the dentition (Figs. 8–5 and 8–6). Lesions of the gingiva, palate, and mucobuccal fold may occur from other sources of irritation. The individual lesions present as areas of erythema surrounding a central removable, yellow fibrinopurulent membrane. In many instances, the lesion develops a rolled white border of hyperkeratosis immediately adjacent to the area of ulceration.

Traumatic granulomas are not uncommon but are not frequently reported. The lesions occur in people of all ages with a significant male predominance. Most have been reported on the tongue, although cases have been seen on the gingiva, buccal mucosa, floor of mouth, palate, and lip (Fig. 8–7). The lesion may last from 1 week to 8 months. The ulcerations appear very similar to the simple traumatic ulcerations; however, on occasion, underlying proliferative granulation tissue can result in a

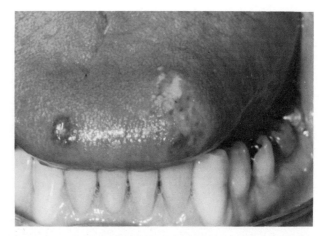

FIGURE 8–6. Traumatic ulceration. Ill-defined ulceration of the anterior dorsal surface of the tongue on the left side. The area of erythema on the patient's right side represents a previous site of injury.

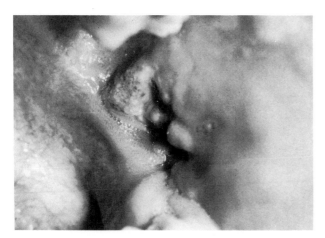

FIGURE 8-7. **Traumatic granuloma.** Irregular, cavitated, and granular area of ulceration of the posterior buccal mucosa on the left side.

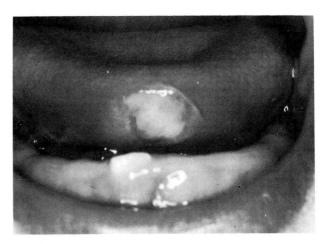

FIGURE 8-9. **Riga-Fede disease.** Newborn with traumatic ulceration of anterior ventral surface of the tongue. Mucosal damage occurred from contact of tongue with adjacent tooth during breast-feeding.

raised lesion similar to a pyogenic granuloma (see p. 371) (Fig. 8-8).

Riga-Fede disease typically presents between 1 week and 1 year of age. The condition often develops in association with natal or neonatal teeth (see p. 64). The anterior ventral surface of the tongue is the most common site of involvement, although the dorsal surface also may be affected (Fig. 8-9). Ventral lesions contact the adjacent mandibular anterior incisors; lesions on the dorsal surface are associated with the maxillary incisors.

The atypical histiocytic granuloma occurs in older people, with most cases developing in patients over age 40. Surface ulceration is present, and an underlying tumefaction is also seen. The tongue and gingiva-alveolar ridge complex are the most common sites, although the mucobuccal fold, buccal mucosa, and lip may be affected (Fig. 8-10).

Histopathologic Features

Simple traumatic ulcerations are covered by a fibrinopurulent membrane that consists of fibrin intermixed with neutrophils. The membrane is of variable thickness.

The adjacent surface epithelium may be normal or may demonstrate slight hyperplasia with or without hyperkeratosis. The ulcer bed consists of granulation tissue that supports a mixed inflammatory infiltrate of lymphocytes, histiocytes, neutrophils, and, occasionally, plasma cells. In patients with traumatic granulomas, the pattern is very similar; however, the inflammatory infiltrate extends into the deeper tissues and exhibits sheets of benign histiocytes intermixed with eosinophils. In addition, the vascular connective tissue deep to the ulceration may become hyperplastic and cause surface elevation.

Atypical histiocytic granulomas exhibit numerous features of the traumatic granuloma, but the deeper tissues are replaced by a highly cellular proliferation of large histiocytic lymphoreticular cells. The infiltrate is pleomorphic, and mitotic features are somewhat common. Intermixed with the large atypical cells are mature lymphocytes and eosinophils. The infiltrate is so worrisome on light microscopy that immunohistochemical studies are often required to rule out the possibility of lymphoma by demonstrating a polyclonal mixture of B lymphocytes, T lymphocytes, and histiocytes.

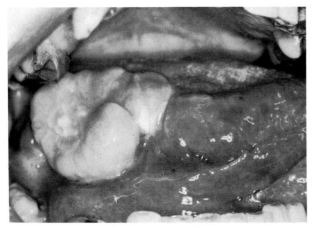

FIGURE 8-8. **Traumatic granuloma.** Ulceration of lateral border of the tongue on the right side. The surface of the ulcer developed proliferative granulation tissue that resembles a pyogenic granuloma.

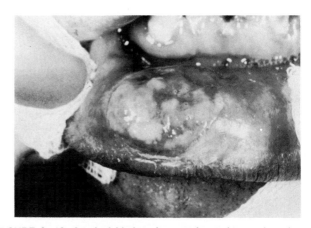

FIGURE 8-10. **Atypical histiocytic granuloma.** Large ulceration of the lower labial mucosa with underlying tumefaction. (Courtesy of Dr. Gregory R. Erena.)

Treatment and Prognosis

For traumatic ulcerations that have an obvious source of injury, the irritating cause should be removed. Dyclonine HCl or hydroxypropyl cellulose films can be applied for temporary pain relief. If the cause is not obvious or if a patient does not respond to therapy, biopsy is indicated. Rapid healing after a biopsy is typical even with large traumatic granulomas. Recurrence is not expected.

The use of corticosteroids in the management of traumatic ulcerations is controversial. Some clinicians have suggested that use of such medications may delay healing. In spite of this, other investigators have reported success using corticosteroids to treat chronic traumatic ulcerations.

Although extraction of the anterior primary teeth is not recommended, this procedure has resolved the ulcerations in Riga-Fede disease. The teeth should be retained if they are stable. Construction of a protective shield or discontinuation of nursing is usually sufficient to allow resolution.

ELECTRICAL/THERMAL BURNS

Electrical burns to the oral cavity are fairly common, constituting approximately 5 percent of all burn admissions to hospitals. Two types of electrical burns can be seen: contact and arc.

Contact burns require a good ground and involve electrical current passing through the body from the point of contact to the ground site. The electric current can cause cardiopulmonary arrest and may be fatal. Most electrical burns affecting the oral cavity are the **arc** type, in which the saliva acts as a conducting medium and an electrical arc flows between the electrical source and the mouth. Extreme heat, up to 3000°C, is possible with resultant significant tissue destruction. Most cases result from chewing on the female end of an extension cord or from biting through a live wire.

Most **thermal burns** of the oral cavity arise from ingestion of hot foods or beverages. The microwave oven has been associated with an increased frequency of thermal burns because of its ability to produce a food that is cool on the outside but extremely hot in the interior.

Clinical Features

Most electrical burns occur in children younger than age 4. The lips are most frequently affected, and the commissure is commonly involved.

Initially, the burn appears as a painless, charred, yellow area that exhibits little to no bleeding (Fig. 8–11). Significant edema often develops within a few hours and may persist up to 12 days. Beginning on the fourth day, the affected area becomes necrotic and begins to slough. Bleeding may develop during this period from exposure of the underlying vital vasculature, and the presence of this complication should be closely monitored. The adjacent mucobuccal fold, the tongue, or both may also be involved. On occasion, adjacent teeth may become non-

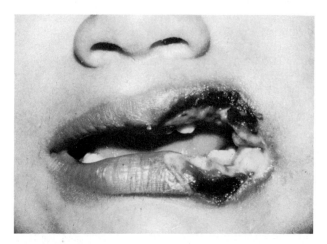

FIGURE 8–11. **Electrical burn.** Yellow charred area of necrosis along the left oral commissure. (Courtesy of Dr. Patricia Hagen.)

vital, with or without necrosis of the surrounding alveolar bone. Malformation of developing teeth has also been documented.

The injuries related to thermal food burns usually present on the palate or posterior buccal mucosa (Fig. 8–12). The lesions appear as zones of erythema and ulceration that often exhibit remnants of necrotic epithelium at the periphery.

Treatment and Prognosis

For patients with electrical burns of the oral cavity, tetanus immunization, if not current, is required. A prophylactic antibiotic, usually penicillin, is given by most clinicians to prevent secondary infection in severe cases. The primary problem with oral burns is contracture of the mouth opening during healing. Without intervention, significant microstomia can develop and may produce such restricted access to the mouth that hygiene and eating become impossible in severe cases. Extensive scarring and disfigurement are typical in untreated patients.

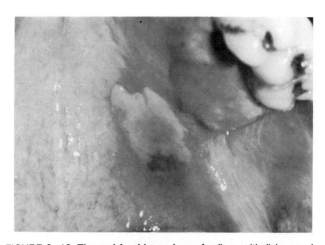

FIGURE 8–12. **Thermal food burn.** Area of yellow epithelial necrosis of the posterior soft palate on the left side. Damage was due to attempted ingestion of hot pizza.

To prevent the disfigurement, an intraoral splint that completely covers the maxilla can be fabricated. Two wings extend extraorally and engage both of the commissures. The wings prevent contracture from developing as the wounds heal. This appliance works best in children over the age of 18 months who have at least eight maxillary teeth for attachment. The splint is worn 24 hours a day for 6 to 12 months except during eating and cleaning. This should be followed by nighttime use for an additional 6 months. Subsequent eruption of teeth necessitates reconstruction of the appliance. Typically, this treatment approach is aesthetically satisfactory, but in severe cases, additional surgical reconstructive therapy may be required.

Most thermal burns are of little clinical consequence and resolve without treatment.

CHEMICAL INJURIES OF THE ORAL MUCOSA

A large number of chemicals and drugs come into contact with the oral tissues. A percentage of these agents are caustic and can cause clinically significant damage.

Patients often can be their own worst enemies. The array of chemicals that have been placed within the mouth in an attempt to resolve oral problems is amazing. Aspirin, sodium perborate, hydrogen peroxide, gasoline, turpentine, rubbing alcohol, and battery acid are just a few of the more interesting examples.

Certain patients, typically children or those under psychiatric care, may hold medications within their mouths rather than swallow them. A surprising number of medications are potentially caustic when held in the mouth long enough. Aspirin and two psychoactive drugs, chlorpromazine and promazine, are well-documented examples.

Over-the-counter medications for mouth pain can compound the problem. Mucosal damage has been documented from many of the topical medicaments sold as treatments for toothache or mouth sores. Products containing phenol, hydrogen peroxide, or eugenol have produced adverse reactions in patients.

Health care practitioners are responsible for the use of many caustic materials. Silver nitrate, formocresol, sodium hypochlorite, paraformaldehyde, chromic acid, trichloroacetic acid, dental cavity varnishes, and acid-etch materials can all cause patient injury. Education and the use of the rubber dam have reduced the frequency of such injuries.

The improper use of aspirin, hydrogen peroxide, silver nitrate, phenol, and certain endodontic materials deserves further discussion because of their frequency of misuse, the severity of related damage, and the lack of adequate documentation of these materials as harmful agents.

Aspirin. Mucosal necrosis from aspirin being held in the mouth is not rare (Fig. 8–13). Aspirin is available not only in the well-known tablets but also as a powder, rinse, gum, and chewable tablets.

Hydrogen Peroxide. Hydrogen peroxide became a popular intraoral medication for prevention of periodontitis

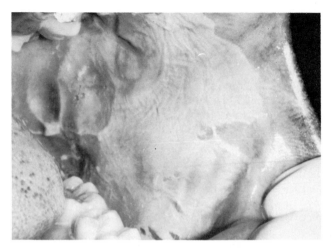

FIGURE 8–13. **Aspirin burn.** Extensive area of white epithelial necrosis of the left buccal mucosa caused by aspirin placement in an attempt to alleviate dental pain.

in the late 1970s. Since that time, mucosal damage has been seen more frequently as a result of this application. Concentrations at 3 percent or greater are most often associated with adverse reactions. Epithelial necrosis has been noted with dilutions as low as 1 percent, and many of the over-the-counter oral medications exceed this concentration (Fig. 8–14).

Silver Nitrate. Silver nitrate remains a popular treatment for aphthous ulcerations because the chemical cautery brings about rapid pain relief by destroying nerve endings. In spite of this, its use should be discouraged. In all cases, the extent of mucosal damage is increased by its use. In some patients, an abnormal reaction is seen with resultant significant damage and enhanced pain. In one report, an application of a silver nitrate stick to a small aphthous ulceration led to a necrotic defect that exceeded 2 × 2 cm and had to be surgically debrided.

Phenol. Phenol has been used occasionally in dentistry as a cavity-sterilizing agent and cauterizing material. It is extremely caustic, and judicious use is required. Over-the-counter agents advertised as "canker sore" treat-

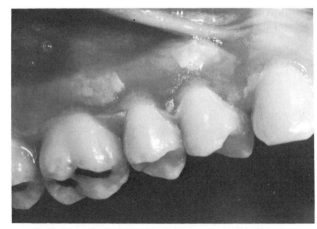

FIGURE 8–14. **Hydrogen peroxide burn.** Extensive epithelial necrosis of the anterior maxillary gingiva secondary to interproximal placement of hydrogen peroxide with cotton swabs.

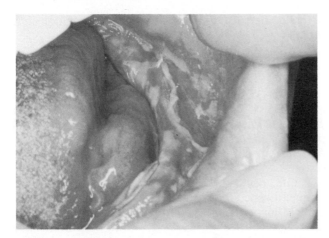

FIGURE 8–15. **Phenol burn.** Extensive epithelial necrosis of the mandibular alveolar mucosa on the left side. Damage resulted from placement of an over-the-counter, phenol-containing, antiseptic-anesthetic gel under a denture. (Courtesy of Dr. Dean K. White.)

ments may contain low concentrations of phenol, often combined with high levels of alcohol. Extensive mucosal necrosis has been seen in patients who placed this material beneath their dentures in attempts to resolve sore spots (Fig. 8–15).

Endodontic Materials. Endodontic materials are especially dangerous because of the possibility of soft tissue damage (Fig. 8–16) or their injection into hard tissue with resultant deep spread and necrosis. Extrusion of filling material containing paraformaldehyde into the periapical tissues has led to significant difficulties, and its use should be discouraged. Sodium hypochlorite produces similar results when injected past the apex. The chances of apical discharge can be reduced by:

- Using a rubber dam
- Avoiding excessive pressure during application
- Keeping the syringe needle away from the apex

Clinical Features

The above-mentioned caustic agents produce similar damage. With short exposure, the affected mucosa exhibits a superficial white, wrinkled appearance. As the duration of exposure increases, the necrosis proceeds and the affected epithelium becomes separated from the underlying tissue and can be easily desquamated. Removal of the necrotic epithelium reveals red, bleeding connective tissue that will subsequently be covered by a yellowish, fibrinopurulent membrane. Mucosa bound to bone is keratinized and more resistant to damage; the non-keratinized movable mucosa is more quickly destroyed.

The use of the rubber dam can dramatically reduce iatrogenic mucosal burns. When cotton rolls are used for moisture control during dental procedures, two problems may occur. On occasion, caustic materials can leak into the cotton roll and be held in place against the mucosa for an extended period, with mucosal injury resulting from the chemical absorbed by the cotton. In addition, oral mucosa can become adherent to dry cotton rolls, and their rapid removal from the mouth can often cause stripping of the epithelium in the area. The latter pattern of mucosal injury has been termed **cotton roll burn (cotton roll stomatitis)** (Fig. 8–17).

Caustic materials injected into bone during endodontic procedures can result in significant bone necrosis, pain, and perforation into soft tissue. Necrotic surface ulceration and edema with underlying areas of soft tissue necrosis may occur adjacent to the site of perforation.

Histopathologic Features

Microscopic examination of the white slough removed from areas of mucosal chemical burns reveals coagulative necrosis of the epithelium, with only the outline of the individual epithelial cells and nuclei remaining (Fig. 8–18). The necrosis begins on the surface and moves basally. The amount of epithelium affected depends on the duration of contact and the concentration of the offending agent. The underlying connective tissue contains a mixture of acute and chronic inflammatory cells.

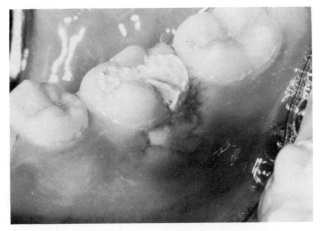

FIGURE 8–16. **Formocresol burn.** Tissue necrosis secondary to leakage of endodontic material between a rubber dam clamp and the tooth.

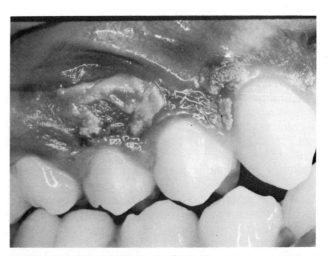

FIGURE 8–17. **Cotton roll burn.** Zone of white epithelial necrosis and erythema of the maxillary alveolar mucosa.

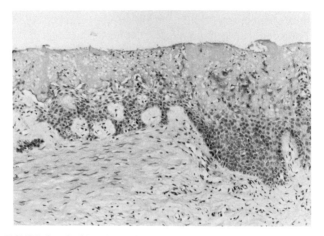

FIGURE 8-18. **Chemical-related epithelial necrosis.** Oral mucosa exhibiting superficial coagulative necrosis of the epithelial cells.

Treatment and Prognosis

The best treatment of chemical injuries is prevention of exposure of the oral mucosa to caustic materials. When using potentially caustic drugs (e.g., aspirin, chlorpromazine), the clinician must instruct the patient to swallow the medication and not allow it to remain in the oral cavity for any significant length of time. Children should not use chewable aspirin immediately before bedtime, and they should rinse after use.

Superficial areas of necrosis typically resolve completely without scarring within 10 to 14 days after discontinuation of the offending agent. Coverage with a protective emollient paste or a hydroxypropyl cellulose film has been used by some clinicians for temporary protection. Topical dyclonine HCl provides excellent but temporary pain relief. When large areas of necrosis are present, such as that related to the use of silver nitrate or accidental intrabony injection of offending materials, surgical debridement and antibiotic coverage are often required to promote healing and prevent spread of the necrosis.

NONINFECTIOUS ORAL COMPLICATIONS OF ANTINEOPLASTIC THERAPY

No systemic anticancer therapy currently available is able to destroy tumor cells without causing the death of at least some normal cells, and tissues with rapid turnover (such as the oral epithelium) are especially susceptible. The mouth is a common site (and one of the most visible) for complications related to cancer therapy. Both radiation therapy and systemic chemotherapy may cause significant oral problems. The more potent the treatment, the greater the risk of complications. Almost 400,000 patients in the United States yearly suffer acute or chronic oral side effects from anticancer treatments. With the advancement of medical practice, these complications are becoming more common as more patients have longer survival times and as intense therapies, such

as bone marrow transplantation, become more commonplace.

Clinical Features

A variety of noninfectious oral complications are regularly seen as a result of both radiation and chemotherapy. Two acute changes, **mucositis** and **hemorrhage**, are the predominant problems associated with chemotherapy, especially in cancers, such as leukemia, that involve high dosages.

Painful acute mucositis and dermatitis are the most frequently encountered side effects of radiation, but several chronic alterations continue to plague patients long after their courses of therapy are completed. Depending on the fields of radiation, the radiation dose, and the age of the patient, the following outcomes are possible:

- Xerostomia
- Loss of taste (hypogeusia)
- Osteoradionecrosis
- Trismus
- Chronic dermatitis
- Developmental abnormalities

Hemorrhage

Intraoral hemorrhage is typically secondary to the thrombocytopenia, which develops from bone marrow suppression. Intestinal or hepatic damage, however, may cause lower vitamin K-dependent clotting factors with resultant increased coagulation times. Conversely, tissue damage related to therapy may cause release of tissue thromboplastin at levels capable of producing potentially devastating disseminated intravascular coagulation (DIC). Oral petechiae and ecchymosis secondary to minor trauma are the most common presentations. Any mucosal site may be affected, but the labial mucosa, tongue, and gingiva are the most frequently involved.

Mucositis

Cases of oral mucositis related to radiation or chemotherapy are similar in their clinical presentations. The manifestations of chemotherapy develop after a few days of treatment; radiation mucositis may begin to appear during the second week of therapy. Both chemotherapy- and radiation-induced mucositis will slowly resolve 2 to 3 weeks after cessation of treatment.

The very earliest manifestation is development of a whitish discoloration from a lack of sufficient desquamation of keratin. This is soon followed by loss of this layer with replacement by atrophic mucosa, which is edematous, erythematous, and friable. Subsequently, areas of ulceration develop with formation of a removable yellowish, fibrinopurulent surface membrane (Figs. 8-19 to 8-23). Pain, burning, and discomfort are significant and can be worsened by eating and by oral hygiene procedures.

Dermatitis

Acute dermatitis of the skin in the fields of radiation is common and varies according to the intensity of the therapy. Patients with mild radiation dermatitis experi-

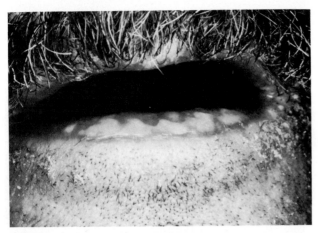

FIGURE 8-19. **Chemotherapy-related epithelial necrosis.** Vermilion border of the lower lip exhibiting epithelial necrosis and ulceration in a patient receiving systemic chemotherapy.

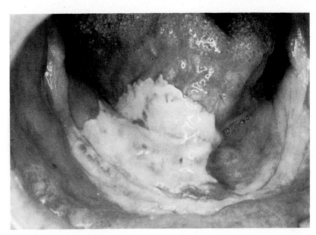

FIGURE 8-22. **Radiation mucositis.** Same patient depicted in Figure 8-21 after initiation of radiation therapy. Note the large, irregular area of epithelial necrosis and ulceration of the anterior floor of the mouth on the patient's right side.

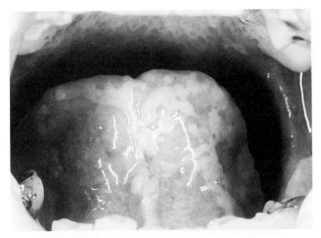

FIGURE 8-20. **Chemotherapy-related epithelial necrosis.** Large, irregular area of epithelial necrosis and ulceration of the anterior ventral surface of the tongue in a patient receiving systemic chemotherapy.

ence erythema, edema, burning, and pruritus. This condition resolves in 2 to 3 weeks following therapy and is replaced by hyperpigmentation and variable hair loss. Moderate radiation causes erythema and edema in combination with erosions and ulcerations. Within 3 months, these alterations resolve and permanent hair loss, hyperpigmentation, and scarring may ensue. Necrosis and deep ulcerations can occur in severe acute reactions.

Radiation dermatitis may also become chronic and may be characterized by dry, smooth, shiny, atrophic, necrotic, telangiectatic, depilated, or ulcerated areas.

Xerostomia

Salivary glands are very sensitive to radiation, and xerostomia is a common complication. Irradiation of the parotid glands produces the most noticeable effect. When a portion of the salivary glands is included in the fields of radiation, the remaining glands undergo compensatory hyperplasia in an attempt to maintain func-

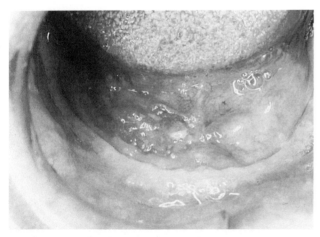

FIGURE 8-21. **Squamous cell carcinoma prior to radiation therapy.** Granular erythroplakia of the floor of the mouth on the patient's right side.

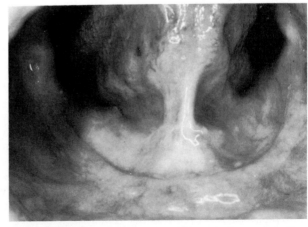

FIGURE 8-23. **Normal oral mucosa after radiation therapy.** Same patient as depicted in Figures 8-21 and 8-22 after completion of therapy. Note resolution of the tumor and the radiation mucositis.

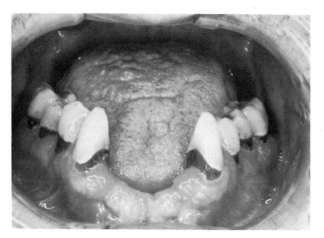

FIGURE 8–24. **Xerostomia-related caries.** Extensive cervical caries of mandibular dentition secondary to radiation-related xerostomia.

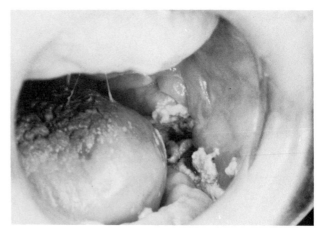

FIGURE 8–25. **Osteoradionecrosis.** Ulceration overlying left body of the mandible with exposure and sequestration of superficial alveolar bone.

tion. When all of the salivary glands are involved, the loss of saliva is progressive, persistent, and irreversible. The changes begin within a week of initiation of radiation therapy, with a dramatic decrease in salivary flow noted during the first 6 weeks of treatment. Even further decreases may be noted for up to 3 years. In addition to the discomfort of a mouth that lacks proper lubrication, diminished flow of saliva leads to a significant decrease of the bactericidal action and self-cleansing properties of saliva. Without intervention, an enormous increase in the caries index (**xerostomia-related caries**) may occur regardless of the patient's past caries history (Fig. 8–24). The decay is predominantly cervical in location and secondary to xerostomia—not a direct effect of the radiation.

Loss of Taste

In patients who receive significant radiation to the oral cavity, a substantial loss of all four tastes *(hypogeusia)* often develops within several weeks. Although these senses return within 4 months for most patients, some patients are left with permanent hypogeusia while others may have persistent *dysgeusia* (altered sense of taste) (see p. 636).

Osteoradionecrosis

Osteoradionecrosis is one of the most serious complications of radiation to the head and neck, but it is seen less frequently today because of better treatment modalities and prevention. Radiation of bone results in permanent damage to the osteocytes and microvasculature system. The altered bone becomes hypoxic, hypovascular, and hypocellular. Osteoradionecrosis is the result of nonhealing, dead bone; infection is not necessarily present. The mandible is involved most frequently, although a few cases have involved the maxilla (Fig. 8–25). Affected areas of bone reveal ill-defined areas of radiolucency that may develop zones of relative radiopacity as the dead bone separates from the residual vital areas (Fig. 8–26). Intractable pain, cortical perforation, fistula formation, surface ulceration, and pathologic fracture may be present (Fig. 8–27).

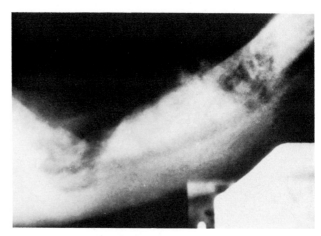

FIGURE 8–26. **Osteoradionecrosis.** Multiple ill-defined areas of radiolucency/radiopacity of the mandibular body.

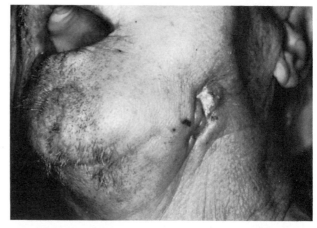

FIGURE 8–27. **Osteoradionecrosis.** Same patient as depicted in Figure 8–25. Note fistula formation of the left submandibular area resulting from osteoradionecrosis of the mandibular body.

The radiation dose is the main factor associated with bone necrosis, although the volume of bone irradiated and the proximity of the maximal dosing both exert an effect. The risk of bone necrosis increases in the presence of:

- Teeth
- Bone trauma
- Periodontal disease
- Concurrent chemotherapy

Postradiation dental extractions should be avoided and are a known risk factor for osteoradionecrosis. In the past, clinicians delayed extractions for 6 months after completion of therapy in the hope that revascularization would decrease the complications. However, bone vascularity actually decreases with time, and delay is not beneficial. Finally, spontaneous osteoradionecrosis can occur without an obvious cause.

Prevention of the bone necrosis is the best course of action. Prior to therapy, all questionable teeth should be extracted or restored, and oral foci of infection should be eliminated; excellent oral hygiene should be initiated and maintained. A healing time of at least 3 weeks between extensive dental procedures and the initiation of radiotherapy significantly decreases the chance of bone necrosis. Extraction of teeth or any bone trauma is strongly contraindicated during radiation therapy. If necessary, hyperbaric oxygen should be used before and after any procedure that may cause bone damage.

Trismus

Trismus may develop and can produce extensive difficulties in regard to access for hygiene and dental treatment. Tonic muscle spasms with or without fibrosis of the muscles of mastication and the temporomandibular joint (TMJ) capsule can cause difficulties in jaw opening. When these structures are heavily radiated, jaw-opening exercises may help to decrease or prevent problems.

Developmental Abnormalities

Antineoplastic therapy during childhood can affect growth and development. The changes vary, according to the age at treatment and the type and severity of therapy. Radiation can alter the facial bones and result in micrognathia, retrognathia, or malocclusion. Developing teeth are very sensitive and can exhibit a number of changes, such as root dwarfism, blunting of roots, dilaceration of roots, incomplete calcification, premature closure of pulp canals in deciduous teeth, enlarged canals in permanent teeth, microdontia, and hypodontia (Figs. 8–28 and 8–29).

Treatment and Prognosis

Mucositis

The pain and discomfort of oral mucositis have been treated with a large number of anesthetics, analgesics, and coating agents. Diphenhydramine, dyclonine HCl, attapulgite (Kaopectate), milk of magnesia, protective emollient paste (Orabase), viscous lidocaine, benzyda-

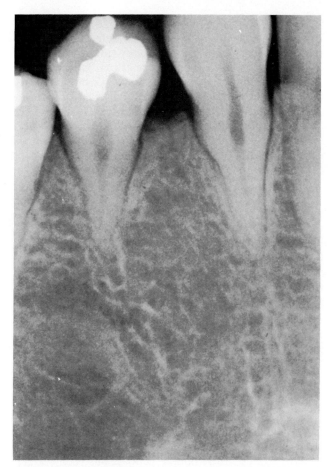

FIGURE 8–28. **Radiation-related dental malformation.** Root dwarfism and spiking of mandibular cuspid and bicuspid secondary to therapeutic radiation during dental formative years.

mine, and systemic analgesics have all been used, but no extensive clinical studies support one approach over the others. Oral viscous lidocaine has caused seizures in children and should be avoided in young patients. Chlorhexidine decreases mucositis and ulceration in patients undergoing intensive chemotherapy but has little effect in those receiving high-dose radiation therapy.

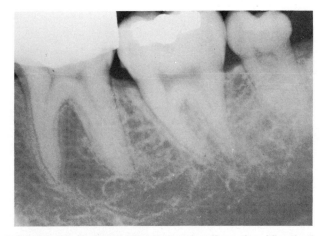

FIGURE 8–29. **Radiation-related dental malformation.** Microdontia of the mandibular third molar and root dwarfism of the first and second molars resulting from therapeutic radiation.

Xerostomia

The problem of chronic xerostomia has been approached through the use of salivary substitutes and sialagogues. Only on rare occasions are all salivary glands destroyed, and the sialagogues show promise because they stimulate the residual functional glands. Sugarless candies and chewing gum are used, but the most efficacious product in controlled clinical studies has been systemic use of the cholinergic drug pilocarpine. To combat xerostomia-related caries, a regimen of daily topical fluoride application should be instituted.

Osteoradionecrosis

Although prevention must be stressed, cases of osteoradionecrosis do occur. Use of hyperbaric oxygen dramatically improves the outcome and is used in combination with antibiotics and local debridement of the infected necrotic bone. Once the diagnosis has been made, therapy must be immediate and aggressive to prevent greater destruction.

ANESTHETIC NECROSIS

Administration of a local anesthetic agent can, on rare occasions, be followed by ulceration and necrosis at the site of injection. This necrosis is thought to result from localized ischemia, although the exact cause is unknown and may vary from case to case. Faulty technique, such as subperiosteal injection or administration of excess solution in tissue firmly bound to bone, has been blamed. The epinephrine contained in many local anesthetics has also received attention as a possible cause of ischemia and secondary necrosis.

Clinical Features

Anesthetic necrosis usually develops several days after the procedure and most commonly presents on the hard palate (Fig. 8–30). A well-circumscribed area of ulceration develops at the site of injection. The ulceration is

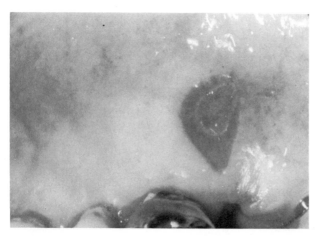

FIGURE 8–30. **Anesthetic necrosis.** Mucosal necrosis of the hard palate secondary to palatal injection with a local anesthetic agent containing epinephrine.

often deep, and on occasion healing may be delayed. One report has documented sequestration of bone at the site of tissue necrosis.

Treatment and Prognosis

Treatment of anesthetic necrosis is usually not required unless the ulceration fails to heal. Minor trauma, such as that caused by performing a cytologic smear, has been reported to induce resolution in these chronic cases. Recurrence is unusual but has been reported in some patients in association with use of epinephrine-containing anesthetics. In these cases, the use of a local anesthetic agent without epinephrine is recommended.

EXFOLIATIVE CHEILITIS (Factitious Cheilitis)

Chronic lip licking, biting, picking, or sucking can cause clinically significant changes on the vermilion border of the lip and, less commonly, on the perioral skin. The most frequently reported pattern is termed **exfoliative cheilitis.** Although other causes, such as cheilitis glandularis, actinic cheilitis, infection, and contact dermatitis, should be ruled out, most cases represent **factitious injuries.** Most patients deny the chronic self-irritation of the area. The patient may be experiencing associated personality disturbances, psychologic difficulties, or stress. In a review of 48 patients with exfoliative cheilitis, 87 percent exhibited psychiatric conditions and 47 percent also demonstrated abnormal thyroid function. There is evidence to suggest that there may be a link between thyroid dysfunction and some psychiatric disturbances.

Clinical Features

A marked female predominance is seen in cases of factitious origin, with most cases affecting those younger than 30 years of age. Mild cases feature chronic dryness, scaling, fissuring, or cracking of the vermilion border of the lip (Fig. 8–31). With progression, the vermilion can become covered with a thickened, yellowish hyperkeratotic crust that can be hemorrhagic or that may exhibit extensive fissuring. When the perioral skin is involved, areas of papular and crusted erythema are noted. The involved skin often forms a semicircle that envelops the affected lip (Fig. 8–32). Both lips or just the lower lip may be involved.

Cheilitis of infectious origin may also be present. The most common presentation of bacterial or fungal infections of the lips is **angular cheilitis** (see p. 166); diffuse primary infection of the entire lip is very unusual. Most diffuse cases represent a secondary candidal infection in areas of low-grade trauma of the vermilion border of the lip (**cheilocandidiasis**).

Rare cases of exfoliative cheilitis may result from photosensitivity or contact allergies to various substances. Phototesting for light sensitivity can be performed by an experienced dermatologist if a correlation with sunlight exposure exists.

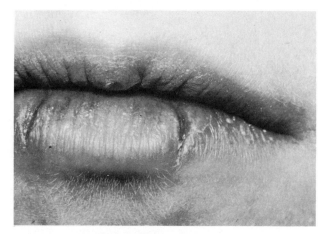

FIGURE 8–31. **Exfoliative cheilitis.** Mild case with scaling and fissuring of the vermilion border of the lower lip.

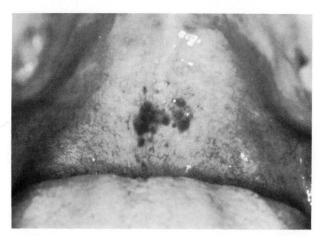

FIGURE 8–33. **Petechiae.** Submucosal hemorrhage of the soft palate caused by violent coughing.

Treatment and Prognosis

In most cases of exfoliative cheilitis, there is no underlying physical, infectious, or allergic cause. Psychotherapy often is combined with mild tranquilization or removal from stress to achieve resolution. Protective moisturizing ointments have been successful in several resistant cases.

Cases that result from candidal infections do not resolve until the chronic trauma is eliminated. Initial topical antifungal agents, antibiotics, or both can be administered to patients in whom chronic trauma is not obvious or is denied. If the condition does not resolve, further investigation is warranted in an attempt to discover the true source of the lip alterations.

SUBMUCOSAL HEMORRHAGE

Everyone has experienced a bruise from minor trauma. This occurs when a traumatic event results in hemorrhage and entrapment of blood within tissues. Different terms are used, depending on the size of the hemorrhage.

1. Minute hemorrhages into skin, mucosa, or serosa are termed **petechiae.**
2. If a slightly larger area is affected, the hemorrhage is a **purpura.**
3. Any accumulation over 2 cm is an **ecchymosis.**
4. If the accumulation of blood within tissue produces a mass, this is a **hematoma.**

Blunt trauma to the oral mucosa often results in hematoma formation. Less well known are petechiae and purpura, which can arise from repeated or prolonged increased intrathoracic pressure (Valsalva maneuver) associated with such activities as repeated coughing, vomiting, convulsions, or giving birth (Fig. 8–33). When considering a diagnosis of traumatic hemorrhage, the clinician should keep in mind that hemorrhages can result from non-traumatic causes, such as thrombocytopenia, disseminated intravascular coagulation (DIC), and a number of viral infections, especially infectious mononucleosis and measles.

Clinical Features

Submucosal hemorrhage appears as a non-blanching flat or elevated zone with a color that varies from red or purple to blue or bluish-black (Fig. 8–34). As would be expected, traumatic lesions are located most frequently on the labial or buccal mucosa. Blunt facial trauma is often responsible, but such injury as minor as cheek biting may produce a hematoma or areas of purpura. Mild pain may be present.

The hemorrhage associated with increased intrathoracic pressure is usually located on the skin of the face and neck and presents as widespread petechiae that clear within 24 to 72 hours. Although it has not been as well documented as the cutaneous lesions, mucosal hemorrhage can be seen in the same setting and most often presents as soft palatal petechiae or purpura.

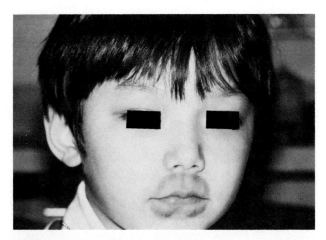

FIGURE 8–32. **Perioral dermatitis.** Perioral crusting and erythema of the skin surface in a child who chronically sucked on both lips.

Treatment and Prognosis

No treatment is required if the hemorrhage is not related to systemic disease, and the areas should resolve

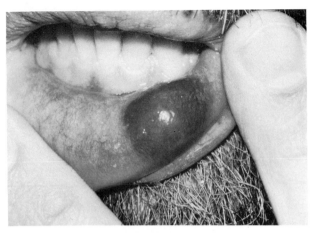

FIGURE 8–34. **Purpura.** Submucosal hemorrhage of the lower labial mucosa on the left side secondary to blunt trauma.

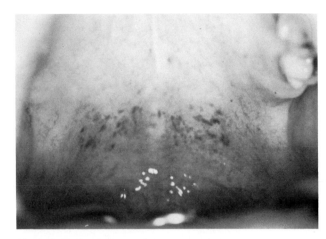

FIGURE 8–35. **Palatal petechiae from fellatio.** Submucosal hemorrhage of the soft palate resulting from the effects of negative pressure.

spontaneously. Large hematomas may require several weeks to resolve. If the hemorrhage occurs secondary to an underlying disorder, treatment is directed toward control of the associated disease.

ORAL TRAUMA FROM SEXUAL PRACTICES

Although orogenital sexual practices are illegal in many jurisdictions, they are extremely common. Among homosexual males and females, orogenital sexual activity is almost universal. For married heterosexual couples under age 25, the frequency has been reported to be as high as 90 percent. Considering the prevalence of these practices, the frequency of associated traumatic oral lesions is surprisingly low.

Clinical Features

The most commonly reported lesion related to orogenital sex is submucosal palatal hemorrhage secondary to fellatio. The lesions present as erythema, petechiae, purpura, or ecchymosis of the soft palate. The areas are often asymptomatic and resolve without treatment in 7 to 10 days (Fig. 8–35). Recurrences are possible with repetition of the inciting (exciting?) event. The erythrocytic extravasation is thought to result from the musculature of the soft palate elevating and tensing against an environment of negative pressure; similar lesions have been induced from forceful sucking on drinking straws and glasses. Forceful thrusting against the vascular soft palate has been suggested as another possible cause.

Oral lesions can also occur from performing cunnilingus. Horizontal ulcerations of the lingual frenum have been reported. As the tongue is thrust forward, the taut frenum rubs or rakes across the incisal edges of the mandibular central incisors. The ulceration created coincides with sharp tooth edges when the tongue is in its most forward position. The lesions resolve in 7 to 10 days but may recur with repeated performances. Linear fibrous hyperplasia has been discovered in the same pattern in individuals who chronically perform the act (Fig. 8–36).

Histopathologic Features

With an appropriate index of suspicion, biopsy is usually not required; however, a biopsy has been performed in some cases of palatal lesions secondary to fellatio. These suction-related lesions reveal subepithelial accumulations of red blood cells that may be extensive enough to separate the surface epithelium from underlying connective tissue. Patchy degeneration of the epithelial basal cell layer can occur. The epithelium classically demonstrates migration of erythrocytes and leukocytes from the underlying lamina propria.

Treatment and Prognosis

No treatment is required, and the prognosis is good. In patients who request assistance, palatal petechiae can be prevented through the use of less negative pressure and avoidance of forceful thrusting. The chance of lingual frenum ulceration can be minimized by smoothing and polishing the rough incisal edges of the adjacent mandibular teeth.

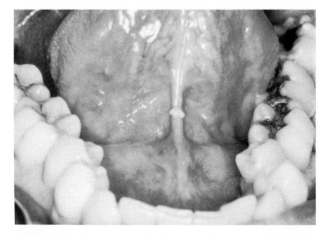

FIGURE 8–36. **Fibrous hyperplasia from repeated cunnilingus.** Linear fibrous hyperplasia of the lingual frenum caused by repeated irritation from lower incisors.

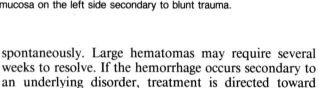

AMALGAM TATTOO AND OTHER LOCALIZED EXOGENOUS PIGMENTATIONS

A number of pigmented materials can be implanted within the oral mucosa, resulting in clinically evident pigmentations. Implantation of dental amalgam (**amalgam tattoo**) occurs most often, with a frequency that far outdistances that for all other materials. "Localized argyrosis" has been used as another name for amalgam tattoo, but this nomenclature is inappropriate because amalgam contains not only silver but also mercury, tin, and other metals.

Amalgam can be incorporated into the oral mucosa in several ways. Previous areas of mucosal abrasion can be contaminated by amalgam dust within the oral fluids. Broken amalgam pieces can fall into extraction sites. If dental floss becomes contaminated with amalgam particles of a recently placed restoration, linear areas of pigmentation can be created in the gingival tissues as a result of hygiene procedures (Fig. 8–37; see Color Figure 47). Amalgam from endodontic retrofill procedures can be left within the soft tissue at the surgical site (Fig. 8–38; see Color Figure 48). Finally, fine metallic particles can be driven through the oral mucosa from the pressure of high-speed air turbine drills.

Theoretically, the use of the rubber dam should decrease the risk, but immediately after removal of the dam, the occlusion is often adjusted with the potential for amalgam contamination of any areas of mucosal damage. Submucosal implantation of pencil graphite, coal and metal dust, fragments of broken carborundum disks, dental burs, and, in the past, charcoal dentifrices, have resulted in similar-appearing areas of discoloration.

Intentional tattooing, which can be found in approximately 25 percent of the world's population, also may be performed in the oral cavity. Although some cases are culturally related, health professionals are also responsi-

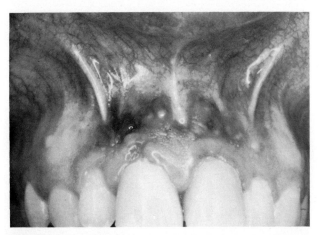

FIGURE 8–38. **Endodontic-related amalgam implantation.** Multifocal areas of mucosal discoloration overlying the maxillary anterior incisors, which have been treated with apical retrofill procedures. See Color Plates.

ble for a number of intentional tattoos for the purpose of demonstrating landmarks, cosmetically disguising disfigured areas, and judging tumor response to antineoplastic therapies. Injudicious intraoral use of these marking agents can cause diffusion of the pigment with discoloration of the adjacent skin surface.

Clinical and Radiographic Features

Amalgam tattoos appear as macules or, rarely, as slightly raised lesions. They may be black, blue, or gray. The borders can be well defined, irregular, or diffuse (Fig. 8–39). Lateral spread may occur for several months after the implantation. In most cases, only one site is affected, although multiple tattoos in a single patient may be present. Any mucosal surface can be involved, but the most common sites are the gingiva, alveolar mucosa, and buccal mucosa (Fig. 8–40).

Periapical radiographs, when taken, are negative in most cases. When metallic fragments are visible radiographically, the clinical area of discoloration typically

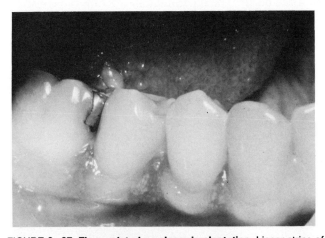

FIGURE 8–37. **Floss-related amalgam implantation.** Linear strips of mucosal pigmentation that align with the interdental papillae. The patient used dental floss on the mandibular first molar immediately after the placement of the amalgam restoration. Because the area was still anesthetized, the patient impaled the floss on the gingiva, then continued forward using the amalgam-impregnated floss in the bicuspid area to create additional amalgam tattoos. See Color Plates.

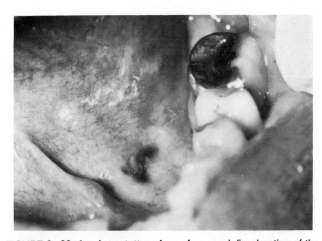

FIGURE 8–39. **Amalgam tattoo.** Area of mucosal discoloration of the floor of the mouth on the patient's left side.

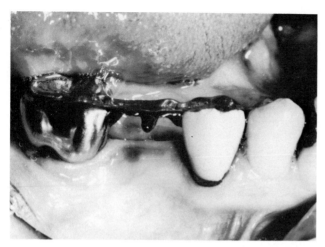

FIGURE 8–40. **Amalgam tattoo.** Area of mucosal discoloration of the mandibular alveolar ridge immediately below the bridge pontic.

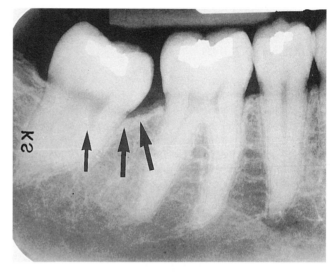

FIGURE 8–42. **Amalgam tattoo.** Radiographic appearance of amalgam tattoo of lingual gingival mucosa adjacent to the mandibular third molar. Note the pinpoint radiopaque metallic fragments overlying the crestal and mesial portions of the root *(arrows)*.

extends beyond the size of the fragment. The fragments are densely radiopaque, varying from several millimeters to pinpoint in size (Figs. 8–41 and 8–42). On occasion, the pattern of the amalgam dispersal has been sufficiently unique to be used as a distinctive characteristic in the identification of unknown deceased individuals.

The pattern of accidental localized foreign body tattoo other than amalgam is diverse and depends on the associated trauma that impacted the material. Mucosal graphite implantation is rarely documented, but it most likely occurs with a higher frequency than indicated by the number of cases reported. Examples in the literature have been presented as grayish areas of mucosal discoloration of the hard palate, the most likely site for pencil-related trauma.

The intentional intraoral tattoos that are not placed by health professionals occur most frequently on the anterior maxillary facial gingiva of Ethiopian women and have been documented at institutions in the United States. In the documented cases, the entire anterior maxillary facial gingiva is given a heavy bluish-black discol-

oration. Occasionally, tattoos are placed on the labial mucosa of adult males in the United States. The pigmentation may be blue or black and usually conveys a vulgar written message.

Histopathologic Features

Microscopic examination of amalgam tattoos reveals scattered fragments of the metal within the connective tissue. Scattered, large, dark, solid fragments or numerous fine, black, or dark-brown granules may be seen (Fig. 8–43). The silver salts of the dental amalgam preferentially stain the reticulin fibers, especially those encircling nerves and vascular channels (Fig. 8–44).

Usually, there is little inflammatory response, but in some instances, significant fibrosis or chronic inflammation can occur. The inflammatory reaction can consist of lymphocytes and histiocytes or foreign-body–type mul-

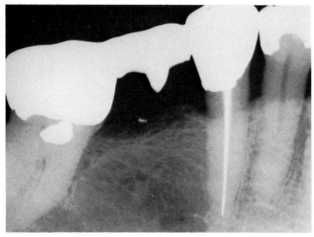

FIGURE 8–41. **Amalgam tattoo.** Radiograph of the same patient depicted in Figure 8–40. Note the radiopaque metallic fragment present at the site of mucosal discoloration.

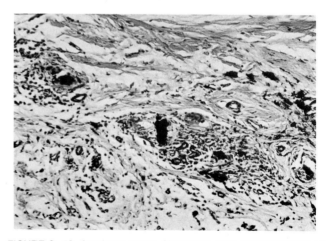

FIGURE 8–43. **Amalgam tattoo.** Numerous dark, solid fragments of amalgam are surrounded by a lymphohistiocytic inflammatory infiltrate.

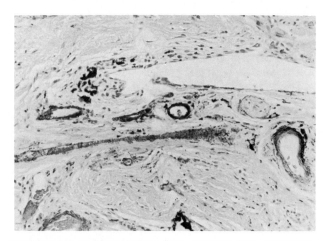

FIGURE 8-44. **Amalgam tattoo.** Dark amalgam stain encircling numerous vascular channels.

tinucleated giant cells. Graphite appears similar microscopically to amalgam; it can be differentiated by its pattern of birefringence after treatment with ammonium sulfide and by the lack of staining of the reticulin fibers. In addition, energy dispersive x-ray microanalysis can be used to identify the type of material present within areas of foreign-body tattoos.

Treatment and Prognosis

To confirm the diagnosis of amalgam tattoo, one can obtain radiographs of the areas of mucosal discoloration in an attempt to demonstrate the metallic fragments. The films should be capable of high detail because many of the fragments are no larger than the point of a pin.

No treatment is required if the fragments can be detected radiographically. If no metallic fragments are found and the lesion cannot be diagnosed clinically, biopsy may be needed to rule out the possibility of melanocytic neoplasia.

SYSTEMIC METALLIC INTOXICATION

Ingestion or exposure to any one of several heavy metals can cause significant systemic and oral abnormalities. Exposure to heavy metals may be massive, resulting in acute reactions, or it may be minimal over a longer period, producing chronic changes. Oral alterations from ingestion of lead, mercury, silver, bismuth, arsenic, and gold are rare but may occur and warrant discussion. Oral complications from excessive zinc, iron, tin, and manganese are extremely rare.

Lead. Little is known about the prevalence of lead poisoning (**plumbism**), but lead is one of the most widespread environmental toxins facing children in the United States. Lead solder was not banned in plumbing until 1986. Homes built before then have the potential for significant water contamination, and one of the pri-

mary causes of lead intoxication in infants is formula preparation using tap water tainted by the metal.

Another significant source of lead poisoning in the young is lead-based paint; children may ingest chips of the paint in older homes or may be exposed to the fumes or dust during sanding and renovation. Adult exposure also occurs and is often related to industry. The potential for exposure exists during handling of lead oxide batteries, in lead processing industries, and from the welding of lead-covered surfaces. Some food and drink containers may also be contaminated with lead.

Mercury. The danger of mercury exposure is well known today. Exposure has occurred in association with the use of mercury in teething powders, cathartic agents, and anthelmintic preparations. A great deal of attention has been directed toward the mercury released from dental amalgams, but no well-documented adverse health effects have been identified except for relatively rare hypersensitivity to mercury. The level of mercury that is released from amalgams does not appear sufficiently high to cause disease.

In spite of the knowledge gained decades ago, scattered problems still arise. Intoxication from chronic household exposure to mercury is still reported secondary to liquid mercury spills that have not been adequately cleaned up. Rare reports of occupation-related incidents in dental offices also occur. As late as 1990, documented cases of mercury intoxication from paint fumes were reported from its incorporation as a preservative in household latex paint.

Silver. Systemic administration of silver was once common, especially in the treatment of gastrointestinal ulcerations, and occasionally silver intoxication resulted. Current examples of silver poisoning are usually restricted to industrial exposure.

Bismuth and Arsenic. Exposure to bismuth and arsenic is mostly historical. The medical use of these metals has dramatically diminished; most current cases arise from occupational exposure. Bismuth was used in the past for treatment of venereal diseases and various dermatoses. Arsenic was used to treat many conditions, especially dermatoses such as psoriasis.

Gold. Gold has been used in medical treatment in the past and continues to be used today in selected cases of active rheumatoid arthritis and other immunologically mediated diseases. In these cases, the side effects are well known and the patients are observed closely by their physician.

Clinical Features

Lead

Lead poisoning results in nonspecific systemic signs and symptoms, thereby making the ultimate diagnosis very difficult. The presentation is extremely variable and is determined by the type of lead (organic or inorganic) and the age of the patient. Patients with acute cases most often present with abdominal colic, which may occur along with anemia, fatigue, irritability, and weakness. Encephalopathy and renal dysfunction also may occur. Chronic exposure causes dysfunction of the nervous system, kidneys, marrow, bone, and joints. Symptoms generally include fatigue, musculoskeletal pain, and headache.

Oral manifestations include ulcerative stomatitis and a gingival *lead line*. The lead line presents as a bluish line along the marginal gingiva resulting from the action of bacterial hydrogen sulfide on lead in the gingival sulcus to produce a precipitate of lead sulfide. Gray areas also may be noted on the buccal mucosa and tongue. Additional manifestations include:

- Tremor of the tongue on thrusting
- Advanced periodontal disease
- Excessive salivation
- A metallic taste

Mercury

Mercury poisoning also may be acute or chronic. With acute cases, abdominal pain, vomiting, diarrhea, thirst, pharyngitis, and gingivitis are typically present. With chronic cases, gastrointestinal upset and numerous neurologic symptoms occur. Oral changes include a metallic taste and ulcerative stomatitis combined with inflammation and enlargement of the salivary glands, gingiva, and tongue. The gingiva may become blue-gray to black. Mercuric sulfide can be generated by the bacterial action on the metal and can cause significant destruction of the alveolar bone with resultant exfoliation of teeth.

Chronic mercury exposure in infants and children is termed **acrodynia (pink disease, Swift disease)**. The children have cold, clammy skin, especially on the hands, feet, nose, ears, and cheeks. An erythematous and pruritic rash is present. Severe sweating, increased lacrimation, irritability, insomnia, photophobia, hypertension, weakness, tachycardia, and gastrointestinal upset also may be present. On occasion, these highly irritable children have torn out patches of their hair. Oral signs include excessive salivation, ulcerative gingivitis, bruxism, and premature loss of teeth. Because mercury salts were formerly used in the processing of felt, hat makers in past centuries were exposed to the metal and experienced similar symptoms, giving rise to the phrase "mad as a hatter."

Silver

Systemic silver intoxication is known as **argyria**. Diffuse grayish-black discoloration of the skin develops primarily in the sun-exposed areas. The sclerae and nails may also be pigmented. The oral cavity may be affected initially and typically presents as a diffuse bluish-black discoloration.

Bismuth

Chronic bismuth exposure can result in a diffuse blue-gray discoloration of the skin. The conjunctiva and oral cavity may also be involved. A blue-gray line along the gingival margin similar to that seen from lead intoxication is the most common intraoral presentation. Bismuth combines with bacterial hydrogen sulfide to form bismuth sulfide, which is irritating locally but not as destructive as mercuric sulfide. Associated ptyalism, burning, stomatitis, and ulceration may be seen.

Arsenic

Prolonged ingestion of arsenic often results in a diffuse macular hyperpigmentation of the skin. The discoloration is due to both the presence of the metal and an increased melanin production. Palmar-plantar hyperkeratosis is also often noted as well as the development of numerous premalignant skin lesions called **arsenical keratoses**. Oral manifestations are rare and typically present as excessive salivation and painful areas of necrotizing ulcerative stomatitis. In the past, extensive dorsal hyperkeratosis of the tongue was seen in patients with syphilis, and this may be related to arsenic therapy used prior to the advent of antibiotic therapy.

Gold

The most common complication of gold therapy is dermatitis, which is often preceded by a warning signal: pruritus. Generalized exfoliative dermatitis with resultant alopecia and loss of nails can be seen.

The second most common adverse reaction to gold is severe oral mucositis, which most frequently involves the buccal mucosa, lateral border of the tongue, palate, and pharynx. A metallic taste often precedes development of the oral lesions and should be considered another warning signal. Therapy with gold rarely can bring about a slate-blue discoloration of sun-exposed skin (**chrysiasis**).

Treatment and Prognosis

The management of heavy metal intoxication involves the use of chelating agents and attempts to limit further exposure to the offending agent. In some cases, a medication may be responsible and can be discontinued, but the source of the metal may be difficult to determine in some instances. Chelating agents that bind and remove the metals are not without their own side effects. They are used primarily in cases of lead and mercury poisoning. Dimercaprol (BAL), dimercaptosuccinic acid, calcium-EDTA, D-penicillamine, and edathamil calcium disodium are examples of chelating agents in current use.

SMOKER'S MELANOSIS

Oral pigmentations are significantly increased in heavy smokers. In one investigation of more than 31,000 whites, 21.5 percent of tobacco smokers exhibited areas of melanin pigmentation compared with 3 percent among those not using tobacco. In another study of an ethnically pigmented population, smokers had more oral surfaces exhibiting melanin pigmentation.

Melanin pigmentation in the skin exerts a well-known protective effect against ultraviolet (UV) damage. Investigations of melanocytes located away from sun-exposed areas have shown the ability of melanin to bind to noxious substances. It has been suggested that melanin production in the oral mucosa of smokers serves as a protective response against some of the harmful substances in tobacco smoke. This has been further substantiated in "reverse" smokers, who smoke with the lit end

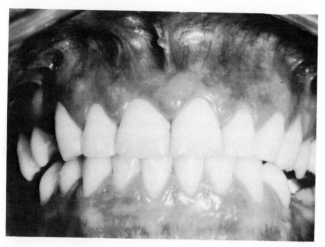

FIGURE 8–45. **Smoker's melanosis.** Light, diffuse melanin pigmentation in a white female who is a heavy smoker. Pigmentary changes are limited to the anterior facial gingiva. See Color Plates.

of the cigarette inside the mouth and who demonstrate heavy melanin pigmentation of the palate. In some reverse smokers, areas of melanocytes are lost and zones of depigmented red mucosa can develop. Cancer is found in 12 percent of patients with these red zones, further delineating the probable protective effects of melanocytes against toxic substances.

Clinical Features

Smoker's melanosis most commonly affects the anterior labial alveolar mucosa. Most people affected by this condition are cigarette users (Fig. 8–45; see Color Figure 49). In contrast, pipe smokers frequently exhibit pigmentations located on the commissural and buccal mucosae. Reverse smokers show alterations of the hard palate.

The areas of pigmentation increase significantly during the first year of smoking and return to normal within 3 years after cessation of smoking. A higher frequency is seen in females, and it has been suggested that female sex hormones exert a synergistic effect when combined with smoking.

Histopathologic Features

Biopsy specimens of affected areas in people with smoker's melanosis reveal an increased melanin pigmentation of the basal cell layer of the surface epithelium, similar to a melanotic macule (see p. 274). In addition, collections of incontinent melanin pigmentation are seen free within the superficial connective tissue and in scattered melanophages.

Diagnosis

The diagnosis can be made by correlating the smoking history with the clinical presentation and medical history. Other causes of melanin pigmentation, such as

trauma, neurofibromatosis, Peutz-Jeghers syndrome, drug-related pigmentation, endocrine disturbances, hemochromatosis, chronic pulmonary disease, and racial pigmentation should be ruled out.

Treatment and Prognosis

Cessation of smoking results in gradual disappearance of the areas of related pigmentation over a 3-year period. Biopsy should be considered when the pigmentation is in unexpected locations, such as the hard palate, or when there are clinically unusual changes, such as increased melanin density or surface elevation.

DRUG-RELATED DISCOLORATIONS OF THE ORAL MUCOSA

An expanding number of medications have been implicated as a cause of oral mucosal discolorations. Although many medications stimulate melanin production by melanocytes, deposition of drug metabolites is responsible for the color change in others. These pigmentary alterations have been associated with use of phenolphthalein, minocycline, tranquilizers, antimalarial medications, estrogen, chemotherapeutic agents, and some medications used in the treatment of patients with acquired immunodeficiency syndrome (AIDS).

The antimalarial agents that are most frequently implicated are chloroquine, hydrochloroquine, quinidine, and quinacrine; chlorpromazine represents the most frequently implicated tranquilizer. Besides treating malaria, these medications are used for many other disorders, including lupus erythematosus and rheumatoid arthritis.

Oral mucosal pigmentation associated with chemotherapeutic medications is most commonly associated with use of doxorubicin, busulfan, cyclophosphamide, or 5-fluorouracil. Although idiopathic hyperpigmentation may also occur, AIDS patients receiving zidovudine (AZT), clofazimine, or ketoconazole have demonstrated increased melanin pigmentation.

Clinical Features

The clinical presentations of pigmentations related to drug use vary. Most agents produce a diffuse melanosis of the skin and mucosal surfaces, but others may cause a more unique pattern. As in many cases of increased melanin pigmentation, females are more sensitive, most likely as a result of an interaction with sex hormones.

Use of phenolphthalein as a laxative has been associated with numerous small, well-circumscribed areas of hyperpigmentation on the skin. Similar areas of oral mucosal melanosis also can occur.

Long-term use of minocycline, a semisynthetic derivative of tetracycline, results in discoloration of the bone and developing teeth. The affected bone appears dark-green and causes a blue-gray discoloration of the translucent oral mucosa. The most noticeable zone is a linear band on the facial attached gingiva near the mucogingival junction.

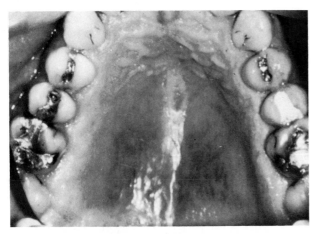

FIGURE 8-46. **Chlorpromazine pigmentation.** Diffuse grayish pigmentation of the hard palate.

The classic presentation of intraoral pigmentation from use of antimalarial medications or tranquilizers is a bluish-black discoloration limited to the hard palate (Fig. 8-46). In addition, the intake of antimalarial medications occasionally may lead to a more diffuse brown melanosis of the oral mucosa and skin.

Estrogen, chemotherapeutic agents, and medications used in the treatment of AIDS patients may result in a diffuse brown melanosis of the skin and mucosal surfaces. Any mucosal surface may be involved, but the attached gingiva and buccal mucosa are affected most frequently. The pattern and appearance of the oral mucosal involvement are similar to those seen in racial pigmentation.

Treatment and Prognosis

Although the discolorations of the oral mucosa may be aesthetically displeasing, they cause no long-term problems. In most instances, discontinuing the medication results in gradual fading of the areas of hyperpigmentation.

TRAUMATIC OSSEOUS AND CHONDROMATOUS METAPLASIA (Cutright Lesion)

In denture wearers, flabby edentulous alveolar ridges may occur from fibrous hyperplasia in areas of extensive alveolar resorption. In histopathologic reviews of this excess fibrous material, the presence of bone or cartilage separate from the underlying periosteum occasionally can be found within the collagen. Although cartilaginous rests are known to exist in the area of the nasopalatine duct, most of the bone and cartilage found in these flabby ridges is thought to represent **osseous and chondromatous metaplasia** from mechanical irritation of the denture. This theory is supported by the occurrence of metaplastic changes in the posterior regions and overlying the mandibular alveolar ridge where cartilaginous rests are not present.

Clinical and Radiographic Features

Alveolar atrophy with secondary fibrous hyperplasia overlying the alveolar ridges occurs predominantly in the anterior maxilla as a result of the pressure of complete maxillary dentures. It is more severe when natural dentition is present in the anterior mandible. Consequently, most cases of osseous and chondromatous metaplasia have been discovered in the soft tissue overlying the anterior maxillary alveolar ridge. The anterior mandible is a distant second in frequency. Posterior maxillary and mandibular lesions are infrequent.

The clinical appearance varies from raised, reddened, ulcerated areas to firm, movable, polyp-like lesions. Radiographs may occasionally demonstrate areas of radiopacity separate from the underlying alveolar ridge.

A similar but different pattern of cartilage or cellular bone development occurs along the crest of thin atrophic alveolar ridges. The patient presents with an extremely tender and localized area of the alveolar ridge that may reveal an enlargement (Fig. 8-47). These changes also appear secondary to mechanical trauma and represent localized areas of periosteal hyperplasia in which the superficial zones of the periosteum demonstrate metaplastic cartilage or bone.

Histopathologic Features

The fibrous connective tissue removed from flabby ridges varies in density and completely surrounds the areas of metaplastic bone or cartilage (Fig. 8-48). Chondroid metaplasia may be characterized by either hyaline cartilage or fibrocartilage, and it usually appears cytologically benign (Fig. 8-49). In some instances, the cartilage may be atypical, with significant pleomorphism and multiple nuclei within a single chondrocyte. In osseous metaplasia, the bone is predominantly woven in appearance, often with osteoid rimming, but with rare osteoblasts. The cartilage and bone found overlying thin atrophic ridges appear similar but are located along the superficial edge of the periosteum. The cellular periosteum is thick-

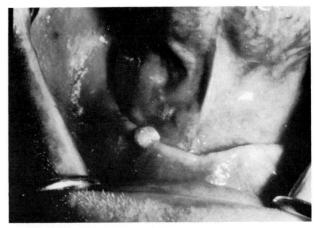

FIGURE 8-47. **Periosteal hyperplasia with osseous and chondromatous metaplasia.** Tender, elevated nodule along the thin crest of the mandibular alveolar ridge. (Courtesy of Dr. Steven Tucker.)

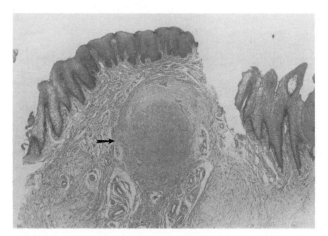

FIGURE 8–48. **Chondromatous metaplasia.** Circumscribed area of hyaline cartilage (*arrow*) completely surrounded by fibrous connective tissue of the maxillary alveolar ridge.

ened in this location and often forms an elevated spire-like projection.

Benign cartilage proliferations are rare in the jaws; therefore, in microscopically atypical cases of chondromatous metaplasia, misdiagnosis as chondrosarcoma is possible, especially if an inadequate patient history is provided.

Treatment and Prognosis

The flabby ridges can be recontoured and the dentures reconstructed. Thin ridges may be recontoured or supplemented with graft material to improve shape and to alleviate the symptoms associated with the localized periosteal hyperplasia.

ANTRAL PSEUDOCYSTS

Antral pseudocysts are common findings on panoramic radiographs. They present as dome-shaped, faintly

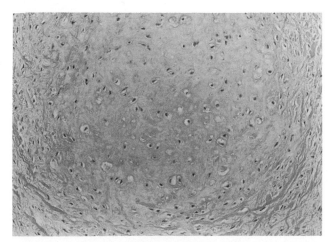

FIGURE 8–49. **Chondromatous metaplasia.** Higher-power photomicrograph of metaplastic cartilage depicted in Figure 8–48. Note the numerous chondrocytes surrounded by hyaline matrix and located within lacunae.

radiopaque lesions arising from the floor of the maxillary sinus. In the past, these sinus changes were incorrectly termed **sinus mucoceles** because previous investigators thought that the lesions resulted from mucus extravasation similar to that seen in salivary glands of soft tissue. In fact, it appears that no comparable mucus extravasation occurs in the maxillary sinus. In two excellent articles by Gardner, the differences between antral pseudocysts, retention cysts, and sinus mucoceles have finally been delineated.

Antral Pseudocyst. "Antral pseudocyst" is the best term for the dome-shaped lesion of the sinus floor. The process usually consists of an inflammatory exudate (serum, not mucin) that has accumulated under the maxillary sinus mucosa and caused a sessile elevation. The exudate is surrounded by connective tissue, and the epithelial lining of the sinus is superior to the fluid. Reviews of large numbers of radiographs have determined the prevalence, which varies from 1.5 to 10 percent of the population. The cause of the inflammatory infiltrate has not been definitively determined, but in a radiographic review, most cases showed a possible source from an adjacent odontogenic infection. Primary irritation of the sinus lining, such as that seen from a sinus infection, can also theoretically result in the subperiosteal inflammatory infiltrate.

Sinus Mucoceles. True sinus mucoceles are accumulations of mucin that are completely encased by epithelium. They occur in two situations.

One type of sinus mucocele occurs after trauma or surgery to the sinus; this type is best known as a **surgical ciliated cyst** or **postoperative maxillary cyst**. A portion of the sinus lining becomes separated from the main body of the sinus and forms an epithelium-lined cavity into which mucin is secreted. The cyst most frequently originates after a Caldwell-Luc operation but may arise from difficult extraction of a maxillary tooth in which the floor of the maxillary sinus is damaged.

The second type of sinus mucocele arises from an obstruction of the sinus ostium, thereby blocking normal drainage. This blocked sinus then acts like a separate cyst-like structure lined by epithelium and filled with mucin.

Sinus mucoceles enlarge in size as the intraluminal pressure increases and can distend the walls of the sinus and erode through bone, often clinically mimicking malignancy of antral origin.

Retention Cysts. Retention cysts of the maxillary sinus arise from the partial blockage of a duct of the seromucous glands or from an invagination of the respiratory epithelium. The mucin is surrounded by epithelium, and no extravasation occurs. Most retention cysts are located around the ostium or within antral polyps. The majority are small and not evident clinically.

Clinical and Radiographic Features

Many symptoms have been attributed to "sinus mucoceles"; however, because of the confusion between pseudocysts and true mucoceles, it is unclear which symptoms are associated with pseudocysts and which are related to true sinus mucoceles. Most pseudocysts are

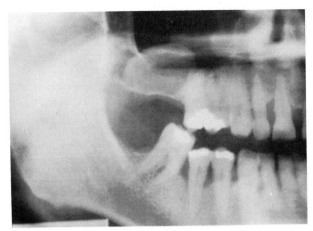

FIGURE 8-50. **Antral pseudocyst.** Dome-shaped radiopacity within the maxillary sinus.

asymptomatic. As true sinus mucoceles enlarge and expand bone, symptoms may develop and vary according to the location and the degree of expansion and destruction.

Radiographically, the pseudocyst classically appears as a dome-shaped and slightly radiopaque lesion on the intact floor of the maxillary sinus (Fig. 8-50). When the maxillary sinus is involved by a true sinus mucocele, the entire sinus will be cloudy. As the lesion enlarges, the walls of the sinus may become thinned and eventually eroded. Surgical ciliated cysts are spherical lesions that are separate from the sinus and lack the dome-shaped appearance of pseudocysts. As these postoperative cysts enlarge, they too can lead to perforation of the sinus walls. Retention cysts rarely reach a size that would produce detectable radiographic changes.

Treatment and Prognosis

Pseudocysts of the maxillary sinus are harmless, and no treatment is necessary. The adjacent teeth should be thoroughly evaluated, and any foci of infection should be eliminated. A few clinicians prefer to confirm their radiographic impression and rule out a tumor through drainage of the inflammatory exudate. Removal by means of a Caldwell-Luc operation should be performed on any radiographically diagnosed lesion that produces significant expansion or is definitively associated with symptoms such as headache.

True sinus mucoceles, including surgical ciliated cysts, are expansile and destructive lesions that should be surgically eliminated.

CERVICOFACIAL EMPHYSEMA

Cervicofacial emphysema arises from the introduction of air into subcutaneous or fascial spaces of the face and neck. The forced air may spread through the spaces to the retropharyngeal and mediastinal areas. The first case was reported almost 100 years ago and occurred as a result of blowing into a bugle a short time after tooth extraction.

Cervicofacial emphysema of dental origin may arise in several ways:

- Following the use of compressed air by the clinician
- After difficult or prolonged extractions
- As a result of increased intraoral pressure (e.g., sneezing, blowing) following an oral surgical procedure
- From no obvious cause

Introduction of air within tissue has been seen following a large number of dental procedures, but most instances involve either surgical extraction of teeth, osteotomies, significant trauma, or the use of air or water syringes. In addition, the prevalence has increased as a result of the use of air-driven handpieces during oral surgery. Conservative surgical flap design without extension into fascial planes and limited use of air-driven handpieces during surgical procedures may minimize the chance of occurrence.

Clinical and Radiographic Features

More than 90 percent of cases of cervicofacial emphysema develop during surgery or within the first postoperative hour. Cases with delayed onset are associated with increased postoperative pressure created by the patient. The initial change is one of soft tissue enlargement from the presence of the air in deeper tissues (Fig. 8-51). Pain

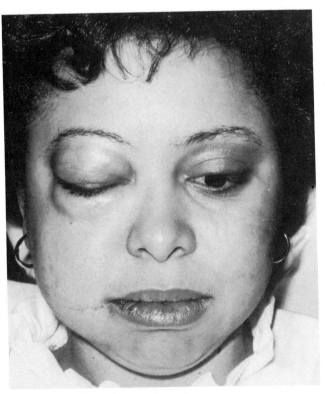

FIGURE 8-51. **Cervicofacial emphysema.** Periorbital and facial enlargement caused by use of an air-driven handpiece during third molar removal.

is usually minimal, and crepitus is detected easily on gentle palpation. Subsequently, the enlargement increases and spreads because of secondary inflammation and edema. Variable pain, facial erythema, and mild fever may occur. Significant spread into the mediastinum can result in dysphonia, dysphagia, or dyspnea. Cardiac auscultation often reveals crepitus synchronous with the heart beat (*Hamman's crunch*) in cases with mediastinal involvement. Pneumomediastinum can be confirmed on chest radiographs by observing displacement of the mediastinal pleura.

Treatment and Prognosis

Broad-spectrum antibiotic coverage is recommended in all dental-related cases. The entrapped air is gradually removed by the body over a 2- to 5-day period. Most cases resolve spontaneously without significant difficulty. Rare cases of respiratory distress have been noted, and assisted ventilation was required.

MYOSPHERULOSIS

Placement of topical tetracycline in a petrolatum base into a surgical site may occasionally result in an unique foreign-body reaction, known as **myospherulosis**. The resultant histopathologic pattern is most unusual and initially was mistakenly thought to represent a previously undescribed endosporulating fungus.

Clinical and Radiographic Features

Myospherulosis may occur at any site within soft tissue or bone where the antibiotic has been placed. The initial report described involvement of the arms, legs, and gluteal and scapular regions. Most cases in the dental literature have occurred within bone at previous extraction sites where an antibiotic had been placed in an attempt to prevent alveolar osteitis. Most cases have occurred within mandibular surgical sites, although maxillary and oral soft tissue examples have been documented.

The involved area may exhibit swelling, or it may be discovered as an asymptomatic and circumscribed radiolucency in a previous extraction site (Fig. 8–52). In some cases, pain and purulent drainage have resulted. On exploration of the lesion, a black, greasy, tar-like material is found.

Histopathologic Features

The histopathologic pattern is unique and the result of a tissue interaction with both the petroleum base and the tetracycline. Dense collagenous tissue is intermixed with a granulomatous inflammatory response showing macrophages and multinucleated giant cells. Within the connective tissue are multiple cyst-like spaces that contain numerous brown- to black-staining spherules (Fig. 8–53). The collections of spherules are sometimes surrounded by an outer membrane known as a "parent body," forming structures that resemble a "bag of marbles." The spherules represent red blood cells that have

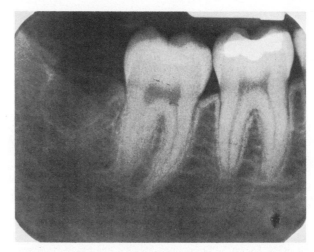

FIGURE 8–52. Myospherulosis. Radiolucency has persisted following extraction of the mandibular third molar. An antibiotic ointment was placed at the time of initial surgery. (Courtesy of Dr. Tony Traynham.)

been altered by the medication. The unusual dark coloration is due to the degradation of hemoglobin.

Treatment and Prognosis

Myospherulosis is treated by surgical removal of the foreign material and associated tissue. Histopathologic examination of the altered tissue provides the definitive diagnosis. Recurrence is not expected.

A similar clinical and radiographic pattern has been seen in association with the use of powdered tetracycline in a polymer dressing. Although somewhat different histopathologically, this formulation also leads to a granulomatous foreign-body reaction. Because of complications associated with both formulations, the practice of applying topical antibiotics to oral wounds should be approached with caution, and other methods of delivery should be considered. If topical antibiotics are used, they should be accompanied by close follow-up to ensure appropriate clinical and radiographic evidence of healing of the surgical site.

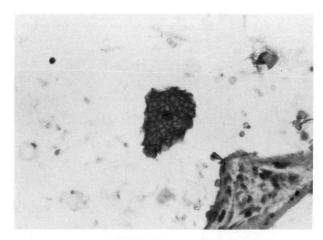

FIGURE 8–53. Myospherulosis. Collection ("parent body") of brown-staining spherules in a cyst-like space.

REFERENCES

Linea Alba

Kashani HG, Mackenzie IC, Kerber PE. Cytology of linea alba using a filter imprint technique. Clin Prev Dent 2:21–24, 1980.

Wood NK, Goaz PW. Differential Diagnosis of Oral Lesions, 4th ed. St. Louis, Mosby–Year Book, 1991, pp 114–115.

Morsicatio Buccarum

Bouquot JE. Common oral lesions found during a mass screening examination. J Am Dent Assoc 112:50–57, 1986.

Hjørting-Hansen E, Holst E. Morsicatio mucosae oris and suctio mucosae oris: An analysis of oral mucosal changes due to biting and sucking habits. Scand J Dent Res 78:492–499, 1970.

Kocsard E, et al. Morsicatio buccarum. Br J Dermatol 74:454–457, 1962.

Sewerin I. A clinical and epidemiologic study of morsicatio buccarum/labiorum. Scand J Dent Res 79:73–80, 1971.

Schiödt M, Larsen V, Bessermann M. Oral findings in glassblowers. Community Dent Oral Epidemiol 8:195–200, 1980.

Van Wyk CW, Staz J, Farman AG. The chewing lesion of the cheeks and lips: Its features and the prevalence among a selected group of adolescents. J Dent 5:193–199, 1977.

Traumatic Ulcerations

Bhaskar SN, Lilly GE. Traumatic granuloma of the tongue (human and experimental). Oral Surg Oral Med Oral Pathol 18:206–218, 1964.

El-Mofty SK, et al. Eosinophilic ulcer of the oral mucosa: Report of 38 new cases with immunohistochemical observations. Oral Surg Oral Med Oral Pathol 75:716–722, 1993.

Elzay RP. Traumatic ulcerative granuloma with stromal eosinophilia (Riga-Fede's disease and traumatic eosinophilic granuloma). Oral Surg Oral Med Oral Pathol 55:497–506, 1983.

Eversole LR, et al. Atypical histiocytic granuloma: Light microscopic, ultrastructural, and histochemical findings in an unusual pseudomalignant reactive lesion of the oral cavity. Cancer 55:1722–1729, 1985.

Kabani S, et al. Atypical lymphohistiocytic infiltrate (pseudolymphoma) of the oral cavity. Oral Surg Oral Med Oral Pathol 66:587–592, 1988.

Regezi JA, et al. Oral traumatic granuloma: Characterization of the cellular infiltrate. Oral Surg Oral Med Oral Pathol 75:723–727, 1993.

Rodriguez JCV, et al. Atypical histiocytic granuloma of the tongue: Case report. Br J Oral Maxillofac Surg 29:350–352, 1991.

Sklavounou A, Laskaris G. Eosinophilic ulcer of the oral mucosa. Oral Surg Oral Med Oral Pathol 58:431–436, 1984.

Wright JM, Rankin KV, Wilson JW. Traumatic granuloma of the tongue. Head Neck Surg 5:363–366, 1983.

Electrical Burns

Colcleugh RG, Ryan JE. Splinting electrical burns of the mouth in children. Plast Recontr Surg 58:239–241, 1976.

Czerepak CS. Oral splint therapy to manage electrical burns of the mouths in children. Clin Plast Surg 11:685–692, 1984.

Gormley MB, et al. Thermal trauma: A review of 22 electrical burns of the lip. J Oral Surg 30:531–533, 1972.

Leake JE, Curtin JW. Electrical burns of the mouth in children. Clin Plast Surg 11:669–683, 1986.

Thomson HG, Juckes AW, Farmer AW. Electrical burns to the mouth in children. Plast Reconstr Surg 35:466–477, 1965.

Oral Adverse Reactions to Chemicals

Baruchin AM, et al. Burns of the oral mucosa: Report of 6 cases. J Craniomaxillofac Surg 19:94–96, 1991.

Buck IF, et al. The treatment of intraoral chemical burns. J Oral Ther 2:101–106, 1965.

Fanibunda KB. Adverse response to endodontic material containing paraformaldehyde. Br Dent J 157:231–235, 1984.

Fletcher PD, Wyman BS, Scopp IW. Acute necrotizing ulcerative gingivitis—sequelae following treatment with silver nitrate. N Y J Dent 46:122–124, 1976.

Frost DE, Barkmeier WW, Abrams H. Aphthous ulcer—a treatment complication. Oral Surg Oral Med Oral Pathol 45:863–869, 1978.

Gatot A, et al. Effects of sodium hypochlorite on soft tissues after its inadvertent injection beyond the root apex. J Endod 17:573–574, 1991.

Maron FS. Mucosal burn resulting from chewable aspirin: Report of case. J Am Dent Assoc 119:279–280, 1989.

Rees TD, Orth CF. Oral ulcerations with use of hydrogen peroxide. J Periodontol 57:689–692, 1986.

Noninfectious Complications of Antineoplastic Therapy

Dreizen S. Description and incidence of oral complications. Consensus Development Conference on Oral Complications of Cancer Therapies: Diagnosis, Prevention, and Treatment. NCI Monogr 9:11–15, 1990.

Ferretti GA, et al. Oral antimicrobial agents—chlorhexidine. Consensus Development Conference on Oral Complications of Cancer Therapies: Diagnosis, Prevention, and Treatment. NCI Monogr 9:51–55, 1990.

Friedman RB. Osteoradionecrosis: Causes and prevention. Consensus Development Conference on Oral Complications of Cancer Therapies: Diagnosis, Prevention, and Treatment. NCI Monogr 9:145–149, 1990.

Greenspan D. Management of salivary dysfunction. Consensus Development Conference on Oral Complications of Cancer Therapies: Diagnosis, Prevention, and Treatment. NCI Monogr 9:159–161, 1990.

Holmes S. The oral complications of specific anticancer therapy. Int J Nurs Stud 28:343–360, 1991.

Miaskowski C. Management of mucositis during therapy. Consensus Development Conference on Oral Complications of Cancer Therapies: Diagnosis, Prevention, and Treatment. NCI Monogr 9:95–98, 1990.

Anesthetic Necrosis

Carroll MJ. Tissue necrosis following a buccal infiltration. Br Dent J 149:209–210, 1980.

Giunta J, et al. Postanesthetic necrotic defect. Oral Surg Oral Med Oral Pathol 40:590–593, 1975.

Schaffer J, Calman HI, Levy B. Changes in the palate color and form (Case 9). Dent Radiogr Photogr 39:3–6, 19–22, 1966.

Exfoliative Cheilitis

Blanton PL, Hurt WC, Largent MD. Oral factitious injuries. J Periodontol 48:33–37, 1977.

Brooke RI. Exfoliative cheilitis. Oral Surg Oral Med Oral Pathol 45:52–55, 1978.

Crotty CP, Dicken CH. Factitious lip crusting. Arch Dermatol 117:338–340, 1981.

Gaffoor PMA. Perioral contact dermatitis: A case report. Cutis 33:280, 1984.

Reade PC, Sim R. Exfoliative cheilitis—a factitious disorder? Int J Oral Maxillofac Surg 15:313–317, 1986.

Tyldesley WR. Exfoliative cheilitis. Br J Oral Surg 10:357–359, 1973.

Thomas JR, Greene SL, Dicken CH. Factitious cheilitis. J Am Acad Dermatol 8:368–372, 1983.

Submucosal Hemorrhage

Alcalay J, Ingber A, Sandbank M. Mask phenomenon: Postemesis facial purpura. Cutis 38:28, 1986.

Kravitz P. The clinical picture of "cough purpura", benign and nonthrombocytopenia eruption. Va Med 106:373–374, 1979.

Wilkin JK. Benign parturient purpura. JAMA 239:930, 1978.

Wood NK, Goaz PW. Differential Diagnosis of Oral Lesions, 4th ed. St. Louis, Mosby–Year Book, 1991, p 65.

Oral Trauma from Sexual Practices

Damm DD, White DK, Brinker CM. Variations of palatal erythema secondary to fellatio. Oral Surg Oral Med Oral Pathol 52:417–421, 1981.

Elam AL. Sexually related trauma: A review. Ann Emerg Med 15:576–584, 1986.

Farman AG, Van Wyk CW. The features of non-infectious oral lesions caused by fellatio. J Dent Assoc S Africa 32:53–55, 1977.

Leider AS. Intraoral ulcers of questionable origin. J Am Dent Assoc 92:1177–1178, 1976.

Mader CL. Lingual frenum ulcer resulting from orogenital sex. J Am Dent Assoc 103:888–890, 1981.

Terezhalmy GT. Oral manifestations of sexually related diseases. Ear Nose Throat J 62:287–296, 1983.

Van Wyk CW. Oral lesions caused by habits. Forensic Sci 7:41–49, 1976.

Localized Exogenous Pigmentations

Buchner A, Hansen LS. Amalgam pigmentation (amalgam tattoo) of the oral mucosa: A clinicopathologic study of 268 cases. Oral Surg Oral Med Oral Pathol 49:139–147, 1980.

Daley TD, Gibson D. Practical applications of energy dispersive x-ray microanalysis in diagnostic oral pathology. Oral Surg Oral Med Oral Pathol 69:339–344, 1990.

Mani NJ. Gingival tattoo: A hitherto undescribed mucosal pigmentation. Quintessence Int 16:157–159, 1985.

Müller H, van der Velden/Samderubun EM. Tattooing in maxillofacial surgery. J. Craniomaxillofac Surg 16:382–384, 1988.

Peters E, Gardner DG. A method of distinguishing between amalgam and graphite in tissue. Oral Surg Oral Med Oral Pathol 62:73–76, 1986.

Slabbert H, Ackermann GL, Altini M. Amalgam tattoo as a means for person identification. J Forensic Odontostomatol 9:17–23, 1991.

Weathers DR, Fine RM. Amalgam tattoo of oral mucosa. Arch Dermatol 110:727–728, 1974.

Systemic Metal Intoxication

Agocs MM, et al. Mercury exposure from interior latex paint. N Engl J Med 323:1096–1101, 1990.

Cohen MM. Stomatologic alterations in childhood. Part II. ASDC J Dent Child 44:327–335, 1977.

Dummett CO. Oral mucosal discolorations related to pharmacotherapeutics. J Oral Ther 1:106–110, 1964.

Dummett CO. Systemic significance of oral pigmentation and discoloration. Postgrad Med 49(1):78–82, 1971.

Gordon NC, et al. Lead poisoning: A comprehensive review and report of a case. Oral Surg Oral Med Oral Pathol 47:500–512, 1979.

Granstein RD, Sober AJ. Drug- and heavy metal-induced hyperpigmentation. J Am Acad Dermatol 5:1–18, 1981.

Iyer K, et al. Mercury poisoning in a dentist. Arch Neurol 33:788–790, 1976.

Shannon MW, Graef JW. Lead intoxication in infancy. Pediatrics 89:87–90, 1992.

Smoker's Melanosis

Axéll T, Hedin CA. Epidemiologic study of excessive oral melanin pigmentation with special reference to the influence of tobacco habits. Scand J Dent Res 90:434–442, 1982.

Brown FH, Houston GD. Smoker's melanosis: A case report. J Periodontol 62:524–527, 1991.

Hedin CA. Smokers' melanosis. Arch Dermatol 113:1533–1538, 1977.

Hedin CA, Axéll T. Oral melanin pigmentation in 467 Thai and Malaysian people with special emphasis on smoker's melanosis. J Oral Pathol Med 20:8–12, 1991.

Hedin CA, Larsson Å. The ultrastructure of the gingival epithelium in smokers' melanosis. J Periodontal Res 19:177–190, 1984.

Hedin CA, et al. Melanin depigmentation of the palatal mucosa in reverse smokers: A preliminary study. J Oral Pathol Med 21:440–444, 1992.

Drug-Related Discolorations of the Oral Mucosa

Birek C, Main JHP. Two cases of oral pigmentation associated with quinidine therapy. Oral Surg Oral Med Oral Pathol 66:59–61, 1988.

Cale AE, Freedman PD, Lumerman H. Pigmentation of the jawbones and teeth secondary to minocycline hydrochloride therapy. J Periodontol 59:112–114, 1988.

Dummett CO. Oral mucosal discolorations related to pharmacotherapeutics. J Oral Ther Pharm 1:106–110, 1964.

Granstein RD, Sober AJ. Drug- and heavy metal-induced hyperpigmentation. J Am Acad Dermatol 5:1–18, 1981.

Hood AF. Cutaneous side effects of cancer chemotherapy. Med Clin North Am 70:187–209, 1986.

Langford A, et al. Oral hyperpigmentation in HIV-infected patients. Oral Surg Oral Med Oral Pathol 67:301–307, 1989.

Levy H. Chloroquine-induced pigmentation: Case reports. S Afr Med J 62:735–737, 1982.

Pérusse R, Morency R. Oral pigmentation induced by Premarin. Cutis 48:61–64, 1991.

Traumatic Osseous and Chondromatous Metaplasia

Cutright DE. Osseous and chondromatous metaplasia caused by dentures. Oral Surg Oral Med Oral Pathol 34:625–633, 1972.

Lello GE, Makek M. Submucosal nodular chondrometaplasia in denture wearers. J Prosthet Dent 54:237–240, 1985.

Magnusson BC, Engström H, Kahnberg K-E. Metaplastic formation of bone and chondroid in flabby ridges. Br J Oral Maxillofac Surg 24:300–305, 1986.

Antral Pseudocysts

Allard RHB, van der Kwast WAM, van der Waal I. Mucosal antral cysts: Review of the literature and report of a radiographic survey. Oral Surg Oral Med Oral Pathol 51:2–9, 1981.

Gardner DG. Pseudocysts and retention cysts of the maxillary sinus. Oral Surg Oral Med Oral Pathol 58:561–567, 1984.

Gardner DG, Gullane PJ. Mucoceles of the maxillary sinus. Oral Surg Oral Med Oral Pathol 62:538–543, 1986.

Gregory GT, Shafer WG. Surgical ciliated cysts of the maxilla: Report of cases. J Oral Surg 16:251–253, 1958.

Halstead CL. Mucosal cysts of the maxillary sinus: Report of 75 cases. J Am Dent Assoc 87:1435–1441, 1973.

Kaneshiro S, et al. The postoperative maxillary cyst: Report of 71 cases. J Oral Surg 39:191–198, 1981.

Paparella MM. Mucosal cyst of the maxillary sinus: Diagnosis and management. Arch Otolaryngol 77:650–657, 1963.

Zizmor J, Noyek AM, Chapnik JS. Mucocele of the paranasal sinuses. Can J Otolaryngol 3(Suppl 1):1–30, 1974.

Cervicofacial Emphysema

Horowitz I, Hirshberg A, Freedman A. Pneumomediastinum and subcutaneous emphysema following surgical extraction of mandibular third molars: Three case reports. Oral Surg Oral Med Oral Pathol 63:25–28, 1987.

Kullaa-Mikkonen A, Mikkonen M. Subcutaneous emphysema. Br J Oral Surg 20:200–202, 1982.

Monsour PA, Savage NW. Cervicofacial emphysema following dental procedures. Aust Dent J 34:403–406, 1989.

Reznick JB, Ardary WC. Cervicofacial subcutaneous air emphysema after dental extraction. J Am Dent Assoc 120:417–419, 1990.

Myospherulosis

Dunlap CL, Barker BF. Myospherulosis of the jaws. Oral Surg Oral Med Oral Pathol 50:238–243, 1980.

Lynch DP, Newland JR, McClendon JL. Myospherulosis of the oral hard and soft tissues. J Oral Maxillofac Surg 42:349–355, 1984.

Moore JW, Brekke JH. Foreign body giant cell reaction related to placement of tetracycline-treated polylactic acid: Report of 18 cases. J Oral Maxillofac Surg 48:808–812, 1990.

Wallace ML, Neville BW. Myospherulosis: Report of a case. J Periodontol 61:55–57, 1990.

9

Allergies and Immunologic Diseases

RECURRENT APHTHOUS STOMATITIS
(Recurrent Aphthous Ulcerations; Canker Sores)

Recurrent aphthous stomatitis is one of the most common oral mucosal pathologic conditions. The reported prevalence in the general population varies from 5 to 66 percent, with a mean of 20 percent. The hypotheses of its pathogenesis are numerous. As soon as one investigator claims to have discovered the definitive cause, a subsequent report discredits the first. Different subgroups of patients appear to have different causes for the occurrence of aphthae. These factors suggest a disease process that may be induced by a variety of etiologic agents, each of which is capable of producing the disease in certain subgroups of patients. To state it simply, the causation appears to be "different things in different people."

The literature points to an immunologic basis that appears to be a primary cause in some and a secondary cause in others. Analysis of the peripheral T lymphocytes in patients with aphthae shows a decreased ratio of T-helper (CD4+) cells to T-suppressor/cytotoxic (CD8+) cells. When aphthae have been investigated locally in oral mucosa, increased percentages of CD8+ cytotoxic cells have been seen. Evidence of the destruction of the oral mucosa mediated by these lymphocytes is strong, but the initiating cause is elusive. The following all have been reported to be responsible in certain subgroups of patients (and each discounted in other subgroups!):

- Allergies
- Genetic predisposition
- Hematologic abnormalities
- Hormonal influences
- Infectious agents
- Nutritional imbalances
- Trauma
- Stress

When all the various subgroups are combined, the various causations cluster into three categories:

- Primary immunodysregulation
- Decrease of the mucosal barrier
- Increase in antigenic exposure

One or more of these three factors may be involved in subgroups of patients.

Primary immunodysregulation is supported by several investigators who have associated certain histocompatibility antigen (HLA) types with subgroups of patients with aphthous stomatitis. HLA-B12, B51, and Cw7 are some of the numerous types that have been mentioned; as expected, however, these findings are not present consistently. Interestingly, the predominantly mucocutaneous form of Behçet's disease (Behçet's syndrome) (see p. 239) exhibits significant aphthous-like oral ulcerations and also has been associated with HLA-B12. Two other disorders—Crohn's disease (see p. 620) and celiac disease—have been associated with certain HLA types and exhibit an increased frequency of aphthous-like ulcerations.

Stress, with its presumed effects on the immune system, directly correlates with the presence of aphthous stomatitis in some groups. In studies of professional students, recurrences clustered around stressful periods of the academic year, and periods of vacation were associated with a low frequency of lesions. Aphthous-like ulcerations have occurred in patients with systemic immunodysregulations. Patients with cyclic neutropenia (see p. 424) occasionally have cycles of aphthous-like ulcerations that correspond to the periods of severe immunodysregulation. Resolution of the neutropenia terminates the cycle of ulcerations. Finally, patients with acquired immunodeficiency syndrome (AIDS) have an increased frequency of severe aphthous stomatitis (see p. 204). This is not surprising when one considers the relatively increased percentage of CD8+ cells, which occurs as a result of the reduction in CD4+ T lymphocytes in that disease.

The mucosal barrier appears to be important in the prevention of aphthous stomatitis, and this might explain the almost exclusive location of aphthous stomatitis on non-keratinized mucosa. Numerous factors that can decrease the mucosal barrier increase the frequency of occurrence; conversely, those associated with an increased mucosal barrier have been correlated with decreased ulcerations. Certainly, trauma can decrease the mucosal barrier locally and has been associated with aphthae. In addition to their effects on the hematologic system, most of the nutritional abnormalities associated with aphthae also cause a decreased relative thickness of the oral mucosa (B_{12}, folate, and iron). Although the effects of tobacco byproducts on the immune system are unclear, the use of tobacco products has been associated with increased keratinization of the oral mucosa and a decreased frequency of aphthae. In a small subset of female patients, a negative association was reported between the occurrence of aphthae and the luteal phase of the menstrual cycle, a period of mucosal proliferation and keratinization. In addition, these same patients often experience ulcer-free periods during pregnancy.

An antigenic stimulus appears to be the primary initiating factor in the immune-mediated cytotoxic destruction of the mucosa in many patients. Numerous antigens have been explored; as expected, however, no one answer is true in all subgroups of patients. Microbiologic agents, such as the L forms of streptococci, herpes simplex virus, varicella-zoster virus, adenovirus, and cytomegalovirus, have been implicated. It is known that patients can exhibit herpesvirus within the epithelium without having a productive infection, and small subgroups of patients have attacks of aphthous stomatitis that coincide with asymptomatic viral shedding and elevated viral titers. Finally, other investigators have discovered subgroups of patients who respond well to a strict elimination diet or the removal of specific foods thought to be allergenic by patch testing.

There are three clinical variations of aphthous stomatitis:

- Minor
- Major
- Herpetiform

Minor aphthous ulcerations are the most common and represent the form present in up to 80 percent of those affected. **Major aphthous ulcerations** (also known historically as **Sutton's disease** or **periadenitis mucosa necrotica recurrens** [PMNR]) occur in approximately 10 percent of the patients. The remaining patients have **herpetiform aphthous ulcerations**. The minor and major forms most likely represent variations of the same process, although herpetiform aphthae demonstrate a more unique pattern. Some investigators differentiate the herpetiform variant because of supposed evidence of a viral cause, but the proof is weak and does not justify its distinction from the other aphthous ulcerations. Some authors include Behçet's disease as an additional variation of aphthous stomatitis, but this multisystem disorder is more complex and is considered later in this chapter.

Clinical Features

Minor Aphthous Ulcerations

Patients with minor aphthous ulcerations experience the fewest recurrences, and the individual lesions exhibit the shortest duration of the three variants. The ulcers arise almost exclusively on non-keratinized mucosa. The lesions may be preceded by prodromal symptoms of burning, itching, or stinging, with the development of an erythematous macule. The macule develops an ulceration that is covered by a yellowish-white, removable fibrinopurulent membrane and is encircled by an erythematous halo (Fig. 9–1). Classically, the ulcerations measure between 3 to 10 mm in diameter and heal without scarring in 7 to 14 days (Fig. 9–2; see Color Figure 50). From one to five lesions may be present during each episode, and the pain often is out of proportion for the size of the ulceration. The buccal and labial mucosae are the most commonly involved sites, followed by the ventral surface of the tongue, mucobuccal fold, floor of the mouth, and soft palate (Fig. 9–3; see Color Figure 51). Involvement of keratinized mucosa (hard palate, gingiva, dorsal surface of the tongue, and vermilion border) is

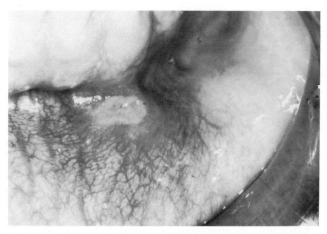

FIGURE 9–1. **Minor aphthous ulceration.** Erythematous halo encircling a yellowish ulceration of the mandibular anterior mucolabial fold.

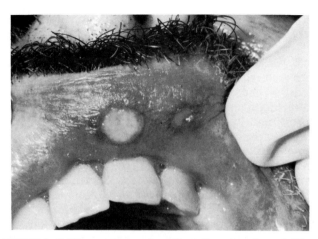

FIGURE 9-2. **Minor aphthous ulcerations.** Two ulcerations of different size located on the maxillary labial mucosa. See Color Plates.

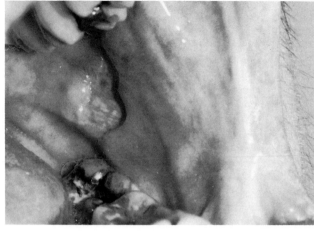

FIGURE 9-4. **Major aphthous ulceration.** Large, deep, and irregular ulceration of the posterior buccal mucosa. Note extensive scarring of the anterior buccal mucosa from previous ulcerations.

rare and usually represents extension from adjacent non-keratinized epithelium. These ulcerations usually begin in childhood or adolescence, and the recurrence rate is highly variable, ranging from one ulceration every few years up to two episodes per month.

Major Aphthous Ulcerations

Major aphthous ulcerations are larger than minor aphthae and demonstrate the longest duration per episode. The number of lesions usually is intermediate between that seen in the minor and herpetiform variants. The ulcerations are deeper than the minor variant, measure from 1 to 3 cm in diameter, take from 2 to 6 weeks to heal, and may cause scarring (Fig. 9-4). The number of lesions varies from 1 to 10. Any oral surface area may be affected but the labial mucosa, soft palate, and tonsillar fauces are the most commonly affected sites (Fig. 9-5). The onset of major aphthae is after puberty, and recurrent episodes may continue to develop for up to 20 years or more.

Herpetiform Aphthous Ulcerations

Herpetiform aphthous ulcerations demonstrate the greatest number of lesions and the most frequent recurrences. The individual lesions are small, averaging 1 to 3 mm in diameter, and as many as 100 may be present in a single recurrence. Because of their small size and large number, the lesions bear a superficial resemblance to a primary herpes simplex virus infection; thus, they are termed (rather confusingly) *herpetiform*. It is common for individual lesions to coalesce into larger irregular ulcerations (Fig. 9-6). The ulcerations heal within 7 to 10 days, but the recurrences tend to be closely spaced. Many patients are almost constantly affected for periods as long as 3 years. Although the non-keratinized movable mucosa is most frequently affected, any oral mucosal surface may be involved. There is a female predominance, and typically the onset is in adulthood.

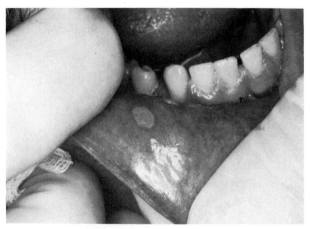

FIGURE 9-3. **Minor aphthous ulceration.** Single ulceration of the lower labial mucosa. See Color Plates. (Courtesy of Dr. Dean K. White.)

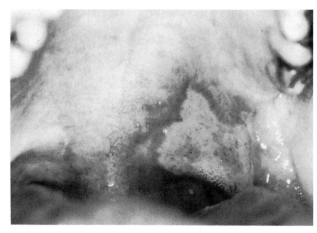

FIGURE 9-5. **Major aphthous ulceration.** Large, irregular ulceration of the soft palate.

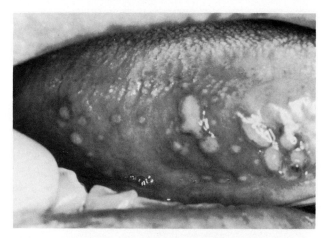

FIGURE 9–6. **Herpetiform aphthous ulcerations.** Numerous pinhead ulcerations of the ventral surface of the tongue, several of which have coalesced into larger, more irregular areas of ulceration.

Histopathologic Features

The histopathologic picture of aphthous stomatitis is characteristic but not pathognomonic. The early ulcerative lesions demonstrate a central zone of ulceration, which is covered by a fibrinopurulent membrane. Deep to the area of ulceration, the connective tissue exhibits an increased vascularity and a mixed inflammatory cellular infiltrate that consists of lymphocytes, histiocytes, and polymorphonuclear leukocytes. The epithelium at the margin of the lesion demonstrates spongiosis and numerous mononuclear cells in the basilar third. A band of lymphocytes intermixed with histiocytes is present in the superficial connective tissue and surrounding deeper blood vessels.

Diagnosis

The diagnosis is made from the clinical presentation and from exclusion of other diseases that can present with ulcerations that closely resemble aphthae. Because the histopathologic features are nonspecific, a biopsy is useful only in eliminating differential possibilities and is not beneficial in arriving at the definitive diagnosis.

Treatment and Prognosis

The mainstay of therapy for all three forms of aphthous stomatitis is topical corticosteroids, and the list of possible choices is long. Most patients with diffuse minor or herpetiform aphthae respond well to betamethasone syrup or 0.01 percent dexamethasone elixir used as a mouth rinse. Patients with localized ulcerations can be successfully treated with 0.05 percent fluocinonide gel. Adrenal suppression does not occur with the appropriate use of these medications. Major aphthous ulcerations are more resistant to therapy and often warrant more potent corticosteroids. The individual lesions may be injected with triamcinolone acetonide or covered with 0.05 percent betamethasone dipropionate gel or 0.05 percent clobetasol propionate ointment. Triamcinolone tablets also can be dissolved directly over the lesions. In resistant cases, systemic corticosteroids may be required to supplement the topical medications and gain control.

Many other medications have been used in an attempt to resolve the disease. Included within the list of therapies are chemical cauterizing agents, topical 5-aminosalicylic acid, vitamins, hydrogen peroxide, chlorhexidine, tetracycline, LongoVital, dapsone, monoamine oxidase (MAO) inhibitors, colchicine, thalidomide, levamisole, sodium cromoglycate (cromolyn), gamma globulin, carbenoxolone sodium, acyclovir, and amlexanox.

All the aforementioned therapies merely "beat back brush fires" and do not resolve the underlying problem. Recurrences often continue, although breaking up the cycle may induce longer disease-free intervals between attacks. To go beyond the management of individual recurrences is difficult, expensive, and often frustrating. In spite of this, patients with severe or frequent recurrences should be offered the opportunity to investigate the underlying causes. The search should concentrate on disorders demonstrating immunodysregulation, a decreased mucosal barrier, or an elevated antigenic stimulus. Such a systemic evaluation might include an investigation for systemic diseases associated with aphthouslike ulcerations, a hematologic evaluation, patch tests for antigen stimuli, and an elimination diet for possible offending foods. Therapeutic trials might be instituted against the viruses and bacteria that have been implicated in subsets of patients with aphthous stomatitis. The investigator should explain to the patient that the underlying causation is diverse; even with the most exhaustive search, the answer may be elusive. In spite of this, discovery of an underlying abnormality that can be specifically treated often leads to permanent resolution or dramatic improvement in the course of the recurrences.

BEHÇET'S SYNDROME (Behçet's Disease)

The combination of chronic ocular inflammation and orogenital ulcerations was reported as early as the era of the ancient Greeks, but it was not delineated until 1937, when a Turkish dermatologist, Hulusi Behçet, described the disease that bears his name. Although no clear causation has been established, **Behçet's syndrome** has an immunogenetic basis because of strong associations with certain HLA types. As in aphthous stomatitis, the disorder appears to be an immunodysregulation that may be primary or secondary to one or more triggers. Investigators have correlated attacks to a number of environmental antigens, including bacteria (especially streptococci), viruses, pesticides, and heavy metals.

HLA-Bw51 (a part of HLA-B5) has been closely linked to Behçet's disease, and the frequency of both the disease and haplotype is high in Turkey, Japan, and the Eastern Mediterranean countries. This distribution appears correlated to the ancient "silk route" traveled by the Turks. Sexual reproduction between immigrants and locals along the route appears to have spread the genetic vulnerability.

Behçet's syndrome may affect the mouth, genitals, skin, joints, eyes, and central nervous system. Four types have been described, depending on the major sites of involvement:

1. The *ocular* form is common in Japan and Middle Eastern countries and is closely associated with HLA-B5.
2. The *mucocutaneous* form is associated with HLA-B12 and is more frequently seen in the United States and Europe.
3. The *arthritic* form appears to correlate with HLA-B27.
4. The *neurologic* form does not relate to a specific HLA.

Oral mucosal involvement is common to all four types. With long-term follow-up, each type may progress to the other types.

Clinical Features

Oral involvement is an important component of Behçet's disease and the first manifestation in 25 to 75 percent of the cases. Oral lesions occur at some point during the disease in 99 percent of the patients and typically precede other sites of involvement.

The lesions are similar to aphthous ulcerations and demonstrate the same duration and frequency. In spite of this, investigators have shown several statistically significant clinical variations that are different from typical aphthous ulcerations and may be used to increase the index of suspicion for Behçet's disease. When compared with patients with aphthae, a larger percentage of those with Behçet's disease demonstrate six or more ulcerations. The lesions commonly involve the soft palate and oropharynx, which usually are infrequent sites for the occurrence of routine aphthae. The individual lesions vary in size, have ragged borders, and are surrounded by a larger zone of diffuse erythema (Fig. 9–7).

The genital lesions are similar in appearance to the oral ulcerations. They occur in 75 percent of the patients

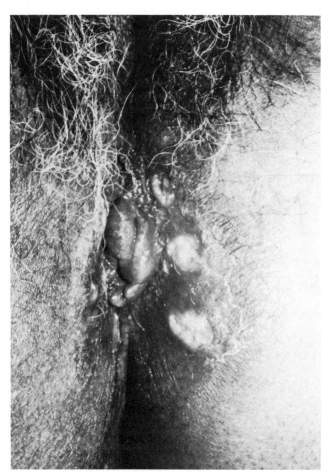

FIGURE 9–8. **Behçet's syndrome.** Numerous irregular ulcerations of the labia majora and perineum. (From Helm TN, Camisa C, Allen C, Lowder C: Clinical features of Behçet's disease. Oral Surg Oral Med Oral Pathol 72:30–34, 1991.)

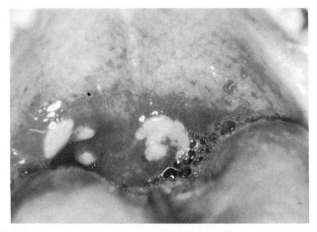

FIGURE 9–7. **Behçet's syndrome.** Diffuse erythema surrounding numerous irregular ulcerations of the soft palate. (From Helm TN, Camisa C, Allen C, Lowder C: Clinical features of Behçet's disease. Oral Surg Oral Med Oral Pathol 72:30–34, 1991.)

and present on the vulva, vagina, glans penis, scrotum, and perianal area (Fig. 9–8). These lesions recur less frequently than do the oral ulcerations, are deeper, and tend to heal with scarring. The genital ulcerations cause more symptoms in males than in females, and may be discovered only by a routine examination in females.

Common cutaneous lesions include erythematous papules, vesicles, pustules, pyoderma, folliculitis, acneiform eruptions, and erythema nodosum-like lesions. From a diagnostic standpoint, one of the most important skin manifestations is the presence of positive "pathergy." One or 2 days after the injection of an inert substance (e.g., sterile saline), a tuberculin-like skin reaction or sterile pustule develops (Fig. 9–9). This skin hyperreactivity (pathergy) appears to be unique to Behçet's disease and is present in 40 to 88 percent of patients with this disorder.

Ocular involvement is present in up to 90 percent of the cases and is more frequent and severe in males. Recurrent uveitis, hypopyon, and iridocyclitis are the most common manifestations. Severe pain and blindness may result.

Arthritis is one of the more common minor manifestations of the disease and is usually self-limiting and

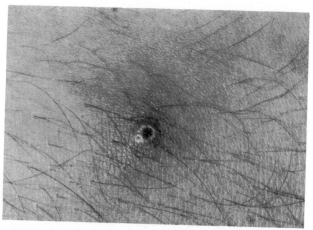

FIGURE 9-9. **Behçet's syndrome.** Sterile pustule of the skin that developed 1 day after injection of saline. This reaction is termed cutaneous pathergy.

non-deforming. The knees, wrists, elbows, and ankles are affected most frequently.

Central nervous system (CNS) involvement is not common but, when present, is associated with a poor prognosis. From 10 to 25 percent of the patients demonstrate CNS involvement, and the alterations produced result in a number of changes that include paralysis and severe dementia.

Other alterations may be seen that involve the gastrointestinal, hematologic, pulmonary, muscular, and renal systems. These most likely occur secondary to vasculitis and create a variety of clinical presentations.

Diagnosis

No laboratory finding is diagnostic of Behçet's disease. The International Study Group for Behçet's Disease established specific criteria for the diagnosis. The patient must have oral ulcerations that have recurred at least three times in 1 year. In addition to the oral manifestations, the patients must have two of the following:

- Recurrent genital ulceration
- Appropriate ocular lesions observed by an ophthalmologist
- Appropriate cutaneous lesions or positive pathergy test read by a physician 24 to 48 hours after injection

Histopathologic Features

The histopathologic features are not specific for Behçet's disease and can be seen in many disorders, including aphthous stomatitis. The pattern most frequently seen is called **leukocytoclastic vasculitis.** The ulceration is similar in appearance to that seen in aphthous stomatitis, but the small blood vessels classically demonstrate intramural invasion by neutrophils, karyorrhexis of neutrophils, extravasation of red blood cells, and fibrinoid necrosis of the vessel wall.

Treatment and Prognosis

The oral lesions of Behçet's disease can be treated with a tetracycline-containing rinse or topical corticosteroids (see aphthous ulcerations, p. 239). The genital lesions also may be controlled with topical corticosteroids. Systemic corticosteroids are reserved for severe cases. Oral lesions resistant to steroids have been managed successfully with thalidomide. Azathioprine and cyclosporine are used for the ocular lesions, and colchicine is effective in reducing the erythema nodosum–like lesions and arthralgia.

Behçet's disease presents with a highly variable course. A relapsing and remitting pattern is typical, with attacks becoming more intermittent after 5 to 7 years. In the absence of CNS disease or significant vascular complications, the prognosis is generally good.

SARCOIDOSIS

Sarcoidosis is a multisystem granulomatous disorder of unknown cause. The evidence implicates improper degradation of antigenic material with the formation of non-caseating granulomatous inflammation. The nature of the antigen is unknown, and probably several different antigens may be responsible. Sensitive polymerase chain reaction and DNA/RNA *in situ* hybridization techniques have detected abnormally high levels of mycobacterial DNA in bronchoalveolar lavage material from patients with sarcoidosis. The inappropriate defense response may result from prolonged or heavy antigenic exposure, an immunodysregulation (genetic or secondary to other factors) that prevents an adequate cell-mediated response, a defective regulation of the initial immune reaction, or a combination of all three of these factors. Future studies are needed to confirm a definitive relationship between sarcoidosis and any infectious agent.

Clinical Features

Sarcoidosis has a worldwide distribution but is more commonly recognized in the developed world. In North America, blacks are affected 10 times more frequently than whites. There is a slight female predominance, and the disease typically arises between 20 and 40 years of age.

Sarcoidosis most commonly presents acutely over a period of days to weeks, and the symptoms are variable. Common clinical symptoms include dyspnea, dry cough, chest pain, fever, malaise, fatigue, arthralgia, and weight loss. Less frequently, sarcoidosis arises insidiously over months to years, without significant symptoms; when clinically evident, pulmonary symptoms are most common. Approximately 20 percent of patients have no symptoms, and the disease is discovered on routine chest radiographs.

Although any organ may be affected, the lungs, lymph nodes, skin, eyes, and salivary glands are the predominant sites. Lymphoid tissue is involved in almost all cases. The mediastinal and paratracheal lymph nodes are commonly involved, and patients frequently present

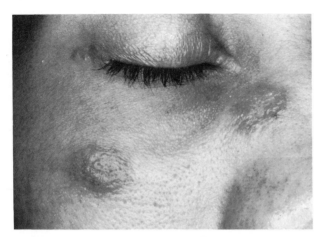

FIGURE 9-10. **Sarcoidosis.** Violaceous indurated plaques of the right malar area and bridge of nose. (Courtesy Dr. George Blozis.)

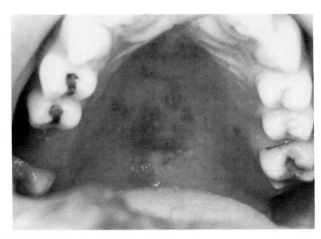

FIGURE 9-11. **Sarcoidosis.** Multiple erythematous macules of the hard palate. (Courtesy of Dr. George Blozis.)

with bilateral hilar lymphadenopathy on chest radiographs. Granulomatous inflammation of the skin is seen about 25 percent of the time and often presents as chronic, violaceous, indurated lesions, which frequent the nose, ears, lips, and face (Fig. 9-10). Symmetric, elevated, indurated, purplish plaques also are seen commonly on the limbs, back, and buttocks. Scattered, nonspecific, tender erythematous nodules, known as **erythema nodosum**, frequently occur on the lower legs.

Ocular involvement is noted in 25 percent of the cases and may present as uveitis or secondary glaucoma. Involvement of the lacrimal glands often produces keratoconjunctivitis sicca; the salivary glands can be altered similarly, with resultant clinical enlargement and xerostomia. Significant enlargement can occur in any major or minor salivary gland. Removal of intraoral mucoceles that occur in the salivary glands affected by the granulomatous process has led to the initial diagnosis in some cases. The salivary gland enlargement, xerostomia, and keratoconjunctivitis sicca can combine to mimic Sjögren's syndrome (see p. 332). Virtually any organ system may be involved.

Two distinctive clinical syndromes are associated with acute sarcoidosis. **Löfgren's syndrome** consists of erythema nodosum, bilateral hilar lymphadenopathy, and arthralgia. Patients with **Heerfordt's syndrome (uveoparotid fever)** have parotid enlargement, anterior uveitis of the eye, facial paralysis, and fever.

If salivary gland and lymph node involvement are excluded, clinically evident oral manifestations in sarcoidosis are uncommon. Any oral mucosal site can be affected, most often presenting as a submucosal mass, an isolated papule, or an area of granularity. The mucosal lesions may be normal in color, brownish-red, violaceous, or hyperkeratotic (Figs. 9-11 and 9-12). Bony involvement is rare and can mimic periodontal disease. Most reported cases represent lesions found in patients with known sarcoidosis, although rare reports have documented the diagnosis of systemic sarcoidosis, with the initial lesions discovered in the oral cavity.

Histopathologic Features

Microscopic examination of sarcoidosis presents a classic picture of granulomatous inflammation. Tightly clustered aggregates of epithelioid histiocytes are present with a surrounding rim of lymphocytes. Intermixed within the histiocytes are scattered Langhans or foreign body-type giant cells (Fig. 9-13). The granulomas often contain laminated basophilic calcifications, known as *Schaumann bodies*, or stellate inclusions, known as *asteroid bodies*. Neither structure is specific for sarcoidosis. Special stains for fungal and bacterial organisms are negative. No polarizable, dissolvable, or pigmented foreign material can be detected.

Diagnosis

The diagnosis is established by the clinical and radiographic presentations, the histopathologic appearance, and the presence of negative findings with both special

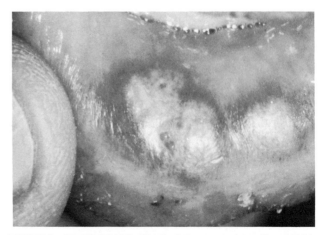

FIGURE 9-12. **Sarcoidosis.** Erythematous macules with central hyperkeratosis of the lower labial mucosa.

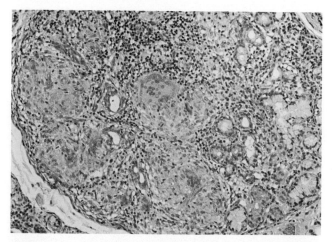

FIGURE 9–13. **Sarcoidosis.** Photomicrograph of a labial minor salivary gland demonstrating granulomatous inflammation characterized by circumscribed collections of histiocytes, lymphocytes, and multinucleated giant cells.

stains and cultures for organisms. Elevated serum angiotensin-converting enzyme (ACE) levels and appropriate documentation of pulmonary involvement strongly support the diagnosis. Other laboratory abnormalities that may be seen include eosinophilia; leukopenia; anemia; thrombocytopenia; and elevated serum alkaline phosphatase level, erythrocyte sedimentation rate, serum calcium concentration, and urinary calcium level.

A skin test for sarcoidosis, the *Kveim* test, can be performed by intradermally injecting a sterilized suspension of human sarcoid tissue. Within 4 to 6 weeks, papulonodular lesions develop in affected patients. A biopsy is done to confirm granulomatous inflammation. The test is accurate in 50 to 85 percent of patients with sarcoidosis but is largely of historical interest because the clinical presentation and demonstration of granulomatous inflammation are adequate for the diagnosis in most cases. Skin testing may be considered in atypical cases or when the biopsy is difficult or the histopathologic findings are negative.

Minor salivary gland biopsy has been promoted as a diagnostic aid in suspected cases of sarcoidosis (see Fig. 9–13). Investigators have documented success rates between 38 and 58 percent. The misdiagnosis of Sjögren's syndrome from minor salivary gland biopsy specimens has been reported in patients with sarcoidosis. Previously, biopsy of the parotid was avoided because of the fear of salivary fistula formation and damage to the facial nerve. These concerns have been reduced through biopsy of the posterior superficial lobe of the parotid gland, and confirmation of sarcoidosis has been reported in 93 percent of patients from this procedure.

Treatment and Prognosis

In approximately 60 percent of patients with sarcoidosis, the symptoms resolve spontaneously within 2 years without treatment. Another 20 percent of those affected can be treated successfully with corticosteroids. Those with significant involvement or disease that hinders normal function are candidates for corticosteroid treatment. In 10 to 20 percent of those affected with sarcoidosis, resolution does not occur even with treatment. Central nervous system and chronic extrathoracic involvement are associated with a poor response to therapy. Approximately 4 to 10 percent of patients die of pulmonary, cardiac, or central nervous system complications.

OROFACIAL GRANULOMATOSIS

As the name implies, **orofacial granulomatosis** refers to the presence of granulomatous inflammation in the oral and facial regions. The diagnosis is one of exclusion after the elimination of the systemic processes capable of producing orofacial granulomatous lesions (Table 9–1). On occasion, patients initially diagnosed as having orofacial granulomatosis over time will have signs or symptoms diagnostic of one of the processes listed in Table 9–1. At that time, the diagnosis is altered to the appropriate systemic disease.

The disorder is somewhat analogous to aphthous stomatitis, in that the causation is idiopathic but appears to represent an abnormal immune reaction; the reaction may be primary or, most likely, secondary to one or more of a large number of factors. Genetic predisposition appears to contribute in a percentage of the patients. Local conditions that have been reported to result in orofacial granulomatosis include bacterial infections; viral infections; and allergic reactions to food, additives, or other materials. The literature implies that each of these items may be responsible for the process in different subsets of patients, and all must be considered in the search for the causation of an individual case of orofacial granulomatosis.

Clinical Features

The clinical presentation of orofacial granulomatosis is highly variable. By far, the most frequent site of involvement is the lips. The labial tissues demonstrate a nontender, persistent swelling that may involve one or both lips (Fig. 9–14). On rare occasions, superficial amber vesicles, resembling lymphangiomas, are found. When these signs are combined with facial paralysis and a fissured tongue, the clinical presentation is called **Melkersson-Rosenthal syndrome** (Figs. 9–15 and 9–16). Involvement of the lips alone is called **cheilitis granulomatosa (of Miescher).** Some consider cheilitis granulo-

Table 9–1. SYSTEMIC PROCESSES ASSOCIATED WITH ORAL GRANULOMATOUS INFLAMMATION

Chronic granulomatous disease
Crohn's disease
Hairy cell leukemia
Mycobacterial infection
Sarcoidosis

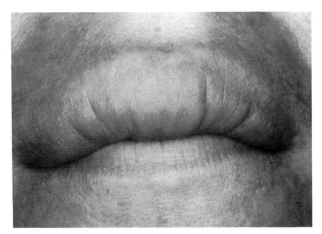

FIGURE 9–14. **Orofacial granulomatosis (cheilitis granulomatosa).** Nontender, persistent enlargement of the upper lip. (Courtesy of Allen CM, Camisa C. Diseases of the mouth and lips. *In:* Principles of Dermatology. Edited by Sams WM, Lynch P. New York, Churchill Livingstone, 1990, p 931.)

matosa an oligosymptomatic form of Melkersson-Rosenthal syndrome, but it appears best to include all of these under the term orofacial granulomatosis. In addition to labial edema, swelling of other parts of the face is common.

Intraoral sites also can be affected, and the predominant lesions are edema, ulcers, and papules. The tongue may present with fissures, edema, paresthesia, erosions, or taste alteration. The gingiva can develop swelling, erythema, pain, or erosions. The buccal mucosa often presents with a cobblestone appearance of edematous mucosa. Linear hyperplastic folds may occur in the mucobuccal fold, with linear ulcerations present in the base of these folds (Fig. 9–17). The palate may have papules or large areas of hyperplastic tissue. Hyposalivation rarely is reported.

Histopathologic Features

Edema is present in the superficial lamina propria with dilation of lymphatic vessels and scattered lymphocytes

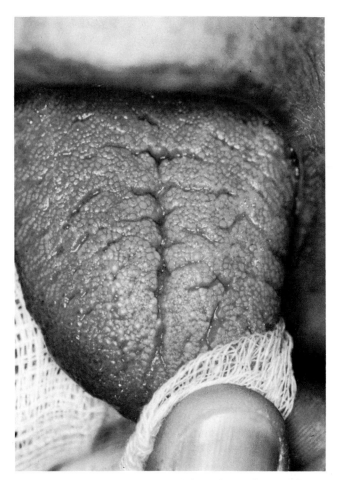

FIGURE 9–16. **Melkersson-Rosenthal syndrome.** Same patient as depicted in Figure 9–15. Note numerous furrows on the dorsal surface of the tongue. (Courtesy of Dr. Richard Ziegler.)

seen diffusely and in clusters. Fibrosis may be present in long-term lesions. Scattered aggregates of non-caseating granulomatous inflammation, consisting of lymphocytes and epithelioid histiocytes, are present, with or without multinucleated giant cells (Fig. 9–18). Typically, the

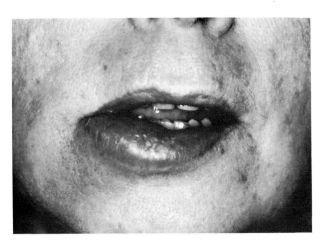

FIGURE 9–15. **Melkersson-Rosenthal syndrome.** Persistent enlargement of the lower lip. (Courtesy of Dr. Richard Ziegler.)

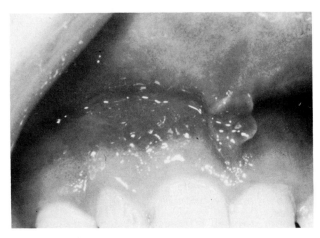

FIGURE 9–17. **Orofacial granulomatosis.** Hyperplastic mucosa of the anterior maxillary mucobuccal fold. (Courtesy of Dr. Greg W. Dimmich.)

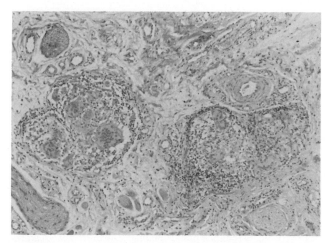

FIGURE 9–18. **Orofacial granulomatosis.** Labial biopsy specimen demonstrating scattered aggregates of histiocytes, lymphocytes, and multinucleated giant cells.

granulomas are not as well formed or as discrete as those seen in sarcoidosis. Special stains for fungal organisms and acid-fast bacteria are negative. No dissolvable, pigmented, or polarizable foreign material should be present. When the lesions are confined to the gingiva, the search for foreign material should be extensive because many cases of granulomatous gingivitis are due to subtle collections of foreign material (see p. 127).

Diagnosis

As mentioned, the definitive diagnosis of orofacial granulomatosis is one of exclusion. After histopathologic elimination of causation from a foreign body or microorganisms, the diagnosis is made by the exclusion of other disorders known to be associated with orofacial granulomas. The systemic processes listed in Table 9–1 must be ruled out. In patients with no intestinal symptoms, Crohn's disease still has been demonstrated in up to 37 percent of the patients with unexplained oral or facial granulomatous inflammation. Some investigators believe that esophagogastroduodenoscopy, ileocolonoscopy, and small bowel radiographs are mandatory. Others perform a complete intestinal investigation only in the presence of malabsorption or serologic evidence of Crohn's disease (elevated erythrocyte sedimentation rate or low serum albumin, calcium, folate, and iron levels). Sarcoidosis is unlikely in the presence of a normal chest radiograph and normal levels of serum angiotensin-converting enzyme (ACE). Chronic granulomatous disease can be ruled out with the neutrophil nitroblue tetrazolium reduction test.

Treatment and Prognosis

There are two tiers of therapy for orofacial granulomatosis:

- Searching for the causation
- Treating the lesions

Antiviral and antibacterial medications, patch testing, and elimination diets have been used in an attempt to elucidate the probable cause. Each approach has produced positive results in different subsets of patients.

An association between orofacial granulomatosis and dental foci of infection has been documented. This should not be totally unexpected because similar significant edematous swellings of the skin, known as **elephantiasis nostras** also have been reported to occur from streptococcal lymphangitis. One group of investigators showed resolution of up to 60 percent of cases of orofacial granulomatosis from the elimination of oral foci of infection.

The individual lesions have been treated with a host of medications with variable results. Intralesional corticosteroids, radiotherapy, salazosulfapyridine (sulfasalazine), hydroxychloroquine sulfate, methotrexate, dapsone, clofazimine, metronidazole, and numerous other antibiotics have already been used. Currently, systemic and intralesional corticosteroids are administered successfully to control the progression of this disease by the greatest number of investigators. Because of the natural variability of the disease's progression and the occurrence of spontaneous remissions, therapies are difficult to assess. In the absence of a response to other therapies, surgical recontouring has been used by some but carries a considerable risk of recurrence.

The prognosis is highly variable. No therapy has proved to be the "silver bullet" in resolving the individual lesions. In many cases, lesions resolve spontaneously with or without therapy; in others, they continue to progress in spite of a myriad of therapeutic attempts to stop the progression. The "lucky" subset of patients includes those who have found an initiating causation and have resolved their problems by the exclusion of the offending agent.

WEGENER'S GRANULOMATOSIS

Wegener's granulomatosis is a well-recognized, although uncommon, disease process of unknown cause. The initial description of the syndrome by Wegener included necrotizing granulomatous lesions of the respiratory tract, necrotizing glomerulonephritis, and systemic vasculitis of small arteries and veins. Hypotheses about the cause of the disease include an abnormal immune reaction secondary to a nonspecific infection or an aberrant hypersensitivity response to an inhaled antigen. A possible hereditary predisposition has been mentioned in some cases.

Before the current treatment modalities were initiated, the disorder was uniformly fatal. The disease begins as a localized process, which may become more widely disseminated if left untreated. Most patients respond favorably to treatment; consequently, early diagnosis and appropriate therapy are critical.

Clinical Features

Wegener's granulomatosis can involve almost every organ system in the body. Classically, patients initially present with involvement of the upper and lower respiratory tract; if the condition remains untreated, renal involvement typically develops. Subsets of patients exhibit a protracted superficial phenomenon in which lesions are present in the skin and mucosa but further dissemination is slow to occur. In addition, other patients can exhibit a limited form of Wegener's granulomatosis in which there is involvement of the respiratory system without rapid development of renal lesions. These different clinical patterns highlight the variability of the clinical aggressiveness that can occur in patients with Wegener's granulomatosis.

Purulent nasal drainage, chronic sinus pain, nasal ulceration, congestion, and fever are frequent findings from upper respiratory involvement. Persistent otitis media, sore throat, and epistaxis also are reported. With progression, destruction of the nasal septum can result in a saddle nose deformity. Patients with lower respiratory involvement may be asymptomatic, or they may present with dry cough, hemoptysis, dyspnea, or chest pain. Renal involvement usually occurs late in the disease process and is the most frequent cause of death. The glomerulonephritis results in proteinuria and red blood cells casts. Occasionally, the eyes, ears, and skin also are involved.

Oral lesions are seen in about 6 percent of those affected; occasionally, the oral changes may be the only clinically evident finding. The most characteristic oral manifestation is *strawberry gingivitis*. This most distinctive pattern of gingival alteration appears to be an early manifestation of Wegener's granulomatosis and has been documented before renal involvement in most cases. The affected gingiva demonstrates a florid and granular hyperplasia. The surface forms numerous short bulbous projections, which are hemorrhagic and friable; this red bumpy surface is responsible for the strawberry-like appearance (Fig. 9–19; see Color Figure 52). The buccal surfaces are more frequently affected, and the alterations are classically confined to the attached gingiva. The process appears to begin in the interdental region and dem-

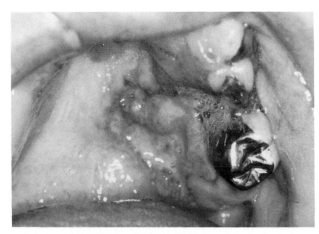

FIGURE 9–20. **Wegener's granulomatosis.** Deep, irregular ulceration of the hard palate on the left side. (From Allen CM, Camisa C, Salewski C, Weiland JE. Wegener's granulomatosis: Report of three cases with oral lesions. J Oral Maxillofac Surg 49:294–298, 1991.)

onstrates lateral spread to adjacent areas. At the time of diagnosis, the involvement may be localized or generalized to multiple quadrants. Destruction of underlying bone with the development of tooth mobility has been reported.

Oral ulceration may also be a manifestation of Wegener's granulomatosis. Unlike the strawberry gingiva, the ulcerations do not form a pattern that is unique. These lesions are clinically nonspecific and may occur on any mucosal surface (Fig. 9–20). In contrast to the gingival changes, the oral ulcerations are diagnosed at a later stage of the disease, with more than 60 percent of the affected patients demonstrating renal involvement.

Other less common oral manifestations include sinusitis-related toothache, arthralgia of the temporomandibular joint, jaw claudication, palatal ulceration from nasal extension, and poorly healing extraction sites. Enlargement of one or more major salivary glands from primary involvement of the granulomatous process also has been reported. The glandular involvement also appears early in the course of the disease and may lead to early diagnosis and treatment.

Histopathologic Features

Wegener's granulomatosis presents with a pattern of mixed inflammation centered around blood vessels. Involved vessels demonstrate transmural inflammation, often with areas of heavy neutrophilic infiltration, necrosis, and nuclear dust (leukocytoclastic vasculitis). The connective tissue adjacent to the vessel has an inflammatory cellular infiltrate, which contains a variable mixture of histiocytes, lymphocytes, eosinophils, and multinucleated giant cells (Fig. 9–21). Special stains for organisms are negative, and no foreign material can be found. In oral biopsy specimens, the oral epithelium may demonstrate pseudoepitheliomatous hyperplasia and subepithelial abscesses. Vasculitis may be difficult to demonstrate in the oral specimens, and the histopathologic presentation may be one of ill-defined collections of

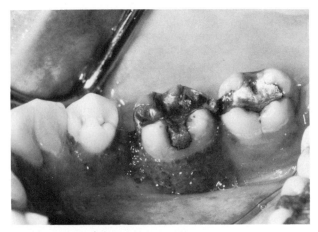

FIGURE 9–19. **Wegener's granulomatosis.** Hemorrhagic and friable gingiva (strawberry gingivitis) of the lingual mandible, which demonstrates numerous short bulbous projections. The area developed within 10 days after removal of similar lesions, which affected the entire facial gingiva of the anterior maxilla. See Color Plates.

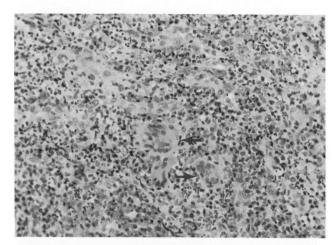

FIGURE 9–21. **Wegener's granulomatosis.** Connective tissue containing proliferation of numerous vascular channels and a heavy inflammatory infiltrate consisting of lymphocytes, neutrophils, eosinophils, and multinucleated giant cells (*arrows*).

epithelioid histiocytes intermixed with eosinophils, lymphocytes, and multinucleated giant cells. In addition, the lesions of strawberry gingivitis typically demonstrate prominent vascularity with extensive red blood cell extravasation (Fig. 9–22).

Diagnosis

The diagnosis of Wegener's granulomatosis is made from the combination of the clinical presentation and the microscopic finding of necrotizing and granulomatous vasculitis. Radiographic evaluation of the chest and sinuses is recommended to document possible involvement of these areas. The serum creatinine and urinalysis results are used to rule out significant renal alterations.

A laboratory marker for Wegener's granulomatosis has been identified. Indirect immunofluorescence for serum antibodies directed against cytoplasmic components of

neutrophils has been used to support a diagnosis of Wegener's granulomatosis. There are two reaction patterns of these antineutrophil cytoplasm antibodies (ANCA):

- Perinuclear (p-ANCA)
- Cytoplasmic (c-ANCA)

Cytoplasmic localization (c-ANCA) is the most useful and is present in 90 to 95 percent of cases of acute generalized Wegener's granulomatosis. This positivity drops to 60 percent in early localized forms of the disease. When positive, a finding of c-ANCA confirms the diagnosis; when the immunologic studies are negative, the diagnosis of Wegener's granulomatosis is not ruled out.

Treatment and Prognosis

The mean survival of untreated patients with disseminated classic Wegener's granulomatosis is 5 months; 80 percent of the patients are dead at 1 year and 90 percent, within 2 years. However, the prognosis is better for the limited and superficial forms of the disease.

The drugs of choice are cyclophosphamide and prednisone, but this approach is not without serious potential side effects. Trimethoprim-sulfamethoxazole has been used successfully in localized cases and when the immunosuppressive regimen has failed. Low-dose methotrexate and corticosteroids also have been used in patients whose disease is not immediately life-threatening or has not responded appropriately to cyclophosphamide.

Treatment has a profound effect on the progression of the disease. With appropriate therapy, prolonged remission is typical and cure is often attainable when the disease is diagnosed and appropriately treated while the involvement is localized. The c-ANCA levels can be used to follow the disease activity. Patients appear less likely to have relapses if their antineutrophilic antibodies disappear during treatment; in contrast, patients whose levels of antibodies persist are at greater risk for relapse.

ALLERGIC MUCOSAL REACTIONS TO SYSTEMIC DRUG ADMINISTRATION

The use of medications is not without potential intraoral complications. The list of offending medications and their resultant side effects appears almost endless. In a short and highly beneficial article, Mathews listed more than 150 frequently prescribed medications and related them to 46 oral and perioral side effects associated with their use.

An allergic reaction of the oral mucosa to the systemic administration of a medication is called **stomatitis medicamentosa**. Besides **erythema multiforme**, several different patterns of oral mucosal disease can be seen:

- Anaphylactic stomatitis
- Intraoral fixed drug eruptions
- Lichenoid drug reactions
- Lupus erythematosus–like eruptions

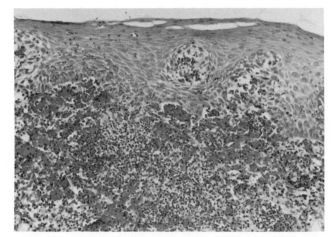

FIGURE 9–22. **Wegener's granulomatosis.** Gingival biopsy specimen showing a mixed inflammatory cellular infiltrate obscured by extensive extravasation of red blood cells.

- Pemphigus-like drug reactions
- Nonspecific vesiculoulcerative lesions

Anaphylactic stomatitis arises after the allergen enters the circulation and binds to IgE–mast cell complexes. Although systemic anaphylactic shock can result, localized alterations also occur. Fixed drug eruptions are inflammatory alterations of the mucosa or skin that recur at the same site after the administration of any allergen, often a medication.

The vast number of medications capable of producing anaphylactic stomatitis precludes their listing, but common culprits are antibiotics (especially penicillin) and sulfa drugs. Medications reported to be associated with fixed drug eruptions are listed in Table 9–2; lichenoid drug eruptions, in Table 9–3; lupus erythematosus–like drug eruptions, in Table 9–4; pemphigus-like drug reactions, in Table 9–5; and nonspecific vesiculoerosive eruptions, in Table 9–6.

Clinical Features

The patterns of mucosal alterations associated with the systemic administration of medications are varied, almost as much as the number of drugs that result in these changes. Anaphylactic stomatitis may occur alone or in conjunction with urticarial skin lesions or other signs and symptoms of anaphylaxis (e.g., hoarseness, respiratory distress, and vomiting). The affected mucosa may exhibit multiple zones of erythema or numerous aphthous-like ulcerations (Figs. 9–23 and 9–24). Mucosal fixed drug eruptions present as localized areas of erythema and edema, which can develop into vesiculoerosive lesions and are located most frequently on the labial mucosa. Lichenoid, lupus-like, and pemphigus-like drug reactions resemble their namesakes clinically, histopathologically, and immunologically. These latter chronic drug reactions may involve any mucosal surface, but the most common sites are the posterior buccal mucosa and the lateral borders of the tongue (Figs. 9–25 and 9–26). Bilateral and symmetric lesions are fairly common.

Diagnosis

A detailed medical history must be obtained, and the patient should be closely questioned concerning the use of both prescription and over-the-counter medications.

Table 9–2. MEDICATIONS ASSOCIATED WITH MUCOSAL FIXED DRUG ERUPTIONS

Analgin
Barbiturates
Co-trimoxazole
Dapsone
Phenazone derivatives
Phenolphthalein
Salicylates
Sulfonamides
Tetracycline

Table 9–3. DRUGS ASSOCIATED WITH LICHENOID ERUPTIONS

Allopurinol	Palladium
Arsenicals	Para-aminosalicylic acid
Bismuth	Penicillamine
Chloroquine	Phenothiazines
Chlorothiazide	Propranolol
Chlorpropamide	Quinacrine
Dapsone	Quinidine
Furosemide	Spironolactone
Gold salts	Streptomycin
Hydroxychloroquine	Tetracycline
Mercury	Tolbutamide
Methyldopa	Triprolidine

Table 9–4. DRUGS ASSOCIATED WITH LUPUS ERYTHEMATOSUS–LIKE ERUPTIONS

Carbamazepine	Methyldopa
Chlorpromazine	Penicillamine
Ethosuximide	Primidone
Gold	Procainamide
Griseofulvin	Quinidine
Hydantoins	Reserpine
Hydralazine	Streptomycin
Isoniazid	Thiouracils
Lithium	Trimethadione

Table 9–5. DRUGS ASSOCIATED WITH PEMPHIGUS-LIKE ERUPTIONS

Alpha-mercaptopropionyl glycine
Ampicillin
Captopril
Cephalexin
Ethambutol
Glibenclamide
Gold
Heroin
Ibuprofen
Penicillamine
Phenobarbital
Phenylbutazone
Piroxicam
Practolol
Propranolol
Pyritinolchlorhydrate
Rifampin
Thiopromine

Table 9–6. DRUGS ASSOCIATED WITH NONSPECIFIC VESICULOEROSIVE LESIONS

Indomethacin
Gold salts
Meprobamate
Methyldopa
Naproxen
Penicillamine
Phenylbutazone
Propranolol
Spironolactone
Thiazide diuretics
Tolbutamide

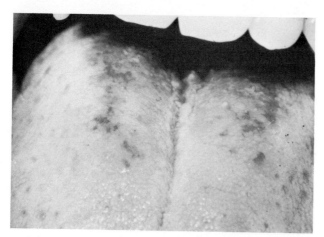

FIGURE 9-23. **Allergic mucosal reaction to systemic administration of gold.** Multiple erythematous macules of the dorsal surface of the tongue.

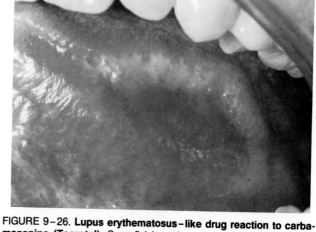

FIGURE 9-26. **Lupus erythematosus-like drug reaction to carbamazepine (Tegretol).** Superficial erosion with peripheral hyperkeratosis of the lateral border of the tongue on the left side. Similar lesions were also present on the right lateral border of the tongue and bilaterally on the buccal mucosa.

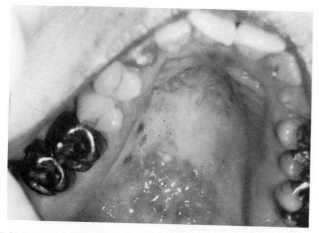

FIGURE 9-24. **Allergic mucosal reaction to systemic administration of gold.** Same patient as depicted in Figure 9-23. Note multiple areas of erythema and erosion of the hard palate.

Once a suspected offending medication is discovered, a temporal relationship between the drug's use and the mucosal alteration must be established. The association may be acute and obvious, or the onset of the oral lesions may be delayed. If more than one medication is suspected, serial elimination of the medications should be performed until the offending agent is discovered.

Treatment and Prognosis

The responsible medication should be discontinued and, if necessary, replaced with another that provides a similar therapeutic result. Localized acute reactions can be resolved with topical corticosteroids. When systemic manifestations are present, anaphylactic stomatitis often warrants systemic administration of adrenaline (epinephrine), corticosteroids, or antihistamines. Chronic oral lesions often resolve on cessation of the offending drug, but topical corticosteroids may sometimes be required for complete resolution. If discontinuation of the medication is contraindicated, palliative care can be provided; corticosteroids, however, often are ineffective as long as the offending medication is continued.

ALLERGIC CONTACT STOMATITIS
(Stomatitis Venenata)

The list of agents reported to cause **allergic contact stomatitis** reactions in the oral cavity is extremely diverse. Numerous foods, chewing gums, dentifrices, mouthwashes, topical anesthetics, restorative metals, acrylic denture materials, dental impression materials, and denture adhesive preparations have been mentioned. Two compounds, cinnamon and amalgam, demonstrate clinical and histopathologic patterns that are sufficiently unique to justify separate descriptions.

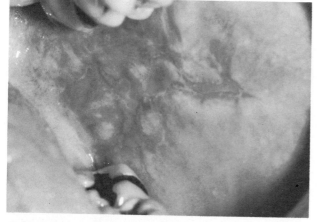

FIGURE 9-25. **Lichenoid drug reaction to allopurinol.** Irregular area of superficial erosion of the left buccal mucosa. Lesions were also present on the contralateral buccal mucosa and bilaterally on the lateral borders of the tongue.

Although the oral cavity is exposed to a wide variety of antigens, the frequency of a true allergic reaction to any one antigen from this contact appears to be rare. This was verified in a prospective study of 13,325 dental patients in which only 7 acute and 15 chronic cases of adverse effects were attributed to dental materials. The oral mucosa is much less sensitive than the surface of the skin, probably because:

- The period of contact is often brief
- The saliva dilutes and removes many antigens
- The anatomy of the mucosa allows rapid dispersal and absorption of antigens

If the skin has been sensitized originally, the mucosa may or may not demonstrate future clinical sensitization. In contrast, if the mucosa is sensitized initially, the skin usually demonstrates similar changes with future exposure.

In reviews of patients referred to allergy clinics with a preliminary diagnosis of hypersensitivity to dental materials, a small minority were definitively diagnosed as being allergic to a dental material. Positive skin test results to dental materials are insufficient for diagnosis because of the aforementioned lesser reactivity of the oral mucosa. Positive allergic history and skin tests become relevant only after a good state of oral health has been obtained with no periodontal, endodontic, or occlusal problems. (Many symptoms thought to be caused by allergies to dental materials were due to primary dental pathologic conditions.)

Clinical Features

Allergic contact stomatitis can be acute or chronic. Of those cases diagnosed, there is a distinct female predominance of both forms.

In patients with acute contact stomatitis, burning is the most frequent symptom. The appearance of the affected mucosa is variable, from a mild and barely visible erythema to a brilliantly erythematous lesion with or without edema. Vesicles are rarely seen and, when present, rapidly rupture to form areas of erosion (Fig. 9–27).

In chronic cases, the affected mucosa typically is in contact with the causative agent and may be erythematous or white and hyperkeratotic. Periodically, erosions may develop within the affected zones. Some allergens, especially toothpastes, can cause widespread erythema, with desquamation of the superficial layers of the epithelium (Fig. 9–28). In addition, the alterations may spread past the vermilion wet line to produce cheilitis or perioral dermatitis. Rarely, symptoms identical to orolingual paresthesia can be present without any clinically evident signs.

Diagnosis

The diagnosis of acute contact stomatitis is usually straightforward because of the temporal relationship between the use of the agent and the resultant eruption. The diagnosis of chronic contact stomatitis is much more difficult. Most investigators require good oral health,

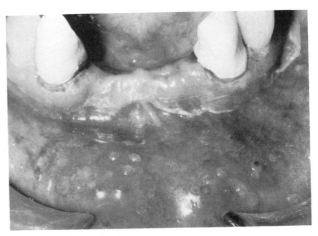

FIGURE 9–27. **Allergic contact stomatitis to aluminum chloride.** Mucosal erythema and vesicles of the lower labial mucosa caused by use of aluminum chloride on gingival retraction cord.

elimination of all other possible causes and visible oral signs, together with a positive history of allergy and a positive skin test result to the suspected allergen. If allergic contact stomatitis is strongly suspected but skin test results are negative, direct testing of the oral mucosa can be attempted. The antigen can be placed on the mucosa

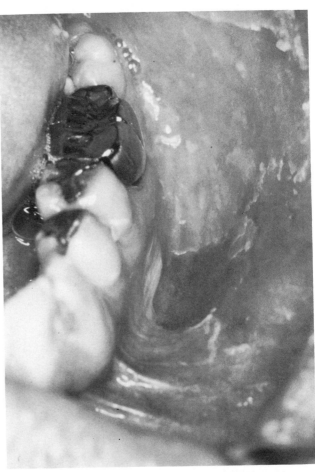

FIGURE 9–28. **Allergic contact stomatitis to toothpaste.** Erythematous mucosa with superficial epithelial desquamation.

in a mixture with Orabase or in a rubber cup, which is fixed to the mucosa.

Treatment and Prognosis

In mild cases of acute contact stomatitis, removal of the suspected allergen is all that is required. In more severe cases, antihistamine therapy, which is combined with topical anesthetics, such as dyclonine HCl, usually is beneficial. Chronic reactions respond to removal of the antigenic source and application of a topical steroid, such as fluocinonide gel or dexamethasone elixir.

CONTACT STOMATITIS FROM ARTIFICIAL CINNAMON FLAVORING

Mucosal abnormalities secondary to the use of artificially flavored cinnamon products are fairly common, but the range of changes has not been widely recognized until recently. Cinnamon oil is used as a flavoring agent in confectionery, ice cream, soft drinks, alcoholic beverages, processed meats, gum, candy, toothpaste, mouthwashes, and even dental floss. Concentrations of the flavoring are up to 100 times that in the natural spice. The reactions are documented most commonly in those products associated with prolonged or frequent contact, such as candy, chewing gum, and toothpaste.

Clinical Features

The clinical presentations of contact stomatitis vary somewhat, according to the medium of delivery. Toothpaste results in a more diffuse pattern; the signs associated with chewing gum and candy are more localized. Pain and burning are common symptoms in all cases.

The gingiva is the most frequent site affected by toothpaste, often resembling "plasma cell gingivitis" (see p. 126), and presenting with enlargement, edema, and erythema. Erythematous mucositis, occasionally combined with desquamation and erosion, has been reported on the buccal mucosa and tongue. Exfoliative cheilitis and perioral dermatitis also may occur.

Reactions from chewing gum and candy are more localized and typically do not affect the lip vermilion or perioral skin. Most of the lesions appear on the buccal mucosa and lateral borders of the tongue. Buccal mucosal lesions often are oblong patches that are aligned along the occlusal plane (Fig. 9–29; see Color Figure 53). Individual lesions have an erythematous base but often are predominantly white as a result of hyperkeratosis of the surface epithelium. Ulceration within the lesions may occur. Hyperkeratotic examples often exhibit a ragged surface and occasionally may resemble the pattern seen in morsicatio (see p. 211). Lingual involvement may become extensive and spread to the dorsal surface (Fig. 9–30). Significant thickening of the surface epithelium can occur and may raise clinical concern for hairy leukoplakia (see p. 202) or carcinoma (Fig. 9–31).

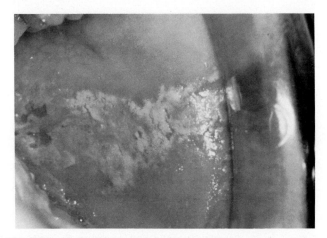

FIGURE 9–29. **Contact stomatitis from cinnamon flavoring.** Oblong area of sensitive erythema with overlying shaggy hyperkeratosis. See Color Plates.

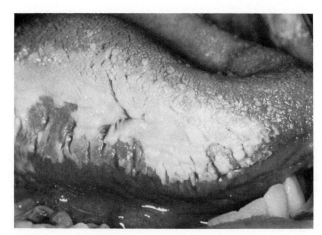

FIGURE 9–30. **Contact stomatitis from cinnamon flavoring.** Sensitive and thickened hyperkeratosis of the lateral and dorsal surface of the tongue on the right side.

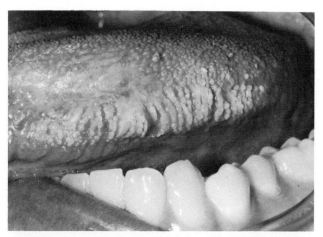

FIGURE 9–31. **Contact stomatitis from cinnamon flavoring.** Left lateral border of the tongue demonstrating linear rows of hyperkeratosis that resemble oral hairy leukoplakia.

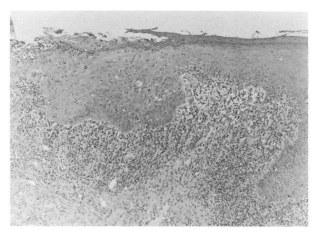

FIGURE 9–32. **Contact stomatitis from cinnamon flavoring.** Oral mucosa demonstrating neutrophilic exocytosis and significant interface mucositis.

Histopathologic Features

Usually, the epithelium in contact stomatitis from artificial cinnamon flavoring is acanthotic, often with elongated rete ridges and thinning of the suprapapillary plates. Hyperkeratosis and extensive neutrophilic exocytosis are commonly present. The superficial lamina propria demonstrates a heavy chronic inflammatory cell infiltrate that consists predominantly of lymphocytes. This infiltrate often obscures the epithelium-connective tissue interface (Fig. 9–32). A characteristic feature is the presence of an obvious perivascular infiltrate of lymphocytes, with occasional plasma cells and rare eosinophils, which extends well below the superficial inflammatory infiltrate (Fig. 9–33).

Diagnosis

With a high index of suspicion and a knowledge of the variations of the clinical pattern, the diagnosis of contact stomatitis often can be made from the clinical appearance and the history of cinnamon use. Often, biopsies are performed for atypical or extensive cases because of the differential diagnosis, which includes several significant vesiculoerosive and neoplastic conditions. The histopathologic features are not specific but are sufficient to raise a high index of suspicion in an oral and maxillofacial pathologist who is familiar with the pattern.

Treatment and Prognosis

Typically, the signs and symptoms disappear within 1 week after the discontinuation of the cinnamon product. If the patient resumes intake of the product, the lesions reappear, usually within 24 hours.

CHRONIC ORAL MUCOSAL CONTACT REACTIONS TO DENTAL AMALGAM

Since the 19th century, when dental amalgam began to have widespread use, the material has been associated in the lay press with almost every medical ailment known to man. Such accusations tend to occur in cycles. In spite of intense scrutiny, there is insufficient evidence to suggest that mercury from amalgam has a significant adverse effect on health. An investigation of patients with concerns associated with their amalgam restorations reveals that most of their complaints can be associated with oral, dental, or medical problems unrelated to the restorations.

A review of the ill effects of mercury in dental amalgam demonstrates that the occurrence of toxicity is negligible, but a small percentage (1 to 2 percent) of those who are allergic to mercury can react to the mercury released from dental amalgams. The frequency of adverse effects to dental amalgam is estimated to be one case per million. Acute hypersensitivity reactions typically appear 2 to 24 hours after the removal and replacement of dental amalgam, and the symptoms disappear after 10 to 14 days.

Rarely, chronic reactions also can occur and may be from hypersensitivity or a chronic toxic reaction. When the reaction is related to hypersensitivity, the most frequent antigen is mercury or a mercury compound; rarely is tin, zinc, copper, or silver responsible. Some investigators have called these alterations "galvanic lesions" and have suggested that the changes develop from electrical currents developed between restorative metals. However, neither clinical nor experimental studies support the electrogalvanic hypothesis of origin.

The lesions appear clinically and histopathologically similar to lichen planus (see p. 572) but demonstrate a difference in evolution. When patients with true oral lichen planus are examined, no evidence of a significantly increased hypersensitivity to dental restorative materials can be found, and these patients do not respond to the removal of their amalgams.

However, within the population of patients with conditions previously diagnosed as lichenoid lesions, there is a subgroup whose lesions do not migrate and involve only the mucosa directly in contact with dental amalgams. These lesions resolve rapidly after removal of adjacent amalgams and should be diagnosed as a **contact lichenoid reaction** to amalgam, not as true lichen planus.

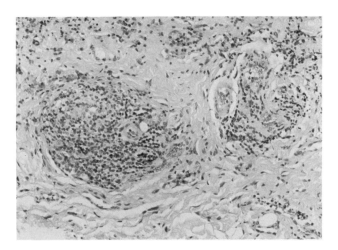

FIGURE 9–33. **Contact stomatitis from cinnamon flavoring.** Perivascular inflammatory infiltrate consisting predominantly of lymphocytes and plasma cells.

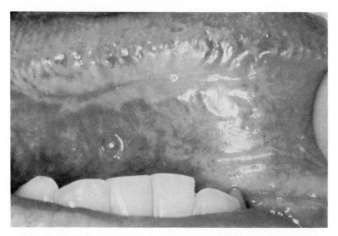

FIGURE 9-34. **Oral mucosal contact reaction to dental amalgam.** Hyperkeratotic lesion with a peripheral radiating pattern on the lateral border of the tongue on the right side; the altered mucosa contacted the amalgams of the adjacent mandibular molar teeth. The lesion remained in the same location for 5 years and periodically became erosive and symptomatic. Smoothing and polishing of the adjacent restorations had no effect.

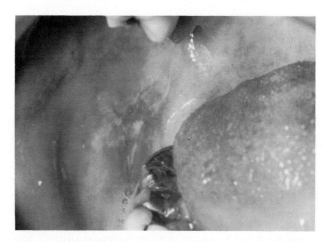

FIGURE 9-36. **Oral mucosal contact reaction to dental amalgam.** Radiating pattern of hyperkeratotic striae on the posterior buccal mucosa that contacts a large distobuccal amalgam of the permanent mandibular second molar.

Clinical Features

The most commonly affected sites in contact reactions to amalgam are the posterior buccal mucosa and the ventral surface of the lateral borders of the tongue. Gingival cuffs adjacent to subgingival amalgams also may be affected. The lesions are confined to the area of contact and may be white or erythematous with or without peripheral striae (Figs. 9-34 and 9-35). Most patients have no symptoms, but periodic erosion may be noted.

Diagnosis

The diagnosis usually is made from the clinical appearance of the lesions, the lack of migration, and the correlation to adjacent amalgams (Fig. 9-36). Appropriate skin test findings will be positive if the lesion is secondary to hypersensitivity and negative if it is related to direct toxicity.

Histopathologic Features

Biopsy material from contact reactions to amalgam exhibits numerous features of lichen planus. The surface epithelium may be hyperkeratotic, atrophic, or ulcerated. Areas of hydropic degeneration of the basal cell layer are often present. The superficial lamina propria contains a dense band-like chronic inflammatory cellular infiltrate predominantly of lymphocytes, but there may be scattered plasma cells. On occasion, deeper lymphoid aggregates may be noted.

Treatment and Prognosis

Local measures, such as improved oral hygiene, smoothing, polishing, and recontouring, should be attempted before more aggressive measures because clinically similar lesions have been noted as a result of surface plaque accumulation. If this is unsuccessful, the amalgam in question should be replaced with porcelain or composite resin. This therapeutic approach is the most conservative, and many teeth with the offending amalgam have large buccal extensions and would benefit from restoration replacement. Some investigators have reported recurrence after replacement with composite resin, but others believe that this phenomenon is due to subsequent plaque accumulation and not true recurrence. A biopsy is recommended if the clinical diagnosis is in question or if the mucosal changes do not respond to the recommended therapy.

ANGIOEDEMA (Angioneurotic Edema; Quincke's Disease)

Angioedema is a diffuse edematous swelling of the soft tissues that most commonly involves the subcutaneous and submucosal connective tissues but may affect the gastrointestinal or respiratory tract, occasionally with fatal results. The disorder has been referred to as **Quincke's disease** after the clinician who initially related the changes to an alteration in vascular permeability.

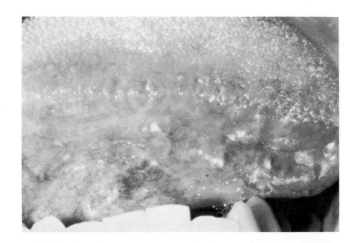

FIGURE 9-35. **Oral mucosal contact reaction to dental amalgam.** Same patient as depicted in Figure 9-34 14 days after removal of adjacent amalgams. Note total resolution of the mucosal alterations.

The outdated term **angioneurotic edema** has also been used because these lesions were once thought to be the result of nervous stimulation.

Knowledge of the mechanisms of angioedema has increased significantly. These advances have allowed us to appreciate the fact that the disorder is much more complicated than originally thought, but such insights have directly influenced therapeutic approaches. The most common cause is mast cell degranulation, which leads to histamine release and the typical clinical alterations. IgE-mediated hypersensitivity reactions due to drugs, foods, plants, dust, and inhalants produce mast cell degranulation and are fairly common. Contact allergic reactions to foods, cosmetics, topical medications, and even dental rubber dams have also been responsible. Mast cell degranulation can even result from physical stimuli, such as heat, cold, exercise, emotional stress, solar exposure, and significant vibration.

An unusual pattern of drug reaction that can produce severe forms of angioedema that are not mediated by IgE is the type associated with use of the antihypertensive drugs called angiotensin-converting enzyme (ACE) inhibitors. These medications result in angioedema secondary to increased levels of bradykinin and do not respond well to antihistamines. The angioedema may arise within hours or years after the initial use of the drug. Attacks precipitated by dental procedures have been reported in long-term users of ACE inhibitors.

In addition, angioedema can result from activation of the complement pathway. This may be hereditary or acquired. Two rare autosomal dominant hereditary forms are seen. Type I arises from a quantitative reduction in the inhibitor that prevents the transformation of C1 to C1 esterase. Without adequate levels of this inhibitor (C1-INH), C1 esterase cleaves C4 and C2 and results in angioedema. Type II exhibits normal levels of C1-INH, but the inhibitor is dysfunctional.

The acquired type of C1-INH deficiency is seen in association with certain types of lymphoproliferative diseases or in patients who develop specific autoantibodies. The lymphoid proliferation increases the consumption of C1-INH, and the autoantibodies prevent binding of C1-INH to C1. In both the acquired and hereditary forms of abnormal C1-INH activity, minor trauma, such as a dental procedure, can precipitate an attack.

Finally, angioedema has been seen in the presence of high levels of antigen-antibody complexes (i.e., lupus erythematosus and viral and bacterial infections) and in patients with grossly elevated peripheral blood eosinophil counts.

Clinical Features

Angioedema is characterized by the relatively rapid onset of soft, nontender tissue swelling, which may be

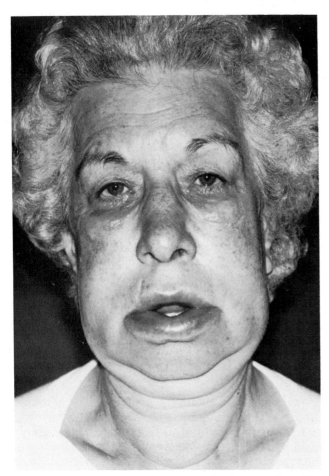

FIGURE 9–37. **Angioedema.** Soft, nontender tissue swelling of the face arose relatively rapidly after dental treatment.

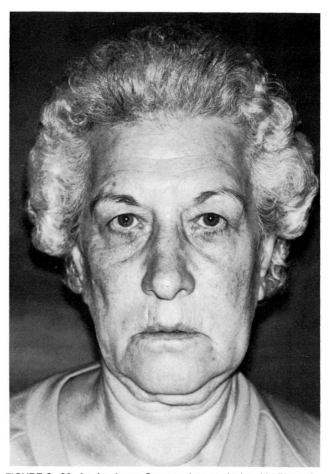

FIGURE 9–38. **Angioedema.** Same patient as depicted in Figure 9–37 after resolution of edematous facial enlargement.

solitary or multiple. Involvement of the skin and mucous membranes can cause enlargements, which may measure up to several centimeters in diameter (Figs. 9–37 and 9–38). The sites of dermatologic involvement include the face, hands, arms, legs, genitals, and buttocks. Although pain is unusual, itching is common and erythema may be present. The enlargement typically resolves over 24 to 72 hours.

Involvement of the respiratory and gastrointestinal systems occurs mainly in the hereditary forms. In these forms, most affected patients become symptomatic during the second decade of life and then follow a highly variable frequency of recurrences. Most attacks occur without apparent reason. Gastrointestinal symptoms may mimic surgical emergencies and include continuous pain, vomiting, and rarely watery diarrhea. Respiratory involvement centers around the upper airway (pharynx and larynx) and is potentially life-threatening from closure of the airway, with hoarseness and difficulty in swallowing or breathing being important signs. Laryngeal involvement also is not unusual in cases related to ACE inhibitors.

Perioral and periorbital involvement is typical of allergic angioedema. In addition, allergic angioedema and the type that is related to ACE inhibitors frequently demonstrate intraoral involvement, which can affect the lips, tongue, uvula, floor of mouth, or facial cheek areas.

Diagnosis

In cases of allergic causation, the diagnosis of angioedema is often made from the clinical presentation in conjunction with the known antigenic stimulus. When multiple antigenic exposures occur, the diagnosis of the offending agent can be difficult and involves dietary diaries and antigenic testing.

Those patients whose conditions cannot be related to antigenic exposure or medications should be evaluated for the presence of adequate functional C1-INH. In the hereditary types, both forms exhibit normal levels of C1 and decreased levels of *functional* C1-INH. Type I demonstrates a decreased quantity of C1-INH; type II exhibits normal levels of the inhibitor (but it is not functional). Both acquired forms demonstrate low levels of both C1-INH and C1.

Treatment and Prognosis

The treatment of angioedema usually consists of oral antihistamines. If the attack is not controlled or if laryngeal involvement is present, intramuscular epinephrine should be administered. If the epinephrine does not stop the attack, intravenous corticosteroids and antihistamines should be given. Cases of angioedema related to ACE inhibitors are not IgE-mediated and may not respond to antihistamines and corticosteroids. Because the airway may have to be opened, affected patients are kept under close observation until the swelling begins to subside.

Those cases related to C1-INH deficiency do not respond to antihistamines, corticosteroids, or adrenergic drugs. Intubation and tracheostomy may be required for laryngeal involvement. Fresh freeze-dried plasma has been used, but some investigators do not recommend its use because there is a risk of transmitting infection and it replaces not only C1-INH but also potentially harmful C1 esterase, C1, C2, and C4. C1-INH concentrate and esterase inhibiting drugs (aprotinin or tranexamic acid) are the treatments of choice for acute attacks.

Because acute attacks of hereditary angioedema are not only unpleasant but also potentially life-threatening, prevention is paramount. Patients should avoid violent physical activity and trauma. Medical prophylaxis is recommended before any dental and surgical procedure. All patients should carry medical warning cards that state the diagnosis and list elementary precautions.

Prophylaxis for C1-INH deficiency is recommended in patients who have more than three attacks a year. Androgens induce hepatic synthesis of C1-INH, and either of the attenuated androgens, danazol or stanozolol, is used for both the hereditary forms and the acquired type that is related to lymphoproliferative disorders. The autoimmune acquired type is best prevented through the use of corticosteroids.

References

Recurrent Aphthous Stomatitis

Bagán JV, et al. Recurrent aphthous stomatitis. A study of the clinical characteristics of lesions in 93 cases. J Oral Pathol Med 20:395–397, 1991.

Brice SL, Jester JD, Huff JC. Recurrent aphthous stomatitis. Curr Probl Dermatol 3:107–127, 1991.

Brooke RI, Sapp JP. Herpetiform ulceration. Oral Surg Oral Med Oral Pathol 42:182–188, 1976.

Challacombe SJ, et al. HLA antigens in recurrent oral ulceration. Arch Dermatol 113:1717–1719, 1977.

Hay KD, Reade PC. The use of an elimination diet in the treatment of recurrent aphthous ulceration of the oral cavity. Oral Surg Oral Med Oral Pathol 57:504–507, 1984.

Nolan A, et al. Recurrent aphthous ulceration: Vitamin B₁, B₂ and B₆ status and response to replacement therapy. J Oral Pathol Med 20:389–391, 1991.

Nolan A, et al. Recurrent aphthous ulceration and food sensitivity. J Oral Pathol Med 20:473–475, 1991.

Pedersen A, et al. T-lymphocyte subsets in recurrent aphthous ulceration. J Oral Pathol Med 18:59–60, 1989.

Pedersen A, et al. Peripheral lymphocyte subpopulations in recurrent aphthous ulceration. Acta Odontol Scand 49:203–206, 1991.

Pedersen A, Hougen HP, Kenrad B. T-lymphocyte subsets in oral mucosa of patients with recurrent aphthous ulceration. J Oral Pathol Med 21:176–180, 1992.

Pedersen A, Hornsleth A. Recurrent aphthous ulceration: A possible clinical manifestation of reactivation of varicella zoster or cytomegalovirus infection. J Oral Pathol Med 22:64–68, 1993.

Porter SR, Scully C. Aphthous stomatitis—an overview of aetiopathogenesis and management. Clin Exp Dermatol 16:235–243, 1991.

Porter S, Scully C. Recurrent aphthous stomatitis: The efficacy of replacement therapy in patients with underlying hematinic deficiencies. Ann Dent 51:14–16, 1992.

Savage NW, Seymour GJ, Kruger BJ. T-lymphocyte subset changes in recurrent aphthous stomatitis. Oral Surg Oral Med Oral Pathol 60:175–181, 1985.

Vincent SD, Lilly GE. Clinical, historic, and therapeutic features of aphthous stomatitis. Literature review and open clinical trial employing steroids. Oral Surg Oral Med Oral Pathol 74:79–86, 1992.

Wray D, Graykowski EA, Notkins AL. Role of mucosal injury in initiating recurrent aphthous stomatitis. Br Med J 283:1569–1570, 1981.

Behçet's Syndrome (Behçet's Disease)

Arbesfeld SJ, Kurban AK. Behçet's disease: New perspectives on an enigmatic syndrome. J Am Acad Dermatol 19:767–779, 1988.

Eisenbud L, Horowitz I, Kay B. Recurrent aphthous stomatitis of the Behçet's type: Successful treatment with thalidomide. Oral Surg Oral Med Oral Pathol 64:289–292, 1987.

Helm TN, et al. Clinical features of Behçet's disease: Report of four cases. Oral Surg Oral Med Oral Pathol 72:30–34, 1991.

International Study Group for Behçet's Disease. Criteria for diagnosis for Behçet's disease. Lancet 335:1078–1080, 1990.

Lehner T, et al. An immunogenetic basis for the tissue involvement in Behçet's syndrome. Immunology 37:895–900, 1979.

Lehner T, Welsh KI, Batchelor JR. The relationship of HLA-B and DR phenotypes to Behçet's syndrome, the recurrent oral ulceration and the class of immune complexes. Immunology 47:581–587, 1982.

Mizushima Y. Behçet's disease. Curr Opin Rheumatol 3:32–35, 1991.

O'Duffy JD. Meeting the diagnostic challenge of Behçet's disease. Cleve Clin J Med 60:13–14, 1993.

Yazici H, Barnes CG. Practical treatment recommendations for pharmacotherapy of Behçet's syndrome. Drugs 42:796–804, 1991.

Sarcoidosis

Cohen DM, Reinhardt RA. Systemic sarcoidosis presenting with Horner's syndrome and mandibular paresthesia. Oral Surg Oral Med Oral Pathol 53:577–581, 1982.

Gold RS, Sager E. Oral sarcoidosis: Review of the literature. J Oral Surg 34:237–244, 1976.

Hildebrand J, Plezia RA, Rao SB. Sarcoidosis: Report of two cases with oral involvement. Oral Surg Oral Med Oral Pathol 69:217–222, 1990.

Marx RE, Hartman KS, Rethman KV. A prospective study comparing incisional labial to incisional parotid biopsies in the detection and confirmation of sarcoidosis, Sjögren's disease, sialosis and lymphoma. J Rheumatol 15:621–629, 1988.

Melsom RD, et al. Sarcoidosis in a patient presenting with clinical and histologic features of primary Sjögren's syndrome. Ann Rheum Dis 47:166–168, 1988.

Mendelsohn SS, Field EA, Woolgar J. Sarcoidosis of the tongue. Clin Exp Dermatol 17:47–48, 1992.

O'Connor CM, FitzGerald MX. Speculations on sarcoidosis. Respir Med 86:277–282, 1992.

Saboor SA, Johnson NM. Sarcoidosis. Br J Hosp Med 48:293–302, 1992.

Tozman ECS. Sarcoidosis: Clinical manifestations, epidemiology, therapy, and pathophysiology. Curr Opin Rheumatol 3:155–159, 1991.

Orofacial Granulomatosis

Allen CM, et al. Cheilitis granulomatosa: Report of six cases and review of the literature. J Am Acad Dermatol 23:444–450, 1990.

Fox R, Sharp D, Evans I. Orofacial granulomatosis (editorial). Lancet 338:20–21, 1991.

Ghandour K, Issa M. Oral Crohn's disease with late intestinal disease. Oral Surg Oral Med Oral Pathol 72:565–567, 1991.

Glickman LT, et al. The surgical management of Melkersson-Rosenthal syndrome. Plast Reconstr Surg 89:815–821, 1992.

Lamey P-J, Lewis MAO. Oral medicine in practice: Orofacial allergic reactions. Br Dent J 168:59–63, 1990.

Meisel-Stosiek M, Hornstein OP, Stosiek N. Family study of Melkersson-Rosenthal syndrome: Some hereditary aspects of the disease and review of the literature. Acta Derm Venereol (Stockh) 70:221–226, 1990.

Oliver AJ, et al. Monosodium glutamate-related orofacial granulomatosis: Review and case report. Oral Surg Oral Med Oral Pathol 71:560–564, 1991.

Patton DW, et al. Oro-facial granulomatosis: A possible allergic basis. Br J Oral Maxillofac Surg 23:235–242, 1985.

Plauth M, Jenss H, Meyle J. Oral manifestations of Crohn's disease. J Clin Gastroenterol 13:29–37, 1991.

Scully C, et al. Crohn's disease of the mouth: An indicator of intestinal involvement. Gut 23:198–201, 1982.

Wiesenfeld D, et al. Oro-facial granulomatosis—a clinical and pathological analysis. Q J Med 54:101–113, 1985.

Winnie R, DeLuke DM. Melkersson-Rosenthal syndrome: Review of the literature and case report. Int J Oral Maxillofac Surg 21:115–117, 1992.

Worsaae N, et al. Melkersson-Rosenthal and cheilitis granulomatosa: A clinicopathologic study of thirty-three patients with special reference to their oral lesions. Oral Surg Oral Med Oral Pathol 54:404–413, 1982.

Wysocki GP, Brooke RI: Oral manifestations of chronic granulomatous disease. Oral Surg Oral Med Oral Pathol 46:815–819, 1978.

Zimmer WM, et al. Orofacial manifestations of Melkersson-Rosenthal syndrome: A study of 42 patients and review of 220 cases from the literature. Oral Surg Oral Med Oral Pathol 74:610–619, 1992.

Wegener's Granulomatosis

Allen CM, et al. Wegener's granulomatosis: Report of three cases with oral lesions. J Oral Maxillofac Surg 49:294–298, 1991.

Cassan SM, Coles DT, Harrison EG. The concept of limited forms of Wegener's granulomatosis. Am J Med 49:366–379, 1970.

Cohen RE, et al. Gingival manifestations of Wegener's granulomatosis. J Periodontol 61:705–709, 1990.

Eufinger H, Machtens E, Akuamoa-Boateng E. Oral manifestations of Wegener's granulomatosis: Review of the literature and report of a case. Int J Oral Maxillofac Surg 21:50–53, 1992.

Fauci AS, et al. Wegener's granulomatosis: Prospective clinical and therapeutic experience with 85 patients for 21 years. Ann Intern Med 98:76–85, 1983.

Fienberg R. The protracted superficial phenomenon in pathergic (Wegener's) granulomatosis. Hum Pathol 12:458–467, 1981.

Geiger WJ, Garrison KL, Losh DP. Wegener's granulomatosis. Am Fam Physician 45:191–196, 1992.

Handlers JP, et al. Oral features of Wegener's granulomatosis. Arch Otolaryngol 111:267–270, 1985.

Hoffman GS, et al. The treatment of Wegener's granulomatosis with glucocorticoids and methotrexate. Arthritis Rheum 35:1322–1329, 1992.

Napier SS, et al. Strawberry gums: A clinicopathological manifestations diagnostic of Wegener's granulomatosis? J Clin Pathol 46:709–712, 1993.

Parson E, et al. Wegener's granulomatosis: A distinct gingival lesion. J Clin Periodontol 19:64–66, 1992.

Patten SF, Tomecki JT. Wegener's granulomatosis: Cutaneous and oral mucosal disease. J Am Acad Dermatol 28:710–718, 1993.

Specks U, et al. Salivary gland involvement in Wegener's granulomatosis. Arch Otolaryngol Head Neck Surg 117:218–223, 1991.

Vanhauwaert BG, et al. Salivary gland involvement as initial presentation of Wegener's disease. Postgrad Med J 69:643–645, 1993.

Walton EW. Giant-cell granuloma of the respiratory tract (Wegener's granulomatosis). Br Med J 2:265–270, 1958.

Mucosal Reactions to Systemic Drug Administration

Eversole LR. Allergic stomatitides. J Oral Med 34:93–102, 1979.

Felder RS, Millar SB, Henry RH. Oral manifestations of drug therapy. Spec Care Dent 8:119–124, 1988.

Jain VK, Dixit VB, Archana. Fixed drug eruption of the oral mucous membrane. Ann Dent 50:9–11, 1991.

Kane M, Zacharczenko N. Oral side effects of drugs. N Y State Dent J 59:37–40, 1993.

Matthews TG. Medication side effects of dental interest. J Prosthet Dent 64:219–226, 1990.

Paterson AJ, et al. Pemphigus vulgaris precipitated by glibenclamide therapy. J Oral Pathol Med 22:92–95, 1993.

Potts AJC, Hamburger J, Scully C. The medication of patients with oral lichen planus and the association of nonsteroidal anti-inflammatory drugs with erosive lesions. Oral Surg Oral Med Oral Pathol 64:541–543, 1987.

Robertson WD, Wray D. Ingestion of medication among patients with oral keratosis including lichen planus. Oral Surg Oral Med Oral Pathol 74:183–185, 1992.

Wright JM. Oral manifestations of drug reactions. Dent Clin North Am 28:529–543, 1984.

Allergic Contact Stomatitis

Beacham BE, Kurgansky D, Gould WM. Circumoral dermatitis and cheilitis caused by tartar control dentrifices. J Am Acad Dermatol 22:1029–1032, 1990.

Burrows D. Hypersensitivity to mercury, nickel and chromium in relation to dental materials. Int Dent J 36:30–34, 1986.

Dutrée-Meulenberg ROGM, Kozel MMA, van Joost T. Burning mouth syndrome: A possible etiologic role for local contact hypersensitivity. J Am Acad Dermatol 26:935–940, 1992.

Eversole LR. Allergic stomatitides. J Oral Med 34:93–102, 1979.

Fisher AA. Contact stomatitis, glossitis, and cheilitis. Otolaryngol Clin North Am 7:827–843, 1974.

Fisher AA. Reactions of the mucous membrane to contactants. Clin Dermatol 5:123–136, 1987.

Kallus T, Mjör IA. Incidence of adverse effects of dental materials. Scand J Dent Res 99:236–240, 1991.

Stenman E, Bergman M. Hypersensitivity reactions to dental materials in a referred group of patients. Scand J Dent Res 97:76–83, 1989.

van Loon LAJ, Bos JD, Davidson CL. Clinical evaluation of fifty-six patients referred with symptoms tentatively related to allergic contact stomatitis. Oral Surg Oral Med Oral Pathol 74:572–575, 1992.

Cinnamon-Induced Contact Stomatitis

Allen CM, Blozis GG. Oral mucosal reactions to cinnamon-flavored chewing gum. J Am Dent Assoc 116:664–667, 1988.

Drake TE, Maibach HI. Allergic contact dermatitis and stomatitis caused by a cinnamic aldehyde-flavored toothpaste. Arch Dermatol 112:202–203, 1976.

Lamey P-J, Ress TD, Forsyth A. Sensitivity reaction to the cinnamon-aldehyde component of toothpaste. Br Dent J 168:115–118, 1990.

Mihail RC. Oral leukoplakia caused by cinnamon food allergy. J Otolaryngol 21:366–367, 1992.

Millard L. Acute contact sensitivity to a new toothpaste. J Dent 1:168–170, 1973.

Miller RL, Gould AR, Bernstein ML. Cinnamon-induced stomatitis venenata. Clinical and characteristic histopathologic features. Oral Surg Oral Med Oral Pathol 73:708–716, 1992.

Tyne G, Young DW, Ferguson MM. Contact stomatitis caused by toothpaste. N Z Dent J 85:124–126, 1989.

Oral Mucosal Contact Reaction to Dental Amalgam

Bergman M. Side-effects of amalgam and its alternatives: Local, systemic and environmental. Int Dent J 40:4–10, 1990.

Bolewska J, et al. Oral mucosal lesions related to silver amalgam restorations. Oral Surg Oral Med Oral Pathol 70:55–58, 1990.

Eversole LR, Ringer M. The role of dental restorative materials in the pathogenesis of oral lichen planus. Oral Surg Oral Med Oral Pathol 57:383–387, 1984.

Hietanen J, et al. No evidence of hypersensitivity to dental restorative metals in oral lichen planus. Scand J Dent Res 95:320–327, 1987.

Holmstrup P. Reaction of the oral mucosa related to silver amalgam: A review. J Oral Pathol Med 20:1–7, 1991.

Holmstrup P. Oral mucosa and skin reactions related to amalgam. Adv Dent Res 6:120–124, 1992.

Hugoson A. Results obtained from patients referred for the investigation of complaints related to oral galvanism. Swed Dent J 10:15–28, 1986.

Jameson MW, et al. Mucosal reactions to amalgam restorations. J Oral Rehabil 17:293–301, 1990.

Kaaber S. Allergy to dental materials with special reference to the use of amalgam and polymethylmethacrylate. Int Dent J 40:359–365, 1990.

Meurman JH, Porko C, Murtomaa H. Patients complaining about amalgam-related symptoms suffer more often from illnesses and chronic craniofacial pain than their controls. Scand J Dent Res 98:167–172, 1990.

Angioedema

Angostoni A, Cicardi M. Hereditary and acquired C1-inhibitor deficiency: Biological and clinical characteristics in 235 patients. Medicine 71:206–215, 1992.

Atkinson JC, Frank MM. Oral manifestations and dental management of patients with hereditary angioedema. J Oral Pathol Med 20:139–142, 1991.

Blinkhorn AS, Leggate EM. An allergic reaction to rubber dam. Br Dent J 156:402–403, 1984.

Greaves M, Lawlor F. Angioedema: Manifestations and management. J Am Acad Dermatol 25:155–165, 1991.

Mattingly G, Rodu B, Alling R. Quincke's disease: Nonhereditary angioneurotic edema of the uvula. Oral Surg Oral Med Oral Pathol 75:292–295, 1993.

Megerian CA, Arnold JE, Berer M. Angioedema: 5 years' experience, with a review of the disorder's presentation and treatment. Laryngoscope 102:256–260, 1992.

Peacock ME, et al. Angioedema as a complication in periodontal surgery: Report of a case. J Periodontol 62:643–645, 1991.

Thompson T, Frable MAS. Drug-induced, life-threatening angioedema revisited. Laryngoscope 103:10–12, 1993.

10

Epithelial Pathology

ORAL SQUAMOUS PAPILLOMA

The **squamous papilloma** is a benign proliferation of stratified squamous epithelium, presumably induced by human papillomavirus (HPV). HPV encompasses a group of double-stranded DNA viruses of the papovavirus subgroup A, which can become totally integrated with the DNA of the host cell. At present, there are more than 64 known HPV subtypes and many are associated with lesions of the head and neck. These viruses can often be identified by *in situ* hybridization, immunohistochemical analysis, and polymerase chain reaction (PCR) techniques, but they are not visible with routine histopathologic staining. Viral subtypes HPV-6 and HPV-11 have been identified in up to 50 percent of oral papillomas.

The exact mode of transmission is unknown. In contrast to other HPV-induced lesions, the viruses in this lesion appear to have an extremely low virulence and infectivity rate. A latency or incubation period of 3 to 12 months has been suggested.

Squamous papillomas make up approximately 3 percent of oral lesions that are submitted for biopsy and are found in four of every 1000 adults. Although some authors have speculated that papillomas develop predominantly in children, epidemiologic studies seem to confirm that they can arise at any age.

Clinical Features

Oral squamous papilloma most commonly is diagnosed in people 30 to 50 years of age and appears with equal frequency in both men and women. Sites of predilection include the tongue and soft palate, but any oral surface may be affected. This lesion is, in fact, the most common of the soft tissue masses arising from the tongue and palate.

The squamous papilloma is a soft, painless, usually pedunculated exophytic lesion with numerous finger-like surface projections that impart a "cauliflower" or wart-like appearance (Fig. 10–1; see Color Figure 54). Projections may be pointed (Fig. 10–2). Lesions may be white, slightly red, or normal in color, depending on the amount of surface keratinization (Fig. 10–3). Papillomas are usually solitary and typically enlarge rapidly to a maximum size of about 0.5 cm, with little or no change thereafter. However, lesions as large as 3.0 cm in greatest diameter have been reported.

It is sometimes difficult to distinguish this lesion clinically from verruca vulgaris (see p. 262) or condyloma acuminatum (see p. 263). In addition, extensive coalescing papillary lesions (papillomatosis) of the oral mucosa may be seen in several skin disorders, including nevus unius lateris, acanthosis nigricans, and focal dermal hypoplasia syndrome (Goltz-Gorlin syndrome).

Histopathologic Features

The papilloma is characterized by a proliferation of keratinized stratified squamous epithelium arrayed in finger-like projections with fibrovascular connective tissue cores (Fig. 10–4). The connective tissue cores may

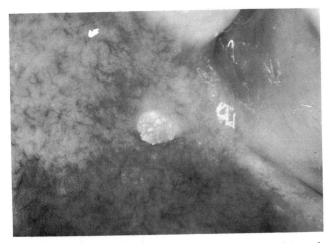

FIGURE 10-1. **Squamous papilloma.** An exophytic lesion of the soft palate with multiple short, white surface projections. See Color Plates.

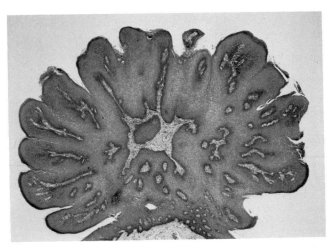

FIGURE 10-4. **Squamous papilloma.** Low-power view showing a pedunculated squamous epithelial proliferation. There are multiple papillary projections with fibrovascular connective tissue cores.

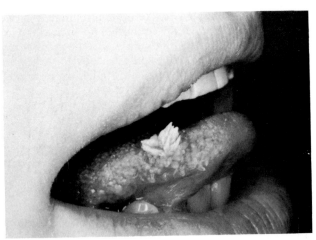

FIGURE 10-2. **Squamous papilloma.** A pedunculated lingual mass with numerous long, pointed, and white surface projections. Note the smaller projections around the base of the lesion.

show chronic inflammatory changes, depending on the amount of trauma sustained by the lesion. The keratin layer may be thick in lesions with a whiter clinical appearance, and the epithelium typically shows a normal maturation pattern (Fig. 10-5). Occasional papillomas

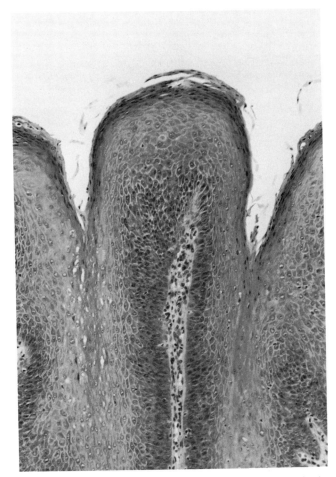

FIGURE 10-5. **Squamous papilloma.** The tip of a papillary projection shows mature stratified squamous epithelium with a slightly thickened parakeratin surface layer.

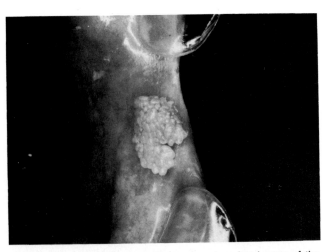

FIGURE 10-3. **Squamous papilloma.** A pedunculated mass of the buccal commissure, exhibiting quite short or blunted surface projections and minimal white coloration.

demonstrate basilar hyperplasia and mitotic activity, which can be mistaken for mild epithelial dysplasia.

Treatment and Prognosis

Conservative surgical excision, including the base of the lesion, is adequate treatment for a patient with squamous papilloma, and recurrence is unlikely. Frequently, lesions have been left untreated for years with no reported transformation into malignancy, continuous enlargement, or dissemination to other parts of the oral cavity. Squamous papillomas of the larynx behave differently from their oral counterparts. Laryngeal lesions tend to recur more often after therapy and are more likely to be multiple and continuously proliferative.

SINONASAL PAPILLOMAS

Papillomas of the sinonasal tract are benign, localized proliferations of the respiratory mucosa of this region. This mucosa gives rise to three histomorphologically distinct papillomas:

- Fungiform
- Inverted
- Cylindrical cell

In addition, a keratinizing papilloma, similar to the oral squamous papilloma, may occur in the nasal vestibule.

Collectively, **sinonasal papillomas** represent 5 to 10 percent of all tumors of the nasal and paranasal region. Approximately 50 percent arise from the mucosa of the lateral nasal wall; the remainder predominantly involve the maxillary and ethmoid sinuses and the nasal septum. Multiple lesions may be present.

The cause of sinonasal papillomas remains controversial and unclear. Some authorities say that these lesions represent neoplasms; others consider them to be a reactive hyperplasia secondary to a variety of environmental stimulants, including:

- Allergy
- Chronic bacterial or viral (HPV-11) infection
- Tobacco smoking

Patients with sinonasal papillomas are not prone to have papillomas in other anatomic sites.

Fungiform (Septal, Squamous, Exophytic) Papilloma

The **fungiform papilloma** bears some similarity to the oral squamous papilloma, although it has a somewhat more aggressive biologic behavior and more varied epithelial types. It represents 50 percent of all sinonasal papillomas.

Clinical Features

The fungiform papilloma arises almost exclusively on the nasal septum and is twice as common in men as in women. It occurs primarily in people 20 to 50 years of age. Typically, it presents with unilateral nasal obstruction or epistaxis and appears as a pink or tan, broad-based nodule with papillary or warty surface projections.

Histopathologic Features

The fungiform papilloma has a microscopic appearance similar to that of an oral squamous papilloma, although the stratified squamous epithelium covering the finger-like projections seldom is keratinized. Respiratory epithelium or "transitional" epithelium (intermediate between squamous and respiratory) may be seen in some lesions. Mucous (goblet) cells and intraepithelial microcysts containing mucus are often present. Mitoses are infrequent, and dysplasia is rare. The underlying connective tissue consists of delicate fibrous tissue with a minimal inflammatory component, unless it is irritated.

Treatment and Prognosis

Complete surgical excision is the treatment of choice for fungiform papillomas. Recurrence is common, developing in approximately one third of all cases, although this may be due to incomplete excision. Most authorities consider this lesion to have minimal or no premalignant character.

Inverted Papilloma

Approximately 45 percent of sinonasal papillomas are **inverted papillomas**. This variant has a greater potential for local destruction and sometimes is associated with malignant change.

Clinical and Radiographic Features

The inverted papilloma seldom occurs in patients younger than 20 years of age; the median age is 55 years. A strong male predilection is noted. This lesion arises predominantly from the lateral nasal cavity wall or a paranasal sinus, usually the antrum. Typically, an inverted papilloma presents with unilateral nasal obstruction, but it may cause pain, epistaxis, purulent discharge, or local deformity. The papilloma appears as a soft, pink or tan, polypoid or nodular growth with numerous blunted surface projections.

Pressure erosion of the underlying bone is usually present and may be visible radiographically as an irregular radiolucency. Primary sinus lesions may be distinguishable only as a soft tissue radiodensity or mucosal thickening on radiographs; sinus involvement generally represents extension from the nasal cavity. Magnetic resonance imaging (MRI) can help to identify the extent of the lesion (Fig. 10-6).

Histopathologic Features

Microscopically, the inverted papilloma is characterized by squamous epithelial proliferation into the sub-

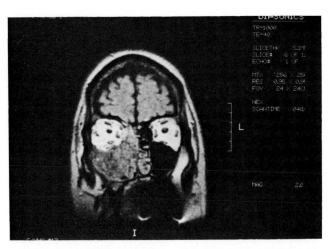

FIGURE 10–6. Inverted papilloma. T1-weighted coronal magnetic resonance image (MRI) showing a tumor of the right lateral nasal fossa. The tumor fills the right maxillary and ethmoid sinuses and involves the floor of the orbit. (Courtesy of Dr. Pamela Van Tassel.)

mucosal stroma (Fig. 10–7). The basement membrane remains intact, and the epithelium appears to be "pushing" into underlying connective tissue. Goblet (mucous) cells and mucin-filled microcysts frequently are noted within the epithelium. Keratin production is uncommon, but surface keratinization may be seen. Mitoses may be noted within the basilar or parabasilar cells, and varying degrees of dysplasia may be seen. The stroma may consist of dense fibrous or loose myxomatous connective tissue with or without inflammatory cells. Destruction of underlying bone frequently is noted.

Treatment and Prognosis

The inverted papilloma has a significant growth potential and, if neglected, may extend into the nasopharynx, middle ear, orbit, or cranial base. In some studies, recurrence after conservative surgical excision has been

reported in nearly 75 percent of all cases. The recommended treatment, therefore, is a lateral rhinotomy and *en bloc* excision of the involved lateral nasal wall. The mucosa of the adjacent paranasal sinus also is removed. With this procedure, the recurrence rate is still 14 to 30 percent of cases. Usually, the lesions reappear within 2 years of surgery. Because recurrences can happen much later, long-term follow-up is essential.

The inverted papilloma also is associated with malignancy, usually **squamous cell carcinoma**, in 3 to 24 percent of cases. In such an eventuality, of course, the lesion is treated as a malignancy, typically with more radical surgery with or without adjunctive radiotherapy.

Cylindrical Cell Papilloma (Oncocytic Schneiderian Papilloma)

Cylindrical cell papillomas account for only 3 to 5 percent of sinonasal papillomas. This lesion is considered by some authorities to be a variant of the **inverted papilloma** because of the similarity in clinical and histopathologic features.

Clinical Features

Cylindrical cell papilloma typically occurs in adults 20 to 50 years of age. There is a strong male predominance, with a predilection for the lateral nasal cavity wall. It presents with unilateral nasal obstruction and appears as a beefy-red or brown nodule with numerous blunted surface projections.

Histopathologic Features

Microscopically, the cylindrical cell papilloma demonstrates both endophytic and exophytic growth. Surface papillary projections are covered by a multilayered columnar epithelium that is three to eight cells thick. The typical cell has a small, dark nucleus with eosinophilic, occasionally granular cytoplasm that is similar to that of an oncocyte. Cilia may be seen on the surface, and there are numerous intraepithelial microcysts filled with mucin, neutrophils, or both. The epithelium overlies a fibrovascular connective tissue that extends as a core into each of the surface projections.

Treatment and Prognosis

Cylindrical cell papilloma is treated in the same manner as inverted papilloma (see previous topic). The potential for recurrence and malignant transformation seems to be lower than that of the inverted papilloma.

VERRUCA VULGARIS (Common Wart)

Verruca vulgaris is a benign, virus-induced, focal hyperplasia of stratified squamous epithelium. The associated viruses are HPV-2, HPV-4, and HPV-40. Verruca vulgaris is contagious and can spread to other parts of

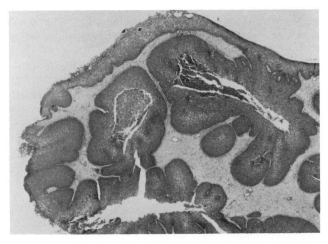

FIGURE 10–7. Inverted papilloma. Low-power photomicrograph showing a squamous epithelial proliferation, with multiple "inverting" islands of epithelium extending into the underlying connective tissue.

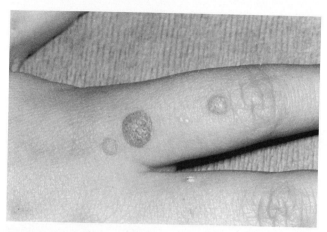

FIGURE 10–8. **Verruca vulgaris.** Several warts on the finger, exhibiting a rough, papillary surface.

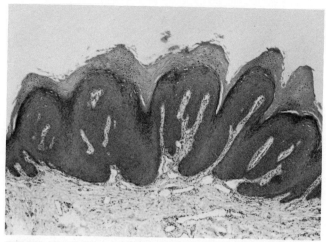

FIGURE 10–10. **Verruca vulgaris.** Numerous pointed and blunted projections are covered by a hyperkeratinized stratified squamous epithelium. A connective tissue core is seen in each projection. Elongated rete ridges at the edge of the lesion converge toward the center.

a person's skin or mucous membranes by way of auto-inoculation. It is uncommon on oral mucosa but extremely common on the skin.

Clinical Features

Verruca vulgaris is frequently discovered in children, but occasional lesions may arise even into middle age. The skin of the hands is the usual site of infection (Fig. 10–8). When the oral mucosa is involved, the lesions are usually found on the vermilion border, labial mucosa, or anterior tongue.

Typically, the lesion presents as a painless papule or nodule with papillary projections or a rough "verruciform" surface (Fig. 10–9). It may be pedunculated or sessile. Cutaneous lesions may be pink, yellow, or white. The oral lesions are almost always white. Verruca vulgaris enlarges rapidly to its maximum size, usually less than 5 mm, and the size remains constant for months or years thereafter unless the lesion is irritated. Multiple or clustered lesions are common.

Histopathologic Features

The verruca vulgaris is characterized by a proliferation of hyperkeratotic stratified squamous epithelium arranged into finger-like or pointed projections with connective tissue cores (Fig. 10–10). The supporting connective tissue often is infiltrated by chronic inflammatory cells. Elongated rete ridges tend to converge toward the center of the lesion, producing a "cupping" effect. A prominent granular cell layer (hypergranulosis) exhibits coarse, clumped keratohyaline granules. Abundant koilocytes are often seen in the superficial spinous layer (Fig. 10–11). Koilocytes are HPV-altered epithelial cells with perinuclear clear spaces and nuclear pyknosis. Eosinophilic intranuclear viral inclusions are sometimes noted within the cells of the granular layer.

Treatment and Prognosis

Skin verrucae are treated effectively by conservative surgical excision or curettage, liquid nitrogen cryotherapy, or topical application of keratinolytic agents (usually containing salicylic acid and lactic acid). Oral lesions are usually surgically excised, or they may be destroyed by cryotherapy or electrosurgery. All destructive or surgical treatments should extend to include the base of the lesion. Recurrence is seen in a small proportion of treated cases. Verrucae do not transform into malignancy, and two thirds disappear spontaneously within 2 years, especially in children.

CONDYLOMA ACUMINATUM
(Venereal Wart)

Condyloma acuminatum is a virus-induced proliferation of stratified squamous epithelium of the genitalia, perianal region, mouth, and larynx. It appears to be associated with HPV-6, HPV-11, HPV-16, and HPV-18 and others. This is considered to be a sexually transmit-

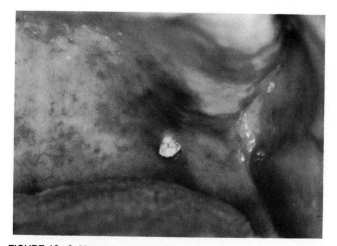

FIGURE 10–9. **Verruca vulgaris.** Exophytic, white, papillary lesion of the lateral soft palate.

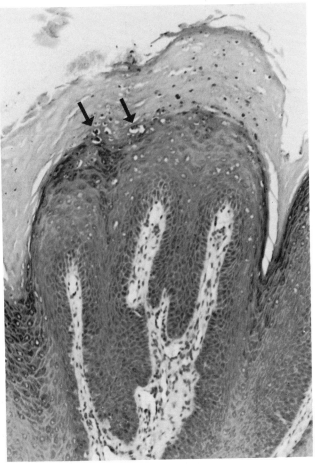

FIGURE 10–11. **Verruca vulgaris.** The epithelium is mature and demonstrates a prominent granular cell layer with coarse, clumped intracellular keratohyaline granules in addition to an excessively thick keratin layer. Koilocytes (*arrows*) are present within the superficial epithelium.

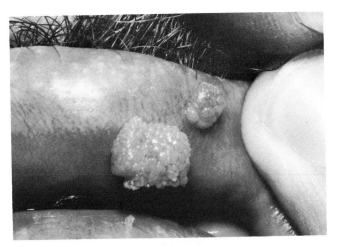

FIGURE 10–12. **Condyloma acuminatum.** Two lesions of the upper lip mucosa exhibit numerous blunted projections. (Courtesy of Dr. Brian Blocher.)

ted disease (STD), with lesions developing at a site of sexual contact or trauma. Condylomata are much more common in the anogenital area than in the mouth and represent about 20 percent of all STDs diagnosed in STD clinics.

The incubation period for a condyloma is 1 to 3 months from the time of sexual contact. Once present, autoinoculation to other sites of trauma is possible.

Clinical Features

Condylomata are usually diagnosed in teen-agers and young adults, but people of all ages are susceptible. Oral lesions most frequently occur on the labial mucosa, soft palate, and lingual frenum. The typical condyloma presents as a sessile, pink, well-demarcated, nontender exophytic mass with short, blunted surface projections (Fig. 10–12). Condylomata tend to be larger than papillomas and are characteristically multiple and clustered. The average lesional size is 1.0 to 1.5 cm, but oral lesions as large as 3 cm have been reported.

Histopathologic Features

Condyloma acuminatum appears as a benign proliferation of acanthotic stratified squamous epithelium

with mildly keratotic papillary surface projections (Fig. 10–13). Thin connective tissue cores support the papillary epithelial projections, which are more blunted and broader than those of squamous papilloma and verruca vulgaris, imparting an appearance of keratin-filled crypts between prominences.

The covering epithelium is mature and differentiated, but the spinous cells sometimes demonstrate pyknotic nuclei surrounded by clear zones (koilocytes), a microscopic feature of HPV infection (Fig. 10–14). Ultrastructural examination reveals virions within the cytoplasm or nuclei of koilocytes, and the virus also can be demonstrated by immunohistochemical analysis, *in situ* hybridization, and polymerase chain reaction (PCR) techniques.

Treatment and Prognosis

Oral condylomata are usually treated by conservative surgical excision. On occasion, topical application of po-

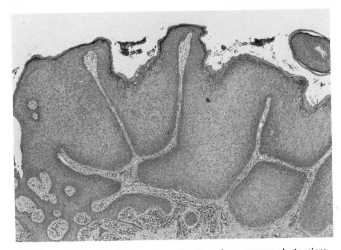

FIGURE 10–13. **Condyloma acuminatum.** Low-power photomicrograph showing acanthotic stratified squamous epithelium with multiple blunted projections.

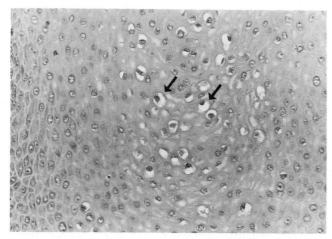

FIGURE 10-14. **Condyloma acuminatum.** High-power photomicrograph demonstrating koilocytes (*arrows*) in the spinous layer.

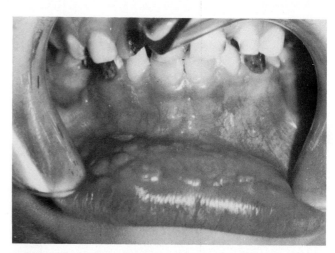

FIGURE 10-15. **Focal epithelial hyperplasia.** Multiple, flat-topped papules and nodules of normal coloration are seen on the lower lip of a child.

dophyllin has been tried. Laser ablation also has been used, but this treatment has raised some question as to the airborne spread of HPV through the aerosolized microdroplets created by the vaporization of lesional tissue. Regardless of the method used, condylomata should be removed because they are contagious and can spread to other oral surfaces as well as to other persons through direct, usually sexual, contact. In the anogenital area, this lesion may demonstrate a premalignant character, especially when infected with HPV-16 and HPV-18, but this has not been demonstrated in oral lesions.

FOCAL EPITHELIAL HYPERPLASIA
(Heck's Disease; Multifocal Papilloma Virus Epithelial Hyperplasia)

Focal epithelial hyperplasia is a virus-induced, localized proliferation of oral squamous epithelium that was first described in Native Americans and Inuits ("Eskimos"). Today, it is known to exist in many populations and ethnic groups and is produced by one of the subtypes of HPV, HPV-13 (and possibly HPV-32). In isolated populations, as many as 39 percent of children may be affected.

Clinical Features

Usually a childhood condition, Heck's disease occasionally affects young and middle-aged adults. There is no gender bias. Sites of greatest involvement include the labial, buccal, and lingual mucosa, but gingival and tonsillar lesions have also been reported.

This disease typically presents as multiple soft, nontender, flattened papules and plaques, which are usually the color of normal mucosa, but they may be pale or, rarely, white (Fig. 10-15). Occasional lesions show a slight papillary surface change (Fig. 10-16). Individual lesions are small (0.3 to 1.0 cm), discrete, and well demarcated, but they frequently cluster so closely together that the entire area takes on a cobblestone or fissured appearance.

Histopathologic Features

The hallmark of focal epithelial hyperplasia is an abrupt and sometimes considerable acanthosis of the oral epithelium (Fig. 10-17). Because the thickened mucosa extends upward, not down into underlying connective tissues, the lesional rete ridges are at the same depth as the adjacent normal rete ridges. The ridges themselves are widened, often confluent, and sometimes club-shaped. Some superficial keratinocytes show a koilocytic change similar to that seen in other HPV infections (see p. 263). Others occasionally demonstrate an altered nucleus that resembles a mitotic figure (mitosoid cell) (Fig. 10-18). These presumably result from viral alteration of the cells. Virus-like particles have been noted ultrastructurally within both cytoplasm and nuclei of cells within the spinous layer, and the presence of HPV has been demonstrated with both DNA *in situ* hybridization and immunohistochemical analysis.

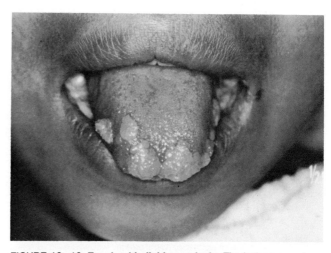

FIGURE 10-16. **Focal epithelial hyperplasia.** The lesions may demonstrate a papillary surface change and paleness, as demonstrated on this child's tongue. (Courtesy of Dr. Román Carlos.)

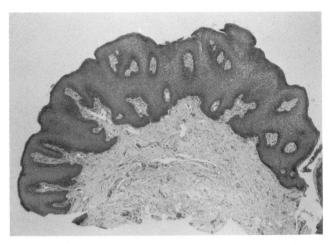

FIGURE 10–17. **Focal epithelial hyperplasia.** Prominent acanthosis of the epithelium with broad and elongated rete ridges. The slightly papillary surface alteration noted here may or may not be present.

Treatment and Prognosis

Spontaneous regression of focal epithelial hyperplasia has been reported after months or years and is inferred from the rarity of the disease in adults. Conservative surgical excision of lesions may be performed for diagnostic or aesthetic purposes. The risk of recurrence after this therapy is minimal, and there is no malignant transformation potential.

MOLLUSCUM CONTAGIOSUM

Molluscum contagiosum is a virus-induced epithelial hyperplasia produced by the molluscum contagiosum virus, a member of the DNA poxvirus group. After an incubation period of 14 to 50 days, infection produces multiple papules of the skin or, rarely, mucous membranes. These remain small for months or years and then spontaneously involute.

During its active phase, the molluscum contagiosum virus is sloughed from a central core in each papule. Routes of transmission include sexual contact (in adults) and such nonsexual contacts (in children and teen-agers) as sharing clothing, wrestling, communal bathing, and swimming. Lesions have a predilection for warm portions of the skin and sites of recent injury, and florid cases have been reported in immunocompromised patients (see p. 206).

Clinical Features

Usually, molluscum contagiosum is seen in children and young adults. The papules almost always are multiple and occur predominantly on the skin of the neck, face (particularly eyelids), trunk, and genitalia. Infrequently, oral involvement occurs, usually on the lips, buccal mucosa, or palate.

Lesions present as pink, smooth-surfaced, sessile, nontender, and non-hemorrhagic papules 2- to 4-mm in diameter (Fig. 10–19). Many show a small central indentation or keratin-like plug from which a curd-like substance can be expressed. Some have a mild inflammatory erythema around them and may be slightly tender.

Histopathologic Features

Molluscum contagiosum appears as a localized lobular proliferation of surface stratified squamous epithelium (Fig. 10–20). The central portion of each lobule is filled with bloated keratinocytes that contain large, intranuclear, basophilic viral inclusions called *molluscum bodies* (Fig. 10–21). These bodies begin as small eosinophilic structures in cells just above the basal layer and increase so much in size as they approach the surface that they frequently become larger than the original size of the invaded cells. A central crater is formed at the surface as stratum corneum cells disintegrate to release their molluscum bodies. These unique features make the diagnosis readily apparent.

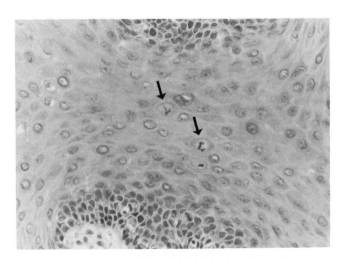

FIGURE 10–18. **Focal epithelial hyperplasia.** Mitosoid cells (*arrows*) contain altered nuclei in this otherwise mature and well-differentiated stratified squamous epithelium.

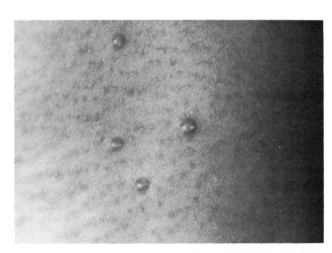

FIGURE 10–19. **Molluscum contagiosum.** Multiple, smooth-surfaced papules, with several demonstrating small keratin-like plugs, are seen on the neck of a child.

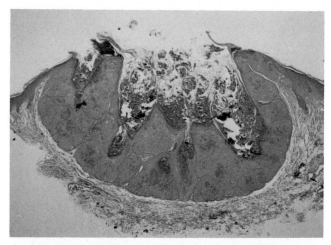

FIGURE 10-20. **Molluscum contagiosum.** Well-defined epidermal proliferation demonstrating a central crater-like depression filled with virally altered keratinocytes.

Treatment and Prognosis

Spontaneous remission occurs within 6 to 9 months in most cases of molluscum contagiosum, but curettage and cryotherapy are effective treatments for papules removed electively. The lesions have no apparent potential to transform into carcinoma and tend not to recur after treatment.

VERRUCIFORM XANTHOMA

Verruciform xanthoma is a hyperplastic condition of unknown etiology. It was first reported on the oral mucosa in 1971 and subsequently has been reported on the skin and vulvar mucosa. It remains a predominantly oral lesion. Although the lesion is characterized by an accumulation of lipid-laden histiocytes and is histopathologically similar to other dermal xanthomas, it appears to have no association with diabetes, hyperlipidemia, or any other metabolic disorder. Some authors suggest that the lesion may represent an unusual reaction to localized epithelial trauma or damage. This hypothesis is supported by cases of verruciform xanthoma that have developed in association with disturbed epithelium (e.g., epidermal nevi, epidermolysis bullosa, epithelial dysplasia, pemphigus vulgaris, and graft-versus-host disease).

Clinical Features

Verruciform xanthoma typically is seen in whites, 40 to 70 years of age. There is a strong female predilection (a 1:2 male-to-female ratio). The most common intraoral locations are the gingiva and alveolar mucosa, but any oral site may be involved.

The lesion appears as a well-demarcated, soft, painless, sessile, slightly elevated mass with a white, yellow-white, or red color and a papillary or roughened ("verruciform") surface (Figs. 10-22 and 10-23; see Color Figure 55). It is usually smaller than 2 cm in greatest diameter;

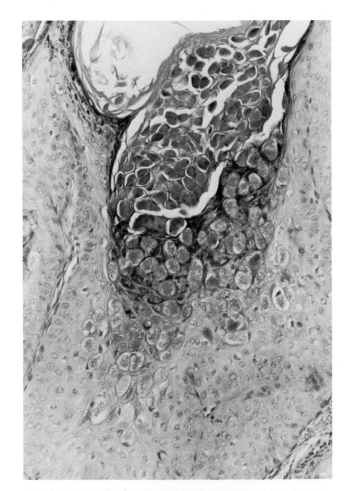

FIGURE 10-21. **Molluscum contagiosum.** Higher-power photomicrograph showing keratinocytes with large, basophilic viral inclusions (molluscum bodies) being sloughed into the central crater *(top)*.

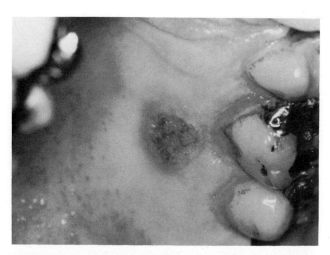

FIGURE 10-22. **Verruciform xanthoma.** A well-demarcated, slightly elevated lesion of the hard palate, which demonstrates a roughened or papillary surface.

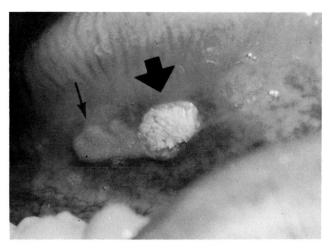

FIGURE 10-23. **Verruciform xanthoma.** A lesion of the ventral tongue exhibits a biphasic appearance. The anterior aspect demonstrates elongated white (well-keratinized) projections *(large arrow).* The posterior aspect demonstrates a surface of yellow, blunted projections *(small arrow).* See Color Plates.

no oral lesion larger than 4 cm has been reported. Multiple lesions have occasionally been described. Clinically, verruciform xanthoma may be similar to squamous papilloma, condyloma acuminatum, or early carcinoma.

Histopathologic Features

Verruciform xanthoma demonstrates papillary, acanthotic surface epithelium covered by a thickened layer of parakeratin. On routine hematoxylin and eosin staining, the keratin layer often exhibits a distinctive orange coloration (Fig. 10-24). Clefts or crypts between the epithelial projections are filled with parakeratin, and rete ridges are elongated to a uniform depth. The most important diagnostic feature is the accumulation of numerous large macrophages with foamy cytoplasm, which are confined to the connective tissue papillae (Fig. 10-

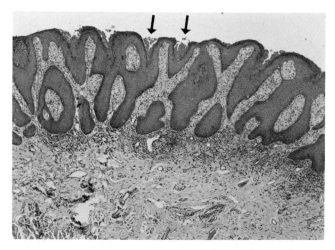

FIGURE 10-24. **Verruciform xanthoma.** A slight papillary appearance is produced by hyperparakeratosis, and the rete ridges are elongated to a uniform depth. Note the parakeratin plugging *(arrows)* between the papillary projections.

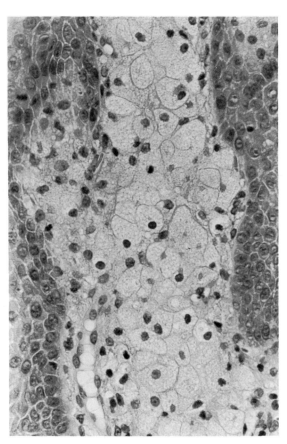

FIGURE 10-25. **Verruciform xanthoma.** Connective tissue papillae are composed almost exclusively of xanthoma cells—large macrophages with foamy cytoplasm.

25). These foam cells, also known as *xanthoma cells,* contain lipid as well as periodic acid-Schiff (PAS)-positive, diastase-resistant granules.

Treatment and Prognosis

The verruciform xanthoma is treated with conservative surgical excision. Recurrence after removal of the lesion is rare, and no malignant transformation has been reported. However, two cases have been reported in which a verruciform xanthoma occurred in association with carcinoma *in situ* or squamous cell carcinoma. This does not necessarily imply that verruciform xanthoma is a potentially malignant lesion but may indicate that hyperkeratotic or dysplastic oral lesions may undergo degenerative changes to form a verruciform xanthoma.

SEBORRHEIC KERATOSIS

Seborrheic keratosis is an extremely common skin lesion of older people and represents an acquired, benign proliferation of epithelial basal cells. The cause is unknown, although there is a positive correlation with chronic sun exposure, sometimes with a hereditary (autosomal dominant) tendency. Seborrheic keratosis does not occur in the mouth.

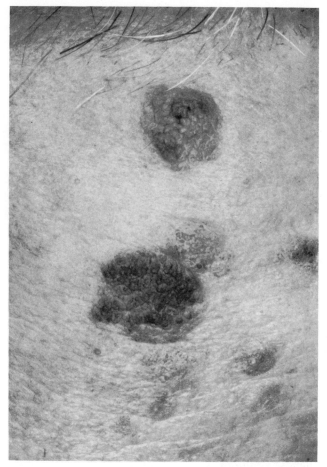

FIGURE 10-26. **Seborrheic keratosis.** Multiple brown plaques of the face of an elderly man exhibit a fissured surface. They had been slowly enlarging for several years.

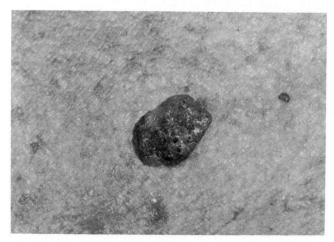

FIGURE 10-27. **Seborrheic keratosis.** Older lesions may become elevated above the skin surface and may demonstrate blunted surface projections, as seen here.

Clinical Features

Seborrheic keratoses begin to arise on the skin of the face, trunk, and extremities during the fourth decade of life, and they become more prevalent with each passing decade. Lesions are usually multiple, beginning as small tan to brown macules that are clinically indistinguishable from actinic lentigines (see p. 272), and which gradually enlarge and elevate (Figs. 10-26 and 10-27). Individual lesions are sharply demarcated plaques and have surfaces that are finely fissured, pitted, or verrucous but may be smooth. They tend to appear "stuck onto" the skin and are usually less than 2 cm in diameter.

Dermatosis papulosa nigra is a form of seborrheic keratosis that occurs in approximately 30 percent of blacks and frequently has an autosomal dominant inheritance pattern. This condition typically presents as multiple, small (1 to 2 mm), dark-brown to black papules scattered about the zygomatic and periorbital region.

Histopathologic Features

Seborrheic keratosis consists of an exophytic proliferation of basilar epithelial cells that exhibit varying degrees of surface keratinization, acanthosis, and papillomatosis (Fig. 10-28). Characteristically, the entire epithelial hy-

perplasia extends upward, above the normal epidermal surface. The lesion usually exhibits deep, keratin-filled invaginations that appear cystic on cross-section; hence, they are called *horn cysts* or *pseudo-horn cysts* (Fig. 10-29). Melanin pigmentation often is seen within the basal layer.

Several histopathologic patterns may be seen in seborrheic keratoses. The most common is the *acanthotic* form, which exhibits little papillomatosis and marked acanthosis with minimal surface keratinization. The *hyperkeratotic* form is characterized by prominent papillomatosis and hyperkeratosis with minimal acanthosis. The *adenoid* form consists of interlacing strands of lesional cells with little hyperkeratosis or papillomatosis. The lesions of dermatosis papulosa nigra are predominantly of the adenoid and acanthotic types.

Chronic trauma may alter these histopathologic features, and the lesion known as **inverted follicular keratosis of Helwig** is thought to represent an irritated seborrheic keratosis. This lesion shows a mild degree of

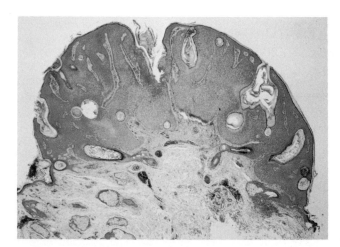

FIGURE 10-28. **Seborrheic keratosis.** The acanthotic form demonstrates considerable acanthosis, surface hyperkeratosis and numerous pseudocysts. The epidermal proliferation extends upward, above the normal epidermal surface.

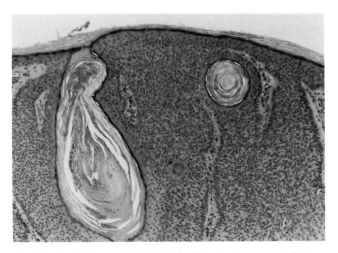

FIGURE 10–29. **Seborrheic keratosis.** Pseudocysts are actually keratin-filled invaginations, as seen toward the left in this high-power photomicrograph. The surrounding epithelial cells are basaloid in appearance.

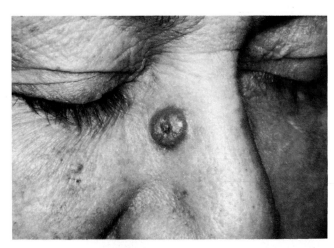

FIGURE 10–30. **Keratoacanthoma.** A nontender, well-demarcated nodule of the skin of the nose in an older woman. The nodule demonstrates a central keratin plug.

proliferation into the connective tissue as well as a chronic inflammatory cell infiltrate adjacent to the lesion. Squamous metaplasia of the lesional cells results in whorled epithelial patterns called "squamous eddies." Occasionally, irritated seborrheic keratoses have been confused histopathologically with well-differentiated squamous cell carcinoma.

Treatment and Prognosis

Except for aesthetic purposes, seborrheic keratoses are seldom removed. Cryotherapy with liquid nitrogen or simple curettage is the treatment of choice for lesions that are removed. Although the lesion has no malignant potential, other more significant skin lesions may develop in areas contiguous to it. The sudden appearance of numerous seborrheic keratoses with pruritus has been associated with internal malignancy, a rare event called the *Leser-Trélat sign.*

KERATOACANTHOMA ("Self-Healing" Carcinoma; Pseudocarcinoma)

Keratoacanthoma is a self-limiting, epithelial proliferation with a strong clinical and histopathologic similarity to well-differentiated **squamous cell carcinoma.** In fact, some authorities consider it to represent an extremely well-differentiated form of squamous cell carcinoma. Cutaneous lesions presumably arise from the infundibulum of hair follicles. Intraoral lesions have been reported, but they are rare; obviously, a different theory is required to explain their origin.

The cause of this lesion is unknown, but sun damage and human papillomavirus, possibly subtypes HPV-26 or HPV-37, have been proposed. The association with sun damage is suggested by the fact that most solitary lesions are found on sun-exposed skin, predominantly in the elderly. Also, keratoacanthoma-like lesions have

been produced in animals by the cutaneous application of carcinogens.

There appears to be a hereditary predisposition for multiple lesions, and the lesions occur with increased frequency in immunosuppressed patients and in the **Muir-Torre syndrome** (sebaceous neoplasms, keratoacanthomas, and gastrointestinal carcinomas).

Clinical Features

Keratoacanthoma rarely occurs in patients before 45 years of age and shows a male predilection. Almost 95 percent of solitary lesions are found on sun-exposed skin, and 8 percent of all cases are found on the outer edge of the vermilion border of the lips. The lesions affect the upper and lower lips with equal frequency.

Keratoacanthoma presents as a firm, nontender, well-demarcated, sessile, dome-shaped nodule with a central plug of keratin (Figs. 10–30 and 10–31), although in-

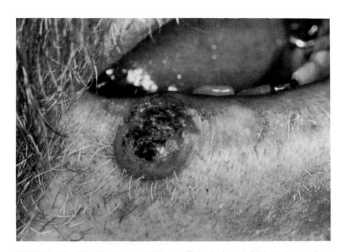

FIGURE 10–31. **Keratoacanthoma.** This lesion, which is located at the outer edge of the vermilion border of the lip, demonstrates a prominent core or plug of keratin.

traoral keratoacanthomas may lack the central plug. The outer portion of the nodule has a normal texture and color but may be erythematous. The central keratin plug is yellowish, brown, or black and has an irregular, crusted, often verruciform surface.

Rapid enlargement is typical, with the lesion usually attaining a diameter of 1 to 2 cm within 6 weeks. This critical feature helps to distinguish it from the more slowly enlarging squamous cell carcinoma. Most lesions regress spontaneously within 6 to 12 months of onset, frequently leaving a depressed scar in the area.

Occasional patients demonstrate large numbers of keratoacanthomas. One multiple-lesion variant may be hereditary and manifested in early life, with the lesions not likely to involve spontaneously (*Ferguson Smith* type). Another variant manifests as hundreds of small papules of the skin and upper digestive tract (*eruptive Grzbowski* type) and may be associated with internal malignancy.

Histopathologic Features

Keratoacanthoma warrants excisional or large incisional biopsy with inclusion of adjacent, clinically normal epithelium for proper histopathologic interpretation; this is because the overall pattern of the tumor is diagnostically more important than the appearance of individual cells. The cells appear mature, although considerable *dyskeratosis* (abnormal or premature keratin production) is typically seen in the form of deeply located individually keratinizing lesional cells and keratin pearls similar to those found in well-differentiated squamous cell carcinoma (see p. 302).

The surface epithelium at the lateral edge of the tumor appears normal; at the lip of the central crater, however, an acute angle is formed between the overlying epithelium and the lesion (Fig. 10–32). The crater is filled with keratin, and the epithelium at the base of the crater proliferates downward. This action often elicits a pronounced chronic inflammatory cell response (Fig.

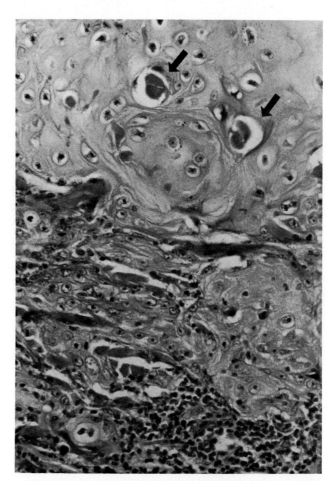

FIGURE 10–33. **Keratoacanthoma.** Stratified squamous epithelial cells are mature and well-differentiated, but exhibit individual cell keratinization (dyskeratosis) deep in the lesion (*arrows*). The connective tissue demonstrates a chronic inflammatory response (*bottom*).

10–33). Downward proliferation normally does not extend below the level of the sweat glands in skin lesions, and underlying muscle seldom is involved in oral lesions. Late-stage lesions show considerably more keratinization of the deeper aspects of the tumor than do early lesions.

Treatment and Prognosis

Despite the propensity of keratoacanthoma to involute of its own accord, surgical excision of large lesions usually is indicated for optimal aesthetic appearance because significant scarring may otherwise occur. After excision, 2 percent of treated patients experience recurrence. Aggressive behavior and malignant transformation into carcinoma have been reported in a few keratoacanthomas, but the close histopathologic similarities between this lesion and squamous cell carcinoma make it difficult to rule out the possibility of misinterpretation of the microscopic sections.

SEBACEOUS HYPERPLASIA

Sebaceous hyperplasia is a common benign skin lesion of unknown etiology that frequently affects the facial

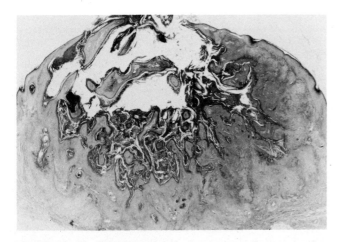

FIGURE 10–32. **Keratoacanthoma.** Low-power microscopic view demonstrating the extensive downward proliferation of the lesion and the acute angle formed by epithelium at the lip of the central keratin-filled crater.

skin. The major significance of this entity is its clinical similarity to more serious facial tumors, such as basal cell carcinoma.

Clinical Features

Cutaneous sebaceous hyperplasia usually affects adults older than 40 years of age. It occurs most commonly on the skin of the face, especially the cheeks and forehead, and is characterized by one or more soft, nontender papules with white, yellow, or normal coloration (Fig. 10–34). Lesions usually are umbilicated, with a small central depression, representing the area where the ducts of the involved sebaceous lobules terminate. Most lesions are smaller than 5 mm in greatest diameter and take considerable time to reach even this small size.

Compression of the lesion usually causes *sebum*, the thick yellow-white product of the sebaceous gland, to be expressed in the central depressed area. This feature may help clinically to distinguish sebaceous hyperplasia from basal cell carcinoma. An oral counterpart, which probably has no relation to the skin lesion, is characterized by a white-to-yellow papule or nodular mass with a "cauliflower" appearance, usually of the buccal mucosa.

Histopathologic Features

Histopathologically, sebaceous hyperplasia is characterized by a collection of enlarged but otherwise normal sebaceous gland lobules grouped around one or more centrally located sebaceous ducts (Fig. 10–35).

Treatment and Prognosis

No treatment is necessary for sebaceous hyperplasia except for aesthetic reasons or unless basal cell carcinoma cannot be eliminated from the clinical differential diagnosis of cutaneous lesions. Excisional biopsy is curative.

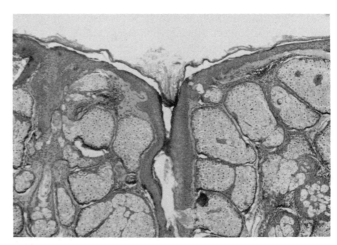

FIGURE 10–35. **Sebaceous hyperplasia.** Sebaceous glands are enlarged and more numerous than normal, but they demonstrate no other pathologic changes. Note the central sebaceous duct, from which sebum may be expressed.

ACTINIC LENTIGO (Lentigo Solaris; Solar Lentigo; Age Spot; Liver Spot; Senile Lentigo)

Actinic lentigo is a benign, freckle-like lesion that results from chronic ultraviolet light damage to the skin. It is found in more than 90 percent of whites older than 70 years of age and is rarely seen before age 40. It does not occur within the mouth but is seen frequently on the facial skin.

Clinical Features

Actinic lentigo is common on the dorsa of the hands, on the face, and on the arms of elderly whites (Figs. 10–36 and 10–37). It is typically multiple, but individual lesions appear as uniformly pigmented brown to tan macules with well-demarcated but irregular borders. Al-

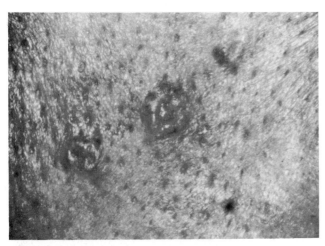

FIGURE 10–34. **Sebaceous hyperplasia.** Multiple soft papules of the mid-face are umbilicated and small. Sebum can often be expressed from the central depressed area.

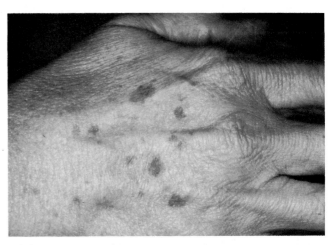

FIGURE 10–36. **Actinic lentigines.** Multiple lesions on the sun-exposed skin of the hand of an elderly person. Lesions are brown macules with irregular borders.

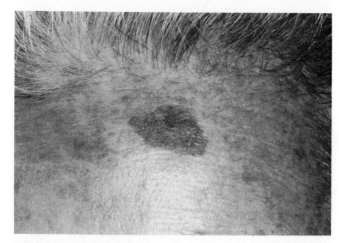

FIGURE 10–37. **Actinic lentigo.** Large, flat, evenly pigmented lesion on the forehead of an elderly man.

though the lesions may reach more than 1 cm or greater in diameter, most examples are smaller than 5 mm. Adjacent lesions may coalesce, and new ones continuously arise with age. Unlike ephelides (freckles), no change in the intensity of color is seen with a variation in exposure to ultraviolet light.

Histopathologic Features

Rete ridges are elongated and club-shaped in actinic lentigines, with thinning of the epithelium above the connective tissue papillae (Fig. 10–38). The ridges sometimes seem to coalesce with one another. Within each rete ridge, melanin-laden basilar cells are intermingled with excessive numbers of heavily pigmented melanocytes.

Treatment and Prognosis

No treatment is required for actinic lentigo except for aesthetic reasons. Topical retinoic acid can reduce the

color intensity in some cases. Actinic lentigo does not undergo malignant transformation, and if removed, does not recur. New lesions, however, can arise in adjacent skin at any time.

LENTIGO SIMPLEX

Lentigo simplex is one of several forms of benign cutaneous melanocytic hyperplasia of unknown etiology. It usually occurs on skin that is not exposed to sunlight, but it may occur on any skin surface and at any age. Its color intensity does not change with variations in sun exposure. Lentigo simplex is clinically similar to the common freckle (ephelis). Freckles, however, are found predominantly on sun-exposed skin, become more pronounced with increased sun exposure, and represent merely an increase in local melanin production rather than an increase in the number of productive melanocytes.

Some investigators believe that lentigo simplex may represent the earliest stage of another common skin lesion, the **melanocytic nevus** (see p. 276). Oral lesions have been reported but are rare and may be examples of oral melanotic macules (see p. 274).

Clinical Features

Lentigo simplex usually occurs in children but may occur at any age. The typical lesion is a sharply demarcated macule smaller than 5 mm in diameter, with a uniformly tan to dark-brown color (Fig. 10–39). It is usually a solitary lesion, although in some patients several may be scattered on the skin of the trunk and extremities. Lentigo simplex reaches its maximum size in a matter of months and may remain unchanged indefinitely thereafter.

Clinically, individual lesions of lentigo simplex are indistinguishable from junctional nevi. With multiple lesions, conditions such as lentiginosis profusa, Peutz-Jeghers syndrome (see p. 550), and the multiple

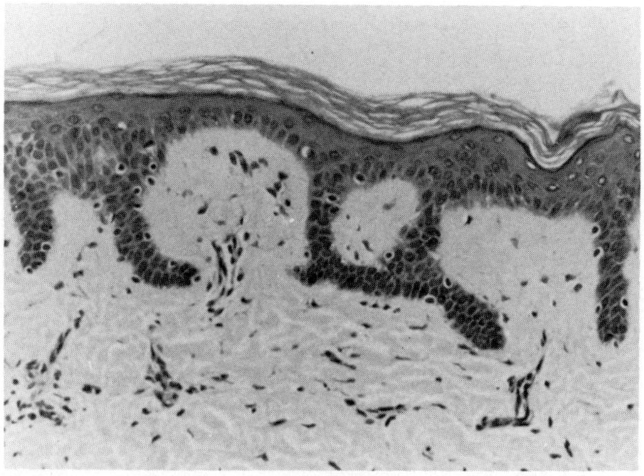

FIGURE 10–38. **Actinic lentigo.** Rete ridges are elongated and occasionally intertwining. Pigmented melanocytes (with clear cytoplasm) are excessive and commingled with melanin-laden basilar cells.

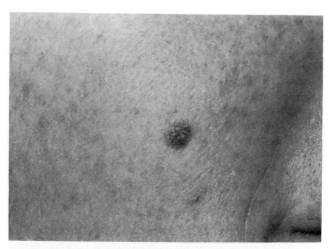

FIGURE 10–39. **Lentigo simplex.** A sharply demarcated lesion of uniform brown coloration is seen on the mid-face.

lentigines syndrome (LEOPARD* syndrome) must be considered as diagnostic possibilities.

Histopathologic Features

Lentigo simplex shows an increased number of benign melanocytes within the basal layer of the epidermis, and these are often clustered at the tips of the rete ridges. Abundant melanin is distributed among the melanocytes and basal keratinocytes as well as within melanophages of the papillary dermis.

Treatment and Prognosis

No treatment is required for lentigo simplex, except for aesthetic reasons. Conservative surgical excision is curative, and no malignant transformation potential has been documented for lesions not removed.

ORAL MELANOTIC MACULE
(Focal Melanosis)

The **oral melanotic macule** is an oral mucosal lesion of unknown etiology that represents a focal increase in melanin deposition and possibly a concomitant increase in the number of melanocytes. Unlike the cutaneous ephelis (freckle), the melanotic macule is not dependent on sun exposure and typically does not show the elongated rete ridges of actinic lentigo (see p. 272). Some authorities have questioned the purported lack of an association with actinic irradiation for the melanotic macule located on the vermilion border and prefer to consider it a distinct entity (**labial melanotic macule**).

Clinical Features

The oral melanotic macule occurs at any age and in both men and women; however, biopsy samples demonstrate a 2:1 female predilection. The average age of patients is 43 years at the time of diagnosis. The vermilion zone of the lower lip is the most common site of occurrence (33 percent), followed by the buccal mucosa, gingiva, and palate.

The typical lesion appears as a solitary (17 percent are multiple), well-demarcated, uniformly tan to dark-brown, asymptomatic, round or oval macule with a diameter of 7 mm or smaller (Figs. 10–40 and 10–41). Occasional lesions may be blue or black. Lesions are not reported to enlarge after diagnosis, which suggests that the maximum dimension is achieved rather rapidly and remains constant thereafter.

Histopathologic Features

The oral melanotic macule is characterized by an increase in the amount of melanin, and perhaps melano-

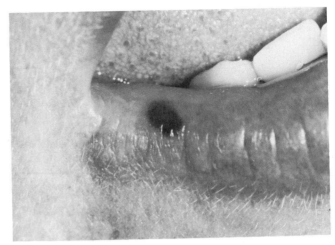

FIGURE 10–40. **Oral melanotic macule.** A single small, uniformly pigmented brown macule on the lower lip vermilion.

cytes, in the basal and parabasal layers of an otherwise normal stratified squamous epithelium (Fig. 10–42). Melanin also may be seen free or within melanophages in the subepithelial connective tissue (melanin incontinence).

Treatment and Prognosis

No treatment is usually required for the labial melanotic macule except for aesthetic considerations. The intraoral melanotic macule has no malignant transformation potential, but an early melanoma can have a similar clinical appearance. For this reason, oral pigmented macular lesions of recent onset, large size, irregular pigmentation, unknown duration, or recent enlargement should be excised and examined histopathologically.

ORAL MELANOACANTHOMA
(Melanoacanthosis)

Oral melanoacanthoma is a benign and uncommon acquired pigmentation of the oral mucosa characterized

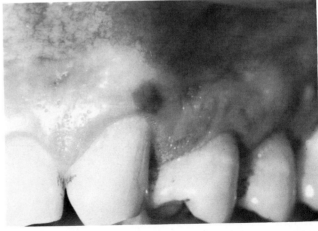

FIGURE 10–41. **Oral melanotic macule.** A well-demarcated brown macule of the gingival mucosa.

---

*Lentigines [multiple], electrocardiographic abnormalities, ocular hypertelorism, pulmonary stenosis, abnormalities of genitalia, retardation of growth, and deafness [sensorineural].

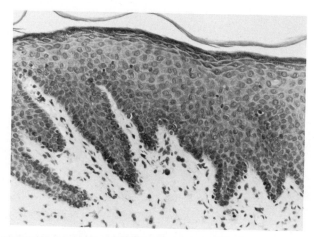

FIGURE 10–42. **Oral melanotic macule.** Excessive melanin is confined to the basal and parabasal layers of an otherwise unremarkable stratified squamous epithelium. Occasional melanin may be seen within underlying connective tissues (pigment incontinence). The pictured lesion demonstrates "elongated" rete ridges and a keratin layer because it was removed from the attached gingiva; these are not lesional changes.

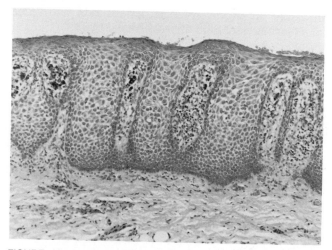

FIGURE 10–44. **Oral melanoacanthoma.** Low-power photomicrograph showing acanthosis of the epithelium. Spongiosis is demonstrated by intercellular spaces between the keratinocytes.

by dendritic melanocytes dispersed throughout the epithelium. The lesion appears to be a reactive process and is unrelated to the melanoacanthoma of skin.

Clinical Features

Oral melanoacanthoma is seen almost exclusively in blacks, shows a female predilection, and is most common during the third and fourth decades of life. The buccal mucosa is the most common site of occurrence. The lesion is smooth, flat, or slightly raised, and dark-brown to black in color (Fig. 10–43). Lesions often demonstrate a rapid increase in size and occasionally reach a diameter of several centimeters within a period of a few weeks.

Histopathologic Features

The oral melanoacanthoma is characterized by numerous benign dendritic melanocytes (cells that normally are confined to the basal cell layer) scattered throughout the lesional epithelium (Figs. 10–44 and 10–45). Basal layer melanocytes are also present in increased numbers. Spongiosis and mild acanthosis are typically noted. In addition, eosinophils and a mild to moderate chronic inflammatory cell infiltrate are usually seen within the underlying connective tissue.

Treatment and Prognosis

Because of the alarming growth rate of oral melanoacanthoma, incisional biopsy usually is indicated in order to rule out the possibility of melanoma. Once the diagnosis has been established, no further treatment is

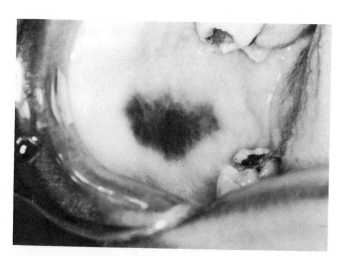

FIGURE 10–43. **Oral melanoacanthoma.** A smooth, darkly pigmented macule of the buccal mucosa is seen in a young adult. (Courtesy of Dr. John M. Wright, Jr.)

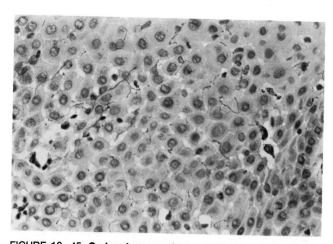

FIGURE 10–45. **Oral melanoacanthoma.** High-power view showing numerous dendritic melanocytes extending between the spinous epithelial cells.

necessary. In several instances, lesions have undergone spontaneous resolution after incisional biopsy.

ACQUIRED MELANOCYTIC NEVUS
(Nevocellular Nevus; Mole)

The generic term "nevus" refers to malformations of the skin (and mucosa) thought to be congenital or developmental in nature. Nevi may arise from the surface epithelium or any of a variety of underlying connective tissues. The most commonly recognized nevus is the **acquired melanocytic nevus**, or common mole—so much so, that the simple term "nevus" is often used synonymously for these pigmented lesions. However, many other types of developmental nevi also are recognized, including:

- Epidermal nevus
- Nevus sebaceus
- Nevus flammeus (see p. 392)
- Basal cell nevus (nevoid basal cell carcinoma; see p. 501)
- White sponge nevus (see p. 542)

The acquired melanocytic nevus represents a benign, localized proliferation of cells from the neural crest, often called "nevus cells." Although there is little debate as to their neural crest origin and their ability to produce melanin, various authorities are divided on the issue of whether these cells represent melanocytes or are merely "first cousins" of melanocytes. These melanocytic cells migrate to the epidermis during development, and acquired melanocytic nevi may first begin to appear shortly after birth. The acquired melanocytic nevus is probably the most common of all human "tumors," and white adults have an average of 10 to 40 cutaneous nevi per person. Intraoral lesions occur but are not common.

Clinical Features

Acquired melanocytic nevi begin to develop on the skin during childhood, and most cutaneous lesions are present before 35 years of age. They occur in both men and women, although women usually have a few more than men. Racial differences are seen. Whites have more nevi than Orientals (Asians) or blacks. Most lesions are distributed above the waist, and the head and neck region is a common site of involvement.

Acquired melanocytic nevi evolve through several clinical stages, which tend to correlate with specific histopathologic features. The earliest presentation (known microscopically as a **junctional nevus**) is that of a sharply demarcated, brown or black macule, typically less than 6 mm in diameter. Although this lesional appearance may persist into adulthood, more often the nevus cells proliferate over a period of years to produce a slightly elevated, soft papule with a relatively smooth surface (**compound nevus**). The degree of pigmentation becomes less; most lesions appear brown or tan. As time passes, the nevus gradually loses its pigmentation, the surface may become somewhat papillomatous, and hairs may be seen growing from the center of the lesion (**intradermal**

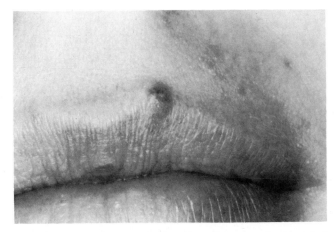

FIGURE 10–46. **Melanocytic (intradermal) nevus.** A pigmented, well-demarcated, dome-shaped papule is seen at the edge of the vermilion border of the upper lip.

nevus) (Figs. 10–46 and 10–47). However, the nevus usually remains less than 6 mm in diameter. Ulceration is not a feature unless the nevus is situated in an area where it is easily traumatized by a belt or bra strap, for example. Throughout the adult years, many acquired melanocytic nevi tend to involute and disappear; therefore, fewer of these lesions can be detected in elderly people.

Intraoral melanocytic nevi are distinctly uncommon. Most arise on the palate or gingiva, although any oral mucosal site may be affected. Intraoral melanocytic nevi have an evolution and appearance similar to skin nevi, although mature lesions typically do not demonstrate a papillary surface change. The lesion may or may not show some degree of melanin pigmentation (Fig. 10–48). Approximately two thirds of intraoral examples are found in females; the average age at diagnosis is 35.

Histopathologic Features

The acquired melanocytic nevus is characterized by a benign, unencapsulated proliferation of small, ovoid cells

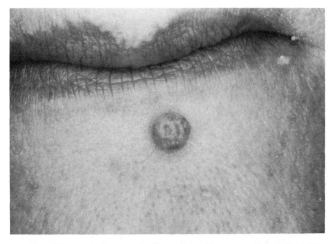

FIGURE 10–47. **Melanocytic (intradermal) nevus.** Several coarse hairs are seen to project from this pigmented papule of the skin of the lower lip.

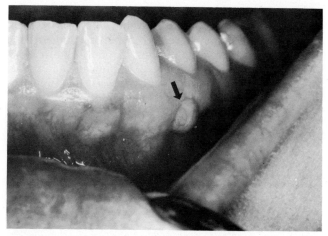

FIGURE 10–48. **Intramucosal melanocytic nevus.** This intramucosal nevus (*arrow*) of the mandibular gingiva is non-pigmented. (Courtesy of Dr. Richard Lee.)

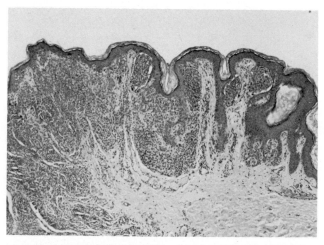

FIGURE 10–50. **Compound nevus.** Low-power view of a skin lesion showing sheets of nevus cells within the dermis along with nests of nevus cells in the basilar epithelium.

(nevus cells). The lesional cells have small, uniform nuclei and a moderate amount of eosinophilic cytoplasm with indistinct cell boundaries. These cells demonstrate a variable capacity to produce melanin, particularly in the superficial aspects of the lesion, although they typically lack the dendritic processes that melanocytes possess. A characteristic microscopic feature is that the superficial nevus cells tend to be organized into small, round aggregates *(thèques).*

Melanocytic nevi are classified histopathologically according to their stage of development, which is evidenced by the relationship of the nevus cells to the surface epithelium and underlying connective tissue. In the early stages, *thèques* of nevus cells are found only along the basal cell layer of the epithelium, especially at the tips of the rete ridges. Because the lesional cells are found at the "junctional" zone between the epithelium and the connective tissue, this stage is known as a **junctional nevus** (Fig. 10–49). As the nevus cells proliferate, groups of

these cells begin to drop off into the underlying dermis or lamina propria. Because cells are now present both along the junctional area and within the underlying connective tissue, the lesion then is called a **compound nevus** (Figs. 10–50 and 10–51).

In the later stages, nests of nevus cells are no longer found within the epithelium but are found only within the underlying connective tissue. Because of the connective tissue location of the lesional cells, on the skin, this stage is called an **intradermal nevus**. The intraoral counterpart is called an **intramucosal nevus** (Figs. 10–52 and 10–53). Zones of differentiation often are seen throughout the lesion. The superficial cells typically appear larger and epithelioid with abundant cytoplasm, frequent intracellular melanin, and a tendency to occur in *thèques*. Nevus cells of the middle portion of the lesion have less cytoplasm, are seldom pigmented, and appear much like lymphocytes. Deeper nevus cells appear elongated and spindle-shaped, much like Schwann cells or fibroblasts. Some authorities classify these variations as type A

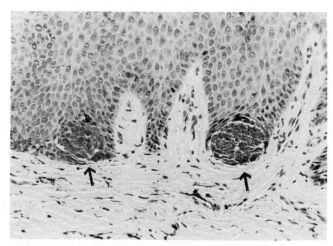

FIGURE 10–49. **Junctional nevus.** Melanin-laden nevus cells are seen to produce well-demarcated nests or *thèques* (*arrows*) along the basal cell layer of the epithelium. Stippled incontinent melanin pigment is present in the lamina propria, but no nevus cells are present in the connective tissue.

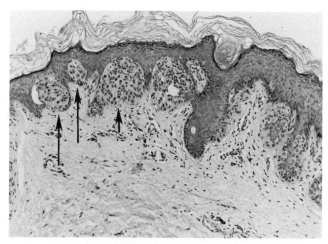

FIGURE 10–51. **Compound nevus.** Higher-power view of the same lesion depicted in Figure 10–50. Note the area with junctional nesting (*long arrows*) and early dermal involvement (*short arrow*).

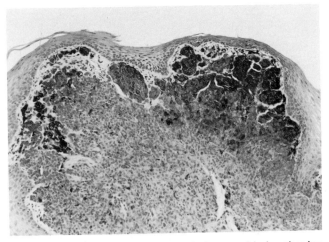

FIGURE 10-52. **Intramucosal nevus.** Oral mucosal lesion showing numerous nevus cells within the lamina propria. The cells are close to the surface, but no junctional nesting is present in the overlying epithelium. The superficial nevus cells stain darker because they contain more melanin pigment.

(epithelioid), type B (lymphocyte-like), and type C (spindle-shaped) nevus cells.

Most intraoral melanocytic nevi are classified microscopically as intramucosal nevi. However, this probably simply reflects the age (average, 35 years) at which most oral nevi undergo biopsy and diagnosis because these lesions would have earlier evolved through junctional and compound stages.

Treatment and Prognosis

No treatment is indicated for a cutaneous melanocytic nevus unless it is cosmetically unacceptable, is chronically irritated by clothing, or shows clinical evidence of a change in size or color. By midlife, cutaneous melanocytic nevi tend to regress, so that by age 90 very few remain. If removal is elected, conservative surgical excision is the treatment of choice; recurrence is unlikely.

At least some skin melanomas arise from longstanding or irritated nevi of the skin. Overall, the risk of transformation of a particular acquired melanocytic nevus to melanoma is approximately one in one million. However, because oral melanocytic nevi clinically can mimic an early melanoma, it is generally advised that biopsy be performed for intraoral pigmented lesions, especially because of the extremely poor prognosis for oral melanoma (see p. 312).

VARIANTS OF MELANOCYTIC NEVUS

Congenital Melanocytic Nevus

Congenital melanocytic nevus affects approximately 1 percent of newborns in the United States. This entity usually is divided into two types: small (<20 cm in diameter) and large (>20 cm in diameter). Approximately 15 percent of congenital nevi are found in the head and neck area, but intraoral involvement appears to be rare.

Clinical Features

Small congenital melanocytic nevi may be similar in appearance to acquired melanocytic nevi, but they are frequently larger in diameter (Fig. 10-54; see Color Figure 56). The large congenital melanocytic nevus classically appears as a brown to black plaque, often with a rough surface or multiple nodular areas. However, the clinical appearance often changes with time. Early lesions may be flat and light tan, becoming elevated, rougher, and darker with age. A common feature is the presence of *hypertrichosis* (excess hair) within the lesion, which may become more prominent with age (**giant hairy nevus**). The large congenital nevus also sometimes is referred to as **bathing trunk nevus** or **garment nevus** because it gives the appearance of the patient wearing an article of clothing.

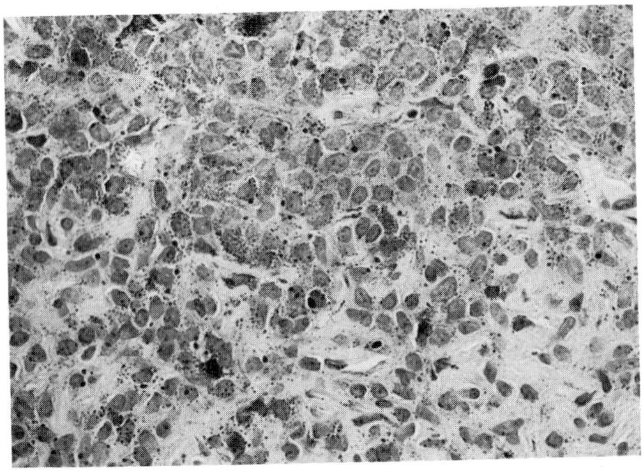

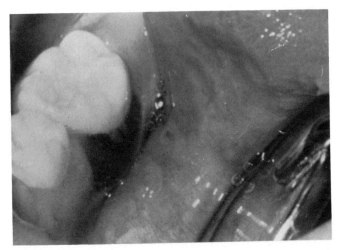

FIGURE 10-54. **Congenital melanocytic nevus.** Deeply pigmented lesion of the lingual mandibular gingiva in a 3-year-old child. See Color Plates.

FIGURE 10-53. **Intramucosal nevus.** High-power view of the same lesion depicted in Figure 10-52. Note ovoid nevus cells, which contain stippled melanin pigment.

The histopathologic appearance of the congenital melanocytic nevus is similar to that of the acquired melanocytic nevus; sometimes a small congenital nevus cannot be distinguished microscopically from an acquired nevus. Both congenital and acquired lesions consist of nevus cells, which may be noted in a junctional, compound, or intradermal pattern. The congenital nevus is usually of the compound or intradermal type. In contrast to acquired melanocytic nevi, congenital melanocytic nevi often show extension of nevus cells into the deeper levels of the dermis, with splaying of cells between collagen bundles. In addition, congenital nevus cells are often seen intermingled with neurovascular bundles in the reticular dermis as well as surrounding normal adnexal skin structures (e.g., hair follicles and sebaceous glands). Large congenital melanocytic nevi may show extension of nevus cells into the subcutaneous fat.

Treatment and Prognosis

Many congenital melanocytic nevi are excised for aesthetic purposes. In addition, 5 to 10 percent of large congenital nevi may undergo malignant transformation into melanoma. Whenever feasible, therefore, these lesions should be completely removed by conservative surgical excision. Close follow-up is required for lesions not removed.

Halo Nevus

Halo nevus is a melanocytic nevus that has a pale hypopigmented border or "halo" of the surrounding epithelium, apparently as a result of nevus cell destruction by the immune system. The halo develops because the melanocytes adjacent to the nevus also are attacked by the immune cells. The cause of the immune attack is unknown, but regression of the nevus usually results.

Clinical Features

The halo nevus is typically an isolated process associated with a pre-existing acquired melanocytic nevus. It is most common on the skin of the trunk during the second decade of life. The lesion typically appears as a central pigmented papule or macule, surrounded by a uniform, 2- to 3-mm zone of hypopigmentation. Sometimes this peripheral zone is much wider.

Histopathologic Features

Histopathologically, the halo nevus differs from the routine acquired melanocytic nevus only in the presence of an intense chronic inflammatory cell infiltrate, which surrounds and infiltrates the nevus cell population.

Treatment and Prognosis

Usually, treatment is not required for halo nevus because it eventually will regress entirely. If treatment is elected, conservative surgical removal is curative and recurrence is unlikely.

Spitz Nevus (Benign Juvenile Melanoma; Spindle and Epithelioid Cell Nevus)

Spitz nevus is an uncommon type of melanocytic nevus that shares many histopathologic features with melanoma. It was, in fact, first described as a "juvenile melanoma." The distinctly benign biologic behavior of the lesion was first emphasized by Spitz in 1948.

Clinical Features

The Spitz nevus typically develops on the skin of the extremities or the face during childhood. It presents as a solitary, dome-shaped, pink to reddish-brown papule, usually smaller than 6 mm in greatest diameter. The young age at presentation and the relatively small size of the Spitz nevus are features that may be useful in clinically distinguishing it from a melanoma.

Histopathologic Features

The Spitz nevus has the overall microscopic architecture of a compound nevus, showing a zonal differentiation from the superficial to deep aspects of the lesion, as well as lateral symmetry. Lesional cells are either *spindle-shaped* or *epithelioid*, and the two types may be admixed. The epithelioid cells may be multinucleated and appear somewhat bizarre, often lacking cell cohesiveness. Mitotic figures, all normal in appearance, may be seen in the superficial aspects of the lesion. Ectatic superficial blood vessels, which probably impart much of the reddish color of some lesions, are seen frequently.

Treatment and Prognosis

Conservative surgical excision is the treatment of choice for a Spitz nevus. There is little chance of recurrence after the nevus is removed.

Blue Nevus (Dermal Melanocytoma; Jadassohn-Tièche Nevus)

Blue nevus is a benign proliferation of dermal melanocytes, usually deep within subepithelial connective tissue. Two types of blue nevus are recognized: the *common* blue nevus and the *cellular* blue nevus. The common blue nevus is the second most frequent melanocytic nevus encountered in the mouth.

The blue color of this melanin-producing lesion can be explained by the *Tyndall effect*, which relates to the interaction of light with particles in a colloidal suspension. In the case of a blue nevus, the melanin particles are deep to the surface, so that the light reflected back has to pass through the overlying tissue. Colors with long wavelengths (reds and yellows) tend to be more readily absorbed by the tissues; the shorter-wavelength blue light is more likely to be reflected back to the observer's eyes.

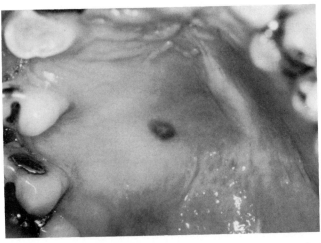

FIGURE 10–55. **Blue nevus.** A well-circumscribed, deep-blue macular lesion is seen on palatal mucosa. See Color Plates.

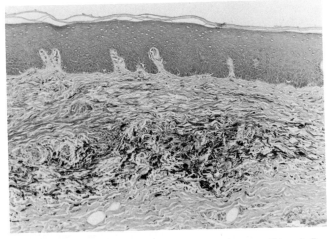

FIGURE 10–56. **Blue nevus.** Abundant melanin is seen within spindle-shaped melanocytes located relatively deep within the lamina propria and parallel to the surface epithelium.

Clinical Features

The common blue nevus may affect any cutaneous or mucosal site, but it has a predilection for the dorsa of the hands and feet, the scalp, and the face. Oral lesions are found most commonly on the palate. The lesion usually occurs in children and young adults, and a female predilection is seen. It presents as a macular or dome-shaped, blue or blue-black lesion smaller than 1 cm in diameter (Fig. 10–55; see Color Figure 57).

The cellular blue nevus is much less common and usually develops during the second to fourth decades of life, but it may be congenital. More than 50 percent of cellular blue nevi arise in the sacrococcygeal or buttock region, although they may be seen on other cutaneous or mucosal surfaces. Clinically, this nevus appears as a slow-growing blue-black papule or nodule that sometimes attains a size of 2 cm or more.

Histopathologic Features

Histopathologically, the common blue nevus consists of a collection of elongated, slender melanocytes with branching dendritic extensions, located within the dermis or lamina propria (Figs. 10–56 and 10–57). These cells usually align themselves parallel to the surface epithelium. The cellular blue nevus appears as a well-circumscribed, highly cellular aggregation of plump, melanin-producing spindle cells within the dermis or submucosa. More typical pigmented dendritic spindle cells are seen at the periphery of the lesional tissue. Occasionally, a blue nevus is found in conjunction with an overlying melanocytic nevus, in which case the term **combined nevus** is used.

Treatment and Prognosis

If clinically indicated, conservative surgical excision is the treatment of choice for the blue nevus of the skin. Recurrence is minimal with this treatment. Malignant transformation to melanoma is rare but has been reported. However, because an oral blue nevus clinically can mimic an early melanoma, it is usually advised that a biopsy be done for intraoral pigmented lesions, especially because of the extremely poor prognosis for oral melanoma (see p. 312).

LEUKOPLAKIA (Leukokeratosis; Erythroleukoplakia)

Oral leukoplakia ("white patch") is defined by the World Health Organization as "a white patch or plaque that cannot be characterized clinically or pathologically as any other disease." The term is strictly a clinical one and does not imply a specific histopathologic tissue alteration.

The definition of leukoplakia is unusual in that it makes the diagnosis dependent not so much on definable appearances as on the *exclusion* of other lesions, which present as oral white plaques. Such lesions as **lichen planus, morsicatio (chronic cheek bite), frictional keratosis, tobacco pouch keratosis, nicotine stomatitis, leu-**

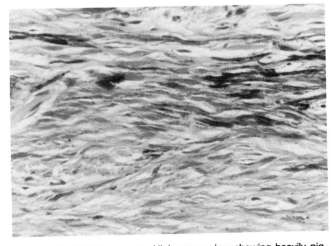

FIGURE 10–57. **Blue nevus.** High-power view showing heavily pigmented spindle-shaped cells.

koedema, and **white sponge nevus** must be ruled out before a clinical diagnosis of leukoplakia can be made. As with most oral white lesions, the clinical color results from a thickened surface *keratin* layer (which appears white when wet) or a thickened *spinous* layer, which masks the normal vascularity (redness) of the underlying connective tissue.

Definitions

Although leukoplakia is not associated with a specific histopathologic diagnosis, it typically is considered to be a precancerous or premalignant lesion. When the outcome of a large number of leukoplakic lesions is reviewed, the frequency of transformation into malignancy is greater than the risk associated with normal or unaltered mucosa. Because there is considerable misunderstanding of this concept, the following definitions are used throughout the chapter.

- **Precancerous lesion (precancer, premalignancy)**—a benign, morphologically altered tissue that has a greater than normal risk of malignant transformation
- **Precancerous condition**—a disease or patient habit that does not necessarily alter the clinical appearance of local tissue but is associated with a greater than normal risk of precancerous lesion or cancer development in that tissue
- **Malignant transformation potential**—the risk of cancer being present in a precancerous lesion or condition, either at initial diagnosis or in the future, usually expressed in percentages. The potential for mucosa without precancerous lesions or conditions is called "normal"
- **Relative risk**—a specific epidemiologic measure of the association between exposure to a particular factor and the risk of acquiring a disease, expressed as a ratio of the incidence or prevalence of a disease among those exposed and those not exposed to the factor

Incidence and Prevalence

Although leukoplakia is considered a premalignant lesion, the use of the clinical term in no way suggests that histopathologic features of epithelial dysplasia are present in all lesions. Dysplastic epithelium or frankly invasive carcinoma is, in fact, found in only 5 to 25 percent of biopsy samples of leukoplakia. The precancerous nature of leukopakia has been established—not so much on the basis of this association or on the fact that more than one third of oral carcinomas have leukoplakia in close proximity—as on the results derived from clinical investigations that followed numerous leukoplakic lesions for long periods. The latter studies suggest a malignant transformation potential of 4 percent (estimated lifetime risk). Specific clinical subtypes or phases, mentioned later, are associated with potential rates as high as 47 percent. These figures may be artificially low because many lesions are surgically removed at the beginning of follow-up.

Leukoplakia is by far the most common oral precancer. It represents 85 percent of such lesions, except in

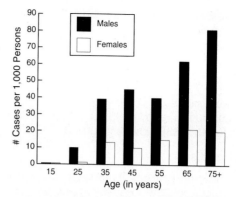

FIGURE 10–58. Leukoplakia. Age-specific prevalence for oral leukoplakia (number of new cases per 1000 adults examined at various ages) demonstrates increasing prevalence with increasing age, especially for men.

populations in whom smokeless tobacco use is popular (see p. 288). It is also the most common chronic lesion of oral mucosa, affecting 3 percent of white adults. There is a strong male predilection (70 percent), except in regional populations in which women use tobacco products more than men. A slight decrease in the proportion of affected males, however, has been noted over the past half century. The disease is diagnosed more frequently now than in the past, probably because of an enhanced awareness on the part of health professionals rather than because of a real increase in incidence.

This precancer usually affects adults older than 40 years of age. Prevalence increases rapidly with age, especially for males, and an alarming 8 percent of men older than 70 years of age are affected (Fig. 10–58). The average age of affected persons—60 years—is similar to the average age for patients with oral cancer, although in some studies it occurs about 5 years earlier than cancer.

Etiology

The cause of leukoplakia remains unknown, although hypotheses abound.

Tobacco

The habit of tobacco smoking appears most closely associated with leukoplakia development. More than 80 percent of patients with leukoplakia are smokers. When large groups of adults are examined, smokers are much more likely to have leukoplakia than nonsmokers. Heavier smokers have greater numbers of lesions and larger lesions than do light smokers, especially after many years of tobacco abuse. Also, a large proportion of leukoplakias in persons who stop smoking either disappear or become smaller within the first year of habit cessation.

The smokeless tobacco habit produces a somewhat different result. It often leads to a clinically distinctive white oral plaque called **tobacco pouch keratosis.** This lesion probably is not a true leukoplakia (see p. 288).

Alcohol

Alcohol, which seems to have a strong synergistic effect with tobacco relative to oral cancer production, has not been associated with leukoplakia. People who excessively use mouth rinses with an alcohol content greater than 25 percent may have grayish buccal mucosal plaques, but these are not considered true leukoplakias.

Ultraviolet Radiation

Ultraviolet radiation is accepted as an etiologic factor for leukoplakia of the lower lip vermilion. This is usually associated with **actinic cheilosis** (see p. 293).

Microorganisms

Several microorganisms have been implicated in the etiology of leukoplakia. *Treponema pallidum*, for example, produces glossitis in the late stage of syphilis, with or without the arsenic therapy in popular use prior to the advent of modern antibiotics. The tongue is stiff and frequently has extensive dorsal leukoplakia. Tertiary syphilis is rare today, but oral infections by another microorganism, *Candida albicans*, are not. *Candida* can colonize the nonviable parakeratinized surface cells of the oral mucosa, often producing a thick, granular plaque having a mixed white and red coloration. The terms **candidal leukoplakia** and **candidal hyperplasia** have been used to describe such lesions, and biopsy may show dysplastic or hyperplastic histopathologic changes. It is not known whether this yeast produces dysplasia or secondarily infects previously altered epithelium, but some of these lesions disappear or become less extensive after antifungal therapy.

Human papillomavirus (HPV), in particular subtypes HPV-16 and HPV-18, has been identified in some oral leukoplakias. These are the same HPV subtypes associated with uterine cervical carcinomas and a few oral carcinomas. Such viruses, unfortunately, also can be found in normal oral epithelial cells, and so their presence is perhaps no more than coincidental. It may be significant, however, that HPV-16 has been shown to induce dysplasia-like changes in normally differentiating squamous epithelium in an otherwise sterile *in vitro* environment.

Trauma

Finally, several keratotic lesions, which until recently had been viewed as variants of leukoplakia, are now considered not to be precancers. **Nicotine stomatitis** is a generalized white plaque that seems to be a hyperkeratotic response to the heat generated by tobacco smoking rather than a response to the carcinogens within the smoke (see p. 291). Its malignant transformation potential is so low as to be about the same as that of normal palatal mucosa. Also, chronic mechanical irritation can produce a white macule with a roughened keratotic surface. Although the resulting lesion is clinically similar to true leukoplakia, such a lesion is now thought to be no more than a normal hyperplastic response, similar to a callus on the skin. Keratoses of this type are readily reversible after elimination of the trauma, and such obviously traumatic lesions as linea alba (see p. 211), morsicatio (see p. 211), and toothbrush gingival "abrasion" have never been documented to have transformed into malignancy. A nonspecific, trauma-induced white plaque, then, should be diagnosed as **frictional keratosis**

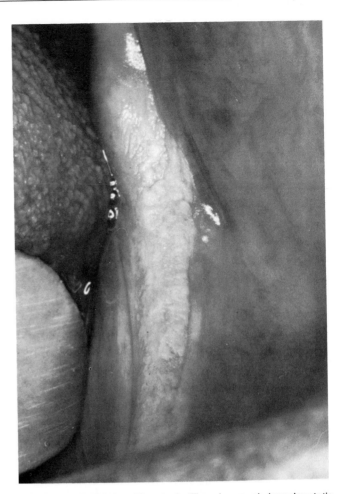

FIGURE 10–59. **Frictional keratosis.** There is a rough, hyperkeratotic change to the posterior mandibular alveolar ridge ("ridge keratosis") because this area is now edentulous and becomes traumatized from mastication. Such frictional keratoses should resolve if the source of irritation can be eliminated and should not be mistaken for true leukoplakia.

(Fig. 10–59) and differentiated from the group of oral precancers.

Clinical Features

Approximately 70 percent of oral leukoplakias are found on the lip vermilion, buccal mucosa, and gingiva. Lesions on the tongue, lip vermilion, and oral floor, however, account for more than 90 percent of those that show dysplasia or carcinoma. Individual lesions may have a varied clinical appearance and tend to change over time. Early and mild lesions present as slightly elevated gray or gray-white plaques, which may appear somewhat translucent, fissured, or wrinkled and are typically soft and flat (Fig. 10–60). They usually have sharply demarcated borders but occasionally blend gradually into normal mucosa.

Mild or **thin leukoplakia**, which shows no evidence of dysplasia on biopsy, may disappear or continue unchanged. For tobacco smokers who do not reduce their habit, as many as two thirds of such lesions slowly extend laterally, become thicker and acquire a distinctly white

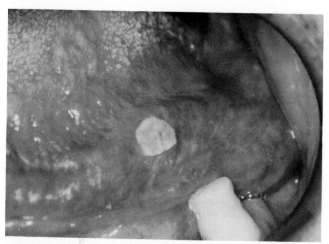

FIGURE 10-60. **Early or thin leukoplakia.** This early lesion of the ventral tongue is smooth, white, and well demarcated from the surrounding normal mucosa.

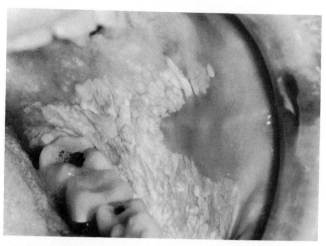

FIGURE 10-62. **Homogeneous or thick leukoplakia.** Extensive buccal mucosa lesion with an uneven whiteness and fissures. Moderate epithelial dysplasia was noted on histopathologic evaluation, and squamous cell carcinoma later developed in this area.

appearance. The affected mucosa may become leathery to palpation, and fissures may deepen and become more numerous. At this stage or phase, the lesion is often called a **homogeneous** or **thick leukoplakia** (Figs. 10-61 and 10-62). Most thick, smooth lesions remain indefinitely at this stage. Some, perhaps as many as one third, regress or disappear, and a few become even more severe. The latter develop surface irregularities and are then called **granular** or **nodular leukoplakia** (Fig. 10-63). Some lesions become exophytic and demonstrate sharp or blunt projections and have been called **verrucous** or **verruciform leukoplakia** (Fig. 10-64).

A special form of leukoplakia (**proliferative verrucous leukoplakia,** or PVL), has recently been described, characterized by the development of roughened surface projections (Fig. 10-65). The relationship of PVL to cases described as verrucous leukoplakia is uncertain. PVL presents as extensive, irregular white plaques, which tend to slowly spread and involve multiple oral mucosal sites.

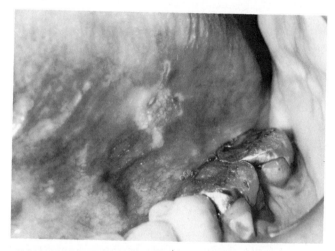

FIGURE 10-63. **Granular leukoplakia.** Focal leukoplakic lesion with a rough, granular surface on the posterior lateral border of the tongue. Biopsy of the lesion revealed an early invasive squamous cell carcinoma.

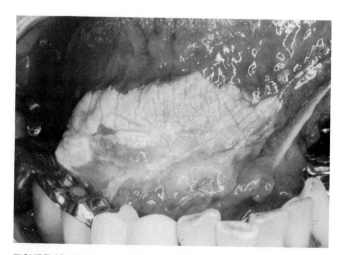

FIGURE 10-61. **Homogeneous or thick leukoplakia.** A lesion of the ventral tongue demonstrates an intense whiteness with numerous intertwining fissures. Surrounding areas of thin leukoplakia are also present.

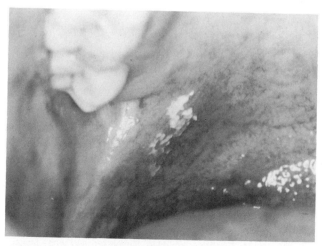

FIGURE 10-64. **Verruciform leukoplakia.** This lateral soft palate lesion exhibits several pointed projections on the surface.

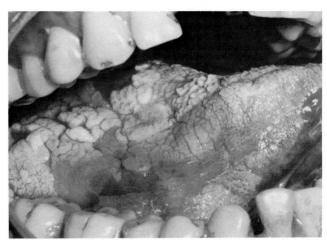

FIGURE 10-65. **Proliferative verrucous leukoplakia.** An extensive papillary and thickened lesion covers much of the lateral tongue, with extreme fissuring and variable whiteness.

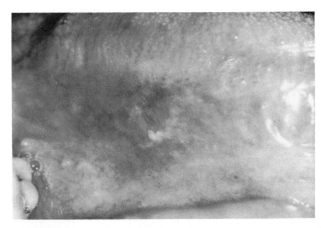

FIGURE 10-67. **Erythroleukoplakia.** Mixed red and white lesion of the lateral border of the tongue. Biopsy revealed carcinoma *in situ*. See Color Plates.

Although the lesions typically begin as simple, flat hyper-keratoses that are indistinguishable from ordinary leuko-plakic lesions, PVL exhibits persistent growth, eventually becoming exophytic and verrucous in nature. As the lesions progress, they may go through a stage indistinguishable from **verrucous carcinoma** (see p. 304), but they later usually develop dysplastic changes and transform into full-fledged squamous cell carcinomas. These lesions rarely regress despite therapy. PVL is unusual among the leukoplakia variants in having a strong female predilection (1:4 male-to-female ratio).

Leukoplakia may become dysplastic, even invasive, with no change in its clinical appearance, but some lesions eventually demonstrate scattered patches of redness, called **erythroplakia** (see p. 288). Such areas usually represent sites in which epithelial cells are so immature that they can no longer produce keratin. This intermixed red-and-white lesion, called **erythroleukoplakia** or **speckled leukoplakia**, represents a pattern of leukoplakia particularly susceptible to malignant transformation (Figs. 10-66 and 10-67; see Color Figures 58 and 59).

Of course, many leukoplakic lesions present with a mixture of the above-mentioned phases or subtypes. Because it is important to perform a biopsy of the lesional site with the greatest potential to contain dysplastic cells, Figures 10-68 (see Color Figure 60) and 10-69 provide a clinical and graphic representation of such a lesion. Biopsy sites should be taken from areas with clinical lesional appearances that are most similar to those toward the right in Figure 10-69.

Histopathologic Features

Microscopically, leukoplakia is characterized by a thickened keratin layer of the surface epithelium (hyperkeratosis) and/or a thickened spinous layer (acanthosis) (Fig. 10-70). Some leukoplakias demonstrate surface hyperkeratosis but show atrophy or thinning of the underlying epithelium. Frequently, chronic inflammatory cells are noted within the subjacent connective tissue.

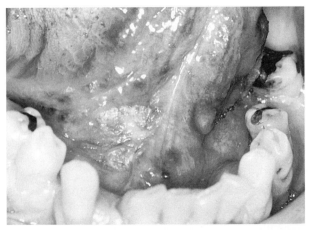

FIGURE 10-66. **Erythroleukoplakia.** Rough red and white lesion in the floor of the mouth. Biopsy revealed invasive squamous cell carcinoma. See Color Plates.

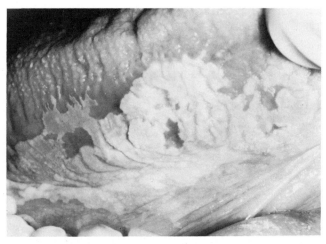

FIGURE 10-68. **Leukoplakia.** Extensive ventral and lateral tongue lesion containing multiple areas representing the various possible phases or clinical appearances; compare with Figure 10-69. See Color Plates.

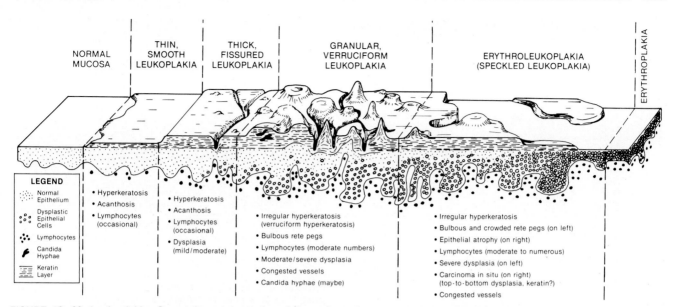

NORMAL
MUCOSA

THIN,
SMOOTH
LEUKOPLAKIA

THICK,
FISSURED
LEUKOPLAKIA

GRANULAR,
VERRUCIFORM
LEUKOPLAKIA

ERYTHROLEUKOPLAKIA
(SPECKLED LEUKOPLAKIA)

ERYTHROPLAKIA

LEGEND

Normal
Epithelium

Dysplastic
Epithelial
Cells

Lymphocytes

Candida
Hyphae

Keratin
Layer

• Hyperkeratosis
• Acanthosis
• Lymphocytes
(occasional)

• Hyperkeratosis
• Acanthosis
• Lymphocytes
(occasional)
• Dysplasia
(mild/moderate)

• Irregular hyperkeratosis
(verruciform hyperkeratosis)
• Bulbous rete pegs
• Lymphocytes (moderate numbers)
• Moderate/severe dysplasia
• Congested vessels
• Candida hyphae (maybe)

• Irregular hyperkeratosis
• Bulbous and crowded rete pegs (on left)
• Epithelial atrophy (on right)
• Lymphocytes (moderate to numerous)
• Severe dysplasia (on left)
• Carcinoma in situ (on right)
(top-to-bottom dysplasia, keratin?)
• Congested vessels

FIGURE 10-69. **Leukoplakia.** Composite representation of the various phases or clinical appearances of oral leukoplakia, with anticipated underlying histopathologic changes. Lesions have increasing malignant transformation potentials as their appearances approach those toward the right. (Modified from Bouquot JE, Gnepp DR: Laryngeal precancer—a review of the literature, commentary and comparison with oral leukoplakia. Head Neck 13:488–497, 1991. © Courtesy of John Wiley & Sons, Inc.)

The keratin layer may consist of orthokeratin (hyperorthokeratosis), parakeratin (hyperparakeratosis), or a combination of both. In orthokeratin, the epithelium demonstrates a granular cell layer and the nuclei are lost in the keratin layer. In parakeratin, there is no granular cell layer and the epithelial nuclei are retained in the keratin layer.

Verrucous leukoplakia has papillary or pointed surface projections of varying keratin thickness and broad, blunted rete ridges. It may be difficult to differentiate it from early verrucous carcinoma.

PVL shows a variable microscopic appearance, depending on the stage of the lesions. Early PVL appears as a benign hyperkeratosis that is indistinguishable from other simple, benign leukoplakic lesions. With time, the condition progresses to a papillary, exophytic proliferation that is similar to localized lesions of verrucous leukoplakia or what is sometimes termed "verrucous hyperplasia." In later stages, this papillary proliferation exhibits downgrowth of well-differentiated squamous epithelium with broad, blunt rete ridges. This epithelium demonstrates invasion into the underlying lamina propria; at this stage, it is indistinguishable from verrucous carcinoma. In the final stages, the invading epithelium becomes less differentiated, transforming into a full-fledged squamous cell carcinoma. Because of the variable clinical and histopathologic appearance of PVL, careful correlation of the clinical and microscopic findings is required for diagnosis.

Most leukoplakic lesions demonstrate no dysplasia on biopsy. Evidence of atypical changes is found in only 5 to 25 percent of cases if all oral sites are considered. When present, these dysplastic changes typically begin in the basilar and parabasilar portions of the epithelium. The more dysplastic the epithelium becomes, the more the atypical epithelial changes extend to involve the entire thickness of the epithelium. The histopathologic alterations of dysplastic epithelial cells are similar to those of squamous cell carcinoma and include the following:

1. Enlarged nuclei and cells.
2. Large and prominent nucleoli.
3. Increased nuclear/cytoplasmic ratio.
4. Hyperchromatic (excessively dark-staining) nuclei.
5. Pleomorphic (abnormally shaped) nuclei and cells.
6. Dyskeratosis (premature keratinization of individual cells).
7. Increased mitotic activity (excessive numbers of mitoses).
8. Abnormal mitotic figures (tripolar or star-shaped mitoses or mitotic figures above the basal layer).

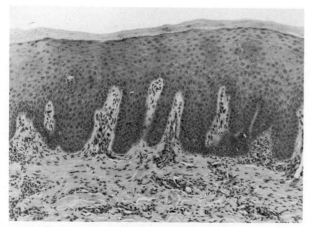

FIGURE 10-70. **Hyperkeratosis and acanthosis.** A thickened surface layer of keratin is the hallmark of leukoplakia. Acanthosis, as seen here, also is a frequent occurrence.

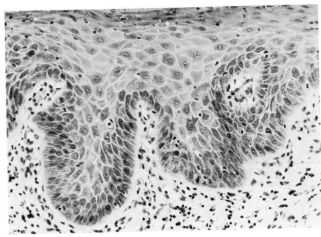

FIGURE 10-71. **Mild epithelial dysplasia.** Hyperchromatic and slightly pleomorphic nuclei are noted in the basal and parabasal cell layers of this stratified squamous epithelium.

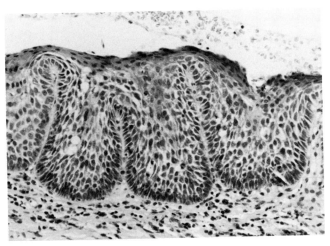

FIGURE 10-73. **Severe epithelial dysplasia.** Cellular crowding and disordered arrangement are noted throughout most of the epithelial thickness, although slight maturation and flattening of the cells appears to be present at the epithelial surface.

In addition, histomorphologic alteration of the epithelium may be seen as:

1. Bulbous or teardrop-shaped rete ridges.
2. Loss of polarity (lack of progressive maturation toward the surface).
3. Keratin or epithelial pearls (spheres of dyskeratotic cells).
4. Loss of typical cellular cohesiveness.

When epithelial dysplasia is present, the pathologist provides a descriptive adjective relating to its "severity" or intensity. *Mild* epithelial dysplasia refers to alterations limited principally to the basal and parabasal layers (Fig. 10-71). *Moderate* epithelial dysplasia demonstrates involvement from the basal layer to the midportion of the spinous layer (Fig. 10-72). *Severe* epithelial dysplasia demonstrates alterations from the basal layer to a level above the midpoint of the epithelium (Figs. 10-73 and 10-74).

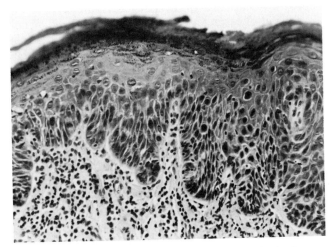

FIGURE 10-72. **Moderate epithelial dysplasia.** Dysplastic changes extend to the midpoint of the epithelium and are characterized by nuclear hyperchromatism, pleomorphism, and cellular crowding. Hyperorthokeratosis is noted on the epithelial surface along with a prominent granular cell layer.

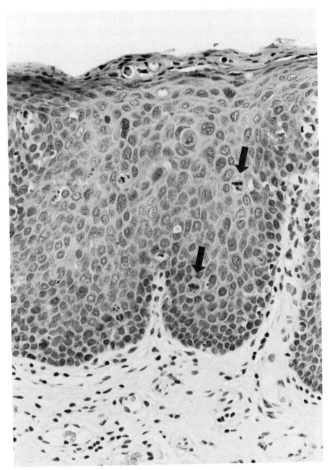

FIGURE 10-74. **Severe epithelial dysplasia.** Epithelial cells are seen to mature very little as they progress toward the hyperparakeratotic surface. The cells demonstrate crowded, pleomorphic nuclei, and mitotic figures (*arrows*) are noted above their normal basilar location.

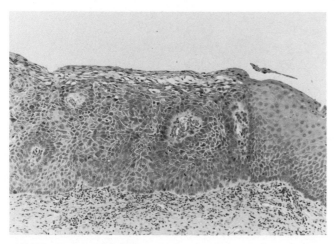

FIGURE 10-75. **Carcinoma *in situ*.** Dysplastic changes extend throughout the entire thickness of the epithelium. Note the abrupt transition with the normal epithelium at the right of the photomicrograph.

When the entire thickness of the epithelium is involved, the term **carcinoma *in situ*** is used. Carcinoma *in situ* is defined as dysplastic epithelial cells that extend from the basal layer to the surface of the mucosa ("top-to-bottom" change, Fig. 10-75). There may or may not be a thin layer of parakeratin on the surface. The epithelium may be hyperplastic or atrophic. This entity is considered by some authorities to be a precancerous lesion; others believe that it represents a genuine malignancy discovered prior to invasion. Regardless of the concept preferred, the important feature of carcinoma *in situ* is that no invasion has occurred, despite the fact that the atypical epithelial cells look exactly like those of squamous cell carcinoma (see p. 302). Without invasion, the most serious aspect of malignant transformation, metastasis, cannot occur. In this light, it should be mentioned that keratin pearl formation is rare in carcinoma *in situ* and may indicate the presence of a focus of invasive squamous cell carcinoma in the adjacent tissue.

Treatment and Prognosis

Because leukoplakia represents a clinical term only, the first step in treatment is to arrive at a definitive histopathologic diagnosis. Therefore, a biopsy is mandatory and will guide the course of treatment. Tissue obtained for biopsy, moreover, should be taken from the clinically most "severe" areas of involvement (with features toward the right side of Fig. 10-69). Multiple biopsies of large or multiple lesions may be required.

Leukoplakia exhibiting moderate epithelial dysplasia or worse warrants complete destruction or removal, if possible. The management of leukoplakia exhibiting less severe change is guided by the size of the lesion and the response to more conservative measures, such as smoking cessation.

Complete removal can be accomplished with equal effectiveness by surgical excision, electrocautery, cryosurgery, or laser ablation. Long-term follow-up after removal is extremely important because recurrences are frequent and because additional leukoplakias may develop.

Leukoplakia not exhibiting dysplasia often is not excised, but clinical evaluation every 6 months is recommended because of the possibility of progression toward epithelial dysplasia. Additional biopsies are recommended if smoking continues or if the clinical changes increase in severity.

Overall, 4 percent of oral leukoplakias become squamous cell carcinomas after diagnosis, according to follow-up studies. As previously stated, this figure, and those mentioned later, may be artificially low because so many followed cases are treated early in an investigation. Not to do so, of course, raises certain ethical questions, and hence more accurate data may never become available. Other confounding features of leukoplakia follow-up investigations include variations in diagnostic definitions and periods of observation. Typically, the latter extend for 5 to 10 years, but several studies have observed patients with lesions for more than 20 years, one study for more than half a century.

With these caveats in mind, follow-up investigations have demonstrated that carcinomatous transformation usually occurs 2 to 4 years after the onset of the white plaque, but it may occur within months or after decades. Transformation does not appear to depend on the age of the affected patient.

Although dysplasia may be present in any leukoplakia, each clinical appearance or phase of leukoplakia has a different malignant transformation potential. Thin leukoplakia seldom becomes malignant without demonstrating a clinical change. Homogeneous, thick leukoplakia undergoes malignant transformation in 1 to 7 percent of cases. Once the surface becomes granular or verruciform, the malignant transformation potential becomes 4 to 15 percent. Erythroleukoplakia carries an average transformation potential of 28 percent, but the rates have varied from 18 to 47 percent in different investigations.

The increased frequency of transformation of the different phases of leukoplakia is related closely to the degree of dysplasia present. The greater the clinical severity, the greater the chance of significant dysplasia and malignant transformation. Estimates of the malignant potential for histopathologically proven dysplastic lesions are, unfortunately, open to question because so many are excised completely. Thus, their true biologic behavior in an unaltered state may not be fully appreciated. Nevertheless, lesions diagnosed as moderate and severe dysplasia have malignant transformation potentials of 4 to 11 percent and 20 to 35 percent, respectively.

In addition to the clinical and histopathologic appearance at diagnosis, several factors may increase the risk for cancer in leukoplakic lesions. These include persistence over several years, occurrence in a female patient, occurrence in a nonsmoker, and occurrence on the oral floor or ventral tongue. Leukoplakia of the latter two locations has shown malignant transformation in 16 to 39 percent of all cases and 47 percent of those occurring in females.

Some smoking-related leukoplakias with no or minimal dysplasia may disappear or diminish in size within 3 months after the patient stops smoking. Thus, habit cessation is recommended. Also, high doses of isotretinoin (13-*cis*-retinoic acid, a form of vitamin A) followed by a course of low-dose isotretinoin or beta-carotene have been reported to reduce or eliminate some leukoplakic lesions in short-term studies. Toxic reactions to systemic retinoids are frequent, however, as is lesion recurrence after the conclusion of therapy. This chemoprevention and treatment of leukoplakia is still experimental but could become a recommended therapy if further research confirms its efficacy and safety.

ERYTHROPLAKIA (Erythroplasia; Erythroplasia of Queyrat)

As with leukoplakia, **erythroplakia** is defined as a red patch that cannot be clinically or pathologically diagnosed as any other condition. The term "erythroplasia" was originally used by Queyrat to describe a precancerous red lesion that develops on the penis. Oral erythroplakia is clinically and histopathologically similar to the genital process. Almost all true erythroplakias demonstrate significant dysplasia, carcinoma *in situ*, or invasive squamous cell carcinoma. The cause of erythroplakia is unknown, but it is presumed to be the same as that of oral squamous cell carcinoma.

The prevalence of the clinical entity oral erythroplakia is unknown, but leukoplakia was observed 77 times more often than erythroplakia in one large population study. The average annual incidence for microscopically proven oral carcinoma *in situ* was 1.2 per 100,000 population (2.0 in males and 0.5 in females), according to one investigation.

This entity may also occur in conjunction with leukoplakia (see p. 280) and has been found concurrently with a large proportion of early invasive oral carcinomas. Although erythroplakia is less common than leukoplakia, it has a much greater potential for the discovery at biopsy of significant dysplasia or for the development of invasive malignancy.

Clinical Features

Erythroplakia is predominantly a disease of older men, with a peak prevalence in 65- to 74-year-olds. The floor of mouth, the tongue, and the soft palate are the most common sites of involvement, and multiple lesions may be present.

The altered mucosa presents as a well-demarcated erythematous macule or plaque with a soft, velvety texture (Fig. 10–76; see Color Figure 61). It is usually asymptomatic and may be associated with an adjacent leukoplakia (erythroleukoplakia; see Figs. 10–66 and 10–67). Nonspecific mucositis, candidiasis, or vascular lesions may clinically mimic erythroplakia, and biopsy is often required to distinguish between them.

Histopathologic Features

According to one large clinicopathologic investigation, 90 percent of erythroplakic lesions histopathologically

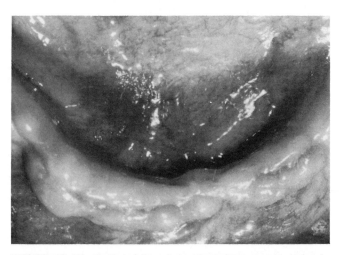

FIGURE 10–76. Erythroplakia. An erythematous macular lesion is seen on the right floor of the mouth with no associated leukoplakia. Biopsy showed early invasive squamous cell carcinoma. See Color Plates.

represent either severe epithelial dysplasia, carcinoma *in situ*, or superficially invasive squamous cell carcinoma. The epithelium shows a lack of keratin production and often is atrophic, but it may be hyperplastic. This lack of keratinization, especially when combined with epithelial thinness, allows the underlying microvasculature to show through, thereby explaining the red color. The underlying connective tissue often demonstrates chronic inflammation.

Treatment and Prognosis

Red lesions of the oral mucosa, especially those of the oral floor and ventral or lateral tongue, should be viewed with suspicion, and a biopsy should be performed. If a source of irritation can be identified and removed, biopsy of such a lesion may be delayed for 2 weeks to allow a clinically similar inflammatory lesion time to regress.

As with leukoplakia, the treatment of erythroplakia is guided by the definitive diagnosis obtained by biopsy. Lesions exhibiting significant dysplasia must be completely removed or destroyed by the methods used for leukoplakia (see p. 287). It is best, however, to preserve most of the specimen for microscopic examination because of the possibility that a focal invasive carcinoma might be missed in the initial biopsy material. Recurrence and multifocal oral mucosal involvement are common with erythroplakia; hence, long-term follow-up is suggested for treated patients.

SMOKELESS TOBACCO USE AND TOBACCO POUCH KERATOSIS (Snuff Pouch; Snuff Dipper's Lesion; Tobacco Pouch; Spit Tobacco Keratosis)

The habit of chewing coarsely cut tobacco leaves (chewing tobacco) or holding finely ground tobacco leaves (snuff) in the mandibular vestibule was once almost universal in the United States and is still common among certain populations around the world, most notably in India and Southeast Asia. Either habit is referred to as **smokeless tobacco use** or **spit tobacco use**. The latter term is preferred by the federal government in its attempt to diminish the appeal of the habit. At present, the proportion of adult men in the United States who regularly use spit tobacco approximates 6 percent. The proportion is as high as 21 percent in some southeastern states. The habit is started early in life, usually at 9 to 15 years of age, and rarely is initiated after 20 years of age.

Clinical Features

Several health and addiction hazards may be associated with the use of spit tobacco because of the ready absorption of nicotine through the oral mucosa. A variety of local oral alterations also are found in chronic users. One of the most common local changes is a characteristic painless loss of gingival and periodontal tissues in the area of tobacco contact. This gingival "recession" frequently includes destruction of the facial surface of the alveolar bone and correlates well with the quantity of daily use and the duration of the smokeless tobacco habit.

Dental caries also has been reported to be more prevalent in spit tobacco users, perhaps because of the high sugar content of some brands; other reports dispute caries susceptibility. Long-term use may lead to localized or generalized wear of occlusal and incisal surfaces, especially in persons employed in dusty environments. A brown-black extrinsic "tobacco" stain typically is found on the enamel and cementum surfaces of the teeth adjacent to the tobacco. In addition, halitosis is a frequent finding in chronic users.

A characteristic, precancerous white plaque, **tobacco pouch keratosis**, also is produced commonly on the mucosa in direct contact with snuff or chewing tobacco. In Western cultures, it affects 15 percent of chewing tobacco users and 60 percent of snuff users. The development of this lesion is influenced by the brand of tobacco used, an early onset of spit tobacco use, the total hours of daily use, the amount of tobacco consumed daily, and the number of sites routinely used for tobacco placement. In India, tobacco pouch keratosis is much more prevalent, presumably because of the increased hours of daily use and the use of different tobacco leaves combined in a quid with such other products as betel leaves, areca nuts, and slaked lime (see text on **oral submucous fibrosis**, p. 291).

Tobacco pouch keratosis in Western cultures usually is noted in young adult men and in men older than 65 years of age. In some populations, the prevalence is higher among older women. The lesion is confined to areas in direct contact with spit tobacco. It is typically a thin, gray or gray-white, almost "translucent," plaque with a border that blends gradually into the surrounding mucosa. Sometimes mild peripheral erythema is present (Fig. 10-77).

The altered mucosa typically has a soft velvety feel to light palpation, and stretching of the mucosa often reveals a distinct "pouch" caused by flaccidity in the

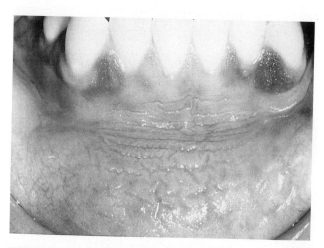

FIGURE 10-77. Tobacco pouch keratosis, mild. A soft, fissured, gray-white lesion of the lower lip mucosa located in the area of chronic snuff placement. The gingival melanosis is racial pigmentation and not associated with the keratosis.

chronically stretched tissues in the area of tobacco placement. Because the tobacco is not in the mouth during a clinical examination, the usually stretched mucosa appears fissured or rippled, in a fashion resembling the sand on a beach after an ebbing tide. Induration, ulceration, and pain are not associated with this lesion.

Tobacco pouch keratosis usually takes 1 to 5 years to become white or gray-white. In many users, this color change never develops. Once it occurs, however, the keratosis typically remains unchanged indefinitely unless the daily tobacco contact time is altered. In some cases, the white lesion gradually becomes thickened to the point of appearing leathery or nodular (Fig. 10-78).

Histopathologic Features

The histopathologic appearance of tobacco pouch keratosis is not specific. The squamous epithelium is hyperkeratinized and acanthotic, with or without intracellular vacuolization or "edema" of glycogen-rich superficial cells (Fig. 10-79). Parakeratin "chevrons" may be seen as pointed projections above or within superficial epithelial layers. Increased subepithelial vascularity and vessel engorgement are often seen. In some cases, an unusual deposition of amorphous eosinophilic material is noted within the subjacent connective tissue and salivary glands. Epithelial dysplasia is uncommon in tobacco pouch keratosis.

Treatment and Prognosis

Chronic use of smokeless tobacco is considered to be carcinogenic. The clinical appearance of tobacco pouch keratosis, however, is distinct enough and the malignant transformation potential is low enough so that biopsy is needed for only the more severe lesions, that is, those demonstrating an intense whiteness, a granular or verruciform clinical appearance, ulceration, mass formation, induration, or hemorrhage. Obviously, treatment would

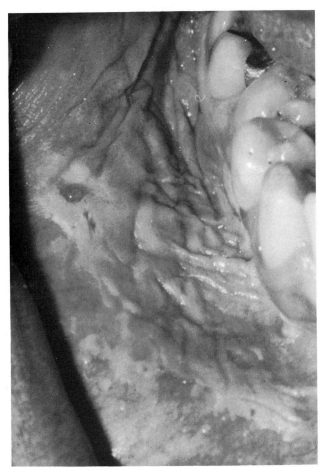

FIGURE 10–78. **Tobacco pouch keratosis, severe.** A somewhat leathery, white, fissured plaque of the posterior mandibular vestibule, which is located in the area of chronic chewing tobacco placement.

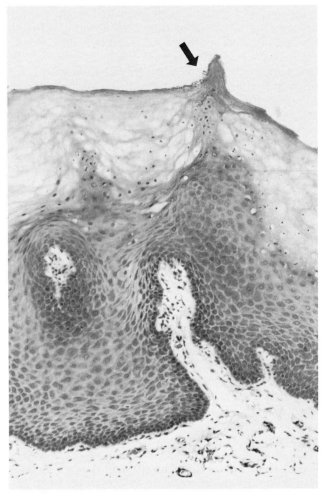

FIGURE 10–79. **Tobacco pouch keratosis.** The epithelium exhibits hyperkeratosis with parakeratin "chevrons" (*arrow*). No dysplastic changes are present.

then depend on the histopathologic diagnosis. Without microscopic evidence of dysplasia or malignancy, keratoses are not treated. Alternating the tobacco chewing sites between the left and right sides will eliminate or reduce the keratotic lesion but may result in epithelial alteration or gingival and periodontal difficulties in two sites rather than one.

The oral cancer risk in chronic smokeless tobacco users may be about four times greater than that in nonusers. Squamous cell carcinoma is the most common malignancy resulting from this habit, but an uncommon and unique low-grade oral malignancy (**verrucous carcinoma**) is specifically associated with spit tobacco use (see p. 304). Verrucous carcinoma is so seldom seen in nonusers that it has been called the "snuff dipper's cancer." The malignant transformation potential of long-term spit tobacco use is probably less than 0.05 percent per annum or 0.4 percent over a lifetime.

Significantly, habit cessation almost always leads to a normal mucosal appearance within 1 to 2 weeks (Figs. 10–80 and 10–81). Lesions that remain after 1 month without smokeless tobacco contact should be considered to be true leukoplakias and should be sampled for biopsy and managed accordingly.

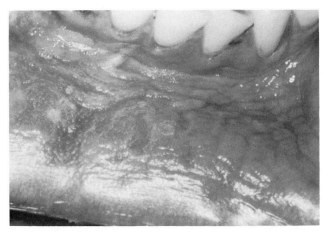

FIGURE 10–80. **Tobacco pouch keratosis.** A moderately severe lesion of the lower anterior vestibule and lip in a 15-year-old male demonstrates a gray-white surface change and fissuring. The patient had been placing snuff in the area for several years.

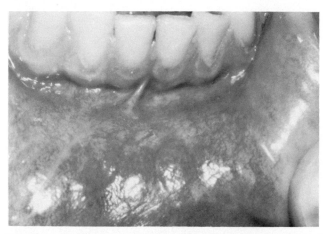

FIGURE 10-81. **Tobacco pouch keratosis.** The same area pictured in Figure 10-80 two weeks after cessation of the tobacco habit. The mucosa has returned to an almost normal appearance.

ORAL SUBMUCOUS FIBROSIS

Oral submucous fibrosis is a chronic, progressive, scarring, high-risk precancerous condition of the oral mucosa seen primarily on the Indian subcontinent and in Southeast Asia. It has been linked to the chronic placement in the mouth of a betel quid and is found in 0.4 percent of India's villagers. Villagers habitually chew betel quids from an early age, frequently for 16 to 24 hours daily. A quid typically consists of areca nut and slaked lime, usually with tobacco, wrapped in a betel leaf. The slaked lime acts to release an alkaloid from the areca nut, producing a feeling of euphoria and well-being in the user.

The condition is characterized by a mucosal rigidity of varied intensity caused by a fibroelastic modification of the superficial connective tissue. The submucosal changes may be a response to the areca nut; the epithelial alterations and carcinogenesis may be the result of tobacco contact.

Clinical Features

Oral submucous fibrosis is often first noted in young adult tobacco, areca, and betel users, whose chief complaint is an inability to open the mouth *(trismus)*, often accompanied by mucosal pain associated with spicy foods. In advanced cases, the jaws may actually be inseparable.

Vesicles, petechiae, melanosis, xerostomia, and a generalized oral burning sensation are usually the first signs and symptoms. The buccal mucosa, retromolar area, and soft palate are the most commonly affected sites. The mucosa in these regions develops a blotchy, marble-like pallor and a progressive stiffness of subepithelial tissues. When the tongue is involved, it becomes rather immobile, frequently diminished in size, and often devoid of papillae. Submucosal fibrous bands are palpable on the buccal mucosa, soft palate, and labial mucosa of fully developed cases. Leukoplakia or a thick keratosis is often superimposed on the surface mucosa.

Histopathologic Features

Oral submucous fibrosis is characterized by the submucosal deposition of extremely dense and avascular collagenous connective tissue with variable numbers of chronic inflammatory cells. Epithelial changes include hyperkeratosis with marked epithelial atrophy. Epithelial dysplasia without carcinoma is found in 10 to 15 percent of cases submitted for biopsy, and carcinoma is found in at least 6 percent of sampled cases.

Treatment and Prognosis

Unlike tobacco pouch keratosis, oral submucous fibrosis does not regress with habit cessation. Patients with mild cases may be treated with intralesional corticosteroids to reduce the symptoms; surgical splitting of the fibrous bands may improve mouth opening and mobility in the later stages of the disease. Frequent evaluation for development of oral squamous cell carcinoma is essential because a 17-year malignant transformation rate of 8 percent has been determined for betel quid users in India.

NICOTINE STOMATITIS (Nicotine Palatinus; Smoker's Palate)

Once a common mucosal change of the hard palate, **nicotine stomatitis** has become less common as cigar and pipe smoking have lost popularity. Although this lesion is a white keratotic change obviously associated with tobacco smoking, it does not appear to have a premalignant nature, perhaps because it develops in response to heat rather than the chemicals in tobacco smoke. Because pipe smoking generates more heat on the palate than other forms of smoking, nicotine stomatitis has most often been associated with this habit. Similar changes can also be produced by the long-term use of extremely hot beverages.

In some South American and Southeast Asian cultures, hand-rolled cigarettes and cigars are smoked with the lit end held within the mouth. This "reverse smoking" habit produces a pronounced palatal keratosis, or **reverse smoker's palate**, which is definitely a premalignant lesion.

Clinical Features

Nicotine stomatitis most commonly is found in men older than 45 years of age. With long-term tobacco use, the palatal mucosa becomes diffusely gray or white; numerous slightly elevated papules are noted, usually with punctate red centers (Figs. 10-82 and 10-83; see Color Figure 62). Such papules represent inflamed and metaplastically altered minor salivary gland duct orifices. The mucosa that covers the papules frequently appears whiter than the surrounding epithelium.

The palatal keratin may become so thickened that a fissured or "dried mud" appearance is imparted. The whiteness usually involves marginal gingiva and interdental papillae, and leukoplakia of the buccal mucosa is

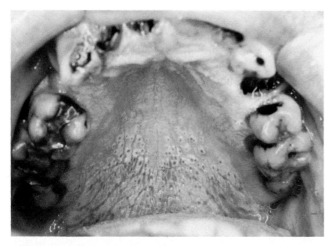

FIGURE 10-82. **Nicotine stomatitis.** This extensive leathery, white change of the hard palate in a pipe smoker is sprinkled throughout with numerous red papules, which represent inflamed salivary duct openings. The gingival mucosa also is keratotic.

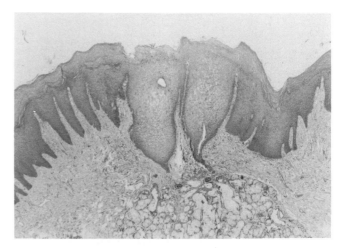

FIGURE 10-84. **Nicotine stomatitis.** There is hyperkeratosis and acanthosis of the palatal epithelium. Note the squamous metaplasia of the superficial aspects of involved salivary ducts as they extend toward the epithelial surface.

occasionally seen. A heavy brown or black "tobacco" stain may be present on the teeth.

Histopathologic Features

Nicotine stomatitis is characterized by hyperkeratosis and acanthosis of the palatal epithelium and mild, patchy, chronic inflammation of subepithelial connective tissue and mucous glands (Fig. 10-84). Squamous metaplasia of the excretory ducts is seen as they approach the mucosal surface, and an inflammatory exudate may be noted within the lumina of the ducts. In cases with papular elevation, the metaplastic duct also exhibits hyperplasia. The degree of epithelial hyperplasia and hyperkeratosis correlates positively with the duration and the amount of smoking. Epithelial dysplasia rarely is seen.

Treatment and Prognosis

Nicotine stomatitis is completely reversible, even when it has been present for many decades. The palate returns to normal, usually within 1 to 2 weeks of smoking cessation. Although this is not a precancerous lesion and no treatment is needed, the patient nevertheless should be encouraged to stop smoking, and other high-risk areas should be examined closely. Any white lesion of the palatal mucosa that persists after 1 month of habit cessation should be considered a true leukoplakia and managed accordingly.

ACTINIC KERATOSIS (Solar Keratosis)

Actinic keratosis is a common cutaneous premalignant lesion that is caused by cumulative ultraviolet radiation to sun-exposed skin, especially in fair-skinned people. It is found on the skin of more than 50 percent of all persons with significant lifetime sun exposure. Although the exact incidence of malignant transformation is unknown, 13%-25% of affected patients will develop squamous cell carcinoma from at least one of their actinic keratoses. A similar phenomenon, **actinic cheilosis**, is associated with sun damage to the lower lip vermilion (see next topic).

Clinical Features

Actinic keratosis seldom is found in patients younger than 40 years of age. The face and neck, the dorsum of the hands, the forearms, and the scalp of bald-headed men are the most common sites of occurrence. Individual lesions are irregular scaly plaques, which vary in color from normal to white, gray, or brown, and may be superimposed on an erythematous background (Fig. 10-85). The keratotic scale peels off with varying degrees of difficulty. Palpation reveals a "sandpaper," roughened texture, and some lesions can be felt more easily than

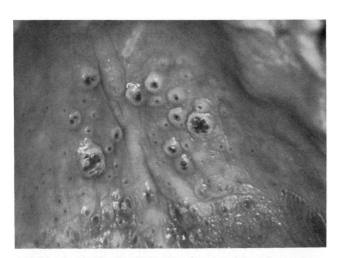

FIGURE 10-83. **Nicotine stomatitis.** Closeup of the inflamed ductal openings of involved salivary glands of the hard palate. Note the white keratotic ring at the lip of many of the inflamed ducts. See Color Plates.

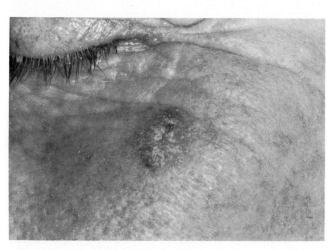

FIGURE 10–85. **Actinic keratosis.** A plaque of the skin of the face with a rough, "sandpaper"-like surface.

they can be seen. Typically, a lesion is smaller than 7 mm in diameter but may reach a size of 2 cm, usually with a minimal elevation above the surface of the skin. Occasional lesions, however, produce so much keratin that a "horn" may be seen arising from the central area. Such **keratin** or **cutaneous horns** also may be produced by other skin lesions, such as verruca vulgaris or seborrheic keratosis.

Histopathologic Features

Histopathologically, actinic keratosis is characterized by hyperparakeratosis and acanthosis (Fig. 10–86). Teardrop-shaped rete ridges typically extend down from the epithelium; by definition, some degree of epithelial dysplasia is present (Fig. 10–87). Suprabasilar acantholysis may be seen, as may melanosis and a lichenoid inflammatory infiltrate. The dermis exhibits a band of pale basophilic change, which probably represents sun-damaged collagen and elastic fibers (**solar elastosis**). Variable numbers of chronic inflammatory cells typically are present.

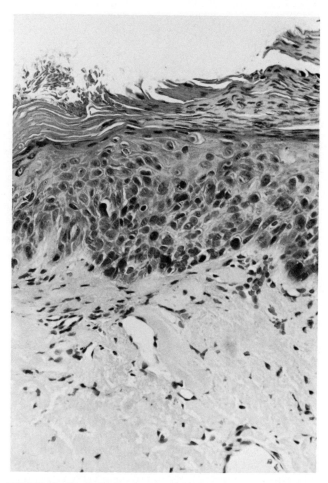

FIGURE 10–87. **Actinic keratosis.** High-power view of the specimen depicted in Figure 10–86. Note the hyperchromatism and pleomorphism of the epidermal cells.

Treatment and Prognosis

The annual rate of malignant transformation for actinic keratosis ranges from 0.01 to 0.24 percent. Because of its precancerous nature, it is usually recommended that actinic keratosis be destroyed by cryotherapy with liquid nitrogen, topical application of 5-fluorouracil, curettage, electrodesiccation, or surgical excision. Recurrence is rare, but additional lesions frequently arise in adjacent sun-damaged skin. Long-term follow-up, therefore, is recommended.

ACTINIC CHEILOSIS (Actinic Cheilitis)

Actinic cheilosis is a diffuse, premalignant alteration of the lower lip vermilion that results from long-term or excessive exposure to the ultraviolet component of solar radiation. It appears to be a problem confined predominantly to light-complexioned people with a tendency to sunburn easily. It is similar to **actinic keratosis** of the skin (see previous topic) in its pathophysiologic and biologic behavior.

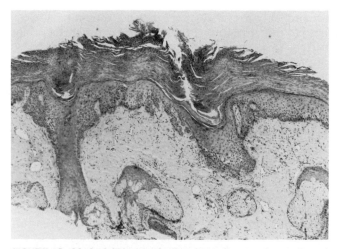

FIGURE 10–86. **Actinic keratosis.** An extremely excessive amount of parakeratin is noted on the epidermal surface.

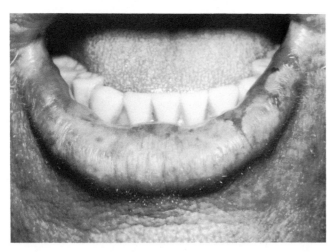

FIGURE 10–88. **Actinic cheilosis.** An irregular mottling of the surface mucosa mixes areas of pallor, erythema, and keratotic whiteness. Several small erosions and ulcerations are also seen.

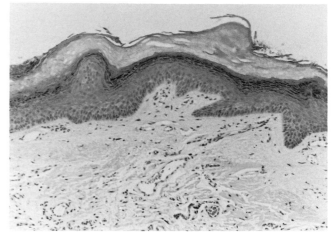

FIGURE 10–90. **Actinic cheilosis.** The epithelium is atrophic but markedly hyperkeratotic. Solar elastosis produces a somewhat amorphous appearance to the superficial connective tissue.

Clinical Features

Actinic cheilosis seldom occurs in persons younger than 45 years of age. It has a strong male predilection, with a male-to-female ratio as high as 10:1 in some studies.

The lesion develops so slowly that patients often are not aware of a change. The earliest clinical changes include atrophy of the lower lip vermilion border, characterized by a smooth surface and blotchy pale areas (Fig. 10–88). Blurring of the margin between the vermilion zone and the cutaneous portion of the lip is typically seen (Fig. 10–89; see Color Figure 63). As the lesion progresses, rough, scaly areas develop on the drier portions of the vermilion. These same areas may appear as leukoplakic lesions, especially when they extend near the wet line of the lip. The patient may report that the scaly material can be peeled off with some difficulty, only to re-form again within a few days.

With further progression, chronic focal ulceration may develop in one or more sites, especially at places of mild

trauma from cigarettes or pipe stems. Such ulcerations may last for months and often suggest progression to early squamous cell carcinoma.

Histopathologic Features

Actinic cheilosis is usually characterized by an atrophic stratified squamous epithelium, often demonstrating marked keratin production (Fig. 10–90). Varying degrees of epithelial dysplasia may be encountered. A mild chronic inflammatory cell infiltrate commonly is present subjacent to the dysplastic epithelium. The underlying connective tissue invariably demonstrates an amorphous, acellular, basophilic change known as **solar** (actinic) **elastosis**, presumably a result of an ultraviolet light–induced alteration of collagen and elastic fibers.

Treatment and Prognosis

Many of the changes associated with actinic cheilosis are probably irreversible, but patients should be encouraged to use lip balms with sunscreens in order to prevent further degeneration. Areas of induration, thickening, ulceration, or leukoplakia should be submitted for biopsy to rule out carcinoma. In severe cases without malignancy, a lip shave procedure (vermilionectomy) may be performed. The vermilion mucosa is removed, and either a portion of the intraoral labial mucosa is pulled forward, or the wound is allowed to heal by secondary intention. Long-term follow-up is recommended if a vermilionectomy is not performed. Of course, if a carcinoma is identified, the involved lip is treated accordingly.

Squamous cell carcinoma, usually well differentiated, develops in 6 to 10 percent of actinic cheilosis cases reported from medical centers. Such malignant transformation seldom occurs before 60 years of age, with the resulting carcinoma typically enlarging slowly and metastasizing only at a late stage.

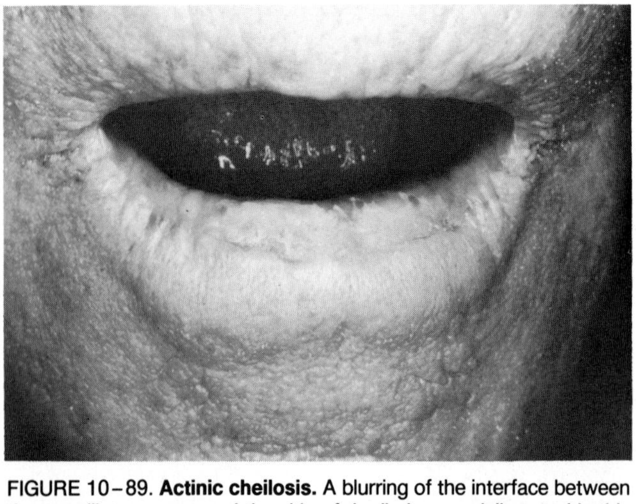

FIGURE 10–89. **Actinic cheilosis.** A blurring of the interface between the vermilion mucosa and the skin of the lip is especially noted in this case. See Color Plates.

SQUAMOUS CELL CARCINOMA

In approximately one of every three Americans now living, a malignancy will develop at some point. In 1993, more than 1,170,000 persons in the United States had at least one malignancy in addition to the 700,000 persons diagnosed with non-melanoma skin carcinomas. Although 52 percent of affected persons now survive their disease, in the United States cancer nevertheless causes 1400 deaths each day of the year and accounts for 20 percent of all deaths. Also, the current annual death rate from non-dermal cancers (170 per 100,000 persons) has increased by 19 percent since 1930, partially because of a considerable increase in the incidence of lung cancer and partially because people are now less likely to die at an early age of other common disorders, such as cardiovascular disease and infection.

Oral cancer accounts for less than 3 percent of all cancers in the United States, but it is the sixth most common cancer in males and the 12th most common in females. More than 90 percent of all oral malignancies are squamous cell carcinomas. Within the adult white population of the United States, oral carcinoma is one of the 25 most common oral mucosal lesions detected, and approximately 21,000 new cases are diagnosed annually. Slightly more than 6000 Americans die of this disease each year. Incidence and mortality rates, however, vary considerably between different races, genders, and age groups.

As with so many carcinomas, the risk of intraoral cancer increases with increasing age, especially for males. The annual incidence rate (the number of newly diagnosed cases per 100,000 persons each year) for this disease is 7.7 in the United States, although many texts report an 11 to 15 per 100,000 rate because of the inadvertent inclusion of pharyngeal and vermilion cancers with the intraoral cases. White men have a higher risk after 65 years of age than do any other group, but the highest incidence in middle age is seen in African-American men (Fig. 10–91). The intraoral cancer incidence, furthermore, is increasing dramatically over time for African-American males while decreasing slightly for all other population subgroups. Females, whether white or non-white, have a much lower incidence than males at all age levels. The overall male-to-female gender ratio is 3:1.

Carcinoma of the lip vermilion is somewhat different from intraoral carcinoma. It has a pathophysiology more akin to squamous cell carcinoma of the sun-exposed skin. The average annual incidence rate for white males in the United States is 4 per 100,000, but the rate increases dramatically with age, to almost 30 per 100,000 for men older than 75 years of age. There has been a considerable decrease in the incidence of this cancer in white males in the United States during the 20th century. Few females or non-white males have lip carcinomas, and there has been little change in the incidence over time for these groups.

Outside the United States, exceptionally wide differences in annual incidence and mortality rates for oral carcinoma are found. These rates vary by as much as 20-fold between different countries. Many of these differences are undoubtedly due to differing population habits, life expectancies, preventive education, and the quality of medical records in various countries. Despite the difficulties involved in interpreting such data, however, the data have been helpful in identifying potential etiologic factors.

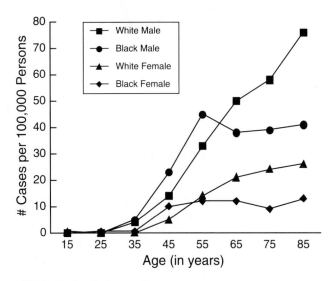

FIGURE 10–91. **Oral carcinoma.** Age-specific incidence rates for intraoral squamous cell carcinoma (number of new cases diagnosed per 100,000 persons each year). Separate rates are provided for white and black males and females in the United States.

Etiology of Oral Cancer

The cause of oral squamous cell carcinoma is multifactorial. No single causative agent or factor (carcinogen) has been clearly defined or accepted, but both extrinsic and intrinsic factors may be at work. It is likely that more than a single factor is needed to produce such a malignancy (cocarcinogenesis). *Extrinsic* factors include such external agents as tobacco smoke, alcohol, syphilis, and sunlight (vermilion cancers only). *Intrinsic* factors include systemic or generalized states, such as general malnutrition or iron-deficiency anemia. Heredity does not appear to play a major etiologic role in oral carcinoma.

Tobacco Smoking

Tobacco smoking reached its greatest popularity in the United States during the 1940s, when at least 65 percent of white males smoked and other population subgroups were beginning to smoke in large numbers. Today only 25 percent of adults in the United States smoke cigarettes, and these numbers are expected to diminish to 15 to 20 percent over the next three decades. Unfortunately, remaining smokers appear to be the heavier users, and, therefore, the effects on the mouth may be even greater than the typical effects noted in the past.

Much indirect clinical evidence implicates the habit of tobacco smoking in the development of oral squamous cell carcinoma. The proportion of smokers (80 percent) among patients with oral carcinomas is two to three times greater than that in the general population. The risk for a second primary carcinoma of the upper aerodigestive tract is two to six times greater for treated patients with oral cancer who continue to smoke than for those who quit after diagnosis.

In addition, case-control studies have shown that pipe and cigar smoking carries a greater oral cancer risk than does cigarette smoking and that the relative risk (smoker's risk for oral cancer compared with that of a nonsmoker) is dose-dependent for cigarette smokers. It is at least 5.0 for persons who smoke 40 cigarettes daily. The risk, furthermore, increases the longer the person smokes.

The greatest risk of all probably is found in certain isolated Indian and South American cultures in which the practice of "reverse smoking" is popular, especially among women. In reverse smoking, the burning end of a handmade cigar or cigarette is held inside the mouth. This habit considerably elevates one's risk for oral cancer. Where reverse smoking is practiced, as many as 50 percent of all oral malignancies are found on the hard palate, a site usually spared by this disease in the United States.

Smokeless (Spit) Tobacco

Smokeless or "spit" tobacco use in Western cultures is considered to increase a chronic user's risk for oral carcinoma by a factor of four (relative risk = 4). This apparent increased risk, which is based on a single epidemiologic (case-control) study of female textile workers, is supported by clinicopathologic investigations that have found an abnormal male-to-female sex ratio for oral carcinoma (greater than 1:1.5) in geographic areas where the habit is more popular among women than among men and by the fact that approximately 50 percent of all oral cancers in spit tobacco users occur at the site where the tobacco is habitually placed.

Alcohol

Alcohol consumption and abuse, in and of itself, has not been proven to be capable of initiating an oral cancer, and oral cancer has not yet been produced by the systemic or topical application of alcohol in animals. This habit does, however, appear to be a significant potentiator or promoter for other etiologic factors, especially tobacco, and its effects are significant when it is understood that most heavy drinkers are also heavy smokers.

Case-control studies have concluded that the risk is dose-dependent and time-dependent, and the combination of alcohol and tobacco abuse over long periods may increase a person's risk for oral cancer by more than 15 times (relative risk = 15). In this light, it may be significant that the lowest oral cancer incidence in the United States is found in Utah, where 75 percent of the population follow Mormon doctrines that forbid the use of tobacco and alcohol.

Indirect evidence for alcohol's role in oral cancer production includes the fact that approximately one third of male patients with oral cancer are heavy alcohol users; less than 10 percent of the general population can be classified as such. Cirrhosis of the liver, likewise, is found in at least 20 percent of male patients with oral cancer.

Radiation

The effects of ultraviolet radiation on the lips are discussed elsewhere (**actinic cheilosis,** see p. 293), but it is well-known that another form of radiation, *x-irradiation*, decreases immune reactivity and produces abnormalities in chromosomal material. It should not seem surprising, then, that radiotherapy to the head and neck area may increase the risk of the later development of a new primary oral malignancy, either a carcinoma or a sarcoma. This effect is dose-dependent, but even low-dose radiotherapy for benign entities may increase the local risk to some extent. However, the small amount of radiation from routine diagnostic dental radiographs has not been associated with oral mucosal carcinomas.

Iron Deficiency

Iron deficiency, especially the severe, chronic form known as the **Plummer-Vinson** or **Paterson-Kelly syndrome** (see p. 603), is associated with an elevated risk for squamous cell carcinoma of the esophagus, oropharynx, and posterior mouth. Malignancies also develop at an earlier age than in patients without iron-deficiency anemia. People who are deficient in iron tend to have impaired cell-mediated immunity, and iron is essential to the normal functioning of epithelial cells of the upper digestive tract. In deficiency states, these epithelial cells turn over more rapidly and produce an atrophic or immature mucosa. Intertwining fibrous bands of scar tissue within the esophagus of severely affected patients may also result. Patients with such esophageal webbing seem to be especially susceptible to malignant transformation.

Vitamin A Deficiency

Vitamin A deficiency produces excessive keratinization of the skin and mucous membranes, and it has been suggested that the vitamin may play a protective or preventive role in oral precancer and cancer. Blood levels of retinol and the amounts of dietary beta-carotene ingested are believed by some to be inversely proportional to the risk of oral squamous cell carcinoma and leukoplakia. Long-term therapy with retinoic acids and beta-carotene also have been associated with a regression of at least some leukoplakic lesions and a concomitant reduction in the severity of dysplasia within such lesions.

Syphilis

Syphilis has long been accepted as having a strong association with the development of dorsal tongue carcinoma. The relative risk ratio approximates four. Conversely, a person with a lingual carcinoma is five times more likely to have a positive Wassermann test result than those without such cancers. The arsenicals and heavy metals that were used to treat syphilis before the advent of modern antibiotics have carcinogenic properties themselves and may be responsible for cancer development in this disease; regardless of the pathophysiologic mechanism at work, however, syphilis-associated oral malignancies are rare today because the infection typically is diagnosed and treated before the onset of the tertiary stage.

Candidal Infection

Hyperplastic candidiasis (see p. 167) frequently is cited as an oral precancerous condition. Because this lesion presents as a white plaque that cannot be rubbed off, it also has been called **candidal leukoplakia**. Unfortunately, it is difficult, both clinically and histopathologically, to distinguish between a true hyperplastic candidiasis and a pre-existing leukoplakia with superimposed candidiasis. Experimentally, some strains of *Candida albicans* can produce hyperkeratotic lesions of the dorsal rat tongue without any other contributing factor. In other studies, certain strains have been shown to produce *nitrosamines*, chemicals that have been implicated in carcinogenesis. Certainly, some candidal strains may have the potential to promote the development of oral cancer; to date, however, the evidence to suggest this role is largely circumstantial.

Oncogenic Viruses

Oncogenic viruses may play a major role in a wide variety of cancers, although no virus has definitively been proven to cause oral cancer so far. However, retroviruses, adenoviruses, herpes simplex viruses (HSV), and human papillomaviruses (HPV) all have been suggested as playing a possible role in the development of oral carcinomas. It appears that HPV is the only one still implicated, not only in oral lesions but also in carcinomas of the pharyngeal tonsils, larynx, esophagus, uterine cervix, vulva, and penis. HPV subtypes 16, 18, 31, and 33 are the strains most closely associated with dysplasia and squamous cell carcinoma.

HSV, especially type 2, once was thought to produce a large proportion of cancers of the uterine cervix, and it has been suggested as an etiologic factor in oral carcinoma. Epidemiologic evidence now suggests that it may be no more than a common companion infection in persons with HPV infections and that the latter virus plays a much more important carcinogenic role than does HSV. Currently, the evidence gathered to prove a causal relationship between HSV and oral carcinoma is considered insufficient.

Immunosuppression

Immunosuppression may play a role in the development of at least some malignancies of the upper aerodigestive tract. Without effective immunologic surveillance and attack, it is thought that newly created malignant cells cannot be recognized and destroyed at an early stage. Persons with acquired immunodeficiency syndrome (AIDS) and those who are undergoing immunosuppressive therapy for malignancy or organ transplantation may be at slightly increased risk for oral squamous cell carcinoma as well as other head and neck malignancies.

Oncogenes and Tumor-Suppressor Genes

Oncogenes and tumor-suppressor genes are chromosomal components that are capable of being acted on by a variety of etiologic agents. Normal genes or *proto-oncogenes* may be transformed into activated oncogenes in certain malignancies through the actions of viruses, irradiation, or chemical carcinogens. Once oncogenes are activated, they may stimulate the production of an excessive amount of new genetic material through amplification or overexpression of the involved gene. Oncogenes probably are involved in the initiation as well as the progression of a wide variety of neoplasms, including oral squamous cell carcinoma.

Tumor-suppressor genes, on the other hand, allow tumor production indirectly when they become inactivated or mutated. Thus far, abnormalities of the *ras, myc,* and c-*erb*B oncogenes, and the p53 and E-cadherin tumor-suppressor genes, have been identified in oral carcinomas, although the significance of these findings is unclear.

Clinical and Radiographic Features

Persons with oral squamous cell carcinoma are most often older men who have been aware of an alteration in an oral cancer site for 4 to 8 months before seeking professional help (8 to 24 months among lower socioeconomic groups). There is minimal pain during the early growth phase, and this may explain the delay in seeking professional care. If the health care professional does not have a high index of suspicion, an additional several weeks may elapse before a biopsy is performed.

Oral squamous cell carcinoma has a varied clinical presentation, including:

- Exophytic (mass-forming)
- Endophytic (ulcerating)
- Leukoplakic (white patch)
- Erythroplakic (red patch) or erythroleukoplakic

The *leukoplakic* and *erythroplakic* examples are probably early cases that have not yet produced a mass or ulceration, and the clinical features are identical to those described for premalignant leukoplakic and erythroplakic lesions (see pp. 280 and 288). These mucosal surface changes typically are destroyed by the developing exophytic or endophytic carcinoma, but many cases are diagnosed prior to their complete destruction (Fig. 10–92).

An *exophytic* lesion typically has an irregular or papillary surface and a color that varies from normal to red to white, depending on the amount of keratin produced (Figs. 10–93 [see Color Figure 64] and 10–94). The surface is often ulcerated, and the tumor feels hard ("indurated") on palpation (Fig. 10–95).

Endophytic carcinomas typically have a depressed, irregularly shaped, ulcerated, central area with a surrounding "rolled" border of normal, red, or white mucosa (Figs. 10–96 and 10–97). The rolled border results from invasion of the tumor downward and laterally under adjacent epithelium. This appearance is not unique to oral carcinoma because granulomatous lesions, such as deep fungal infections, tuberculosis, tertiary syphilis, oral lesions of Crohn's disease, and chronic traumatic ulcers, may look similar.

Destruction of underlying bone, when present, may be painful or completely painless and appears on radio-

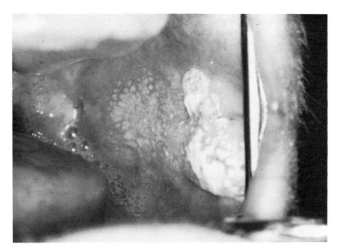

FIGURE 10–92. **Squamous cell carcinoma.** A buccal lesion with a granular, erythematous surface is destroying the prior leukoplakic lesion from which it appeared to arise. Only the anteriormost portion of the white precancerous lesion remains.

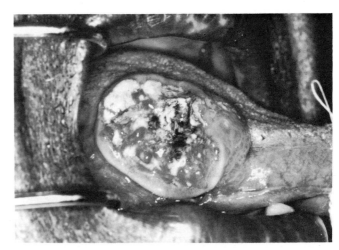

FIGURE 10–95. **Squamous cell carcinoma.** A posterior lateral tongue lesion is exophytic but also demonstrates extensive surface ulceration and nodularity. Such lesions are sometimes referred to as "fungating" carcinomas.

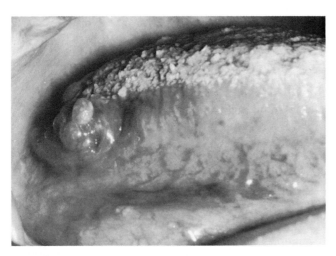

FIGURE 10–93. **Squamous cell carcinoma.** An exophytic lesion of the posterior lateral tongue demonstrates surface nodularity and minimal surface keratin production. It is painless and indurated. See Color Plates.

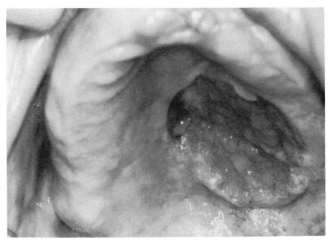

FIGURE 10–96. **Squamous cell carcinoma.** An ulcerated or endophytic lesion of the hard palate demonstrates rolled borders and a necrotic ulcer bed. This cancer was painless, even though it had partially destroyed underlying palatal bone.

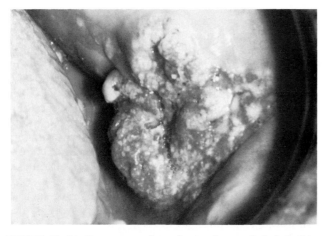

FIGURE 10–94. **Squamous cell carcinoma.** An exophytic buccal lesion shows a roughened and irregular surface with areas of erythema admixed with small areas of white keratosis. Surface ulceration is evident.

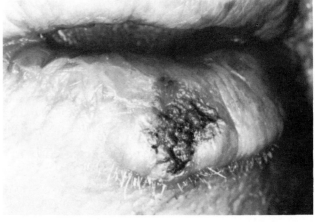

FIGURE 10–97. **Squamous cell carcinoma.** Rolled borders are evident in this crusted ulceration of the lower lip vermilion. Induration extended beyond the visible limits of the rolled borders.

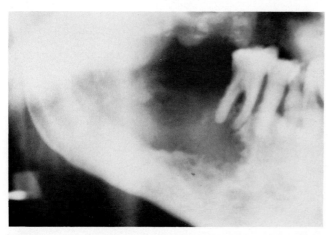

FIGURE 10-98. **Squamous cell carcinoma.** Bone involvement is characterized by an irregular, "moth-eaten" radiolucency with ragged margins—an appearance similar to that of osteomyelitis.

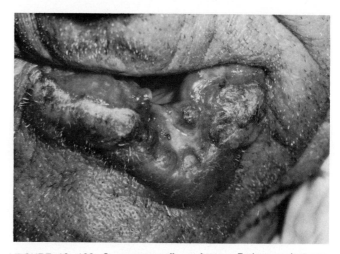

FIGURE 10-100. **Squamous cell carcinoma.** Patient neglect can result in extensive involvement, even in a readily visible site such as the lip vermilion. This ulcerating lesion of the lower lip had been present for more than a year prior to diagnosis.

graphs as a "moth-eaten" radiolucency with ill-defined or ragged margins, an appearance similar to osteomyelitis (Fig. 10-98). Carcinoma also can extend for many centimeters along a nerve without breaking away to form a true metastasis (perineural invasion).

Lip vermilion carcinoma typically is found in persons who have experienced chronic ultraviolet radiation. Seventy percent of affected individuals have outdoor occupations. It usually is associated with **actinic cheilosis** (see p. 293). It is seldom seen in persons with darkly pigmented skin. Cancers frequently arise at the site where a cigarette, cigar, or pipe stem is held by the patient, and almost 90 percent of lesions are located on the lower lip.

The typical vermilion carcinoma is a crusted, oozing, nontender, indurated ulceration that is often less than 1 cm in greatest diameter when discovered (Figs. 10-97 and 10-99). The tumor is characterized by a slow growth rate, and most patients have been aware of a "problem" in the area for 12 to 16 months before a formal diagnosis is made. Metastases are a late event, with fewer than 2 percent of patients presenting at diagnosis with metastatically involved lymph nodes, usually those in the submental region. Although this tumor is typically diagnosed and treated at an early stage, patient neglect can result in considerable destruction of normal tissue (Fig. 10-100).

The frequency of carcinoma of the lip vermilion varies considerably among population groups. During the 20th century, this lesion has decreased from the most frequent "oral" cancer to a less common one because the population in the United States no longer includes large numbers of outdoor white laborers. Overall, intraoral carcinoma is diagnosed approximately four times more frequently than vermilion carcinoma.

The most common site of intraoral carcinoma involvement is the tongue, usually the posterior lateral and ventral surfaces. The oral floor is affected almost as frequently in males but is involved much less commonly in females. Other sites of involvement, in descending order of frequency, are: soft palate, gingiva, buccal mucosa, labial mucosa, and hard palate.

Carcinoma of the tongue accounts for more than 50 percent of intraoral cancers in population studies in the United States (Figs. 10-63, 10-93, 10-95, 10-101 [see Color Figure 65], and 10-102). Two thirds of lingual carcinomas present as painless, indurated masses or ulcers of the posterior lateral border; 20 percent occur on anterior lateral or ventral surfaces, and only 4 percent occur on the dorsum. The tongue especially is the site of involvement in young patients and, in fact, is the site of the only congenital oral squamous cell carcinoma reported.

Carcinoma of the oral floor represents 35 percent of all intraoral cancers in epidemiologic surveys and appears to be increasing in frequency among females. It occurs a decade earlier in females than in males but is still usually a disease of elderly people. Of all intraoral carcinomas, oral floor lesions are the most likely to arise from a pre-existing leukoplakia or erythroplakia (Figs. 10-66, 10-76, and 10-103; see Color Figure 66). It is also the

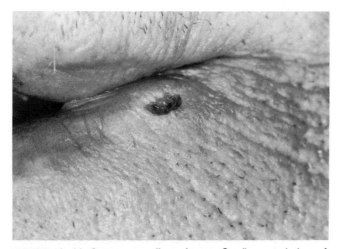

FIGURE 10-99. **Squamous cell carcinoma.** Small, crusted ulcer of the lower lip vermilion.

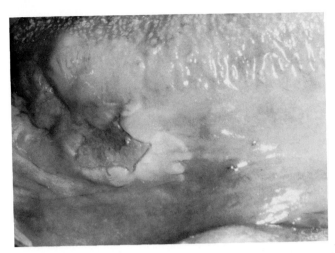

FIGURE 10–101. **Squamous cell carcinoma.** Ulcerated lesion with surrounding leukoplakia on the posterior lateral and ventral tongue. See Color Plates.

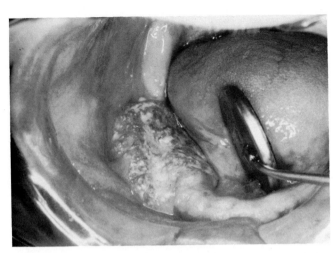

FIGURE 10–104. **Squamous cell carcinoma.** An exophytic lesion with an irregular and pebbled surface has a linear indentation along its facial aspect resulting from pressure from the patient's lower denture. Underlying alveolar bone was extensively destroyed. See Color Plates.

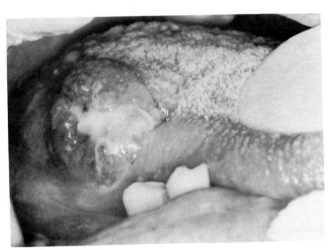

FIGURE 10–102. **Squamous cell carcinoma.** Ulcerated, exophytic mass of the posterior lateral border of the tongue.

oral site most often associated with second primary malignancies of other aerodigestive tract sites or of distant organs. The most common site of involvement is the midline near the frenum.

Gingival and alveolar carcinoma usually is painless and most frequently arises from keratinized mucosa in a posterior mandibular site (Fig. 10–104; see Color Figure 67). This tumor has a special propensity to mimic the benign inflammatory changes and lesions that are so common to the gingiva. The cancer may become clinically evident after tooth extraction. These cancers appear similar to the hyperplastic granulation tissue that arises from the socket. When the cancer develops in an edentulous area, it may give rise to a mass that "wraps around" a denture flange and superficially resembles inflammatory fibrous hyperplasia (epulis fissuratum). If the tumor is adjacent to a tooth (Fig. 10–105), it may mimic periodontal disease or a pyogenic granuloma. Gingival carci-

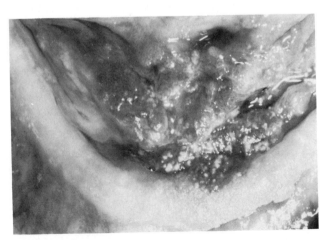

FIGURE 10–103. **Squamous cell carcinoma.** Oral floor lesions are typically ulcerated or present as an admixed red and white pebbled surface change, as depicted here. See Color Plates.

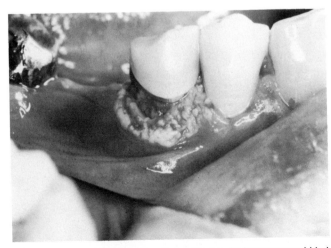

FIGURE 10–105. **Squamous cell carcinoma.** An innocuous pebbled surface change of the attached and marginal gingiva was interpreted as an inflammatory change until multifocal white keratoses occurred.

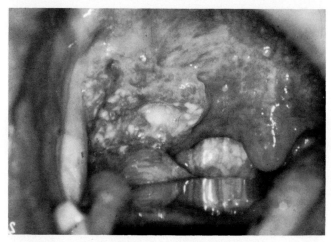

FIGURE 10–106. **Squamous cell carcinoma.** Large, ulcerated lesion of the right lateral soft palate.

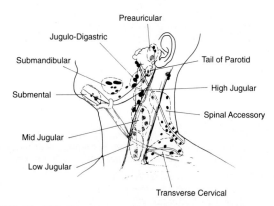

FIGURE 10–107. **Squamous cell carcinoma, metastatic spread.** Diagram demonstrating potential sites for metastatic spread of oral carcinoma to regional lymph nodes.

nomas often invade into the periodontal ligament, destroying the surrounding bone structure and causing tooth mobility. Of all the intraoral carcinomas, this one is least associated with tobacco smoking and has the greatest predilection for females.

Carcinoma of the soft palate and oropharyngeal mucosa has the same basic clinical appearance as do oral carcinomas, except that, in this more posterior location, the patient often is unaware of its presence and the diagnosis may be delayed. Tumor size typically is greater than that of oral carcinomas of other sites, and the proportion of cases with cervical and distant metastases at diagnosis is higher (Fig. 10–106). Three of every four oropharyngeal carcinomas arise from the tonsillar area or soft palate; most of the others originate on the base of the tongue. The initial symptoms are usually pain or difficulty in swallowing (*dysphagia*). The pain may be dull or sharp and frequently is referred to the ear.

As a general rule, the more posterior or inferior the oropharyngeal tumor location, the larger the lesion and the greater the chance for lymphatic spread by the time of diagnosis. A soft palate lesion may present as a localized tumor, but 80 percent of posterior oropharyngeal wall lesions have metastasized or extensively involved surrounding structures by the time of diagnosis.

Metastasis

The metastatic spread of oral squamous cell carcinoma is largely through the lymphatics to the ipsilateral cervical lymph nodes (Fig. 10–107). A cervical lymph node that contains a metastatic deposit of carcinoma is usually firm to stony hard, nontender, and enlarged (Fig. 10–108). If the malignant cells have perforated the capsule of the node and invaded into surrounding tissues, the node will feel "fixed," or not easily movable.

Occasionally, contralateral or bilateral metastatic deposits are seen, and approximately 2 percent of patients have distant ("below the clavicles") metastases at diagnosis. The most common sites of distant metastasis are the lungs, liver, and bones, but any part of the body may be affected.

Carcinoma of the lower lip and oral floor tends to travel to the submental nodes; tumors from the posterior portions of the mouth travel to the superior jugular and digastric nodes. Lymphatic drainage from the oropharynx leads to the jugulodigastric chain of lymph nodes or to the retropharyngeal nodes, and metastatic deposits from oropharyngeal carcinomas are usually found there.

Metastasis is not an early event in oral carcinoma, but because of delay in the diagnosis, approximately 21 percent of patients present at diagnosis with cervical metastases, according to epidemiologic studies (60 percent in reports from medical centers). Oropharyngeal cancer, on the other hand, is prone to early metastasis. More than 50 percent of all affected persons in population studies present with positive cervical nodes at diagnosis, and one in ten already have distant metastases by that time.

Staging

Tumor size and the extent of metastatic spread of oral squamous cell carcinoma are the best indicators of the patient's prognosis. Quantifying these clinical parameters

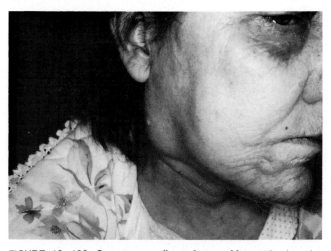

FIGURE 10–108. **Squamous cell carcinoma.** Metastatic deposits within cervical lymph nodes present as firm, painless enlargements, as seen in this patient with metastasis to a superior jugular node from a posterior lateral tongue carcinoma.

Table 10–1. TUMOR-NODE-METASTASIS (TNM) STAGING SYSTEM FOR ORAL CARCINOMA

Primary Tumor Size (T)

TX	No available information on primary tumor
T0	No evidence of primary tumor
T1S	Only carcinoma *in situ* at primary site
T1	Tumor is less than 2 cm in greatest diameter
T2	Tumor is 2 to 4 cm in greatest diameter
T3	Tumor is more than 4 cm in greatest diameter
T4	Massive tumor greater than 4 cm in diameter with involvement of antrum, pterygoid muscles, base of tongue, or skin

Regional Lymph Node Involvement (N)

NX	Nodes could not be or were not assessed
N0	No clinically positive nodes
N1	Single clinically positive homolateral node less than 3 cm in diameter
N2	Single clinically positive homolateral node 3 to 6 cm in diameter or multiple clinically positive homolateral nodes, none more than 6 cm in diameter
N2a	Single clinically positive homolateral node 3 to 6 cm in diameter
N2b	Multiple clinically positive homolateral nodes, none more than 6 cm in diameter
N3	Massive homolateral node(s), bilateral nodes, or contralateral node(s)
N3a	Clinically positive homolateral node(s), one more than 6 cm in diameter
N3b	Bilateral clinically positive nodes
N3c	Contralateral clinically positive node(s)

Involvement by Distant Metastases (M)

MX	Distant metastasis was not assessed
M0	No evidence of distant metastasis
M1	Distant metastasis is present

is called "staging" the disease. Table 10–1 summarizes the most popular staging protocol, the tumor-node-metastasis (TNM) system. Individualized TNM systems are used for most human cancers. Each system is used exclusively for a specific anatomic site and a specific tumor type.

Each specific TNM system depends on three basic clinical features:

- The size, in centimeters, of the tumor itself (T)
- The presence and type of spread to the local lymph nodes (N)
- The presence or absence of distant metastasis (M)

The various TNM aspects are tallied together to determine the appropriate stage. The higher the stage classification, the worse the prognosis (Table 10–2). In other

Table 10–2. TNM CLINICAL STAGING CATEGORIES FOR ORAL SQUAMOUS CELL CARCINOMA

Stage	TNM Classification	Five-Year Survival Rate
Stage I	T1N0M0	85%
Stage II	T2N0M0	66%
Stage III	T3N0M0, *or* T1, T2, or T3, N1M0	41%
Stage IV	Any T4 lesion, *or* Any N2 or N3 lesion, *or* Any M1 lesion	9%

words, a stage IV lesion is associated with a much worse prognosis than a stage I lesion. Most head and neck staging protocols do not use histopathologic findings beyond those needed for a determination of the diagnosis.

Histopathologic Features

Squamous cell carcinoma arises from dysplastic surface epithelium and is characterized histopathologically by invasive islands and cords of malignant epithelial cells, which demonstrate differentiation toward a squamous morphology. When the tumor is fortuitously sampled at the earliest moment of invasion, the adjectives "superficially invasive" or "microinvasive" are often used.

Whether the tumor is superficially or deeply invasive, lesional cells generally show abundant eosinophilic cytoplasm with large nuclei and an increased nuclear-cytoplasmic ratio. Varying degrees of cellular and nuclear pleomorphism are seen. The normal product of squamous epithelium is keratin, and "keratin pearls" are produced by islands of squamous epithelium, which mature to form a centrally located, round focus of keratin. Single cells also may undergo individual cell keratinization.

Histopathologic evaluation of the degree to which these tumors resemble their parent tissue (squamous epithelium) and produce their normal product (keratin) is called "grading." Lesions are graded on a three-point (grades I to III) or a four-point (grades I to IV) scale. The less differentiated tumors receive the higher numerals. The histopathologic grade of a tumor is related somewhat to its biologic behavior. In other words, a tumor that closely resembles its tissue of origin seems to grow at a slightly slower pace and metastasize at a later time in its course. Such a tumor is called "low-grade," "grade I," or "well-differentiated" squamous cell carcinoma (Figs. 10–109 to 10–111). In contrast, a tumor with much cellular and nuclear pleomorphism with little or no kera-

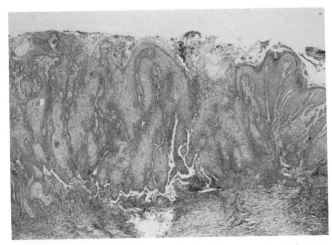

FIGURE 10–109. Well-differentiated squamous cell carcinoma. Low-power photomicrograph showing markedly hyperplastic surface epithelium with a papillary, hyperkeratotic surface and superficial invasion into the lamina propria.

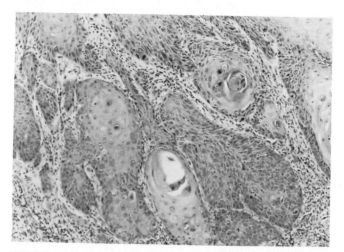

FIGURE 10–110. **Well-differentiated squamous cell carcinoma.** Higher-power view of the same lesion seen in Figure 10–109. Note invading islands of well-differentiated squamous epithelium with focal keratin pearl formation.

tin production may be difficult to identify as having an origin from squamous epithelium. Such a tumor often enlarges rapidly, metastasizes early in its course, and is termed "high-grade," "grade III/IV," "poorly differentiated," or "anaplastic" (Fig. 10–112). A tumor with a microscopic appearance somewhere between these two extremes is labeled a "moderately differentiated" carcinoma (Fig. 10–113).

To a certain extent, the grading of squamous cell carcinoma is a subjective process, depending on the area of the tumor sampled and the individual pathologist's criteria for evaluation. Clinical staging seems to correlate much better with the prognosis in most instances.

The diagnosis of squamous cell carcinoma almost always is made with routine light microscopy. Special studies that use monoclonal antibodies directed against cytokeratins may be helpful in distinguishing high-grade or poorly differentiated squamous cell carcinomas from other malignancies.

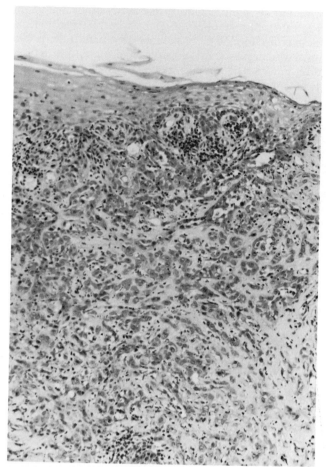

FIGURE 10–112. **Poorly differentiated squamous cell carcinoma.** Cords of poorly differentiated epithelial cells seem to be streaming downward from the surface epithelium. If the surface origin were not observable, it might be difficult to diagnose this lesion as a squamous cell carcinoma.

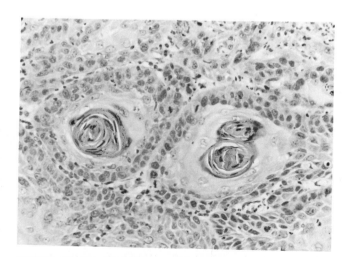

FIGURE 10–111. **Well-differentiated squamous cell carcinoma.** High-power view showing two keratin pearls.

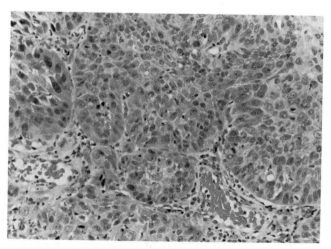

FIGURE 10–113. **Moderately differentiated squamous cell carcinoma.** Although no keratinization is seen in this high-power view, these malignant cells are still easily recognizable as being of squamous epithelial origin.

Squamous cell carcinoma, like many other malignancies, can induce numerous changes in the surrounding stroma. Occasionally, considerable dense collagen is laid down (desmoplastic or scirrhous change), but more typically new small blood vessels (angiogenesis) and a chronic inflammatory (immunologic) cell infiltrate of variable intensity are present.

Treatment and Prognosis

The treatment of intraoral squamous cell carcinoma is guided by the clinical stage of the disease and consists of wide ("radical") surgical excision, radiation therapy, or a combination of surgery and radiation therapy. The tumor's location may influence the treatment plan. Oropharyngeal lesions usually receive radiation therapy. A variety of chemotherapeutic agents are used as adjunctive therapy; some can temporarily reduce the size of a tumor mass, but none has improved survival rates significantly.

Vermilion carcinomas usually are treated by surgical excision, typically a wedge resection, with excellent results. Only 8 percent recur, and 5-year survival rates are 95 to 100 percent. In one study that evaluated all vermilion cancers diagnosed in a population over six decades, not one patient died of his or her disease. Squamous cell carcinoma of the upper lip vermilion appears to have a different biologic behavior than do those of the lower lip. The 5-year survival rate is only 58 percent, and 25 percent of lesions recur after treatment. Fortunately, upper lip carcinomas are considerably less common than lower vermilion carcinomas.

For smaller intraoral carcinomas, a single modality usually is chosen. Patients with larger lesions or lesions with clinically palpable lymph nodes typically require combined therapy. With suspected local lymph node metastasis, either a radical or modified radical neck dissection is performed. Radical neck dissection is essentially an *en bloc* removal of all fibrofatty tissues of the lateral triangle of the neck, including the superior, middle, and inferior jugular nodes; the supraclavicular group of nodes; and variable portions of the surrounding musculature.

The prognosis for survival from oral cancer depends on tumor stage (see Table 10-2). The 5-year disease-free survival rate for intraoral carcinoma is 76 percent if metastasis has not occurred by the time of diagnosis (stage I and II), 41 percent when the cervical nodes are involved (stage III), and only 9 percent when metastasis below the clavicle is present (stage IV).

The overall 5-year survival rate for intraoral carcinoma in whites in the United States has increased from 45 percent in 1960 to 55 percent today. During the same period, however, the rate for African-Americans decreased from 36 to 32 percent. The latter trend is thought to result from a combination of delayed diagnosis and inadequate initial therapy and is partially responsible for an 8 percent increase in the oral and pharyngeal cancer-related mortality rate in African-Americans since 1960. The oral cancer mortality rate for whites has decreased by 20 percent since that time.

Multiple Carcinomas

Patients with one carcinoma of the mouth or throat are at increased risk for additional concurrent (synchronous) or later (metachronous) primary surface epithelial malignancies of the upper aerodigestive tract, the esophagus, the lungs, and other sites. This risk has been estimated to be as low as 6 percent and as high as 44 percent in affected individuals. The highest figures are associated with those patients who continue to smoke after therapy. Overall, in 9 to 25 percent of patients with oral carcinomas, additional mouth or throat malignancies develop.

In patients with more than one upper aerodigestive tract malignancy, approximately one third of the tumors arise simultaneously. Of the rest, the second lesion usually develops within 3 years after the initial cancer. This tendency toward the development of multiple mucosal cancers, sometimes called "field cancerization," may reflect diffuse exposure to local carcinogens, a process that perhaps increases the malignant transformation potential of all exposed epithelial cells.

VERRUCOUS CARCINOMA
(Snuff Dipper's Cancer)

Verrucous carcinoma is a low-grade variant of oral squamous cell carcinoma. It was first reported in 1948 as a spit tobacco–associated malignancy, but it has since been diagnosed at several extraoral sites, including laryngeal, vaginal, and rectal mucosa and skin from the breast, axilla, ear canal, and soles of the feet. Tumors from anatomic sites other than the mouth are apparently unrelated to tobacco use. Several investigators have identified human papillomavirus (HPV) subtypes HPV-16 and HPV-18 in oral verrucous carcinoma, but the significance of this is unclear.

Verrucous carcinoma represents 1 to 10 percent of all oral squamous cell carcinomas, depending on the local popularity of spit tobacco use. The only epidemiologic assessment of this tumor in a Western culture reported an incidence rate of one oral lesion per 1 million population each year. The population studied was a middle-class, white, midwestern community. It is likely that the incidence is higher in the southeastern United States or in other areas where spit tobacco use is more common.

Most verrucous carcinomas arise from the oral mucosa in people who chronically use chewing tobacco or snuff, typically in areas where the tobacco is placed habitually. As many as 20 percent of the oral lesions are diagnosed in nonusers, but the common practice of patients denying tobacco habits makes the exact figure difficult to assess. In spit tobacco users, a regular squamous cell carcinoma is 25 times more likely to develop than this low-grade variant.

Clinical Features

Verrucous carcinoma is found predominantly in men older than 55 years of age (average age, 65 to 70 years). In

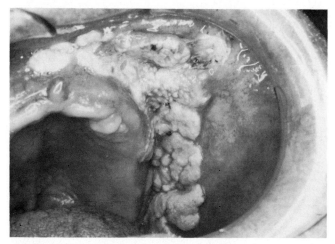

FIGURE 10-114. **Verrucous carcinoma.** Extensive papillary, white lesion of the maxillary vestibule. See Color Plates.

areas where women are frequent users of spit tobacco, however, females may predominate. The most common sites of oral mucosal involvement include the mandibular vestibule, the buccal mucosa, and the hard palate. The site of occurrence often corresponds to the site of chronic tobacco placement. In cultural groups who keep spit tobacco in the maxillary vestibule or under the tongue, this site is the most commonly involved.

Oral verrucous carcinoma is usually extensive by the time of diagnosis, and it is not unusual for a tumor to be present in the mouth for 2 to 3 years prior to the diagnosis. The lesion appears as a diffuse, well-demarcated, painless, thick plaque with papillary or verruciform surface projections (Figs. 10-114 [see Color Figure 68] and 10-115). Because of the papillary projections, many of these carcinomas probably were reported in the past as **oral florid papillomatosis.** Lesions typically are white but also may appear erythematous or pink. The color depends on the amount of keratin produced and the degree of host inflammatory response to the tumor. **Leuko-**

plakia or **tobacco pouch keratosis** may be seen on adjacent mucosal surfaces.

Histopathologic Features

Verrucous carcinoma has a deceptively benign microscopic appearance. It is characterized by wide and elongated rete ridges that appear to "push" into the underlying connective tissue (Fig. 10-116). Lesions usually show abundant keratin (usually parakeratin) production and a papillary or verruciform surface. Parakeratin typically fills the numerous clefts or crypts ("parakeratin plugging") between the surface projections (Fig. 10-117). These projections may be long and pointed or short and blunted. The lesional epithelial cells generally show a normal maturation pattern with no significant degree of cellular atypia (Fig. 10-118). There is frequently an intense infiltrate of chronic inflammatory cells in the subjacent connective tissue.

The histopathologic diagnosis of verrucous carcinoma requires an adequate incisional biopsy. Because the individual cells are not very dysplastic, the pathologist must evaluate the overall histomorphologic configuration of the lesion to arrive at an appropriate diagnosis. Adequate sampling also is important because as many as 20 percent of these lesions may have a routine squamous cell carcinoma develop concurrently within the verrucous carcinoma.

Treatment and Prognosis

Because metastasis is an extremely rare event in verrucous carcinomas, the treatment of choice is surgical excision without radical neck dissection. The surgery generally need not be as extensive as that required for a routine squamous cell carcinoma of a similar size. With this treatment, 90 percent of patients are disease-free after 5 years, although 8 percent require at least one additional surgical procedure during that time. The treatment failures usually occur in patients with the most extensive involvement or in those unable to tolerate extensive sur-

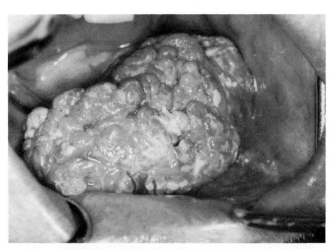

FIGURE 10-115. **Verrucous carcinoma.** Large, exophytic, papillary mass of the mandibular alveolar ridge.

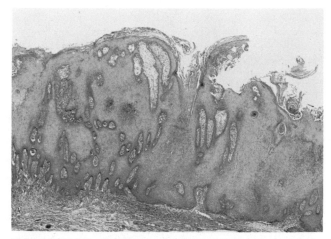

FIGURE 10-116. **Verrucous carcinoma.** Low-power photomicrograph showing marked epithelial hyperplasia with a rough, papillary surface.

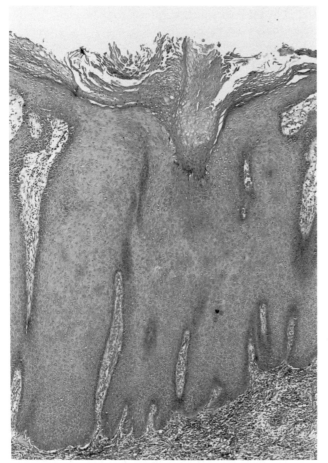

FIGURE 10-117. **Verrucous carcinoma.** Higher-power view demonstrating prominent hyperparakeratosis on the epithelial surface and hyperplasia of the rete ridges. Note how the keratin invaginates downward into the epithelium (parakeratin plugging).

gery because of unrelated systemic diseases. An additional cause of treatment failure is the initial inability to identify a focal squamous cell carcinoma arising concurrently within the less aggressive lesion.

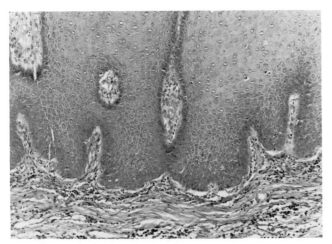

FIGURE 10-118. **Verrucous carcinoma.** High-power view showing the "pushing" nature of the rete ridges without significant cellular atypia.

Radiotherapy is effective, but has been less popular because of published reports of poorly differentiated or anaplastic carcinoma developing within the lesion after radiotherapy. A recent analysis suggests that this threat is seriously overexaggerated. Chemotherapy may temporarily reduce the size of a verrucous carcinoma, but it is not considered a definitive, stand-alone treatment.

SPINDLE CELL CARCINOMA
(Sarcomatoid Squamous Cell Carcinoma; Polypoid Squamous Cell Carcinoma)

Spindle cell carcinoma is a rare variant of squamous cell carcinoma characterized by dysplastic surface squamous epithelium in conjunction with an invasive spindle cell element, which may be indistinguishable from connective tissue sarcomas or other spindle cell malignancies at the level of the light microscope.

In the past, this was thought to be a "collision" tumor between a carcinoma and sarcoma, but most authorities now consider the spindle cells to be simply an anaplastic type of carcinoma cell. Electron microscopy and immunohistochemical analysis support the concept that these lesional cells are of epithelial origin with the ability to produce mesenchymal intermediate filaments.

About one third of spindle cell carcinoma cases have occurred after radiotherapy for oral squamous cell carcinoma, but the numbers are too few to explain the complete pathogenesis of the disease. The remaining two thirds of cases arise spontaneously and for no known reason.

Clinical Features

The mean age at diagnosis for spindle cell carcinoma is 57 years (range, 29 to 93 years). There is no sex predilection. The neoplasm occurs predominantly in the upper aerodigestive tract, especially the larynx, oral cavity, and esophagus. Within the mouth, the lower lip, lateral posterior tongue, and alveolar ridges are common sites, but other areas may be involved.

Unlike most oral cancers, the spindle cell carcinoma typically presents as a pedunculated, polypoid mass, but it may occasionally appear as a sessile, granular mass or an ulcer (Fig. 10-119). Pain and paresthesia are prominent features. The tumors grow rapidly and tend to metastasize early. Lower lip lesions seem to have a special propensity to travel along nerves to the mental foramen or the mandibular canal.

Histopathologic Features

The spindle cell carcinoma is composed predominantly of fascicles of anaplastic spindle-shaped cells. Some spindle cells may appear as obvious epithelial elements. Others have a strong connective tissue appearance, even to the point of producing osteoid-like extracellular material. Numerous mitotic figures often can be seen. The overall picture is similar to that of an anaplas-

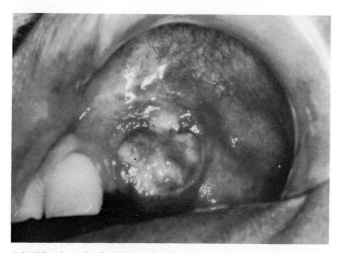

FIGURE 10–119. **Spindle cell carcinoma**. Ulcerated mass of the maxillary alveolar ridge. (Courtesy of Dr. Michael Robinson.)

tic fibrosarcoma except for the often inconspicuous squamous element.

The squamous component usually consists of carcinoma *in situ* of the overlying surface epithelium but may present as islands of dysplastic squamous epithelium within the spindle cells (Fig. 10–120). Direct transition between the two cell types may be seen, usually at the level of the basal layer of the surface mucosa, and is necessary for the diagnosis, according to some experts. Metastatic lesions may show only spindle cells, only squamous cells, or a combination of spindle and squamous cells.

Serial sections may be needed in order to find areas of unequivocal squamous cell carcinoma, and immunohistochemical techniques may be particularly useful in distinguishing this tumor from mesenchymal spindle cell malignancies. The lesional cells of mesenchymal tumors typically produce vimentin but not cytokeratin. Spindle cell carcinoma cells produce cytokeratin and may or may not produce vimentin.

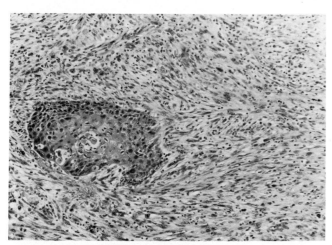

FIGURE 10–120. **Spindle cell carcinoma**. An island of malignant squamous epithelial cells *(left)* can be seen within a poorly differentiated spindle cell proliferation.

Treatment and Prognosis

The treatment of choice for spindle cell carcinomas is radical surgery, with neck dissection when clinically positive nodes are present. Radiotherapy and chemotherapy are ineffective. The 5-year disease-free survival rate is approximately 30 percent for oral lesions. This is somewhat worse than the prognosis for the tumor when it occurs in other anatomic sites, but it is similar to the prognosis for high-grade oral squamous cell carcinomas. Surprisingly, tumor size seems to have little effect on the prognosis, although there is some evidence that the microscopic depth of invasion is a strong prognostic indicator in oral lesions.

ADENOSQUAMOUS CARCINOMA

Adenosquamous carcinoma is a rare variant of squamous cell carcinoma, which is characterized histopathologically by a combination of adenocarcinoma and squamous cell carcinoma. The adenoid (glandular) pattern has been clearly demonstrated in metastatic deposits. Some authorities consider this carcinoma to be merely a high-grade **mucoepidermoid carcinoma** (see p. 349). The cause is unknown.

Clinical Features

Cases of adenosquamous carcinoma have been reported from the tongue, oral floor, and other mucosal surfaces, usually in older adults. There is no sex predilection. The clinical appearance is that of a painless, nodular, broad-based mass with or without surface ulceration. Eighty percent of patients have metastatic deposits within the neck nodes at diagnosis.

Histopathologic Features

Adenosquamous carcinoma presents as an admixture of a surface squamous cell carcinoma and an underlying glandular adenocarcinoma. Intracytoplasmic mucin is noted by mucicarmine staining in all cases, making differentiation from mucoepidermoid carcinoma difficult but helping to distinguish adenosquamous carcinoma from forms of squamous cell carcinoma that exhibit a pseudoglandular pattern of degeneration.

Treatment and Prognosis

Radical surgical excision, with or without radiation therapy, is the treatment of choice for patients with adenosquamous carcinomas, but the prognosis is poor.

CARCINOMA OF THE MAXILLARY SINUS

Carcinoma of the maxillary sinus or antrum is an uncommon malignancy of unknown etiology. It does not

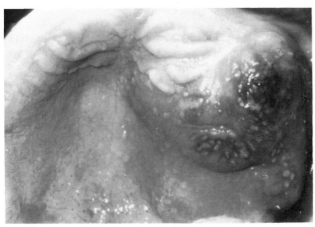

FIGURE 10-121. **Carcinoma of the maxillary sinus.** The tumor has produced a bulge of the posterior maxillary alveolar ridge and is beginning to ulcerate through the surface mucosa.

appear to be related to sinusitis, nasal polyps, or tobacco use. Most lesions remain asymptomatic for long periods while the tumor grows to fill the sinus and may not be diagnosed until they perforate through the surrounding bone.

Clinical and Radiographic Features

Typically, carcinoma of the maxillary sinus is a disease of elderly people. There is a slight predilection for males. Affected patients generally complain of a chronic unilateral nasal stuffiness or notice an ulceration or mass of the hard palate or alveolar bone (Fig. 10-121). When the second division of the trigeminal nerve is involved, intense pain or paresthesia of the mid-face or maxilla may occur, simulating toothache-like symptoms. Teeth in the area of the tumor may become loosened, and dental radiographs often reveal a "moth-eaten" destruction of the lamina dura and surrounding bone. A panoramic radiograph shows a cloudy sinus with destruction of its bony wall, although the extent of the tumor is visualized best by computed tomography (CT).

If the tumor perforates the lateral wall of the sinus, unilateral facial swelling and pain may be present. If the extension is medial, nasal obstruction or hemorrhage usually occur. Extension superiorly results in displacement or protrusion of the eyeball. When metastasis is present at diagnosis, it is usually to the ipsilateral submandibular and cervical lymph nodes; distant metastasis is uncommon.

Histopathologic Features

Although the antrum is lined by respiratory epithelium, almost all maxillary sinus carcinomas are squamous cell carcinomas, usually moderately or poorly differentiated.

Treatment and Prognosis

Carcinoma confined within the maxillary sinus is treated by hemimaxillectomy; those that have perforated through the surrounding bone are treated by radiotherapy or combined radical surgery and radiotherapy. Even with radical treatment, however, the prognosis is poor. Only 10 to 30 percent of patients survive 5 years after therapy. The presence of metastatic deposits in local lymph nodes reduces the survival rate to less than 8 percent, as does involvement of the pterygopalatine fossa. With or without cervical node involvement, death usually occurs from local destruction and the inability to control the primary disease.

NASOPHARYNGEAL CARCINOMA

Nasopharyngeal carcinoma is a malignancy that arises from the lining epithelium of the nasopharynx. This lesion is rare in most areas of the world. The annual incidence is less than one case per 100,000 population. In southern Chinese males, however, the incidence is a startling 20 to 55 cases per 100,000. Among southern Chinese males who migrate to the United States, the incidence is intermediate, which suggests an environmental etiologic agent. Diets deficient in vitamin C, infection with Epstein-Barr virus, and consumption of salt fish

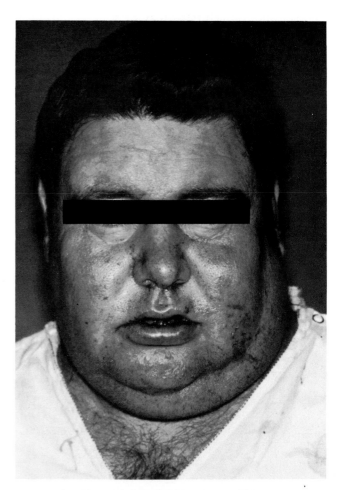

FIGURE 10-122. **Nasopharyngeal carcinoma.** This patient initially presented with metastatic carcinoma in the left lateral neck. Further evaluation revealed a primary tumor of the nasopharynx. (Courtesy of Dr. D. E. Kenady.)

that contains carcinogenic nitrosamines all have been implicated as contributory factors.

Clinical Features

Although nasopharyngeal carcinoma may occur at any age, the mean age at the time of diagnosis is 50 to 55 years. The less-differentiated lesions tend to occur in younger individuals. In fact, virtually all nasopharyngeal carcinomas in people younger than 40 years of age are undifferentiated carcinomas.

For nearly 60 percent of patients affected by nasopharyngeal carcinoma, the first sign of disease is an enlarged cervical lymph node, which represents metastasis (Fig. 10-122). The primary lesion, which usually arises from the lateral nasopharyngeal wall, often is small and difficult to detect, even when the area is examined endoscopically. When the carcinoma cannot be visualized, multiple, systematic biopsy sampling of nasopharyngeal mucosa may be necessary for tumor identification and diagnosis.

Unilateral serous otitis media and hearing loss from an obstructed eustachian tube occur in nearly 50 percent of affected patients. Epistaxis, nasal obstruction, and pain may be present. In this anatomic site, the tumor may invade through the foramen lacerum into the brain, producing central nervous system (CNS) symptoms.

Histopathologic Features

Microscopic examination of a nasopharyngeal carcinoma typically shows one of three histopathologic patterns:

- Squamous cell carcinoma (keratinizing squamous cell carcinoma)
- Nonkeratinizing carcinoma
- Undifferentiated (poorly differentiated or anaplastic) carcinoma

The histopathologic findings of the first group are identical to those of squamous cell carcinoma of other sites. Evidence of keratinization must be seen at the light microscopic level.

Nonkeratinizing carcinoma is a poorly differentiated tumor of squamous epithelium with no keratin production. Islands of malignant cells are well demarcated from a surrounding fibrovascular connective tissue stroma.

The third group, **undifferentiated carcinoma**, consists of malignant epithelial cells with essentially no differentiation. Lesional cells usually have large vesicular nuclei with prominent nucleoli and little cytoplasm. The margin between the clusters of lesional cells and the supporting stroma is blurred. Tumor cells are often intermixed with the lymphoid cells normal to this anatomic site (Fig. 10-123). The term "lymphoepithelioma" has been used to describe this lesion because it was once thought to be a malignancy that originated conjointly from local epithelial and lymphoid tissues. This terminology should be discouraged, however, because the lymphoid tissue is not part of the neoplastic process. Such undifferentiated tumors may be difficult to distinguish from lymphoma by light microscopy alone, and immunohistochemical studies often are used to demonstrate cytokeratins within the carcinoma cells.

Treatment and Prognosis

Because of the inaccessibility of the nasopharynx and the high frequency of metastasis at diagnosis, nasopharyngeal carcinoma is treated most frequently with radiotherapy to the nasopharynx and neck, usually combined with chemotherapy (cyclophosphamide, methotrexate, and bleomycin). The prognosis ranges from good to poor, depending on the stage of the disease. For stage I patients, a 100 percent 5-year survival rate has been demonstrated. Stage II is associated with a 67 percent 5-year survival rate; stage III, 44 percent; and stage IV, 34 percent.

BASALOID SQUAMOUS CARCINOMA
(Basaloid Squamous Cell Carcinoma)

Basaloid squamous carcinoma is strictly a lesion of the upper aerodigestive tract mucosa and represents the newest of the squamous cell carcinoma variants to be accepted. It has a tendency to arise in the hypopharynx and base of the tongue, but several oral lesions have been reported.

Clinical Features

Basaloid squamous carcinoma occurs predominantly in men, in persons 40 to 85 years of age, and in abusers of alcohol and smoked tobacco. It clinically presents as a fungating mass or ulcer and may be painful or interfere with swallowing (dysphagia). Almost 80 percent of patients have cervical metastases at the time of diagnosis.

Histopathologic Features

As its name connotes, basaloid squamous carcinoma has two microscopic components. The first is a superficial, well-differentiated or moderately differentiated

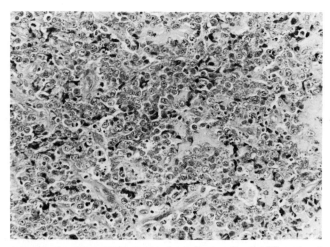

FIGURE 10-123. **Nasopharyngeal carcinoma.** Poorly differentiated tumor exhibiting sheets of rounded tumor cells that resemble lymphoid tissue.

squamous cell carcinoma, often with surface ulceration, a multifocal origin, and areas of carcinoma *in situ*. The second, deeper component is an invasive basaloid epithelium arranged in islands, cords, and gland-like lobules. It appears similar to basal cell carcinoma, adenoid cystic carcinoma, basal cell adenocarcinoma, or neuroendocrine carcinoma. The interface between the two components typically is sharp and distinct, but transition from squamous to basaloid cells may occasionally be seen. Basaloid cells and islands of cells often are surrounded by mucoid-like stroma (basal lamina material).

Treatment and Prognosis

Basaloid squamous carcinoma is an aggressive malignancy. Affected patients have a mean survival time of only 23 months. Surgery followed by radiotherapy is the recommended treatment, usually with adjuvant chemotherapy for the distant metastases.

BASAL CELL CARCINOMA (Basal Cell Epithelioma; Rodent Ulcer)

Basal cell carcinoma is a locally invasive, slowly spreading primary epithelial malignancy that arises from the basal cell layer of the skin and its appendages. About 85 percent of cases are found on the skin of the head and neck. Approximately 500,000 new cases of basal cell carcinoma are diagnosed annually in the United States, representing 80 percent of all skin cancers, and the number of new cases is increasing by 3 to 7 percent each year. These cancers result from chronic exposure to ultraviolet radiation. Oral lesions have been reported but are usually considered to be cases of misdiagnosed salivary or odontogenic neoplasms.

Clinical Features

Basal cell carcinoma is a disease of adult whites, especially those with fair complexions. Although most patients are older than 40 years of age at the time of diagnosis, some lesions are detected as early as the second decade of life, particularly in patients with red hair and blue eyes.

The most common form of this lesion, the **nodulo-ulcerative basal cell carcinoma**, begins as a firm, painless papule that slowly enlarges and gradually develops a central depression with an umbilicated appearance. One or more telangiectatic blood vessels usually are seen coursing over the rolled border surrounding the central depression (Fig. 10–124; see Color Figure 69). When the lesion is pressed, a characteristic pearly opalescent quality is discerned. Ulceration often develops in the central depressed area (Fig. 10–125), and the patient may give a history of intermittent bleeding followed by healing. Untreated lesions continue to enlarge slowly, with ulceration and destruction of underlying structures, hence their historical name, **rodent ulcer.** Destruction of underlying bone or cartilage may occur, but metastasis is extremely rare.

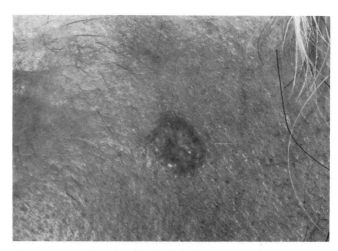

FIGURE 10–124. Basal cell carcinoma. Early noduloulcerative basal cell carcinoma of the facial skin showing raised, rolled borders and a central depression. Fine, telangiectatic blood vessels can be seen on the surface. See Color Plates.

Several other clinicopathologic varieties of this tumor have also been described. **Pigmented basal cell carcinoma** is seen occasionally and represents a noduloulcerative tumor colonized by benign melanocytes (Fig. 10–126; see Color Figure 70). The melanin production imparts a tan, brown, black, or even bluish color to the lesion, and usually the pigment is not distributed uniformly, as it would be in a melanocytic nevus.

Sclerosing (morpheaform) basal cell carcinoma is an insidious lesion that often mimics scar tissue. The overlying skin appears pale and atrophic, and the lesion is firm to palpation with poorly demarcated borders. A slight elevation may be noted at the edges of the tumor. Often a great deal of invasion has occurred before the patient becomes aware of a problem.

The **superficial basal cell carcinoma** occurs primarily on the skin of the trunk. Often, lesions are multiple and present as well-demarcated, erythematous, scaly patches that may be mistaken clinically for psoriasis. A fine, elevated, "thread-like" border is seen at the margins.

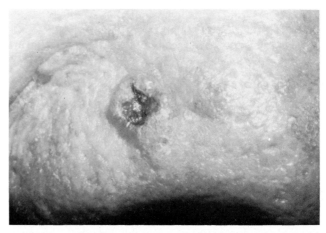

FIGURE 10–125. Basal cell carcinoma. Noduloulcerative lesion of the nose demonstrating a central crusted area of ulceration.

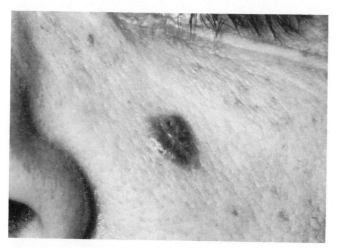

FIGURE 10–126. **Basal cell carcinoma.** Pigmented basal cell carcinoma of the cheek. See Color Plates.

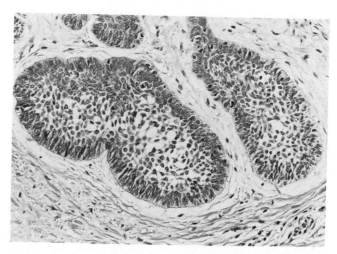

FIGURE 10–128. **Basal cell carcinoma.** High-power view showing islands of hyperchromatic, basaloid epithelial cells demonstrating palisading of the peripheral nuclei.

Some investigators believe that the basal cell carcinoma associated with the **nevoid basal cell carcinoma syndrome** (see p. 501) should be placed in a separate category. These lesions develop in both sun-exposed and protected areas of the skin and may number in the hundreds on a single patient. Frequently, the tumors associated with this syndrome do not produce a significant degree of tissue destruction.

Histopathologic Features

The noduloulcerative, pigmented, and syndrome-related basal cell carcinomas consist of uniform, dark-staining basaloid cells with oval nuclei and relatively little cytoplasm (Figs. 10–127 and 10–128). The cells are arranged into well-demarcated islands and strands, which appear to arise from the basal cell layer of the overlying epidermis and invade into the underlying dermal connective tissue. Epithelial islands typically demonstrate palisading of the peripheral cells; frequently, a

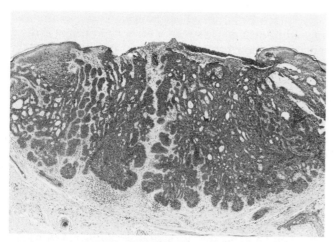

FIGURE 10–127. **Basal cell carcinoma.** Low-power photomicrograph showing ulceration of the epidermal surface associated with an invading tumor of hyperchromatic epithelial cells.

clear zone of retraction is seen between the epithelial islands and the connective tissue. Although most of these neoplasms show no differentiation, some exhibit areas of keratin production, sebaceous differentiation, or interlacing strands of lesional cells that resemble duct formation ("adenoid").

Pigmented basal cell carcinoma demonstrates dendritic melanocytes within tumor islands, and melanophages may be seen in the surrounding stroma. Sclerosing basal cell carcinoma is characterized by infiltrating thin strands of basaloid tumor cells set in a densely collagenous background. Superficial basal cell carcinoma includes lobules of tumor cells that drop from the epidermis in a multifocal pattern. Occasionally, basal cell carcinoma is seen admixed with an independent primary squamous cell carcinoma of the skin. The resulting "collision" tumor is called **basosquamous carcinoma**. Some authorities consider the basosquamous carcinoma to be a simple basal cell carcinoma with abundant squamous metaplasia.

Treatment and Prognosis

The treatment of a patient with a basal cell carcinoma often depends on the size and site of the lesion. Radical surgical excision and radiation therapy may control large or aggressive lesions. For relatively small lesions (<1 cm), routine surgical excision or electrodesiccation and curettage are generally adequate. These methods result in a cure rate of 95 to 98 percent. For larger lesions, sclerosing-type lesions, recurrent lesions, or lesions situated near embryonic planes of fusion (along which these tumor cells tend to invade), a procedure called Mohs micrographic surgery should be used. This technique essentially uses frozen-section evaluation of specially mapped and marked surgical specimens to determine whether tumor tissue has been left behind. If it has, the surgeon can return immediately to that particular area and remove more tissue, repeating the process until the patient is free of disease.

Recurrence of a properly treated basal cell carcinoma is uncommon, and metastasis is exceptionally rare. In patients with uncontrolled or uncontrollable disease, death is usually the result of local invasion into vital structures. However, with early detection and the advent of Mohs surgery, such an outcome is unusual today.

Patients with a history of basal cell carcinoma must be evaluated periodically. There is a 30 percent chance of a second lesion developing within 3 years of the treatment of the initial tumor.

MERKEL CELL CARCINOMA (Merkel Cell Tumor; Neuroendocrine Carcinoma of Skin; Small Cell Carcinoma of Skin; Trabecular Carcinoma of Skin)

The **Merkel cell carcinoma**, first described in 1972, is a rare but aggressive primary malignancy of the skin. Lesional cells contain cytoplasmic granules that resemble the neurosecretory granules found within the epidermal Merkel cells of touch receptor regions. Intraoral and lip vermilion cases have been reported but are rare.

Clinical Features

Merkel cell carcinoma typically presents in elderly people. It occurs primarily on the sun-exposed areas of fair-skinned individuals, most commonly (75 percent) on the skin of the face. The tumor usually appears as a slowly enlarging dome-shaped nodule with a smooth surface, demonstrating prominent surface vessels or telangiectases. It is red or violaceous and ranges in size from 0.5 to 5.0 cm. Ulceration rarely is seen. Occasional lesions grow rapidly, and 25 percent demonstrate local metastasis at diagnosis, belying its innocuous clinical appearance.

Histopathologic Features

Merkel cell carcinoma consists of infiltrating sheets and anastomosing strands of moderately sized, uniform, undifferentiated basophilic cells in the dermis and subcutaneous fat (Fig. 10-129). Pseudoglandular, trabecular, and cribriform ("Swiss cheese") patterns may be seen. The surface epithelium usually is intact and otherwise unremarkable unless secondarily ulcerated by the tumor. Mitotic figures are abundant, and tumor cells have prominent nuclei, scant cytoplasm, and indistinct cell borders. Intracytoplasmic argyrophilic granules may be demonstrated by the Grimelius stain.

At times, this entity is difficult to differentiate histopathologically from amelanotic melanoma, metastatic esthesioneuroblastoma, metastatic small cell carcinoma of the lung, malignant lymphoma, and other undifferentiated malignancies. In this situation, a panel of immunohistochemical studies should be used to exclude these other diagnostic possibilities. Careful physical examination of the patient also may provide useful diagnostic information.

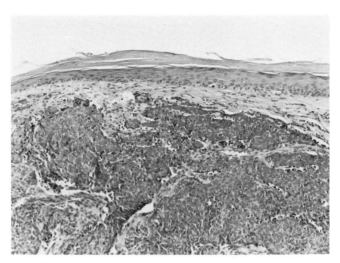

FIGURE 10-129. **Merkel cell carcinoma.** A sheet of undifferentiated basophilic cells is seen beneath the epidermal surface.

Treatment and Prognosis

Merkel cell carcinoma is treated with wide local excision, which may be combined with lymph node dissection when clinically palpable nodes are found. The addition of postoperative radiotherapy improves the prognosis.

Although no long-term studies are available, the prognosis for Merkel cell carcinoma is guarded. Local recurrence develops in one third of cases, regional metastases occur in one half to two thirds of cases, and distant metastases (predominantly to liver, bones, and brain) occur in more than one third of cases. At least 25 to 45 percent of patients will die of their disease.

MELANOMA (Malignant Melanoma; Melanocarcinoma)

Melanoma is a malignant neoplasm of melanocytic origin that arises from a benign melanocytic lesion or *de novo* from melanocytes within otherwise normal skin or mucosa. Although most melanomas occur on the skin, they may develop at any site where melanocytes are present. Damage from ultraviolet radiation is considered a major causative factor, as suggested by the fact that the incidence of melanoma increases for light-complexioned populations as they approach the equator, but chronic sun exposure does not seem to be as significant as it is for other cutaneous cancers, such as basal and squamous cell carcinoma. Acute sun damage may be of greater etiologic importance than chronic exposure in melanoma.

The risk of melanoma development is two to eight times greater when a relative has a history of the cancer. Additional risk factors include a fair complexion and light hair, a tendency to sunburn easily, a history of painful or blistering sunburns in childhood, an indoor occupation with outdoor recreational habits, a personal history of melanoma, and a personal history of dysplastic or congenital nevus.

Melanoma is the third most common skin cancer. It accounts for 5 percent of cutaneous malignancies. Most deaths that are due to skin cancer, however, are caused by melanoma. In the United States, 32,000 new cases are diagnosed each year, and 6800 persons die of the disease. The average annual incidence for skin melanomas (9.3 per 100,000 males and 8.7 per 100,000 females) has been increasing dramatically over the past several decades. Today, it is estimated that the lifetime risk for melanoma development in a white person in the United States is one in 100.

Almost 25 percent of cutaneous melanomas arise in the head and neck area, 40 percent occur on the extremities, and most of the rest occur on the trunk.

Oral mucosal melanoma is rare in the United States. It occurs in only one of every two million persons annually, but it is more frequent in Japan and Uganda.

Clinical Features

Most melanomas are seen in white adults; the average age of affected persons is 50 to 55 years. Cases are rather evenly distributed over the 30- to 80-year age bracket, and a few melanomas occur in the second and third decades of life. Four clinicopathologic types of melanoma have been described:

- Lentigo maligna melanoma
- Superficial spreading melanoma
- Nodular melanoma
- Acral lentiginous melanoma

Melanomas tend to exhibit two directional patterns of growth: the *radial* growth phase and the *vertical* growth phase. In the early stages of melanoma development, the radial growth phase tends to predominate in lentigo maligna, superficial spreading, and acral lentiginous melanomas. In these lesions, the malignant melanocytes tend to spread horizontally through the basal layer of the epidermis. Eventually, however, the malignant cells begin to invade the underlying connective tissue, thus initiating the vertical growth phase. With nodular melanoma, the radial growth phase is very short or nonexistent and the vertical growth phase predominates.

Because many clinical similarities exist between melanoma and its benign counterpart, the **melanocytic nevus**, an "ABCD" system of evaluation has been developed to help distinguish a melanoma clinically from a melanocytic nevus. Melanoma characteristically exhibits:

- **A**symmetry, because of its uncontrolled growth pattern
- **B**order irregularity, often with notching
- **C**olor variegation, which varies from shades of brown to black, white, red, and blue, depending on the amount and depth of melanin pigmentation
- **D**iameter greater than 6 mm (which is the diameter of a pencil eraser)

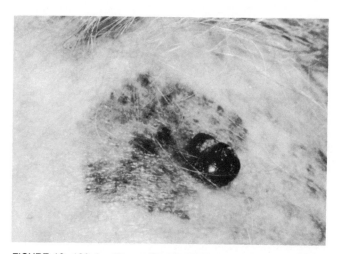

FIGURE 10–130. **Lentigo maligna melanoma.** A slowly evolving lesion of the facial skin in an elderly man. The "ABCD" warning signs of melanoma are demonstrated. The lesion is **a**symmetric, has an irregular **b**order, has **c**olor variegation, and is much larger in **d**iameter than a pencil eraser.

Lentigo Maligna Melanoma

Lentigo maligna melanoma, which accounts for 5 percent of cutaneous melanomas, develops from a precursor lesion called **lentigo maligna (Hutchinson's freckle).** Lentigo maligna occurs almost exclusively on the sun-exposed skin of fair-complexioned elderly persons, particularly in the mid-facial region, and probably represents a melanoma *in situ* or melanoma in a purely radial growth phase. Lentigo maligna essentially exhibits all the clinical features of melanoma.

The lesion presents as a large, slowly expanding (radial growth phase) macule with irregular borders and a variety of colors, including tan, brown, black, and even white (Fig. 10–130). Patients usually indicate that the lesion has been present and has slowly expanded laterally for years. The average duration of the radial growth phase is 15 years. The appearance of nodularity within the lentigo maligna signals the onset of the invasive or vertical growth phase and the transition to lentigo maligna melanoma.

Superficial Spreading Melanoma

Superficial spreading melanoma is the most common clinicopathologic form of melanoma, representing 70 percent of cutaneous lesions (Fig. 10–131; see Color Figure 71). The most common sites are the interscapular area of males and the back of the legs of females. This form of melanoma presents as a macule with a variety of potential colors (tan, brown, gray, black, blue, white, or pink). Typically, the lesion is smaller than 3 cm in greatest diameter at diagnosis, but it may be several times that size. Many lesions are slightly elevated. Clinically, invasion is indicated by the appearance of surface nodules or induration, and usually occurs within 1 year of discovery of the precursor macule. Satellite macules or nodules of malignant cells may develop around the primary lesion.

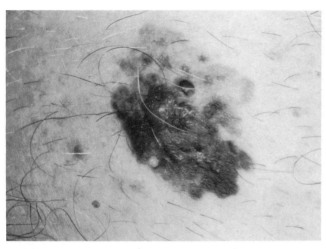

FIGURE 10–131. **Superficial spreading melanoma.** This lesion also demonstrates the ABCD warning signs of melanoma: **a**symmetry, **b**order irregularity, **c**olor variegation, and **d**iameter larger than a pencil eraser. See Color Plates.

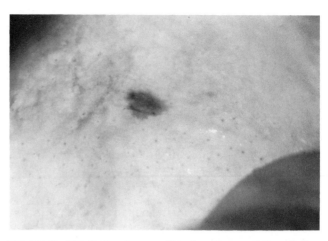

FIGURE 10–132. **Oral melanoma.** This discrete area of pigmentation, measuring approximately 5 mm in diameter, was discovered on the posterior hard palate of this middle-aged woman during an oral examination. Biopsy revealed melanoma *in situ*.

Nodular Melanoma

Nodular melanoma represents 15 percent of cutaneous melanomas, and one third of such lesions develop in the head and neck area. Nodular melanoma is thought to begin almost immediately in the vertical growth phase and, therefore, presents typically as a nodular elevation that rapidly invades into the connective tissue. Nodular melanoma is usually a deeply pigmented exophytic lesion, although sometimes the melanoma cells are so poorly differentiated that they no longer can produce melanin, resulting in a nonpigmented **amelanotic melanoma.**

Acral Lentiginous Melanoma

Acral lentiginous melanoma is the most common form of melanoma in blacks, and it is also the most common form of **oral melanoma.** It typically develops on the palms of the hands, soles of the feet, subungual area, and mucous membranes. It begins as a darkly pigmented, irregularly marginated macule, which later develops a papular invasive growth phase.

As mentioned earlier, oral melanoma is rare in the United States, making up less than 1 percent of all melanomas. Affected persons are usually in their sixth or seventh decade of life. Four of every five oral melanomas are found on the hard palate and maxillary gingiva or alveolar mucosa. A lesion typically begins as a brown to black macule with irregular borders (Figs. 10–132 and 10–133; see Color Figure 72). The macule extends laterally, and thickened areas develop as the vertical growth is initiated. Ulceration soon follows.

Histopathologic Features

With cutaneous and oral melanomas, atypical melanocytes initially are seen at the epithelial-connective tissue junction. From here, they have the potential to proliferate throughout the epithelium, laterally along the basal cell layer and downward into the connective tissue. In the early stages of the neoplasm, atypical melanocytes are seen either scattered singly among the basal epithelial cells or as nests within the basal cell layer. The atypical melanocytes usually are larger than normal melanocytes and have varying degrees of nuclear pleomorphism and hyperchromatism.

With superficial spreading melanoma, "pagetoid spread" is often seen. Large melanoma cells infiltrate the surface epithelium singly or in nests (Fig. 10–134). The resulting microscopic pattern is called pagetoid because it resembles an intraepithelial adenocarcinoma known as Paget's disease of skin.

The spreading of the lesional cells along the basal layer constitutes the radial growth phase of the neoplasm. Such lateral spread of cells within the epithelium, which occurs before invasion into the underlying connective tissue, is characteristically seen in superficial spreading melanoma, lentigo maligna melanoma, and acral lentiginous melanoma. In acral lentiginous melanomas,

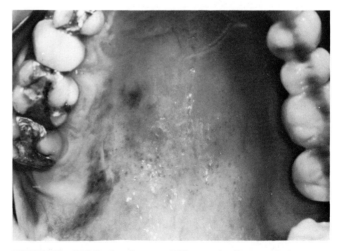

FIGURE 10–133. **Oral melanoma.** Diffuse, splotchy area of pigmentation of the lateral hard palate. See Color Plates.

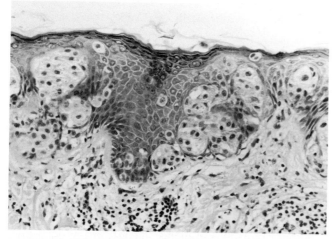

FIGURE 10–134. **Superficial spreading melanoma.** The radial growth phase is characterized by the spread of atypical melanocytes along the basilar portion of the epidermis. Also note the presence of individual melanocytes invading the higher levels of the epidermis.

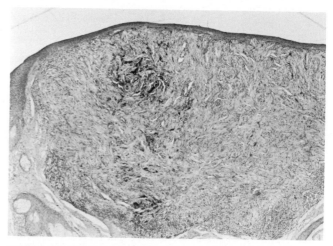

FIGURE 10–136. **Nodular melanoma.** A nodular tumor is seen invading the dermis without the presence of lateral radial growth in the overlying epidermis.

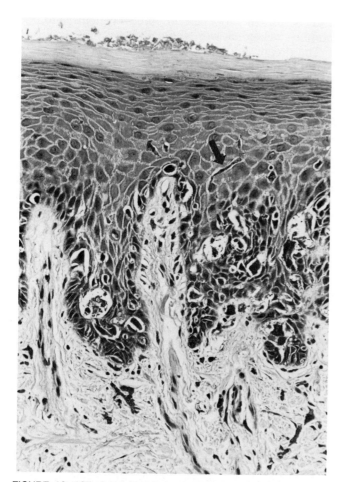

FIGURE 10–135. **Acral lentiginous melanoma.** This palatal melanoma demonstrates numerous atypical melanocytes in the basilar portion of the epithelium. Some of these melanocytes have prominent dendritic processes (*arrow*).

many of the melanocytes have prominent dendritic processes (Fig. 10–135).

When malignant melanocytes are observed invading the connective tissue, the vertical growth phase has taken place. In nodular melanomas, this vertical growth phase occurs early in the course of the tumor. No radial growth of cells can be observed in the overlying epithelium beyond the edge of the invasive tumor (Fig. 10–136). The invasive melanoma cells usually appear either spindle-shaped or epithelioid and infiltrate the connective tissue as loosely aggregated cords or sheets of pleomorphic cells (Fig. 10–137).

In most instances, the lesional cells of melanoma contain fine melanin granules, but they may demonstrate no melanin production (amelanotic melanoma). A lack of melanin production may cause diagnostic confusion at the light microscopic level because melanoma can mimic a variety of undifferentiated tumors. Immunohisto-

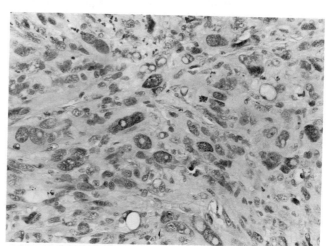

FIGURE 10–137. **Melanoma.** The cells of this invasive melanoma are mostly spindle-shaped and demonstrate marked pleomorphism. If melanin pigment is absent, such poorly differentiated tumors may be difficult to distinguish from other malignant neoplasms.

Table 10–3. TWO CLASSIFICATION SYSTEMS* USED TO MEASURE DEPTH OF INVASION IN CUTANEOUS MELANOMA

Clark's Definition of Level of Tumor Invasion	Clark's Classification	Breslow's Depth of Invasion (mm)†	Estimated 10-Year Survival Rate	
			Clark	Breslow
Cells confined to epithelium	Level I	N/A	96%	N/A
Cells penetrating papillary dermis	Level II	0.0–0.75 mm	96%	98%
Cells filling papillary dermis	Level III	0.76–1.69 mm	90%	89%
Cells extending into reticular dermis	Level IV	1.70–3.59 mm	67%	67%
Cells invading subcutaneous fat	Level V	> 3.6 mm	26%	43%

*The Clark and Breslow classifications are the most widely used systems for prognostic purposes.
†Breslow's depth is measured from the top of the granular cell layer.

chemical studies for S-100 and HMB-45 reactivity may be beneficial in distinguishing such melanomas from other malignancies.

Treatment and Prognosis

Microscopic measurement of the depth of invasion is an important component of the histopathologic evaluation of melanoma because of its correlation with the prognosis. The Clark system of measurement assigns a "level" to the lesion that depends on the deepest anatomic cutaneous region that has been invaded by tumor cells. The more recent Breslow classification, however, appears to show a more accurate correlation with the prognosis and is based on the actual measurement of the distance from the top of the granular cell layer to the deepest identifiable point of tumor invasion (Table 10–3). Patients also are staged clinically in a fashion similar to patients with squamous cell carcinoma.

Surgical excision is the only curative treatment. The extent of the excision is still somewhat controversial. Older literature suggests that surgical margins of 3 to 5 cm around the tumor are necessary to achieve control, regardless of the size of the lesion. More recent studies indicate that a 1-cm margin is adequate for small, early tumors. For larger, more deeply invasive tumors, wide surgical excision still is recommended. Surgical removal of regional lymph nodes is recommended for lesions with a histopathologic depth of invasion that exceeds 1.24 mm. Radiation therapy, chemotherapy, and immunotherapy show no significant impact on survival to date.

Melanomas that are detected early and removed before metastasis has developed (stage I) are associated with an 89 percent 5-year survival rate and an 81 percent 10-year survival rate. Melanomas that have metastasized to local lymph nodes at the time of diagnosis (stage II) are associated with a 61 percent 5-year survival rate and a 47 percent 10-year survival rate. If disseminated disease is present at the time of diagnosis (stage III), the tumor is virtually always fatal. Overall, the 10-year survival rate is 79 percent. Survivability is much improved relative to that of past decades, primarily as a result of public education. Currently, the clinical features of melanoma are so widely known that many lesions are discovered and treated at an early stage.

Other factors may influence the outcome of the disease besides the depth of invasion. For reasons that are unclear, melanomas affecting certain cutaneous sites seem to carry a worse prognosis compared with those of a similar depth of invasion at other sites. The areas with a worse prognosis are designated "BANS" (interscapular area of the Back, posterior upper Arm, posterior and lateral Neck, and Scalp). In addition, the prognosis is better for patients younger than 50 years of age and for women. Follow-up of patients treated for melanoma is important not only to monitor for metastatic disease but also because, in 3 to 5 percent of these patients, a second primary melanoma will eventually develop.

The prognosis for **oral melanoma** is extremely poor. Only 4 to 20 percent of affected patients survive for 5 years or more. Radical surgical removal is the treatment of choice; hemimaxillectomy is done for lesions that invade the overlying maxillary bone.

REFERENCES

Squamous Papilloma

Abbey LM, Page DG, Sawyer DR. The clinical and histopathologic features of a series of 464 oral squamous cell papillomas. Oral Surg Oral Med Oral Pathol 49:419–428, 1980.
Batsakis JG, Raymond AK, Rice DH. The pathology of head and neck tumors: Papillomas of the upper aerodigestive tract, part 18. Head Neck Surg 5:332–344, 1983.
Bouquot JE, Gundlach KKH. Oral exophytic lesions in 23,616 white Americans over 35 years of age. Oral Surg Oral Med Oral Pathol 62:284–291, 1986.
Miller CS, White DK, Royse DD. *In situ* hybridization analysis of human papillomavirus in orofacial lesions using a consensus biotinylated probe. Am J Dermatopathol 15:256–259, 1993.

Sinonasal Papillomas

Barnes L, Bedetti C. Oncocytic Schneiderian papilloma: A reappraisal of cylindrical cell papilloma of the sinonasal tract. Hum Pathol 15:344–351, 1984.
Bielamowicz S, Calcaterra TC, Watson D. Inverting papilloma of the head and neck: The UCLA update. Otolaryngol Head Neck Surg 109:71–76, 1993.
Buchwald C, et al. The presence of human papillomavirus in sinonasal papillomas, demonstrated by polymerase chain reaction with consensus primers. Hum Pathol 24:1354–1356, 1993.
Hyams VJ. Papillomas of the nasal cavity and paranasal sinuses: A clinicopathological study of 315 cases. Ann Otol Rhinol Laryngol 80:192–206, 1971.

Judd R, et al. Sinonasal papillomas and human papillomavirus: Human papillomavirus 11 detected in fungiform Schneiderian papillomas by *in situ* hybridization and the polymerase chain reaction. Hum Pathol 22:550–556, 1991.

Kusakari J, et al. Clinical report: Cylindrical cell papilloma of the paranasal sinus. Arch Otorhinolaryngol 244:246–248, 1987.

Lasser A, Rothfeld PR, Shapiro RS. Epithelial papilloma and squamous cell carcinoma of the nasal cavity and paranasal sinuses: A clinicopathological study. Cancer 38:2503–2510, 1976.

Lawson W, et al. Inverted papilloma: An analysis of 87 cases. Laryngoscope 99:1117–1124, 1989.

Verruca Vulgaris

Adler-Storthz K, et al. Identification of human papillomavirus types in oral verruca vulgaris. J Oral Pathol 15:230–233, 1986.

Eversole LR, Laipis PJ, Green TL. Human papillomavirus type 2 DNA in oral and labial verruca vulgaris. J Cutan Pathol 14:319–325, 1987.

Green TL, Eversole LR, Leider AS. Oral and labial verruca vulgaris: Clinical, histologic, and immunohistochemical evaluation. Oral Surg Oral Med Oral Pathol 62:410–416, 1986.

Premoli-de-Percoco G, et al. Detection of human papillomavirus-related oral verruca vulgaris among Venezuelans. J Oral Pathol Med 22:113–116, 1993.

Condyloma Acuminatum

Barone R, et al. Prevalence of oral lesions among HIV-infected intravenous drug abusers and other risk groups. Oral Surg Oral Med Oral Pathol 69:169–173, 1990.

Greenspan D, et al. Unusual HPV types in oral warts in association with HIV infection. J Oral Pathol 17:482–488, 1988.

Silverman S Jr, et al. Oral findings in people with or at high risk for AIDS: A study of 375 homosexual males. J Am Dent Assoc 112:187–192, 1986.

Zunt SL, Tomich CE. Oral condyloma acuminatum. J Dermatol Surg Oncol 15:591–594, 1989.

Focal Epithelial Hyperplasia

Archard HO, Heck JW, Stanley HR. Focal epithelial hyperplasia: An unusual mucosal lesion found in Indian children. Oral Surg Oral Med Oral Pathol 20:201–212, 1965.

Carlos R, Sedano HO. Multifocal papilloma virus epithelial hyperplasia. Oral Surg Oral Med Oral Pathol 77:631–635, 1994.

Harris AM, van Wyk CW. Heck's disease (focal epithelial hyperplasia): A longitudinal study. Community Dent Oral Epidemiol 21:82–85, 1993.

Padayachee A, van Wyk CW. Human papillomavirus (HPV) DNA in focal epithelial hyperplasia by *in situ* hybridization. J Oral Pathol Med 20:210–214, 1991.

Witkop CJ Jr, Niswander JD. Focal epithelial hyperplasia in Central and South American Indians and Ladinos. Oral Surg Oral Med Oral Pathol 20:213–217, 1965.

Molluscum Contagiosum

Laskaris G, Sklavounou A. Molluscum contagiosum of the oral mucosa. Oral Surg Oral Med Oral Pathol 58:688–691, 1984.

Whitaker SB, Wiegand SE, Budnick SD. Intraoral molluscum contagiosum. Oral Surg Oral Med Oral Pathol 72:334–336, 1991.

Verruciform Xanthoma

Allen CM, Kapoor N. Verruciform xanthoma in a bone marrow transplant recipient. Oral Surg Oral Med Oral Pathol 75:591–594, 1993.

Barr RJ, Plank CJ. Verruciform xanthoma of the skin. J Cutan Pathol 7:422–428, 1980.

Neville B. The verruciform xanthoma: A review and report of eight new cases. Am J Dermatopathol 8:247–253, 1986.

Nowparast B, Howell FV, Rick GM. Verruciform xanthoma: A clinicopathologic review and report of fifty-four cases. Oral Surg Oral Med Oral Pathol 51:619–625, 1981.

Seborrheic Keratosis

Ellis DL, Yates RA. Sign of Leser-Trélat. Clin Dermatol 11:141–148, 1993.

Fujisawa H, et al. Differentiation disorders of keratinocytes in seborrheic keratosis (acanthotic type). J Dermatol 18:635–638, 1991.

Ho VCY, McLean DI. Benign epithelial tumors. *In*: Dermatology in General Medicine, 4th ed. Edited by Fitzpatrick TB, et al. New York, McGraw-Hill, 1993, pp 855–858.

Wade TR, Ackerman AB. The many faces of seborrheic keratoses. J Dermatol Surg Oncol 5:378–382, 1979.

Wilborn WH, Dismukes DE, Montes LF. Seborrheic keratoses. J Cutan Pathol 5:373–375, 1978.

Keratoacanthoma

Eversole LR, Leider AS, Alexander G. Intraoral and labial keratoacanthoma. Oral Surg Oral Med Oral Pathol 54:663–667, 1982.

Fahmy A, et al. Muir-Torre syndrome: Report of a case and reevaluation of the dermatopathologic features. Cancer 49:1898–1903, 1982.

Goldschmidt H, Sherwin WK. Radiation therapy of giant aggressive keratoacanthomas. Arch Dermatol 129:1162–1165, 1993.

Jaber PW, Cooper PH, Greer KE. Generalized eruptive keratoacanthoma of Grzybowski. J Am Acad Dermatol 29:299–304, 1993.

Rook A, Whimster I. Keratoacanthoma—a thirty year retrospect. Br J Dermatol 100:41–47, 1979.

Schwartz RA. Keratoacanthoma. J Am Acad Dermatol 30:1–19, 1994.

Young SK, Larsen PE, Markowitz NR. Generalized eruptive keratoacanthoma. Oral Surg Oral Med Oral Pathol 62:422–426, 1986.

Sebaceous Hyperplasia

Daley TD. Intraoral sebaceous hyperplasia: Diagnostic criteria. Oral Surg Oral Med Oral Pathol 75:343–347, 1993.

De Villez RL, Roberts LC. Premature sebaceous gland hyperplasia. J Am Acad Dermatol 6:933–935, 1982.

Graham-Brown RAC, McGibbon DH, Sarkany I. A papular plaque-like eruption on the face due to naevoid sebaceous gland hyperplasia. Clin Exp Dermatol 8:379–382, 1983.

Rosian R, Goslen JB, Brodell RT. The treatment of benign sebaceous hyperplasia with the topical application of bichloracetic acid. J Dermatol Surg Oncol 17:876–879, 1991.

Actinic Lentigo

Beacham BE. Solar-induced epidermal tumors in the elderly. Am Fam Physician 42:153–160, 1990.

Griffiths CEM, et al. Topical tretinoin (retinoic acid) treatment of hyperpigmented lesions associated with photoaging in Chinese and Japanese patients: A vehicle-controlled trial. J Am Acad Dermatol 30:76–84, 1994.

Holzle E. Pigmented lesions as a sign of photodamage. Br J Dermatol 127:48–50, 1992.

Mehregan AH. Lentigo senilis and its evolutions. J Invest Dermatol 65:429–433, 1975.

Montagna W, Hu F, Carlisle K. A reinvestigation of solar lentigines. Arch Dermatol 116:1151–1154, 1980.

Rafal ES, et al. Topical tretinoin (retinoic acid) treatment for liver spots associated with photodamage. N Engl J Med 326:368–374, 1992.

Rhodes AR. Benign neoplasias, hyperplasias and dysplasias of melanocytes. *In*: Dermatology in General Medicine, 4th ed. Edited by Fitzpatrick TB, et al. New York, McGraw-Hill, 1993, pp 1056–1060.

Lentigo Simplex

Buchner A, et al. Melanocytic hyperplasia of the oral mucosa. Oral Surg Oral Med Oral Pathol 71:58–62, 1991.

Coleman WP, et al. Nevi, lentigines and melanomas in blacks. Arch Dermatol 116:548–551, 1980.

Gorlin RJ, Andersen RC, Blaw M. Multiple lentigines syndrome. Am J Dis Child 117:652–662, 1969.

Rhodes AR. Benign neoplasias, hyperplasias and dysplasias of melanocytes. *In*: Dermatology in General Medicine, 4th ed. Edited by Fitzpatrick TB, et al. New York, McGraw-Hill, 1993, pp 1048–1052.

Oral Melanotic Macule

Axéll T. A prevalence study of oral mucosal lesions in an adult Swedish population. Odontol Revy (Brazil) 27(36):1–103, 1976.

Bouquot JE. Common oral lesions found during a mass screening examination. J Am Dent Assoc 112:50–57, 1986.

Buchner A, Hansen LS. Melanotic macule of the oral mucosa: A clinicopathologic study of 105 cases. Oral Surg Oral Med Oral Pathol 48:244–249, 1979.

Kaugars GE, et al. Oral melanotic macules: A review of 353 cases. Oral Surg Oral Med Oral Pathol 76:59–61, 1993.

Page LR, et al. The oral melanotic macule. Oral Surg Oral Med Oral Pathol 44:219–226, 1977.

Sexton FM, Maize JC. Melanotic macules and melanoacanthomas of the lip; a comparative study with census of the basal melanocyte population. Am J Dermatopathol 9:438–444, 1987.

Spann CR, Owen LG, Hodge SJ. The labial melanotic macule. Arch Dermatol 123:1029–1031, 1987.

Watkins KV, et al. Benign focal melanotic lesions of the oral mucosa. J Oral Med 39:91–96, 118, 1984.

Weathers DR, et al. The labial melanotic macule. Oral Surg Oral Med Oral Pathol 42:196–205, 1976.

Oral Melanoacanthoma

Goode RK, et al. Oral melanoacanthoma: Review of the literature and report of ten cases. Oral Surg Oral Med Oral Pathol 56:622–628, 1983.

Tomich CE, Zunt SL. Melanoacanthosis (melanoacanthoma) of the oral mucosa. J Dermatol Surg Oncol 16:231–236, 1990.

Witt JC, et al. Rapidly expanding pigmented lesion of the buccal mucosa. J Am Dent Assoc 117:620–622, 1988.

Melanocytic Nevus

Brener MD, Harrison BD. Intraoral blue nevus: Report of a case. Oral Surg Oral Med Oral Pathol 28:326–330, 1969.

Buchner A, Hansen LS. Pigmented nevi of the oral mucosa: A clinicopathologic study of 36 new cases and review of 155 cases from the literature: Part I: A clinicopathologic study of 36 new cases. Oral Surg Oral Med Oral Pathol 63:566–572, 1987.

Buchner A, Hansen LS. Pigmented nevi of the oral mucosa: A clinicopathologic study of 36 new cases and review of 155 cases from the literature. Part II: Analysis of 191 cases. Oral Surg Oral Med Oral Pathol 63:676–682, 1987.

Buchner A, et al. Melanocytic nevi of oral mucosa: A clinicopathologic study of 130 cases from northern California. J Oral Pathol Med 19:197–201, 1990.

Casso EM, Grin-Jorgensen CM, Grant-Kels JM. Spitz nevi. J Am Acad Dermatol 27:901–913, 1992.

Castilla EE, da Graça Dutra M, Orioli-Parreiras IM. Epidemiology of congenital pigmented naevi: I. Incidence rates and relative frequencies. Br J Dermatol 104:307–315, 1981.

Cochran AJ, et al. Nevi, other than dysplastic and Spitz nevi. Semin Diagn Pathol 10:3–17, 1993.

Frank SB, Cohen HJ. The halo nevus. Arch Dermatol 89:367–373, 1964.

Rhodes AR. Benign neoplasms, hyperplasias and dysplasias of melanocytes. In: Dermatology in General Medicine, 4th ed. Edited by Fitzpatrick TB, et al. New York, McGraw-Hill, 1993, pp 996–1048.

Rhodes AR, et al. A histologic comparison of congenital and acquired nevomelanocytic nevi. Arch Dermatol 121:1266–1273, 1985.

Stenn KS, Arons M, Hurwitz S. Patterns of congenital nevocellular nevi: A histologic study of thirty-eight cases. J Am Acad Dermatol 9:388–393, 1983.

Temple-Camp CRE, Saxe N, King H. Benign and malignant cellular blue nevus: A clinicopathological study of 30 cases. Am J Dermatopathol 10:289–296, 1988.

Weedon D, Little JH. Spindle and epithelioid cell nevi in children and adults: A review of 211 cases of the Spitz nevus. Cancer 40:217–225, 1977.

Leukoplakia

Bánóczy J. Follow-up studies in oral leukoplakia. J Maxillofac Surg 5:69–75, 1977.

Baric JM, et al. Influence of cigarette, pipe, and cigar smoking, removable partial dentures, and age on oral leukoplakia. Oral Surg Oral Med Oral Pathol 54:424–429, 1982.

Bernstein ML. Oral mucosal white lesions associated with excessive use of Listerine mouthwash: Report of two cases. Oral Surg Oral Med Oral Pathol 46:781–785, 1978.

Bouquot JE. Epidemiology. In: Pathology of the Head and Neck. Edited by Gnepp DR. New York, Churchill Livingstone, 1988, pp 263–314.

Bouquot JE. Reviewing oral leukoplakia—clinical concepts for the 1990s. J Am Dent Assoc 122:80–82, 1991.

Bouquot JE, Gnepp DR. Laryngeal precancer—a review of the literature, commentary and comparison with oral leukoplakia. Head Neck 13:488–497, 1991.

Bouquot JE, Gorlin RJ. Leukoplakia, lichen planus and other oral keratoses in 23,616 white Americans over the age of 35 years. Oral Surg Oral Med Oral Pathol 61:373–381, 1986.

Bouquot JE, Weiland LH, Kurland LT. Leukoplakia and carcinoma in situ synchronously associated with invasive oral/oropharyngeal carcinoma in Rochester, Minnesota, 1935–1984. Oral Surg Oral Med Oral Pathol 65:199–207, 1988.

Bouquot JE, Whitaker SB. Oral leukoplakia—rationale for diagnosis and prognosis of its clinical subtypes or "phases." Quintessence Int 25:133–140, 1994.

Crissman JD, et al. Preinvasive lesions of the upper aerodigestive tract: Histologic definitions and clinical implications (a symposium). Pathol Annu 22:311–352, 1987.

Crissman JD, Zarbo RJ. Dysplasia, in situ carcinoma, and progression to invasive squamous cell carcinoma of the upper aerodigestive tract. Am J Surg Pathol 13(Suppl 1):5–16, 1989.

Field EA, Field JK, Martin MV. Does Candida have a role in oral epithelial neoplasia? J Med Vet Mycol 27:277–294, 1989.

Garewal HS, et al. Response of oral leukoplakia to beta-carotene. J Clin Oncol 8:1715–1720, 1990.

Gassenmaier A, Hornstein OP. Presence of papillomavirus DNA in benign and precancerous oral leukoplakias and squamous cell carcinomas. Dermatologica 176:224–233, 1988.

Gupta PC, et al. Incidence rates of oral cancer and natural history of oral precancerous lesions in a 10-year follow-up study of Indian villagers. Community Dent Oral Epidemiol 8:283–333, 1980.

Hansen LS, Olson JA, Silverman S. Proliferative verrucous leukoplakia: A long-term study of thirty patients. Oral Surg Oral Med Oral Pathol 60:285–298, 1985.

Kashima HK, et al. Human papillomavirus in squamous cell carcinoma, leukoplakia, lichen planus, and clinically normal epithelium of the oral cavity. Ann Otol Rhinol Laryngol 99:55–61, 1990.

Kaugars GE, Burns JC, Gunsolley JC. Epithelial dysplasia of the oral cavity and lips. Cancer 62:2166–2170, 1988.

Krogh P, et al. Yeast species and biotypes associated with oral leukoplakia and lichen planus. Oral Surg Oral Med Oral Pathol 63:48–54, 1987.

Mehta FS, et al. Incidence of oral leucoplakias among 20,358 Indian villagers in a 7-year period. Br J Cancer 333:549–554, 1976.

O'Grady JF, Reade PC. Candida albicans as a promoter of oral mucosal neoplasia. Carcinogenesis 13:783–786, 1992.

Pindborg JJ. Oral precancer. In: Surgical Pathology of the Head and Neck. Edited by Barnes L. New York, Marcel Dekker, 1985, pp 279–301.

Pindborg JJ, Daftary DK, Mehta FS. A follow-up study of sixty-one oral dysplastic precancerous lesions in Indian villagers. Oral Surg Oral Med Oral Pathol 43:383–390, 1977.

Roed-Petersen B. Effect on oral leukoplakia of reducing or ceasing tobacco smoking. Acta Derm Venereol (Stockh) 62:164–167, 1982.

Schwimmer E. Die idiopathischen Schleimhautplauques der Mundhohle (Leukoplakia buccalis). Arch Dermatol Syph 9:511–570, 1877.

Shafer WG. Oral carcinoma in situ. Oral Surg Oral Med Oral Pathol 39:227–238, 1975.

Shear M, Pindborg JJ. Verrucous hyperplasia of the oral mucosa. Cancer 46:1855–1862, 1980.

Silverman S Jr, Gorsky M, Lozada F. Oral leukoplakia and malignant transformation: A follow-up study of 257 patients. Cancer 53:563–568, 1984.

Waldron CA, Shafer WG. Leukoplakia revisited: A clinicopathologic study of 3256 oral leukoplakias. Cancer 36:1386–1392, 1975.

Erythroplakia

Amagasa T, et al. A study of the clinical characteristics and treatment of oral carcinoma *in situ*. Oral Surg Oral Med Oral Pathol 60:50–55, 1985.

Bouquot JE, Gnepp DR. Epidemiology of carcinoma *in situ* of the upper aerodigestive tract. Cancer 61:1685–1690, 1988.

Bouquot JE, Kurland LT, Weiland LH. Carcinoma *in situ* of the upper aerodigestive tract: Incidence, time trends, and follow-up in Rochester, Minnesota, 1935–1984. Cancer 61:1691–1698, 1988.

Crissman JD, Zarbo RJ. Dysplasia, in situ carcinoma, and progression to invasive squamous cell carcinoma of the upper aerodigestive tract. Am J Surg Pathol 13(Suppl 1):5–16, 1989.

Mashberg A, Samit AM. Early detection, diagnosis, and management of oral and oropharyngeal cancer. CA Cancer J Clin 39:67–88, 1989.

Mincer HH, Coleman SA, Hopkins KP. Observations on the clinical characteristics of oral lesions showing histologic epithelial dysplasia. Oral Surg Oral Med Oral Pathol 33:389–399, 1972.

Shafer WG, Waldron CA. Erythroplakia of the oral cavity. Cancer 36:1021–1028, 1975.

Tobacco Pouch Keratosis

Axéll T, Mörnstad H, Sundström B. The relation of the clinical picture to the histopathology of snuff dipper's lesions in a Swedish population. J Oral Pathol 5:229–236, 1976.

Bouquot JE, Glover ED, Schroeder KL. Leukoplakia and smokeless tobacco keratosis are two separate precancers. *In*: Oral Oncology. Vol 2. Edited by Varma AD. Delhi, MacMillan India, 1991, pp 67–69.

Greer RO, et al. Smokeless tobacco–associated oral changes in juvenile, adult and geriatric patients: Clinical and histomorphologic features. Gerodontics 2:87–98, 1986.

Greer RO Jr, Eversole LR, Crosby LK. Detection of human papillomavirus-genomic DNA in oral epithelial dysplasias, oral smokeless tobacco–associated leukoplakias, and epithelial malignancies. J Oral Maxillofac Surg 48:1201–1205, 1990.

Gregory RL, et al. Effect of smokeless tobacco use in humans on mucosal immune factors. Arch Oral Biol 36:25–31, 1991.

Hirsch J-M, Heyden G, Thilander H. A clinical, histomorphological and histochemical study on snuff-induced lesions of varying severity. J Oral Pathol 11:387–398, 1982.

Kaugars GE, et al. The prevalence of oral lesions in smokeless tobacco users and an evaluation of risk factors. Cancer 70:2579–2585, 1992.

Kaugars GE, Mehailescu WL, Gunsolley JC. Smokeless tobacco use and oral epithelial dysplasia. Cancer 64:1527–1530, 1989.

Koop CE. The Health Consequences of Using Smokeless Tobacco: A Report of the Advisory Committee to the Surgeon General. NIH publication no. 86-2874. Bethesda, Md, U.S. Department of Health and Human Services, 1986.

Schroeder KL. Oral and systemic concerns with smokeless tobacco. *In*: Clark's Clinical Dentistry. Edited by Hardin JF. Philadelphia, JB Lippincott, 1989.

Stotts RC, Schroeder KL, Burns DM. Smokeless Tobacco and Health. NIH publication no. 92-3461. Bethesda, Md, National Institutes of Health, 1992.

Oral Submucous Fibrosis

Canniff JP, Harvey W, Harris M. Oral submucous fibrosis: Its pathogenesis and management. Br Dent J 160:429–434, 1986.

Maher R, et al. Role of areca nut in the causation of oral submucous fibrosis: A case-control study in Pakistan. J Oral Pathol Med 23:65–69, 1994.

Morawetz G, et al. Oral submucous fibrosis. Int J Oral Maxillofac Surg 16:609–614, 1987.

Murti PR, et al. Smokeless tobacco use in India: Effects on oral mucosa. *In*: Smokeless Tobacco and Health. Edited by Stotts RC, Schroeder KL, Burns DM. NIH publication no. 92-3461. Bethesda, Md, National Institutes of Health, 1992.

Nicotine Stomatitis

Quigley LF Jr, et al. Reverse smoking and its oral consequences in Caribbean and South American peoples. J Am Dent Assoc 69:427–442, 1964.

Rossie KM, Guggenheimer J. Thermally induced "nicotine" stomatitis: A case report. Oral Surg Oral Med Oral Pathol 70:597–599, 1990.

Saunders WH. Nicotine stomatitis of the palate. Ann Otol Rhinol Laryngol 67:618–627, 1958.

Schwartz DL. Stomatitis nicotina of the palate: Report of two cases. Oral Surg Oral Med Oral Pathol 20:306–315, 1965.

Actinic Keratosis

Ackerman AB. What is the boundary that separates a thick solar keratosis and a thin squamous cell carcinoma? Am J Dermatopathol 6:306, 1984.

Brownstein MH, Rabinowitz AD. The precursors of cutaneous squamous cell carcinoma. Int J Dermatol 18:1–16, 1979.

Marks VJ. Actinic keratosis: A premalignant skin lesion. Otolaryngol Clin North Am 26:23–35, 1993.

Vitasa BC, et al. Association of nonmelanoma skin cancer and actinic keratosis with cumulative solar ultraviolet exposure in Maryland watermen. Cancer 65:2811–2817, 1990.

Wade TR, Ackerman AB. The many faces of solar keratoses. J Dermatol Surg Oncol 4:730–734, 1978.

Actinic Cheilosis

Cataldo E, Doku HC. Solar cheilitis. J Dermatol Surg Oncol 7:989–993, 1981.

Johnson TM, et al. Carbon dioxide laser treatment of actinic cheilitis: Clinicohistopathologic correlation to determine the optimal depth of destruction. J Am Acad Dermatol 27:737–740, 1992.

Picascia DD, Robinson JK. Actinic cheilitis: A review of the etiology, differential diagnosis, and treatment. J Am Acad Dermatol 17:255–264, 1987.

Schmitt CK, Folsom TC. Histologic evaluation of degenerative changes of the lower lip. J Oral Surg 26:51–56, 1968.

Squamous Cell Carcinoma

Ahlbom HE. Simple achlorhydric anaemia, Plummer-Vinson syndrome, and carcinoma of the mouth, pharynx, and oesophagus in women. Br Med J 2:331–333, 1936.

American Cancer Society. Cancer Facts & Figures—1993. Atlanta, Ga, American Cancer Society, 1993, pp 1–23.

Anneroth G, Hansen LS, Silverman S Jr. Malignancy grading in oral squamous cell carcinoma: 1. Squamous cell carcinoma of the tongue and floor of mouth: Histologic grading in the clinical evaluation. J Oral Pathol 15:162–168, 1986.

Baker SR, Krause CJ. Carcinoma of the lip. Laryngoscope 90:19–27, 1980.

Ballantyne AJ, McCarten AB, Ibanez ML. The extension of cancer of the head and neck through peripheral nerves. Am J Surg 106:651–667, 1963.

Beahrs OH, et al. Manual for Staging of Cancer, 4th ed. Philadelphia, JB Lippincott, 1992, pp 27–30.

Black RJ, Gluckman JL, Shumrick DA. Multiple primary tumours of the upper aerodigestive tract. Clin Otolaryngol 8:277–281, 1983.

Blot WJ, et al. Smoking and drinking in relation to oral and pharyngeal cancer. Cancer Res 48:3282–3287, 1988.

Bouquot JE. Epidermoid carcinoma of the palate and tonsil. *In*: Surgical Pathology of the Head and Neck. Edited by Barnes L. New York, Marcel Dekker, 1985, pp 353–356, 391–392.

Bouquot JE. Common oral lesions found during a mass screening examination. J Am Dent Assoc 112:50–57, 1986.

Bouquot JE. Epidemiology. *In*: Pathology of the Head and Neck. Edited by Gnepp DR. New York, Churchill Livingstone, 1988, pp 263–314.

Bouquot JE, Weiland LH, Kurland LT. Metastases to and from the upper aerodigestive tract in the population of Rochester, Minnesota, 1935–1984. Head Neck 11:212–218, 1989.

Brugere J, et al. Differential effects of tobacco and alcohol in cancer of the larynx, pharynx, and mouth. Cancer 57:391–395, 1986.

Carter RL, et al. Patterns and mechanisms of bone invasion by squamous carcinomas of the head and neck. Am J Surg 146:451–455, 1983.

Chang K-W, et al. High prevalence of human papillomavirus infection and possible association with betel quid chewing and smoking in oral epidermoid carcinomas in Taiwan. J Med Virol 28:57–61, 1989.

Chen JK, et al. Changing trends in oral cancer in the United States, 1935 to 1985: A Connecticut study. J Oral Maxillofac Surg 49: 1152–1158, 1991.

Choi SY, Kahyo H. Effect of cigarette smoking and alcohol consumption in the aetiology of cancer of the oral cavity, pharynx and larynx. Int J Epidemiol 20:878–885, 1991.

Cox MF, Scully C, Maitland N. Viruses in the aetiology of oral carcinoma? Examination of the evidence. Br J Oral Maxillofac Surg 29:381–387, 1991.

Day GL, Blot WJ. Second primary tumors in patients with oral cancer. Cancer 70:14–19, 1992.

deVries N, Gluckman JL. Multiple Primary Tumors of the Head and Neck. Berlin, Georg Thieme Verlag, 1990.

Dimitroulis G, Reade P, Wiesenfeld D. Referral patterns of patients with oral squamous cell carcinoma. Eur J Cancer B Oral Oncol 28B:23–27, 1992.

Douglas CW, Gammon MD. Reassessing the epidemiology of lip cancer. Oral Surg Oral Med Oral Pathol 57:631–642, 1984.

Field JK. Oncogenes and tumour-suppressor genes in squamous cell carcinoma of the head and neck. Eur J Cancer B Oral Oncol 28B:67–76, 1992.

Fry HJB. Syphilis and malignant disease: A serological study. Br J Hyg 29:313–322, 1929.

Hibbert J, et al. Prognostic factors in oral squamous carcinoma and their relation to clinical staging. Clin Otolaryngol 8:197–203, 1983.

Hoffmann D, Hecht SS. Nicotine-derived N-nitrosamines and tobacco-related cancer: Current status and future directions. Cancer Res 45:935–944, 1985.

Joynson DH, et al. Defect of cell-mediated immunity in patients with iron-deficiency anaemia. Lancet 2:1058–1059, 1972.

Karja J, et al. Oral cancer in children under 15 years of age: A clinicopathological and virological study. Acta Otolaryngol Suppl (Stockh) 449:145–149, 1988.

Kleinman DV, et al. Cancer of the Oral Cavity and Pharynx: A Statistics Review Monograph, 1973–1987. NIH Monograph. Bethesda, Md, National Institute of Dental Research, 1992.

Krogh P, Hald B, Holmstrup P. Possible mycological etiology of oral mucosal cancer: Catalytic potential of infecting Candida albicans and other yeasts in production of N-nitrosobenzylmethylamine. Carcinogenesis 8:1543–1548, 1987.

Larsson P-A, et al. Reactivity against herpes simplex virus in patients with head and neck cancer. Int J Cancer 49:14–18, 1991.

Levin ML, Kress LC, Goldstein H. Syphilis and cancer: Reported syphilis prevalence among 7,761 cancer patients. N Y State J Med 42:1737–1745, 1942.

Lindqvist C, Teppo L. Epidemiological evaluation of sunlight as a risk factor of lip cancer. Br J Cancer 37:983–989, 1978.

Maitland NJ, et al. Detection of human papillomavirus DNA in biopsies of human oral tissue. Br J Cancer 56:245–250, 1987.

Mashberg A, Samit AM. Early detection, diagnosis, and management of oral and oropharyngeal cancer. CA Cancer J Clin 39:67–88, 1989.

Mattson ME, Winn DM. Smokeless tobacco: Association with increased cancer risk. NCI Monogr No. 8, pp 13–16, 1989.

Notani PN, Jayant K. Role of diet in upper aerodigestive tract cancers. Nutr Cancer 10:103–113, 1987.

Owens W, et al. Multiple cytogenetic aberrations in squamous cell carcinomas of the head and neck. Eur J Cancer B Oral Oncol 28B:17–21, 1992.

Papac RJ. Distant metastases from head and neck cancer. Cancer 53:342–345, 1984.

Park N-H, et al. Synergism of herpes simplex virus and tobacco-specific N'-nitrosamines in cell transformation. J Oral Maxillofac Surg 49:276–281, 1991.

Quenelle DJ, Crissman JD, Shumrick DA. Tonsil carcinoma—treatment results. Laryngoscope 89:1842–1846, 1979.

Rollo J, et al. Squamous carcinoma of the base of the tongue: A clinicopathologic study of 81 cases. Cancer 47:333–342, 1981.

Rothman K, Keller A. The effect of joint exposure to alcohol and tobacco on risk of cancer of the mouth and pharynx. J Chronic Dis 25:711–716, 1972.

Sankaranarayanan R. Oral cancer in India: An epidemiologic and clinical review. Oral Surg Oral Med Oral Pathol 69:325–330, 1990.

Schantz SP, et al. Natural killer cell activity and head and neck cancer: A clinical assessment. J Natl Cancer Inst 77:869–875, 1986.

Schou G, Storm HH, Jensen OM. Second cancer following cancers of the buccal cavity and pharynx in Denmark, 1943–1980. Monogr Natl Cancer Inst 68:253–276, 1985.

Scully C. The immunology of cancer of the head and neck with particular reference to oral cancer. Oral Surg Oral Med Oral Pathol 53: 157–169, 1982.

Scully C. Viruses and oral squamous carcinoma. Eur J Cancer B Oral Oncol 28B:57–59, 1992.

Shafer WG. Initial mismanagement and delay in diagnosis of oral cancer. J Am Dent Assoc 90:1262–1264, 1964.

Shikhani AH, et al. Multiple primary malignancies in head and neck cancer. Arch Otolaryngol Head Neck Surg 112:1172–1179, 1986.

Silverman S Jr. Early diagnosis of oral cancer. Cancer 62:1796–1799, 1988.

Silverman S Jr, Griffith M. Smoking characteristics of patients with oral carcinoma and the risk for second oral primary carcinoma. J Am Dent Assoc 85:637–640, 1972.

Snow GB, et al. Prognostic factors of neck node metastasis. Clin Otolaryngol 7:185–192, 1982.

Sundström B, Mörnstad H, Axéll T. Oral carcinomas associated with snuff dipping: Some clinical and histological characteristics of 23 tumours in Swedish males. J Oral Pathol 11:245–251, 1982.

Syrjänen SM, Syrjänen KJ, Happonen R-P. Human papillomavirus (HPV) DNA sequences in oral precancerous lesions and squamous cell carcinoma demonstrated by in situ hybridization. J Oral Pathol 17:273–278, 1988.

Thumfart W, et al. Chronic mechanical trauma in the aetiology of oro-pharyngeal carcinoma. J Maxillofac Surg 6:217–221, 1978.

Trell E, et al. Carcinoma of the oral cavity in relation to aryl hydrocarbon hydroxylase inducibility, smoking and dental status. Int J Oral Surg 10:93–99, 1981.

Watts JM. The importance of the Plummer-Vinson syndrome in the aetiology of carcinoma of the upper gastro-intestinal tract. Postgrad Med J 37:523–533, 1961.

Watts SL, Brewer EE, Fry TL. Human papillomavirus DNA types in squamous cell carcinomas of the head and neck. Oral Surg Oral Med Oral Pathol 71:701–707, 1991.

Willen R, et al. Squamous cell carcinoma of the gingiva: Histological classification and grading of malignancy. Acta Otolaryngol 79:146–154, 1975.

Winn DM. Smokeless tobacco and cancer: The epidemiologic evidence. CA Cancer J Clin 38:236–243, 1988.

Winn DM, Blot WJ. Second cancer following cancers of the buccal cavity and pharynx in Connecticut, 1935–1982. Monogr Natl Cancer Inst 68:25–48, 1985.

Winn DM, et al. Diet in the etiology of oral and pharyngeal cancer among women from the southern United States. Cancer Res 44:1216–1222, 1984.

Wong DTW. Amplification of the c-erbB1 oncogene in chemically-induced oral carcinomas. Carcinogenesis 8:1963–1965, 1987.

Wynder EL, et al. Oral cancer and mouthwash use. J Natl Cancer Inst 70:255–260, 1983.

Yeudall WA. Human papillomaviruses and oral neoplasia. Eur J Cancer B Oral Oncol 28B:61–66, 1992.

Verrucous Carcinoma

Ackerman LV. Verrucous carcinoma of the oral cavity. Surgery 23:670–678, 1948.

Batsakis JG, et al. The pathology of head and neck tumors: Verrucous carcinoma, part 15. Head Neck Surg 5:29–38, 1982.

Guitart J, et al. Human papillomavirus-induced verrucous carcinoma of the mouth: Case report of an aggressive tumor. J Dermatol Surg Oncol 19:875–877, 1993.

Kamath VV, et al. Oral verrucous carcinoma: An analysis of 37 cases. J Craniomaxillofacial Surg 17:309–314, 1989.

McCoy JM, Waldron CA. Verrucous carcinoma of the oral cavity: A review of forty-nine cases. Oral Surg Oral Med Oral Pathol 52:623–629, 1981.

Medina JE, Dichtel W, Luna MA. Verrucous-squamous carcinomas of the oral cavity: A clinicopathologic study of 104 cases. Arch Otolaryngol 110:437–440, 1984.

Tornes K, et al. Oral verrucous carcinoma. Int J Oral Surg 14:485–492, 1985.

Spindle Cell Carcinoma

Batsakis JG, Rice DH, Howard DR. The pathology of head and neck tumors: Spindle cell lesions (sarcomatoid carcinomas, nodular fasciitis, and fibrosarcoma) of the aerodigestive tracts, part 14. Head Neck Surg 4:499–513, 1982.

Benninger MS, et al. Head and neck spindle cell carcinoma: An evaluation of current management. Cleve Clin J Med 59:479–482, 1992.

Ellis GL, Corio RL. Spindle cell carcinoma of the oral cavity: A clinicopathologic assessment of fifty-nine cases. Oral Surg Oral Med Oral Pathol 50:523–534, 1980.

Ellis GL, et al. Spindle-cell carcinoma of the aerodigestive tract: An immunohistochemical analysis of 21 cases. Am J Surg Pathol 11:335–342, 1987.

Adenosquamous Carcinoma

Banks ER, Cooper PH. Adenosquamous carcinoma of the skin: A report of 10 cases. J Cutan Pathol 18:227–234, 1991.

Gerughty RM, Hennigar GB, Brown FM. Adenosquamous carcinoma of the nasal, oral and laryngeal cavities: A clinicopathologic survey of ten cases. Cancer 22:1140–1155, 1968.

Martinez-Madrigal F, et al. Oral and pharyngeal adenosquamous carcinoma: A report of four cases with immunohistochemical studies. Eur Arch Otorhinolaryngol 248:255–258, 1991.

Carcinoma of the Maxillary Sinus

Batsakis JG, Rice DH, Solomon AR. The pathology of head and neck tumors: Squamous and mucous-gland carcinomas of the nasal cavity, paranasal sinuses, and larynx, part 6. Head Neck Surg 2:497–508, 1980.

Giri SP, et al. Management of advanced squamous cell carcinomas of the maxillary sinus. Cancer 69:657–661, 1992.

Gullane PJ, Conley J. Cancer of the maxillary sinus: A correlation of the clinical course with orbital involvement, pterygoid erosion or pterygopalatine invasion and cervical metastases. J Otolaryngol 12:141–145, 1983.

Kenady DE. Cancer of the paranasal sinuses. Surg Clin North Am 66:119–131, 1986.

Sakata K, et al. Analysis of the results of combined therapy for maxillary carcinoma. Cancer 71:2715–2722, 1993.

Nasopharyngeal Carcinoma

Dickson RI. Nasopharyngeal cancer: An evaluation of 209 patients. Laryngoscope 91:333–354, 1981.

Epstein JB, Jones CK. Presenting signs and symptoms of nasopharyngeal carcinoma. Oral Surg Oral Med Oral Pathol 75:32–36, 1993.

Hopkin N, et al. Cancer of the paranasal sinuses and nasal cavities: Part I: Clinical features. J Laryngol Otol 98:585–595, 1984.

McNicoll W, et al. Cancer of the paranasal sinuses and nasal cavities: Part II: Results of treatment. J Laryngol Otol 98:707–718, 1984.

Mills SE, Fechner RE. "Undifferentiated" neoplasms of the sinonasal region: Differential diagnosis based on clinical, light microscopic, immunohistochemical, and ultrastructural features. Semin Diagn Pathol 6:316–328, 1989.

Saemundsen AK, et al. Epstein-Barr virus in nasopharyngeal and salivary gland carcinomas of Greenland Eskimoes. Br J Cancer 46:721–728, 1982.

Zheng X, Christensson B, Drettner B. Studies on etiological factors of nasopharyngeal carcinoma. Acta Otolaryngol (Stockh) 113:455–457, 1993.

Basaloid Squamous Carcinoma

Banks ER, et al. Basaloid squamous cell carcinoma of the head and neck: A clinicopathologic and immunohistochemical study of 40 cases. Am J Surg Pathol 16:939–946, 1992.

Batsakis JG, el Naggar A. Basaloid-squamous carcinomas of the upper aerodigestive tract. Ann Otol Rhinol Laryngol 98:919–920, 1989.

Luna MA, et al. Basaloid squamous carcinoma of the upper aerodigestive tract: Clinicopathologic and DNA flow cytometric analysis. Cancer 66:537–542, 1990.

Basal Cell Carcinoma

Cannon CR, Hayne S. Basosquamous carcinoma of the head and neck. Ear Nose Throat J 69:822–824, 1990.

Gutierrez MM, Mora RG. Nevoid basal cell carcinoma syndrome: A review and case report of a patient with unilateral basal cell nevus syndrome. J Am Acad Dermatol 15:1023–1030, 1986.

Miller SJ. Biology of basal cell carcinoma, part 1. J Am Acad Dermatol 24:1–13, 1991.

Miller SJ. Biology of basal cell carcinoma, part 2. 24:161–175, 1991.

Nguyen AV, Whitaker DC, Frodel J. Differentiation of basal cell carcinoma. Otolaryngol Clin North Am 26:37–56, 1993.

Preston DS, Stern RS. Nonmelanoma cancers of the skin. N Engl J Med 327:1649–1662, 1992.

Roenigk RK, et al. Trends in the presentation and treatment of basal cell carcinomas. J Dermatol Surg Oncol 12:860–865, 1986.

v. Domarus H, Stevens PJ. Metastatic basal cell carcinoma: Report of five cases and review of 170 cases in the literature. J Am Acad Dermatol 10:1043–1060, 1984.

Merkel Cell Carcinoma

Marenda SA, Otto RA. Adnexal carcinomas of the skin. Otolaryngol Clin North Am 26:87–116, 1993.

Ratner D, et al. Merkel cell carcinoma. J Am Acad Dermatol 29:143–156, 1993.

Rice RD Jr, et al. Merkel cell tumor of the head and neck: Five new cases with literature review. Arch Otolaryngol Head Neck Surg 119:782–786, 1993.

Sidhu GS, et al. Merkel cell neoplasms: Histology, electron microscopy, biology, and histogenesis. Am J Dermatopathol 2:101–119, 1980.

Wick MR, et al. Primary neuroendocrine carcinomas of the skin (Merkel cell tumors): A clinical, histologic, and ultrastructural study of thirteen cases. Am J Clin Pathol 79:6–13, 1983.

Melanoma

Barnhill RL, Mihm MC Jr. The histopathology of cutaneous malignant melanoma. Semin Diagn Pathol 10:47–75, 1993.

Berthelsen A, et al. Melanomas of the mucosa in the oral cavity and the upper respiratory passages. Cancer 54:907–912, 1984.

Langford FP, et al. Lentigo maligna melanoma of the head and neck. Laryngoscope 103:520–524, 1993.

Medina JE. Malignant melanoma of the head and neck. Otolaryngol Clin North Am 26:73–85, 1993.

Rapini RP, et al. Primary malignant melanoma of the oral cavity: A review of 177 cases. Cancer 55:1543–1551, 1985.

Ringborg U, et al. Cutaneous malignant melanoma of the head and neck: Analysis of treatment results and prognostic factors in 581 patients: A report from the Swedish Melanoma Study Group. Cancer 71:751–758, 1993.

Smyth AG, et al. Malignant melanoma of the oral cavity—an increasing clinical diagnosis? Br J Oral Maxillofac Surg 31:230–235, 1993.

Stern SJ, Guillamondegui OM. Mucosal melanoma of the head and neck. Head Neck 13:22–27, 1991.

Umeda M, Shimada K. Primary malignant melanoma of the oral cavity—its histological classification and treatment. Br J Oral Maxillofac Surg 32:39–47, 1994.

11

Salivary Gland Pathology

MUCOCELE (Mucus Extravasation Phenomenon; Mucus Escape Reaction)

The **mucocele** is a common lesion of the oral mucosa that results from rupture of a salivary gland duct and spillage of mucin into the surrounding soft tissues. This spillage is often the result of local trauma, although there is no known history of trauma in many cases. Unlike the salivary duct cyst (see p. 325), the mucocele is not a true cyst because it lacks an epithelial lining. Some authors, however, have included true salivary duct cysts in their reported series of "mucoceles." Because these two entities exhibit distinctly different clinical and histopathologic features, they are discussed as separate topics in this chapter.

Clinical Features

Mucoceles typically present as dome-shaped mucosal swellings that can range from 1 or 2 mm to several centimeters in size (Figs. 11–1 to 11–3; see Color Figure 73). They are most common in children and young adults, perhaps because younger people are more likely to experience trauma that induces mucin spillage. However, mucoceles have been reported in patients of all ages, including newborn infants and older people. The spilled mucin below the mucosal surface often imparts a bluish translucent hue to the swelling, although deeper mucoceles may be normal in color. The lesion characteristically is fluctuant, but some mucoceles feel firmer to palpation. The reported duration of the lesion can vary from a few days to several years; most patients report that the lesion has been present for several weeks. Many patients relate a history of a recurrent swelling that may periodically rupture and release its fluid contents.

The lower lip is the most common site for the mucocele, accounting for at least 75 percent of all cases. Mucoceles are usually found lateral to the midline. Less common sites include the buccal mucosa, anterior ventral tongue, and floor of mouth (ranula). Mucoceles rarely develop on the upper lip. This is in contradistinction to salivary gland tumors, which are not unusual in the upper lip but are distinctly uncommon in the lower lip.

The palate and retromolar area are also uncommon sites for mucoceles. However, one interesting variant, the **superficial mucocele**, does develop in these areas and along the posterior buccal mucosa. Superficial mucoceles present as single or multiple tense vesicles that measure 1 to 4 mm in diameter (Fig. 11–4). The lesions often burst, leaving shallow, painful ulcers that heal within a few days. Repeated episodes at the same location are not unusual. Some patients relate the development of the lesions to mealtimes. The vesicular appearance is created by the superficial nature of the mucin spillage, which causes a separation of the epithelium from the connective tissue. The pathologist must be aware of this lesion and should avoid mistaking it microscopically for a vesiculobullous disorder, especially cicatricial (mucous membrane) pemphigoid.

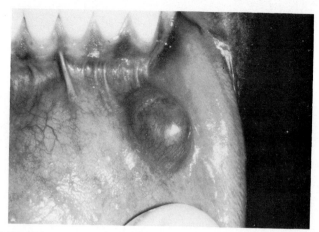

FIGURE 11–1. **Mucocele.** Blue-pigmented nodule on the lower lip. See Color Plates.

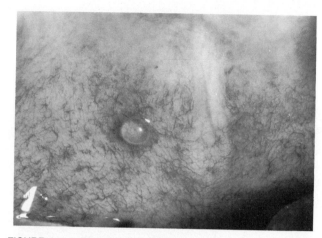

FIGURE 11–4. **Superficial mucocele.** Vesicle-like lesion on the soft palate.

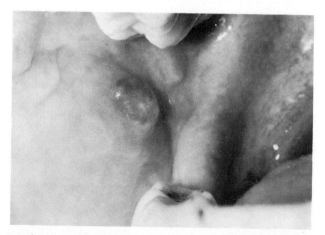

FIGURE 11–2. **Mucocele.** Nodule on the posterior buccal mucosa.

Histopathologic Features

On microscopic examination, the mucocele shows an area of spilled mucin surrounded by a granulation tissue response (Figs. 11–5 and Fig. 11–6). The inflammation includes numerous neutrophils and foamy histiocytes. In some cases, a ruptured salivary duct may be identified feeding into the area. The adjacent minor salivary glands often contain a chronic inflammatory cell infiltrate and dilated ducts.

Treatment and Prognosis

Some mucoceles are short-lived lesions that rupture and heal by themselves. Many lesions, however, are chronic in nature, and local surgical excision is necessary. To minimize the risk of recurrence, when the area is excised, the surgeon should remove any adjacent minor salivary glands that may be feeding into the lesion. The excised tissue should be submitted for microscopic examination to confirm the diagnosis and rule out the possibility of a salivary gland tumor. The prognosis is excellent, although occasional mucoceles will recur, necessitating re-excision, especially if the feeding glands are not removed.

RANULA

Ranula is a term used for mucoceles that occur in the floor of the mouth. The name is derived from the Latin word *rana*, which means frog, because the swelling may resemble the appearance of a frog's translucent underbelly. The term ranula has also been used to describe other similar swellings in the floor of the mouth, including true salivary duct cysts, dermoid cysts, and cystic hygromas. However, the term is best used for mucus escape reactions (mucoceles). Although the source of mucin spillage is usually the sublingual gland, ranulas may arise from the submandibular duct or, possibly, from minor salivary glands in the floor of the mouth.

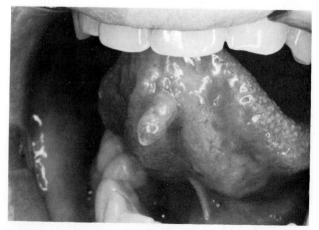

FIGURE 11–3. **Mucocele.** Exophytic lesion on the anterior ventral tongue.

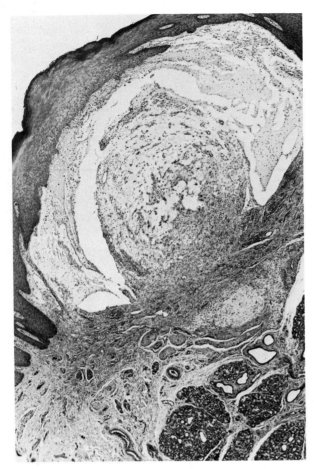

FIGURE 11–5. **Mucocele.** Mucin-filled cyst-like cavity below the mucosal surface.

Clinical Features

The ranula presents as a blue, dome-shaped, fluctuant swelling in the floor of the mouth (Fig. 11–7; see Color Figure 74). Deeper lesions may be normal in color. Ranulas tend to be larger than mucoceles in other oral locations; they can develop into large masses, measuring many centimeters in diameter that fill the floor of mouth

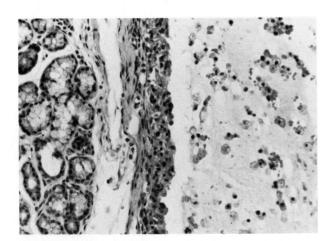

FIGURE 11–6. **Mucocele.** Spilled mucin (*right*) surrounded by granulation tissue containing foamy histiocytes and neutrophils. Salivary acini are visible at left.

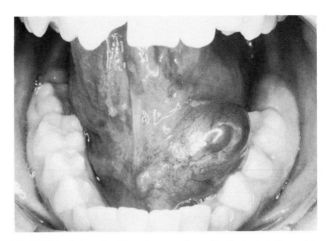

FIGURE 11–7. **Ranula.** Blue-pigmented swelling in the left floor of the mouth. See Color Plates. (Courtesy of Dr. George Blozis.)

and elevate the tongue. The ranula is usually located lateral to the midline, a feature that may help to distinguish it from a midline dermoid cyst (see p. 30). Like other mucoceles, ranulas may rupture and may release their mucin contents, only to re-form.

An unusual clinical variant, the **plunging** or **cervical ranula**, occurs when the spilled mucin dissects through the mylohyoid muscle and produces swelling within the neck (Fig. 11–8). A concomitant swelling in the floor of mouth may or may not be present. If no lesion is produced in the mouth, the clinical diagnosis of ranula may not be suspected.

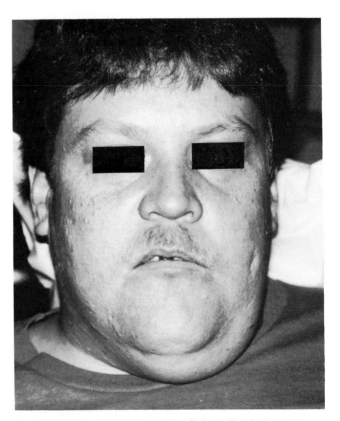

FIGURE 11–8. **Plunging ranula.** Soft swelling in the neck.

Histopathologic Features

The microscopic appearance of a ranula is similar to that of a mucocele in other locations. The spilled mucin elicits a granulation tissue response that contains foamy histiocytes and neutrophils.

Treatment and Prognosis

Treatment of the ranula consists of marsupialization and/or removal of the feeding sublingual gland. Marsupialization (exteriorization) entails removal of the roof of the intraoral lesion, potentially allowing the sublingual gland ducts to re-establish communication with the oral cavity. However, this procedure is often unsuccessful, and some authors emphasize that removal of the offending gland is the most important consideration in preventing a recurrence of the ranula. If the gland is removed, meticulous dissection of the lining of the lesion may not be necessary for the lesion to resolve, even for the plunging ranula.

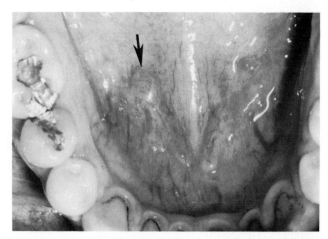

FIGURE 11–9. **Salivary duct cyst.** Nodular swelling (*arrow*) overlying Wharton's duct. See Color Plates.

SALIVARY DUCT CYST (Mucus Retention Cyst; Mucus Duct Cyst; Sialocyst)

The **salivary duct cyst** is an epithelium-lined cavity that arises from salivary gland tissue. Unlike the more common mucocele (see p. 322), it is a true cyst because it is lined by epithelium. The cause of such cysts is uncertain. Some cases may represent ductal dilatation secondary to ductal obstruction (such as a mucus plug), which creates increased intraluminal pressure. Other cases may represent true cysts that are separate from the adjacent salivary ducts.

Clinical Features

Salivary duct cysts usually occur in adults and can arise within either the major or minor glands. Cysts of the major glands are most common within the parotid gland, presenting as slowly growing, asymptomatic swellings. Intraoral cysts can occur at any minor gland site, but most frequently they develop in the floor of mouth, buccal mucosa, and lips (Fig. 11–9; see Color Figure 75). They often look like mucoceles and are characterized by a soft, fluctuant swelling that may appear bluish, depending on the depth of the cyst below the surface. Some cysts may feel relatively firm to palpation. Cysts in the floor of the mouth often arise adjacent to the submandibular duct and sometimes have an amber color.

Histopathologic Features

The lining of the salivary duct cyst is variable and may consist of cuboidal, columnar, or atrophic squamous epithelium surrounding thin or mucoid secretions in the lumen (Figs. 11–10 and 11–11). In some cases (especially those due to ductal obstruction), the epithelium may undergo oncocytic metaplasia, often demonstrating papillary folds into the cystic lumen, somewhat reminis-

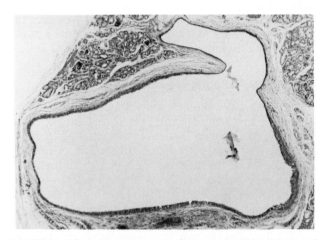

FIGURE 11–10. **Salivary duct cyst.** Cystic cavity with adjacent salivary acini.

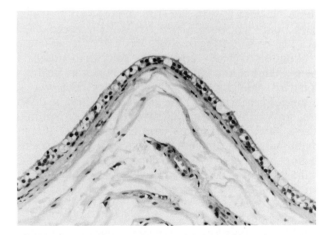

FIGURE 11–11. **Salivary duct cyst.** High-power view of cystic lining demonstrating cuboidal to columnar epithelium with scattered mucin-producing cells.

cent of a small Warthin's tumor (see p. 344) but without the prominent lymphoid stroma. If this proliferation is extensive enough, these lesions are sometimes diagnosed as **papillary cystadenoma**, although it seems likely that most are not true neoplasms.

Treatment and Prognosis

Salivary duct cysts are treated by conservative surgical excision. For cysts in the major glands, partial or total removal of the gland may be necessary. The lesion should not recur.

SIALOLITHIASIS (Salivary Calculi; Salivary Stones)

Sialoliths are calcified structures that develop within the salivary ductal system. They are believed to arise from deposition of calcium salts around a nidus of debris within the duct lumen. This debris may include inspissated mucus, bacteria, ductal epithelial cells, or foreign bodies. The cause of sialoliths is unknown; their development is not related to any systemic derangement in calcium-phosphorus metabolism.

Clinical and Radiographic Features

Sialoliths most often develop within the ductal system of the submandibular gland; the formation of stones within the parotid gland system is distinctly less frequent. The long, tortuous path of the submandibular (Wharton's) duct and the thicker, mucoid secretions of this gland may be responsible for its greater tendency to form salivary calculi. Sialoliths can also form within the minor salivary glands, most often within the glands of the upper lip or buccal mucosa. Salivary stones can occur at almost any age, but they are most common in young and middle-aged adults.

Major gland sialoliths most frequently present with episodic pain or swelling of the affected gland, especially at mealtime. The severity of the symptoms varies, depending on the degree of obstruction and the amount of resultant back pressure produced within the gland. If the stone is located toward the terminal portion of the duct, a hard mass may be palpated beneath the mucosa (Fig. 11–12; see Color Figure 76).

Sialoliths typically appear as radiopaque masses on x-ray examination, although not all stones are visible on standard radiographs, which is perhaps related to the degree of calcification of the lesion. They may be discovered anywhere along the length of the duct or within the gland itself. Stones in the terminal portion of the submandibular duct are best demonstrated with an occlusal radiograph (Fig. 11–13). On panoramic or periapical radiographs, the calcification may appear superimposed on the mandible and care must be exercised not to confuse it with an intrabony lesion (Fig. 11–14). Multiple parotid stones can radiographically mimic calcified parotid lymph nodes, such as might occur in tuberculosis.

Minor gland sialoliths are often asymptomatic but may produce local swelling or tenderness of the affected

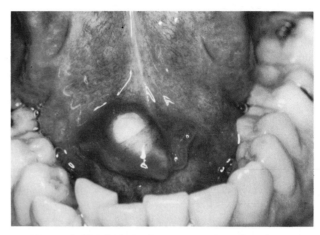

FIGURE 11–12. **Sialolithiasis.** Hard mass at the orifice of Wharton's duct. See Color Plates.

gland (Fig. 11–15). A small radiopacity can often be demonstrated with a soft tissue radiograph (Fig. 11–16).

Histopathologic Features

On gross examination, sialoliths appear as hard masses that are round, oval, or cylindrical. They are typically yellow, although they may be white or yellowish-brown. Submandibular stones tend to be larger than those of the parotid or minor glands. Sialoliths are usually solitary, although occasionally two or more stones may be discovered at surgery.

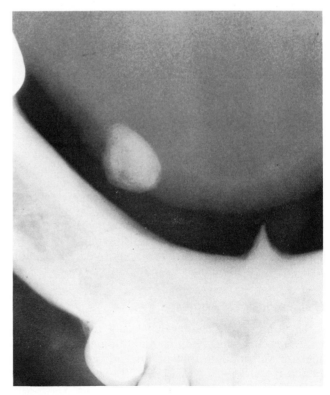

FIGURE 11–13. **Sialolithiasis.** Occlusal radiograph demonstrating radiopaque stone in Wharton's duct.

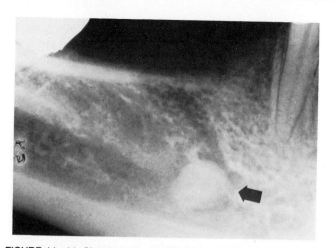

FIGURE 11–14. **Sialolithiasis.** Periapical film of the same sialolith as depicted in Figure 11–13. A radiopacity (*arrow*) is superimposed on the mandible. Care must be taken not to confuse such lesions with intrabony pathosis.

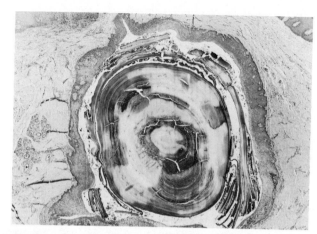

FIGURE 11–17. **Sialolithiasis.** Intraductal calcified mass showing concentric laminations. The duct exhibits squamous metaplasia.

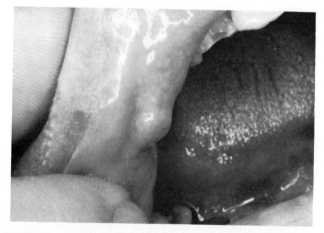

FIGURE 11–15. **Sialolithiasis.** Minor salivary gland sialolith presenting as a hard nodule in the upper lip.

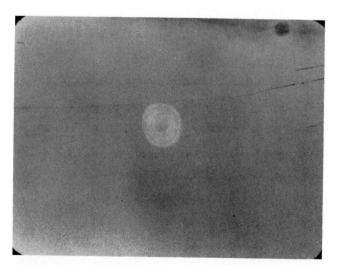

FIGURE 11–16. **Sialolithiasis.** Soft tissue radiograph of the same lesion depicted in Figure 11–15. A laminated calcified mass is revealed.

Microscopically, the calcified mass exhibits concentric laminations that may surround a nidus of amorphous debris (Fig. 11–17). If the associated duct is also removed, it often demonstrates squamous, oncocytic, or mucous cell metaplasia. Periductal inflammation is also evident. The ductal obstruction often leads to an acute or chronic sialadenitis of the feeding gland.

Treatment and Prognosis

Small sialoliths of the major glands can sometimes be treated conservatively by gentle massage of the gland in an effort to milk the stone toward the duct orifice. Sialagogues (drugs that stimulate salivary flow), moist heat, and increased fluid intake may also promote passage of the stone. Larger sialoliths usually need to be removed surgically. If significant inflammatory damage has occurred within the feeding gland, the gland may need to be removed. Minor gland sialoliths are best treated by surgical removal, including the associated gland.

SIALADENITIS

Inflammation of the salivary glands (**sialadenitis**) can arise from various infectious and noninfectious causes (see elsewhere in this text). The most common viral infection is **mumps** (see p. 196), although a number of other viruses can also involve the salivary glands, including Coxsackie A, ECHO, choriomeningitis, parainfluenza, and cytomegalovirus (in neonates). Most bacterial infections arise as a result of ductal obstruction or decreased salivary flow, allowing retrograde spread of bacteria throughout the ductal system. Blockage of the duct can be caused by sialolithiasis (see previous topic), congenital strictures, or compression by an adjacent tumor. Decreased flow can result from dehydration, debilitation, or medications that inhibit secretions.

One of the more common causes of sialadenitis is recent surgery (especially abdominal surgery), after which an acute parotitis ("surgical mumps") may arise because the patient has been kept without food or fluids

(NPO) and has received atropine during the surgical procedure. Other medications that produce xerostomia as a side effect can also predispose patients to such an infection. Most cases of acute bacterial sialadenitis are due to *Staphylococcus aureus* but they also may arise from streptococci or pneumococci. Noninfectious causes of salivary inflammation include Sjögren's syndrome (see p. 332), sarcoidosis (see p. 241), radiation therapy (see p. 219), and various allergens.

Clinical and Radiographic Features

Acute bacterial sialadenitis is most common in the parotid gland and is bilateral in 20 to 25 percent of cases. The affected gland is swollen and painful, and the overlying skin may be erythematous (Fig. 11–18). An associated low-grade fever as well as trismus may be present. A purulent discharge is often observed from the duct orifice when the gland is massaged.

Recurrent or persistent ductal obstruction, most commonly due to sialoliths, can lead to a chronic sialadenitis. Periodic swelling and pain occur within the affected gland, usually developing at mealtime when salivary flow is stimulated. Sialography often demonstrates sialectasia (ductal dilatation), proximal to the area of obstruction (Fig. 11–19). Chronic sialadenitis can also occur in the minor glands, possibly as a result of blockage of ductal flow or local trauma.

A new form of salivary inflammation, **subacute necrotizing sialadenitis**, has been described in young males. The lesion involves the minor salivary glands of the palatal area. It presents as a painful nodule, typically 1 cm or less in size, that is covered by intact, erythematous mucosa. Unlike necrotizing sialometaplasia (see p. 335), the lesion does not ulcerate or slough necrotic tissue. An infectious cause has been hypothesized.

Histopathologic Features

In patients with acute sialadenitis, accumulation of neutrophils is observed within the ductal system and acini. Chronic sialadenitis is characterized by scattered or

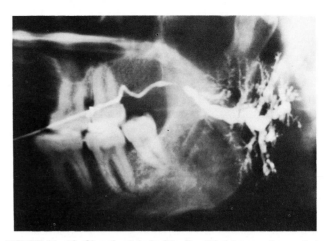

FIGURE 11–19. **Chronic sialadenitis.** Parotid sialogram demonstrating ductal dilatation proximal to an area of obstruction. (Courtesy of Dr. George Blozis.)

patchy infiltration of the salivary parenchyma by lymphocytes and plasma cells. Atrophy of the acini is common, as is ductal dilatation (Fig. 11–20). If associated fibrosis is present, the term **chronic sclerosing sialadenitis** is used.

Subacute necrotizing sialadenitis is characterized by a heavy mixed inflammatory infiltrate consisting mainly of histiocytes and neutrophils. There is loss of most of the acinar cells, and many of the remaining ones exhibit necrosis. The ducts tend to be atrophic and do not show hyperplasia or squamous metaplasia.

Treatment and Prognosis

The treatment of acute sialadenitis includes appropriate antibiotic therapy and rehydration of the patient to stimulate salivary flow. Although this regimen is usually sufficient, surgical drainage may be needed if there is abscess formation.

The management of chronic sialadenitis depends on the severity and duration of the condition. Early cases

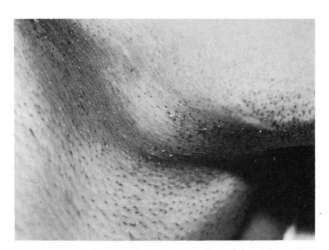

FIGURE 11–18. **Sialadenitis.** Tender swelling of the submandibular gland.

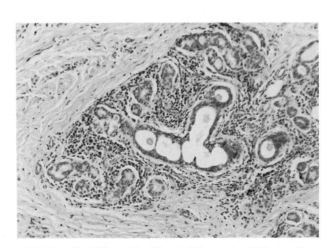

FIGURE 11–20. **Sialadenitis.** Chronic inflammatory infiltrate with associated acinar atrophy and ductal dilatation.

that develop secondary to ductal blockage may respond to removal of the sialolith or other obstruction. If sialectasia is present, the dilated ducts can lead to stasis of secretions and predispose the gland to further sialolith formation. If sufficient inflammatory destruction of the salivary tissue has occurred, surgical removal of the affected gland may be necessary.

Subacute necrotizing sialadenitis is a self-limiting condition that usually resolves within 2 weeks of diagnosis without treatment.

CHEILITIS GLANDULARIS

Cheilitis glandularis is a rare inflammatory condition of the minor salivary glands. The cause is uncertain, although several etiologic factors have been suggested, including actinic damage, tobacco, syphilis, poor hygiene, and heredity.

Clinical Features

Cheilitis glandularis characteristically occurs on the lower lip, although there are also purported cases involving the upper lip and palate. Affected individuals present with swelling and eversion of the lower lip as a result of hypertrophy and inflammation of the glands (Fig. 11–21). The openings of the minor salivary ducts are inflamed and dilated, and pressure on the glands may produce mucopurulent secretions from the ductal openings. The condition has most often been reported in middle-aged and older men, although cases have also been described in women and children. However, some of the childhood cases may represent other entities, such as exfoliative cheilitis (see p. 222).

Historically, cheilitis glandularis has been classified into three types, based on the severity of the disease:

1. Simple.
2. Superficial suppurative (Baelz's disease).
3. Deep suppurative (cheilitis glandularis apostematosa).

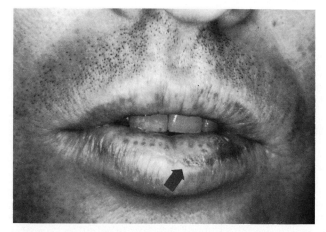

FIGURE 11–21. **Cheilitis glandularis.** Prominent lower lip with inflamed openings of the minor salivary gland ducts. An early squamous cell carcinoma has developed on the patient's left side just lateral to the midline (*arrow*). (Courtesy of Dr. George Blozis.)

The latter two types represent progressive stages of the disease with bacterial involvement and are characterized by increasing inflammation, suppuration, ulceration, and swelling of the lip.

Histopathologic Features

The microscopic findings of cheilitis glandularis are not specific and usually consist of chronic sialadenitis and ductal dilatation. Concomitant dysplastic changes may be observed in the overlying surface epithelium in some cases.

Treatment and Prognosis

The treatment of choice in most cases of cheilitis glandularis consists of a vermilionectomy (lip shave), which usually produces a satisfactory cosmetic result. A significant percentage of cases (18 to 35 percent) have been associated with the development of squamous cell carcinoma of the overlying epithelium of the lip. Because actinic damage has been implicated in many cases of cheilitis glandularis, this same solar radiation is also probably responsible for the malignant degeneration.

SIALORRHEA

Sialorrhea, or excessive salivation, is an uncommon condition that has various causes. Minor sialorrhea may result from local irritations, such as aphthous ulcers or ill-fitting dentures. Patients with new dentures often experience excess saliva production until they become accustomed to the prosthesis. Sialorrhea is a well-known clinical feature of rabies and heavy metal poisoning (see p. 227). It may also occur as a consequence of certain medications, such as lithium and cholinergic agonists.

Drooling can be a problem for patients who are mentally retarded, who have a neurologic disorder such as cerebral palsy, or who have undergone surgical resection of the mandible. In these instances, the drooling is probably not due to overproduction of saliva but to poor neuromuscular control.

Clinical Features

The excess saliva production typically produces drooling and choking, which may cause social embarrassment. In children with mental retardation or cerebral palsy, the uncontrolled salivary flow may lead to macerated sores around the mouth, chin, and neck that can become secondarily infected. The constant soiling of clothes and bed linens can be a significant problem for the parents and caretakers of these patients.

An interesting type of supersalivation of unknown cause has been described called **idiopathic paroxysmal sialorrhea**. Individuals with this condition experience short episodes of excessive salivation lasting from 2 to 5 minutes. These episodes are associated with a prodrome of nausea or epigastric pain.

Treatment and Prognosis

Some causes of sialorrhea are transitory or mild, and no treatment is needed. For persistent severe drooling, however, therapeutic intervention may be indicated. Anticholinergic medications can decrease saliva production but may produce unacceptable side effects. Transdermal scopolamine has been tried with some success, but it should not be used in children younger than age 10. Speech therapy can be used to improve neuromuscular control, but patient cooperation is necessary.

Several surgical techniques have been successfully used to control severe drooling in individuals with poor neuromuscular control:

- Submandibular gland excision plus parotid duct ligation
- Relocation of the parotid ducts
- Relocation of the submandibular ducts
- Bilateral tympanic neurectomy with sectioning of the chorda tympani

In ductal relocation, the ducts are repositioned posteriorly to the tonsillar fossa, thereby redirecting salivary flow and minimizing drooling. The use of bilateral tympanic neurectomy and sectioning of the chorda tympani destroys parasympathetic innervation to the glands, reducing salivary secretions and possibly inducing xerostomia. However, this procedure also produces a loss of taste to the anterior two thirds of the tongue.

XEROSTOMIA

Xerostomia refers to a subjective sensation of a dry mouth. A number of factors may play a role in its pathogenesis, including salivary gland aplasia, aging, smoking, mouth breathing, local radiation therapy (see p. 219), Sjögren's syndrome (see p. 332), and human immunodeficiency virus (HIV) infection (see p. 206). A wide variety of medications may produce xerostomia as a side effect (Table 11–1).

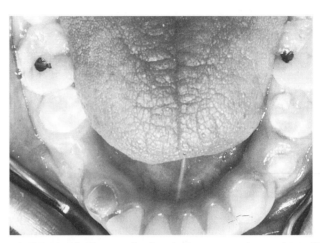

FIGURE 11–22. **Xerostomia.** Dry, leathery tongue in a patient with aplasia of the salivary glands.

Clinical Features

Xerostomia affects women more frequently than men, and it is also more common in older people. This dryness may be due to decreasing glandular secretions as a function of age, but this is often difficult to prove because so many older patients take medications that may induce xerostomia.

Examination of the patient typically demonstrates a reduction in salivary secretions, and the residual saliva appears either foamy or thick and "ropey." The mucosa appears dry, and the dorsal tongue is often fissured with atrophy of the filiform papillae (Fig. 11–22). The patient may complain of difficulty with mastication and swallowing and may even indicate that food adheres to the oral membranes during eating. The clinical findings, however, do not always correspond to the patient's symptoms. Some patients who complain of dry mouth may appear to have adequate salivary flow and oral moistness. Conversely, some patients who clinically appear to have a dry mouth have no complaints. The lack of saliva production can be confirmed by measuring both resting and stimulated salivary flow.

There is an increased prevalence of oral candidiasis in patients with xerostomia because of the reduction in the cleansing and antimicrobial activity normally provided by saliva. In addition, these patients are more prone to dental decay, especially cervical and root caries. This problem has more often been associated with radiation therapy, and it is sometimes called "radiation-induced caries" but should more appropriately be called "xerostomia-related caries" (see p. 220).

Treatment and Prognosis

The treatment of xerostomia is difficult and often unsatisfactory. Artificial salivas are available and may help make the patient more comfortable, as may continuous sips of water throughout the day. In addition, sugarless candy can be used in an effort to stimulate salivary flow. Pilocarpine has shown great promise as a sialagogue. If the dryness is secondary to the patient's medication, dis-

Table 11–1. MEDICATIONS THAT MAY PRODUCE XEROSTOMIA	
Class of Drug	**Example**
Antihistamines	Diphenhydramine Chlorpheniramine
Decongestants	Pseudoephedrine
Antidepressants	Amitriptyline
Antipsychotics	Phenothiazine derivatives Haloperidol
Antihypertensives	Reserpine Methyldopa Chlorothiazide Furosemide
Anticholinergics	Atropine

continuation or dose modification in consultation with the patient's physician may be considered or a substitute drug can be tried.

Because of the increased potential for dental caries, frequent dental visits are recommended. Office and daily home fluoride applications can be used to help prevent decay, and chlorhexidine mouth rinses minimize plaque buildup.

BENIGN LYMPHOEPITHELIAL LESION

In the late 1800s, Johann von Mikulicz-Radecki described the case of a patient with an unusual bilateral painless swelling of the lacrimal glands and all of the salivary glands. Histopathologic examination of the involved glands showed an intense lymphocytic infiltrate with features that are today recognized microscopically as the **benign lymphoepithelial lesion**. This clinical presentation became known as **Mikulicz's disease**, and clinicians began using this term to describe a variety of cases of bilateral parotid and lacrimal enlargement. However, many of these cases were not examples of benign lymphoepithelial lesions microscopically but represented salivary and lacrimal involvement by other disease processes, such as tuberculosis, sarcoidosis, and lymphoma. These cases of parotid-lacrimal enlargement secondary to other diseases were later recognized as being different and termed **Mikulicz's syndrome**, with the term **Mikulicz's disease** reserved for cases associated with benign lymphoepithelial lesions. However, these two terms have become so confusing and ambiguous that they should no longer be used.

Many cases of so-called Mikulicz's disease may be examples of what is now more commonly known as **Sjögren's syndrome** (see next topic). Sjögren's syndrome is an autoimmune disease that may produce bilateral salivary and lacrimal enlargement with microscopic features of benign lymphoepithelial lesion. However, not all benign lymphoepithelial lesions are necessarily associated with the clinical disease complex of Sjögren's syndrome.

Clinical Features

Most benign lymphoepithelial lesions develop as a component of Sjögren's syndrome. Those not associated with Sjögren's syndrome are usually unilateral, although occasional bilateral examples are seen. Sometimes benign lymphoepithelial lesions occur in association with other salivary gland pathologic conditions, such as sialoliths and benign or malignant epithelial tumors.

The benign lymphoepithelial lesion most often develops in adults, with a mean age of 50 years. From 60 to 80 percent of cases occur in women. Eighty percent of cases occur in the parotid gland, with infrequent examples also reported in the submandibular gland and minor salivary glands. The lesion usually presents as a firm, diffuse swelling of the affected gland that sometimes is dramatic in size. It may be asymptomatic or associated with mild pain.

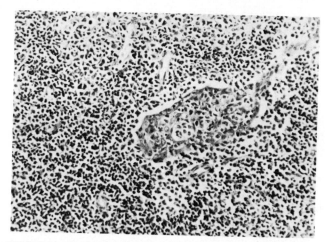

FIGURE 11–23. **Benign lymphoepithelial lesion.** Lymphocytic infiltrate of the parotid gland with an associated epimyoepithelial island.

Histopathologic Features

Microscopic examination of the benign lymphoepithelial lesion shows a heavy lymphocytic infiltrate associated with the destruction of the salivary acini (Fig. 11–23). Germinal centers may or may not be seen. Although the acini are destroyed, the ductal epithelium persists. The ductal cells and surrounding myoepithelial cells become hyperplastic, forming highly characteristic groups of cells, known as "epimyoepithelial islands," throughout the lymphoid proliferation. These epimyoepithelial islands can be helpful in distinguishing the lesion from lymphoma.

Treatment and Prognosis

Although the benign lymphoepithelial lesion frequently necessitates surgical removal of the involved gland, the prognosis in most cases is good. However, individuals with benign lymphoepithelial lesions have an increased risk for lymphoma, either within the affected gland or in an extrasalivary site. Although the exact risk is uncertain, one study showed the risk in patients with Sjögren's syndrome to be more than 40 times higher than expected in the general population. The management of patients with Sjögren's syndrome is discussed in the next section.

In addition, a rare malignant counterpart of this lesion, called a **malignant lymphoepithelial lesion** or **lymphoepithelial carcinoma**, represents a poorly differentiated salivary carcinoma with a prominent lymphoid stroma. Most of these lesions have occurred in Eskimos (Inuits) and Asians. Most of these tumors appear to arise *de novo* as carcinomas, although some cases (especially in non-Inuits) have been reported to develop from a prior benign lymphoepithelial lesion. Because of the strong ethnic association of this tumor, attempts have been made to determine a common etiologic agent. Most of this speculation has centered around the Epstein-Barr virus, although definite proof has not been established. The prognosis for these carcinomas appears guarded, although Asian patients have had a better survival rate.

SJÖGREN'S SYNDROME

Sjögren's syndrome is a chronic, systemic autoimmune disorder that principally involves the salivary and lacrimal glands, resulting in xerostomia (dry mouth) and xerophthalmia (dry eyes). The effects on the eye are often called **keratoconjunctivitis sicca** (*sicca* = dry), and the clinical presentation of both xerostomia and xerophthalmia is also sometimes called the **sicca syndrome**. Two forms of the disease are recognized:

- *Primary* Sjögren's syndrome (sicca syndrome alone; no other autoimmune disorder is present)
- *Secondary* Sjögren's syndrome (the patient manifests sicca syndrome in addition to another associated autoimmune disease)

The cause of Sjögren's syndrome is unknown. Although it is not a hereditary disease *per se*, there is evidence of a genetic influence. Relatives of affected patients have an increased frequency of other autoimmune diseases. In addition, certain histocompatibility antigens (HLA) are found with greater frequency in patients with Sjögren's syndrome. HLA-DRw52 is associated with both forms of the disease; HLA-B8 and HLA-DR3 are seen with increased frequency in the primary form of the disease. It has been suggested that viruses, such as Epstein-Barr virus, may play a pathogenetic role in Sjögren's syndrome, but evidence for this appears speculative.

Clinical and Radiographic Features

Sjögren's syndrome is not a rare condition. Although the exact prevalence is unknown, it has been estimated to occur in 0.5 percent of the population of the United States. Between 80 and 90 percent of cases occur in females. It is predominantly seen in middle-aged adults, but rare examples have been described in children.

When the condition is associated with another connective tissue disease, it is called secondary Sjögren's syndrome. It can be associated with almost any other autoimmune disease, but the most common associated disorder is rheumatoid arthritis. About 15 percent of patients with rheumatoid arthritis have Sjögren's syndrome. In addition, secondary Sjögren's syndrome may develop in 30 percent of patients with systemic lupus erythematosus.

The principal oral symptom is xerostomia, which is caused by decreased salivary secretions, but the severity of this dryness can vary widely from patient to patient. The saliva may appear frothy, with a lack of the usual pooling saliva in the floor of the mouth. Affected patients may complain of difficulty in swallowing, altered taste, or difficulty in wearing dentures. The tongue often becomes fissured and exhibits atrophy of the papillae (Fig. 11–24). The oral mucosa may be red and tender, usually as a result of secondary candidiasis. Related denture sore mouth and angular cheilitis are common. The lack of salivary cleansing action predisposes the patient to dental decay, especially cervical caries.

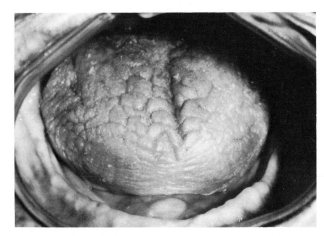

FIGURE 11–24. **Sjögren's syndrome.** Dry and fissured tongue. (Courtesy of Dr. David Schaffner.)

From one third to one half of patients have diffuse, firm enlargement of the major salivary glands during the course of their disease (Fig. 11–25). This swelling is usually bilateral, may be nonpainful or slightly tender, and may be intermittent or persistent in nature. The greater the severity of the disease, the greater the likelihood of this salivary enlargement. In addition, the re-

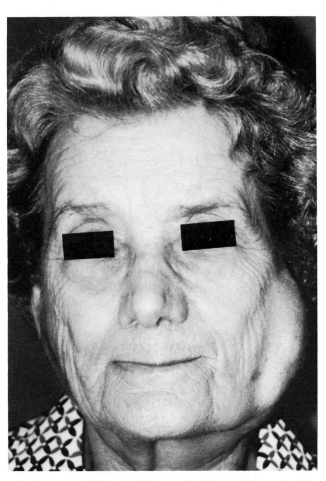

FIGURE 11–25. **Sjögren's syndrome.** Benign lymphoepithelial lesion of the parotid gland. (Courtesy of Dr. David Schaffner.)

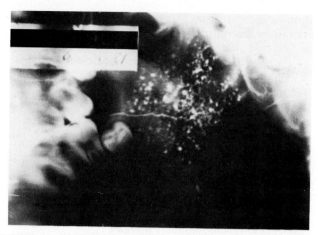

FIGURE 11–26. **Sjögren's syndrome.** Parotid sialogram demonstrating atrophy and punctate sialectasia ("fruit-laden, branchless tree"). (Courtesy of Dr. George Blozis.)

duced salivary flow places these individuals at increased risk for retrograde bacterial sialadenitis.

Although it is not diagnostic, sialographic examination often reveals punctate sialectasia and lack of normal arborization of the ductal system, typically demonstrating a "fruit-laden, branchless tree" pattern (Fig. 11–26). Scintigraphy with radioactive technetium-99m pertechnetate characteristically shows decreased uptake and delayed emptying of the isotope.

The term keratoconjunctivitis sicca describes not only the reduced tear production by the lacrimal glands but also the pathologic effect on the epithelial cells of the ocular surface. As in xerostomia, the severity of xerophthalmia can vary widely from one patient to the next. The lacrimal inflammation causes a decrease of the aqueous layer of the tear film; however, mucin production is normal and may result in a mucoid discharge. Patients often complain of a scratchy, gritty sensation or the perceived presence of a foreign body in the eye. Defects of the ocular surface epithelium develop and can be demonstrated with rose bengal dye. Vision may become blurred, and sometimes there is an aching pain. The ocular manifestations are least severe in the morning on wakening and become more pronounced as the day progresses.

A simple means to confirm the decreased tear secretion is the Schirmer test. Standardized strips of sterile filter paper are hooked over the margins of the lower lids so that their tabbed ends rest just inside the lower lid. The degree of tear absorption by the filter paper can then be measured. Values below 5 mm (after a 5-minute period) are highly suggestive of keratoconjunctivitis sicca, and values from 0 to 2 mm strongly confirm a dry eye state.

Sjögren's syndrome is a systemic disease, and various other body tissues can also be affected by the inflammatory process. The skin is often dry, as are the nasal and vaginal mucosae. Fatigue is fairly common, and depression can sometimes occur. Other possible associated problems include lymphadenopathy, primary biliary cirrhosis, Raynaud's phenomenon, interstitial nephritis, interstitial lung fibrosis, vasculitis, and peripheral neuropathies.

Laboratory Values

In patients with Sjögren's syndrome, the erythrocyte sedimentation rate is high and serum immunoglobulin levels, especially IgG, are typically elevated. A variety of autoantibodies can be produced, and although none of these is specifically diagnostic, their presence can be another helpful clue to the diagnosis. A positive rheumatoid factor (RF) is found in 75 percent of cases, regardless of whether the patient has rheumatoid arthritis. Antinuclear antibody (ANA) is also present in most patients. Two particular nuclear autoantibodies—anti-SS-A (anti-Ro) and anti-SS-B (anti-La)—are frequently found, especially in those with primary Sjögren's syndrome. Salivary duct autoantibodies can also sometimes be demonstrated, usually in secondary Sjögren's syndrome. Because these are infrequent in primary cases, however, they are believed to occur as a secondary phenomenon rather than playing a primary role in pathogenesis.

Histopathologic Features

The basic microscopic finding in Sjögren's syndrome is a lymphocytic infiltration of the salivary glands with destruction of the acinar units. If the major glands are enlarged, microscopic examination usually shows progression to a benign lymphoepithelial lesion (see previous topic), with characteristic epimyoepithelial islands in a background lymphoid stroma. Lymphocytic infiltration of the minor glands also occurs, although epimyoepithelial islands are rarely seen in this location.

Biopsy of the minor salivary glands of the lower lip has become a useful test in the diagnosis of Sjögren's syndrome. A 1.5- to 2.0-cm incision is made on clinically normal lower labial mucosa, parallel to the vermilion border and lateral to the midline, allowing the harvest of five or more accessory glands. These glands are then examined histopathologically for the presence of focal chronic inflammatory aggregates (50 or more lymphocytes and plasma cells). These aggregates should be adjacent to normal-appearing acini and should be found consistently in most of the glands in the specimen. The finding of more than one focus of 50 or more cells within a 4-mm² area of glandular tissue is considered supportive of the diagnosis of Sjögren's syndrome (Fig. 11–27). The greater the number of foci (up to ten or confluent foci), the greater the correlation with this diagnosis. The focal nature of this chronic inflammation among otherwise normal acini is a highly suggestive pattern; in contrast, the finding of scattered inflammation with ductal dilatation and fibrosis (chronic sclerosing sialadenitis) does not support the diagnosis of Sjögren's syndrome.

Other authors have advocated incisional biopsy of the parotid gland through a posterior auricular approach instead of a labial salivary gland biopsy. One study has shown this technique to be more sensitive in demonstrating inflammatory changes that support the diagnosis of

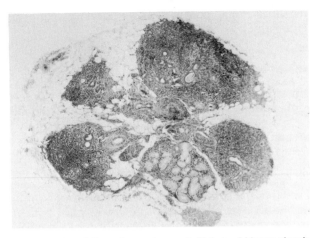

FIGURE 11–27. **Sjögren's syndrome.** Labial gland biopsy showing multiple lymphocytic foci.

Sjögren's syndrome; however, other authors think that this technique confers no increased benefit over labial gland biopsy. Parotid biopsy may enable one to evaluate an enlarged gland for the development of lymphoma and rule out the possibility of sialadenosis or sarcoidosis.

Treatment and Prognosis

The treatment of the patient with Sjögren's syndrome is mostly supportive. The dry eyes are best managed by periodic use of artificial tears. In addition, attempts can be made to conserve the tear film through the use of sealed glasses to prevent evaporation. Sealing the lacrimal punctum at the inner margin of the eyelids also can be helpful by blocking of the normal drainage of any lacrimal secretions into the nose.

Artificial salivas are available for the treatment of xerostomia; sugarless candy or gum can help to keep the mouth moist. Sialagogues, such as pilocarpine, can be useful to stimulate salivary flow if enough functional salivary tissue still remains. Medications known to diminish secretions should be avoided, if at all possible. Because of the increased risk of dental caries, daily fluoride applications may be indicated in dentulous patients. Antifungal therapy is often needed to treat secondary candidiasis.

Patients with Sjögren's syndrome have an increased risk for lymphoma, up to 40 times higher than the normal population. These tumors are predominantly non-Hodgkin's B-cell lymphomas and may initially arise within the salivary glands or within lymph nodes. These malignancies may be difficult to distinguish clinically and microscopically from the extensive, benign enlargements of the salivary glands or lymph nodes that develop in some patients (pseudolymphomas).

SIALADENOSIS (Sialosis)

Sialadenosis is an unusual noninflammatory disorder characterized by asymptomatic salivary gland enlargement, particularly involving the parotid glands. The con-

dition is almost always associated with an underlying systemic problem, including:

- Hormonal disorders (especially diabetes mellitus)
- Alcoholism
- Anorexia nervosa
- Bulimia
- Malnutrition
- Drug reactions

These conditions may result in dysregulation of the autonomic innervation of the salivary acini, producing clinical enlargement.

Clinical and Radiographic Features

Most cases of sialadenosis present as a slowly evolving, painless swelling of the parotid glands (Fig. 11–28). The condition is usually bilateral but can also be unilateral. Decreased salivary secretion may occur. Sialography demonstrates a "leafless tree" pattern, which is thought to be caused by compression of the finer ducts by hypertrophic acinar cells.

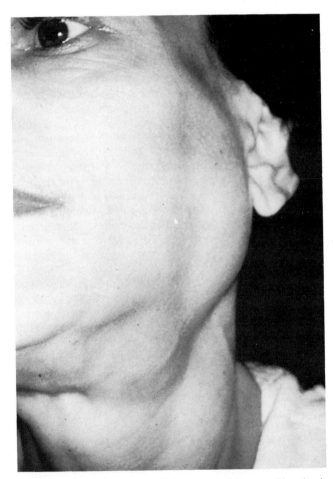

FIGURE 11–28. **Sialadenosis.** Enlargement of the parotid and submandibular glands secondary to alcoholism. (Courtesy of Dr. George Blozis.)

Histopathologic Features

Microscopic examination reveals hypertrophy of the acinar cells, sometimes two to three times greater than normal size. The nuclei are displaced to the cell base, and the cytoplasm is engorged with zymogen granules. In cases associated with longstanding diabetes or alcoholism, there may be acinar atrophy and fatty infiltration. Inflammation is not observed.

Treatment and Prognosis

The clinical management of sialadenosis is often unsatisfactory because it is closely related to the control of the underlying cause. Mild examples may cause few problems. If the swelling becomes a cosmetic concern, partial parotidectomy may be considered as a last resort.

ADENOMATOID HYPERPLASIA OF THE MINOR SALIVARY GLANDS

Clinical Features

Adenomatoid hyperplasia is a rare lesion of the minor salivary glands characterized by localized swelling that mimics a neoplasm. This pseudotumor most often occurs on the hard or soft palate, although it also has been reported in other oral minor salivary gland sites. It is most common in the fourth to sixth decades of life. Most of these lesions present as sessile, painless masses that may be soft or firm to palpation. They are usually normal in color, although a few lesions are red or bluish.

Histopathologic Features

Microscopic examination demonstrates lobular aggregates of normal-appearing mucous acini that are greater in number than normally would be found in the area (Fig. 11–29). These glands also sometimes appear to be increased in size. In some instances, the glands are situated close to the mucosal surface.

Treatment and Prognosis

Because the clinical presentation of adenomatoid hyperplasia mimics a tumor, biopsy is necessary to establish the diagnosis. Once the diagnosis has been established, no further treatment is indicated and the lesion should not recur.

NECROTIZING SIALOMETAPLASIA

Necrotizing sialometaplasia is an uncommon, locally destructive inflammatory condition of the salivary glands. Although the cause is uncertain, most authors believe it is the result of ischemia of the salivary tissue, which leads to local infarction. The importance of this lesion rests in the fact that it mimics a malignant process, both clinically and microscopically.

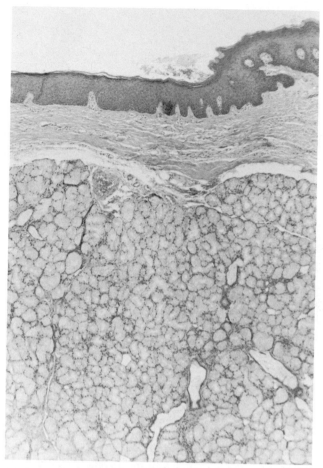

FIGURE 11–29. Adenomatoid hyperplasia. Palatal biopsy showing hyperplasia of mucous acini.

A number of potential predisposing factors have been suggested, including:

- Traumatic injuries
- Dental injections
- Ill-fitting dentures
- Upper respiratory infections
- Adjacent tumors
- Previous surgery

It has been suggested that these factors may play a role in compromising the blood supply to the involved glands, resulting in ischemic necrosis. However, many cases occur without any known predisposing factors.

Clinical Features

Necrotizing sialometaplasia most frequently develops in the palatal salivary glands; more than 75 percent of all cases occur on the posterior palate. The hard palate is more often affected than the soft palate. About two thirds of palatal cases are unilateral, with the rest being bilateral or midline in location. Necrotizing sialometaplasia has also been reported in other minor salivary gland sites and, occasionally, in the parotid gland. The submandib-

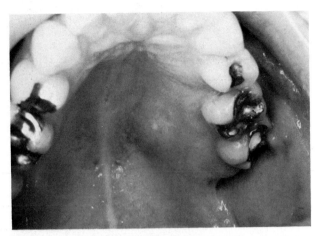

FIGURE 11–30. Necrotizing sialometaplasia. Early lesion demonstrating swelling of the posterior lateral hard palate. (From Allen CM, Camisa C. Diseases of the mouth and lips. *In:* Principles of Dermatology. Edited by Sams WM, Lynch P. New York, Churchill Livingstone 1990, pp 913–941.)

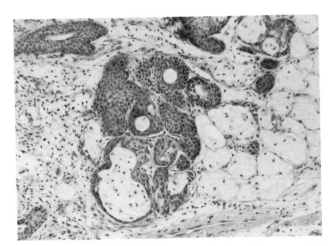

FIGURE 11–32. Necrotizing sialometaplasia. Necrotic mucous acini (*right*) and adjacent ductal squamous metaplasia (*center*).

ular and sublingual glands are rarely affected. Although it can occur at almost any age, necrotizing sialometaplasia is most common in adults; the mean age of onset is 46 years. Males are affected nearly twice as often as females.

The condition presents initially as a non-ulcerated swelling, often associated with pain or paresthesia (Fig. 11–30). Within 2 to 3 weeks, necrotic tissue sloughs out, leaving a crater-like ulcer that can range from less than 1 cm to more than 5 cm in diameter (Fig. 11–31). The patient may report that "a part of my palate fell out." At this point, the pain often subsides. In rare instances, there can be destruction of the underlying palatal bone.

Histopathologic Features

The microscopic appearance of necrotizing sialometaplasia is characterized by acinar necrosis in early lesions, followed by associated squamous metaplasia of the salivary ducts (Fig. 11–32). Although the mucous acinar cells are necrotic, the overall lobular architecture of the involved glands is still preserved—a helpful histopatho-

logic clue. There may be liberation of mucin, with an associated inflammatory response. The squamous metaplasia of the salivary ducts can be striking and produce a pattern that is easily misdiagnosed as squamous cell carcinoma or mucoepidermoid carcinoma. This mistaken impression may be further compounded by the frequent association of pseudoepitheliomatous hyperplasia of the overlying epithelium. In most cases, however, the squamous proliferation has a bland cytologic appearance.

Treatment and Prognosis

Because of the worrisome clinical presentation of necrotizing sialometaplasia, biopsy is usually indicated to rule out the possibility of malignant disease. Once the diagnosis has been established, no specific treatment is indicated or necessary. The lesion typically resolves on its own accord, with an average healing time of 5 to 6 weeks.

SALIVARY GLAND TUMORS

General Considerations

Tumors of the salivary glands constitute an important area in the field of oral and maxillofacial pathology. Although such tumors are uncommon, they are by no means rare. The annual incidence of salivary gland tumors around the world ranges from about 1 to 6.5 cases per 100,000 people. Although mesenchymal (e.g., hemangioma) and metastatic tumors can occur within the salivary glands, the discussion in this chapter is limited to primary epithelial neoplasms.

An often bewildering array of different salivary tumors have been identified and categorized. In addition, the classification scheme is a dynamic one that changes as we learn more about these lesions. Table 11–2 includes most of the currently recognized tumors. Some of the tumors on this list are not specifically discussed because their rarity places them outside the scope of this book.

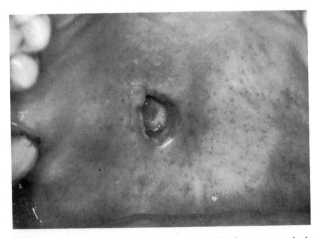

FIGURE 11–31. Necrotizing sialometaplasia. Later-stage lesion showing crater-like defect of the posterior palate.

Table 11–2. CLASSIFICATION OF SALIVARY GLAND TUMORS

Benign

Pleomorphic adenoma (mixed tumor)
Myoepithelioma
Basal cell adenoma
Canalicular adenoma
Warthin's tumor (papillary cystadenoma lymphomatosum)
Oncocytoma
Sebaceous adenoma
Sebaceous lymphadenoma
Ductal papillomas
    Sialadenoma papilliferum
    Intraductal papilloma
    Inverted ductal papilloma
Papillary cystadenoma

Malignant

Malignant mixed tumors
    Carcinoma ex pleomorphic adenoma
    Carcinosarcoma
    Metastasizing mixed tumor
Mucoepidermoid carcinoma
Acinic cell adenocarcinoma
Adenoid cystic carcinoma
Polymorphous low-grade adenocarcinoma
Basal cell adenocarcinoma
Epithelial-myoepithelial carcinoma
Salivary duct carcinoma
Sebaceous carcinoma
Sebaceous lymphadenocarcinoma
Clear cell carcinoma
Oncocytic carcinoma
Squamous cell carcinoma
Malignant lymphoepithelial lesion (lymphoepithelial carcinoma)
Small cell carcinoma
Adenocarcinoma, not otherwise specified

A number of investigators have published their findings on salivary gland neoplasia, but a comparison of these studies is often difficult. Some studies have been limited to only the major glands or have not included all the minor salivary gland sites. In addition, the ever evolving classification system makes an evaluation of some older studies difficult, especially when we try to compare them with more recent analyses. (For example, the polymorphous low-grade adenocarcinoma was first identified in 1983, but we now recognize that it is one of the more common malignancies in the minor glands.) Notwithstanding these difficulties, it is still helpful to compare these studies because they give us a good overview of salivary neoplasia in general. An evaluation of various studies shows fairly consistent trends (with minor variations) with regard to salivary gland tumors.

Tables 11–3 and 11–4 summarize four large series of primary epithelial salivary gland tumors, analyzed by sites of occurrence and frequency of malignancy, respectively. Some variations between studies may represent differences in diagnostic criteria, geographic differences, or referral bias in the cases seen. (Some centers may tend to see more malignant tumors on referral from other sources.)

The most common site for salivary gland tumors is the parotid gland, accounting for 64 to 80 percent of all cases. Fortunately, a relatively low percentage of parotid tumors are malignant, ranging from 15 to 32 percent. Overall, it can be stated that two thirds to three quarters of all salivary tumors occur in the parotid and two thirds to three quarters of these parotid tumors are benign.

Table 11–5 summarizes five large, well-known series of parotid neoplasms. The pleomorphic adenoma is overwhelmingly the most common tumor (53 to 77 percent of all cases in the parotid gland). Warthin's tumors are also fairly common; they account for 6 to 14 percent of cases. A variety of malignant tumors occur, with the mucoepidermoid carcinoma appearing to be the most frequent overall. However, two studies from Great Britain show a significantly lower prevalence of this tumor, possibly indicative of a geographic difference, especially compared with reports of cases from the United States.

From 8 to 11 percent of all salivary tumors occur in the submandibular gland, but the frequency of malignancy in this gland is almost double that of the parotid gland, ranging from 37 to 45 percent. However, as shown in Table 11–6, the pleomorphic adenoma is still the most common tumor and makes up 44 to 68 percent of all neoplasms. Unlike its occurrence in the parotid gland, Warthin's tumor is unusual in the submandibular gland, making up no more than 1 to 2 percent of all tumors. Adenoid cystic carcinoma is the most common malignancy, ranging from 12 to 27 percent of all cases.

Tumors of the sublingual gland are rare, comprising no more than 1 percent of all salivary neoplasms. However, 70 to 90 percent of sublingual tumors are malignant.

Tumors of the various smaller minor salivary glands make up 9 to 23 percent of all tumors, which makes this group the second most common site for salivary neoplasia. Table 11–7 summarizes the findings of three major surveys of minor gland tumors. Unfortunately, a relatively high proportion (almost 50 percent) of these have been malignant in most studies. Excluding rare sublingual tumors, it can be stated that "the smaller the gland, the greater the likelihood of malignancy for a salivary gland tumor."

Table 11–3. SITES OF OCCURRENCE OF PRIMARY EPITHELIAL SALIVARY GLAND TUMORS

| Author (Year) | No. of Cases | Site of Occurrence (%) | | | |
		Parotid	*Submandibular*	*Sublingual*	*Minor*
Eveson and Cawson (1985)	2,410	73%	11%	0.3%	14%
Seifert et al. (1986)	2,579	80%	10%	1%	9%
Spiro (1986)	2,807	70%	8%	(Included with minor gland tumors)	22%
Ellis et al. (1991)	13,749	64%	10%	0.3%	23%

Table 11–4. FREQUENCY OF MALIGNANCY FOR SALIVARY TUMORS AT DIFFERENT SITES

Author (Year)	No. of Cases	Percentage of Cases That Are Malignant			
		Parotid	*Submandibular*	*Sublingual*	*Minor*
Eveson and Cawson (1985)	2,410	15%	37%	86%	46%
Seifert et al. (1986)	2,579	20%	45%	90%	45%
Spiro (1986)	2,807	25%	43%	(Included with minor gland tumors)	82%
Ellis et al. (1991)	13,749	32%	41%	70%	49%

Table 11–5. PAROTID TUMORS

	Ellis et al. (United States, 1991)	Eveson and Cawson (Great Britain, 1985)	Thackray and Lucas (Great Britain, 1974)	Eneroth (Sweden, 1971)	Foote and Frazell (United States, 1953)
Total No. of Cases	8,222	1,756	651	2,158	764
Benign Tumors					
Pleomorphic adenoma	53.0%	63.3%	72.0%	76.8%	58.5%
Warthin's tumor	7.7%	14.0%	9.0%	4.7%	6.5%
Oncocytoma	1.9%	0.9%	0.6%	1.0%	0.1%
Basal cell adenoma	1.4%	—	—	—	—
Other benign tumors	3.7%	7.1% (Includes all "other monomorphic adenomas")	1.8%	—	0.7%
TOTAL	67.7%	85.3%	83.4%	82.5%	65.8%
Malignant Tumors					
Mucoepidermoid carcinoma	9.6%	1.5%	2.3%	4.1%	11.8%
Acinic cell adenocarcinoma	8.6%	2.5%	1.2%	3.1%	2.7%
Adenoid cystic carcinoma	2.0%	2.0%	3.3%	2.3%	2.1%
Malignant mixed tumor	2.5%	3.2%	4.1%	1.5%	6.0%
Squamous cell carcinoma	2.1%	1.1%	1.0%	0.3%	3.4%
Other malignant tumors	7.5%	4.4%	4.7%	6.3%	8.1%
TOTAL	32.3%	14.7%	16.6%	17.5%	34.2%

Table 11–6. SUBMANDIBULAR TUMORS

	Ellis et al. (United States, 1991)	Eveson and Cawson (Great Britain, 1985)	Thackray and Lucas (Great Britain, 1974)	Eneroth (Sweden, 1971)	Foote and Frazell (United States, 1953)
Total No. of Cases	1235	257	60	170	107
Benign Tumors					
Pleomorphic adenoma	53.3%	59.5%	68.0%	60.0%	43.9%
Warthin's tumor	1.3%	0.8%	1.7%	2.4%	0.0%
Oncocytoma	1.5%	0.4%	0.0%	0.6%	0.0%
Basal cell adenoma	1.0%	—	—	—	—
Other benign tumors	1.7%	1.9% (Includes all "other monomorphic adenomas")	0.0%	—	0.0%
TOTAL	58.8%	62.6%	69.7%	62.9%	43.9%
Malignant Tumors					
Mucoepidermoid carcinoma	9.1%	1.6%	0.0%	3.5%	7.5%
Acinic cell adenocarcinoma	2.7%	0.4%	0.0%	0.6%	0.0%
Adenoid cystic carcinoma	11.7%	16.8%	17.0%	15.3%	15.9%
Malignant mixed tumor	3.5%	7.8%	1.7%	1.8%	10.3%
Squamous cell carcinoma	3.4%	1.9%	3.3%	7.1%	12.1%
Other malignant tumors	10.8%	8.9%	8.3%	8.8%	10.3%
TOTAL	41.2%	37.4%	30.3%	37.1%	56.1%

Table 11-7. MINOR SALIVARY GLAND TUMORS

	Ellis et al. (1991)	Waldron et al. (1988)	Eveson and Cawson (1985)
Total No. of Cases	3355	426	336
Benign Tumors			
Pleomorphic adenoma	38.1%	40.8%	42.6%
"Monomorphic" adenoma (canalicular and basal cell adenoma)	4.5%	10.8%	11.0%
Other benign tumors	8.8%	5.9%	—
TOTAL	51.3%	57.5%	53.6%
Malignant Tumors			
Mucoepidermoid carcinoma	21.5%	15.3%	8.9%
Acinic cell adenocarcinoma	3.5%	3.5%	1.8%
Adenoid cystic carcinoma	7.7%	9.4%	13.1%
Malignant mixed tumor	1.7%	1.4%	7.1%
Polymorphous low-grade adenocarcinoma	2.2%	11.0%	—
Other malignant tumors	12.1%	1.9%	15.2%
TOTAL	48.7%	42.5%	46.4%

As observed in the major glands, the pleomorphic adenoma is the most common minor gland tumor and accounts for about 40 percent of all cases. The mucoepidermoid carcinoma and adenoid cystic carcinoma have generally been considered the two most common malignancies, although the recently delineated polymorphous low-grade adenocarcinoma is also becoming recognized as one of the more common minor gland tumors.

The palate is the most frequent site for minor salivary gland tumors, with 42 to 54 percent of all cases found there (Table 11-8). Most of these occur on the posterior lateral hard or soft palate, where the greatest concentration of glands is. Table 11-9 shows the relative prevalence of various tumors on the palate. The lips are the second most common location for minor gland tumors (21 to 22 percent of cases), followed by the buccal mucosa (11 to 15 percent of cases). Labial tumors are significantly more common in the upper lip, which accounts for 77 to 89 percent of all lip tumors (Table 11-10). Although mucoceles are commonly found on the lower lip, this is a surprisingly rare site for salivary gland tumors.

Significant differences in the percentage of malignancies and the relative frequency of various tumors can be noted for different minor salivary gland sites. As shown in Table 11-11, 42 to 50 percent of tumors of the palate and buccal mucosa sites are malignant, similar to the overall prevalence of malignancy in all minor salivary gland sites combined. In the upper lip, however, only 14

to 25 percent of tumors are malignant because of the high prevalence of the canalicular adenoma, which has a special affinity for this location. In contrast, although lower lip tumors are uncommon, 50 to 86 percent are malignant — mostly mucoepidermoid carcinomas. Up to 91 percent of retromolar tumors are malignant, also because of a predominance of mucoepidermoid carcinomas. Unfortunately, most tumors in the floor of the mouth and tongue are also malignant.

Pleomorphic Adenoma
(Benign Mixed Tumor)

The **pleomorphic adenoma**, or **benign mixed tumor**, is easily the most common salivary neoplasm. It accounts for 53 to 77 percent of parotid tumors, 44 to 68 percent of submandibular tumors, and 38 to 43 percent of minor gland tumors.

Pleomorphic adenomas are derived from a mixture of ductal and myoepithelial elements. A remarkable microscopic diversity can exist from one tumor to the next and in different areas of the same tumor. The terms pleomorphic adenoma and mixed tumor both represent attempts to describe this tumor's unusual histopathologic features, but neither term is entirely accurate. Although the basic tumor pattern is highly variable, the individual cells are rarely "pleomorphic." (However, focal minor atypia is

Table 11-8. LOCATION OF MINOR SALIVARY GLAND TUMORS

Author (Year)	No. of Cases	Palate	Lips	Buccal	Retromolar	Floor of Mouth	Tongue	Other
Eveson and Cawson (1985)	336	54%	21%	11%	1%	—	4%	8%
Waldron et al. (1988)	426	42%	22%	15%	5%	5%	1%	9%
Ellis et al. (1991)	3355	44%	21%	12%	2%	3%	5%	12%

Table 11-9. PALATAL SALIVARY GLAND TUMORS

	Ellis et al. (1991)	Waldron et al. (1988)	Eveson and Cawson (1985)
Total No. of Cases	1478	181	183
Benign Tumors			
Pleomorphic adenoma	48.2%	51.9%	47.0%
Other benign tumors	5.0%	6.0%	6.0%
TOTAL	53.2%	58.0%	53.0%
Malignant Tumors			
Mucoepidermoid carcinoma	20.7%	9.9%	9.3%
Acinic cell adenocarcinoma	1.4%	1.7%	1.1%
Adenoid cystic carcinoma	8.3%	10.5%	15.3%
Malignant mixed tumor	2.4%	2.2%	8.2%
Polymorphous low-grade adenocarcinoma	3.0%	16.0%	—
Other malignant tumors	11.0%	1.7%	13.1%
TOTAL	46.8%	42.0%	47.0%

Table 11-10. LOCATION OF LABIAL SALIVARY GLAND TUMORS

Author (Year)	No. of Cases	Upper Lip	Lower Lip
Eveson and Cawson (1985)	71	89%	11%
Waldron et al. (1988)	93	85%	15%
Neville et al. (1988)	103	84%	16%
Ellis et al. (1991)	536	77%	23%

acceptable.) Likewise, even though the tumor often has a prominent mesenchyme-appearing "stromal" component, it is not truly a "mixed" neoplasm that is derived from more than one germ layer.

Clinical Features

Regardless of the site of origin, the pleomorphic adenoma typically presents as a painless, slowly growing, firm mass (Figs. 11-33 and 11-34). The patient may be aware of the lesion for many months or years before seeking a diagnosis. The tumor can occur at any age but is most common in young adults between the ages of 30 and 50. There is a slight female predilection.

Most pleomorphic adenomas of the parotid gland occur in the superficial lobe and present as a swelling overlying the mandibular ramus in front of the ear. Facial nerve palsy and pain are rare. Initially, the tumor is movable but becomes less mobile as it grows larger. If neglected, the lesion can grow to grotesque proportions. About 10 percent of parotid mixed tumors develop within the deep lobe of the gland beneath the facial nerve (Fig. 11-35). Sometimes these lesions grow in a medial direction between the ascending ramus and stylomandibular ligament, resulting in a dumbbell-shaped tumor that presents as a mass of the lateral pharyngeal wall or soft palate.

The palate is the most common site for minor gland mixed tumors, accounting for approximately 60 percent of intraoral examples. This is followed by the upper lip (20 percent) and buccal mucosa (10 percent). Palatal tumors almost always are found on the posterior lateral aspect of the palate, presenting as smooth-surfaced, dome-shaped masses (Figs. 11-36 and 11-37). If the tumor is traumatized, secondary ulceration may occur. Because of the tightly bound nature of the hard palate mucosa, tumors in this location are not movable, although those in the lip or buccal mucosa frequently are mobile.

Histopathologic Features

The pleomorphic adenoma is typically a well-circumscribed, encapsulated tumor (Fig. 11-38). However, the capsule may be incomplete or show infiltration by tumor

Table 11-11. INTRAORAL MINOR SALIVARY GLAND TUMORS: PERCENTAGE MALIGNANT BY SITE

Author (Year)	Palate	Upper Lip	Lower Lip	Buccal	Retromolar	Floor of Mouth	Tongue
Eveson and Cawson (1985)	47%	25%	50%	50%	60%	—	92%
Waldron et al. (1988)	42%	14%	86%	46%	91%	80%	75%
Ellis et al. (1991)	47%	22%	60%	50%	90%	88%	86%

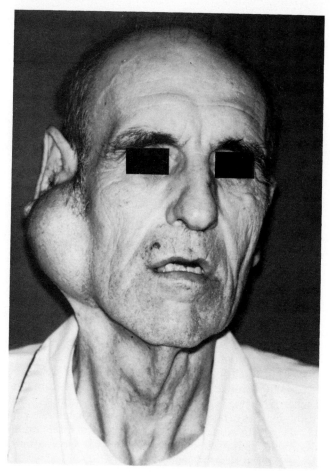

FIGURE 11–33. **Pleomorphic adenoma.** Slowly growing tumor of the parotid gland.

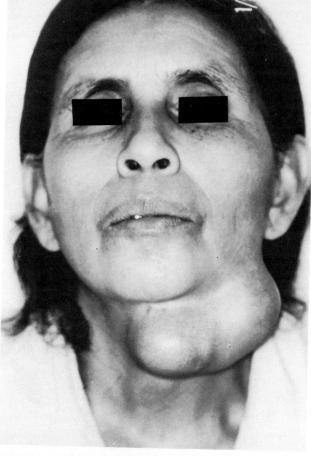

FIGURE 11–34. **Pleomorphic adenoma.** Tumor of the submandibular gland. (Courtesy of Dr. Román Carlos.)

cells. This lack of complete encapsulation is more common for minor gland tumors, especially along the superficial aspect of palatal tumors beneath the epithelial surface.

The tumor is composed of a mixture of glandular epithelium and myoepithelial cells within a mesenchyme-like background. The ratio of the epithelial elements and the mesenchyme-like component is highly variable among different tumors. Some tumors may consist almost entirely of background "stroma." Others are highly cellular with little background alteration.

The epithelium often forms ducts and cystic structures or may occur as islands or sheets of cells. Keratinizing squamous cells and mucus-producing cells can also be seen. Myoepithelial cells often make up a large percentage of the tumor cells and have a variable morphology, sometimes appearing angular or spindled. Some myoepithelial cells are rounded and demonstrate an eccentric nucleus and eosinophilic hyalinized cytoplasm, thus resembling plasma cells (Fig. 11–39). These characteristic plasmacytoid myoepithelial cells are more prominent in tumors arising in the minor glands. Occasionally, a tumor is composed entirely of myoepithelial cells with no ductal elements. Such tumors are often called **myoepitheliomas**, although they probably represent one end of the spectrum of mixed tumors.

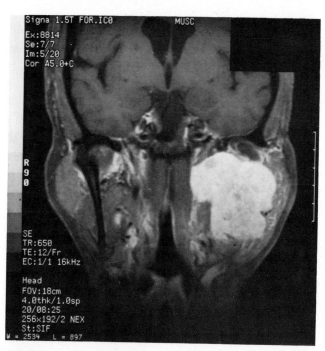

FIGURE 11–35. **Pleomorphic adenoma.** T1-weighted, fat-suppressed, contrast-enhanced coronal magnetic resonance image (MRI) of a tumor of the deep lobe of the parotid gland. (Courtesy of Dr. Joel Curé.)

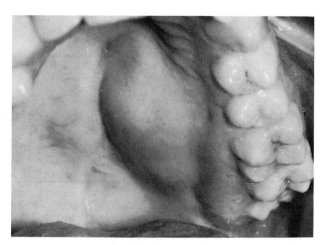

FIGURE 11–36. **Pleomorphic adenoma.** Palatal mass in a 23-year-old woman.

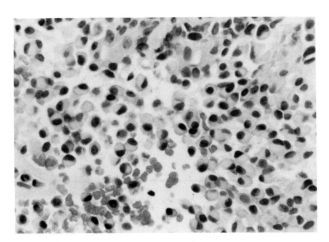

FIGURE 11–39. **Pleomorphic adenoma.** Plasmacytoid myoepithelial cells.

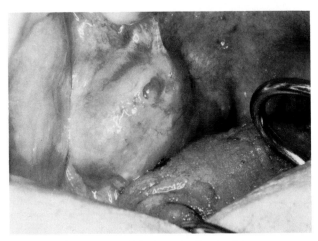

FIGURE 11–37. **Pleomorphic adenoma.** Tumor of the pterygomandibular area.

The highly characteristic "stromal" changes are believed to be produced by the myoepithelial cells. Extensive accumulation of mucoid material may occur between the tumor cells resulting in a myxomatous background (Fig. 11–40). Vacuolar degeneration of cells in these areas can produce a chondroid appearance (Fig. 11–41). With some tumors, the stroma exhibits an eosinophilic, hyalinized change (Fig. 11–42). Occasionally, fat or osteoid is also seen.

Treatment and Prognosis

Pleomorphic adenomas are best treated by surgical excision. For lesions in the superficial lobe of the parotid gland, superficial parotidectomy with identification and preservation of the facial nerve is recommended. Local enucleation should be avoided because the entire tumor may not be removed or the capsule may be violated,

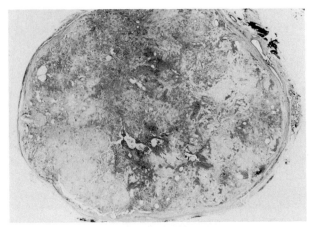

FIGURE 11–38. **Pleomorphic adenoma.** Low-power view showing a well-circumscribed, encapsulated tumor mass. Even at this power, the variable microscopic pattern of the tumor is evident.

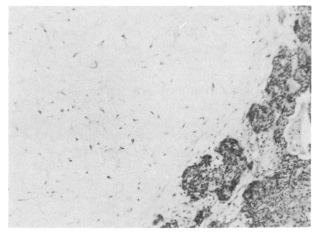

FIGURE 11–40. **Pleomorphic adenoma.** Ductal structures (*right*) with associated myxomatous background (*left*).

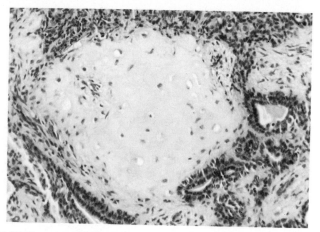

FIGURE 11–41. **Pleomorphic adenoma.** Chondroid material with adjacent ductal epithelium.

resulting in seeding of the tumor bed. For tumors of the deep lobe of the parotid, total parotidectomy is usually necessary, also with preservation of the facial nerve, if possible. Submandibular tumors are best treated by total removal of the gland with the tumor. Tumors of the hard palate are usually excised down to periosteum, including the overlying mucosa. In other oral sites, the lesion often enucleates easily through the incision site.

With adequate surgery, the prognosis is excellent, with a cure rate of more than 95 percent. The risk of recurrence appears to be lower for tumors of the minor glands. Conservative enucleation of parotid tumors often results in recurrence, with management of these cases made difficult as a result of multifocal seeding of the primary tumor bed. Multiple recurrences in such cases are not unusual. Malignant degeneration is a potential complication, resulting in a carcinoma ex pleomorphic adenoma (see p. 353). The risk of malignant transformation is probably small but may occur in as many as 5 percent of all cases.

Oncocytoma (Oxyphilic Adenoma)

The **oncocytoma** is a benign salivary gland tumor composed of large epithelial cells known as oncocytes. It is a rare neoplasm, representing no more than 1 percent of all salivary tumors.

Clinical Features

The oncocytoma is predominantly a tumor of older adults, with a peak prevalence in the eighth decade of life. A slight female predilection has been observed but may not be significant. Oncocytomas occur primarily in the major salivary glands, especially the parotid gland, which accounts for about 80 percent of all cases. Oncocytomas of the minor salivary glands are exceedingly rare.

The tumor presents as a firm, slowly growing, painless mass that rarely exceeds 4 cm in diameter. Parotid oncocytomas are usually found in the superficial lobe and are clinically indistinguishable from other benign tumors.

Histopathologic Features

The oncocytoma is usually a well-circumscribed tumor that is composed of sheets of large, polyhedral cells (oncocytes) with abundant granular, eosinophilic cytoplasm (Fig. 11–43). Sometimes these cells form an alveolar or glandular pattern. The cells have centrally located nuclei that can vary from small and hyperchromatic to large and vesicular. Little stroma is present, usually in the form of thin fibrovascular septa. A mild, chronic inflammatory cell infiltrate may be noted.

The granularity of the cells is created by an overabundance of mitochondria, which can be demonstrated by electron microscopy. These granules can also be identified on light microscopic examination with a phosphotungstic acid–hematoxylin (PTAH) stain. The cells also contain glycogen, as evidenced by their positive staining with the periodic acid–Schiff (PAS) technique but by negative PAS staining after digestion with diastase.

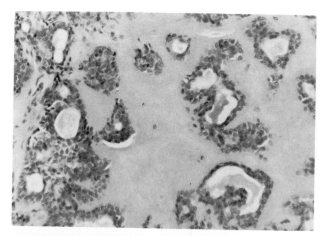

FIGURE 11–42. **Pleomorphic adenoma.** Ductal structures with hyalinized background alteration.

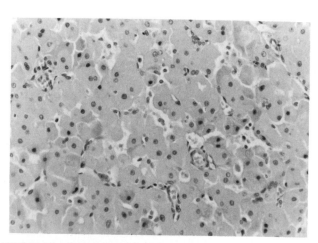

FIGURE 11–43. **Oncocytoma.** Sheet of large, eosinophilic oncocytes.

Oncocytomas may contain variable numbers of cells with a clear cytoplasm. In rare instances, these clear cells may compose most of the lesion and create difficulty in distinguishing the tumor from other clear cell salivary gland tumors that have a low-grade malignant potential.

Treatment and Prognosis

Oncocytomas are best treated by surgical excision. In the parotid gland, this usually entails partial parotidectomy (lobectomy) to avoid violation of the tumor capsule. The facial nerve should be preserved whenever possible. For tumors in the submandibular gland, treatment consists of total removal of the gland. Oncocytomas of the oral minor salivary glands should be removed with a small margin of normal surrounding tissue.

The prognosis after removal is good, with a low rate of recurrence. However, oncocytomas of the sinonasal glands can be locally aggressive and have been considered to be low-grade malignancies. Rare examples of histopathologically malignant oncocytomas (**oncocytic carcinoma**) also have been reported. These carcinomas have a relatively poor prognosis.

Oncocytosis

Oncocytosis is a rarely biopsied condition characterized by focal proliferations of oncocytes within salivary gland tissue. Unlike the oncocytoma, oncocytosis is considered a metaplastic process rather than a neoplastic one. However, it may mimic a neoplasia, both clinically and microscopically.

Clinical Features

Oncocytosis is primarily found in the parotid gland, although in rare instances it may involve the submandibular or minor salivary glands. It is often an incidental finding in otherwise normal salivary gland tissue but occasionally may be extensive enough to produce clinical swelling. Focal oncocytosis can also be a feature of other salivary gland tumors. As with other oncocytic proliferations, oncocytosis occurs most frequently in older adults.

Histopathologic Features

Microscopic examination reveals focal collections of oncocytes within salivary gland tissue or a salivary tumor. These enlarged cells are polyhedral and demonstrate abundant granular, eosinophilic cytoplasm as a result of the proliferation of mitochondria. On occasion, these cells may have a clear cytoplasm from the accumulation of glycogen (Fig. 11–44). The multifocal nature of the proliferation may be confused with that of a metastatic tumor, especially when the oncocytes are clear in appearance.

Treatment and Prognosis

Oncocytosis is a benign condition and is often discovered only as an incidental finding. No further treatment is necessary, and the prognosis is excellent.

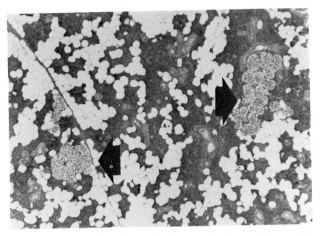

FIGURE 11–44. **Oncocytosis.** Multifocal collections of clear oncocytes (*arrows*) in the parotid gland.

Warthin's Tumor (Papillary Cystadenoma Lymphomatosum)

Warthin's tumor is a benign neoplasm that occurs almost exclusively in the parotid gland. Although it is much less common than the pleomorphic adenoma, it represents the second most common benign parotid tumor, accounting for 5 to 14 percent of all parotid neoplasms. The name **adenolymphoma** also has been used for this tumor, but this term should be avoided because it overemphasizes the lymphoid component and may give the mistaken impression that the lesion is a type of lymphoma.

The pathogenesis of these tumors is uncertain. The best known hypothesis suggests that they arise from heterotopic salivary gland tissue found within parotid lymph nodes. However, it has also been suggested that these tumors may develop from a proliferation of salivary gland ductal epithelium that is associated with secondary formation of lymphoid tissue. Several studies have demonstrated a strong association between the development of this tumor and smoking. Smokers have an eightfold greater risk for Warthin's tumor than do nonsmokers.

Clinical Features

Warthin's tumor usually presents as a slowly growing, painless, nodular mass of the parotid gland (Fig. 11–45). It may be firm or fluctuant to palpation. The tumor most frequently occurs in the tail of the parotid near the angle of the mandible and may be noted for many months before the patient seeks a diagnosis. One unique feature is the tendency of Warthin's tumor to occur bilaterally, which has been noted in 5 to 14 percent of cases. Most of these bilateral tumors do not occur simultaneously but are metachronous (occurring at different times).

In rare instances, Warthin's tumor has been reported within the submandibular gland or minor salivary glands. However, because the lymphoid component is often less pronounced in these extraparotid sites, caution should be exercised by the pathologist to avoid overdiagnosis of a lesion better classified as a papillary cystade-

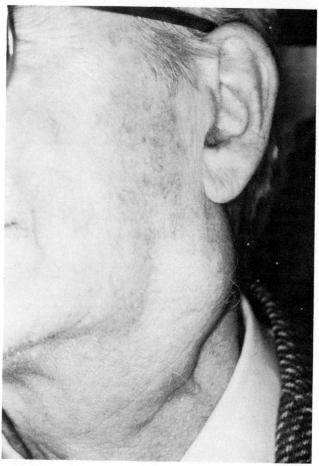

FIGURE 11–45. **Warthin's tumor.** Mass in the tail of the parotid gland. (Courtesy of Dr. George Blozis.)

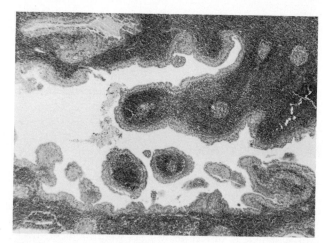

FIGURE 11–46. **Warthin's tumor.** Low-power view showing a papillary cystic tumor with a lymphoid stroma.

The epithelium is oncocytic in nature, forming uniform rows of cells surrounding cystic spaces. The cells have abundant, finely granular eosinophilic cytoplasm and are arranged in two layers. The inner luminal layer consists of tall columnar cells with centrally placed pyknotic nuclei. Beneath this is a second layer of cuboidal or polygonal cells with more vesicular nuclei. The lining epithelium demonstrates multiple papillary infoldings that protrude into the cystic spaces. Focal areas of squamous metaplasia or mucous cell prosoplasia may be seen. The epithelium is supported by a lymphoid stroma that frequently shows germinal center formation.

Treatment and Prognosis

Surgical removal is the treatment of choice for patients with Warthin's tumor. The procedure is usually easily accomplished because of the superficial location of the tumor. Some surgeons prefer local resection with minimal surrounding tissue; others opt for superficial parotidectomy to avoid violating the tumor capsule and because a tentative diagnosis may not be known preoperatively.

noma or salivary duct cyst with oncocytic ductal metaplasia.

Warthin's tumor most often occurs in older adults, with a peak prevalence in the sixth and seventh decades of life. Most studies show a decided male predilection, with some early studies demonstrating a male-to-female ratio up to 10 to 1. However, more recent investigations show a more equal sex ratio. Because Warthin's tumors have been associated with cigarette smoking, this changing sex ratio may be a reflection of the increased prevalence of smoking in females over the past few decades. This association with smoking may also help explain the frequent bilaterality of the tumor because any tumorigenic effects of smoking might be manifested in both parotids.

Histopathologic Features

Warthin's tumor has one of the most distinctive histopathologic patterns of any tumor in the body. Although the term **papillary cystadenoma lymphomatosum** is cumbersome, it accurately describes the salient microscopic features.

The tumor is composed of a mixture of ductal epithelium and a lymphoid stroma (Figs. 11–46 and 11–47).

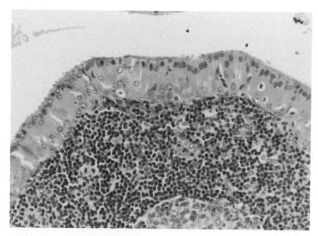

FIGURE 11–47. **Warthin's tumor.** High-power view of epithelial lining showing double row of oncocytes with adjacent lymphoid stroma.

A 6 to 12 percent recurrence rate has been reported. Many authors, however, believe that the tumor is frequently multicentric in nature; therefore, it is difficult to determine whether these are true recurrences or secondary tumor sites. Malignant Warthin's tumors (**carcinoma ex papillary cystadenoma lymphomatosum**) have been reported but are exceedingly rare.

Monomorphic Adenoma

The term **monomorphic adenoma** was originally used to describe a group of benign salivary gland tumors demonstrating a more uniform histopathologic pattern than the common pleomorphic adenoma. In some classification schemes, a variety of tumors were included under the broad heading of monomorphic adenoma, including Warthin's tumor, oncocytoma, basal cell adenoma, and canalicular adenoma. Other authors have used this term more specifically as a synonym just for the basal cell adenoma or canalicular adenoma. Because of its ambiguous nature, the term monomorphic adenoma should probably be avoided, and each of the tumors mentioned should be referred to by its more specific name.

Canalicular Adenoma

The **canalicular adenoma** is an uncommon tumor that almost exclusively occurs in the minor salivary glands. Because of its uniform microscopic pattern, the canalicular adenoma has also been called a "monomorphic adenoma," but because this term has also been applied to other tumors, its use should probably be discontinued. Likewise, the term **basal cell adenoma** sometimes has been used synonymously for this tumor but should be avoided because it refers to a separate tumor with different clinical features (see next topic).

Clinical Features

The canalicular adenoma shows a striking predilection for the upper lip, with 75 percent or more occurring in this one location. It represents the first or second most common tumor (along with pleomorphic adenoma) of the upper lip. The buccal mucosa is the second most common site. Occurrence in other minor salivary glands is uncommon, and canalicular adenomas of the parotid gland are rare.

The tumor nearly always occurs in older adults, with a peak prevalence in the seventh decade of life. There is a definite female predominance, ranging from 1.2 to 1.8 females for each male.

The canalicular adenoma presents as a slowly growing, painless mass that ranges from several millimeters to 2 cm (Fig. 11-48). It may be firm or somewhat fluctuant to palpation. The overlying mucosa may be normal in color or bluish and can be mistaken for a mucocele. However, mucoceles of the upper lip are rare. In some instances, the lesion has been noted to be multifocal, with multiple separate tumors discovered in the upper lip.

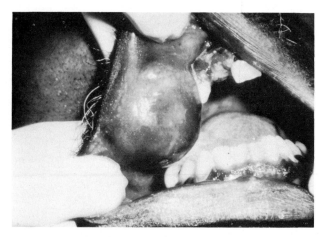

FIGURE 11-48. **Canalicular adenoma.** Mass in the upper lip. (Courtesy of Dr. John Fantasia.)

Histopathologic Features

The microscopic pattern of canalicular adenoma is "monomorphic" in nature. This pattern is characterized by single-layered cords of columnar or cuboidal epithelial cells with deeply basophilic nuclei (Fig. 11-49). In some areas, adjacent parallel rows of cells may be seen, resulting in a bilayered appearance of the tumor cords. These cells enclose ductal structures, sometimes in the form of long "canals." Larger cystic spaces are often created, and the epithelium may demonstrate papillary projections into the cystic lumina. The tumor cells are supported by a loose connective tissue stroma with prominent vascularity. Unlike the appearance in pleomorphic adenomas, stromal alterations, such as chondroid metaplasia, do not occur. The tumor is often surrounded by a thin, fibrous capsule, although incipient foci of additional tumors are sometimes observed in the surrounding salivary gland tissue.

Treatment and Prognosis

The canalicular adenoma is best treated by local surgical excision. Recurrence is uncommon and may be related to cases that are multifocal in nature.

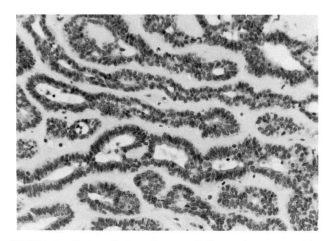

FIGURE 11-49. **Canalicular adenoma.** Uniform columnar cells forming canal-like ductal structures.

Basal Cell Adenoma

The **basal cell adenoma** is a benign salivary tumor that derives its name from the basaloid appearance of the tumor cells. It is an uncommon neoplasm that represents only 1 percent of all salivary tumors. Because of its uniform histopathologic appearance, it has often been classified as one of the monomorphic adenomas. However, as mentioned previously, this term should probably be avoided because of its imprecise and often confusing definition. Also, ultrastructural and immunohistochemical studies have shown that basal cell adenomas are not necessarily composed of only one cell type but sometimes of a combination of salivary ductal epithelium and myoepithelial cells. The basal cell adenoma shows some histopathologic similarity to the canalicular adenoma; in the past, these two terms have been used synonymously. However, histopathologic and clinical differences can be noted that warrant that they be considered as distinct entities.

Clinical Features

Unlike the canalicular adenoma, the basal cell adenoma is primarily a tumor of the parotid gland, with around 75 percent of all cases occurring there. However, the minor glands represent the second most common site, specifically the glands of the upper lip and buccal mucosa. The tumor can occur at any age but is most common in middle-aged and older adults, with a peak prevalence in the seventh decade of life. The tumor appears to be more common in females, with some studies showing as high as a 2:1 female-to-male ratio.

Clinically, the basal cell adenoma presents as a slowly growing, freely movable mass similar to a pleomorphic adenoma. Most tumors are less than 3 cm in diameter. Parotid tumors are usually located within the superficial lobe of the gland.

One subtype, the **membranous basal cell adenoma**, deserves separate mention. This form of the tumor appears to be hereditary, often occurring in combination with skin appendage tumors, such as **dermal cylindromas** and **trichoepitheliomas**. Multiple bilateral tumors may develop within the parotids. Because these tumors often bear a histopathologic resemblance to the skin tumors, they have also been called **dermal analogue tumors**.

Histopathologic Features

The basal cell adenoma is usually encapsulated or well circumscribed. The most common subtype is the solid variant, which consists of multiple islands and cords of epithelial cells that are supported by a small amount of fibrous stroma. The peripheral cells of these islands are palisaded and cuboidal to columnar in shape, similar to the microscopic appearance of basal cell carcinoma. These peripheral cells are frequently hyperchromatic; the central cells of the islands tend to have paler staining nuclei. The central cells occasionally form eddies or keratin pearls.

The trabecular subtype demonstrates narrow cord-like epithelial strands (Fig. 11-50). The tubular subtype is

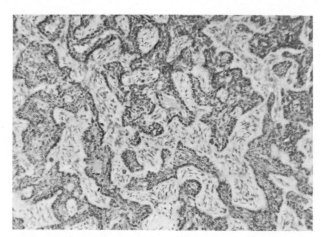

FIGURE 11-50. **Basal cell adenoma.** Parotid tumor showing cords of basaloid cells arranged in a trabecular pattern.

characterized by the formation of small, round, duct-like structures. Frequently, a mixture of histopathologic subtypes is seen.

The membranous basal cell adenoma exhibits multiple large lobular islands of tumor that are molded together in a jigsaw fashion. These islands are surrounded by a thick layer of hyaline material, which represents reduplicated basement membrane. Similar hyaline droplets also are often found among the epithelial cells. The microscopic appearance is similar to that of a dermal cylindroma, one of the skin tumors with which it is often associated.

Treatment and Prognosis

The treatment of basal cell adenoma is similar to that of pleomorphic adenoma and consists of complete surgical removal. Recurrence is rare for most histopathologic subtypes. However, the membranous subtype has a 25 to 37 percent recurrence rate, possibly related to its multifocal nature. Malignant transformation of a previously benign basal cell adenoma is rare. There is an uncommon malignant basaloid tumor, **basal cell adenocarcinoma**, however, that may arise *de novo* in the salivary glands.

Ductal Papillomas (Sialadenoma Papilliferum; Intraductal Papilloma; Inverted Ductal Papilloma)

A number of salivary gland tumors can be characterized microscopically by a papillomatous pattern, the most common being Warthin's tumor (papillary cystadenoma lymphomatosum). The **sialadenoma papilliferum**, **intraductal papilloma**, and **inverted ductal papilloma** are three rare salivary tumors that also show unique papillomatous features.

Clinical Features

The sialadenoma papilliferum most commonly arises from the minor salivary glands, especially on the palate, although it has also been reported in the parotid gland. It is usually seen in older adults and has a 2:1 male-to-female ratio. The tumor presents as an exophytic, papillary surface growth that is clinically similar to the common squamous papilloma.

The intraductal papilloma is an ill-defined lesion that has often been confused with other salivary gland lesions, such as the papillary cystadenoma. It usually occurs in adults and is most common in the minor salivary glands (especially on the lips), where it presents as a submucosal swelling.

The inverted ductal papilloma is the rarest of these tumors and has been seen only in the minor salivary glands of adults. The lower lip/mandibular vestibule is the most common location. The lesion usually presents as an asymptomatic submucosal nodule.

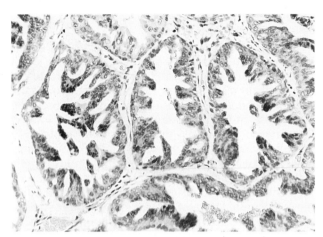

FIGURE 11–52. **Sialadenoma papilliferum.** Higher-power view of cystic areas lined by papillomatous epithelium.

Histopathologic Features

At low power, the sialadenoma papilliferum is somewhat similar to the squamous papilloma, exhibiting multiple exophytic papillary projections that are covered by stratified squamous epithelium. This epithelium is contiguous with a proliferation of papillomatous ductal epithelium found below the surface and extending downward into the deeper connective tissues (Fig. 11–51). Multiple ductal lumina are formed, which are characteristically lined by a double-rowed layer of cells consisting of a luminal layer of tall columnar cells and a basilar layer of smaller cuboidal cells (Fig. 11–52). These ductal cells often have an oncocytic appearance. An inflammatory infiltrate of plasma cells, lymphocytes, and neutrophils is characteristically present. Because of their microscopic similarity, this tumor has been considered to be an analogue of the cutaneous syringocystadenoma papilliferum.

The intraductal papilloma exhibits a dilated, unicystic structure that is located below the mucosal surface. It is lined by a single or double row of cuboidal or columnar epithelium, which has multiple arborizing papillary projections into the cystic lumen. In contrast, the inverted

ductal papilloma is composed primarily of a proliferation of squamoid epithelium with multiple thick, bulbous papillary projections that fill the ductal lumen (Fig. 11–53). This epithelium may be contiguous with the overlying mucosal epithelium, communicating with the surface through a small pore-like opening. Although

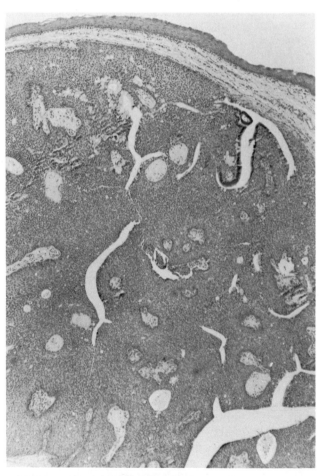

FIGURE 11–53. **Inverted ductal papilloma.** Submucosal papillary intraductal proliferation consisting of squamous and mucous cells.

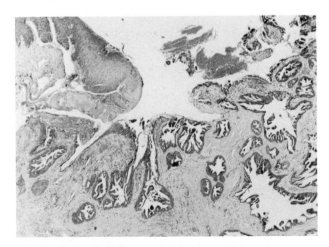

FIGURE 11–51. **Sialadenoma papilliferum.** Surface tumor forming multiple cystic structures with a papillomatous lining.

the tumor is primarily squamous in nature, the luminal lining cells of the papillary projections are often cuboidal or columnar in shape, with scattered mucus-producing cells.

Treatment and Prognosis

All three forms of ductal papilloma are best treated by conservative surgical excision. Recurrence is rare.

Mucoepidermoid Carcinoma

The **mucoepidermoid carcinoma** is one of the most common salivary gland malignancies. Because of its highly variable biologic potential, it was originally called *mucoepidermoid tumor*. The term recognized one subset that acted in a malignant fashion and a second group that appeared to behave in a benign fashion with favorable prognosis. However, it was later recognized that even low-grade tumors occasionally could exhibit malignant behavior; therefore, the term mucoepidermoid carcinoma is the preferred designation.

Clinical Features

Most studies show that the mucoepidermoid carcinoma is the most common malignant salivary gland neoplasm. In the United States, it makes up 10 percent of all major gland tumors and 15 to 21 percent of minor gland tumors. However, British studies have shown a much lower relative frequency, with mucoepidermoid carcinoma accounting for only 1 to 2 percent of major gland neoplasms and 9 percent of minor gland tumors. Perhaps a true geographic difference exists in the prevalence of this lesion.

The tumor occurs fairly evenly over a wide age range, extending from the second to seventh decades of life. Rarely is it seen in the first decade of life. However, mucoepidermoid carcinoma is the most common malignant salivary gland tumor in children. A slight female predilection has been noted.

The mucoepidermoid carcinoma is most common in the parotid gland and usually presents as an asymptomatic swelling. Most patients are aware of the lesion for a year or less, although some report a mass of many years' duration. Pain or facial nerve palsy may develop, usually in association with high-grade tumors. The minor glands constitute the second most common site, especially the palate (Fig. 11–54; see Color Figure 77). Minor gland tumors also typically appear as asymptomatic swellings, which are sometimes fluctuant and have a blue or red color that can be mistaken clinically for a mucocele. Although the lower lip, floor of mouth, tongue, and retromolar pad areas are uncommon locations for salivary gland neoplasia, the mucoepidermoid carcinoma is the most common salivary tumor in each of these sites (Fig. 11–55). Intraosseous tumors (discussed next) may also develop in the jaws.

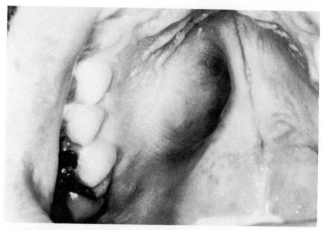

FIGURE 11–54. **Mucoepidermoid carcinoma.** Blue-pigmented mass of the posterior lateral hard palate. See Color Plates. (Courtesy of Dr. James F. Drummond.)

Histopathologic Features

As its name implies, the mucoepidermoid carcinoma is composed of a mixture of mucus-producing cells and epidermoid or squamous cells (Figs. 11–56 to 11–58). The mucous cells vary in shape but contain abundant foamy cytoplasm that stains positively with mucin stains. The epidermoid cells are characterized by squamoid features, often demonstrating a polygonal shape, intercellular bridges, and, rarely, keratinization. In addition, a third type of cell is typically present—the intermediate cell. This cell is basaloid in appearance and is believed to be a progenitor of the mucous and epidermoid cells. Some tumors also show variable numbers of clear cells, which sometimes can predominate the microscopic picture (Fig. 11–59). An associated lymphoid infiltrate is not unusual and may be so prominent in some cases that the lesion can be mistaken for a metastatic tumor within a lymph node.

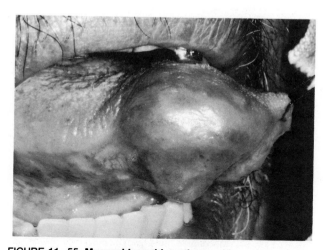

FIGURE 11–55. **Mucoepidermoid carcinoma.** Mass of the tongue.

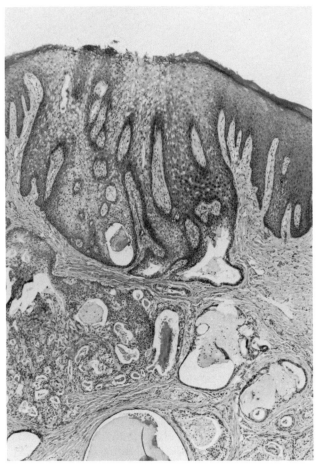

FIGURE 11–56. **Mucoepidermoid carcinoma.** Low-power view of a moderately well-differentiated tumor below the mucosal surface. Involvement of the terminal portion of the salivary ducts is well demonstrated.

Mucoepidermoid carcinomas can be categorized into one of three histopathologic grades on the basis of:

- The amount of cyst formation
- The degree of cytologic atypia
- The relative numbers of mucous, epidermoid, and intermediate cells

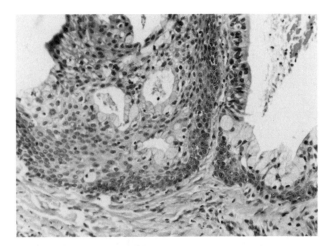

FIGURE 11–57. **Mucoepidermoid carcinoma.** High-power view showing a mixture of squamous cells and mucus-producing cells.

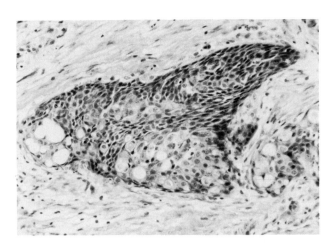

FIGURE 11–58. **Mucoepidermoid carcinoma.** High-grade tumor demonstrating an island of pleomorphic squamous cells with occasional mucin-producing cells.

Low-grade tumors show prominent cyst formation, minimal cellular atypia, and a relatively high proportion of mucous cells.

High-grade tumors consist of solid islands of squamous and intermediate cells, which can demonstrate considerable pleomorphism and mitotic activity. Mucus-producing cells may be infrequent, and the tumor can sometimes be difficult to distinguish from squamous cell carcinoma.

Intermediate-grade tumors show features that fall between those of the low-grade and high-grade neoplasms. Cyst formation occurs but is less prominent than that observed in low-grade tumors. All three major cell types are present, but the intermediate cells usually predominate. Cellular atypia may or may not be observed.

Treatment and Prognosis

The treatment of mucoepidermoid carcinoma is predicated by the location, histopathologic grade, and clinical stage of the tumor. Early-stage tumors of the parotid can often be treated by subtotal parotidectomy with preservation of the facial nerve. Advanced tumors may necessitate total removal of the parotid gland with sacrifice of

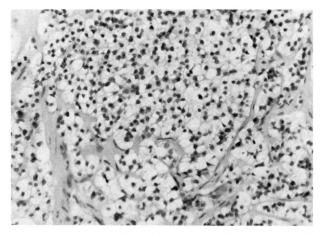

FIGURE 11–59. **Mucoepidermoid carcinoma.** Clear cell mucoepidermoid carcinoma.

the facial nerve. Submandibular gland tumors are treated by total removal of the gland. Mucoepidermoid carcinomas of the minor glands are usually treated by assured surgical excision. For low-grade neoplasms, only a modest margin of surrounding normal tissue may need to be removed, but high-grade or large tumors warrant wider resection, similar to that required for squamous cell carcinomas. If there is underlying bone destruction, the involved bone must be excised.

Radical neck dissection is indicated for patients with clinical evidence of metastatic disease and also may be considered for patients with larger or high-grade tumors. Postoperative radiation therapy may also be helpful for more aggressive tumors.

The prognosis depends on the grade and stage of the tumor. Patients with low-grade tumors have a good prognosis. Local recurrences or regional metastases are uncommon, and more than 90 percent of patients are cured. The outlook for patients with high-grade tumors is guarded, with only 30 percent of patients surviving. As would be expected, the prognosis for those with intermediate-grade tumors falls between that for low- and high-grade tumors.

The prognosis is better in children than in older people. Submandibular gland tumors are associated with a poorer outlook than those in the parotid gland. For tumors arising at the base of the tongue, the cure rate is also low.

Intraosseous Mucoepidermoid Carcinoma (Central Mucoepidermoid Carcinoma)

On rare occasions, salivary gland tumors arise centrally within the jaws. The most common and best recognized intraosseous salivary tumor is the **intraosseous mucoepidermoid carcinoma**. However, other salivary tumors have been reported to develop within the jaws, including adenoid cystic carcinoma, benign and malignant mixed tumors, adenocarcinoma, acinic cell adenocarcinoma, and monomorphic adenoma.

Several hypotheses have been proposed to explain the pathogenesis of intraosseous salivary tumors. One theory suggests that they may arise from ectopic salivary gland tissue that was developmentally entrapped within the jaws. However, such ectopic salivary tissue is rarely discovered in other biopsy specimens from the jaws and, therefore, seems an unlikely source. Some maxillary tumors may arise from glands of the sinus lining, but this is often difficult to prove or disprove. The most likely source for most intraosseous tumors is odontogenic epithelium. Mucus-producing cells are common in odontogenic cyst linings, especially dentigerous cysts (see p. 493). Also, many intraosseous mucoepidermoid carcinomas develop in association with impacted teeth or odontogenic cysts.

Clinical and Radiographic Features

Intraosseous mucoepidermoid carcinomas are most common in middle-aged adults and demonstrate a slight

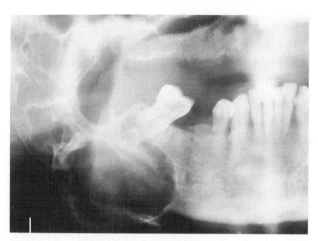

FIGURE 11–60. **Intraosseous mucoepidermoid carcinoma.** Multilocular lesion of the posterior mandible. (Courtesy of Dr. Joseph F. Finelli.)

female predilection. They are three times more common in the mandible than in the maxilla and are most often seen in the molar-ramus area. The most frequent presenting symptom is cortical swelling, although some lesions may be discovered as incidental findings on radiographs. Pain, trismus, and paresthesia are less frequently reported.

Radiographs usually reveal either a unilocular or multilocular radiolucency with well-defined borders (Fig. 11–60). Some cases are associated with an unerupted tooth and, therefore, may clinically suggest an odontogenic cyst or tumor.

Histopathologic Features

The microscopic appearance of intraosseous mucoepidermoid carcinoma is similar to that of its soft tissue counterpart. Most tumors are low-grade lesions, although high-grade mucoepidermoid carcinomas have also been reported within the jaws.

Treatment and Prognosis

The primary treatment modality for patients with intraosseous mucoepidermoid carcinoma is surgery; adjunct radiation therapy is also sometimes used. Radical surgical resection offers a better chance for cure than do more conservative procedures, such as enucleation or curettage. The local recurrence rate with conservative treatment is 40 percent in contrast to 13 percent for more radical treatment. Metastasis has been reported in about 12 percent of cases.

The overall prognosis is fairly good; around 10 percent of patients die, usually as a result of local recurrence of the tumor.

Acinic Cell Adenocarcinoma

The **acinic cell adenocarcinoma** is a salivary gland malignancy with cells that show serous acinar differentiation. Because many of these tumors act in a non-aggressive fashion and are associated with a good prognosis, this neoplasm was formerly called *acinic cell tumor*, a nonspecific designation that did not indicate whether the lesion was benign or malignant. However, because some of these tumors do metastasize or recur and cause death, it is generally agreed today that acinic cell adenocarcinoma should be considered a low-grade malignancy.

Clinical Features

The acinic cell adenocarcinoma is most common in the parotid gland, a logical finding because this is the largest gland and one that is composed entirely of serous elements. Most studies have shown that this neoplasm makes up 1 to 3 percent of all parotid tumors, although one study showed it represented 8.6 percent of all parotid tumors (see Table 11–4). It is much less common in the submandibular gland, where it composes less than 1 percent of all tumors in most studies. The acinic cell adenocarcinoma accounts for 2 to 4 percent of all tumors in the oral minor salivary glands, with the buccal mucosa, lips, and palate being the most common sites (Fig. 11–61).

The tumor occurs over a broad age range, with a relatively even peak prevalence stretching from the second to the seventh decades of life; the mean age is in the mid-40s. Approximately 60 percent of cases occur in women. The tumor usually presents as a slowly growing mass, and the lesion is often present for many months or years before a diagnosis is made. The tumor may be otherwise asymptomatic, although associated pain or tenderness are sometimes reported. Facial nerve paralysis is an infrequent but ominous sign for parotid tumors.

Histopathologic Features

Acinic cell adenocarcinomas are highly variable in their microscopic appearance. The tumor often is well circumscribed and sometimes may even appear encapsulated; however, some tumors exhibit an infiltrative growth pattern. The most characteristic cell is one with features of the serous acinar cell, with abundant granular

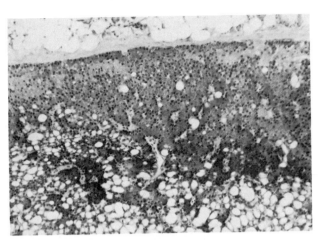

FIGURE 11–62. **Acinic cell adenocarcinoma.** Parotid tumor demonstrating sheet of granular, basophilic serous acinar cells.

basophilic cytoplasm and a round, darkly stained eccentric nucleus. These cells are fairly uniform in appearance, and mitotic activity is uncommon. Other cells may resemble intercalated duct cells, and some tumors also have cells with a clear, vacuolated cytoplasm.

Several growth patterns may be seen. The *solid* variety consists of numerous well-differentiated acinar cells arranged in a pattern that resembles normal parotid gland tissue (Figs. 11–62 and 11–63). In the *microcystic* variety, multiple small cystic spaces are created that may contain some mucinous or eosinophilic material. In the *papillary-cystic* variety, larger cystic areas are formed that are lined by epithelium having papillary projections into the cystic spaces (Fig. 11–64). The *follicular* variety has an appearance similar to that of thyroid tissue. A lymphoid infiltrate is not unusual, sometimes with germinal center formation.

Treatment and Prognosis

Acinic cell adenocarcinomas confined to the superficial lobe of the parotid gland are best treated by lobec-

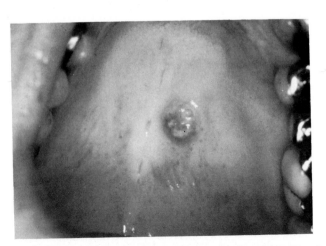

FIGURE 11–61. **Acinic cell adenocarcinoma.** Small, nodular mass of the hard palate. (Courtesy of Dr. Rick Canaan.)

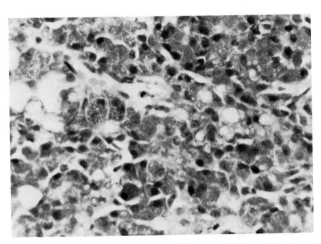

FIGURE 11–63. **Acinic cell adenocarcinoma.** High-power view of serous cells with basophilic, granular cytoplasm.

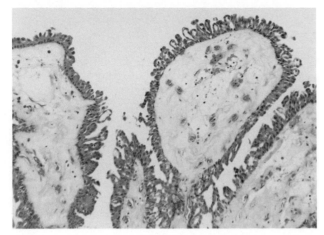

FIGURE 11–64. **Acinic cell adenocarcinoma.** Papillary-cystic variant.

tomy; for those in the deep lobe, total parotidectomy is usually necessary. The facial nerve may need to be sacrificed if it is involved by tumor. Submandibular tumors are managed by total removal of the gland, and minor gland tumors are treated with assured surgical excision. Lymph node dissection is not indicated unless there is clinical evidence of metastatic disease. Adjunctive radiation therapy may be considered for uncontrolled local disease.

The acinic cell adenocarcinoma is associated with one of the better prognoses of any of the malignant salivary gland tumors. Approximately one third of patients have recurrences locally, and metastases develop in 10 to 15 percent of patients. From 6 to 26 percent of patients die of their disease. The prognosis for minor gland tumors is better than that for tumors arising in the major glands.

Malignant Mixed Tumors (Carcinoma ex Pleomorphic Adenoma; Carcinoma ex Mixed Tumor; Carcinosarcoma; Metastasizing Mixed Tumor)

Malignant mixed tumors represent malignant counterparts to the benign mixed tumor or pleomorphic adenoma. These uncommon neoplasms represent 2 to 6 percent of all salivary tumors and can be divided into three categories:

1. Carcinoma ex pleomorphic adenoma (carcinoma ex mixed tumor).
2. Carcinosarcoma.
3. Metastasizing mixed tumor.

The most common of these is the **carcinoma ex pleomorphic adenoma**, which is characterized by malignant transformation of the epithelial component of a previously benign pleomorphic adenoma. The **carcinosarcoma** is a rare "mixed" tumor in which both the epithelial and stromal components are malignant. The **metastasizing mixed tumor** has histopathologic features that are identical to the common pleomorphic adenoma

(mixed tumor). In spite of its benign appearance, however, the lesion metastasizes. The metastatic tumor also has a benign microscopic appearance, usually similar to that of the primary lesion.

Clinical Features

Carcinoma ex Pleomorphic Adenoma

There is fairly convincing evidence that the carcinoma ex pleomorphic adenoma represents a malignant transformation within what was previously a benign neoplasm. First of all, the mean age of patients with this tumor is about 15 years older than that for the benign pleomorphic adenoma. It is most common in middle-aged and older adults, with a peak prevalence in the sixth to eighth decades of life. In addition, patients may report that a mass has been present for many years, sometimes undergoing a recent rapid growth with associated pain or ulceration. However, some tumors may have a short duration. The histopathologic features, which are discussed later, also support malignant transformation of a benign pleomorphic adenoma.

Eighty percent of cases of carcinoma ex pleomorphic adenoma have been reported within the major glands, primarily the parotid gland (Fig. 11–65). Nearly two thirds of minor salivary gland cases occur on the palate

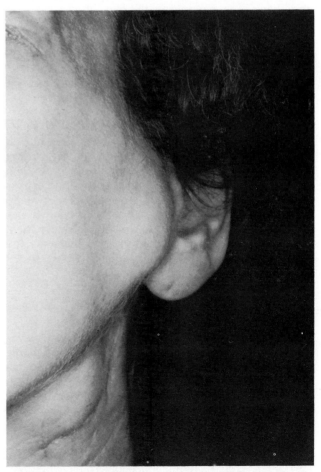

FIGURE 11–65. **Carcinoma ex pleomorphic adenoma.** Mass of the parotid gland.

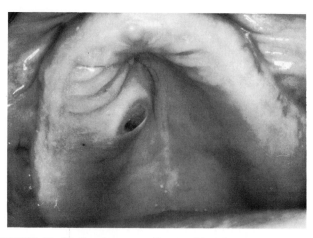

FIGURE 11-66. **Carcinoma ex pleomorphic adenoma.** Painful, ulcerated mass of the palate.

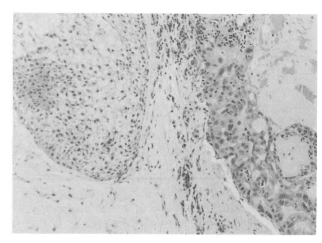

FIGURE 11-67. **Carcinoma ex pleomorphic adenoma.** Medium-power view demonstrating atypical, malignant cells (*right*) arising within a benign mixed tumor (*left*).

(Fig. 11-66). There is a slight female predilection. Although pain or recent rapid growth is not unusual, many cases present as a painless mass that is indistinguishable from a benign tumor. Parotid tumors may produce facial nerve palsy.

Carcinosarcoma

The carcinosarcoma is an extremely rare tumor. Most cases have been reported in the parotid gland, but the lesion has also been seen in the submandibular gland and minor salivary glands. The clinical signs and symptoms are similar to those of the carcinoma ex pleomorphic adenoma. Some patients have a previous history of a benign pleomorphic adenoma, although other cases appear to arise *de novo*.

Metastasizing Mixed Tumor

The metastasizing mixed tumor is also quite rare. As with other malignant mixed tumors, most cases originate in the parotid gland, but the primary tumor also may occur in the submandibular gland or minor salivary glands. Metastases have most frequently been found in the bones or lungs, but they can also occur in other sites, such as regional lymph nodes or the liver. Most patients have a history of a benign mixed tumor, which may have been excised many years earlier.

Histopathologic Features

Carcinoma ex Pleomorphic Adenoma

The carcinoma ex pleomorphic adenoma shows a variable microscopic appearance. Areas of typical benign pleomorphic adenoma usually can be found and may constitute most or only a small portion of the lesion. Within the tumor are areas of malignant degeneration of the epithelial component, characterized by cellular pleomorphism and abnormal mitotic activity (Figs. 11-67 and 11-68). This change is most often in the form of a poorly differentiated adenocarcinoma, but other patterns also can develop, including mucoepidermoid carcinoma, adenoid cystic carcinoma, and polymorphous low-grade

adenocarcinoma. The malignant component often has an infiltrative growth pattern, although sometimes it is discovered as a small focus within the center of an encapsulated mixed tumor.

Carcinosarcoma

The carcinosarcoma is a biphasic tumor, demonstrating both carcinomatous and sarcomatous areas. The epithelial component usually consists of a poorly differentiated adenocarcinoma or an undifferentiated carcinoma. The sarcomatous portion often predominates the tumor and is usually in the form of chondrosarcoma but also may show characteristics of osteosarcoma, fibrosarcoma, liposarcoma, or malignant fibrous histiocytoma. Some lesions have evidence of an origin from a benign mixed tumor.

Metastasizing Mixed Tumor

The metastasizing mixed tumor has microscopic features of a benign pleomorphic adenoma, within both the primary and metastatic sites. Malignant histopathologic changes are not observed.

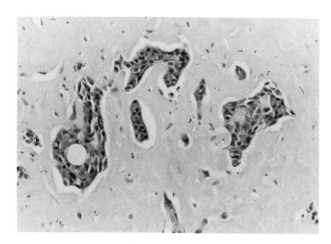

FIGURE 11-68. **Carcinoma ex pleomorphic adenoma.** Islands of hyperchromatic epithelial cells in a densely hyalinized background matrix.

Treatment and Prognosis

Invasive carcinoma ex pleomorphic adenoma and carcinosarcoma are usually best treated by wide excision, possibly in conjunction with local lymph node dissection and adjunctive radiation therapy. The prognosis is guarded, with 50 percent of all patients experiencing local recurrence or metastases and dying. However, in cases of carcinoma ex pleomorphic adenoma in which the malignant component is contained within the tumor capsule, the prognosis is similar to that for benign mixed tumor.

The treatment for a metastasizing mixed tumor consists of surgical excision of both the primary tumor and metastatic sites, but nearly 50 percent of all patients die of their metastatic disease.

Adenoid Cystic Carcinoma

The **adenoid cystic carcinoma** is one of the more common and best recognized salivary malignancies. Because of its distinctive histopathologic features, it was originally called a *cylindroma*, and this term is still used sometimes as a synonym for this neoplasm. However, use of the term cylindroma should probably be avoided today because the same term is used for a skin adnexal tumor that has a markedly different clinical presentation and prognosis.

Clinical and Radiographic Features

The adenoid cystic carcinoma can occur in any salivary gland site, but approximately 50 percent develop within the minor salivary glands. The palate is the most common site for minor gland tumors (Fig. 11–69). The remaining tumors are mostly found in the parotid and submandibular glands, with a fairly even distribution between these two sites. On an individual basis, however, a striking difference can be seen among the various glands. In the parotid gland, the adenoid cystic carcinoma is relatively rare, constituting only 2 to 3 percent of

all tumors. In the submandibular gland, this tumor accounts for 12 to 17 percent of all tumors and is the most common malignancy. It is also relatively common among palatal salivary neoplasms; it represents 8 to 15 percent of all such tumors. The lesion is most common in middle-aged adults and is rare in people younger than age 20. There is a fairly equal sex distribution, although some studies have shown a slight female predilection.

The adenoid cystic carcinoma usually presents as a slowly growing mass. Pain is a common and important finding, occasionally occurring early in the course of the disease before there is a noticeable swelling. Patients often complain of a constant, low-grade, dull ache, which gradually increases in intensity. Facial nerve paralysis may develop with parotid tumors. Palatal tumors can be smooth-surfaced or ulcerated. Tumors arising in the palate or maxillary sinus may show radiographic evidence of bone destruction.

Histopathologic Features

The adenoid cystic carcinoma is composed of a mixture of ductal cells and myoepithelial cells that can have a varied arrangement (Fig. 11–70). Three major patterns are recognized: (1) cribriform, (2) tubular, and (3) solid. Usually a combination of these is seen, and the tumor is classified on the basis of the predominant pattern.

The *cribriform pattern* is the most classic and best recognized appearance (Fig. 11–71), characterized by islands of basaloid epithelial cells that contain multiple cylindrical, cyst-like spaces resembling Swiss cheese. These spaces often contain a mildly basophilic mucoid material, a hyalinized eosinophilic product, or a combined mucoid-hyalinized appearance. Sometimes the hyalinized material also surrounds these cribriform islands, or small strands of tumor are found embedded within this hyalinized "stroma." The tumor cells are small and cuboidal, exhibiting deeply basophilic nuclei and little cytoplasm. These cells are fairly uniform in appearance, and mitotic activity is rarely seen.

In the *tubular pattern*, the tumor cells are similar but

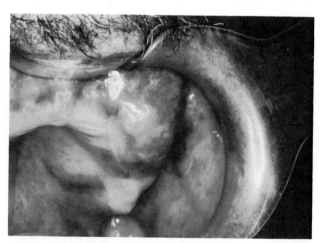

FIGURE 11–69. **Adenoid cystic carcinoma.** Painful mass of the hard palate and maxillary alveolar ridge. (Courtesy of Dr. George Blozis.)

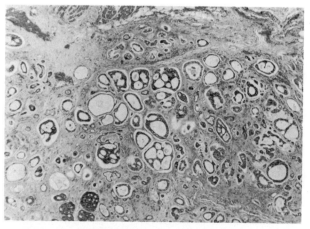

FIGURE 11–70. **Adenoid cystic carcinoma.** Islands of hyperchromatic cells forming tubular and cribriform structures.

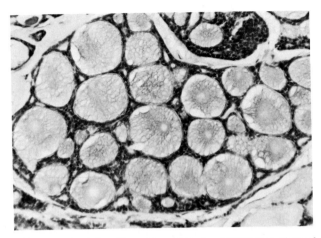

FIGURE 11–71. **Adenoid cystic carcinoma.** High-power view of tumor cells forming a cribriform ("Swiss cheese") pattern.

occur as multiple small ducts or tubules within a hyalinized stroma. The tubular lumina can be lined by one to several layers of cells, and sometimes both a layer of ductal cells and myoepithelial cells can be discerned.

The *solid variant* consists of larger islands or sheets of tumor cells that demonstrate little tendency toward duct or cyst formation. Unlike the cribriform and tubular patterns, cellular pleomorphism and mitotic activity, as well as focal necrosis in the center of the tumor islands, may be observed.

A highly characteristic feature of adenoid cystic carcinoma is its tendency to show perineural invasion, which probably corresponds to the common clinical finding of pain in these patients. Sometimes the cells appear to have a swirling arrangement around nerve bundles (Fig. 11–72). However, perineural invasion is not pathognomonic for adenoid cystic carcinoma; it also may be seen in other salivary malignancies, especially polymorphous low-grade adenocarcinomas.

Treatment and Prognosis

Adenoid cystic carcinoma is a relentless tumor that is prone to local recurrence and eventual distant metas-

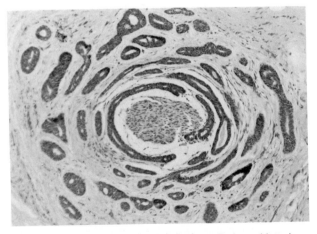

FIGURE 11–72. **Adenoid cystic carcinoma.** Perineural invasion.

tasis. Surgical excision is usually the treatment of choice, and adjunct radiation therapy may slightly improve patient survival in some cases. Because metastasis to regional lymph nodes is uncommon, radical neck dissection is typically not indicated. Because of the poor overall prognosis, regardless of treatment, clinicians should be cautioned against needlessly aggressive and mutilating surgical procedures for large tumors or cases already showing metastases.

Because the tumor is prone to late recurrence and metastasis, the 5-year survival rate has little significance and does not equate to a "cure." The 5-year survival rate may be as high as 70 percent, but this rate continues to decrease over time. By 20 years, only 20 percent of patients are still alive. Tumors with a solid histopathologic pattern are associated with a worse outlook than those with a cribriform or tubular arrangement. With respect to site, the prognosis is poorest for tumors arising in the maxillary sinus and submandibular gland. Most studies have shown that perineural invasion has little effect on the prognosis.

Death usually results from local recurrence or distant metastases. Tumors of the palate or maxillary sinus may eventually invade upward to the base of the brain. Metastatic spread most commonly occurs to the lungs and bones.

Polymorphous Low-Grade Adenocarcinoma (Lobular Carcinoma; Terminal Duct Carcinoma)

The **polymorphous low-grade adenocarcinoma** is a recently recognized type of salivary malignancy that was first described in 1983. Before its identification as a distinct entity, this tumor was categorized as a pleomorphic adenoma, an unspecified form of adenocarcinoma, or sometimes included with adenoid cystic carcinoma. Once recognized, however, it was realized that this tumor possesses distinct clinicopathologic features and is one of the more common minor salivary gland malignancies.

Clinical Features

The polymorphous low-grade adenocarcinoma is almost exclusively a tumor of the minor salivary glands, except when it composes the malignant component of a carcinoma ex pleomorphic adenoma. Sixty percent occur on the hard or soft palate (Fig. 11–73; see Color Figure 78), with the upper lip and buccal mucosa being the next most common locations. It is most common in older adults, having a peak prevalence in the sixth to eighth decades of life. Two thirds of all cases occur in females.

The tumor most often presents as a painless mass that may have been present for a long time with slow growth. Occasionally, it is associated with bleeding or discomfort.

Histopathologic Features

The tumor cells of polymorphous low-grade adenocarcinomas have a deceptively uniform appearance, with a

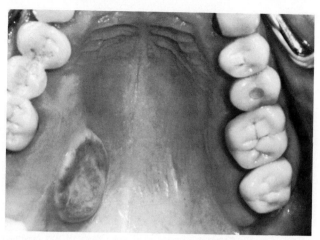

FIGURE 11–73. **Polymorphous low-grade adenocarcinoma.** Ulcerated mass of the posterior lateral hard palate. See Color Plates.

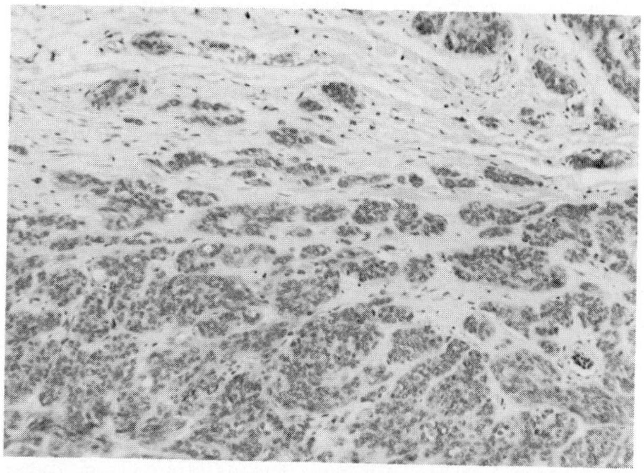

FIGURE 11–75. **Polymorphous low-grade adenocarcinoma.** Pale-staining cells forming islands and infiltrating cords.

cuboidal to columnar shape and ovoid to spindle-shaped nuclei. These nuclei are usually pale-staining, although they can be more basophilic in some areas. The cells can exhibit different growth patterns, hence, the "polymorphous" term. The cells may grow in a solid pattern or form cords, ducts, or larger cystic spaces. In some tumors, a cribriform pattern can be produced that

mimics adenoid cystic carcinoma. Mitotic figures are uncommon.

At low power, the tumor sometimes appears well circumscribed (Fig. 11–74). However, the peripheral cells are usually infiltrative, invading the adjacent tissue in a single-file fashion (Fig. 11–75). Extension into underlying bone or skeletal muscle may be observed. The stroma is often mucoid in nature, or it may demonstrate hyalinization. Perineural invasion is common—another feature that may cause the tumor to be mistaken for adenoid cystic carcinoma (Fig. 11–76). However, a distinction between these two tumors is important because of their vastly different prognoses.

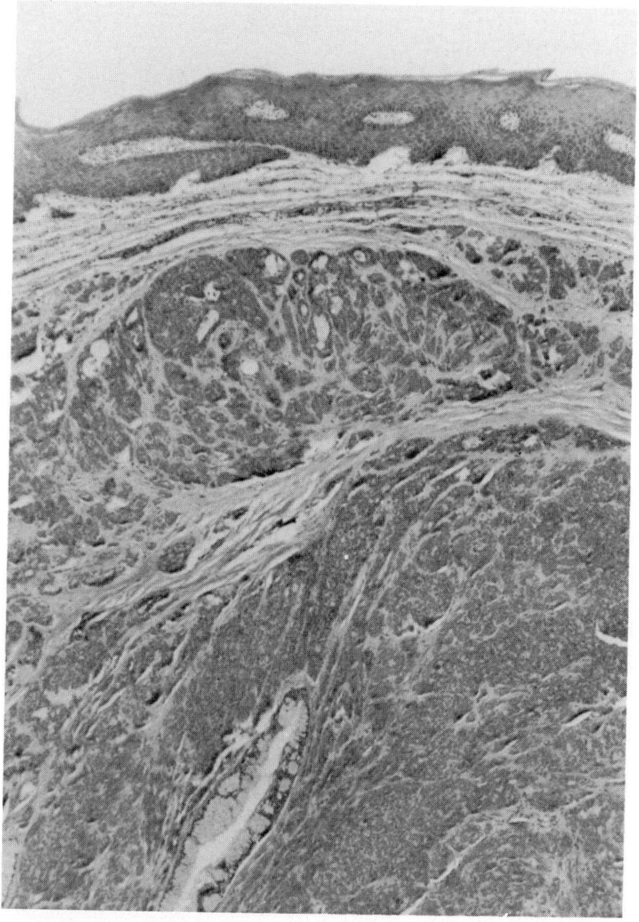

Treatment and Prognosis

The polymorphous low-grade adenocarcinoma is best treated by wide surgical excision, sometimes including resection of the underlying bone. Metastasis to regional lymph nodes may occur but is uncommon. Distant spread appears rare. Radical neck dissection seems unwarranted unless there is clinical evidence of cervical metastases.

FIGURE 11–74. **Polymorphous low-grade adenocarcinoma.** Low-power view showing cellular tumor below the mucosal surface.

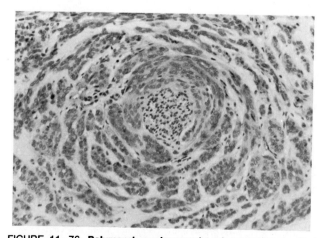

FIGURE 11–76. **Polymorphous low-grade adenocarcinoma.** Perineural invasion.

The overall prognosis appears to be relatively good, with around 80 percent of cases reported to be free of tumor after treatment. Recurrent disease has been reported in nearly one fourth of all patients but can usually be controlled with re-excision. Death due to tumor is rare but may occur secondary to direct extension into vital structures. Perineural invasion does not appear to affect the prognosis.

Salivary Adenocarcinoma, Not Otherwise Specified

In spite of the wide variety of salivary gland malignancies that have been specifically identified and categorized, some tumors still defy the existing classification schemes. These tumors are usually designated as **salivary adenocarcinomas, not otherwise specified (NOS)**.

Clinical and Histopathologic Features

Because these adenocarcinomas represent such a diverse group of neoplasms, it is difficult to generalize about their clinical and microscopic features. Like most salivary tumors, they appear to be most common in the parotid gland, followed by the minor glands and the submandibular gland (Figs. 11–77 and 11–78). They

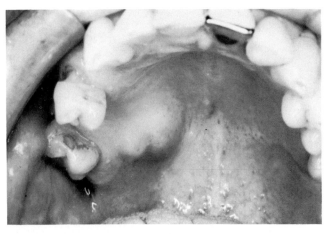

FIGURE 11–78. **Salivary adenocarcinoma.** Mass of the posterior lateral hard palate.

may present as asymptomatic masses or cause pain or facial nerve paralysis. The microscopic appearance is highly variable but demonstrates features of a glandular malignancy with evidence of cellular pleomorphism, an infiltrative growth pattern, or both. These tumors exhibit a wide spectrum of differentiation, ranging from well-differentiated, low-grade neoplasms to poorly differentiated, high-grade malignancies.

As these tumors are studied more, it should be possible to classify some of them into separate, specific categories and allow more definitive analyses of their clinical and microscopic features.

Treatment and Prognosis

The prognosis for salivary adenocarcinoma (NOS) is guarded, but patients with early-stage, well-differentiated tumors appear to have a better outcome.

REFERENCES

Mucocele

Cataldo E, Mosadomi A. Mucoceles of the oral mucous membrane. Arch Otolaryngol 91:360–365, 1970.
Eveson JW. Superficial mucoceles: Pitfall in clinical and microscopic diagnosis. Oral Surg Oral Med Oral Pathol 66:318–322, 1988.
Jensen JL. Superficial mucoceles of the oral mucosa. Am J Dermatopathol 12: 88–92, 1990.
Standish SM, Shafer WG. The mucus retention phenomenon. J Oral Surg 17:15–22, 1959.

Ranula

de Visscher JGAM, van der Wal KGH, de Vogel PL. The plunging ranula: Pathogenesis, diagnosis and management. J Craniomaxillofac Surg 17:182–185, 1989.
Galloway RH, et al. Pathogenesis and treatment of ranula: Report of three cases. J Oral Maxillofac Surg 47:299–302, 1989.
McClatchy KD, et al. Plunging ranula. Oral Surg Oral Med Oral Pathol 57:408–412, 1984.
Quick CA, Lowell SH. Ranula and the sublingual salivary glands. Arch Otolaryngol 103:397–400, 1977.

Salivary Duct Cyst

Eversole LR. Oral sialocysts. Arch Otolaryngol 113:51–56, 1987.

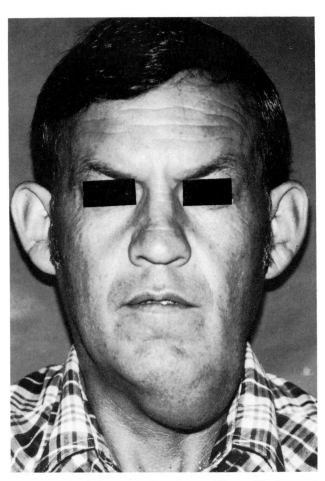

FIGURE 11–77. **Salivary adenocarcinoma.** "Clear cell" adenocarcinoma of the submandibular gland.

Sialolithiasis

Jensen JL, et al. Minor salivary gland calculi: A clinicopathologic study of forty-seven new cases. Oral Surg Oral Med Oral Pathol 47:44–50, 1979.

Levy DM, ReMine WH, Devine KD. Salivary gland calculi: Pain, swelling associated with eating. JAMA 181:1115–1119, 1962.

Narang R, Dixon RA. Surgical management of submandibular sialadenitis and sialolithiasis. Oral Surg Oral Med Oral Pathol 43:201–210, 1977.

Sialadenitis

Blitzer A. Inflammatory and obstructive disorders of salivary glands. J Dent Res 66(Suppl):675–679, 1987.

Johnson A. Inflammatory conditions of the major salivary glands. Ear Nose Throat J 68:94–102, 1989.

Werning JT, Waterhouse JP, Mooney JW. Subacute necrotizing sialadenitis. Oral Surg Oral Med Oral Pathol 70:756–759, 1990.

Cheilitis Glandularis

Cohen DM, Green JG, Diekmann SL. Concurrent anomalies: Cheilitis glandularis and double lip: Report of a case. Oral Surg Oral Med Oral Pathol 66:397–399, 1988.

Doku HC, Shklar G, McCarthy PL. Cheilitis glandularis. Oral Surg Oral Med Oral Pathol 20:563–571, 1965.

Oliver ID, Pickett AB. Cheilitis glandularis. Oral Surg Oral Med Oral Pathol 49:526–529, 1980.

Swerlick RA, Cooper PH. Cheilitis glandularis: A re-evaluation. J Am Acad Dermatol 10:466–472, 1984.

Sialorrhea

Lew KM, Younis RT, Lazar RH. The current management of sialorrhea. Ear Nose Throat J 70:99–105, 1991.

Lieblich S. Episodic supersalivation (idiopathic paroxysmal sialorrhea): Description of a new clinical syndrome. Oral Surg Oral Med Oral Pathol 68:159–161, 1989.

Talmi YP, Finkelstein Y, Zohar Y. Reduction of salivary flow with transdermal scopolamine. A four-year experience. Otolaryngol Head Neck Surg 103:615–618, 1990.

Xerostomia

Epstein JB, Scully C. The role of saliva in oral health and the causes and effects of xerostomia. J Can Dent Assoc 58:217–221, 1992.

Epstein JB, Stevenson-Moore P, Scully C. Management of xerostomia. J Can Dent Assoc 58:140–143, 1992.

Fox PC, et al. Pilocarpine treatment of salivary gland hypofunction and dry mouth (xerostomia). Arch Intern Med 151:1149–1152, 1991.

Johnson JT, et al. Oral pilocarpine for post-irradiation xerostomia in patients with head and neck cancer. N Engl J Med 329:390–395, 1993.

Sreebny LM, Valdini A. Xerostomia: A neglected symptom. Arch Intern Med 147:1333–1337, 1987.

Benign Lymphoepithelial Lesion

Bridges AJ, England DM. Benign lymphoepithelial lesion: Relationship to Sjögren's syndrome and evolving malignant lymphoma. Semin Arthritis Rheum 19:201–208, 1989.

Chaudhry AP, et al. Light and ultrastructural features of lymphoepithelial lesions of the salivary glands in Mikulicz's disease. J Pathol 146:239–250, 1986.

Gleeson MJ, Cawson RA, Bennett MH. Benign lymphoepithelial lesion: A less than benign disease. Clin Otolaryngol 11:47–51, 1986.

Kassan S, et al. Increased risk of lymphoma in sicca syndrome. Ann Intern Med 89:888–892, 1978.

Nagao K, et al. A histopathologic study of benign and malignant lymphoepithelial lesions of the parotid gland. Cancer 52:1044–1052, 1983.

Penfold CN. Mikulicz syndrome. J Oral Maxillofac Surg 43:900–905, 1985.

Saw D, et al. Malignant lymphoepithelial lesion of the salivary gland. Hum Pathol 17:914–923, 1986.

Sjögren's Syndrome

Daniels TE. Labial salivary gland biopsy in Sjögren's syndrome: Assessment as a diagnostic criterion in 362 suspected cases. Arthritis Rheum 27:147–156, 1984.

Daniels TE, Fox PC. Salivary and oral components of Sjögren's syndrome. Rheum Dis Clin North Am 18:571–589, 1992.

Fox RI, Kang H-I. Pathogenesis of Sjögren's syndrome. Rheum Dis Clin North Am 18:517–538, 1992.

Friedlaender MH. Ocular manifestations of Sjögren's syndrome: Keratoconjunctivitis sicca. Rheum Dis Clin North Am 18:591–608, 1992.

Lindvall AM, Jonsson R. The salivary gland component of Sjögren's syndrome: An evaluation of diagnostic methods. Oral Surg Oral Med Oral Pathol 62:32–42, 1986.

Marx RE, Hartman KS, Rethman KV. A prospective study comparing incisional labial to incisional parotid biopsies in the detection and confirmation of sarcoidosis, Sjögren's disease, sialosis and lymphoma. J Rheumatol 15:621–629, 1988.

Saito T, et al. Relationship between sialographic findings of parotid glands and histopathologic finding of labial glands in Sjögren's syndrome. Oral Surg Oral Med Oral Pathol 72:675–680, 1991.

Scully C. Sjögren's syndrome: Clinical and laboratory features, immunopathogenesis, and management. Oral Surg Oral Med Oral Pathol 62:510–523, 1986.

Sialadenosis

Batsakis JG. Pathology consultation: Sialadenosis. Ann Otol Rhinol Laryngol 97:94–95, 1988.

Chilla R. Sialadenosis of the salivary glands of the head. Studies on the physiology and pathophysiology of parotid secretion. Adv Otorhinolaryngol 26:1–38, 1981.

Hasler JF. Parotid enlargement: A presenting sign in anorexia nervosa. Oral Surg Oral Med Oral Pathol 53:567–573, 1982.

Russotto SB. Asymptomatic parotid gland enlargement in diabetes mellitus. Oral Surg Oral Med Oral Pathol 52:594–598, 1981.

Adenomatoid Hyperplasia

Arafat A, Brannon RB, Ellis GL. Adenomatoid hyperplasia of mucous salivary glands. Oral Surg Oral Med Oral Pathol 52:51–55, 1981.

Buchner A, et al. Adenomatoid hyperplasia of minor salivary glands. Oral Surg Oral Med Oral Pathol 71:583–587, 1991.

Giansanti JS, Baker GO, Waldron CA. Intraoral, mucinous, minor salivary gland lesions presenting clinically as tumors. Oral Surg Oral Med Oral Pathol 32:918–922, 1971.

Necrotizing Sialometaplasia

Abrams AM, Melrose RJ, Howell FV. Necrotizing sialometaplasia: A disease simulating malignancy. Cancer 32:130–135, 1973.

Brannon RB, Fowler CB, Hartman KS. Necrotizing sialometaplasia: A clinicopathologic study of sixty-nine cases and review of the literature. Oral Surg Oral Med Oral Pathol 72:317–325, 1991.

Sneige N, Batsakis JG. Necrotizing sialometaplasia. Ann Otol Rhinol Laryngol 101:282–284, 1992.

Salivary Gland Tumors: General Considerations

Ellis GL, Auclair PL, Gnepp DR. Surgical Pathology of the Salivary Glands. Philadelphia, WB Saunders, 1991.

Eneroth C-M. Salivary gland tumors in the parotid gland, submandibular gland, and the palate region. Cancer 27:1415–1418, 1971.

Eveson JW, Cawson RA. Salivary gland tumours: A review of 2410 cases with particular reference to histological types, site, age, and sex distribution. J Pathol 146:51–58, 1985.

Eveson JW, Cawson RA. Tumours of the minor (oropharyngeal) salivary glands: A demographic study of 336 cases. J Oral Pathol 14:500–509, 1985.

Foote FW, Frazell EL. Tumors of the major salivary glands. Cancer 6:1065–1113, 1953.

Neville BW, et al. Labial salivary gland tumors. Cancer 61:2113–2116, 1988.

Seifert G, et al. WHO international histological classification of tumours: Tentative histological classification of salivary gland tumours. Pathol Res Pract 186:555–581, 1990.

Seifert G, et al. Diseases of the Salivary Glands. Pathology—Diagnosis —Treatment—Facial Nerve Surgery. New York, George Thieme Verlag, 1986.

Spiro RH. Salivary neoplasms: Overview of a 35-year experience with 2,807 patients. Head Neck Surg 8:177–184, 1986.

Thackray AC, Lucas RB. Tumors of the Major Salivary Glands. Atlas of Tumor Pathology, 2nd Series, Fascicle 10. Washington, DC, Armed Forces Institute of Pathology, 1974.

Waldron CA, El-Mofty SK, Gnepp DR. Tumors of the intraoral minor salivary glands: A demographic and histologic study of 426 cases. Oral Surg Oral Med Oral Pathol 66:323–333, 1988.

Pleomorphic Adenoma

Chau MNY, Radden BG. A clinical-pathologic study of 53 intraoral pleomorphic adenomas. Int J Oral Maxillofac Surg 18:158–162, 1989.

Maynard JD. Management of pleomorphic adenoma of the parotid. Br J Surg 75:305–308, 1988.

Myssiorek D, Ruah CB, Hybels RL. Recurrent pleomorphic adenomas of the parotid gland. Head Neck 12:332–336, 1990.

Nigro MF Jr, Spiro RH. Deep lobe parotid tumors. Am J Surg 134:523–527, 1977.

Sciubba JJ, Brannon R. Myoepithelioma of salivary glands: Report of 23 cases. Cancer 47:562–572, 1982.

Oncocytoma

Brandwein MS, Huvos AG. Oncocytic tumors of major salivary glands: A study of 68 cases with follow-up of 44 patients. Am J Surg Pathol 15:514–528, 1991.

Damm DD, et al. Benign solid oncocytoma of intraoral minor salivary glands. Oral Surg Oral Med Oral Pathol 67:84–86, 1989.

Ellis GL. "Clear cell" oncocytoma of salivary gland. Human Pathol 19:862–867, 1988.

Goode RK, Corio RL. Oncocytic adenocarcinoma of salivary glands. Oral Surg Oral Med Oral Pathol 65:61–66, 1988.

Palmer TJ, et al. Oncocytic adenomas and oncocytic hyperplasia of salivary glands: A clinicopathological study of 26 cases. Histopathology 16:487–493, 1990.

Oncocytosis

Tkeda Y. Diffuse hyperplastic oncocytosis of the parotid gland. Int J Oral Maxillofac Surg 15:765–768, 1986.

Warthin's Tumor

Batsakis JG. Carcinoma ex papillary cystadenoma lymphomatosum. Malignant Warthin's tumor. Ann Otol Rhinol Laryngol 96:234–235, 1987.

Dietert SE. Papillary cystadenoma lymphomatosum (Warthin's tumor) in patients in a general hospital over a 24-year period. Am J Clin Pathol 63:866–875, 1975.

Fantasia JE, Miller AS. Papillary cystadenoma lymphomatosum arising in minor salivary glands. Oral Surg Oral Med Oral Pathol 52:411–416, 1981.

Kotwall CA. Smoking as an etiologic factor in the development of Warthin's tumor of the parotid gland. Am J Surg 164:646–647, 1992.

Monk JS Jr, Church JS. Warthin's tumor: A high incidence and no sex predominance in central Pennsylvania. Arch Otolaryngol Head Neck Surg 118:477–478, 1992.

van der Wal JE, Davids JJ, van der Waal I. Extraparotid Warthin's tumours—report of 10 cases. Br J Oral Maxillofac Surg 31:43–44, 1993.

Zappia JJ, Sullivan MJ, McClatchey KD. Unilateral multicentric Warthin's tumors. J Otolaryngol 20:93–96, 1991.

Canalicular Adenoma

Daley TD, Gardner DG, Smout MS. Canalicular adenoma: Not a basal cell adenoma. Oral Surg Oral Med Oral Pathol 57:181–188, 1984.

Fantasia JE, Neville BW. Basal cell adenomas of the minor salivary glands. Oral Surg Oral Med Oral Pathol 50:433–440, 1980.

Gardner DG, Daley TD. The use of the terms monomorphic adenoma, basal cell adenoma, and canalicular adenoma as applied to salivary gland tumors. Oral Surg Oral Med Oral Pathol 56:608–615, 1983.

Khullar SM, Best PV. Adenomatosis of minor salivary glands: Report of a case. Oral Surg Oral Med Oral Pathol 74:783–787, 1992.

Nelson JF, Jacoway JR. Monomorphic adenoma (canalicular type): Report of 29 cases. Cancer 31:1511–1513, 1973.

Neville BW, et al. Labial salivary gland tumors. Cancer 61:2113–2116, 1988.

Basal Cell Adenoma

Batsakis JG, Brannon RB. Dermal analogue tumours of major salivary glands. J Laryngol Otol 95:155–164, 1981.

Batsakis JG, Luna MA, El-Naggar AK. Basaloid monomorphic adenomas. Ann Otol Rhinol Laryngol 100:687–690, 1991.

Dardick I, et al. Salivary gland monomorphic adenoma: Ultrastructural, immunoperoxidase, and histogenetic aspects. Am J Pathol 115:334–348, 1984.

Ellis GL, Wiscovitch JG. Basal cell adenocarcinomas of the major salivary glands. Oral Surg Oral Med Oral Pathol 69:461–469, 1990.

Luna MA, Tortoledo ME, Allen M. Salivary dermal analogue tumors arising in lymph nodes. Cancer 59:1165–1169, 1987.

Nagao K, et al. Histopathologic studies of basal cell adenoma of the parotid gland. Cancer 50:736–745, 1982.

Pogrel MA. The intraoral basal cell adenoma. J Craniomaxillofac Surg 15:372–375, 1987.

Salivary Papillomas

Abbey LM. Solitary intraductal papilloma of the minor salivary glands. Oral Surg Oral Med Oral Pathol 40:135–140, 1975.

Abrams AM, Finck FM. Sialadenoma papilliferum: A previously unreported salivary gland tumor. Cancer 24:1057–1063, 1969.

Fantasia JE, Nocco CE, Lally ET. Ultrastructure of sialadenoma papilliferum. Arch Pathol Lab Med 110:523–527, 1986.

van der Wal JE, van der Waal I. The rare sialadenoma papilliferum: Report of a case and review of the literature. Int J Oral Maxillofac Surg 21:104–106, 1992.

White DK, et al. Inverted ductal papilloma: A distinctive lesion of minor salivary gland. Cancer 49:519–524, 1982.

Mucoepidermoid Carcinoma

Auclair PL, Goode RK, Ellis GL. Mucoepidermoid carcinoma of intraoral salivary glands. Cancer 69:2021–2030, 1992.

Batsakis JG, Luna MA. Histopathologic grading of salivary gland neoplasms: I. Mucoepidermoid carcinomas. Ann Otol Rhinol Laryngol 99:835–838, 1990.

Evans HL. Mucoepidermoid carcinoma of salivary glands: A study of 69 cases with special attention to histologic grading. Am J Clin Pathol 81:696–701, 1984.

Spiro RH, et al. Mucoepidermoid carcinoma of salivary gland origin: A clinicopathologic study of 367 cases. Am J Surg 136:461–468, 1978.

Stewart FW, Foote FW, Becker WF. Muco-epidermoid tumors of salivary glands. Ann Surg 122:820–844, 1945.

Intraosseous Mucoepidermoid Carcinoma

Brookstone MS, Huvos AG. Central salivary gland tumors of the maxilla and mandible: A clinicopathologic study of 11 cases with an analysis of the literature. J Oral Maxillofac Surg 50:229–236, 1992.

Browand BC, Waldron CA. Central mucoepidermoid tumors of the jaws. Oral Surg Oral Med Oral Pathol 40:631–643, 1975.

Waldron CA, Koh ML. Central mucoepidermoid carcinoma of the jaws: Report of four cases with analysis of the literature and discussion of the relationship to mucoepidermoid, sialodontogenic, and glandular odontogenic cysts. J Oral Maxillofac Surg 48:871–877, 1990.

Acinic Cell Adenocarcinoma

Batsakis JG, Luna MA, El-Naggar AK. Histopathologic grading of salivary gland neoplasms: II. Acinic cell carcinomas. Ann Otol Rhinol Laryngol 99:929–933, 1990.

Chen S-Y, et al. Acinic cell adenocarcinoma of minor salivary glands. Cancer 42:678–685, 1978.

Ellis GL, Corio RL. Acinic cell adenocarcinoma: A clinicopathologic analysis of 294 cases. Cancer 52:542–549, 1983.

Hamper K, et al. Acinic cell carcinoma of the salivary glands: The prognostic relevance of DNA cytophotometry in a retrospective study of long duration (1965–1987). Oral Surg Oral Med Oral Pathol 69:68–75, 1990.

Lewis JE, Olsen KD, Weiland LH. Acinic cell carcinoma: Clinicopathologic review. Cancer 67:172–179, 1991.

Perzin KH, LiVolsi VA. Acinic cell carcinomas arising in salivary glands: A clinicopathologic study. Cancer 44:1434–1457, 1979.

Malignant Mixed Tumor

LiVolsi VA, Perzin KH. Malignant mixed tumors arising in salivary glands I: Carcinomas arising in benign mixed tumor: A clinicopathologic study. Cancer 39:2209–2230, 1977.

Nagao K, et al. Histopathologic studies on carcinoma in pleomorphic adenoma of the parotid gland. Cancer 48:113–121, 1981.

Spiro RH, Huvos AG, Strong EW. Malignant mixed tumor of salivary origin: A clinicopathologic study of 146 cases. Cancer 39:388–396, 1977.

Tortoledo ME, Luna MA, Batsakis JG. Carcinomas ex pleomorphic adenoma and malignant mixed tumors. Arch Otolaryngol 110:172–176, 1984.

Adenoid Cystic Carcinoma

Batsakis JG, Luna MA, El-Naggar A. Histopathologic grading of salivary gland neoplasms: III. Adenoid cystic carcinomas. Ann Otol Rhinol Laryngol 99:1007–1009, 1990.

Hamper K, et al. Prognostic factors for adenoid cystic carcinoma of the head and neck: A retrospective evaluation of 96 cases. J Oral Pathol Med 19:101–107, 1990.

Perzin KH, Gullane P, Clairmont AC. Adenoid cystic carcinomas arising in salivary glands: A correlation of histologic features and clinical course. Cancer 42:265–282, 1978.

Spiro RH, Huvos AG. Stage means more than grade in adenoid cystic carcinoma. Am J Surg 164:623–628, 1992.

Szanto PA, et al. Histologic grading of adenoid cystic carcinoma of the salivary glands. Cancer 54:1062–1069, 1984.

van der Wal JE, Snow GB, van der Waal I. Intraoral adenoid cystic carcinoma: The presence of perineural spread in relation to site, size, local extension, and metastatic spread in 22 cases. Cancer 66:2031–2033, 1990.

Polymorphous Low-Grade Adenocarcinoma

Aberle AM, et al. Lobular (polymorphous low-grade) carcinoma of minor salivary glands: A clinicopathologic study of 20 cases. Oral Surg Oral Med Oral Pathol 60:387–395, 1985.

Batsakis JG, et al. Adenocarcinomas of the oral cavity: A clinicopathologic study of terminal duct carcinomas. J Laryngol Otol 97:825–835, 1983.

Colmenero CM, et al. Polymorphous low-grade adenocarcinoma of the oral cavity: A report of 14 cases. J Oral Maxillofac Surg 50:595–600, 1992.

Evans HL, Batsakis JG. Polymorphous low-grade adenocarcinoma of minor salivary glands: A study of 14 cases of a distinctive neoplasm. Cancer 53:935–942, 1984.

Freedman PD, Lumerman H. Lobular carcinoma of intraoral minor salivary glands. Oral Surg Oral Med Oral Pathol 56:157–165, 1983.

Gnepp DR, Chen JC, Warren C. Polymorphous low-grade adenocarcinoma of minor salivary gland: An immunohistochemical and clinicopathologic study. Am J Surg Pathol 12:461–468, 1988.

Salivary Adenocarcinoma

Spiro RH, Huvos AG, Strong EW. Adenocarcinoma of salivary origin: Clinicopathologic study of 204 patients. Am J Surg 144:423–431, 1982.

12

Soft Tissue Tumors

FIBROMA (Irritation Fibroma; Traumatic Fibroma; Focal Fibrous Hyperplasia; Fibrous Nodule)

The **fibroma** is the most common "tumor" of the oral cavity. However, it is doubtful that it represents a true neoplasm in most instances; rather, it is a reactive hyperplasia of fibrous connective tissue in response to local irritation or trauma.

Clinical Features

Although the irritation fibroma can occur anywhere in the mouth, the most common location is the buccal mucosa along the bite line. Presumably, this is a consequence of trauma from biting the cheek (Figs. 12–1 and 12–2; see Color Figure 79). The labial mucosa, tongue, and gingiva also are common sites (Figs. 12–3 and 12–4). The lesion typically presents as a smooth-surfaced pink nodule that is similar in color to the surrounding mucosa. In some cases, the surface may appear white as a result of hyperkeratosis from continued irritation. Most fibromas are sessile, although some are pedunculated. They range in size from tiny lesions that are only a couple of millimeters in diameter to large masses that are several centimeters across; however, most fibromas are 1.5 cm or less in diameter. The lesion usually produces no symptoms unless secondary traumatic ulceration of the surface has occurred. Irritation fibromas are most common in the fourth to sixth decades of life, and the male-to-female ratio is almost 1:2 for cases submitted for biopsy.

Histopathologic Features

Microscopic examination of the irritation fibroma shows a nodular mass of fibrous connective tissue covered by stratified squamous epithelium (Figs. 12–5 and 12–6). This connective tissue usually is dense and collagenized, although in some cases it is looser in nature. The lesion is not encapsulated; the fibrous tissue instead blends gradually into the surrounding connective tissues. The collagen bundles may be arranged in a radiating, circular, or haphazard fashion. The covering epithelium often demonstrates atrophy of the rete ridges because of the underlying fibrous mass. However, the surface may exhibit hyperkeratosis from secondary trauma. Scattered inflammation may be seen, most often beneath the epithelial surface. Usually, this inflammation is chronic in nature and consists mostly of lymphocytes and plasma cells.

Treatment and Prognosis

The irritation fibroma is treated by conservative surgical excision; recurrence is extremely rare. However, it is important to submit the excised tissue for microscopic examination because other benign or malignant tumors may mimic the clinical appearance of a fibroma.

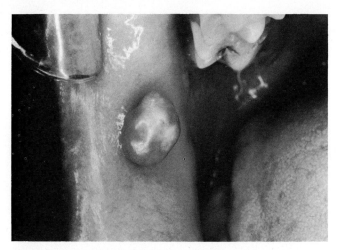

FIGURE 12–1. **Irritation fibroma.** Smooth-surfaced nodule on the buccal mucosa near the commissure.

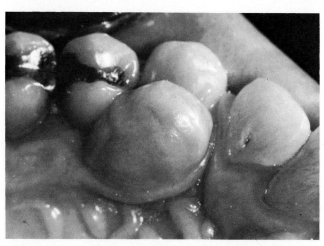

FIGURE 12–4. **Irritation fibroma.** Smooth-surfaced, pink nodular mass of the palatal gingiva between the cuspid and first bicuspid.

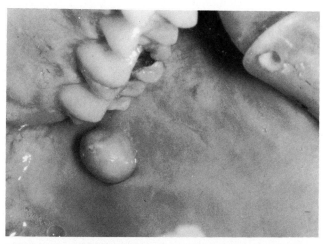

FIGURE 12–2. **Irritation fibroma.** Nodule of the posterior buccal mucosa near the level of the occlusal plane. See Color Plates.

GIANT CELL FIBROMA

The **giant cell fibroma** is a fibrous tumor with distinctive clinicopathologic features. It represents approximately 5 percent of all oral fibrous proliferations submitted for biopsy.

Clinical Features

The giant cell fibroma typically presents as an asymptomatic sessile or pedunculated nodule, usually less than 1 cm in size (Fig. 12–7). The surface of the mass often appears papillary; therefore, the lesion may be mistaken clinically for a papilloma. Compared with the common irritation fibroma, the lesion usually occurs at a younger age. In about 60 percent of cases, the lesion is diagnosed

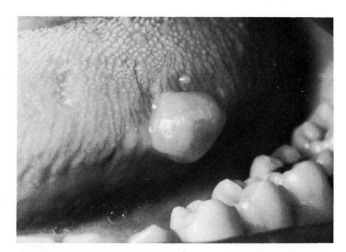

FIGURE 12–3. **Irritation fibroma.** Lesion on the lateral border of the tongue.

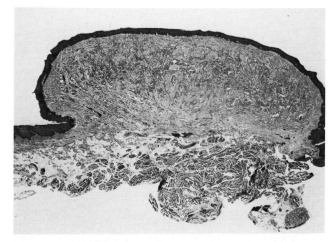

FIGURE 12–5. **Irritation fibroma.** Low-power view showing an exophytic nodular mass of dense fibrous connective tissue.

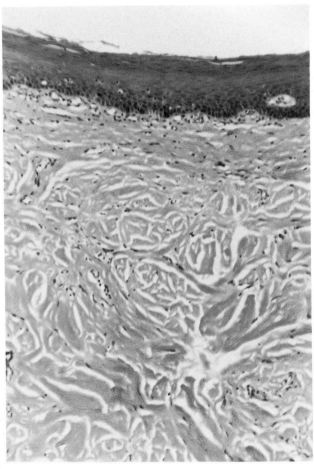

FIGURE 12-6. **Irritation fibroma.** High-power view demonstrating dense collagen beneath the epithelial surface.

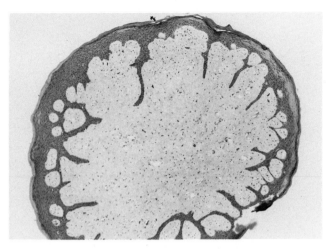

FIGURE 12-8. **Giant cell fibroma.** Low-power view showing a nodular mass of fibrous connective tissue covered by stratified squamous epithelium. Note the elongation of the rete ridges.

Histopathologic Features

Microscopic examination of the giant cell fibroma reveals a mass of vascular fibrous connective tissue, which usually is loosely arranged (Fig. 12-8). The hallmark is the presence of numerous large, stellate fibroblasts within the superficial connective tissue (Fig. 12-9). These cells may contain several nuclei. Frequently, the surface of the lesion is pebbly. The covering epithelium often is thin and atrophic, although the rete ridges may appear narrow and elongated.

Treatment and Prognosis

The giant cell fibroma is treated by conservative surgical excision. Recurrence is rare.

during the first three decades of life. There is a slight female predilection. Nearly 50 percent of all cases occur on the gingiva. The mandibular gingiva is affected twice as often as the maxillary gingiva. The tongue and palate also are common sites.

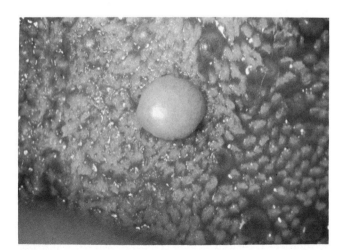

FIGURE 12-7. **Giant cell fibroma.** Exophytic nodule on the dorsum of the tongue.

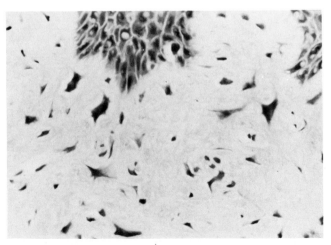

FIGURE 12-9. **Giant cell fibroma.** High-power view showing multiple large stellate-shaped and multinucleated fibroblasts beneath the surface epithelium.

EPULIS FISSURATUM (Inflammatory Fibrous Hyperplasia; Denture Injury Tumor; Denture Epulis)

The **epulis fissuratum** is a tumor-like hyperplasia of fibrous connective tissue that develops in association with the flange of an ill-fitting complete or partial denture. Although the simple term "epulis" sometimes is used synonymously for epulis fissuratum, epulis is actually a generic term that can be applied to any tumor of the gingiva or alveolar mucosa. Therefore, some authors have advocated not using this term, preferring to call these lesions "inflammatory fibrous hyperplasia" or other descriptive names. However, epulis fissuratum is still widely used today, and this term is well understood by virtually all clinicians. Other examples of epulides include the **giant cell epulis (peripheral giant cell granuloma)** (see p. 373), **ossifying fibroid epulis (peripheral ossifying fibroma)** (see p. 374), and **congenital epulis** (see p. 388).

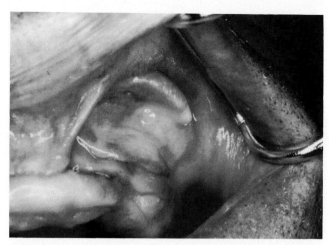

FIGURE 12–11. **Epulis fissuratum.** Several folds of hyperplastic tissue in the maxillary vestibule. (Courtesy of Dr. William Bruce.)

Clinical Features

The epulis fissuratum typically presents as a single or multiple fold(s) of hyperplastic tissue in the alveolar vestibule (Figs. 12–10 to 12–12). Most often, there are two folds of tissue, and the flange of the associated denture fits conveniently into the fissure between the folds. The redundant tissue usually is firm and fibrous, although some lesions appear erythematous and ulcerated similar to the appearance of a pyogenic granuloma. Occasional examples of epulis fissuratum demonstrate surface areas of inflammatory papillary hyperplasia (see next topic). The size of the lesion can vary from localized hyperplasias less than 1 cm in size to massive lesions that involve most of the length of the vestibule. The epulis fissuratum usually develops on the facial aspect of the alveolar ridge, although occasional lesions are seen lingual to the mandibular alveolar ridge (Fig. 12–13).

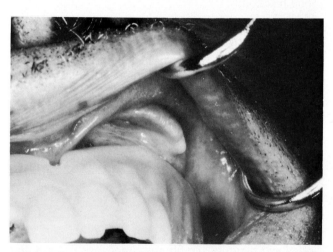

FIGURE 12–12. **Epulis fissuratum.** Same patient as depicted in Figure 12–11. An ill-fitting denture fits into the fissure between two of the folds. (Courtesy of Dr. William Bruce.)

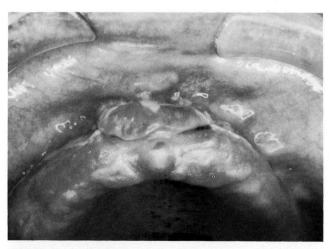

FIGURE 12–10. **Epulis fissuratum.** Hyperplastic fold of tissue in the maxillary labial vestibule.

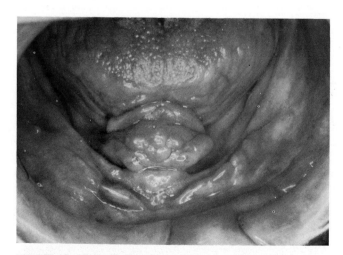

FIGURE 12–13. **Epulis fissuratum.** Redundant folds of tissue arising in the floor of the mouth in association with a mandibular denture.

The epulis fissuratum most often occurs in middle-aged and older adults, as would be expected with a denture-related lesion. It may occur on either the maxilla or mandible. The anterior portion of the jaws is affected much more often than the posterior areas. There is a pronounced female predilection; most studies show that two thirds to three fourths of all cases submitted for biopsy occur in women. The reason for this female predominance is uncertain, although various possibilities have been suggested:

1. Surveys show that more older women wear dentures than men do.
2. Women live longer than men.
3. Women seek dental treatment more frequently, which allows the clinical discovery of lesions.
4. Women wear their dentures more frequently and for longer periods than men do for esthetic reasons.
5. Postmenopausal hormonal changes may make the mucosal lining more susceptible to such a hyperplastic reaction.

Another similar but less common fibrous hyperplasia, often called a **fibroepithelial polyp** or **leaf-like denture fibroma**, occurs on the hard palate beneath a maxillary denture. This characteristic lesion presents as a flattened pink mass that is attached to the palate by a narrow stalk (Fig. 12–14). Usually, the flattened mass is closely applied to the palate and sits in a slightly cupped-out depression. However, it is easily lifted up with a probe, which demonstrates its pedunculated nature (Fig. 12–15). The edge of the lesion often is serrated and resembles a leaf.

Histopathologic Features

Microscopic examination of the epulis fissuratum reveals hyperplasia of the fibrous connective tissue. Often multiple folds and grooves occur where the denture impinges on the tissue (Fig. 12–16). The overlying epithelium frequently is hyperparakeratotic and demonstrates irregular hyperplasia of the rete ridges. In some instances, the epithelium shows inflammatory papillary hyperplasia (see next topic) or pseudoepitheliomatous (pseudocarcinomatous) hyperplasia. Focal areas of ulceration are not unusual, especially at the base of the grooves between the folds. A variable chronic inflammatory infiltrate is present; sometimes, it may include eosinophils or show lymphoid follicles. If minor salivary glands are included in the specimen, they usually show chronic sialadenitis.

In rare instances, the formation of osteoid or chondroid is observed. This unusual-appearing product, known as **osseous and chondromatous metaplasia**, is a reactive phenomenon caused by chronic irritation by the ill-fitting denture (see p. 230). The irregular nature of this bone or cartilage can be microscopically disturbing, and the pathologist should not mistake it for a sarcoma.

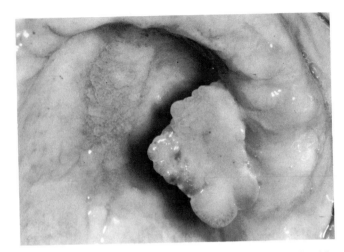

FIGURE 12–15. **Fibroepithelial polyp.** Same lesion as depicted in Figure 12–14; note its pedunculated nature. Because of its flattened appearance with a serrated edge, this lesion also is known as a **leaf-like denture fibroma**.

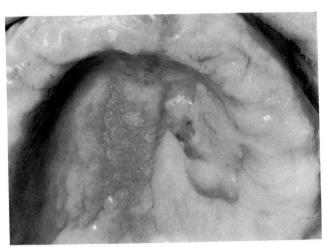

FIGURE 12–14. **Fibroepithelial polyp.** Flattened mass of tissue arising on the hard palate beneath a maxillary denture. Associated inflammatory papillary hyperplasia is visible in the midline.

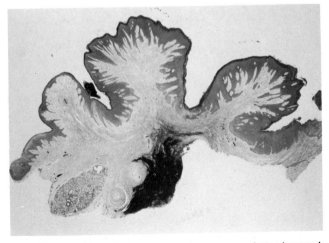

FIGURE 12–16. **Epulis fissuratum.** Low-power photomicrograph demonstrating multiple folds of hyperplastic fibrovascular connective tissue. The overlying epithelium also exhibits hyperplasia of the rete ridges.

The denture-related fibroepithelial polyp has a narrow core of dense fibrous connective tissue covered by stratified squamous epithelium. Like the epulis fissuratum, the overlying epithelium may be hyperplastic.

Treatment and Prognosis

The treatment of the epulis fissuratum or fibroepithelial polyp consists of surgical removal, with microscopic examination of the excised tissue. The ill-fitting denture should be remade or relined to prevent a recurrence of the lesion.

INFLAMMATORY PAPILLARY HYPERPLASIA (Denture Papillomatosis)

Inflammatory papillary hyperplasia is a reactive tissue growth that usually, although not always, develops beneath a denture. Some investigators classify this lesion as part of the spectrum of "denture sore mouth" (see p. 166). Although the exact pathogenesis is unknown, the condition most often appears to be related to:

- An ill-fitting denture
- Poor denture hygiene
- Wearing the denture 24 hours a day

Approximately 20 percent of patients who wear their dentures 24 hours a day have inflammatory papillary hyperplasia. *Candida* also has been suggested as a cause, but any possible role appears uncertain.

Clinical Features

Inflammatory papillary hyperplasia usually occurs on the hard palate beneath a denture base (Figs. 12–17 and 12–18; see Color Figure 80). Early lesions may involve only the palatal vault, although advanced cases cover most of the palate. Less frequently, this hyperplasia develops on the edentulous mandibular alveolar ridge or on

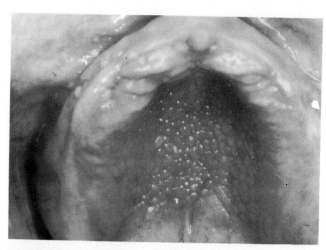

FIGURE 12–18. **Inflammatory papillary hyperplasia.** An advanced case exhibiting more pronounced papular lesions of the hard palate. See Color Plates.

the surface of an epulis fissuratum. On rare occasions, the condition occurs on the palate of a patient without a denture, especially in people who habitually breathe through their mouth or have a high palatal vault.

Inflammatory papillary hyperplasia is usually asymptomatic. The mucosa is erythematous and has a pebbly or papillary surface. Many cases are associated with denture sore mouth.

Histopathologic Features

The mucosa in inflammatory papillary hyperplasia exhibits numerous papillary growths on the surface that are covered by hyperplastic stratified squamous epithelium (Fig. 12–19). In advanced cases, this hyperplasia is pseudoepitheliomatous in appearance, and the pathologist should not mistake it for carcinoma (Fig. 12–20). The connective tissue can vary from loose and edematous to

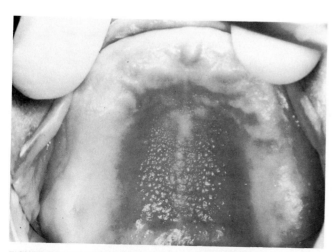

FIGURE 12–17. **Inflammatory papillary hyperplasia.** Erythematous, pebbly appearance of the palatal vault.

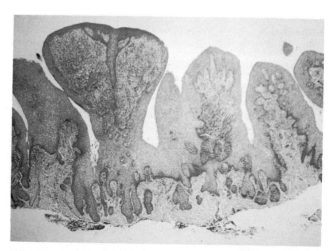

FIGURE 12–19. **Inflammatory papillary hyperplasia.** Low-power view showing fibrous and epithelial hyperplasia resulting in multiple papillary surface projections. Note the pseudoepitheliomatous hyperplasia of the epithelium into the connective tissue at the base of the specimen.

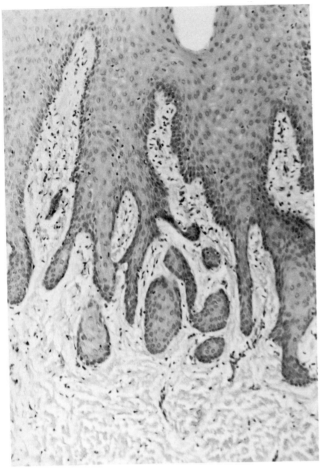

FIGURE 12–20. **Inflammatory papillary hyperplasia.** Higher-power view of the pseudoepitheliomatous hyperplasia of the epithelium. Note the bland appearance of this epithelium, which should not be mistaken for carcinoma.

densely collagenized. A chronic inflammatory cell infiltrate usually is seen, which consists of lymphocytes and plasma cells. Less frequently, polymorphonuclear leukocytes are also present. If underlying salivary glands are present, they often show sclerosing sialadenitis.

Treatment and Prognosis

For very early lesions of inflammatory papillary hyperplasia, removal of the denture may allow the erythema and edema to subside, and the tissues may resume a more normal appearance. For more advanced and collagenized lesions, many clinicians prefer to excise the hyperplastic tissue before fabricating a new denture. Various surgical methods have been used, including:

- Partial thickness or full-thickness surgical blade excision
- Curettage
- Electrosurgery
- Cryosurgery

After healing, the patient should be encouraged to leave the new denture out at night and to keep it clean.

FIBROUS HISTIOCYTOMA

Fibrous histiocytomas are a diverse group of tumors that exhibit both fibroblastic and histiocytic differentiation. Although the cell of origin is still uncertain, it may arise from the tissue histiocyte, which then assumes fibroblastic properties. Because of their variable nature, an array of terms has been used for these lesions, including **dermatofibroma**, **sclerosing hemangioma**, **fibroxanthoma**, and **nodular subepidermal fibrosis**.

Clinical Features

The fibrous histiocytoma can develop almost anywhere in the body. The most common site is the skin of the extremities, where the lesion is called a dermatofibroma. Tumors of the oral and perioral region are uncommon. Although oral tumors can occur at any site, the most frequent location is the buccal mucosa and vestibule. Rare intrabony lesions of the jaws have also been reported. Oral fibrous histiocytomas tend to occur in middle-aged and older adults; cutaneous examples are most frequent in young adults. The tumor usually presents as a painless nodular mass, and can vary in size from a few millimeters to several centimeters in diameter (Fig. 12–21). Deeper tumors tend to be larger.

Histopathologic Features

Microscopically, the fibrous histiocytoma is characterized by a cellular proliferation of spindle-shaped fibroblastic cells with vesicular nuclei (Figs. 12–22 and 12–23). The margins of the tumor often are not sharply defined. The tumor cells are arranged in short, intersecting fascicles, known as a "storiform" pattern because of its resemblance to the irregular, whorled appearance of a straw mat. Rounded histiocyte-like cells, lipid-containing xanthoma cells, or multinucleated giant cells occasionally can be seen, as may scattered lymphocytes. The stroma may demonstrate areas of myxoid change or focal hyalinization.

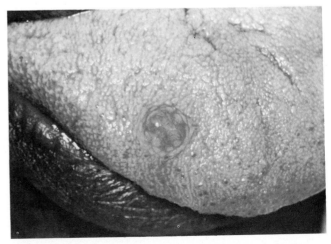

FIGURE 12–21. **Fibrous histiocytoma.** Nodular mass on the dorsum of the tongue.

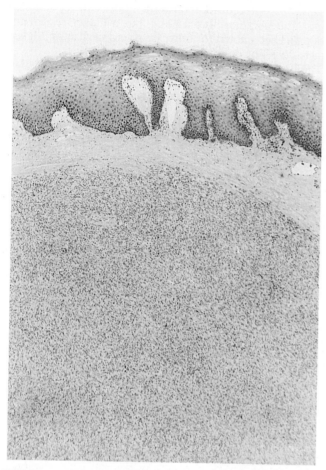

FIGURE 12–22. **Fibrous histiocytoma.** Low-power view showing a cellular tumor separated from the surface epithelium by a zone of fibrous connective tissue (*arrow*).

Treatment and Prognosis

Local surgical excision is the treatment of choice. Recurrence is uncommon, especially for superficial tumors. Larger lesions of the deeper soft tissues have a greater potential to recur.

FIBROMATOSIS AND MYOFIBROMATOSIS

The **fibromatoses** are a broad group of fibrous proliferations. They have a biologic behavior and histopathologic pattern that is intermediate between those of benign fibrous lesions and fibrosarcoma. A number of different forms of fibromatosis are recognized throughout the body, and they often are named on the basis of their particular clinicopathologic features. In the soft tissues of the head and neck, these lesions are frequently called **juvenile aggressive fibromatoses** or **extra-abdominal desmoids.** Similar lesions within the bone have been called **desmoplastic fibromas** (see p. 480).

Myofibromatosis is a similar but less aggressive proliferation that consists of myofibroblasts, i.e., cells with both smooth muscle and fibroblastic features. Such cells are not specific for this lesion, however, since they also can be identified in other fibrous proliferations.

Clinical and Radiographic Features

Soft tissue fibromatosis of the head and neck presents as a firm, painless mass, which may be either rapid or insidious in growth (Fig. 12–24). The lesion usually occurs in children or young adults (mean age, 8 to 11 years), hence, the term **juvenile fibromatosis**. However, rare cases have also been seen in middle-aged adults. The most common oral site is the paramandibular soft tissue region, although the lesion can occur almost anywhere. The tumor can grow to considerable size, resulting in significant facial disfigurement. Destruction of adjacent bone may be observed on radiographs.

Myofibromatosis primarily affects neonates and infants, but it also rarely has been reported in adults. It most frequently arises as a firm mass in the dermis or subcutaneous tissues of the head and neck. Intraosseous examples also have been reported. Myofibromatosis is most often solitary in nature, although multiple lesions may occur.

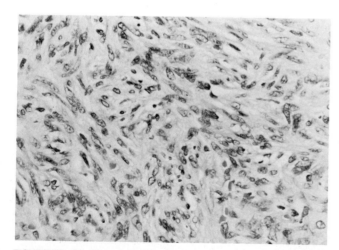

FIGURE 12–23. **Fibrous histiocytoma.** High-power view demonstrating storiform arrangement of spindle-shaped cells with vesicular nuclei.

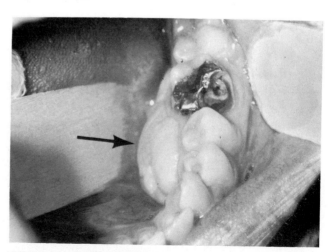

FIGURE 12–24. **Fibromatosis.** Locally aggressive proliferation of fibrous connective tissue (*arrow*).

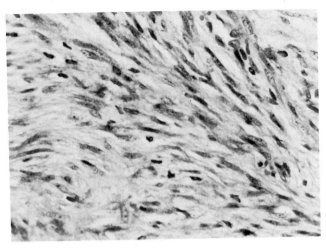

FIGURE 12–25. **Fibromatosis.** Streaming fascicles of fibroblastic cells demonstrating little pleomorphism.

Histopathologic Features

Soft tissue fibromatosis is characterized by a cellular proliferation of spindle-shaped cells that are arranged in streaming fascicles and are associated with a variable amount of collagen (Fig. 12–25). The lesion usually is poorly circumscribed and infiltrates the adjacent tissues. Hyperchromatism and pleomorphism of the cells should not be observed.

Myofibromatosis demonstrates a somewhat similar microscopic pattern (Fig. 12–26). The cells at the periphery often demonstrate marked eosinophilia, which is reminiscent of smooth muscle. Centrally, the lesion is more vascular with a hemangiopericytoma-like appearance.

Treatment and Prognosis

Because of its locally aggressive nature, the preferred treatment for soft tissue fibromatosis is wide excision that includes a generous margin of adjacent normal tis-

sues. A 23 percent recurrence rate has been reported for oral and paraoral fibromatosis, but a higher recurrence rate has been noted for other head and neck sites. Metastasis does not occur.

Solitary lesions of myofibromatosis pursue a benign course, and the patient may need only a biopsy for diagnostic purposes. Spontaneous regression may occur in some cases. The prognosis for multicentric lesions with visceral involvement is less favorable; some infants die soon after birth with symptoms of respiratory distress or diarrhea.

ORAL FOCAL MUCINOSIS

Oral focal mucinosis is an uncommon tumor-like mass that is believed to represent the oral counterpart of **cutaneous focal mucinosis** or a **cutaneous myxoid cyst**. The cause is unknown, although the lesion may result from overproduction of hyaluronic acid by fibroblasts.

Clinical Features

Oral focal mucinosis is most common in young adults and shows a 2 : 1 female-to-male predilection. The gingiva is the most common site; two thirds to three fourths of all cases are found there. The hard palate is the second most common location. The mass rarely appears at other oral sites. The lesion usually presents as a sessile, painless nodular mass that is the same color as the surrounding mucosa (Fig. 12–27). The surface is typically smooth and non-ulcerated, although occasional cases exhibit a lobulated appearance. The size varies from a few millimeters up to 2 cm in diameter. The patient often has been aware of the mass for many months or years before the diagnosis is made.

Histopathologic Features

Microscopic examination of oral focal mucinosis shows a well-localized but non-encapsulated area of

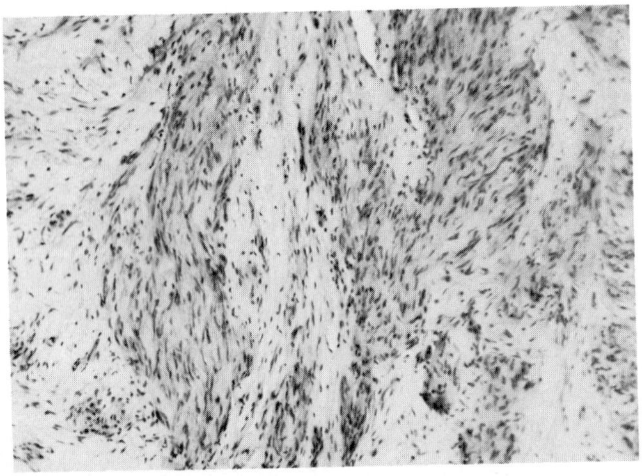

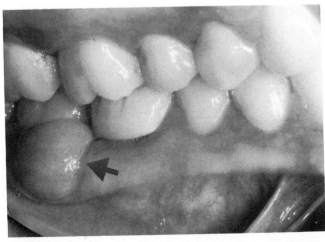

FIGURE 12–26. **Myofibromatosis.** Proliferation of spindle-shaped cells with both fibroblastic and smooth muscle features.

FIGURE 12–27. **Oral focal mucinosis.** Nodular mass arising from the gingiva between the mandibular first and second molars (*arrow*).

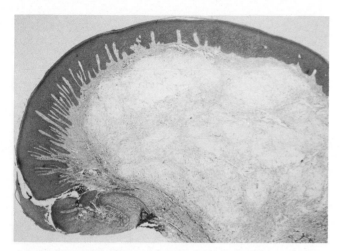

FIGURE 12-28. **Oral focal mucinosis.** Low-power view showing a nodular mass of loose, myxomatous connective tissue.

loose, myxomatous connective tissue surrounded by denser, normal collagenous connective tissue (Figs. 12–28 and 12–29). The lesion usually is found just beneath the surface epithelium and often causes flattening of the rete ridges. The fibroblasts within the mucinous area can be ovoid, fusiform, or stellate, and they may demonstrate

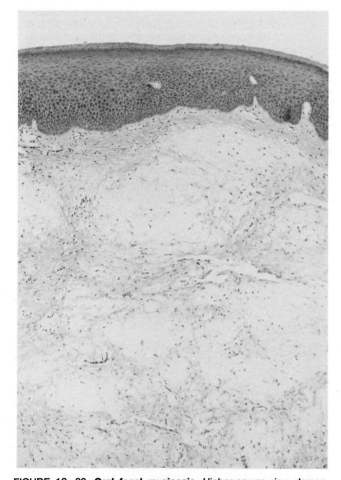

FIGURE 12-29. **Oral focal mucinosis.** Higher-power view demonstrating the myxomatous change to the connective tissue.

delicate, fibrillar processes. Few capillaries are seen within the lesion, especially compared with the surrounding denser collagen. Similarly, no significant inflammation is observed, although a perivascular lymphocytic infiltrate often is noted within the surrounding collagenous connective tissue. No appreciable reticulin is evident within the lesion, and special stains suggest that the mucinous product is hyaluronic acid.

Treatment and Prognosis

Oral focal mucinosis is treated by surgical excision and does not tend to recur.

PYOGENIC GRANULOMA

The **pyogenic granuloma** is a common tumor-like growth of the oral cavity that is considered to be non-neoplastic in nature. Although it originally was thought to be caused by pyogenic organisms, it is now believed to be unrelated to infection. Instead, the pyogenic granuloma is thought to represent an exuberant tissue response to local irritation or trauma. In spite of its name, it is not a true granuloma.

Clinical Features

The pyogenic granuloma presents as a smooth or lobulated mass that usually is pedunculated, although some lesions are sessile (Figs. 12–30 [see Color Figure 81] to 12–32). The surface characteristically is ulcerated and ranges from pink to red to purple, depending on the age of the lesion. Young pyogenic granulomas are highly vascular in appearance; older lesions tend to become more collagenized and pink. They vary from small growths only a few millimeters in size to larger lesions that may measure several centimeters in diameter. Typically, the mass is painless, although it often bleeds easily because of its extreme vascularity. Pyogenic granulomas may exhibit rapid growth, which may create alarm for

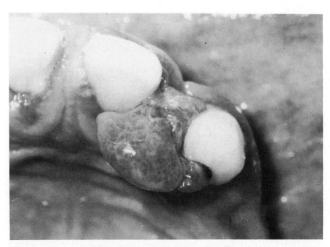

FIGURE 12-30. **Pyogenic granuloma.** Erythematous, hemorrhagic mass arising from the maxillary anterior gingiva. See Color Plates.

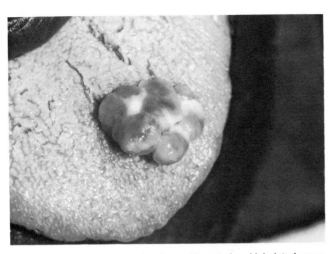

FIGURE 12–31. **Pyogenic granuloma.** Ulcerated and lobulated mass on the dorsum of the tongue.

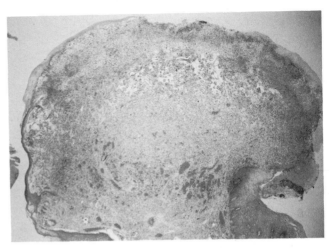

FIGURE 12–33. **Pyogenic granuloma.** Low-power view showing an exophytic mass of granulation-like tissue with an ulcerated surface.

both the patient and clinician, who may fear that the lesion might be malignant.

Oral pyogenic granulomas show a striking predilection for the gingiva, which accounts for 75 percent of all cases. Gingival irritation and inflammation that result from poor oral hygiene may be a precipitating factor in many patients. The lips, tongue, and buccal mucosa are the next most common sites. A history of trauma before the development of the lesion is not unusual, especially for extragingival pyogenic granulomas. Lesions are slightly more common on the maxillary gingiva than the mandibular gingiva; anterior areas are more frequently affected than posterior areas. These lesions are much more common on the facial aspect of the gingiva than the lingual aspect; some extend between the teeth and involve both the facial and lingual gingiva.

Although the pyogenic granuloma can develop at any age, it is most common in children and young adults. Most studies also demonstrate a definite female predilection, possibly due to the vascular effects of female hor-

mones. Pyogenic granulomas of the gingiva frequently develop in pregnant women, so much so, that the terms "pregnancy tumor" or "granuloma gravidarum" are often used. Such lesions may begin to develop during the first trimester, and their incidence increases up through the seventh month of pregnancy. The gradual rise in development of these lesions throughout pregnancy may be related to the increasing levels of estrogen and progesterone as the pregnancy progresses. After pregnancy and the return of normal hormone levels, some of these pyogenic granulomas resolve without treatment or undergo fibrous maturation and resemble a fibroma.

Histopathologic Features

Microscopic examination of pyogenic granulomas shows a highly vascular proliferation that resembles granulation tissue (Figs. 12–33 and 12–34). Numerous small and larger endothelium-lined channels are formed

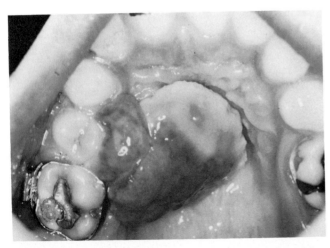

FIGURE 12–32. **Pyogenic granuloma.** Unusually large lesion arising from the palatal gingiva in association with an orthodontic band. The patient was pregnant.

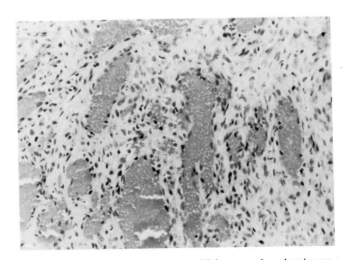

FIGURE 12–34. **Pyogenic granuloma.** High-power view showing engorged capillary blood vessels.

that are engorged with red blood cells. These vessels are sometimes organized in lobular aggregates, and some pathologists require this lobular arrangement for the diagnosis. The surface usually is ulcerated and replaced by a thick fibrinopurulent membrane. A mixed inflammatory cell infiltrate of neutrophils, plasma cells, and lymphocytes is evident. Neutrophils are most prevalent near the ulcerated surface; chronic inflammatory cells are found deeper in the specimen. Older lesions may have areas with a more fibrous appearance. In fact, many gingival fibromas probably represent pyogenic granulomas that have undergone fibrous maturation.

Treatment and Prognosis

The treatment of patients with pyogenic granuloma consists of conservative surgical excision down to periosteum, which usually is curative. The specimen should be submitted for microscopic examination to rule out other more serious diagnoses. For gingival lesions, the adjacent teeth should be thoroughly scaled to remove any source of continuing irritation. Occasionally, the lesion recurs and re-excision is necessary. In rare instances, multiple recurrences have been noted.

For lesions that develop during pregnancy, treatment usually should be deferred unless significant functional or aesthetic problems develop. The recurrence rate is higher for pyogenic granulomas removed during pregnancy, and some lesions will resolve spontaneously after parturition.

PERIPHERAL GIANT CELL GRANULOMA (Giant Cell Epulis)

The **peripheral giant cell granuloma** is a relatively common tumor-like growth of the oral cavity. It probably does not represent a true neoplasm but rather is a reactive lesion caused by local irritation or trauma. In the past, it was often called a peripheral giant cell "reparative" granuloma, but any reparative nature appears doubtful. Current immunohistochemical evidence indicates that the giant cells within the lesion show features of osteoclasts. The peripheral giant cell granuloma bears a close microscopic resemblance to the **central giant cell granuloma** (see p. 453), and some pathologists believe that it may represent a soft tissue counterpart of this central bony lesion.

Clinical and Radiographic Features

The peripheral giant cell granuloma occurs exclusively on the gingiva or edentulous alveolar ridge, presenting as a red or reddish-blue nodular mass (Figs. 12–35 [see Color Figure 82] and 12–36). Most lesions are smaller than 2 cm in diameter, although larger ones are seen occasionally. The lesion can be sessile or pedunculated and may or may not be ulcerated. The clinical appearance is similar to the more common pyogenic granuloma of the gingiva (see p. 371), although the peripheral giant cell granuloma often is more bluish-purple compared with the bright-red of a typical pyogenic granuloma.

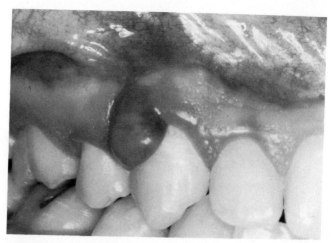

FIGURE 12–35. **Peripheral giant cell granuloma.** Nodular reddish-purple mass of the maxillary gingiva. See Color Plates. (Courtesy of Dr. Lewis Claman.)

Peripheral giant cell granulomas can develop at almost any age but show a peak prevalence in the fifth and sixth decades of life. Approximately 60 percent of cases occur in females. It may develop in either the anterior or posterior regions of the gingiva or alveolar mucosa, and the mandible is affected slightly more often than the maxilla. Although the peripheral giant cell granuloma develops within soft tissue, "cupping" resorption of the underlying alveolar bone sometimes is seen. On occasion, it may be difficult to determine whether the mass arose as a peripheral lesion or as a central giant cell granuloma that eroded through the cortical plate into the gingival soft tissues.

Histopathologic Features

Microscopic examination of a peripheral giant cell granuloma shows a proliferation of multinucleated giant cells within a background of plump ovoid and spindle-shaped mesenchymal cells (Figs. 12–37 and 12–38). The giant cells may contain only a few nuclei or up to several

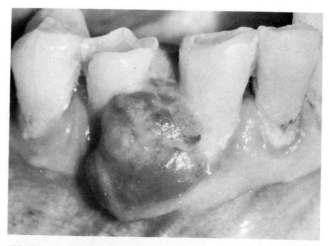

FIGURE 12–36. **Peripheral giant cell granuloma.** Ulcerated mass of the mandibular gingiva.

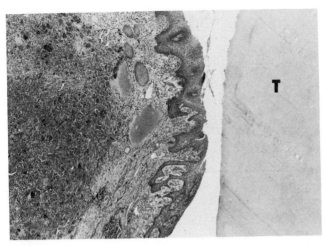

FIGURE 12-37. **Peripheral giant cell granuloma.** Low-power view showing a nodular proliferation of multinucleated giant cells within the gingiva (*left*). The adjacent tooth (T) is on the right.

dozen. Some of these cells may have large, vesicular nuclei; others demonstrate small, pyknotic nuclei. Mitotic figures are fairly common in the background mesenchymal cells. Abundant hemorrhage is characteristically found throughout the mass, which often results in deposits of hemosiderin pigment, especially at the periphery of the lesion.

The overlying mucosal surface is ulcerated in about 50 percent of cases. A zone of dense fibrous connective tissue usually separates the giant cell proliferation from the mucosal surface. Adjacent acute and chronic inflammatory cells are frequently present. Areas of reactive bone formation or dystrophic calcifications are not unusual.

Treatment and Prognosis

The treatment of the peripheral giant cell granuloma consists of local surgical excision down to the underlying bone. The adjacent teeth should be carefully scaled to

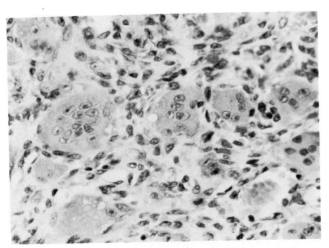

FIGURE 12-38. **Peripheral giant cell granuloma.** High-power view showing several multinucleated giant cells within a background of ovoid and spindle-shaped mesenchymal cells.

remove any source of irritation and to minimize the risk of recurrence. Approximately 10 percent of lesions are reported to recur, and re-excision must be performed. On rare occasions, lesions indistinguishable from peripheral giant cell granulomas have been seen in patients with hyperparathyroidism (see p. 612). They apparently represent the so-called osteoclastic "brown tumors" associated with this endocrine disorder. However, the brown tumors of hyperparathyroidism are much more likely to be intraosseous in location and mimic a central giant cell granuloma.

PERIPHERAL OSSIFYING FIBROMA
(Ossifying Fibroid Epulis; Peripheral Fibroma With Calcification; Calcifying Fibroblastic Granuloma)

The **peripheral ossifying fibroma** is a relatively common gingival growth that is considered to be reactive rather than neoplastic in nature. The pathogenesis of this lesion is uncertain. Because of their clinical and histopathologic similarities, some peripheral ossifying fibromas are thought to develop initially as pyogenic granulomas that undergo fibrous maturation and subsequent calcification. However, not all peripheral ossifying fibromas may develop in this manner. The mineralized product probably has its origin from cells of the periosteum or periodontal ligament.

Considerable confusion has existed over the nomenclature of this lesion, and several terms have been used to describe its variable histopathologic features. In the past, the terms peripheral odontogenic fibroma (see p. 536) and peripheral ossifying fibroma often were used synonymously, but the peripheral odontogenic fibroma is now considered to be a distinct and separate entity. Also, in spite of the similarity in names, the peripheral ossifying fibroma does not represent the soft tissue counterpart of the central ossifying fibroma (see p. 469).

Clinical Features

The peripheral ossifying fibroma occurs exclusively on the gingiva. It presents as a nodular mass, either pedunculated or sessile, that usually emanates from the interdental papilla (Figs. 12-39 and 12-40). The color ranges from red to pink, and the surface is frequently, but not always, ulcerated. The growth probably begins as an ulcerated lesion; older ones are more likely to demonstrate healing of the ulcer and an intact surface. Red, ulcerated lesions often are mistaken for pyogenic granulomas; the pink, non-ulcerated ones are similar clinically to irritation fibromas. Most lesions are less than 2 cm in size, although larger ones occasionally occur. The lesion has often been present for many weeks or months before the diagnosis is made.

The peripheral ossifying fibroma is predominantly a lesion of teen-agers and young adults, with a peak prevalence between the ages of 10 and 19. Almost two thirds of all cases occur in females. There is a slight predilection for the maxillary arch, and more than 50 percent of all

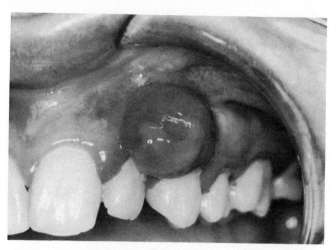

FIGURE 12–39. **Peripheral ossifying fibroma.** Red, ulcerated mass of the maxillary gingiva. Such ulcerated lesions are easily mistaken for a pyogenic granuloma.

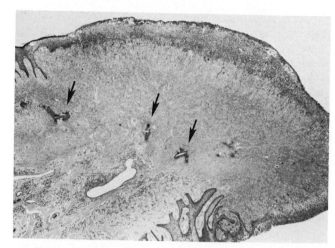

FIGURE 12–41. **Peripheral ossifying fibroma.** Ulcerated gingival mass demonstrating focal early mineralization (*arrows*).

cases occur in the incisor-cuspid region. Usually, the teeth are unaffected; rarely, there can be migration and loosening of adjacent teeth.

Histopathologic Features

The basic microscopic pattern of the peripheral ossifying fibroma is one of a fibrous proliferation associated with the formation of a mineralized product (Figs. 12–41 to 12–43). If the epithelium is ulcerated, the surface is covered by a fibrinopurulent membrane with a subjacent zone of granulation tissue. The deeper fibroblastic component often is cellular, especially in areas of mineralization. In some cases, the fibroblastic proliferation and associated mineralization is only a small component of a larger mass that resembles a fibroma or pyogenic granuloma.

The type of mineralized component is variable and may consist of bone, cementum-like material, or dystrophic calcifications. Frequently, a combination of

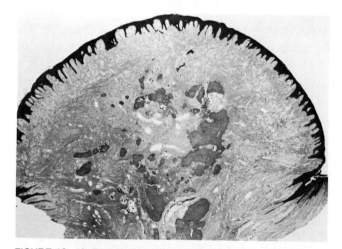

FIGURE 12–42. **Peripheral ossifying fibroma.** Non-ulcerated fibrous mass of the gingiva showing central bone formation.

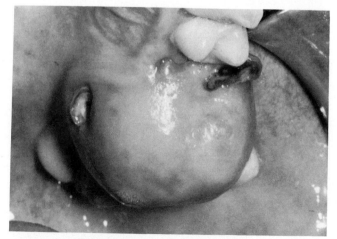

FIGURE 12–40. **Peripheral ossifying fibroma.** Pink, non-ulcerated mass arising from the maxillary gingiva. The remaining roots of the first molar are present.

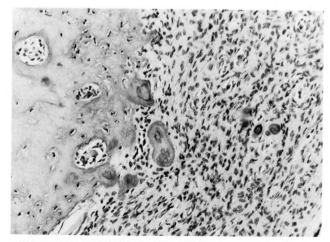

FIGURE 12–43. **Peripheral ossifying fibroma.** High-power view showing formation of bone and droplet calcifications within a cellular fibrous stroma.

products is formed. Usually, the bone is woven and tra-becular in type, although older lesions may demonstrate mature lamellar bone. Trabeculae of unmineralized osteoid are not unusual. Less frequently, ovoid droplets of basophilic cementum-like material are formed. Dystrophic calcifications are characterized by multiple granules, tiny globules, or large, irregular masses of basophilic mineralized material. Such dystrophic calcifications are more common in early, ulcerated lesions; older, non-ulcerated fibromas are more likely to demonstrate well-formed bone or cementum. In some cases, multinucleated giant cells may be found, usually in association with the mineralized product.

Treatment and Prognosis

The treatment of choice for the peripheral ossifying fibroma is local surgical excision with submission of the specimen for histopathologic examination. The mass should be excised down to periosteum because recurrence is more likely if the base of the lesion is allowed to remain. In addition, the adjacent teeth should be thoroughly scaled to eliminate any possible irritants. Although excision usually is curative, a recurrence rate of 16 percent has been reported.

LIPOMA

The **lipoma** is a benign tumor of fat. Although it represents by far the most common mesenchymal neoplasm, most examples occur on the trunk and proximal portions of the extremities. Lipomas of the oral and maxillofacial region are much less frequent. The pathogenesis of lipomas is uncertain, but they appear to be more common in obese people. However, the metabolism of lipomas is completely independent of the normal body fat. If the caloric intake is reduced, lipomas do not decrease in size, although normal body fat may be lost.

Clinical Features

Oral lipomas usually present as soft, smooth-surfaced nodular masses that can be sessile or pedunculated (Fig. 12-44). Typically, the tumor is asymptomatic and often has been noted for many months or years before diagnosis. Most are less than 3 cm in size, but occasional lesions can become much larger. Although a subtle or more obvious yellow hue often is detected clinically, deeper examples may appear pink. The buccal mucosa and buccal vestibule are the most common intraoral sites and account for 50 percent of all cases. Some buccal cases may not represent true tumors, but rather herniation of the buccal fat pad. Less common sites include the tongue, floor of the mouth, and lips. Most patients are 40 years of age or older; lipomas are uncommon in children. Although lipomas elsewhere in the body are reported to be twice as common in females as in males, oral lipomas are characterized by a more equal sex distribution.

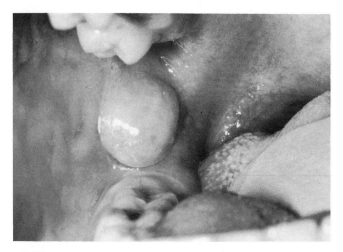

FIGURE 12-44. **Lipoma.** Nodular mass of the posterior buccal mucosa.

Histopathologic Features

Most oral lipomas are composed of mature fat cells that differ little in microscopic appearance from the surrounding normal fat (Figs. 12-45 and 12-46). The tumor usually is well circumscribed and may demon-

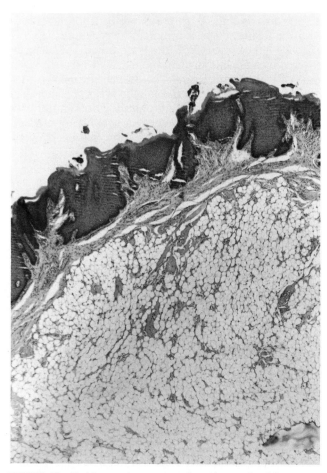

FIGURE 12-45. **Lipoma.** Low-power view of a tumor of the tongue demonstrating a mass of mature adipose tissue.

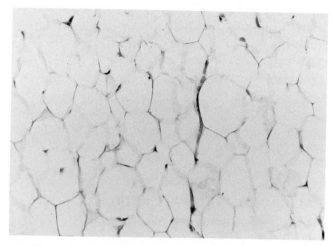

FIGURE 12–46. **Lipoma.** High-power view of the same lesion depicted in Figure 12–45. Note the similarity of the tumor cells to normal fat.

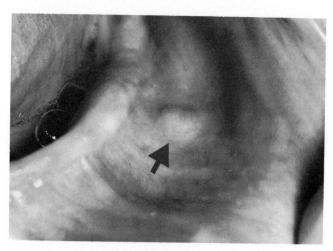

FIGURE 12–47. **Traumatic neuroma.** Painful nodule of the mental nerve as it exits the mental foramen (*arrow*).

strate a thin fibrous capsule. A distinct lobular arrangement of the cells often is seen. On rare occasions, central cartilaginous or osseous metaplasia may occur within an otherwise typical lipoma.

A number of microscopic variants have been described. The most common of these is the **fibrolipoma**, characterized by a significant fibrous component intermixed with the lobules of fat cells. The remaining variants are rare.

The **angiolipoma** consists of an admixture of mature fat and numerous small blood vessels. **Myxoid lipomas** exhibit a mucoid background and may be confused with myxoid liposarcomas. The **spindle cell lipoma** demonstrates variable amounts of uniform-appearing spindle cells in conjunction with a more typical lipomatous component. **Pleomorphic lipomas** are characterized by the presence of spindle cells plus bizarre, hyperchromatic giant cells; they can be difficult to distinguish from a pleomorphic liposarcoma. **Intramuscular (infiltrating) lipomas** often are more deeply situated and have an infiltrative growth pattern that extends between skeletal muscle bundles.

Treatment and Prognosis

Lipomas are treated by conservative local excision, and recurrence is rare. Most microscopic variants do not affect the prognosis. Intramuscular lipomas have a higher recurrence rate because of their infiltrative growth pattern, but this variant is rare in the oral and maxillofacial region.

TRAUMATIC NEUROMA
(Amputation Neuroma)

The **traumatic neuroma** is not a true neoplasm but a reactive proliferation of neural tissue after transection or other damage of a nerve bundle. After a nerve has been damaged or severed, the proximal portion attempts to regenerate and re-establish innervation of the distal segment by the growth of axons through tubes of proliferating Schwann cells. If these regenerating elements encounter scar tissue or otherwise cannot re-establish innervation, a tumor-like mass may develop at the site of injury.

Clinical and Radiographic Features

Traumatic neuromas of the oral mucosa typically present as smooth-surfaced, non-ulcerated nodules. They can develop at any location but are most common in the mental foramen area, tongue, and lower lip (Figs. 12–47 and 12–48). A history of trauma often can be elicited; some lesions arise subsequent to tooth extraction or other oral surgical procedures. Intraosseous examples

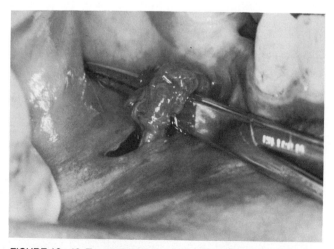

FIGURE 12–48. **Traumatic neuroma.** Note the irregular nodular proliferation along the mental nerve that is being exposed at the time of surgery.

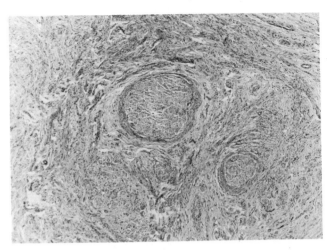

FIGURE 12-49. Traumatic neuroma. Low-power view showing the haphazard arrangement of nerve bundles within the background fibrous connective tissue.

also can occur and may demonstrate a radiolucent defect on oral radiographs.

Traumatic neuromas can occur at any age, but they are diagnosed most often in middle-aged adults. They appear to be slightly more common in females. Although pain traditionally has been considered a hallmark of this lesion, studies indicate that only one fourth to one third of oral traumatic neuromas are painful. This pain can be intermittent or constant and ranges from mild tenderness or burning to severe radiating pain. Neuromas of the mental nerve frequently are painful, especially when palpated or impinged on by a denture.

Histopathologic Features

Microscopic examination of traumatic neuromas shows a haphazard proliferation of mature, myelinated nerve bundles within a fibrous connective tissue stroma that ranges from densely collagenized to myxomatous in nature (Figs. 12-49 and 12-50). An associated mild chronic inflammatory cell infiltrate may be present.

Traumatic neuromas with inflammation are more likely to be painful than those without significant inflammation.

Treatment and Prognosis

The treatment of choice for the patient with a traumatic neuroma is surgical excision, including a small portion of the involved nerve bundle. Most lesions do not recur; in some cases, however, the pain persists or returns at a later date.

PALISADED ENCAPSULATED NEUROMA (Solitary Circumscribed Neuroma)

The **palisaded encapsulated neuroma** is a benign neural tumor with distinctive clinical and histopathologic features. Although it was first recognized only as late as 1972, it represents one of the more common superficial nerve tumors, especially in the head and neck region. The cause is uncertain, but some authors have speculated that trauma may play an etiologic role.

Clinical Features

The palisaded encapsulated neuroma shows a striking predilection for the face, which accounts for approximately 90 percent of reported cases. The nose and cheek are the most common specific sites. The lesion is most frequently diagnosed between the fifth and seventh decades of life, although the tumor often has been present for many months or years. It presents as a smooth-surfaced, painless, dome-shaped papule or nodule that is usually less than 1 cm in diameter. There is no sex predilection.

Oral palisaded encapsulated neuromas are not uncommon, although many are probably diagnosed microscopically as neurofibromas or neurilemomas. The lesion appears most frequently on the hard palate (Fig. 12-51), although it also may occur in other oral locations.

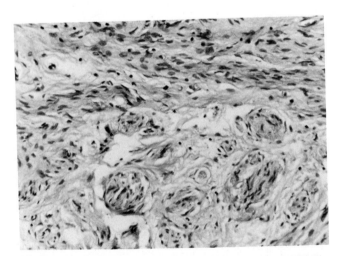

FIGURE 12-50. Traumatic neuroma. High-power view showing irregular nerve bundles within moderately dense fibrous connective tissue.

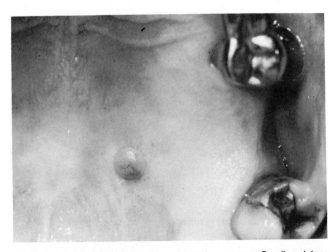

FIGURE 12-51. Palisaded encapsulated neuroma. Small, painless nodule of the lateral hard palate.

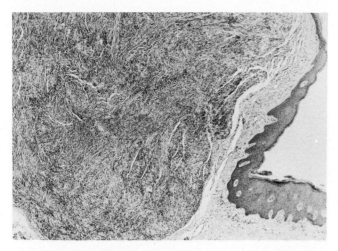

FIGURE 12–52. **Palisaded encapsulated neuroma.** Low-power view showing a well-circumscribed, nodular proliferation of neural tissue.

Histopathologic Features

Palisaded encapsulated neuromas appear well circumscribed and often encapsulated (Fig. 12–52), although this capsule may be incomplete, especially along the superficial aspect of the tumor. Some lesions have a lobulated appearance. The tumor consists of moderately cellular interlacing fascicles of spindle cells that are consistent with Schwann cells (Fig. 12–53). The nuclei are characteristically wavy and pointed, with no significant pleomorphism or mitotic activity. Although the nuclei show a similar parallel orientation within the fascicles, the more definite palisading and *Verocay bodies* typical of the *Antoni A* tissue of a neurilemoma usually are not seen. Special stains reveal the presence of numerous axons within the tumor. Because the tumor is not always encapsulated and the cells usually are not truly palisaded, some pathologists prefer the name **solitary circumscribed neuroma** as a better descriptive term for this lesion.

Treatment and Prognosis

The treatment for the palisaded encapsulated neuroma consists of conservative local surgical excision. Recurrence is rare. However, specific recognition of this lesion is important because it is not associated with neurofibromatosis or multiple endocrine neoplasia type III.

NEURILEMOMA (Schwannoma)

The **neurilemoma** is a benign neural neoplasm of Schwann cell origin. It is relatively uncommon, although 25 to 48 percent of all cases occur in the head and neck region.

Clinical and Radiographic Features

The neurilemoma presents as a slowly growing, encapsulated tumor that typically arises in association with a nerve trunk. As it grows, it pushes the nerve aside. Usually, the mass is asymptomatic, although tenderness or pain may occur in some instances. The lesion is most common in young and middle-aged adults and can range from a few millimeters to several centimeters in size.

The tongue is the most common location for oral neurilemomas, although the tumor can occur almost anywhere in the mouth (Fig. 12–54). On occasion, the tumor arises centrally within bone and may produce bony expansion. Intraosseous examples are most common in the posterior mandible and usually appear as unilocular radiolucencies on radiographs. Pain and paresthesia are not unusual for intrabony tumors.

Histopathologic Features

The neurilemoma usually is an encapsulated tumor that demonstrates two microscopic patterns in varying amounts: *Antoni A* and *Antoni B*. Antoni A tissue is characterized by streaming fascicles of spindle-shaped

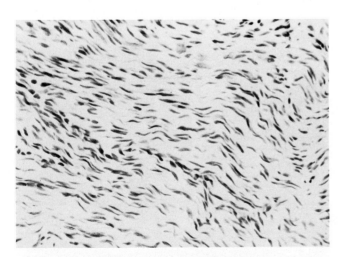

FIGURE 12–53. **Palisaded encapsulated neuroma.** High-power view demonstrating parallel arrangement of spindle-shaped cells consistent with Schwann cells.

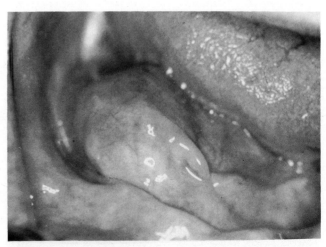

FIGURE 12–54. **Neurilemoma.** Nodular mass in the floor of the mouth. (Courtesy of Dr. Art A. Gonty.)

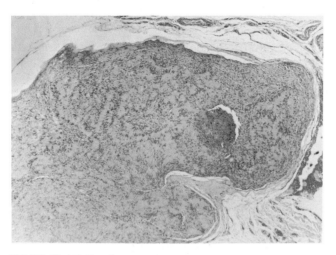

FIGURE 12–55. **Neurilemoma.** Low-power view showing an encapsulated tumor mass.

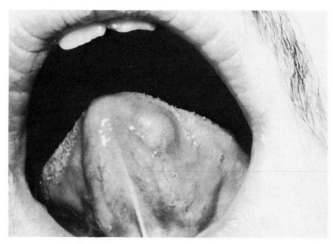

FIGURE 12–57. **Neurofibroma.** Nodular mass of the anterior ventral tongue. (Courtesy of Dr. Lindsey Douglas.)

Schwann cells. These cells often form a palisaded arrangement around central acellular, eosinophilic areas known as *Verocay bodies* (Figs. 12–55 and 12–56). These Verocay bodies consist of reduplicated basement membrane and cytoplasmic processes. Antoni B tissue is less cellular and less organized; the spindle cells are randomly arranged within a loose, myxomatous stroma. Typically, neurites cannot be demonstrated within the tumor mass.

Degenerative changes can be seen in some older tumors (ancient neurilemomas). These changes consist of hemorrhage, hemosiderin, inflammation, fibrosis, and nuclear atypia. However, these tumors are still benign, and the pathologist must be careful not to mistake these alterations for evidence of a sarcoma.

Treatment and Prognosis

The neurilemoma is treated by surgical excision, and the lesion should not recur. Malignant transformation does not occur or is extremely rare.

NEUROFIBROMA

The **neurofibroma** is the most common type of peripheral nerve neoplasm. It arises from a mixture of cell types, including Schwann cells and perineural fibroblasts.

Clinical and Radiographic Features

Neurofibromas can arise as solitary tumors or be a component of neurofibromatosis (discussed next). Solitary tumors are most common in young adults and present as slow-growing, soft, painless lesions that vary in size from small nodules to larger masses. The skin is the most frequent location for neurofibromas, but lesions of the oral cavity are not uncommon (Figs. 12–57 and 12–58). The tongue and buccal mucosa are the most common intraoral sites. On rare occasions, the tumor can arise centrally within bone, where it may produce a well-demarcated or poorly defined unilocular or multilocular radiolucency (Fig. 12–59).

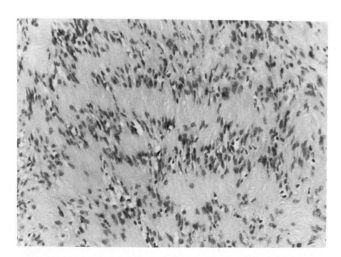

FIGURE 12–56. **Neurilemoma.** High-power view of Antoni A tissue. The Schwann cells form a palisaded arrangement around central acellular zones known as Verocay bodies.

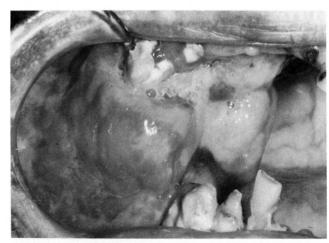

FIGURE 12–58. **Neurofibroma.** Huge tumor involving the maxillary gingiva and hard palate.

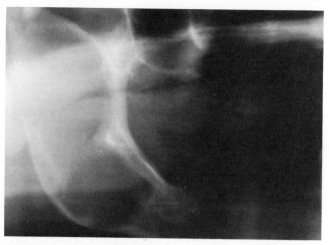

FIGURE 12–59. **Neurofibroma.** Intraosseous tumor filling the right mandibular ramus. (Courtesy of Dr. Paul Allen.)

Histopathologic Features

The solitary neurofibroma often is well circumscribed, especially when the proliferation occurs within the perineurium of the involved nerve. Tumors that proliferate outside of the perineurium may not appear well demarcated and tend to blend with the adjacent connective tissues.

The tumor is composed of interlacing bundles of spindle-shaped cells that often exhibit wavy nuclei (Figs. 12–60 and 12–61). These cells are associated with delicate collagen bundles and variable amounts of myxoid matrix. Mast cells tend to be numerous and can be a helpful diagnostic feature. Sparsely distributed small axons usually can be demonstrated within the tumor tissue by using silver stains.

Treatment and Prognosis

The treatment for solitary neurofibromas is local surgical excision, and recurrence is rare. Any patient with a lesion that is diagnosed as a neurofibroma should be evaluated clinically for the possibility of **neurofibromatosis** (discussed next). Malignant transformation of solitary neurofibromas can occur, although the risk appears to be remote, especially compared with that in patients with neurofibromatosis.

NEUROFIBROMATOSIS (von Recklinghausen's Disease of the Skin)

Neurofibromatosis is a relatively common hereditary condition that is estimated to occur in one of every 3000 births. At least eight forms of neurofibromatosis have been recognized, but the most common form is neurofibromatosis type I (von Recklinghausen's disease of the skin), which accounts for 85 to 90 percent of cases. This form of the disease is inherited as an autosomal dominant trait, although 50 percent of all patients have no family history and apparently represent new mutations. Our discussion is limited to type I neurofibromatosis.

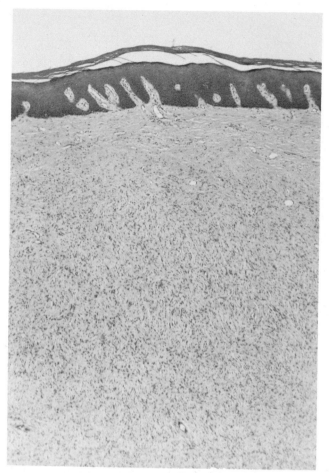

FIGURE 12–60. **Neurofibroma.** Low-power view showing a cellular tumor mass below the epithelial surface.

Clinical and Radiographic Features

Patients with neurofibromatosis have multiple neurofibromas that can occur anywhere in the body but are most common on the skin. The clinical appearance can vary from small papules to larger soft nodules to massive baggy, pendulous masses (*elephantiasis neuromatosa*) on

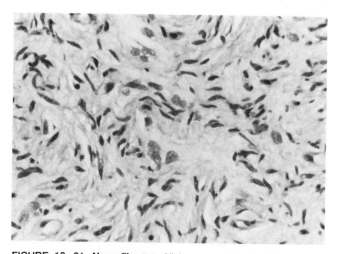

FIGURE 12–61. **Neurofibroma.** High-power view showing spindle-shaped cells with wavy nuclei.

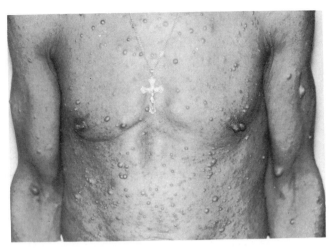

FIGURE 12–62. **Neurofibromatosis.** Multiple tumors of the trunk and arms.

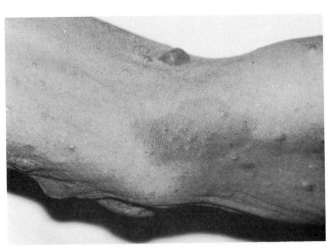

FIGURE 12–64. **Neurofibromatosis.** Same patient as depicted in Figure 12–62. Note the *café au lait* pigmentation on the arm.

the skin (Figs. 12–62 and 12–63). The plexiform variant of neurofibroma, which feels like a "bag of worms," is considered pathognomonic for neurofibromatosis. The tumors may be present at birth, but they often begin to appear during puberty and may continue to develop slowly throughout adulthood. Accelerated growth may be seen during pregnancy. There is a wide variability in the expression of the disease. Some patients have only a few neurofibromas; others have literally hundreds or thousands of tumors. However, two thirds of patients have relatively mild disease.

Another highly characteristic feature is the presence of *café au lait* (coffee with milk) pigmentation on the skin (Fig. 12–64). These spots are smooth-edged, yellow-tan to dark brown macules that vary in diameter from 1 to 2 mm to several centimeters. They usually are present at birth or may develop during the first year of life. The presence of six or more *café au lait* spots greater than 1.5 cm in diameter has been considered pathognomonic of

the disease. Axillary freckling (*Crowe's sign*) is also a highly suggestive sign.

Lisch nodules, translucent brown-pigmented spots on the iris, are found in nearly all affected individuals. Other possible abnormalities may be seen, including central nervous system tumors, macrocephaly, mental deficiency, seizures, short stature, and scoliosis.

In the past, oral lesions were estimated to occur in 4 to 7 percent of cases (Fig. 12–65). However, two studies suggest that oral manifestations may occur in as high as 72 to 92 percent of cases, especially if a detailed clinical and radiographic examination is performed. The most common reported finding is enlargement of the fungiform papillae (in about 50 percent of all affected patients); however, the specificity of this finding for neurofibromatosis is unknown. Only about 25 percent of patients examined in these two studies exhibited actual intraoral neurofibromas. Radiographic findings included enlargement of the mandibular foramen and enlarge-

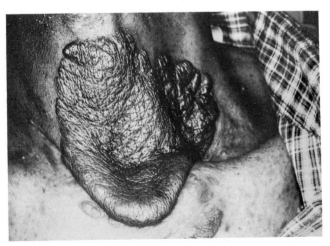

FIGURE 12–63. **Neurofibromatosis.** Baggy, pendulous neurofibroma of the lower neck.

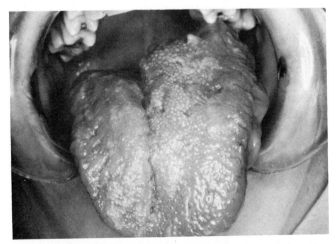

FIGURE 12–65. **Neurofibromatosis.** Intraoral involvement characterized by unilateral enlargement of the tongue.

ment or branching of the mandibular canal, each seen in one fourth to one third of cases.

Treatment and Prognosis

There is no specific therapy for neurofibromatosis, and treatment often is directed toward prevention or management of complications. Facial neurofibromas can be removed for cosmetic purposes. Carbon dioxide laser and dermabrasion have been used successfully for extensive lesions.

One of the most feared complications is the development of cancer, most often **neurofibrosarcoma (malignant schwannoma)**, which occurs in about 5 percent of cases. These tumors are most common on the trunk and extremities, although head and neck involvement occasionally is seen (Figs. 12–66 to 12–68). The prognosis for neurofibrosarcomas associated with neurofibromatosis is poor, with a 5-year survival rate of only 15 percent. Other malignancies also have been associated with neurofibromatosis, including central nervous system tumors, pheochromocytoma, leukemia, rhabdomyosarcoma, and Wilms tumor.

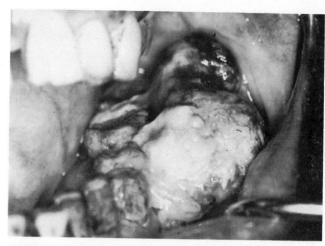

FIGURE 12–67. **Neurofibromatosis.** Same patient as depicted in Figure 12–66. Note the intraoral appearance of neurofibrosarcoma of the mandibular buccal vestibule. The patient eventually died of this tumor. (From Neville BW, Hann J, Narang R, Garen P. Oral neurofibrosarcoma associated with neurofibromatosis type I. Oral Surg Oral Med Oral Pathol 72:456–461, 1991.)

In recent years, there has been considerable interest in Joseph (not John) Merrick, the so-called "Elephant Man." Although Merrick once was mistakenly considered to have neurofibromatosis, it is now generally accepted that his horribly disfigured appearance was not due to neurofibromatosis but that he most likely had a rare condition known as **Proteus syndrome**. Because patients with neurofibromatosis may fear acquiring a similar clinical appearance, they should be reassured that they have a different condition. The phrase "Elephant Man disease" is incorrect, misleading, and should be avoided. Genetic counseling is extremely important for all patients with neurofibromatosis.

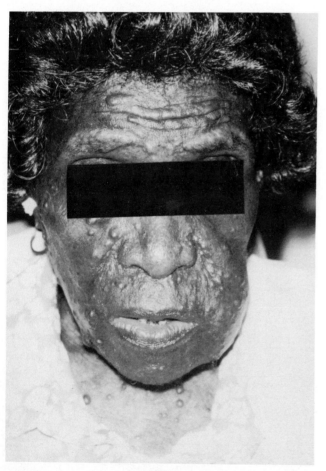

FIGURE 12–66. **Neurofibromatosis.** Neurofibrosarcoma of the left cheek in a patient with type I neurofibromatosis. (From Neville BW, Hann J, Narang R, Garen P. Oral neurofibrosarcoma associated with neurofibromatosis type I. Oral Surg Oral Med Oral Pathol 72:456–461, 1991.)

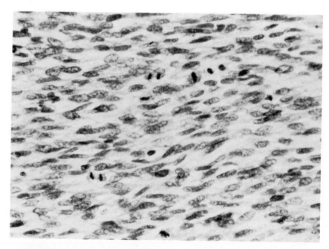

FIGURE 12–68. **Neurofibrosarcoma.** High-power view of an intraoral tumor that developed in a patient with neurofibromatosis. There is a cellular spindle cell proliferation with numerous mitotic figures.

MULTIPLE ENDOCRINE NEOPLASIA
TYPE III (Multiple Endocrine Neoplasia, Type 2B; Multiple Mucosal Neuroma Syndrome)

The **multiple endocrine neoplasia (MEN) syndromes** are a group of rare conditions characterized by tumors or hyperplasias of neuroendocrine origin. For example, patients with MEN type I have benign tumors of the pancreatic islets, adrenal cortex, parathyroid glands, and pituitary gland. MEN type II, also known as MEN type 2A or **Sipple syndrome**, is characterized by the development of adrenal pheochromocytomas and medullary thyroid carcinoma. In addition to pheochromocytomas and medullary thyroid carcinoma, patients with MEN type III (also known as type 2B) have mucosal neuromas that especially involve the oral mucous membranes. Because oral manifestations are most prominent in MEN type III, the remainder of the discussion is limited to this condition.

Clinical and Radiographic Features

MEN type III is inherited as an autosomal dominant trait, although 50 percent of cases represent new mutations. Most affected individuals have a marfanoid body build, characterized by thin, elongated limbs with muscle wasting. The face is narrow, but the lips are characteristically thick and protuberant because of the diffuse proliferation of nerve bundles (Fig. 12–69). The upper eyelid sometimes is everted because of thickening of the tarsal plate. Small, pedunculated neuromas may be observable on the conjunctiva, eyelid margin, or cornea.

Oral mucosal neuromas are usually the first sign of the condition. These present as soft, painless papules or nodules that principally affect the lips and anterior tongue but also may be seen on the buccal mucosa, gingiva, and palate (Fig. 12–70). Bilateral neuromas of the commissural mucosa are highly characteristic.

Pheochromocytomas of the adrenal glands develop in at least 50 percent of all patients and become more prevalent with increasing age. These neuroendocrine tumors are frequently bilateral or multifocal. The tumor cells secrete catecholamines, which result in symptoms such as profuse sweating, intractable diarrhea, headaches, flushing, heart palpitations, and hypertension.

The most significant aspect of this condition is the development of medullary carcinoma of the thyroid gland, which occurs in more than 90 percent of cases. This aggressive tumor arises from the parafollicular cells (C cells) of the thyroid. These cells are responsible for calcitonin production. Medullary carcinoma most often is diagnosed in patients between the ages of 18 and 25 and shows a marked propensity for metastasis. The average age at death from this neoplasm is 21 years.

Laboratory Values

If medullary carcinoma of the thyroid gland is present, serum or urinary levels of calcitonin are elevated. An increase in calcitonin levels may herald the onset of

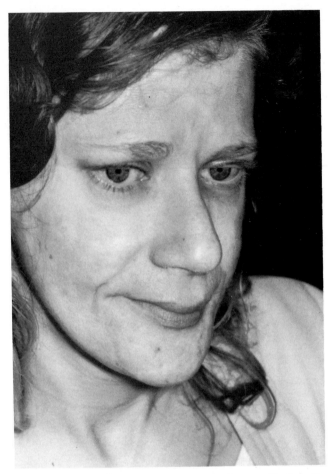

FIGURE 12–69. **Multiple endocrine neoplasia, type III.** Note the narrow face and eversion of the upper eyelids.

the tumor, and calcitonin also can be monitored to detect local recurrences or metastases after treatment. Pheochromocytomas may result in increased levels of vanillylmandelic acid (VMA) and altered epinephrine-norepinephrine ratios.

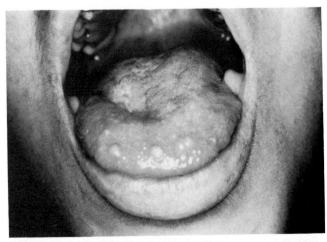

FIGURE 12–70. **Multiple endocrine neoplasia, type III.** Multiple neuromas along the anterior margin of the tongue and bilaterally at the commissures. (Courtesy of Dr. Emmitt Costich.)

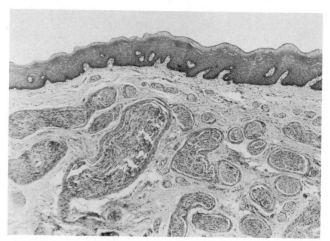

FIGURE 12-71. **Multiple endocrine neoplasia, type III.** Low-power view of an oral mucosal neuroma showing marked hyperplasia of nerve bundles.

Histopathologic Features

The mucosal neuromas are plexiform in nature and characterized by marked hyperplasia of nerve bundles in an otherwise normal or loose connective tissue background (Figs. 12-71 and 12-72). Prominent thickening of the perineurium typically is seen.

Treatment and Prognosis

The prognosis for patients with MEN type III centers around early recognition of the oral features, given the serious nature of the medullary thyroid carcinoma. Some investigators advocate prophylactic removal of the thyroid gland at an early age because medullary carcinoma is almost certain to occur. Once it has developed, this tumor often exhibits an aggressive behavior with a poor prognosis. The patient should also be observed for the development of pheochromocytomas because they may result in a life-threatening hypertensive crisis, especially if surgery with general anesthesia is performed.

MELANOTIC NEUROECTODERMAL TUMOR OF INFANCY

The **melanotic neuroectodermal tumor of infancy** is a rare pigmented neoplasm that usually occurs during the first year of life. It is generally accepted that this lesion is of neural crest origin. In the past, however, a number of tissues were suggested as possible sources of this tumor. These included odontogenic epithelium and retina, which resulted in various older terms for this entity, such as **pigmented ameloblastoma**, **retinal anlage tumor**, and **melanotic progonoma**. Because these names are inaccurate, however, they should no longer be used. Melanotic (pigmented) neuroectodermal tumor of infancy is the preferred term.

Clinical and Radiographic Features

Melanotic neuroectodermal tumor of infancy almost always develops during the first year of life; some patients are affected at birth. There is a striking predilection for the maxilla; two thirds of all reported cases occur there. The lesion is most common in the anterior region of the maxilla, where it classically presents as a rapidly expanding mass that frequently is blue or black (Fig. 12-73). The tumor often destroys the underlying bone and may be associated with displacement of the developing teeth (Fig. 12-74). In some instances, there may be an associated osteogenic reaction, which exhibits a "sun-ray" radiographic pattern that can be mistaken for osteosarcoma. The tumor also can occur at other locations; the skull, mandible, brain, and epididymis or testis are the most frequent extramaxillary sites. There is no apparent sex predilection.

Laboratory Values

High urinary levels of vanillylmandelic acid (VMA) often are found in patients with melanotic neuroectoder-

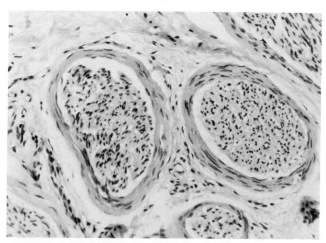

FIGURE 12-72. **Multiple endocrine neoplasia, type III.** High-power view of the same neuroma as depicted in Figure 12-71. Note the prominent thickening of the perineurium.

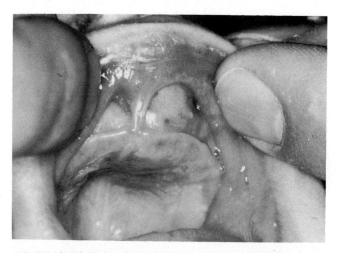

FIGURE 12-73. **Melanotic neuroectodermal tumor of infancy.** Infant with an expansile mass of the anterior maxilla. (From Steinberg B, Shuler C, Wilson S. Melanotic neuroectodermal tumor of infancy: Evidence for multicentricity. Oral Surg Oral Med Oral Pathol 66:666-669, 1988.)

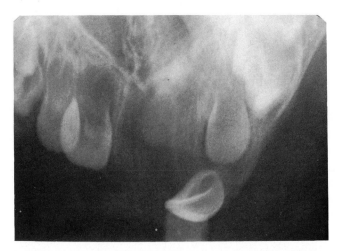

FIGURE 12-74. **Melanotic neuroectodermal tumor of infancy.** Radiolucent destruction of the anterior maxilla associated with displacement of the developing teeth. (From Neville BW, Damm DD, White DK, Waldron CA. Color Atlas of Clinical Oral Pathology. Philadelphia, Lea & Febiger, 1991.)

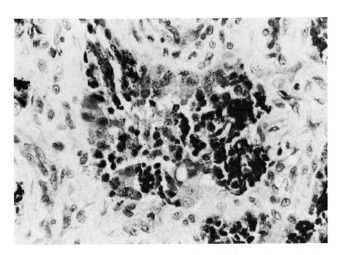

FIGURE 12-76. **Melanotic neuroectodermal tumor of infancy.** High-power view of a tumor nest demonstrating two cell types: small, hyperchromatic round cells and larger epithelioid cells with vesicular nuclei. Some stippled melanin pigment is also present.

mal tumor of infancy. These levels may return to normal once the tumor has been resected. This finding supports the hypothesis of neural crest origin because other tumors from this tissue (e.g., pheochromocytoma and neuroblastoma) often secrete norepinephrine-like hormones that are metabolized to VMA and excreted in the urine.

Histopathologic Features

The tumor consists of a biphasic population of cells that form nests, tubules, or alveolar structures within a dense, collagenous stroma (Figs. 12-75 and 12-76). The alveolar and tubular structures are lined by cuboidal epithelioid cells that demonstrate vesicular nuclei and granules of dark-brown melanin pigment. The second cell type is neuroblastic in appearance and consists of small, round cells with hyperchromatic nuclei and little cytoplasm. These cells grow in loose nests and frequently are surrounded by the larger pigment-producing cells. Mitotic figures are rare.

Treatment and Prognosis

Despite their rapid growth and potential to destroy bone, most melanotic neuroectodermal tumors of infancy are benign. The lesion is best treated by surgical removal. Some clinicians prefer simple curettage, although others advocate that a 5-mm margin of normal tissue be included with the specimen. Recurrence of the tumor has been reported in about 15 percent of cases. In addition, about 6 percent of reported cases have acted in a malignant fashion, resulting in metastasis and death. Although this 6 percent figure is probably high (because unusual malignant cases are more likely to be reported), it does underscore the potential serious nature of this tumor and the need for careful clinical evaluation and follow-up of affected patients.

PARAGANGLIOMA (Carotid Body Tumor; Chemodectoma; Glomus Jugulare Tumor; Glomus Tympanicum Tumor)

The paraganglia are specialized tissues of neural crest origin that are associated with the autonomic nerves and ganglia throughout the body. Some of these cells act as chemoreceptors, such as the carotid body (located at the carotid bifurcation), which can detect changes in blood pH or oxygen tension and subsequently cause changes in respiration and heart rate. Tumors that arise from these structures are known collectively as **paragangliomas**, with the term preferably preceded by the anatomic site at which they are located. Therefore, tumors of the carotid body are appropriately known as **carotid body paragangliomas (carotid body tumors)**; those that develop in the temporal bone and middle ear are called **jugulotympanic paragangliomas**. Jugulotympanic paragangliomas also

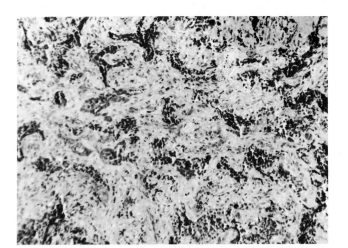

FIGURE 12-75. **Melanotic neuroectodermal tumor of infancy.** Low-power view showing nests of epithelioid cells within a fibrous stroma.

are commonly known as **glomus jugulare tumors**, although some authors prefer to reserve this term only for those examples that arise from the jugular bulb and to use the term **glomus tympanicum tumors** for those that arise in the middle ear.

Clinical and Radiographic Features

Although paragangliomas are rare, the head and neck area is the most common site for these lesions. The most common paraganglioma is the carotid body tumor, which develops at the bifurcation of the internal and external carotid arteries. This tumor usually occurs in middle-aged adults. Most often it presents as a slowly enlarging, painless mass of the upper lateral neck below the angle of the jaw. It is seen more frequently in patients who live at high altitudes, indicating that some cases may arise from chronic hyperplasia of the carotid body in response to lower oxygen levels. Angiography can help to localize the tumor and demonstrate its characteristic vascular nature.

Jugulotympanic paragangliomas are the second most common type of these tumors. They also are most frequent in middle-aged individuals but show a 2:1 female predilection. The most common symptoms include dizziness, tinnitus (a ringing or other noise in the ear), hearing loss, and cranial nerve palsies. Other less common paragangliomas of the head and neck include vagal, nasopharyngeal, laryngeal, and orbital paragangliomas.

Approximately 10 percent of affected patients have multifocal tumors. In 7 to 9 percent of cases, there is a family history of such tumors, with an autosomal dominant inheritance pattern. Hereditary cases have an even greater chance of being multicentric; about one third of these patients have more than one tumor.

Histopathologic Features

The paraganglioma is characterized by round or polygonal epithelioid cells that are organized into nests or *Zellballen* (Fig. 12–77). The overall architecture is similar to that of the normal paraganglia, except the *Zellballen* are usually larger and more irregular in shape. These nests consist primarily of chief cells, which demonstrate centrally located, vesicular nuclei and somewhat granular, eosinophilic cytoplasm. The tumor is typically vascular and may be surrounded by a thin fibrous capsule.

Treatment and Prognosis

The treatment of paragangliomas may include surgery, radiation therapy, or both, depending on the extent and location of the tumor. Localized carotid body paragangliomas often can be treated by surgical excision with maintenance of the vascular tree. If the carotid artery is encased by tumor, it also may need to be resected, followed by vascular grafting. Radiation therapy may be used as adjunctive treatment or for unresectable carotid body tumors.

Although most carotid body paragangliomas are benign and can be controlled with surgery and radiation therapy, vascular complications can lead to considerable surgical morbidity or mortality. In addition, 6 to 9 percent of carotid body paragangliomas metastasize, either to regional lymph nodes or distant sites. Unfortunately, it usually is difficult to predict which tumors will act in a malignant fashion on the basis of their microscopic features. Because such metastases may develop many years after the original diagnosis is made, long-term follow-up is important.

Because of their location near the base of the brain, jugulotympanic paragangliomas are more difficult to manage and often impossible to resect surgically. Therefore, radiation therapy frequently is used as a primary treatment or in conjunction with surgery. Long-term local control is achieved in approximately 75 percent of cases.

GRANULAR CELL TUMOR

The **granular cell tumor** is an uncommon benign soft tissue neoplasm that shows a predilection for the oral cavity. The histogenesis of this lesion has long been debated. Originally, it was believed to be of skeletal muscle origin and was called the **granular cell myoblastoma**. However, more recent investigations do not support a muscle origin but point to a derivation from Schwann cells (**granular cell schwannoma**) or an undifferentiated mesenchymal cell. At present, it seems best to use the noncommittal term **granular cell tumor** for this lesion.

Clinical Features

Granular cell tumors are most common in the oral cavity and on the skin. The single most common site is the tongue, which accounts for one third to one half of all reported cases. Tongue lesions most often occur on the dorsal surface. The buccal mucosa is the second most common intraoral location. The tumor most frequently occurs in the fourth to sixth decades of life and is rare in children. There is a 2:1 female predilection.

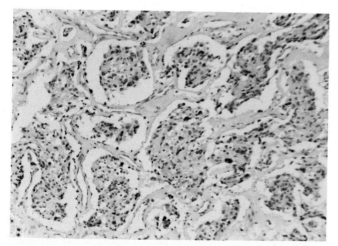

FIGURE 12–77. **Carotid body tumor.** Nested arrangement of tumor cells.

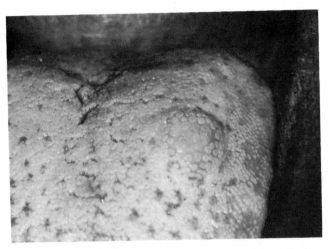

FIGURE 12–78. **Granular cell tumor.** Submucosal nodule on the dorsum of the tongue. See Color Plates.

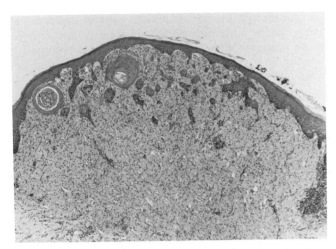

FIGURE 12–80. **Granular cell tumor.** Low-power view showing a nodular mass of granular cells with pseudoepitheliomatous hyperplasia of the overlying epithelium.

The granular cell tumor typically presents as an asymptomatic sessile nodule that is usually 2 cm or less in size (Fig. 12–78; see Color Figure 83). The lesion often has been noted for many months or years, although sometimes the patient is unaware of its presence. The mass usually is pink, although occasional granular cell tumors appear yellow. The granular cell tumor typically is solitary, but some patients have multiple, separate tumors.

Histopathologic Features

The granular cell tumor is composed of large, polygonal cells with abundant pale eosinophilic, granular cytoplasm and small, vesicular nuclei (Fig. 12–79). The cells usually are arranged in sheets, but they also may be found as cords and nests. The cell borders often are indistinct, which results in a syncytial appearance. The lesion is not encapsulated and sometimes appears to infiltrate the adjacent connective tissues. Often, there appears to be a transition from normal adjacent skeletal muscle fibers to granular tumor cells; this finding led

earlier investigators to suggest a muscle origin for this tumor. Less frequently, one may see groups of granular cells that envelop small nerve bundles. Immunohistochemical staining reveals positivity for S-100 protein within the cells—a finding that is supportive, but not diagnostic, of neural origin.

An unusual and significant microscopic finding is the presence of acanthosis or pseudoepitheliomatous (pseudocarcinomatous) hyperplasia of the overlying epithelium, which has been reported in up to 50 percent of all cases (Figs. 12–80 and 12–81). Although this hyperplasia is usually minor in degree, in some cases it may be so striking that it results in a mistaken diagnosis of squamous cell carcinoma and subsequent unnecessary cancer surgery. The pathologist must be aware of this possibility, especially when dealing with a superficial biopsy sample or a specimen from the dorsum of the tongue—an unusual location for oral cancer.

Treatment and Prognosis

The granular cell tumor is best treated by conservative local excision. Recurrence is rare.

CONGENITAL EPULIS (Congenital Epulis of the Newborn)

The **congenital epulis** is a rare soft tissue tumor that occurs exclusively on the alveolar ridges of newborns. It is often known by the redundant term, **congenital epulis of the newborn**. It also has been called **gingival granular cell tumor of the newborn**, but this term should be avoided. Although it bears a light microscopic resemblance to the granular cell tumor (discussed earlier), it exhibits ultrastructural and immunohistochemical differences that warrant its classification as a distinct and separate entity. The histogenesis of this tumor is still uncertain. Studies suggest that it arises from primitive mesenchymal cells that exhibit differentiation toward myofibroblasts or pericytes.

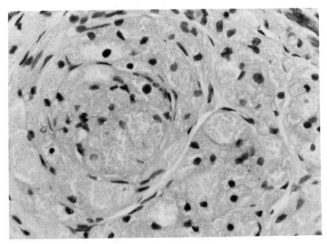

FIGURE 12–79. **Granular cell tumor.** Polygonal cells with indistinct cell borders and abundant granular cytoplasm.

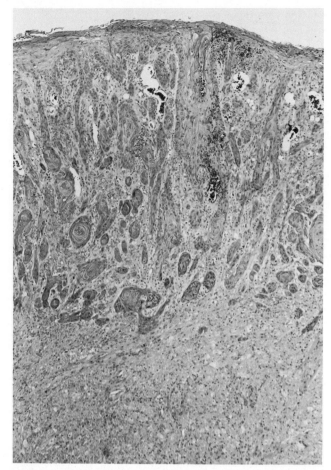

FIGURE 12–81. **Granular cell tumor.** Marked pseudoepitheliomatous hyperplasia overlying a granular cell tumor. Such cases may easily be mistaken for squamous cell carcinoma.

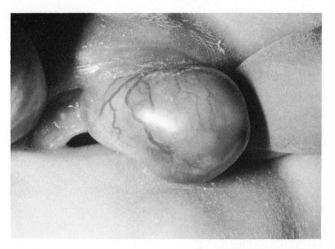

FIGURE 12–82. **Congenital epulis.** Polypoid mass of the anterior maxillary alveolar ridge in a newborn infant.

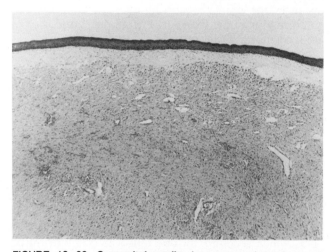

FIGURE 12–83. **Congenital epulis.** Low-power photomicrograph showing a tumor with a narrow zone of loose fibrous connective tissue separating it and the overlying epithelium. Note the atrophy of the rete ridges.

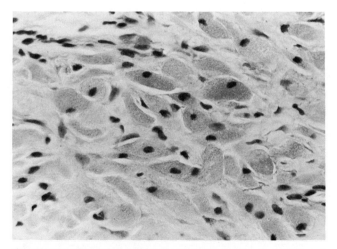

FIGURE 12–84. **Congenital epulis.** High-power view of rounded and elongated cells with abundant granular cytoplasm.

Clinical Features

The congenital epulis presents as a pink to red, smooth-surfaced, polypoid mass on the alveolar ridge of a newborn infant (Fig. 12–82). Most examples are 2 cm or less in size, although lesions as large as 7.5 cm have been reported. Multiple tumors develop in 10 percent of cases.

The tumor is two to three times more common on the maxillary ridge than on the mandibular ridge. It most frequently occurs lateral to the midline in the area of the developing lateral incisor and canine teeth. The congenital epulis shows a striking predilection for females, which suggests a hormonal influence in its development. Nearly 90 percent of cases occur in females.

Histopathologic Features

The congenital epulis is characterized by large, rounded cells with abundant granular, eosinophilic cytoplasm and round to oval, lightly basophilic nuclei (Figs. 12–83 and 12–84). In older tumors, these cells may become elongated and separated by fibrous connective tissue. In contrast to the granular cell tumor, the overlying epithelium never shows pseudoepitheliomatous hyperplasia but typically demonstrates atrophy of the rete ridges. Also, in contradistinction to the granular cell tumor, immunohistochemical stains for S-100 protein give negative results.

Treatment and Prognosis

The congenital epulis usually is treated by surgical excision. The lesion never has been reported to recur, even with incomplete removal.

After birth, the tumor appears to stop growing and may even diminish in size. Eventual complete regression has been reported in a few patients, even without treatment.

HEMANGIOMA

The **hemangioma**, a benign proliferation of blood vessels, is the most common tumor of infancy and childhood, although some cases develop in adults. In many instances, the lesion probably represents a hamartoma or malformation rather than a true neoplasm. Various types are recognized. These include:

- Capillary hemangioma
- Juvenile hemangioma
- Cavernous hemangioma
- Arteriovenous hemangioma (malformation)

Clinical Features

Hemangiomas are primarily tumors of childhood, although some cases develop in adults. They are found in 1.1 to 2.6 percent of newborns. It is estimated that up to 10 to 12 percent of children eventually have one of these tumors. The most common location is the head and neck, which accounts for one fourth to one third of all cases (Figs. 12–85 and 12–86; see Color Figure 84).

Capillary Hemangioma

The most common type is the **capillary hemangioma** —named because of the capillary size of the blood ves-

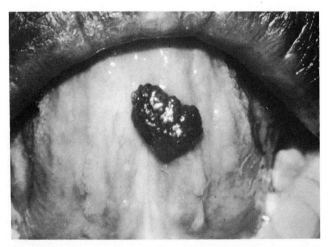

FIGURE 12–85. **Hemangioma.** Exophytic bluish-purple mass on the ventral surface of the tongue. (Courtesy of Dr. Richard Hart.)

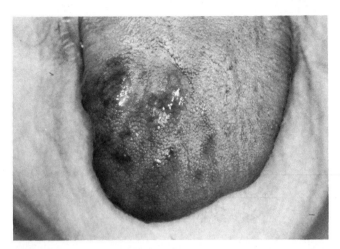

FIGURE 12–86. **Hemangioma.** Mass of the anterior tongue. See Color Plates.

sels. Capillary hemangiomas are three to five times more common in females than males. Because of their bright color, they are sometimes called "strawberry" hemangiomas. The lesion begins on the skin as a flat area of red pigmentation that is noted at birth or during the first few weeks of life. It rapidly proliferates over the next 6 to 12 months and produces an elevated and often lobulated mass that is red to purple. The lesion stabilizes in size and subsequently regresses over the next several years, first evidenced by a darkening in color. By age 7, most capillary hemangiomas have involuted.

Juvenile Hemangioma

The terms **juvenile hemangioma** and **cellular hemangioma** refer to the immature and highly cellular stage of a capillary hemangioma. Such lesions are common in the parotid region and constitute the most common tumor of the parotid gland in children. As the tumor ages, it becomes less cellular and is indistinguishable from the typical capillary hemangioma. Because of their cellular nature, these lesions sometimes have been known as "juvenile hemangioendothelioma," although this term probably should be avoided because hemangioendothelioma also is used to designate other vascular tumors of intermediate malignant potential.

Cavernous Hemangioma

Cavernous hemangiomas are so named because of the larger diameter of the proliferating blood vessels. They show some clinical features similar to the capillary hemangioma, including occurrence in childhood and a predilection for females and the head and neck region. However, they tend to be larger and less circumscribed and more frequently involve deeper structures. Also, unlike the capillary hemangioma, they usually do not undergo regression.

Arteriovenous Hemangioma

Arteriovenous hemangiomas (**arteriovenous malformation** or **arteriovenous fistula**) are vascular malformations

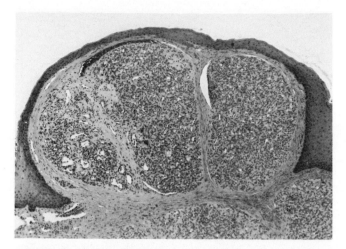

FIGURE 12–87. **Juvenile (cellular) hemangioma.** Low-power photomicrograph showing a cellular mass of vascular endothelial cells arranged in lobular aggregates.

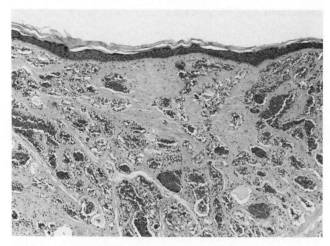

FIGURE 12–89. **Capillary hemangioma.** Low-power view of a vascular tumor forming multiple capillary blood vessels.

caused by abnormal communication between the arterial and venous circulation, bypassing the capillary bed. A thrill or bruit over the mass may be detected, and the overlying skin often feels significantly warmer.

Histopathologic Features

Early capillary (juvenile) hemangiomas are characterized by numerous plump endothelial cells and often indistinct vascular lumina (Figs. 12–87 and 12–88). As the lesion matures, the endothelial cells become flattened, and the small, capillary-sized vascular spaces become more evident (Figs. 12–89 and 12–90). Cavernous hemangiomas exhibit much larger, dilated vessels (Fig. 12–91). Secondary thrombosis and phlebolith formation may occur. Sometimes a mixture of both capillary- and cavernous-sized blood vessels is seen. Arteriovenous hemangiomas demonstrate a mixture of thick-walled arteries and veins, along with capillary vessels.

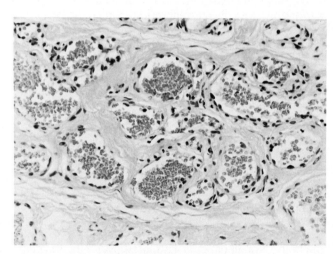

FIGURE 12–90. **Capillary hemangioma.** High-power photomicrograph demonstrating well-formed capillary-sized vessels.

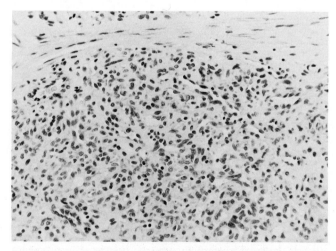

FIGURE 12–88. **Juvenile (cellular) hemangioma.** High-power view showing a highly cellular endothelial proliferation forming occasional indistinct vascular lumina.

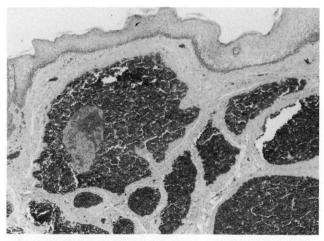

FIGURE 12–91. **Cavernous hemangioma.** Low-power photomicrograph showing multiple large, dilated blood vessels.

Treatment and Prognosis

Because most capillary hemangiomas undergo involution, management often consists of "watchful neglect." Systemic corticosteroids may help to reduce the size of the lesion in some cases. Frequently, surgery is necessary for cavernous hemangiomas and arteriovenous malformations, depending on the size, location, and symptoms associated with the lesion. Laser therapy has become popular as a surgical tool. Embolization also may be used as a primary mode of therapy for large, inaccessible lesions or preoperatively to reduce surgical blood loss. Injection of sclerosing agents, such as sodium morrhuate, has been used in the past but may result in scarring.

STURGE-WEBER ANGIOMATOSIS
(Encephalotrigeminal Angiomatosis; Sturge-Weber Syndrome)

Sturge-Weber angiomatosis is a rare, non-hereditary developmental condition that is characterized by a hamartomatous vascular proliferation, which involves the tissues of the brain and face. It is believed to be caused by the persistence of a vascular plexus around the cephalic portion of the neural tube. This plexus develops during the sixth week of intrauterine development but normally should undergo regression during the ninth week.

Clinical and Radiographic Features

Patients with Sturge-Weber angiomatosis are born with a dermal capillary vascular malformation of the face known as a *port-wine stain* or *nevus flammeus* because of its deep purple color. This port-wine stain usually has a unilateral distribution along one or more segments of the trigeminal nerve. Occasionally, patients have bilateral involvement or additional port-wine lesions elsewhere on the body. Not all patients with facial port-wine nevi have Sturge-Weber angiomatosis. In one study of patients with facial port-wine nevi, only slightly more than 10 percent had Sturge-Weber angiomatosis. Only patients with involvement along the distribution of the ophthalmic branch of the trigeminal nerve were at risk for the full condition (Figs. 12-92 [see Color Figure 85] and 12-93).

In addition to the facial port-wine nevus, affected individuals also have leptomeningeal angiomas that overlie the ipsilateral cerebral cortex. This meningeal angiomatosis usually is associated with a convulsive disorder and often results in mental retardation or contralateral hemiplegia. Radiographs of the skull may reveal gyriform "tram-line" calcifications on the affected side (Fig. 12-94). Ocular involvement may be manifested by glaucoma and vascular malformations of the conjunctiva, episclera, choroid, and retina.

Intraoral involvement in Sturge-Weber angiomatosis is common, resulting in hypervascular changes to the ipsilateral mucosa (Fig. 12-95). The gingiva may exhibit slight vascular hyperplasia or a more massive hemangiomatous proliferation that can resemble a pyogenic granuloma. Such gingival hyperplasia may be attributable to

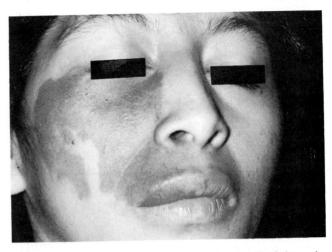

FIGURE 12-92. **Port-wine stain.** "Nevus flammeus" of the malar area in a patient without Sturge-Weber angiomatosis. Unless the vascular lesion includes the region innervated by the ophthalmic branch of the trigeminal nerve, the patient usually does not have central nervous system involvement. See Color Plates.

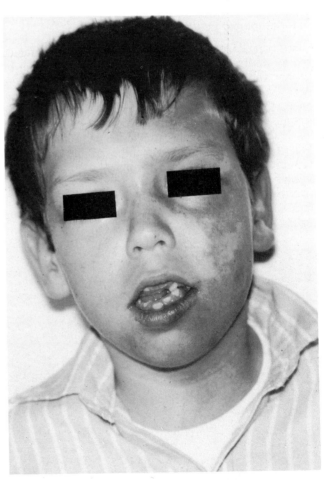

FIGURE 12-93. **Sturge-Weber angiomatosis.** Port-wine stain of the left face, including involvement along the ophthalmic branch of the trigeminal nerve. The patient also was mentally retarded and had a seizure disorder.

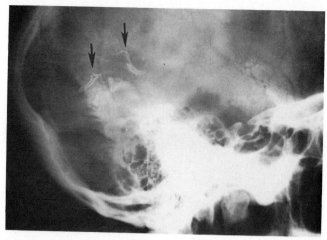

FIGURE 12-94. **Sturge-Weber angiomatosis.** Skull film showing "tram-line" calcifications (arrows). (Courtesy of Dr. Reg Munden.)

the increased vascular component, phenytoin therapy used to control the epileptic seizures, or both. Destruction of the underlying alveolar bone has been reported in rare instances.

Histopathologic Features

The port-wine nevus is characterized by excessive numbers of dilated blood vessels in the mid and deep dermis. The intraoral lesions show a similar vascular dilatation. Proliferative gingival lesions may resemble a pyogenic granuloma.

Treatment and Prognosis

The treatment and prognosis of Sturge-Weber angiomatosis depend on the nature and severity of the possible clinical features. Facial port-wine nevi usually can be improved by using the newer flashlamp-pulsed dye lasers. Neurosurgical removal of angiomatous meningeal lesions may be necessary in some cases.

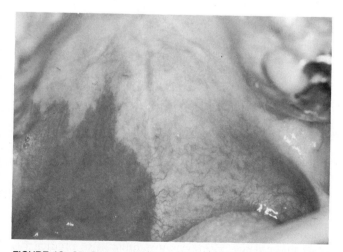

FIGURE 12-95. **Sturge-Weber angiomatosis.** Unilateral vascular involvement of the soft palate.

Great care must be taken when performing surgical procedures in affected areas of the mouth because severe hemorrhage may be encountered. Lasers also may be helpful in the removal of hyperplastic oral lesions.

NASOPHARYNGEAL ANGIOFIBROMA

The **nasopharyngeal angiofibroma** is a rare vascular and fibrous neoplasm that occurs only in the nasopharynx. Although microscopically benign, it frequently exhibits locally destructive and aggressive behavior.

Clinical and Radiographic Features

Nasopharyngeal angiofibromas occur almost exclusively in males. The tumor is exceedingly rare in females —so much so, that the diagnosis in a female should be viewed with skepticism and closely scrutinized. The lesion also shows a striking predilection for adolescents between the ages of 10 and 17 and has often been called the "juvenile" nasopharyngeal angiofibroma. However, rare examples also have been reported in slightly younger and older patients. Because of its almost exclusive occurrence in adolescent boys, a hormonal influence seems likely, although no endocrine abnormalities have been detected.

Nasal obstruction and epistaxis are common early symptoms. From its origin in the soft tissues of the nasopharynx, this destructive tumor can extend into the nasal cavity, paranasal sinuses, orbits, middle cranial fossa, and oral cavity. Computed tomographic (CT) scans and magnetic resonance imaging (MRI) studies are helpful adjuncts in visualizing the extent of the lesion and degree of adjacent tissue destruction. Anterior bowing of the posterior wall of the maxillary sinus is a characteristic feature (Fig. 12-96). Angiograms can be used to confirm the vascular nature of the lesion (Fig. 12-97).

Histopathologic Features

The nasopharyngeal angiofibroma consists of dense fibrous connective tissue that contains numerous dilated, thin-walled blood vessels of variable size (Fig. 12-98). Typically, the vascular component is more prominent at the periphery of the tumor, especially in lesions from younger patients.

Treatment and Prognosis

The primary treatment of nasopharyngeal angiofibroma usually consists of surgical excision through a transantral or transpalatal approach. Preoperative embolization of the tumor is helpful in controlling blood loss. Radiation therapy usually is reserved for recurrent lesions and extensive tumors with unusual vascular supplies or intracranial extension.

The recurrence rate varies but averages about 20 percent. Such recurrences usually are re-treated with further surgery or radiation therapy. The overall patient survival rate is 95 percent. Malignant transformation into fibrosarcoma rarely has been reported and probably is associated with prior radiation therapy.

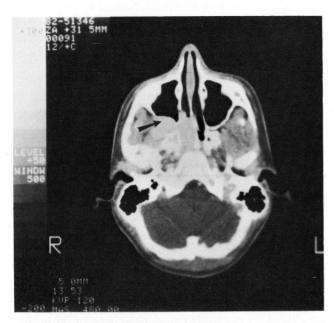

FIGURE 12-96. Nasopharyngeal angiofibroma. A contrasted CT scan showing a tumor of the nasopharynx and pterygopalatine fossa with characteristic anterior bowing of the posterior wall of the right maxillary sinus (*arrow*). (Courtesy of Dr. Pamela Van Tassel.)

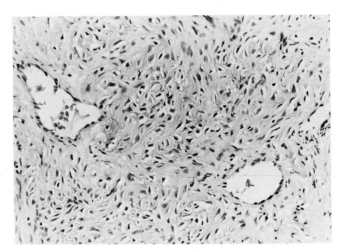

FIGURE 12-98. Nasopharyngeal angiofibroma. Moderately cellular fibrous connective tissue with prominent blood vessels.

HEMANGIOPERICYTOMA

The **hemangiopericytoma** is a rare neoplasm that is derived from pericytes, i.e., cells whose processes encircle the endothelial cells of capillaries. It is most common in the lower extremity, and approximately 16 percent of cases occur in the head and neck region.

Clinical Features

Hemangiopericytomas are seen primarily in adults and are rare in children. There is no sex predilection. The tumor usually presents as a slow-growing, painless mass. Superficial lesions may demonstrate vascular pigmentation.

A distinctive form of hemangiopericytoma (**hemangiopericytoma-like tumor**) occurs in the nasal cavity and paranasal sinuses. The lesion primarily occurs in middle-aged and older adults and usually presents with symptoms of nasal obstruction or epistaxis.

Histopathologic Features

The hemangiopericytoma usually is fairly well circumscribed and exhibits tightly packed cells that surround endothelium-lined vascular channels. The cells are haphazardly arranged and demonstrate round to ovoid nuclei and indistinct cytoplasmic borders. Occasionally, they are spindle-shaped. The blood vessels often show irregular branching, which results in a characteristic "staghorn" and "antlerlike" appearance (Fig. 12-99). A reticulin stain demonstrates a dense reticulin network that surrounds the vessels and individual tumor cells (Fig. 12-100).

The identification of four or more mitoses per ten high-power fields suggests a rapidly growing tumor that is capable of metastasis. The presence of necrosis also suggests malignancy. However, it is difficult to predict microscopically whether a particular tumor will act in a benign or malignant fashion.

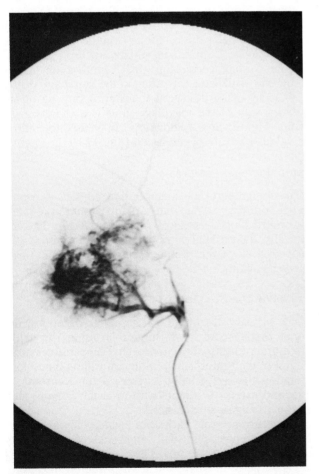

FIGURE 12-97. Nasopharyngeal angiofibroma. A digital subtraction angiogram of the external carotid artery showing the intense vascular blush of the tumor. (Courtesy of Dr. Pamela Van Tassel.)

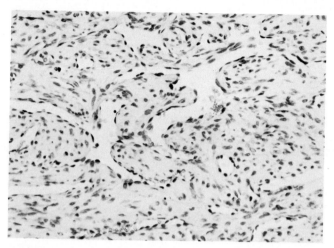

FIGURE 12–99. **Hemangiopericytoma.** "Staghorn" blood vessels with surrounding pericytes.

Sinonasal hemangiopericytomas have a more prominent spindle cell pattern, with the cells arranged in a more orderly fashion. The vascular component is less intricate, and less interstitial collagen is found between the tumor cells.

Treatment and Prognosis

For hemangiopericytomas with a benign histopathologic appearance, local excision is the treatment of choice. More extensive surgery is required for tumors with malignant characteristics. Most tumors appear to behave in a benign fashion, although the reported metastatic rate has varied from 11.7 to 56.5 percent. Local recurrence has been reported in 40 to 50 percent of cases and may develop many years after the primary excision. Recurrence is a worrisome sign because many of these tumors eventually metastasize.

Studies show that patients with sinonasal hemangiopericytomas have a better prognosis than do those with tumors at other sites. Because of its different clinical

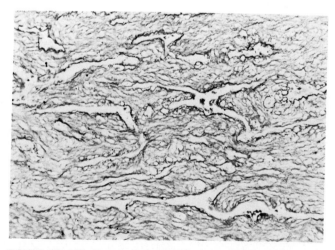

FIGURE 12–100. **Hemangiopericytoma.** Silver stain demonstrating reticulin outlining the blood vessels and surrounding the individual tumor cells.

features, microscopic appearance, and prognosis, some authors prefer to designate it as a hemangiopericytoma-like tumor because they believe that it represents a related but separate entity.

LYMPHANGIOMA

Lymphangiomas are benign, hamartomatous tumors of lymphatic vessels. It is doubtful that they are true neoplasms; instead, they most likely represent developmental malformations that arise from sequestrations of lymphatic tissue that do not communicate normally with the rest of the lymphatic system.

Lymphangiomas often have been classified into one of three types:

1. **Lymphangioma simplex (capillary lymphangioma),** which consists of small, capillary-sized vessels
2. **Cavernous lymphangioma,** which is composed of larger, dilated lymphatic vessels
3. **Cystic lymphangioma (cystic hygroma),** which exhibits large, macroscopic cystic spaces.

However, this classification system is rather arbitrary because all three sizes of vessels often can be found within the same lesion.

The subtypes are probably variants of the same pathologic process, and the size of the vessels may depend on the nature of the surrounding tissues. Cystic lymphangiomas most often occur in the neck and axilla, where the loose adjacent connective tissues allow for more expansion of the vessels. Cavernous lymphangiomas are more frequent in the mouth, where the denser surrounding connective tissue and skeletal muscle limit vessel expansion.

Clinical Features

Lymphangiomas have a marked predilection for the head and neck, which accounts for about 75 percent of all cases (Fig. 12–101). About 50 percent of all lesions are noted at birth, and around 90 percent develop by 2 years of age.

Cervical lymphangiomas are more common in the posterior triangle and typically present as soft, fluctuant masses. They occur less frequently in the anterior triangle, although lesions in this location are more likely to result in respiratory difficulties or dysphagia if they grow large. On occasion, cervical lymphangiomas extend into the mediastinum or upward into the oral cavity. Such tumors can become massive and can measure 15 cm or greater in size. Rapid tumor enlargement may occur secondary to an upper respiratory tract infection, presumably because of increased lymph production, blocked lymphatic drainage, or secondary infection of the tumor.

Oral lymphangiomas may occur at various sites but are most frequent on the anterior two thirds of the tongue, where they often result in macroglossia (Figs. 12–102 [see Color Figure 86] and 12–103). Usually, the tumor is superficial in location and demonstrates a peb-

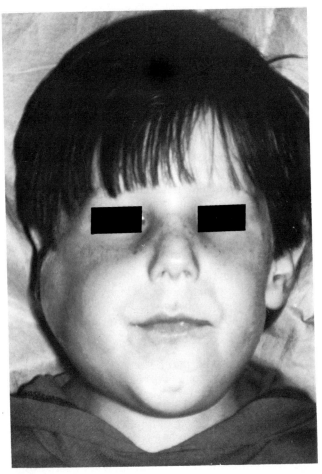

FIGURE 12–101. **Lymphangioma.** Young boy with a cystic hygroma primarily involving the right side of the face. (Courtesy of Dr. Frank Kendrick.)

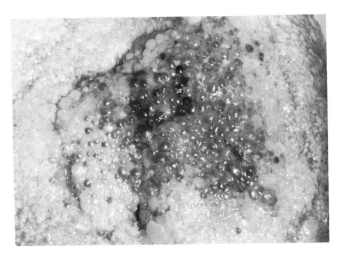

FIGURE 12–103. **Lymphangioma.** Dorsal tongue lesion demonstrating a purple color, which can be due to secondary hemorrhage or an associated hemangiomatous component.

Small lymphangiomas less than 1 cm in size occur on the alveolar ridge in around 4 percent of black neonates. These lesions often occur bilaterally on the mandibular ridge and show a 2:1 male-to-female distribution. Most of these alveolar lymphangiomas apparently resolve spontaneously because they are not observed in older people.

Histopathologic Features

Lymphangiomas are composed of lymphatic vessels that may show marked dilatation (cavernous lymphangioma) (Figs. 12–104 and 12–105) or macroscopic cyst-like structures (cystic hygroma) (Fig. 12–106). The vessels often diffusely infiltrate the adjacent soft tissues and may demonstrate lymphoid aggregates in their walls. The lining endothelium is typically thin, and the spaces contain proteinaceous fluid and occasional lymphocytes. Some channels also may contain red blood cells, which creates uncertainty as to whether they are lymphatic or blood vessels. Although many of these likely represent

bly surface that resembles a cluster of translucent "vesicles." The surface has been likened to the appearance of frog eggs or tapioca pudding. Secondary hemorrhage into the lymphatic spaces may cause some of these "vesicles" to become purple. Deeper tumors present as soft, ill-defined masses.

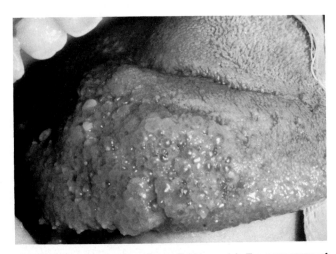

FIGURE 12–102. **Lymphangioma.** Pebbly, vesicle-like appearance of a tumor of the right lateral tongue. See Color Plates.

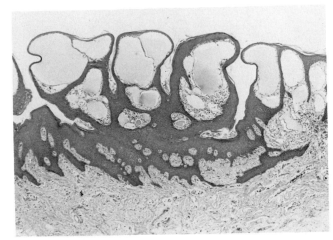

FIGURE 12–104. **Cavernous lymphangioma.** Lesion of the tongue showing a papillary surface with dilated lymphatic vessels just beneath the epithelium.

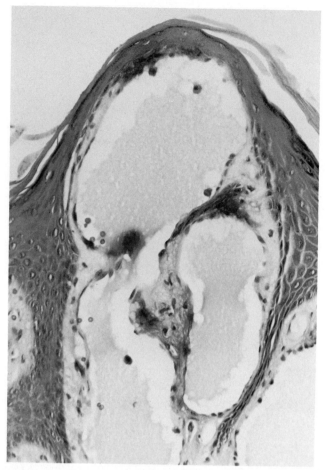

FIGURE 12–105. **Cavernous lymphangioma.** High-power photomicrograph showing a dilated, lymph-filled vessel immediately below the atrophic surface epithelium.

secondary hemorrhage into a lymphatic vessel, some actually may be examples of mixed lymphangioma and hemangioma.

In intraoral tumors, the lymphatic vessels characteristically are located just beneath the epithelial surface and often replace the connective tissue papillae. This superfi-

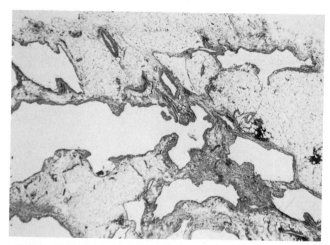

FIGURE 12–106. **Cystic hygroma.** Lesion from the neck showing markedly dilated lymphatic vessels.

cial location results in the translucent, vesicle-like clinical appearance. However, extension of these vessels into the deeper connective tissue and skeletal muscle also may be seen.

Treatment and Prognosis

The treatment of lymphangiomas usually consists of surgical excision, although total removal may not be possible in all cases because of large size or involvement of vital structures. Recurrence is common, especially for cavernous lymphangiomas of the oral cavity, because of their infiltrative nature. Some clinicians do not recommend treatment for nonenlarging lymphangiomas of the tongue because of the difficulty in removal and high recurrence rate. Cystic lymphangiomas of the cervical region are often well circumscribed and have a lower rate of recurrence. Spontaneous regression of lymphangiomas is rare.

Unfortunately, lymphangiomas do not respond to sclerosing agents as hemangiomas do. However, some success with sclerosant therapy for unresectable lymphangiomas has been reported using OK-432, a lyophilized incubation mixture of a low-virulent strain of *Streptococcus pyogenes* with penicillin G potassium, which has lost its streptolysin S–producing ability.

The prognosis is good for most patients, although large tumors of the neck or tongue may result in airway obstruction and death. The mortality rate for cystic hygromas ranges from 2 to 6 percent in most series.

LEIOMYOMA

Leiomyomas are benign neoplasms of smooth muscle that most commonly occur in the uterus, gastrointestinal tract, and skin. Leiomyomas of the oral cavity are rare. Most of these probably have their origin from vascular smooth muscle.

There are three types:

- Solid leiomyomas
- Vascular leiomyomas (angiomyomas or angioleiomyomas)
- Epithelioid leiomyomas (leiomyoblastomas)

Almost all oral leiomyomas are either solid or vascular in type; angiomyomas account for nearly 75 percent of all oral cases.

Clinical Features

The oral leiomyoma can occur at any age and usually presents as a slowly growing, firm mucosal nodule (Fig. 12–107). Most lesions are asymptomatic, although occasional tumors can be painful. Solid leiomyomas typically are normal in color, although angiomyomas may exhibit a bluish hue. The most common sites are the lips, palate, tongue, and cheek, which together account for 80 percent of cases.

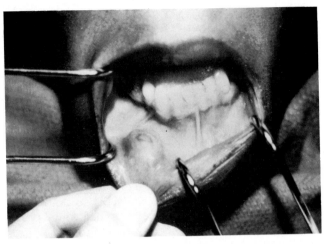

FIGURE 12–107. **Leiomyoma.** Nodular tumor of the lower labial mucosa. (From Damm DD, Neville BW. Oral leiomyomas. Oral Surg Oral Med Oral Pathol 47:343–348, 1979.)

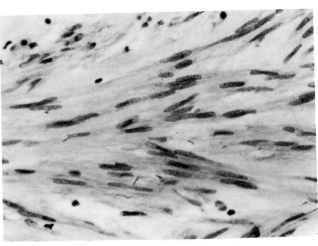

FIGURE 12–109. **Leiomyoma.** High-power view showing spindle-shaped cells with blunt-ended nuclei.

Histopathologic Features

Solid leiomyomas are well-circumscribed tumors that consist of interlacing bundles of spindle-shaped smooth muscle cells (Figs. 12–108 and 12–109). The nuclei are elongated, pale-staining, and blunt-ended. Angiomyomas also are well-circumscribed lesions that demonstrate multiple tortuous blood vessels with thickened walls caused by hyperplasia of their smooth muscle coats (Figs. 12–110 and 12–111). Intertwining bundles of smooth muscle may be found between the vessels, sometimes with intermixed adipose tissue. Mitoses are uncommon in both forms of the tumor.

Special stains may be helpful to confirm the smooth muscle origin if the diagnosis is in doubt. The smooth muscle stains bright-red with the Masson's trichrome stain, and myofibrils may be demonstrated by Mallory's phosphotungstic acid hematoxylin (PTAH) stain.

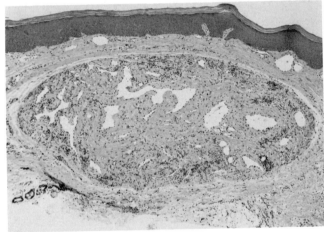

FIGURE 12–110. **Angiomyoma.** Well-circumscribed tumor exhibiting prominent blood vessels.

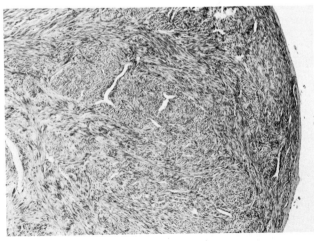

FIGURE 12–108. **Leiomyoma.** Low-power view showing a well-circumscribed cellular mass of spindle-shaped smooth muscle cells.

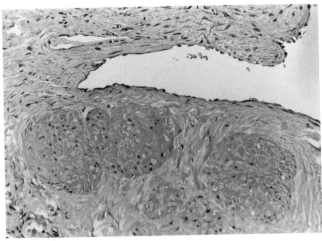

FIGURE 12–111. **Angiomyoma.** High-power view showing bundles of smooth muscle adjacent to a blood vessel.

Treatment and Prognosis

Oral leiomyomas are treated by local surgical excision. The lesion should not recur.

RHABDOMYOMA

Benign neoplasms of skeletal muscle are called **rhabdomyomas**. The term rhabdomyoma also is used to describe a hamartomatous lesion of the heart than often is associated with tuberous sclerosis (see p. 553). Despite the great amount of skeletal muscle throughout the body, benign skeletal muscle tumors are extremely rare. However, these extracardiac rhabdomyomas show a striking predilection for the head and neck. Rhabdomyomas of the head and neck can be subclassified into two categories: adult and fetal.

Clinical Features

Adult Rhabdomyomas

Adult rhabdomyomas of the head and neck occur primarily in middle-aged and older patients, with about 70 percent of cases found in men. The most frequent sites are the pharynx, oral cavity, and larynx; intraoral lesions are most common in the floor of the mouth, soft palate, and base of tongue. The tumor presents as a nodule or mass that can grow to many centimeters in size before discovery (Figs. 12–112 and 12–113). Laryngeal and pharyngeal lesions often lead to airway obstruction. Sometimes, the tumor is multinodular in nature, with two or more discrete nodules found in the same anatomic location. Occasional cases are multicentric, with separate, distinct tumors at different sites.

Fetal Rhabdomyomas

Fetal rhabdomyomas usually occur in young children, although some also develop in adults. A similar male predilection is noted. The most common locations are the face and periauricular region.

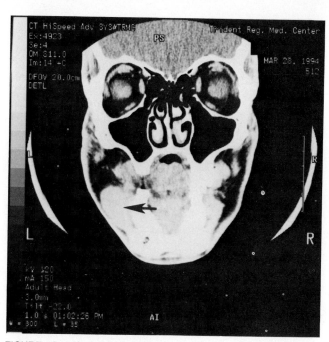

FIGURE 12–113. **Adult rhabdomyoma.** CT scan of the same tumor depicted in Figure 12–112. Note the mass (*arrow*) lateral to the left body of the mandible. (Courtesy of Dr. Craig Little.)

Histopathologic Features

Adult Rhabdomyomas

The adult rhabdomyoma is composed of well-circumscribed lobules of large, polygonal cells, which exhibit abundant granular, eosinophilic cytoplasm (Figs. 12–114 and 12–115). These cells often demonstrate peripheral vacuolization that results in a "spider web" appearance of the cytoplasm. Focal cells with cross-striations can be identified in most cases.

Fetal Rhabdomyomas

The fetal rhabdomyoma has a less mature appearance and consists of a haphazard arrangement of spindle-

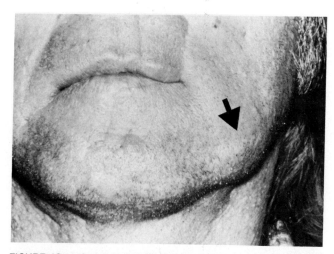

FIGURE 12–112. **Adult rhabdomyoma.** Nodular mass (*arrow*) in the left cheek. (Courtesy of Dr. Craig Little.)

FIGURE 12–114. **Adult rhabdomyoma.** Low-power view showing a uniform tumor composed of rounded and polygonal cells with focal vacuolization.

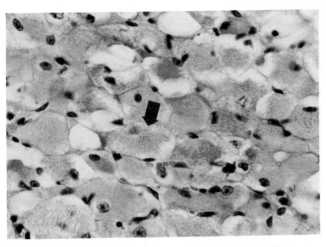

FIGURE 12–115. **Adult rhabdomyoma.** High-power view of the tumor cells, which demonstrate abundant granular, eosinophilic cytoplasm. Note the faint cross-striations in some cells (*arrow*).

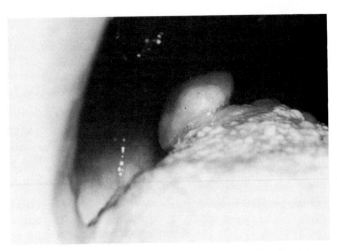

FIGURE 12–116. **Osseous choristoma.** Hard pedunculated nodule on the posterior dorsum of the tongue. (Courtesy of Dr. Michael Meyrowitz.)

shaped muscle cells that sometimes are found within a myxoid stroma. Some tumors may show considerable cellularity and mild pleomorphism, which makes them easily mistaken for rhabdomyosarcomas.

Treatment and Prognosis

The treatment of both variants of rhabdomyoma consists of local surgical excision. Recurrence is uncommon but has been reported in a few cases.

OSSEOUS AND CARTILAGINOUS CHORISTOMAS

A **choristoma** is a tumor-like growth of microscopically normal tissue in an abnormal location. Several different tissue types may occur in the mouth as choristomas. These include gastric mucosa, glial tissue, and tumor-like masses of sebaceous glands. However, the most frequently observed choristomas of the oral cavity are those that consist of bone, cartilage, or both. These lesions sometimes have been called **soft tissue osteomas** or **soft tissue chondromas**, but choristoma is a better term because they do not appear to be true neoplasms.

Clinical Features

Osseous and cartilaginous choristomas show a striking predilection for the tongue, which accounts for 85 percent of cases. The most common location is the posterior tongue near the foramen cecum, although rare examples also have been reported elsewhere on the tongue and at other oral locations. The lesion usually presents as a firm, smooth-surfaced, sessile, or pedunculated nodule between 0.5 and 2.0 cm in diameter (Fig. 12–116). Many patients are unaware of the lesion, although some complain of gagging or dysphagia. More than 70 percent of osseous choristomas have been reported in women.

Histopathologic Features

Microscopic examination of choristomas shows a well-circumscribed mass of dense lamellar bone or mature cartilage that is surrounded by dense fibrous connective tissue (Fig. 12–117). Sometimes a combination of bone and cartilage is formed. The bone has a well-developed haversian canal system and occasionally demonstrates central fatty or hematopoietic marrow.

Treatment and Prognosis

Osseous and cartilaginous choristomas are best treated by local surgical excision. Recurrence has not been reported.

SOFT TISSUE SARCOMAS

Fortunately, **soft tissue sarcomas** are rare in the oral and maxillofacial region and account for less than 1

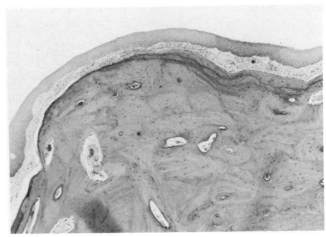

FIGURE 12–117. **Osseous choristoma.** Mass of dense lamellar bone beneath the surface epithelium.

percent of the cancers in this area. Because of their relative rarity, it is beyond the scope of this book to give a complete, detailed discussion of each of these tumors. However, a review of these entities is included below.

Fibrosarcoma

The **fibrosarcoma** is a malignant tumor of fibroblasts. At one time, it was considered one of the most common soft tissue sarcomas. However, the diagnosis of fibrosarcoma is made much less frequently today because of the recognition and separate classification of other spindle cell lesions that have similar microscopic features. The tumor is most common in the extremities; only 10 percent occur in the head and neck region.

Clinical Features

Fibrosarcomas most often present as slowly growing masses that may reach considerable size before they produce pain (Fig. 12–118). They can occur anywhere in the head and neck region. Most frequently, they have been reported in the nose and paranasal sinuses, where they often result in obstructive symptoms. They can occur at any age but are most common in young adults and children.

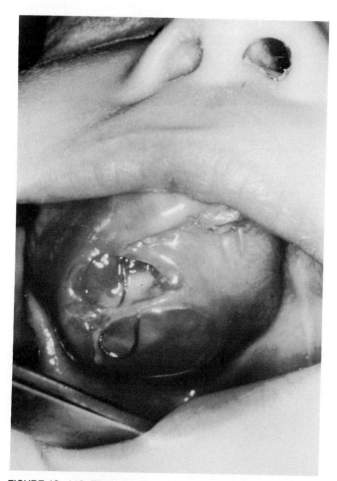

FIGURE 12–118. **Fibrosarcoma.** Child with a large mass of the hard palate and maxillary alveolar ridge. (Courtesy of Dr. John McDonald.)

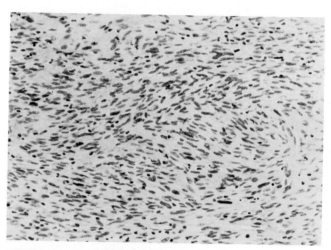

FIGURE 12–119. **Fibrosarcoma.** Cellular mass of spindle-shaped cells demonstrating mild pleomorphism.

Histopathologic Features

Well-differentiated fibrosarcomas consist of fascicles of spindle-shaped cells that classically form a "herringbone" pattern (Fig. 12–119). The cells often show little variation in size and shape, although variable numbers of mitotic figures usually can be identified. In poorly differentiated tumors, the cells are less organized and may appear rounder or ovoid. Mild pleomorphism along with more frequent mitotic activity may be seen. Poorly differentiated tumors tend to produce less collagen than do well-differentiated tumors.

Treatment and Prognosis

The treatment of choice is usually surgical excision, including a wide margin of adjacent normal tissue. Recurrence rates vary from 20 to 60 percent, and 5-year survival rates range from 40 to 70 percent.

Malignant Fibrous Histiocytoma

The **malignant fibrous histiocytoma** is a sarcoma with both fibroblastic and histiocytic differentiation. Although this term was first introduced in 1963, this tumor is now considered to be the most common soft tissue sarcoma in adults. The extremities and retroperitoneum are the most common sites; lesions in the head and neck are rare.

Clinical Features

The malignant fibrous histiocytoma is primarily a tumor of older age groups. The most common complaint is an expanding mass that may or may not be painful or ulcerated. Tumors of the nasal cavity and paranasal sinuses produce obstructive symptoms.

Histopathologic Features

Several histopathologic subtypes have been described. The storiform-pleomorphic type is the most common.

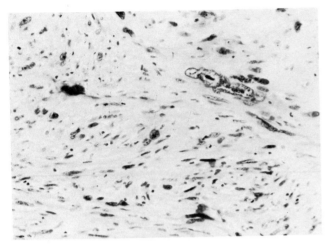

FIGURE 12–120. **Malignant fibrous histiocytoma.** Spindle cell neoplasm demonstrating marked pleomorphism of some of the larger histiocytic cells.

This pattern is characterized by short fascicles of plump spindle cells arranged in a storiform pattern, admixed with areas of pleomorphic giant cells (Fig. 12–120). Myxoid, giant cell, inflammatory, and angiomatoid subtypes also are recognized.

Treatment and Prognosis

The malignant fibrous histiocytoma is an aggressive tumor that usually is treated by radical surgical resection. Approximately 40 percent of patients have local recurrences. A similar percentage have metastases, usually within 2 years. The survival rate for patients with oral tumors appears to be worse than for those with tumors at other body sites.

Liposarcoma

The **liposarcoma** is a malignant neoplasm of fatty origin. It is the second most common soft tissue sarcoma of adult life, after the malignant fibrous histiocytoma. The most common sites are the thigh, retroperitoneum, and inguinal region. Liposarcomas of the head and neck are rare.

Clinical Features

Liposarcomas primarily are seen in adults, with a peak prevalence between the ages of 40 and 60. The tumor typically presents as a soft, slowly growing, ill-defined mass that may appear normal in color or yellow. Pain or tenderness is uncommon; when present, it is usually a late feature. The neck is the most common site for liposarcomas of the head and neck region. The most frequent oral location is the cheek.

Histopathologic Features

Liposarcomas are classified into four histopathologic categories:

1. Myxoid.
2. Round cell.
3. Well-differentiated.
4. Pleomorphic.

The most common of these is the **myxoid liposarcoma**, which accounts for nearly 50 percent of all cases. These tumors demonstrate proliferating lipoblasts within a myxoid stroma that contains a rich capillary network.

The **round cell liposarcoma** is a more aggressive form of myxoid liposarcoma with less differentiated, rounded cells.

Well-differentiated liposarcomas resemble benign lipomas but demonstrate scattered lipoblasts with atypical hyperchromatic nuclei (Fig. 12–121).

Pleomorphic liposarcomas exhibit extreme cellular pleomorphism and bizarre giant cells.

Treatment and Prognosis

Radical excision is the treatment of choice for most liposarcomas. In spite of this, around 50 percent of all tumors recur. The overall 5-year survival rate ranges from 57 to 70 percent. There is a 10-year survival rate of approximately 50 percent. The histopathologic subtype is extremely important in predicting the prognosis; the outlook for round cell and pleomorphic liposarcomas is much worse than for myxoid and well-differentiated tumors.

Neurofibrosarcoma (Malignant Schwannoma; Neurogenic Sarcoma; Malignant Peripheral Nerve Sheath Tumor)

Neurofibrosarcoma is the principal malignancy of peripheral nerve origin. About 50 percent of all cases occur in patients with neurofibromatosis (see p. 381). The lesion is most common on the proximal portions of the extremities and the trunk; it is rare in the head and neck.

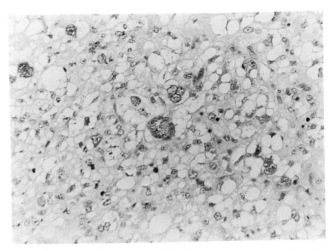

FIGURE 12–121. **Liposarcoma.** Medium-power view showing vacuolated lipoblasts with pleomorphic nuclei.

Clinical and Radiographic Features

Neurofibrosarcomas are most common in young adults. The mean age in patients with neurofibromatosis (29 years) is about one decade younger than in those without this condition (40 years). The tumor presents as an enlarging mass that sometimes exhibits rapid growth. Associated pain or a nerve deficit is common.

Oral tumors may occur anywhere, but the most common sites are the mandible, lips, and buccal mucosa (see Figs. 12–66 and 12–67 on p. 383). Radiographic examination of intraosseous tumors of the mandible may reveal widening of the mandibular canal or the mental foramen, with or without irregular destruction of the surrounding bone.

Histopathologic Features

Microscopic examination of neurofibrosarcomas shows fascicles of atypical spindle-shaped cells, which often resemble the cells of fibrosarcomas (see Fig. 12–68 on p. 383). However, these cells frequently are more irregular in shape with wavy or comma-shaped nuclei. In addition to streaming fascicles, less cellular myxoid areas may also be present. With some neurofibrosarcomas, one can see heterologous elements, which include skeletal muscle differentiation (**malignant Triton tumor**), cartilage, bone, or glandular structures.

A definitive diagnosis of neural origin is often difficult, especially in the absence of neurofibromatosis. Positive immunostaining for S-100 protein is a helpful clue, but this is found in only about 50 percent of all cases.

Treatment and Prognosis

The treatment of neurofibrosarcoma consists primarily of radical surgical excision, possibly along with adjuvant radiation therapy and chemotherapy. The prognosis is poor, especially in patients with neurofibromatosis. The 5-year survival rate in individuals with neurofibromatosis is only 16 percent. For other patients, the 5-year survival rate is 53 percent; this rate drops to 38 percent at 10 years.

Olfactory Neuroblastoma
(Esthesioneuroblastoma)

The **olfactory neuroblastoma** is a rare neuroectodermal neoplasm of the upper nasal vault that shows some similarities to neuroblastomas seen elsewhere in the body. Traditionally, it is believed to arise from the olfactory epithelium.

Clinical and Radiographic Features

Unlike the usual neuroblastoma, the olfactory neuroblastoma is rare in patients younger than the age of 10 years. Instead, it is more common in adults and occurs over a wide age range. The tumor arises high in the nasal cavity close to the cribriform plate. From here it may extend into the adjacent paranasal sinuses (especially the

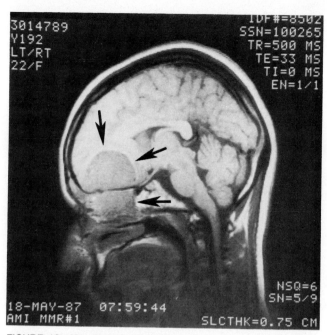

FIGURE 12–122. **Olfactory neuroblastoma.** A T1-weighted sagittal magnetic resonance image (MRI) showing a tumor filling the superior nasal cavity and ethmoid sinus, with extension into the anterior cranial fossa (*arrows*). (Courtesy of Dr. Pamela Van Tassel.)

ethmoid sinus), the orbit, and the anterior cranial fossa (Fig. 12–122). The most common symptoms are nasal obstruction, epistaxis, and pain.

Histopathologic Features

Olfactory neuroblastomas consist of small, round to ovoid basophilic cells that are arranged in sheets and lobules (Fig. 12–123). Rosette and pseudorosette formation as well as areas of delicate neurofibrillary material may be seen.

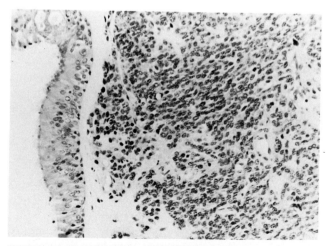

FIGURE 12–123. **Olfactory neuroblastoma.** Sheet of small, basophilic cells adjacent to the sinonasal epithelium (*left*).

Treatment and Prognosis

The treatment of olfactory neuroblastoma consists of surgical excision, often with adjuvant radiation therapy. A combined craniofacial surgical approach frequently is used. Chemotherapy also has been administered, especially in advanced cases.

The prognosis depends on the stage of the disease. For patients with stage A lesions (tumor confined to the nasal cavity), the 5-year survival rate may approach 90 percent. The 5-year survival rate drops to 60 percent for stage B disease (tumor extending into the paranasal sinuses). For stage C disease (tumor extending beyond the nasal cavity and sinuses), the 5-year survival rate has improved to nearly 50 percent or even greater with newer treatment regimens. Death is usually a result of local recurrence; metastasis occurs in approximately 20 percent of cases.

Angiosarcoma

Angiosarcoma is a rare malignancy of vascular endothelium. It may arise from either blood or lymphatic vessels. More than 50 percent of all cases occur in the head and neck region. The scalp and forehead are the most common sites. Oral lesions are quite rare.

The term **hemangioendothelioma** is used to describe vascular tumors with microscopic features intermediate between those of hemangiomas and angiosarcomas. Such tumors also are rare and are considered to be of intermediate malignancy.

Clinical Features

Cutaneous angiosarcomas of the head and neck are most common in elderly patients. Early lesions often resemble a simple bruise, which may lead to a delay in diagnosis. However, the lesion continues to enlarge, which results in an elevated, nodular, or ulcerated surface. Many examples appear multifocal in nature. Oral angiosarcomas have been reported in various locations; the mandible is the most common site (Fig. 12–124).

Histopathologic Features

Angiosarcoma is characterized by an infiltrative proliferation of endothelium-lined blood vessels that form an anastomosing network (Fig. 12–125). The endothelial cells appear hyperchromatic and atypical; they often tend to pile up within the vascular lumina. Increased mitotic activity may be seen.

Treatment and Prognosis

Treatment usually consists of radical surgical excision, radiation therapy, or both. The prognosis for angiosarcoma of the face and scalp is extremely poor, with a reported 5-year survival rate of only 12 percent. Although few oral angiosarcomas have been analyzed, the outlook may be slightly better.

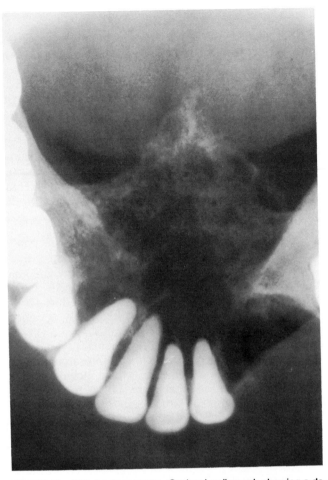

FIGURE 12–124. **Angiosarcoma.** Occlusal radiograph showing a destructive, expansile tumor of the anterior mandible. (Courtesy of Dr. W.C. John.)

Kaposi's Sarcoma

Kaposi's sarcoma is an unusual vascular neoplasm that was first described in 1872 by Moritz Kaposi (correct pronunciation = KOP-osh-ee). Before the advent of the acquired immunodeficiency syndrome (AIDS) epi-

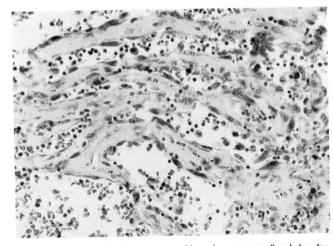

FIGURE 12–125. **Angiosarcoma.** Vascular spaces lined by hyperchromatic and pleomorphic endothelial cells.

demic, it was a rare tumor; however, since the early 1980s it has become quite common because of its propensity to develop in individuals with human immunodeficiency virus (HIV).

The pathogenesis of Kaposi's sarcoma is uncertain, although its multicentricity, geographic distribution, and patient population suggest a viral origin. Cytomegalovirus (CMV) has been suggested as a possible culprit. In fact, some investigators do not believe that it represents a true sarcoma but an infectious process. The lesion most likely arises from endothelial cells, with some evidence of lymphatic origin. Four clinical presentations are recognized:

- Classic
- Endemic (African)
- Iatrogenic immunosuppression-associated
- AIDS-related

The first three forms are discussed here; AIDS-related Kaposi's sarcoma is covered in the section on HIV disease (see p. 203).

Clinical Features

Classic Type

Classic (chronic) Kaposi's sarcoma is primarily a disease of late adult life, and about 90 percent of cases occur in men. It mostly affects individuals of Italian, Jewish, or Slavic ancestry. Multiple bluish-purple macules and plaques are present on the skin of the lower extremities (Fig. 12–126). These lesions grow slowly over many years and develop into painless tumor nodules. Oral lesions are rare and most frequently involve the palate. Approximately one third of patients with classic Kaposi's sarcoma have a history of, or subsequently suffer from, a lymphoreticular malignancy, especially malignant lymphoma.

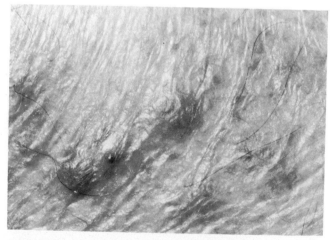

FIGURE 12–126. **Kaposi's sarcoma.** Classic Kaposi's sarcoma in an older man presenting as multiple purple macules and plaques on the lower leg.

Endemic Type

Endemic Kaposi's sarcoma in Africa has been divided into four subtypes:

1. A **benign nodular** type, similar to classic Kaposi's sarcoma, but it occurs in young adults 25 to 40 years old.
2. An **aggressive** or **infiltrative** type, characterized by progressive development of locally invasive lesions that involve the underlying soft tissues and bone.
3. A **florid** form, characterized by rapidly progressive and widely disseminated, aggressive lesions with frequent visceral involvement.
4. A unique **lymphadenopathic** type, occurring primarily in young black African children, and presenting with generalized, rapidly growing tumors of the lymph nodes, occasional visceral organ lesions, and sparse skin involvement.

Iatrogenic Type

Iatrogenic immunosuppression-associated Kaposi's sarcoma most often occurs in recipients of organ transplants. It affects 0.4 percent of renal transplant patients, usually several months to a few years after the transplant. It is probably related to the loss of cellular immunity, which occurs as a result of immunosuppressive drugs. Like classic Kaposi's sarcoma, iatrogenic immunosuppression-associated cases are most common in individuals of Italian, Jewish, and Slavic ancestry. However, the disease may run a more aggressive course.

Histopathologic Features

Kaposi's sarcoma typically evolves through three stages:

- Patch (macular)
- Plaque
- Nodular

The *patch stage* is characterized by a proliferation of miniature vessels. This results in an irregular, jagged vascular network that surrounds pre-existing vessels. Sometimes normal structures, such as hair follicles or pre-existing blood vessels, may appear to protrude into these new vessels ("promontory" sign). The lesional endothelial cells have a bland appearance and may be associated with scattered lymphocytes and plasma cells.

The *plaque stage* demonstrates further proliferation of these vascular channels along with the development of a significant spindle cell component.

In the *nodular stage*, the spindle cells increase to form a nodular tumor-like mass that may resemble a fibrosarcoma or other spindle cell sarcomas (Figs. 12–127 and 12–128). However, numerous extravasated erythrocytes are present, and slit-like vascular spaces may be discerned.

Treatment and Prognosis

The treatment of Kaposi's sarcoma depends on the clinical subtype and stage of the disease. For skin lesions

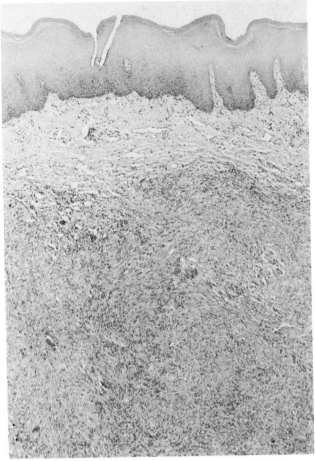

FIGURE 12–127. **Kaposi's sarcoma.** Low-power photomicrograph showing a cellular spindle cell tumor within the connective tissue.

especially vinblastine, also may be helpful. Intralesional injection of chemotherapeutic agents is used to control individual lesions.

The prognosis is variable, depending on the form of the disease and the patient's immune status. The classic form of the disease is slowly progressive; only 10 to 20 percent die of disease after 8 to 10 years. However, 25 percent die of a secondary malignancy, usually of lymphoreticular origin. The benign nodular, endemic African form of the disease is similar in behavior to classic non-African Kaposi's sarcoma. However, the other endemic African forms are more aggressive and the prognosis is poorer. The lymphadenopathic form runs a particularly fulminant course, usually resulting in the death of the patient within 2 to 3 years. In transplant patients, the disease also may be somewhat more aggressive, although the tumors may regress if immunosuppressive therapy is discontinued.

Leiomyosarcoma

The **leiomyosarcoma** is a malignant neoplasm of smooth muscle origin. The most common sites are the uterine wall and gastrointestinal tract. Leiomyosarcomas at other sites are uncommon.

Clinical Features

Leiomyosarcomas are most common in middle-aged and older adults. Tumors in the oral and maxillofacial region are rare but have been reported at various sites (Fig. 12–129). The clinical appearance is nonspecific; usually there is an enlarging mass that may or may not be painful. Secondary ulceration of the mucosal surface may occur.

Histopathologic Features

The microscopic examination of a leiomyosarcoma shows fascicles of spindle-shaped cells with abundant eosinophilic cytoplasm and blunt-ended, cigar-shaped

in the classic form of the disease, radiation therapy (especially electron beam) is often used. Radiation therapy for oral lesions must be approached with caution, because an unusually severe mucositis can develop. Surgical excision can be performed for the control of individual lesions of the skin or mucosa. Systemic chemotherapy,

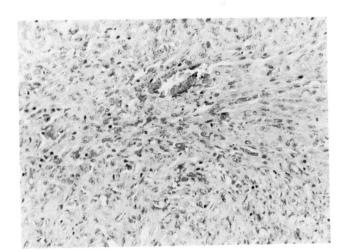

FIGURE 12–128. **Kaposi's sarcoma.** High-power photomicrograph showing spindle cells and poorly defined vascular slits.

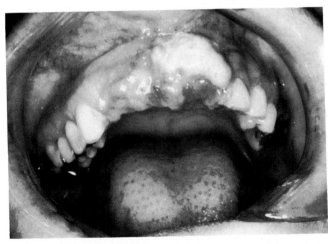

FIGURE 12–129. **Leiomyosarcoma.** Ulcerated mass of the anterior maxillary alveolar ridge. (Courtesy of Dr. Jim Weir.)

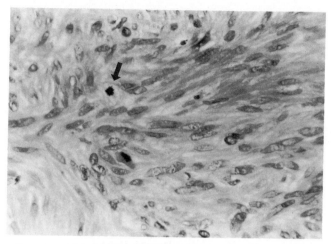

FIGURE 12-130. **Leiomyosarcoma.** High-power view of spindle cell proliferation. Note the mitotic figure (*arrow*).

nuclei (Fig. 12-130). Some tumors may be composed primarily of rounded epithelioid cells that have either eosinophilic or clear cytoplasm (epithelioid leiomyosarcoma). The degree of pleomorphism varies from one tumor to the next, but smooth muscle tumors with the presence of five mitoses per ten high-power fields should be considered malignant. Glycogen usually can be demonstrated within the cells with a periodic acid–Schiff (PAS) stain, and the cell cytoplasm appears bright-red with a Masson's trichrome stain. Longitudinal striations may be seen with a phosphotungstic acid–hematoxylin (PTAH) stain. Immunostaining often reveals the presence of desmin and muscle-specific actin.

Treatment and Prognosis

The treatment of leiomyosarcoma consists primarily of radical surgical excision, sometimes with adjunctive chemotherapy or radiation therapy. The prognosis for oral tumors is poor, with a high rate of local recurrence and distant metastasis.

Rhabdomyosarcoma

Rhabdomyosarcoma, a malignant neoplasm of skeletal muscle origin, is the most common soft tissue sarcoma of children. The most frequent site is the head and neck, which accounts for 40 percent of all cases. The genitourinary tract is the second most common location. Three basic microscopic patterns are recognized:

- Embryonal
- Alveolar
- Pleomorphic

Clinical Features

Rhabdomyosarcoma occurs primarily in the first decade of life, but also is seen in teen-agers and young adults. It is rare in people older than age 45, and approximately 60 percent of all cases occur in males. Embryonal

rhabdomyosarcomas are most common in the first 10 years of life; alveolar rhabdomyosarcomas occur at a median age of 16 years. The median age of patients with pleomorphic rhabdomyosarcomas ranges from 50 to 55 years. Most head and neck lesions are embryonal or alveolar types; pleomorphic rhabdomyosarcomas occur primarily on the extremities.

The tumor most often presents as a painless, infiltrative mass that may grow rapidly (Fig. 12-131). In the head and neck region, the orbit is the most frequent location, followed by the nasal cavity and nasopharynx. The palate is the most frequent intraoral site, and some lesions may appear to arise in the maxillary sinus and break through into the oral cavity. Some embryonal rhabdomyosarcomas that arise within a cavity, such as the vagina or oropharynx, demonstrate an exophytic, polypoid growth pattern that resembles a cluster of grapes. The term **botryoid** (grape-like) **rhabdomyosarcoma** has been used for these lesions (Fig. 12-132).

Histopathologic Features

Embryonal Type

The embryonal rhabdomyosarcoma accounts for about 75 percent of all cases and resembles various stages in the embryogenesis of skeletal muscle. Poorly differentiated examples may be difficult to diagnose and consist of small round or oval cells with hyperchromatic nuclei and indistinct cytoplasm (Fig 12-133). Alternating hypercellular and myxoid zones may be seen. Better-differentiated lesions show round to ovoid rhabdomyoblasts with distinctly eosinophilic cytoplasm and fibrillar material around the nucleus. Cross-striations are rarely

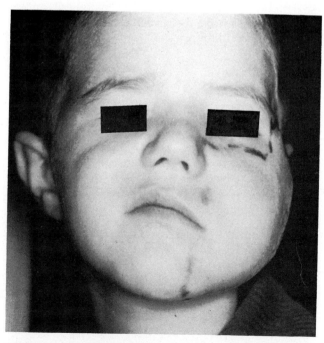

FIGURE 12-131. **Embryonal rhabdomyosarcoma.** Young child with a mass of the left cheek. Marks on the skin have been placed to serve as a guide during radiation therapy. (Courtesy of Dr. George Blozis.)

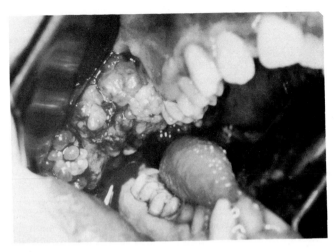

FIGURE 12–132. **Botryoid rhabdomyosarcoma.** Exophytic, polypoid mass arising in the retromolar area. (Courtesy of Dr. John Fantasia.)

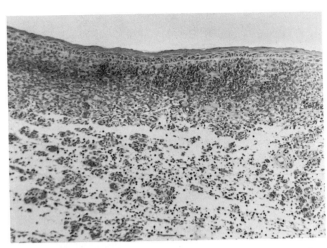

FIGURE 12–134. **Botryoid rhabdomyosarcoma.** Low-power view demonstrating increased cellularity ("cambium layer") just beneath the surface epithelium (*at top*).

found. Some tumors show better-differentiated, elongated, strap-shaped rhabdomyoblasts.

The *botryoid* subtype of embryonal rhabdomyosarcoma is sparsely cellular and has a pronounced myxoid stroma. Increased cellularity, or a so-called cambium layer, usually is seen just beneath the mucosal surface (Figs. 12–134 and 12–135).

Alveolar Type

The alveolar rhabdomyosarcoma is characterized by aggregates of poorly differentiated round to oval cells separated by fibrous septa. These cells demonstrate a central loss of cohesiveness, which results in an alveolar pattern. The peripheral cells of these aggregates adhere to the septal walls in a single layer. The central cells appear to float freely within the alveolar spaces. Mitoses are common, and multinucleated giant cells also may be seen.

Pleomorphic Type

The pleomorphic rhabdomyosarcoma is characterized by loosely arranged and haphazardly oriented cells of variable morphology. Both small and large cells with round or pleomorphic shapes may be present. Deeply eosinophilic cytoplasm may be noted in some cells. Positive immunostains for desmin and myoglobin are helpful in distinguishing these tumors from other pleomorphic sarcomas.

Treatment and Prognosis

Before 1960, the prognosis for a patient with rhabdomyosarcoma was extremely poor, with more than 90 percent of patients dying. With the advent of multimodal therapy during the past several decades, the prognosis has improved dramatically.

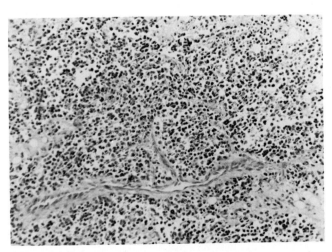

FIGURE 12–133. **Embryonal rhabdomyosarcoma.** Low-power view showing a sheet of small, round cells with hyperchromatic nuclei.

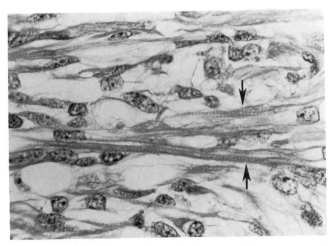

FIGURE 12–135. **Botryoid rhabdomyosarcoma.** High-power view of elongated, strap-shaped rhabdomyoblasts. Note the cross-striations (*arrows*).

Treatment typically consists of local surgical excision followed by multiagent chemotherapy (vincristine, dactinomycin, and sometimes cyclophosphamide). Postoperative radiation therapy is also used, except for localized tumors that have been completely resected at initial surgery. The overall 5-year survival rate is 63 percent; earlier stage neoplasms are associated with an even better prognosis.

Synovial Sarcoma

Synovial sarcoma is an uncommon tumor that occurs primarily in the vicinity of large joints and bursae, especially in the extremities. However, most authorities now agree that the tumor probably does not arise from the synovium. Although it is often para-articular in location, the tumor rarely occurs within the joint capsule. In some instances, it arises in areas without any obvious relationship to synovial structures. Synovial sarcomas of the head and neck are rare, and many of these apparently are unrelated to joint areas.

Clinical Features

Synovial sarcomas most frequently occur in teen-agers and young adults, and there is a slight male predilection. The most common presentation is a gradually enlarging mass that is often associated with pain or tenderness. Tumors in the head and neck region are most common in the paravertebral and parapharyngeal areas. Often, they produce symptoms of dysphagia, dyspnea, or hoarseness. Orofacial tumors most often have been reported in the cheek-parotid region and the base of the tongue.

Histopathologic Features

Classic synovial sarcoma is a biphasic tumor that consists of a combination of spindle cells and epithelial cells (Fig. 12–136). The spindle cells usually predominate and produce a pattern that is similar to fibrosarcoma. Within this spindle cell background are groups of cuboidal to columnar epithelial cells that surround gland-like spaces or form nests, cords, or whorls. Calcifications are seen in around 30 percent of cases.

Less frequently, the tumor is monophasic and consists primarily or entirely of spindle cells. The diagnosis of these tumors is difficult, but most lesions demonstrate at least focal positive immunostaining of spindle cells for cytokeratin or epithelial membrane antigen. Rare examples of monophasic epithelial synovial sarcomas also have been reported.

Treatment and Prognosis

Treatment of synovial sarcoma usually consists of radical surgical excision, possibly with adjunctive radiation therapy or chemotherapy. The prognosis is poor because the tumor has a high rate of recurrence and metastasis. The reported 5-year survival rate ranges from 36 to 51

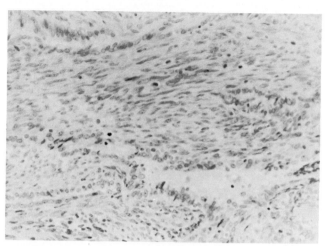

FIGURE 12–136. Synovial sarcoma. Biphasic tumor consisting of spindle cells along with cuboidal to columnar epithelial cells that line gland-like spaces.

percent. However, the 10-year survival rate drops to 11 to 30 percent because of the high rate of late metastases.

Alveolar Soft Part Sarcoma

The **alveolar soft part sarcoma** is a rare neoplasm of uncertain histogenesis. About 25 percent of all cases occur in the head and neck.

Clinical Features

The alveolar soft part sarcoma usually presents as a slowly growing, painless mass. The tumor is most common in young adults and children and shows nearly a 2:1 female predilection. In older patients, the lower extremity is the most frequent location. In younger patients, the head and neck region is the most common site. The orbit and tongue are the most common head and neck locations. For unknown reasons, the right side of the body is affected more frequently.

Histopathologic Features

Alveolar soft part sarcomas are composed of groups of large, polygonal cells that are arranged around central, necrotic alveolar spaces (Fig. 12–137). These cells have abundant granular, eosinophilic cytoplasm and one to several vesicular nuclei. Mitoses are rare. Special stains will reveal PAS-positive, diastase-resistant crystals that are highly characteristic for this tumor. Under the electron microscope, these crystals appear as rhomboid, polygonal, or rod-shaped structures with a regular latticework pattern.

Treatment and Prognosis

Most patients with alveolar soft part sarcomas are treated by radical surgical excision, possibly in conjunction with radiation therapy and chemotherapy. The

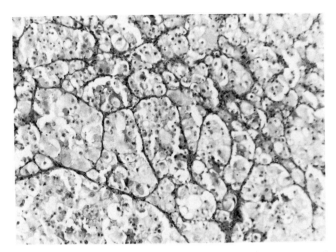

FIGURE 12–137. **Alveolar soft part sarcoma.** Alveolar collections of large, polygonal cells containing abundant granular cytoplasm.

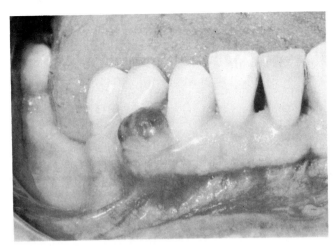

FIGURE 12–138. **Metastatic melanoma.** Pigmented nodule of the mandibular gingiva. See Color Plates.

prognosis is poor because the tumor often metastasizes. The 5-year survival rate is 60 percent, but the 20-year survival rate drops to only 15 percent. The prognosis for children appears to be better than for adults.

METASTASES TO THE ORAL SOFT TISSUES

The metastasis of tumors to the oral cavity is an uncommon phenomenon. Such metastases can occur to bone (see p. 489) or to the oral soft tissues. The mechanism by which tumors can spread to the oral cavity is poorly understood. Primary malignancies from immediately adjacent tissues might be able to spread by a lymphatic route; however, such a mechanism cannot explain metastases from tumors from lower parts of the body, which are almost certainly blood-borne and should be filtered out by the lungs. One possible explanation for blood-borne metastases to the head and neck, especially in the absence of pulmonary metastases, is *Batson's plexus*, a valveless vertebral venous plexus that might allow retrograde spread of tumor cells, bypassing filtration through the lungs.

Clinical Features

The most common site for oral soft tissue metastases is the gingiva, which accounts for slightly more than 50 percent of all cases. This is followed by the tongue, which is the site for 25 percent of cases. The lesion usually presents as a nodular mass that often resembles a hyperplastic or reactive growth, such as a pyogenic granuloma (Figs. 12–138 [see Color Figure 87] to 12–141). Occasionally, the lesion appears as a surface ulceration. Adjacent teeth may become loosened by an underlying destruction of the alveolar bone. The presence of teeth may play an important role in the preference of metastases for the gingiva. Once malignant cells reach the oral cavity, the rich vascular network of inflamed gingival tissues may serve as a fertile site for further growth.

Oral soft tissue metastases are more common in males and are seen most frequently in middle-aged and older adults. Almost any malignancy from any body site is capable of metastasis to the oral cavity, and a wide variety of tumors have been reported to spread to the mouth.

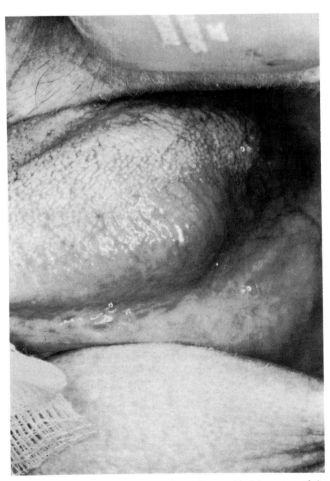

FIGURE 12–139. **Metastatic renal carcinoma.** Nodular mass of the left lateral border of the tongue. (Courtesy of Dr. Mark Bowden.)

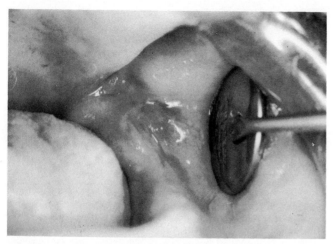

FIGURE 12–140. **Metastatic adenocarcinoma of the colon.** Focal swelling of the left retromolar pad area. (Courtesy of Dr. George Blozis.)

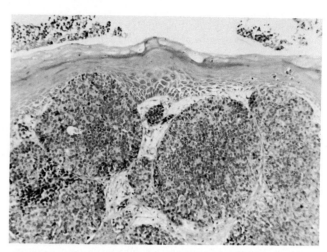

FIGURE 12–142. **Metastatic carcinoma of the lung.** Aggregates of malignant epithelial cells below the surface epithelium.

(However, there is probably a bias in the literature toward reporting more unusual cases.) In the cases reported, lung cancer is responsible for more than one third of all oral soft tissue metastases in men, followed by renal carcinoma and melanoma. Although prostate cancer is common in men, metastases from these tumors have an affinity for bone and rarely occur in soft tissues. For women, breast cancer accounts for 25 percent of all cases, followed by malignancies of the genital organs, lung, bone, and kidney. It is probable that in the future we will see an increased number of metastatic lung cancers in women because today this is the most common cancer killer of women in the United States.

In most cases, the primary tumor already is known when the metastatic lesion is discovered. In some cases, however, the oral lesion is the first sign of the malignant disease.

Histopathologic Features

The microscopic appearance of the metastatic neoplasm should resemble the tumor of origin (Fig. 12–142). Most cases represent carcinomas; metastatic sarcomas to the oral region are rare.

Treatment and Prognosis

The prognosis for patients with metastatic tumors is generally poor because other metastatic sites frequently are also present. Management of the oral lesion is usually palliative and should be coordinated with the patient's overall treatment.

REFERENCES

Fibroma and Giant Cell Fibroma

Barker DS, Lucas RB. Localised fibrous overgrowth of the oral mucosa. Br J Oral Surg 5:86–92, 1967.
Houston GD. The giant cell fibroma: A review of 464 cases. Oral Surg Oral Med Oral Pathol 53:582–587, 1982.
Savage NW, Monsour PA. Oral fibrous hyperplasias and the giant cell fibroma. Austral Dent J 30:405–409, 1985.
Weathers DR, Callihan MD. Giant cell fibroma. Oral Surg Oral Med Oral Pathol 37:374–384, 1974.

Epulis Fissuratum

Buchner A, Begleiter A, Hansen LS. The predominance of epulis fissuratum in females. Quintessence Int 15:699–702, 1984.
Cutright DE. Osseous and chondromatous metaplasia caused by dentures. Oral Surg Oral Med Oral Pathol 34:625–633, 1972.
Cutright DE. The histopathologic findings in 583 cases of epulis fissuratum. Oral Surg Oral Med Oral Pathol 37:401–411, 1974.

Inflammatory Papillary Hyperplasia

Bergendal T, Heimdahl A, Isacsson G. Surgery in the treatment of denture-related inflammatory papillary hyperplasia of the palate. Int J Oral Surg 9:312–319, 1980.
Bhaskar SN, Beasley JD III, Cutright DE. Inflammatory papillary hyperplasia of the oral mucosa: Report of 341 cases. J Am Dent Assoc 81:949–952, 1970.

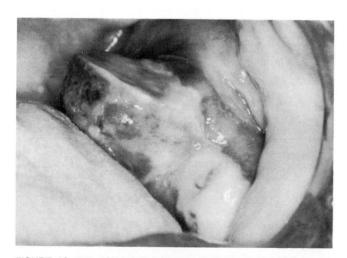

FIGURE 12–141. **Metastatic adenocarcinoma of the colon.** Same patient as depicted in Figure 12–140. Note the marked enlargement of the lesion just 4 weeks later. (Courtesy of Dr. George Blozis.)

Budtz-Jørgensen E. Oral mucosal lesions associated with the wearing of removable dentures. J Oral Pathol 10:65–80, 1981.

Cutright DE. Morphogenesis of inflammatory papillary hyperplasia. J Prosthet Dent 33:380–385, 1975.

Fibrous Histiocytoma

Gray PB, Miller AS, Loftus MJ. Benign fibrous histiocytoma of the oral/perioral regions: Report of a case and review of 17 additional cases. J Oral Maxillofac Surg 50:1239–1242, 1992.

Hoffman S, Martinez MG Jr. Fibrous histiocytomas of the oral mucosa. Oral Surg Oral Med Oral Pathol 52:277–283, 1981.

Thompson SH, Shear M. Fibrous histiocytomas of the oral and maxillofacial regions. J Oral Pathol 13:282–294, 1984.

Fibromatosis and Myofibromatosis

Carr RJ, et al. Infantile fibromatosis with involvement of the mandible. Br J Oral Maxillofac Surg 30:257–262, 1992.

Fowler CB, Hartman KS, Brannon RB. Fibromatosis of the oral and paraoral region. Oral Surg Oral Med Oral Pathol 77:373–386, 1994.

Matthews MS, et al. Infantile myofibromatosis of the mandible. J Oral Maxillofac Surg 48:884–889, 1990.

Speight PM, Dayan D, Fletcher CDM. Adult and infantile myofibromatosis: A report of three cases affecting the oral cavity. J Oral Pathol Med 20:380–384, 1991.

Thompson DH, et al. Juvenile aggressive fibromatosis: Report of three cases and review of the literature. Ear Nose Throat J 70:462–468, 1991.

Vally IM, Altini M. Fibromatoses of the oral and paraoral soft tissues and jaws. Review of the literature and report of 12 new cases. Oral Surg Oral Med Oral Pathol 69:191–198, 1990.

Oral Focal Mucinosis

Buchner A, et al. Oral focal mucinosis. Int J Oral Maxillofac Surg 19:337–340, 1990.

Tomich CE. Oral focal mucinosis: A clinicopathologic and histochemical study of eight cases. Oral Surg Oral Med Oral Pathol 38:714–724, 1974.

Pyogenic Granuloma

Bhaskar SN, Jacoway JR. Pyogenic granuloma—clinical features, incidence, histology, and result of treatment: Report of 242 cases. J Oral Surg 24:391–398, 1966.

Daley TD, Nartey NO, Wysocki GP. Pregnancy tumor: An analysis. Oral Surg Oral Med Oral Pathol 72:196–199, 1991.

Kerr DA. Granuloma pyogenicum. Oral Surg Oral Med Oral Pathol 4:158–176, 1951.

Mills SE, Cooper PH, Fechner RE. Lobular capillary hemangioma: The underlying lesion of pyogenic granuloma: A study of 73 cases from the oral and nasal mucous membranes. Am J Surg Pathol 4:471–479, 1980.

Patrice SJ, Wiss K, Mulliken JB. Pyogenic granuloma (lobular capillary hemangioma): A clinicopathologic study of 178 cases. Pediatr Dermatol 8:267–276, 1991.

Vilmann A, Vilmann P, Vilmann H. Pyogenic granuloma: Evaluation of oral conditions. Br J Oral Maxillofac Surg 24:376–382, 1986.

Peripheral Giant Cell Granuloma

Flanagan AM, et al. The multinucleate cells in giant cell granulomas of the jaw are osteoclasts. Cancer 62:1139–1145, 1988.

Giansanti JS, Waldron CA. Peripheral giant cell granuloma: Review of 720 cases. J Oral Surg 17:787–791, 1969.

Katsikeris N, Kakarantza-Angelopoulou E, Angelopoulos AP. Peripheral giant cell granuloma: Clinicopathologic study of 224 new cases and review of 956 reported cases. Int J Oral Maxillofac Surg 17:94–99, 1988.

Smith BR, Fowler CB, Svane TJ. Primary hyperparathyroidism presenting as a "peripheral" giant cell granuloma. J Oral Maxillofac Surg 46:65–69, 1988.

Peripheral Ossifying Fibroma

Buchner A, Hansen LS. The histomorphologic spectrum of peripheral ossifying fibroma. Oral Surg Oral Med Oral Pathol 63:452–461, 1987.

Kenney JN, Kaugars GE, Abbey LM. Comparison between the peripheral ossifying fibroma and peripheral odontogenic fibroma. J Oral Maxillofac Surg 47:378–382, 1989.

Zain RB, Fei YJ. Fibrous lesions of the gingiva: A histopathologic analysis of 204 cases. Oral Surg Oral Med Oral Pathol 70:466–470, 1990.

Lipoma

Chen S-Y, Fantasia JE, Miller AS. Myxoid lipoma of oral soft tissue: A clinical and ultrastructural study. Oral Surg Oral Med Oral Pathol 57:300–307, 1984.

de Visscher JGAM. Lipomas and fibrolipomas of the oral cavity. J Maxillofac Surg 10:177–181, 1982.

Fujimura N, Enomoto S. Lipoma of the tongue with cartilaginous change: A case report and review of the literature. J Oral Maxillofac Surg 50:1015–1017, 1992.

Garavaglia J, Gnepp DR. Intramuscular (infiltrating) lipoma of the tongue. Oral Surg Oral Med Oral Pathol 63:348–350, 1987.

McDaniel RK, Newland JR, Chiles DG. Intraoral spindle cell lipoma: Case report with correlated light and electron microscopy. Oral Surg Oral Med Oral Pathol 57:52–57, 1984.

Rapidis AD. Lipoma of the oral cavity. Int J Oral Surg 11:30–35, 1982.

Shmookler BM, Enzinger FM. Pleomorphic lipoma: A benign tumor simulating liposarcoma: A clinicopathologic analysis of 48 cases. Cancer 47:126–133, 1982.

Traumatic Neuroma

Peszkowski MJ, Larsson Å. Extraosseous and intraosseous oral traumatic neuromas and their association with tooth extraction. J Oral Maxillofac Surg 48:963–967, 1990.

Sist TC Jr, Greene GW. Traumatic neuroma of the oral cavity: Report of thirty-one new cases and review of the literature. Oral Surg Oral Med Oral Pathol 51:394–402, 1981.

Palisaded Encapsulated Neuroma

Chauvin PJ, et al. Palisaded encapsulated neuroma of oral mucosa. Oral Surg Oral Med Oral Pathol 73:71–74, 1992.

Dakin MC, Leppard B, Theaker JM. The palisaded, encapsulated neuroma (solitary circumscribed neuroma). Histopathology 20:405–410, 1992.

Dover JS, From L, Lewis A. Palisaded encapsulated neuromas: A clinicopathologic study. Arch Dermatol 125:386–389, 1989.

Fletcher CDM. Solitary circumscribed neuroma of the skin (so-called palisaded, encapsulated neuroma): A clinicopathologic and immunohistochemical study. Am J Surg Pathol 13:574–580, 1989.

Megahed M. Palisaded encapsulated neuroma (solitary circumscribed neuroma): A clinicopathologic and immunohistochemical study. Am J Dermatopathol 16:120–125, 1994.

Neurilemoma and Neurofibroma

Ellis GL, Abrams AM, Melrose RJ. Intraosseous benign neural sheath neoplasms of the jaws: Report of seven new cases and review of the literature. Oral Surg Oral Med Oral Pathol 44:731–743, 1977.

Hatziotis JC, Asprides H. Neurilemoma (schwannoma) of the oral cavity. Oral Surg Oral Med Oral Pathol 24:510–526, 1967.

Williams HK, et al. Neurilemmoma of the head and neck. Br J Oral Maxillofac Surg 31:32–35, 1993.

Woodruff JM. The pathology and treatment of peripheral nerve tumors and tumor-like conditions. CA Cancer J Clin 43:290–308, 1993.

Wright BA, Jackson D. Neural tumors of the oral cavity. Oral Surg Oral Med Oral Pathol 49:509–522, 1980.

Neurofibromatosis

D'Ambrosio JA, Langlais RP, Young RS. Jaw and skull changes in neurofibromatosis. Oral Surg Oral Med Oral Pathol 66:391–396, 1988.

Goldberg NS. Neurofibromatosis (von Recklinghausen's disease). *In:* Clinical Dermatology. Edited by Demis DJ. Hagerstown, Md, Harper & Row, 1993.

Neville BW, et al. Oral neurofibrosarcoma associated with neurofibromatosis type I. Oral Surg Oral Med Oral Pathol 72:456–461, 1991.

Riccardi VM, Eichner JE. Neurofibromatosis: Phenotype, Natural History, and Pathogenesis. Baltimore, Johns Hopkins University Press, 1986.

Shapiro SD, et al. Neurofibromatosis: Oral and radiographic manifestations. Oral Surg Oral Med Oral Pathol 58:493–498, 1984.

Multiple Endocrine Neoplasia Type III

Gorlin RJ, Cohen MM Jr, Levin LS. Multiple endocrine neoplasia, type 2B (multiple mucosal neuroma syndrome). *In:* Syndromes of the Head and Neck, 3rd ed. New York, Oxford University Press, 1990, pp 385–392.

Schenberg ME, et al. Multiple endocrine neoplasia syndrome—type 2b: Case report and review. Int J Oral Maxillofac Surg 21:110–114, 1992.

Melanotic Neuroectodermal Tumor of Infancy

Hupp JR, Topazian RG, Krutchkoff DJ. The melanotic neuroectodermal tumor of infancy: Report of two cases and review of the literature. Int J Oral Surg 10:432–446, 1981.

Kapadia SB, et al. Melanotic neuroectodermal tumor of infancy: Clinicopathological, immunohistochemical, and flow cytometric study. Am J Surg Pathol 17:566–573, 1993.

Mosby EL, et al. Melanotic neuroectodermal tumor of infancy: Review of the literature and report of a case. J Oral Maxillofac Surg 50:886–894, 1992.

Pettinato G, et al. Melanotic neuroectodermal tumor of infancy: A reexamination of a histogenetic problem based on immunohistochemical, flow cytometric, and ultrastructural study of 10 cases. Am J Surg Pathol 15:233–245, 1991.

Paraganglioma

Hodge KM, Byers RM, Peters LJ. Paragangliomas of the head and neck. Arch Otolaryngol Head Neck Surg 114:872–877, 1988.

LaMuraglia GM, et al. The current surgical management of carotid body paragangliomas. J Vasc Surg 15:1038–1045, 1992.

Powell S, Peters N, Harmer C. Chemodectoma of the head and neck: Results of treatment in 84 patients. Int J Radiat Oncol Biol Phys 22:919–924, 1992.

Sykes JM, Ossoff RH. Paragangliomas of the head and neck. Otolaryngol Clin North Am 19:755–767, 1986.

Granular Cell Tumor

Fliss DM, et al. Granular cell lesions in head and neck: A clinicopathological study. J Surg Oncol 42:154–160, 1989.

Mirchandani R, Sciubba JJ, Mir R. Granular cell lesions of the jaws and oral cavity: A clinicopathologic, immunohistochemical, and ultrastructural study. J Oral Maxillofac Surg 47:1248–1255, 1989.

Regezi JA, Batsakis JG, Courtney RM. Granular cell tumors of the head and neck. J Oral Surg 37:402–406, 1979.

Stewart CM, et al. Oral granular cell tumors: A clinicopathologic and immunocytochemical study. Oral Surg Oral Med Oral Pathol 65:427–435, 1988.

Congenital Epulis

Damm DD, et al. Investigation into the histogenesis of congenital epulis of the newborn. Oral Surg Oral Med Oral Pathol 76:205–212, 1993.

Lack EE, et al. Gingival granular cell tumors of the newborn (congenital "epulis"): A clinical and pathologic study of 21 patients. Am J Surg Pathol 5:37–46, 1981.

O'Brien FV, Pielou WD. Congenital epulis: Its natural history. Arch Dis Child 46:559–560, 1971.

Tucker MC, et al. Gingival granular cell tumors of the newborn: An ultrastructural and immunohistochemical study. Arch Pathol Lab Med 114:895–898, 1990.

Hemangioma

Bartlett JA, Riding KH, Salkeld LJ. Management of hemangiomas of the head and neck in children. J Otolaryngol 17:111–120, 1988.

Kaban LB, Mulliken JB. Vascular anomalies of the maxillofacial region. J Oral Maxillofac Surg 44:203–213, 1986.

Silverman RA. Hemangiomas and vascular malformations. Pediatr Clin North Am 38:811–834, 1991.

Stal S, Hamilton S, Spira M. Hemangiomas, lymphangiomas, and vascular malformations of the head and neck. Otolaryngol Clin North Am 19:769–796, 1986.

Waner M, Suen JY, Dinehart S. Treatment of hemangiomas of the head and neck. Laryngoscope 102:1123–1132, 1992.

Sturge-Weber Angiomatosis

Enjolras O, Riche MC, Merland JJ. Facial port-wine stains and Sturge-Weber syndrome. Pediatrics 76:48–51, 1985.

Hylton RP. Use of CO_2 laser for gingivectomy in a patient with Sturge-Weber disease complicated by Dilantin hyperplasia. J Oral Maxillofac Surg 44:646–648, 1986.

Sullivan TJ, Clarke MP, Morin JD. The ocular manifestations of the Sturge-Weber syndrome. J Pediatr Ophthalmol Strabismus 29:349–356, 1992.

Wilson S, Venzel JM, Miller R. Angiography, gingival hyperplasia and Sturge-Weber syndrome: Report of case. ASDC J Dent Child 53:283–286, 1986.

Yukna RA, Cassingham RJ, Carr RF. Periodontal manifestations and treatment in a case of Sturge-Weber syndrome. Oral Surg Oral Med Oral Pathol 47:408–415, 1979.

Nasopharyngeal Angiofibroma

Deschler DG, Kaplan MJ, Boles R. Treatment of large juvenile nasopharyngeal angiofibroma. Otolaryngol Head Neck Surg 106:278–284, 1992.

Duvall AJ III, Moreano AE. Juvenile nasopharyngeal angiofibroma: Diagnosis and treatment. Otolaryngol Head Neck Surg 97:534–540, 1987.

Kabot TE, et al. Juvenile nasopharyngeal angiofibroma: An unusual presentation in the oral cavity. Oral Surg Oral Med Oral Pathol 59:453–457, 1985.

Makek MS, Andrews JC, Fisch U. Malignant transformation of a nasopharyngeal angiofibroma. Laryngoscope 99:1088–1092, 1989.

Roberts JK, et al. Results of surgical management of nasopharyngeal angiofibroma: The Cleveland Clinic experience, 1977–1986. Cleve Clin J Med 56:529–533, 1989.

Hemangiopericytoma

Compagno J. Hemangiopericytoma-like tumors of the nasal cavity: A comparison with hemangiopericytoma of soft tissues. Laryngoscope 88:460–469, 1978.

Eichhorn JH, et al. Sinonasal hemangiopericytoma: A reassessment with electron microscopy, immunohistochemistry, and long-term follow-up. Am J Surg Pathol 14:856–866, 1990.

Enzinger FM, Smith BH. Hemangiopericytoma: An analysis of 106 cases. Hum Pathol 7:61–82, 1976.

Philippou S, Gellrich N-C. Hemangiopericytoma of the head and neck region: A clinical and morphological study of three cases. Int J Oral Maxillofac Surg 21:99–103, 1992.

Lymphangioma

Kennedy TL. Cystic hygroma-lymphangioma: A rare and still unclear entity. Laryngoscope 99(Suppl 49):1–10, 1989.

Levin LS, Jorgenson RJ, Jarvey BA. Lymphangiomas of the alveolar ridges in neonates. Pediatrics 58:881–884, 1976.

Ogita S, et al. OK-432 therapy for unresectable lymphangiomas in children. J Pediatr Surg 26:263–270, 1991.

Osborne TE, et al. Surgical correction of mandibulofacial deformities secondary to large cervical cystic hygromas. J Oral Maxillofac Surg 45:1015–1021, 1987.

Ricciardelli EJ, Richardson MA. Cervicofacial cystic hygroma: Patterns of recurrence and management of the difficult case. Arch Otolaryngol Head Neck Surg 117:546–553, 1991.

Wilson S, Gould AR, Wolff C. Multiple lymphangiomas of the alveolar ridge in a neonate: Case study. Pediatr Dent 8:231–234, 1986.

Leiomyoma

Damm DD, Neville BW. Oral leiomyomas. Oral Surg Oral Med Oral Pathol 47:343–348, 1979.

Epivatianos A, Trigonidis G, Papanayotou P. Vascular leiomyoma of the oral cavity. J Oral Maxillofac Surg 43:377–382, 1985.

Leung K-W, Wong DY-K, Li W-Y. Oral leiomyoma: Case report. J Oral Maxillofac Surg 48:735–738, 1990.

Rhabdomyoma

Corio RL, Lewis DM. Intraoral rhabdomyomas. Oral Surg Oral Med Oral Pathol 48:525–531, 1979.

Kapadia SB, et al. Adult rhabdomyoma of the head and neck: A clinicopathologic and immunophenotypic study. Hum Pathol 24:608–617, 1993.

Kapadia SB, et al. Fetal rhabdomyoma of the head and neck: A clinicopathologic and immunophenotypic study. Hum Pathol 24:754–765, 1993.

Neville BW, McConnel FMS. Multifocal adult rhabdomyoma: Report of a case and review of the literature. Arch Otolaryngol 107:175–178, 1981.

Osseous and Cartilaginous Choristomas

Chou L, Hansen LS, Daniels TE. Choristomas of the oral cavity: A review. Oral Surg Oral Med Oral Pathol 72:584–593, 1991.

Krolls SO, Jacoway JR, Alexander WN. Osseous choristomas (osteomas) of the intraoral soft tissues. Oral Surg Oral Med Oral Pathol 32:588–595, 1971.

Tohill MJ, Green JG, Cohen DM. Intraoral osseous and cartilaginous choristomas: Report of three cases and review of the literature. Oral Surg Oral Med Oral Pathol 63:506–510, 1987.

Soft Tissue Sarcomas

Enzinger FM, Weiss SW. Soft Tissue Tumors, 2nd ed. St. Louis, CV Mosby, 1988.

Farhood AI, et al. Soft tissue sarcomas of the head and neck in adults. Am J Surg 160:365–369, 1990.

Freedman AM, Reiman HM, Woods JE. Soft tissue sarcomas of the head and neck. Am J Surg 158:367–372, 1989.

Wanebo HJ, et al. Head and neck sarcoma: Report of the Head and Neck Sarcoma Registry. Head Neck 14:1–7, 1992.

Fibrosarcoma

Mark RJ, et al. Fibrosarcoma of the head and neck: The UCLA experience. Arch Otolaryngol Head Neck Surg 117:396–401, 1991.

Malignant Fibrous Histiocytoma

Barnes L, Kanbour A. Malignant fibrous histiocytoma of the head and neck: A report of 12 cases. Arch Otolaryngol Head Neck Surg 114:1149–1156, 1988.

Bras J, Batsakis JG, Luna MA. Malignant fibrous histiocytoma of the oral soft tissues. Oral Surg Oral Med Oral Pathol 64:57–67, 1987.

Liposarcoma

Eidinger G, Katsikeris N, Gullane P. Liposarcoma: Report of a case and review of the literature. J Oral Maxillofac Surg 48:984–988, 1990.

Saunders JR, et al. Liposarcomas of the head and neck: A review of the literature and addition of four cases. Cancer 43:162–168, 1979.

Neurofibrosarcoma

Bailet JW, et al. Malignant nerve sheath tumors of the head and neck: A combined experience from two university hospitals. Laryngoscope 101:1044–1049, 1991.

DiCerbo M, et al. Malignant schwannoma of the palate: A case report and review of the literature. J Oral Maxillofac Surg 50:1217–1221, 1992.

Ducatman BS, et al. Malignant peripheral nerve sheath tumors: A clinicopathologic study of 120 cases. Cancer 57:2006–2021, 1986.

Olfactory Neuroblastoma

Dulguerov P, Calcaterra T. Esthesioneuroblastoma: The UCLA experience 1970–1990. Laryngoscope 102:843–849, 1992.

Zappia JJ, et al. Olfactory neuroblastoma: The results of modern treatment approaches at the University of Michigan. Head Neck 15:190–196, 1993.

Angiosarcoma

Holden CA, Spittle MF, Jones EW. Angiosarcoma of the face and scalp, prognosis and treatment. Cancer 59:1046–1057, 1987.

Lanigan DT, Hey JH, Lee L. Angiosarcoma of the maxilla and maxillary sinus: Report of a case and review of the literature. J Oral Maxillofac Surg 47:747–753, 1989.

Zachariades N, et al. Primary hemangioendotheliosarcoma of the mandible: Review of the literature and report of case. J Oral Surg 38:288–296, 1980.

Kaposi's Sarcoma

DiGiovanna JJ, Safai B. Kaposi's sarcoma: Retrospective study of 90 cases with particular emphasis on the familial occurrence, ethnic background and prevalence of other diseases. Am J Med 71:779–783, 1981.

Farman AG, Uys PB. Oral Kaposi's sarcoma. Oral Surg Oral Med Oral Pathol 39:288–296, 1975.

Friedman-Kien AE, Saltzman BR. Clinical manifestations of classical, endemic African, and epidemic AIDS-associated Kaposi's sarcoma. J Am Acad Dermatol 22:1237–1250, 1990.

Gottlieb G, Ackerman AB. Kaposi's Sarcoma: A Text and Atlas. Philadelphia, Lea & Febiger, 1988.

Leiomyosarcoma

Freedman PD, Jones AC, Kerpel SM. Epithelioid leiomyosarcoma of the oral cavity: Report of two cases and review of the literature. J Oral Maxillofac Surg 51:928–932, 1993.

Nishi M, Mimura T, Senba I. Leiomyosarcoma of the maxilla. J Oral Maxillofac Surg 45:64–68, 1987.

Rhabdomyosarcoma

Bras J, Batsakis JG, Luna MA. Rhabdomyosarcoma of the oral soft tissues. Oral Surg Oral Med Oral Pathol 64:585–596, 1987.

Maurer HM, et al. The Intergroup Rhabdomyosarcoma Study—I. A final report. Cancer 61:209–220, 1988.

Maurer HM, et al. The Intergroup Rhabdomyosarcoma Study—II. Cancer 71:1904–1922, 1993.

Nakhleh RE, Swanson PE, Dehner LP. Juvenile (embryonal and alveolar) rhabdomyosarcoma of the head and neck in adults: A clinical, pathologic, and immunohistochemical study of 12 cases. Cancer 67:1019–1024, 1991.

Peters E, et al. Rhabdomyosarcoma of the oral and paraoral region. Cancer 63:963–966, 1989.

Synovial Sarcoma

Bukachevsky RP, et al. Synovial sarcoma of the head and neck. Head Neck 14:44–48, 1992.

Miloro M, Quinn PD, Stewart JCB. Monophasic spindle cell synovial sarcoma of the head and neck: Report of two cases and review of the literature. J Oral Maxillofac Surg 52:309–313, 1994.

Shmookler BM, Enzinger FM, Brannon RB: Orofacial synovial sarcoma: A clinicopathologic study of 11 new cases and review of the literature. Cancer 50:269–276, 1982.

Alveolar Soft Part Sarcoma

Lieberman PH, et al. Alveolar soft-part sarcoma: A clinico-pathologic study of half a century. Cancer 63:1–13, 1989.

Takita M-A, et al. Alveolar soft-part sarcoma of the tongue: Report of a case. Int J Oral Maxillofac Surg 19:110–112, 1990.

Metastases to the Oral Soft Tissues

Allen CM, et al. Leiomyosarcoma metastatic to the oral region: Report of three cases. Oral Surg Oral Med Oral Pathol 76:752–756, 1993.

Hirshberg A, Leibovich P, Buchner A. Metastases to the oral mucosa: Analysis of 157 cases. J Oral Pathol Med 22:385–390, 1993.

Zachariades N. Neoplasms metastatic to the mouth, jaws and surrounding tissues. J Craniomaxillofac Surg 17:283–290, 1989.

Hematologic Disorders

LYMPHOID HYPERPLASIA

The lymphoid tissue of the body plays an important role in the recognition and processing of foreign antigens, such as viruses, fungi, and bacteria. In addition, the lymphoid tissue has a protective function through a variety of direct and indirect mechanisms. In responding to antigenic challenges, the lymphoid cells undergo proliferation, thus increasing their numbers, in order to combat the offending agent more effectively. This proliferation results in enlargement of the lymphoid tissue, which is seen clinically as **lymphoid hyperplasia.**

Clinical Features

Lymphoid hyperplasia may affect the lymph nodes, the lymphoid tissue of Waldeyer's ring, or the aggregates of lymphoid tissue that are normally scattered throughout the oral cavity, particularly in the oropharynx, the soft palate, the lateral tongue, and the floor of the mouth. When lymphoid hyperplasia affects the lymph nodes, usually the site that the lymph node drains can be identified as a source of active or recent infection. In the head and neck region, the anterior cervical chain of lymph nodes is most commonly involved, although any lymph node in the area may be affected.

With acute infections, the lymphadenopathy presents as enlarged, tender, relatively soft, freely movable nodules. Chronic inflammatory conditions produce enlarged, rubbery firm, nontender, freely movable nodes. Sometimes these chronic hyperplastic lymph nodes may be difficult to distinguish clinically from lymphoma, and a history of a preceding inflammatory process and lack of progressive enlargement are helpful clues that are consistent with a reactive process. Another condition, however, that should be considered in the differential diagnosis of multiple, enlarged, nontender lymph nodes is human immunodeficiency virus (HIV) infection (see p. 199).

Tonsillar size is variable from one person to the next, but lymphoid tissue is normally prominent in younger individuals, usually reaching its peak size early during the second decade of life and gradually shrinking thereafter. Some patients may have large tonsils, which sometimes seem as if they would occlude the airway (so-called "kissing tonsils"). Often, however, these patients have no symptoms and are unaware of a problem. As long as the large tonsils are symmetric and asymptomatic (Fig. 13–1), it is likely that they are normal for that particular patient. Tonsillar asymmetry is a potentially serious sign that should be evaluated further to rule out the presence of a metastatic tumor or lymphoma.

Hyperplastic intraoral lymphoid aggregates present as discrete, nontender, submucosal swellings, usually less than 1 cm, which may appear normal or dark-pink in color if the aggregate is deeper or may have a creamy yellow-orange hue if the collection of lymphocytes (which are white blood cells) is closer to the surface (Figs. 13–2 and 13–3; see Color Figure 88). Lymphoid hyperplasia commonly involves the posterior lateral tongue, where it may appear somewhat ominous. The enlargement is usually bilaterally symmetric, however, which

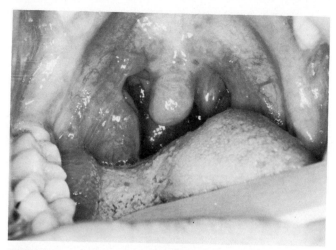

FIGURE 13-1. **Lymphoid hyperplasia.** The large tonsil observed in this patient represents a benign hyperplasia of the lymphoid cells. If significant asymmetry is observed, further investigation may be warranted to rule out the possibility of lymphoma.

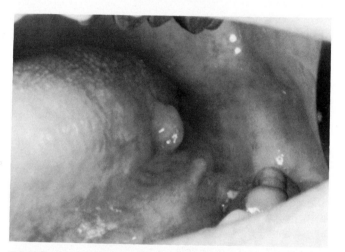

FIGURE 13-2. **Lymphoid hyperplasia.** The smooth-surfaced papule of the posterior lateral tongue represents an enlarged lymphoid aggregate. The lesion exhibits a lighter color as a result of the accumulation of lymphocytes, which are white blood cells. (Courtesy of Dr. Dean White.)

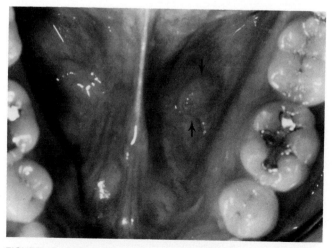

FIGURE 13-3. **Lymphoid hyperplasia.** Lymphoid aggregates (*arrows*) are frequently noted in the floor of the mouth, as in this photograph. See Color Plates.

helps to distinguish the condition from a malignancy. The buccal lymph node may also become hyperplastic and present as a nontender, solitary, freely movable nodule, usually less than 1 cm in diameter, within the substance of the cheek. Infrequently, a more diffuse lymphoid hyperplasia that involves the posterior hard palate is seen, producing a slowly growing, nontender, boggy swelling with an intact mucosal surface and little color change. These palatal lesions may be clinically impossible to distinguish from extranodal lymphoma and would therefore necessitate biopsy.

Histopathologic Features

The microscopic features of lymphoid hyperplasia include sheets of small, well-differentiated lymphocytes with numerous interspersed, sharply demarcated collections of reactive lymphoblasts called *germinal centers.* The cells that comprise the germinal centers are primarily transformed B lymphocytes that may demonstrate numerous mitoses. Macrophages can also be identified by the presence of phagocytized material ("tingible bodies") in their cytoplasm as they engulf nuclear debris from the proliferating lymphocytes.

Treatment and Prognosis

Once the diagnosis of lymphoid hyperplasia is confirmed, no treatment is usually required because it is a completely benign process. For those patients with palatal lymphoid hyperplasia that may interfere with a dental prosthesis, complete excision of the lesion is recommended.

HEMOPHILIA

Hemophilia (*hemo* = blood; *philia* = loving) represents a variety of bleeding disorders associated with a genetic deficiency of any one of the clotting factors of the blood (Table 13-1). This condition was common in the royal families of Europe who carried an X-linked hereditary deficiency of factor VIII; consequently, as a result of

Table 13-1. COMPARISON OF THE MOST COMMONLY ENCOUNTERED INHERITED BLEEDING DISORDERS

Type	Defect	Inheritance	Findings
Hemophilia A (classic hemophilia)	Factor VIII deficiency	X-linked recessive	Abnormal PTT
Hemophilia B (Christmas disease)	Factor IX deficiency	X-linked recessive	Abnormal PTT
von Willebrand's disease	Abnormal von Willebrand's factor; abnormal platelets	Autosomal dominant	Abnormal BT, abnormal PTT

BT, bleeding time; PTT, partial thromboplastin time.

inbreeding, a significant proportion of the male members of these families had hemophilia. In the days before blood transfusions and clotting factor replacement therapy, many of these patients died as a direct result of, or from the complications of, uncontrolled hemorrhage. In the United States, approximately 20,000 people suffer from hemophilia, with 16,000 to 17,000 having **hemophilia A**. Because hemophilia A is the most significant and widely recognized form of hemophilia and accounts for 80 to 85 percent of the bleeding diatheses associated with a specific clotting factor deficiency, most of this discussion centers on that entity.

Other clotting disorders that may be encountered clinically include **hemophilia B (Christmas disease)** and **von Willebrand's disease**. Hemophilia B is characterized by a genetic deficiency of factor IX, and this condition presents in a manner similar to hemophilia A. Von Willebrand's disease is caused by a genetic deficiency of a plasma glycoprotein called *von Willebrand's factor*. This glycoprotein aids in the adhesion of platelets at a site of bleeding, and it also binds to factor VIII, acting as a transport molecule. Von Willebrand's disease is the most common of the inherited bleeding disorders. It affects an estimated 1 in every 800 to 1000 persons. However, many cases of von Willebrand's disease are mild and may be clinically insignificant.

Clinical Features

Hemophilia A is an X-linked disorder. Females typically carry the trait, but it is expressed primarily in males. Approximately 1 in 8000 to 10,000 males are born with this genetic disease. Failure of normal hemostasis after circumcision is typically one of the first signs that a bleeding disorder is present.

The severity of the bleeding disorder depends on the extent of the clotting factor deficiency. Hemophilia A is a heterogeneous disorder that is caused by any one of a variety of mutations associated with the gene for factor VIII. Because the mutations occur at different sites in the factor VIII gene, a clinical spectrum of deficiency of factor VIII is seen. This results in varying degrees of disease expression. Not all patients have an absolute lack of the particular clotting factor; rather, the deficiency may be a percentage of the normal value in a given patient. For example, a patient with only 25 percent of normal factor VIII levels may be able to function normally under most circumstances; one with less than 5 percent commonly manifests a marked tendency to bruise with only minor trauma.

In toddlers, oral lacerations and ecchymoses that involve the lips and tongue are a frequent occurrence as a result of the common falls and bumps experienced by this age group. If not treated appropriately, such lacerations may result in significant blood loss in more severely affected patients. Sometimes deep hemorrhage occurs during normal activity, and may involve the muscles, soft tissues, and weight-bearing joints (hemarthrosis), especially the knees (Fig. 13–4). The result of such uncontrolled bleeding is the formation of scar tissue as the extravasated blood is removed by the body. This often causes a crippling deformity of the knee joints secondary

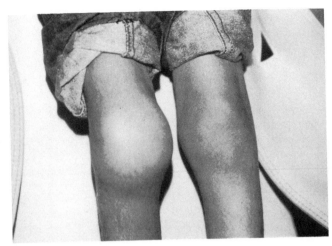

FIGURE 13–4. Hemophilia. The enlargement of the knees of this patient with factor VIII deficiency is due to repeated episodes of bleeding into the joints (hemarthrosis). Inflammation and scarring have resulted.

to arthritis and ankylosis. Sometimes the tissue hemorrhage results in the formation of a tumor-like mass, which has been called *pseudotumor of hemophilia*. Such lesions have been reported in the oral regions.

An increased coagulation time (delay in blood clotting), of course, is the hallmark feature of this group of conditions. Uncontrollable hemorrhage may result from any laceration; this includes surgical incisions, dental extractions, and periodontal curettage (Fig. 13–5). Measurements of the platelet count, bleeding time, prothrombin time (PT), and partial thromboplastin time (PTT) should be ordered as screening tests for any patient with a suspected bleeding disorder.

Treatment and Prognosis

The treatment of clotting factor deficiencies essentially consists of replacement therapy with the appropriate

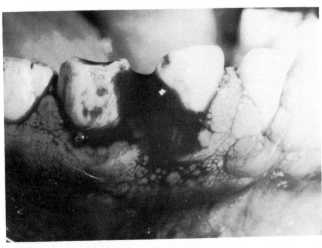

FIGURE 13–5. Hemophilia. Hemorrhage in a patient with factor IX deficiency occurred after routine periodontal curettage.

clotting factor. Whether treatment is instituted depends on the severity of the clotting factor deficiency.

Patients who have greater than 25 percent of normal values of factor VIII may function normally. For patients with mild hemophilia (5 to 25 percent of normal levels of factor VIII), no special treatment is typically required for normal activities. If surgery is to be performed, clotting factor replacement therapy may be indicated.

For patients with severe deficiencies (no detectable factor VIII levels), injections with the clotting factor must be performed as soon as a hemorrhagic episode occurs to prevent such complications as the crippling joint deformities of the knees.

The use of aspirin is strictly contraindicated because of its adverse effect on blood platelet function. Severe hemorrhage may result if aspirin-containing medications are used by these patients. Genetic counseling should be provided to these patients and their families to help them understand the mechanism of inheritance.

Optimal dental care is strongly encouraged for these patients to prevent oral problems that might require surgery. If oral or periodontal surgery is necessary, consultation with the patient's physician is mandatory. The patient is usually prepared for the procedure by the administration of clotting factor just before the surgery. With an extensive surgical procedure, additional doses of clotting factor may be needed subsequently. In addition, epsilon-aminocaproic acid (EACA, an antifibrinolytic agent that inhibits clot degradation) should be given 1 day before the surgery and continued for 7 to 10 days afterward. Alternative therapy for patients who have levels of factor VIII greater than 5 percent of normal is desmopressin acetate, which can be given just before surgery. This drug causes the release of bound factor VIII, which results in a temporary increase in the plasma levels of the clotting factor.

Clotting factor replacement therapy, although it has saved many lives, at the same time has resulted in a tragic complication for many of these patients. Cryoprecipitation, the traditional method of concentrating clotting factors from the serum, has also resulted in the concentration of several viruses, including the hepatitis viruses and human immunodeficiency virus (HIV). Consequently, as many as 80 to 90 percent of hemophiliac patients treated with multiple doses of factor VIII cryoprecipitate are now HIV-positive. The methods of preparing the clotting factors have been modified to eliminate the risk of acquiring HIV from the preparation; however, many hemophiliac patients who have already been infected still face the prospect of acquired immunodeficiency syndrome (AIDS). Recombinant DNA technology now provides a source of factor VIII that is manufactured by inserting the human factor VIII gene into bacteria that then synthesize the protein. Thus, this product can now be manufactured without contamination by any viral organisms.

ANEMIA

Anemia is a general term for either a decrease in the volume of red blood cells (hematocrit) or in the concentration of hemoglobin. This problem can result from a number of factors, including a decreased production of erythrocytes or an increased destruction or loss of erythrocytes. Laboratory studies, such as the red blood cell (RBC) count, hematocrit, hemoglobin concentration, mean corpuscular volume (MCV), mean corpuscular hemoglobin concentration (MCHC), and mean corpuscular hemoglobin (MCH), can help indicate the probable cause of the anemia.

Rather than being a disease itself, anemia is often a sign of an underlying disease, such as renal failure, liver disease, chronic inflammatory conditions, malignancies, or vitamin or mineral deficiencies. The diverse causes and complexity of the problem of anemia are presented in Table 13–2.

Clinical Features

The symptoms of anemia are typically related to the reduced oxygen-carrying capacity of the blood, which is a result of the reduced numbers of erythrocytes. Symptoms such as tiredness, headache, or lightheadedness are often present.

Table 13–2. CAUSES OF ANEMIA

Anemias with Disturbed Iron Metabolism
Iron deficiency anemia
Sideroblastic anemias

Megaloblastic Anemias
Cobalamin (B_{12}) deficiency (pernicious anemia)
Folic acid deficiency

Anemia Associated with Chronic Disorders
Anemia of chronic infection (infective endocarditis, tuberculosis, osteomyelitis, lung abscess, pyelonephritis)
Anemia of inflammatory connective tissue disorders (rheumatoid arthritis, lupus erythematosus, sarcoidosis, temporal arteritis, regional enteritis)
Anemia associated with malignancy
    Secondary to chronic bleeding
    Myelophthisic anemia
Anemia of uremia
Anemia due to endocrine failure
Anemia of liver disease

Hemolytic Anemias
Extrinsic causes
    Splenomegaly
    Red cell antibodies
    Trauma in the circulation
    Direct toxic effects (various microorganisms, copper salts, venom of certain snakes)
Membrane abnormalities
    Spur cell anemia
    Paroxysmal nocturnal hemoglobinuria
    Hereditary spherocytosis
    Hereditary elliptocytosis
Disorders of the interior of the red cell
    Defects in the Embden-Meyerhof pathway
    Defects in the hexose-monophosphate shunt

Disorders of Hemoglobin
Sickle cell anemia
Thalassemias

Pallor of the mucous membranes may be observed in severe cases of anemia. The palpebral conjunctiva is often the site where this paleness is most easily appreciated, but the oral mucosa may show similar signs.

Treatment and Prognosis

The treatment of anemia depends on determining the underlying cause of the anemia and correcting that problem, if possible.

SICKLE CELL ANEMIA

Sickle cell anemia is one of the more severe genetic disorders of hemoglobin synthesis (**hemoglobinopathies**). Because of the mutational substitution of a thymine molecule for an adenine in DNA, the codon is altered to code for the amino acid valine rather than glutamic acid in the beta-globin chain of hemoglobin. This results in a hemoglobin molecule that, in the deoxygenated state, is prone to molecular aggregation and polymerization. Consequently, the red blood cells of patients with sickle cell anemia have a marked tendency to undergo deformation from the normal biconcave disc shape to a rigid and curved, or "sickle" shape. Because the genes for hemoglobin synthesis are codominant, if only one allele is affected, only 50 percent of that patient's hemoglobin will be abnormal. Such a patient is simply a carrier of the sickle cell trait and has no significant clinical manifestations under most everyday conditions. Some sickling may be precipitated under certain conditions, however, particularly with low oxygen tensions associated with exercise or high altitudes.

This abnormal gene has persisted in the human race perhaps because it confers a degree of resistance to the malarial organism. As a result, the gene is seen most frequently in populations, such as African, Mediterranean and Asian, who reside in areas where malaria is endemic. In the United States, nearly 2.5 million people (approximately 8 percent of the black population) carry this trait.

Unfortunately, in patients who inherit two alleles that code for sickle hemoglobin, the red blood cells contain primarily sickle hemoglobin. This results in the condition called **sickle cell disease**. In the United States, about 1 of every 350 blacks is born with this disease. Such patients are often susceptible to the problems associated with abnormal RBC morphology. These problems can be traced directly to the fact that the sickled erythrocytes are more fragile than normal and that they tend to block the capillaries because of their shape and adherence properties. As a result, these patients have a chronic hemolytic anemia as well as many difficulties related to reduced blood flow to organs and tissues, which produces ischemia, infarction, and tissue death.

Clinical and Radiographic Features

Virtually any tissue or organ may be affected in sickle cell disease. The clinical spectrum of involvement can vary tremendously. Approximately one third of patients with sickle cell disease exhibit severe manifestations. Perhaps the most dramatic sign of this disease is the *sickle cell crisis*, a situation in which the sickling of the erythrocytes becomes severe. A crisis may be precipitated by hypoxia, infection, hypothermia, or dehydration; however, for most crises there is no identifiable predisposing factor. Patients who experience a crisis present in extreme pain from ischemia and infarction of the affected tissue. The long bones, lungs, and abdomen are among the most commonly affected sites, and each episode lasts 3 to 10 days. Some patients may experience such crises monthly; others may go for 1 year or longer without problems. Often fever accompanies the crisis; therefore, infection must be considered in the differential diagnosis.

Patients with sickle cell disease are also susceptible to infections, especially those caused by *Streptococcus pneumoniae*, probably because of the destruction of the spleen at an early age by repeated infarctions. Such infections are the most common cause of death among children affected by sickle cell disease in the United States.

Other problems include delayed growth and development in most patients. Impaired kidney function and ocular abnormalities develop secondary to the damage caused by vaso-occlusive episodes in the capillary networks of those organs. If the patient lives long enough, renal failure may eventually develop. In addition, approximately 5 percent of these patients will experience central nervous system damage in the form of a stroke, which occurs at an average age of about 8 years.

The oral radiographic features of sickle cell disease are relatively nonspecific. They consist of a reduced trabecular pattern of the mandible because of the increased hematopoiesis that occurs in the marrow spaces. Occasionally, a "hair-on-end" appearance is seen on the skull radiograph, although this is less prominent than that seen in thalassemia (Fig. 13–6).

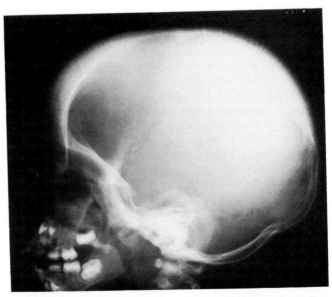

FIGURE 13–6. **Sickle cell anemia**. Lateral skull radiograph reveals an altered trabecular pattern, including a slight degree of "hair-on-end" appearance of the cranial bones. (Courtesy of Dr. Reg Munden.)

Histopathologic Features

In homozygous sickle cell disease, a peripheral blood smear shows a peculiar curved distortion of the erythrocytes, resembling a sickle or boomerang shape.

Treatment and Prognosis

The patient experiencing a sickle cell crisis should be managed with supportive care, including fluids, rest, and appropriate analgesic therapy, usually narcotic preparations. It is important, but often difficult, to rule out the possibility of infection.

As of this writing, 36 states screen for this hemoglobin disorder as part of their newborn infant health care system to identify affected individuals as soon as possible so that appropriate therapy can be instituted. For children with a diagnosis of sickle cell disease, continuous prophylactic penicillin therapy is indicated. In addition, the child should be given polyvalent pneumococcal vaccination. Situations that might precipitate a crisis, such as strenuous exercise, dehydration, or exposure to cold, should be avoided.

When surgery is necessary, local anesthesia, if possible, is usually preferred. If general anesthesia is indicated, precautions should be taken to avoid conditions that might induce a crisis, such as hypoxia, reduced body temperature, or dehydration.

For patients who have either the sickle cell trait or the disease, genetic counseling is appropriate. The prognosis for sickle cell disease is variable because of the wide spectrum of disease activity. Those who are severely affected, however, often are quite disabled because of the many complications of the disease and have a decreased life span.

THALASSEMIA

Thalassemia represents a group of disorders of hemoglobin synthesis that are characterized by reduced synthesis of either the alpha-globin or beta-globin chains of the hemoglobin molecule. As in those with sickle cell trait, people who carry the trait for one of the forms of thalassemia seem to be more resistant to infection by the malarial organism; an increased frequency of these genes is seen in Mediterranean, African, Indian, and Southeast Asian populations.

An understanding of the structure and synthesis of hemoglobin is helpful in explaining the pathophysiology of these conditions. The hemoglobin molecule is a tetramer that is composed of two alpha and two beta chains; if one of the chains is not being made in adequate quantities, the normal amount of hemoglobin cannot be made. Furthermore, the excess globin chains accumulate within the erythrocyte, further compromising the structure and function of the cell. These abnormal erythrocytes are recognized by the spleen and selected for destruction (*hemolysis*). The net result is that the patient has hypochromic, microcytic anemia.

Because two genes code for the beta chain and four genes code for the alpha chain, the degree of clinical severity in these conditions can vary considerably. The severity depends on which specific genetic alteration is present and whether it is heterozygous or homozygous. If the heterozygous state is present, an adequate amount of normal hemoglobin can be made and the affected patient experiences few signs or symptoms. In the homozygous state, however, the problems are often severe or even fatal.

Clinical and Radiographic Features

Beta-Thalassemia

If only one defective gene for the beta-globin molecule is inherited (**thalassemia minor**), no significant clinical manifestations are usually present.

When two defective genes for the beta-globin molecule are inherited, the patient is affected with **thalassemia major**, also called **Cooley's anemia** or **Mediterranean fever**. The disease is usually detected during the first year of life because a severe microcytic, hypochromic anemia develops when fetal hemoglobin synthesis ceases after 3 to 4 months of age. The red blood cells that are produced are extremely fragile and survive for only a few days in the peripheral circulation.

In an attempt to maintain adequate oxygenation, the rate of hematopoiesis is greatly increased, resulting in massive bone marrow hyperplasia, as well as hepatosplenomegaly and lymphadenopathy because of extramedullary hematopoiesis. The bone marrow hyperplasia may affect the jaws especially, producing marked, but painless, enlargement of the mandible and maxilla. This results in a characteristic "chipmunk" facies. Frontal bossing is also present, and a skull radiograph shows a "hair-on-end" appearance of the calvaria (Fig. 13–7).

Without therapy, tissue hypoxia worsens and serious bacterial infections with pneumococcal organisms often develop. Eventually, high-output cardiac failure occurs; many patients die by 1 year of age as a result of infection or heart problems.

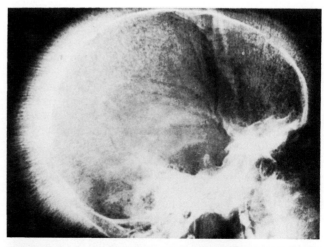

FIGURE 13–7. **Thalassemia**. Lateral skull radiograph depicting the characteristic "hair-on-end" appearance in patients with thalassemia.

Alpha-Thalassemia

Alpha-thalassemia has a broader spectrum of involvement than does beta-thalassemia because there are four alpha-globin genes that may be affected.

With the alteration of only one gene, no disease can be detected. With the inheritance of two altered genes, the condition is known as **alpha-thalassemia trait**; these patients have a mild degree of anemia and microcytosis that usually is not clinically significant.

With three altered genes, the term **Hb (hemoglobin) H disease** is applied. Patients have problems with hemolytic anemia and splenomegaly. In patients with severe hemolysis, splenectomy may be indicated.

The homozygous state, in which all four genes are abnormal, is called **hydrops fetalis**. This condition is typically fatal within a few hours of birth.

Treatment and Prognosis

Thalassemia major is treated today primarily by means of blood transfusions. These should be administered every 2 to 3 weeks to simulate the normal hematologic state. Unfortunately, with repeated blood transfusions, iron overload develops because of the constant infusion of exogenous red blood cells. This was a serious problem in the past when patients died of **hemochromatosis**, an abnormal deposition of iron throughout the tissues of the body. To combat this problem, an iron-chelating agent deferoxamine (also known as desferrioxamine) must be given. If such therapy is used steadfastly, patients with beta-thalassemia may have a relatively normal life span. Bone marrow transplantation has also been used with considerable success for individuals who are relatively young, have little organ damage, and have a histocompatability antigen (HLA)-matched donor.

APLASTIC ANEMIA

Aplastic anemia is a rare, life-threatening hematologic disorder that is characterized by failure of the hematopoietic precursor cells in the bone marrow to produce adequate numbers of all types of blood cells. The hematopoietic stem cells do not seem to undergo normal maturation despite normal or increased levels of cytokines, such as granulocyte-macrophage colony–stimulating factor, which normally induce the production and maturation of several types of white blood cells.

Although the underlying cause is unknown, some cases are associated with exposure to certain environmental toxins (such as benzene), treatment with certain drugs (especially the antibiotic chloramphenicol), or infection with certain viruses (particularly non-A, non-B, non-C hepatitis). The failure of the bone marrow may be due to immunologic abnormalities, perhaps triggered by exposure to drugs or viruses, which target the bone marrow stem cells. A few genetic disorders, such as **Fanconi's anemia** and **dyskeratosis congenita** (see p. 545), also appear to be associated with an increased frequency of aplastic anemia.

Clinical Features

Because all of the formed elements of the blood are decreased in patients with aplastic anemia, the initial symptoms may be related to any one or several of the deficiencies. The erythrocyte deficiency produces signs and symptoms related to a decreased oxygen-carrying capacity of the blood; therefore, patients may experience fatigue, lightheadedness, tachycardia, or weakness. The platelet deficiency (thrombocytopenia) is seen as a marked tendency for bruising and bleeding, which affects a variety of sites. Retinal and cerebral hemorrhages are some of the more devastating manifestations of this bleeding tendency. A deficiency of white blood cells (neutropenia, leukopenia, or granulocytopenia) predisposes the patient to various infections.

The oral findings related to thrombocytopenia include gingival hemorrhage, oral mucosal petechiae, purpura, and ecchymoses. The oral mucosa may appear pale because of the decreased numbers of red blood cells. Oral ulcerations associated with infection, particularly those that involve the gingival tissues, may be present. Minimal erythema is usually associated with the periphery of the ulcers. Gingival hyperplasia has also been reported in association with aplastic anemia.

Histopathologic Features

A bone marrow biopsy specimen usually demonstrates a relatively acellular marrow with fatty infiltration. The histopathologic features of an oral ulceration in a patient with aplastic anemia show numerous microorganisms in addition to a remarkable lack of inflammatory cells in the ulcer bed.

Diagnosis

The diagnosis of aplastic anemia is usually established by laboratory studies. There is a pancytopenia characterized by at least two of the following findings:

- Less than 500 granulocytes/μL
- Less than 20,000 platelets/μL
- Less than 10,000 reticulocytes/μL

Treatment and Prognosis

The course for patients with aplastic anemia is unpredictable. For the milder forms of the disease, spontaneous recovery of the marrow may occur in some instances; progression to severe aplastic anemia may be seen in others. Generally, in severe cases, the chances of spontaneous recovery are slim. If a particular environmental toxin or drug is associated with the process, withdrawal of the offending agent may sometimes result in recovery.

The treatment is initially supportive. Appropriate antibiotics are given for the infections that develop, and transfusions of packed red blood cells or platelets are administered for symptomatic treatment of anemia and bleeding problems, respectively.

Attempts to stimulate the bone marrow have met with

variable success. Androgenic steroids appear to benefit patients with mild disease, but they have little effect on the severe form. Because some cases of aplastic anemia seem to be immunologically mediated, immunomodulatory therapy has been attempted. A combination of anti-lymphocyte globulin, corticosteroids, and cyclosporine produces a response in approximately 70 percent of these patients.

Another approach to therapy is to replace the defective marrow with normal marrow (bone marrow transplantation). This treatment has been gaining acceptance despite the risk of graft-versus-host disease. Patients must be carefully selected; patients younger than 40 years of age and those with an HLA-matched donor have the best prognosis.

Typically, the prognosis for this condition is guarded at best. In the past, in patients with severe aplastic anemia, the mortality rate was greater than 80 percent in the first year after the diagnosis. Today, even if the disease is controlled, the patient remains at risk for recurrent marrow aplasia and is at increased risk for acute leukemia.

NEUTROPENIA

Neutropenia refers to a decrease in the number of the circulating neutrophils below 1500/mm³ in an adult. It is often associated with an increased susceptibility of the patient to bacterial infections. Clinicians must be aware of this disorder because infection of the oral mucosa may be the initial sign of the disease.

The decrease in neutrophils may be precipitated by several mechanisms, most of which involve decreased production or increased destruction of these important inflammatory cells. When infections are noted in infancy and neutropenia is detected, the problem is usually due to a congenital or genetic abnormality, such as **Schwachman-Diamond syndrome**, **dyskeratosis congenita** (see p. 545), **cartilage-hair syndrome**, or **severe congenital neutropenia**. If the neutropenia is detected later in life, it usually represents one of the acquired forms. Many acquired neutropenias have an unknown cause; however, others are clearly associated with various causes. A decreased production of neutrophils and the other formed elements of the blood may result from the destruction of the bone marrow by malignancies such as leukemia (see p. 427) or by metabolic diseases, such as Gaucher's disease (see p. 595) and osteopetrosis (see p. 444).

Many drugs may affect neutrophil production, either through direct toxic effects on the bone marrow progenitor cells or by unknown idiosyncratic mechanisms. Some of these drugs include:

1. Anticancer chemotherapeutic agents (e.g., nitrogen mustard, busulfan, chlorambucil, and cyclophosphamide).
2. Antibiotics (e.g., penicillins and sulfonamides).
3. Phenothiazines.
4. Tranquilizers.
5. Diuretics.

Nutritional deficiencies of vitamin B_{12} or folate, which may be a consequence of malabsorption syndromes, can inhibit neutrophil production.

A variety of viral and bacterial infections not only may reduce production of neutrophils but also seem to increase their destruction, typically at the sites of infection. Viruses that have been implicated include:

- Hepatitis A and B
- Rubella
- Measles
- Respiratory syncytial virus
- Varicella
- Human immunodeficiency virus (HIV)

Numerous bacterial infections, such as typhoid, tuberculosis, brucellosis, and tularemia, may also cause neutropenia. The increased destruction of neutrophils by an autoimmune mechanism also occurs in such disorders as systemic lupus erythematosus (SLE), in which autoantibodies directed against the neutrophil are produced.

Clinical Features

Most patients with neutropenia have some form of bacterial infection rather than a viral or fungal infection, particularly if the other elements of the immune system (lymphocytes, plasma cells, and monocytes) are still intact. *Staphylococcus aureus* and gram-negative organisms seem to cause the most problems for the neutropenic patient. The suppuration and abscess formation normally associated with such infections may be markedly reduced because of the lack of neutrophils. The most common sites of infection include the middle ear, the oral cavity, and the perirectal area. When neutrophil counts drop below 500/mm³, however, pulmonary infections often develop.

The oral lesions of neutropenia consist of ulcerations that usually involve the gingival mucosa, probably because of the heavy bacterial colonization of this area and the chronic trauma that it receives. These ulcers characteristically lack an erythematous periphery.

Histopathologic Features

A biopsy specimen of a neutropenic ulceration usually shows a reduced number or the absence of neutrophils. Bacterial invasion of the host tissue may be apparent in some instances.

Treatment and Prognosis

Infections related to neutropenia are managed with appropriate antibiotic therapy. The patient should be encouraged to maintain optimal oral hygiene to decrease the bacterial load in the oral cavity. Studies using recombinant human granulocyte colony-stimulating factor (G-CSF), a cytokine that promotes the growth and differentiation of neutrophils, have shown remarkable results. Patients with severe neutropenia showed a significant increase in neutrophil counts and resolution of infections after treatment with this agent.

AGRANULOCYTOSIS

Agranulocytosis is a condition in which the cells of the granulocytic series, particularly neutrophils, are absent. As in other disorders of the formed elements of the blood, agranulocytosis may occur as a result of decreased production or increased destruction or use of these cells. Although some cases are idiopathic, most are induced by exposure to one of several drugs. Some drugs, such as the anticancer chemotherapeutic agents, induce agranulocytosis by inhibiting the normal mitotic division and maturation of the hematopoietic stem cells. In other instances, the drugs set off an immunologic reaction that results in the destruction of granulocytes. Rarely, agranulocytosis may be a congenital syndrome (**congenital agranulocytosis, Kostmann syndrome**), which is caused by a decreased level of the cytokine, granulocyte colony-stimulating factor (G-CSF).

Clinical Features

Agranulocytosis typically develops within a few days after a person ingests the offending drug. Because of the lack of granulocytes (especially neutrophils), bacterial infections often develop and patients may show signs and symptoms of malaise, sore throat, swelling, fever, chills, bone pain, pneumonia, and shock. The erythrocyte and platelet counts are usually normal or only slightly depressed.

Oral lesions are common and include necrotizing, deep, punched-out ulcerations of the buccal mucosa, tongue, and palate. The gingivae are especially susceptible to infection, often resembling the pattern of acute necrotizing ulcerative gingivitis (ANUG; see p. 124).

Histopathologic Features

Microscopic examination of a biopsy specimen from one of the oral ulcerations in agranulocytosis characteristically shows abundant bacterial organisms both on the surface and within the tissue. The host inflammatory response is relatively sparse, with few granulocytes, particularly neutrophils, seen in the ulcer bed.

Treatment and Prognosis

If the agranulocytosis is thought to be due to a particular drug, the medication should be discontinued as soon as is reasonably possible. In many instances, the granulocyte count returns to normal within 10 to 14 days after cessation of the offending agent. For patients who have agranulocytosis secondary to cancer chemotherapy, oral hygiene should be meticulous to foster an immaculate oral environment. In addition, the use of chlorhexidine-containing mouth rinses seems to reduce the severity of the oral lesions. Active infections are treated with appropriate antibiotics.

If the agranulocytosis is related to cancer treatment, the white blood cell count usually returns to normal after a period of weeks. For patients whose granulocyte counts do not recover, administration of G-CSF or granulocyte-macrophage–colony-stimulating factor (GM-CSF) may be beneficial. The overall mortality rate for this condition in the past was 20 to 30 percent, although cytokine therapy and the newer broad-spectrum antibiotics have improved the outlook for these patients.

CYCLIC NEUTROPENIA

Cyclic neutropenia is a rare idiopathic hematologic disorder that is characterized by regular periodic reductions in the neutrophil population of the affected patient. Although an autosomal dominant pattern of inheritance has been described in a few cases, most examples of cyclic neutropenia are isolated.

Symptoms usually begin in childhood and tend to correlate with the neutrophil counts. When the neutrophil count is at its nadir (lowest point), the patient experiences problems with infection. As the neutrophil count rises toward normal, the signs and symptoms abate. Very low neutrophil counts usually are present for 3 to 6 days, and blood monocyte levels are typically increased when the neutrophil count is depressed. Even when the neutrophil count is at its peak, the levels are often less than normal.

Clinical Features

The signs and symptoms of cyclic neutropenia occur in rather uniformly spaced episodes, which have a 21-day cycle. Patients typically present with recurrent episodes of fever, anorexia, cervical lymphadenopathy, malaise, pharyngitis, and oral mucosal ulcerations. Other gastrointestinal mucosal areas, including the colon, rectum, and anus, may be affected by recurrent ulcerations.

The oral ulcerations develop on any oral mucosal surface that is exposed to even minor trauma, particularly the lips, tongue, buccal mucosa, and oropharynx (Fig. 13-8). An erythematous halo is variably present at the periphery of the ulcers. The gingiva is the most severely affected region of the oral cavity. Severe periodontal bone loss with marked gingival recession and tooth mobility are also characteristic (Fig. 13-9).

Diagnosis

The diagnosis of cyclic neutropenia should be established by sequential complete blood counts (typically two to three times per week for 8 weeks) to determine whether cycling of the neutrophil levels occurs.

Histopathologic Features

The histopathologic features of cyclic neutropenia are similar to those of the other neutropenic and granulocytopenic ulcerations if the biopsy is performed during the nadir of the neutrophil count.

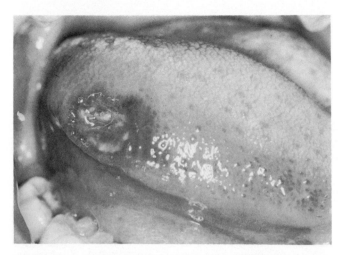

FIGURE 13-8. **Cyclic neutropenia.** Ulceration of the lateral tongue is typical of the lesions associated with cyclic neutropenia. (From Allen CM, Camisa C. Diseases of the mouth and lips. *In*: Principles of Dermatology. Edited by Sams WM, Lynch P. New York, Churchill Livingstone, 1990.)

Treatment and Prognosis

Supportive care for the patient with cyclic neutropenia includes antibiotic therapy for significant infections that might occur while the neutrophil count is at its lowest. Unfortunately, this approach cannot be considered a permanent treatment. Other methods that have been used with marginal success include splenectomy, corticosteroid therapy, and nutritional supplementation. Studies have used the cytokine, human granulocyte colony-stimulating factor (G-CSF), in an attempt to correct the lack of production of neutrophils. These studies have shown a decrease in the time of neutropenia from 5 days to 1 day, which resulted in improvement in the clinical course of the disease. The cycles were reduced from 18-21 days to

11-13 days, and the severity of mucositis and infection was reduced.

Supportive care in the form of optimal oral hygiene should be maintained to reduce the number and severity of oral infections and improve the prognosis of the periodontal structures. Fortunately, for many of these patients, the severity of symptoms related to cyclic neutropenia seems to diminish after the second decade of life, despite the fact that the cycling of the neutrophils continues.

THROMBOCYTOPENIA

Thrombocytopenia is a hematologic disorder that is characterized by a markedly decreased number of circulating blood platelets (formed elements derived from megakaryocyte precursors in the bone marrow). Platelets are necessary for hemostasis and clot formation. A platelet count of 200,000 to 400,000/mm^3 is considered normal. The decrease in platelets may be due to:

- Reduced production
- Increased destruction
- Sequestration in the spleen

Reduced Platelet Production. Reduced production of platelets may be due to various causes, such as infiltration of the bone marrow by malignant cells or the toxic effects of cancer chemotherapeutic drugs. In such instances, decreases in the other formed elements of the blood are also seen.

Increased Platelet Destruction. An increased destruction of platelets may be due to an immunologic reaction, which is often precipitated by any one of more than 100

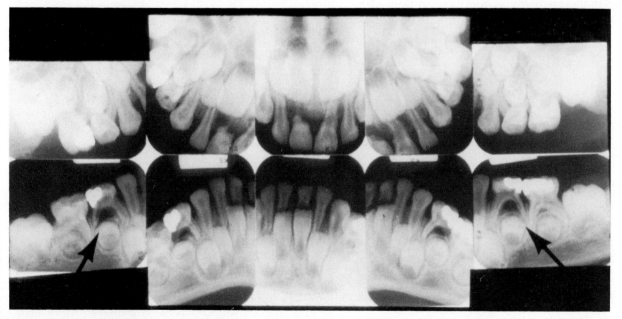

FIGURE 13-9. **Cyclic neutropenia.** Cyclic neutropenia is one of several conditions that may produce premature bone loss, as shown in the interradicular regions (*arrows*) of the mandibular deciduous molar teeth.

different drugs; heparin is one of the most common offending agents. This type of reaction is typically idiosyncratic and, therefore, not related to the dose of the drug. Increased destruction may also occur by non-immunologic means because of an increase in the use of the platelets associated with abnormal blood clot formation. This occurs in patients with conditions such as **thrombotic thrombocytopenic purpura** (TTP).

Sequestration in the Spleen. Under normal conditions, one third of the platelet population is sequestered in the spleen. Consequently, conditions that cause splenomegaly (e.g., portal hypertension secondary to liver disease, splenic enlargement secondary to tumor infiltration, or splenomegaly associated with Gaucher's disease) also cause larger numbers of platelets to be taken out of circulation. Regardless of the cause, the result for the patient is a bleeding problem because normal numbers of platelets are necessary for proper hemostasis.

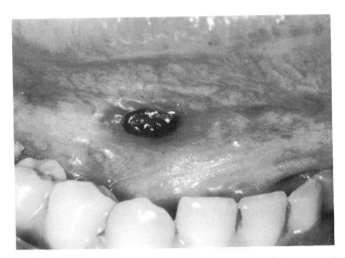

FIGURE 13-11. Thrombocytopenia. Hemorrhage of the ventral tongue secondary to thrombocytopenia.

Clinical Features

Clinical evidence of thrombocytopenia is usually not seen until the platelet levels drop below 100,000/mm³. The severity of involvement is directly related to the extent of platelet reduction. The condition often is initially detected because of the presence of oral lesions. Minor traumatic events are continuously inflicted on the oral mucosa during chewing and swallowing of food. The small capillaries that are damaged during this process normally are sealed off with microscopic thrombi. In a patient with thrombocytopenia, however, the thrombi do not form properly. This results in a leakage of blood from the small vessels. Clinically, this usually produces pinpoint hemorrhagic lesions known as *petechiae*. If a larger quantity of blood is extravasated, an *ecchymosis* or bruise results. With even larger amounts of extravasated blood, a *hematoma* (*hemat* = blood; *oma* = tumor) will develop (Fig. 13-10). Spontaneous gingival hemorrhage often occurs in these patients, as does bleeding from sites of minor trauma (Fig. 13-11).

Similar hemorrhagic events occur throughout the body. With severe thrombocytopenia (<10,000 to 15,000 platelets/mm³), massive bleeding from the gastrointestinal or urinary tract may be fatal. Epistaxis is often present in these patients, and hemoptosis indicates significant pulmonary hemorrhage.

Special types of thrombocytopenia include **idiopathic thrombocytopenic purpura** (ITP) and **thrombotic thrombocytopenic purpura** (TTP). ITP usually presents during childhood, classically following a nonspecific viral infection. The symptoms of thrombocytopenia appear quickly and may be severe. Most cases, however, resolve spontaneously within 4 to 6 weeks, and 90 percent of patients recover by 3 to 6 months.

TTP is a serious disorder of coagulation. It is thought to be caused by some form of endothelial damage, perhaps one that triggers the formation of numerous thrombi within the small blood vessels of the body.

Histopathologic Features

Gingival biopsy is often performed for diagnostic purposes in patients with suspected TTP. Approximately 30 to 40 percent of such biopsy specimens show the presence of fibrin deposits in the small vessels. These deposits are more readily appreciated after staining the tissue section using the periodic acid-Schiff method.

Treatment and Prognosis

If the thrombocytopenia is thought to be drug-related, the drug should be discontinued immediately. In most instances, the platelet count returns to normal after several days. Platelet transfusions and corticosteroid therapy may be necessary if life-threatening hemorrhage occurs. For some forms of thrombocytopenia, such as TTP, the patient's prognosis is relatively guarded. In the past, the condition was almost uniformly fatal, although the outlook has improved since therapy with plasmapheresis or exchange transfusions became available. More than 50 percent of these patients now survive with proper treatment.

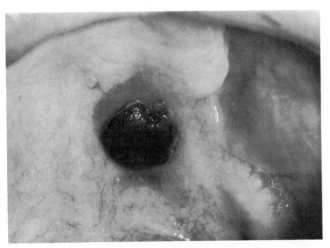

FIGURE 13-10. Thrombocytopenia. This dark palatal lesion represents a hematoma caused by a lack of normal coagulation, characteristic of thrombocytopenia.

POLYCYTHEMIA VERA (Primary Polycythemia; Polycythemia Rubra Vera)

Polycythemia vera is a rare idiopathic hematologic disorder that is best thought of as an increase in the mass of the red blood cells. Uncontrolled production of platelets and granulocytes, however, is also often seen concurrently. The overproduction is thought to be related to the abnormal behavior of a single progenitor marrow stem cell, which begins multiplying without regard to the normal regulatory hormones, such as erythropoietin. This gives rise to a group or clone of unregulated cells that then produce the excess numbers of these formed elements of the blood at two to three times the normal rate. These cells generally function in a normal fashion.

Clinical Features

Polycythemia vera typically affects older adults. The median age at diagnosis is 60 years. Only 5 percent of cases are diagnosed before the age of 40 years. No sex predilection is seen, and the prevalence of the condition is estimated to be 4 to 16 cases per million population.

The initial symptoms of the disease are nonspecific and include:

- Headache
- Weakness
- Dizziness
- Drowsiness
- Visual disturbances
- Sweating
- Weight loss
- Dyspnea
- Epigastric pain

A ruddy complexion may be evident on physical examination. One relatively characteristic complaint, described in about 40 percent of affected patients, is that of generalized pruritus (itching) without evidence of a rash.

The problems caused by thrombus formation, which would be expected with the increased viscosity of the blood and the increased platelet numbers, include cerebrovascular accidents and myocardial infarctions. Hypertension and splenomegaly are also common.

A peculiar peripheral vascular event called *erythromelalgia* affects the hands and feet. Patients experience a painful burning sensation accompanied by erythema and warmth. This may eventually lead to thrombotic occlusion of the vessels that supply the digits. Digital gangrene and necrosis may result. Erythromelalgia is probably caused by excessive platelets, and its onset seems to be precipitated by exercise, standing, or warm temperatures.

Strangely enough, these patients may also have problems with excess hemorrhage. Epistaxis and ecchymoses are often a problem, and gingival hemorrhage has been described.

Treatment and Prognosis

With the initial diagnosis of polycythemia vera, an immediate attempt is made to reduce the red blood cell mass. The first treatment is usually phlebotomy, with as much as 500 mL of blood removed daily. If thrombotic events are an immediate problem, treatment with aspirin should be started. Antihistamines may help to control the symptoms of pruritus.

Long-term management may include intermittent phlebotomy, although myelosuppressive therapy has also been advocated. Each has disadvantages. An increased risk of thrombosis is associated with phlebotomy, and an increased risk of leukemia is associated with some chemotherapeutic drugs. Hydroxyurea is one chemotherapeutic agent that may not pose an increased risk of leukemia, however, because it acts as an antimetabolite and does not appear to have any mutagenic properties. Nevertheless, in 2 to 10 percent of patients with polycythemia vera, acute leukemia ultimately develops.

Overall, the prognosis is fair; patients with polycythemia vera survive an average of 10 to 12 years after the diagnosis. Given the fact that the median age at diagnosis is 60 years, affected patients do not seem to have a markedly higher death rate compared with their unaffected peers.

LEUKEMIA

Leukemia represents several types of malignancies of hematopoietic stem cell derivation. The disease begins with the malignant transformation of one of the stem cells, which initially proliferates in the bone marrow and eventually overflows into the peripheral blood of the affected patient. Problems arise when the leukemic cells crowd out the normal defense cell and erythrocyte precursors.

Leukemias are usually classified according to their histogenesis and clinical behavior. Thus, the broad categories would be *acute* or *chronic* (referring to the clinical course) and *myeloid* or *lymphocytic* (referring to the histogenetic origin).

Myeloid leukemias can differentiate along several different pathways; thus, they produce malignant cells that show features of granulocytes, monocytes, erythrocytes, or megakaryocytes.

Acute leukemias, if untreated, run an aggressive course and often result in the death of the patient within a few months.

Chronic leukemias tend to follow a more indolent course, although the end result is the same.

One of the greatest successes in cancer treatment has been achieved in acute lymphocytic leukemia of childhood, a condition that used to be uniformly fatal but now is often capable of being controlled.

Leukemias are probably caused by a combination of environmental and genetic factors. Certain syndromes are associated with an increased risk. These genetic disorders include:

- Down syndrome
- Bloom syndrome
- Klinefelter syndrome
- Fanconi's anemia
- Wiskott-Aldrich syndrome

In addition, certain types of leukemia show specific chromosomal abnormalities. One of these, **chronic myeloid leukemia**, has a genetic alteration called the Philadelphia chromosome, which represents a translocation of the chromosomal material between the long arms of chromosomes 22 and 9. This rearrangement of the genetic material may occur in such a fashion as to activate a specific oncogene, which results in the uncontrolled proliferation of the leukemic cell.

Some environmental agents are associated with an increased risk. *Benzene* and benzene-like chemicals are well known to have this capability. *Ionizing radiation* has also been implicated; this was documented by the increased frequency of chronic myeloid leukemia in the survivors of the atomic bomb blasts at Hiroshima and Nagasaki during World War II. *Viruses* have also been shown to produce leukemia, although this is not a common finding. The most thoroughly studied is the retrovirus known as human T-cell leukemia/lymphoma virus type 1 (HTLV-1), which is transmitted by contaminated blood from infected to uninfected individuals. This virus can cause a relatively rare form of malignancy of T lymphocytes, which may present as a leukemia or non-Hodgkin's lymphoma (see p. 431). Most cases have been identified in parts of the Caribbean, central Africa, and southwestern Japan.

Clinical Features

If all types of leukemia are considered, this condition occurs at a rate of 13 cases per 100,000 population every year. Slightly more males than females are affected. The myeloid leukemias generally affect an adult population; **acute myeloid leukemia** affects a broader age range, which includes children. **Chronic myeloid leukemia** shows a peak incidence during the third and fourth decades of life. **Chronic lymphocytic leukemia**, the most common type of leukemia, primarily affects elderly adults. **Acute lymphocytic leukemia**, in contrast, almost always occurs in children and represents one of the more common childhood malignancies.

Many of the clinical signs and symptoms of leukemia are related to the marked reduction in the numbers of normal white and red blood cells, a phenomenon that results from the crowding out of the normal hematopoietic stem cells by the malignant proliferation (**myelophthisic anemia**). Because of the reduced red blood cell count and subsequent reduction in oxygen-carrying capacity of the blood, patients complain of fatigue, easy tiring, and dyspnea on mild exertion. The malignant cells may also infiltrate other organs and often cause splenomegaly, hepatomegaly, and lymphadenopathy.

Leukemic patients may also complain of easy bruising and bleeding, problems that are caused by a lack of blood platelets (**thrombocytopenia**), the result of megakaryocytes being crowded out of the marrow. Petechial hemorrhages of the posterior hard palate and the soft palate may be observed, with spontaneous gingival hemorrhage, especially with platelet counts less than 10,000 to 20,000/mm³. Serious hemorrhagic complications may result from bleeding into the central nervous system or the lungs.

A fever associated with infection may be the initial sign of the leukemic process. Perirectal infections, pneumonia, urinary tract infections, and septicemia are common infectious complications. The microorganisms that are typically involved include gram-negative bacteria, gram-positive cocci, and certain *Candida* species.

Ulceration of the oral mucosa is often present as a result of the impaired ability of the host to combat the normal microbial flora. Usually, the gingival mucosa is the most severely affected because of the abundant bacteria normally present around the teeth. The neutropenic ulcers that are produced typically are deep, punched-out lesions with a gray-white necrotic base. Oral candidiasis is often a complication of leukemia, involving the oral mucosa diffusely. Herpetic infections are the most common viral lesions, and these may involve any area of the oral mucosa rather than being confined to the keratinized mucosa, as in immunocompetent patients.

Occasionally, the leukemic cells infiltrate the oral soft tissues and produce a diffuse, boggy, nontender swelling that may or may not be ulcerated. This occurs most frequently with the myelomonocytic types of leukemia, and it may result in diffuse gingival enlargement (Fig. 13–12) or a prominent tumor-like growth (Fig. 13–13). This tumor-like collection of leukemic cells has been termed a **chloroma** because it is often greenish (*chlor* = green; *oma* = tumor) on fresh cut sections. Other oral manifestations include infiltration of the periapical tissues, simulating periapical inflammatory disease both clinically and radiographically.

Histopathologic Features

Microscopic examination of leukemia-affected tissue shows diffuse infiltration and destruction of the normal host tissue by sheets of poorly differentiated cells with either myelomonocytic characteristics or lymphoid features.

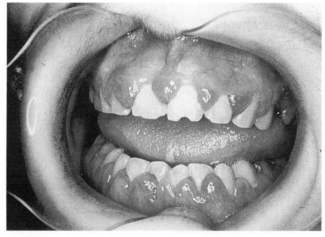

FIGURE 13–12. **Leukemia.** Diffuse gingival enlargement, as depicted in this photograph, may occur in leukemic patients, particularly in those with monocytic leukemia. (Courtesy of Dr. George Blozis.)

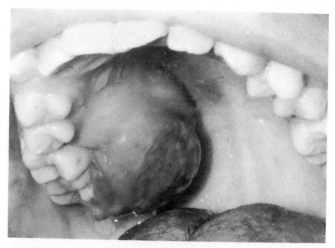

FIGURE 13–13. **Leukemia.** The ulcerated soft tissue nodule of the hard palate represents leukemic cells that have proliferated in this area.

Diagnosis

The diagnosis is usually established by confirming the presence of poorly differentiated leukemic cells in the peripheral blood and bone marrow. Both studies are normally performed because some patients may go through an aleukemic phase in which the atypical cells are absent from the circulation.

Treatment and Prognosis

The treatment of a patient with leukemia consists of various forms of chemotherapy; the type of leukemia dictates the chemotherapeutic regimen. The purpose of chemotherapy is to destroy as many of the atypical cells as possible in a short time, thus inducing a remission. For this reason, this technique has been termed *induction chemotherapy*. Usually, this phase of chemotherapy requires high doses of toxic chemotherapeutic agents; often, the patient experiences a number of unpleasant side effects during treatment. Once remission has been induced, this state must be maintained. This is the purpose of *maintenance chemotherapy*, which typically requires lower doses of chemotherapeutic drugs given over a longer period.

Drug therapy may be combined with radiation therapy to the central nervous system because the chemotherapeutic drugs often do not cross the blood-brain barrier effectively. Therefore, the leukemic cells may survive in this site and cause a relapse of the leukemia. Direct intrathecal infusion of the chemotherapeutic agent may be performed to circumvent the problem of the blood-brain barrier. If this strategy succeeds in inducing a remission, a bone marrow transplant may be considered as a therapeutic option, particularly for the types of leukemia that tend to relapse. Usually, this option is reserved for patients younger than 45 years of age because the success rate is poor in older patients.

Supportive care is often necessary if these patients are to survive their leukemia. For patients with bleeding problems, transfusions with platelets may be necessary. If severe anemia is present, packed red blood cells may be required. Infections, of course, should be evaluated with respect to the causative organism, and appropriate antibiotics must be prescribed. Support must be maintained from an oral perspective because many of these patients experience infections of the oral mucosa during the course of their disease. Optimal oral hygiene should be encouraged, and aggressive investigation of any oral complaint should be performed as soon as possible to prevent potentially serious oral infectious complications.

The prognosis depends on the type of leukemia and the age of the patient. In children with **acute lymphocytic leukemia**, a 50 to 70 percent 5-year survival rate can be expected, with 45 percent being long-term survivors. In an adult with the same diagnosis, however, the 5-year survival rate drops to 10 to 30 percent.

Patients with **acute myeloid leukemia** also have a 5-year survival rate of 10 to 30 percent. Even though an indolent period is experienced with **chronic myeloid leukemia**, eventually the neoplastic cells undergo a process known as *blast transformation*, in which they become less differentiated, proliferate wildly, and cause the patient's death within a short period. Nevertheless, attempts to control this disease by bone marrow transplantation have resulted in 2-year survival rates that average about 60 percent.

Chronic lymphocytic leukemia is considered to be incurable, but its course is highly variable and depends on the stage of the disease. Patients with limited disease have an average survival time of more than 10 years. Those with more advanced disease survive an average of only 2 years.

HODGKIN'S DISEASE
(Hodgkin's Lymphoma)

Hodgkin's disease is classified by most authorities as a malignant lymphoproliferative disorder, although the exact nature of the process is poorly understood. Perhaps one reason why Hodgkin's disease is not easily understood is that, unlike most malignancies, the neoplastic cells ("Reed-Sternberg cells") make up only about 1 to 3 percent of the cells in the enlarged lymph nodes that characterize this condition. Certainly, the disease can cause death if appropriate therapy is not instituted, although the treatment of this malignancy is one of the few major success stories in cancer therapy during the past 20 years. In the United States, Hodgkin's disease is about one fifth as common as non-Hodgkin's lymphoma; approximately 8000 cases are diagnosed annually.

Clinical Features

Hodgkin's disease almost always begins in the lymph nodes, and any lymph node group is susceptible. The most common sites of initial presentation are the cervical and supraclavicular nodes (70 to 75 percent) or the axillary and mediastinal nodes (5 to 10 percent each). The disease initially appears less than 5 percent of the time in the abdominal and inguinal lymph nodes.

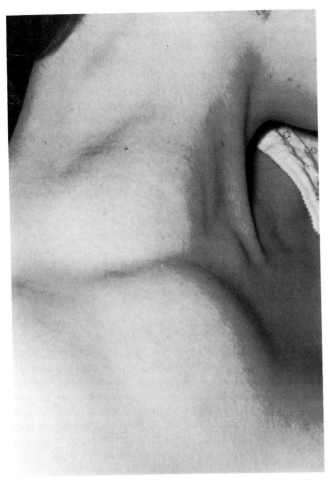

FIGURE 13–14. **Hodgkin's disease.** The prominent supraclavicular and cervical masses represent Hodgkin's disease.

Stage	Defining Features
I	Involvement of a single lymph node region (I) or a single extralymphatic organ or site (I$_E$)
II	Involvement of two or more lymph node regions on the same side of the diaphragm (II) or one or more lymph node regions with an extralymphatic site (II$_E$)
III	Involvement of lymph node regions on both sides of the diaphragm (III) possibly with an extralymphatic organ or site (III$_E$), the spleen (III$_S$), or both III$_{SE}$)
IV	Diffuse or disseminated involvement of one or more extralymphatic organs (identified by symbols), with or without associated lymph node involvement
	A = Absence of systemic signs
	B = Presence of fever, night sweats and/or unexplained loss of 10 percent or more of body weight during the 6-month period before diagnosis

Adapted from DeVita VT, Hubbard SM. Hodgkin's disease. N Engl J Med 328:560–565, 1993.

given patient. The staging procedure typically includes a careful history, physical examination, abdominal and thoracic computed tomographic (CT) scans or magnetic resonance imaging (MRI) studies, chest radiographs, and lymphangiography. Exploratory laparotomy and splenectomy may be necessary if the information that they would provide might have an impact on staging or treatment. A summary of the staging system for Hodgkin's disease is presented in Table 13–3.

Histopathologic Features

At least four histopathologic subtypes of Hodgkin's disease are recognized, although they have certain features in common. These features include effacement of the normal nodal architecture by a diffuse, often mixed, infiltrate of inflammatory cells interspersed with large, Reed-Sternberg cells (Fig. 13–15). The Reed-Sternberg

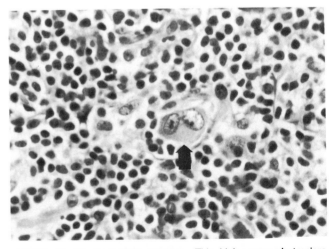

FIGURE 13–15. **Hodgkin's disease.** This high-power photomicrograph shows the characteristic Reed-Sternberg cell (*arrow*) of Hodgkin's disease, identified by its "owl-eye" nucleus.

Overall, a male predilection is observed, and a bimodal pattern is noted with respect to the patient's age at diagnosis. One peak is observed between 15 and 35 years of age; another peak is seen after the age of 50.

The usual presenting sign is the identification by the patient of a persistently enlarging, nontender, discrete mass or masses in one lymph node region (Fig. 13–14). In the early stages, the involved lymph nodes are often rather movable; as the condition progresses, the nodes become more matted and fixed to the surrounding tissues. If it is untreated, the condition spreads to other lymph node groups and eventually involves the spleen and other extralymphatic tissues, such as bone, liver, and lung. Oral involvement has been reported, but it is rare. Other systemic signs and symptoms may be present, such as weight loss, fever, night sweats, and generalized pruritus (itching). The absence of these systemic signs and symptoms is considered to be better in terms of the patient's prognosis, and this information is used in staging the disease. Patients who have no systemic signs are assigned to category A and those with systemic signs, to category B.

The staging of Hodgkin's disease is important for planning treatment and estimating the prognosis for a cell is typically binucleated ("owl eye nuclei"), although it may be multinucleated ("pennies on a plate"), with prominent nucleoli. The pathologist must see Reed-Sternberg cells to make a diagnosis of Hodgkin's disease, although their presence does not automatically imply that diagnosis, because similar cells may be seen in certain viral infections, especially infectious mononucleosis. The histogenetic origin of the Reed-Sternberg cell is still being debated, with some groups presenting evidence for a B-lymphocyte origin and others, for a T-lymphocyte origin.

The four histopathologic subtypes of Hodgkin's disease are:

- Lymphocyte predominant
- Nodular sclerosis
- Mixed cellularity
- Lymphocyte depletion

These names describe the most prominent histopathologic feature of each type, and specific epidemiologic and prognostic characteristics are associated with each type.

Lymphocyte-predominant Hodgkin's lymphoma represents about 2 to 10 percent of all cases. There is a proliferation of small lymphocytes with few Reed-Sternberg cells.

The *nodular sclerosis* subtype makes up 40 to 80 percent of cases and occurs more frequently in females during the second decade of life. This type gets its name from the broad fibrotic bands that extend from the lymph node capsule into the lesional tissue. Reed-Sternberg cells in the nodular sclerosis form appear to reside in clear spaces and, therefore, are referred to as "lacunar cells."

The *mixed cellularity* form constitutes about 20 to 40 percent of the cases and is characterized by a mixture of small lymphocytes, plasma cells, eosinophils, and histiocytes with abundant Reed-Sternberg cells.

The *lymphocyte depletion* subtype, the most aggressive type, makes up 2 to 15 percent of the cases. Numerous bizarre giant Reed-Sternberg cells are present with few lymphocytes.

Treatment and Prognosis

The treatment of Hodgkin's disease depends on the stage of involvement. Patients who have limited disease (stages I and II) are managed almost entirely by local radiation therapy alone. Those who present with stages III or IV disease require chemotherapy; radiation therapy is used conjointly if significant mediastinal involvement is detected. The most widely accepted regimen for treating Hodgkin's disease is known as **MOPP**, which stands for the drugs that are used:

- Mechlorethamine
- Vincristine (Oncovin)
- Procarbazine
- Prednisone

Before modern cancer therapy was developed for Hodgkin's disease, the 5-year survival rate was only 5 percent. The prognosis for this disease is fairly good today; the best treatment results occur in those who present in the early stages. Patients with stages I and II disease have a 90 percent or better 5-year survival rate; those with stage III disease have a 60 to 70 percent 5-year survival; and those with stage IV have a 50 percent survival rate.

The histopathologic subtype also influences the response to therapy. Patients with the lymphocyte predominant and nodular sclerosis forms have the best prognosis; those with the mixed cellularity form have an intermediate prognosis; and those with the lymphocyte depletion form have a poor prognosis. In most instances, however, the stage of disease now plays a more important role in determining the patient's prognosis than does the histopathologic subtype.

NON-HODGKIN'S LYMPHOMA

The **non-Hodgkin's lymphomas** include a diverse and complex group of malignancies of lymphoreticular histogenesis. In most instances, they initially arise within lymph nodes and tend to grow as solid masses. This is in contrast to lymphocytic leukemias (see p. 427), which begin in the bone marrow and are characterized by a large proportion of malignant cells that circulate in the peripheral blood. The non-Hodgkin's lymphomas most commonly originate from cells of the B-lymphocyte series; a T-lymphocyte derivation is less common. Histiocyte-derived lymphomas are even rarer.

In the past, the histomorphology of the lesions was used to classify the tumors as either lymphocytic or histiocytic. With the development of modern immunologic techniques, however, we now know that many of the lesions that had been classified as "histiocytic" in fact represent transformed B lymphocytes. Today, a combination of histopathologic features, immunologic cell surface markers, and gene rearrangement studies are used to diagnose and classify this group of neoplasms. On the basis of these studies, the tumors can be broadly grouped into three categories:

- Low grade
- Intermediate grade
- High grade

These categories are correlated with increasing degrees of aggressiveness, which correspond with their increasingly poor prognosis (Table 13–4). Of patients who are newly diagnosed with lymphoma, 35 to 40 percent will have a low-grade lesion, typically with widely disseminated involvement at the time of diagnosis; 55 to 60 percent will have an intermediate-grade lymphoma; only 5 percent have a high-grade lymphoma.

Approximately 40,000 cases of non-Hodgkin's lymphoma are diagnosed in the United States annually; approximately half of this number will die of the disease each year. The prevalence of lymphoma is increased in patients who have immunologic problems, such as congenital immunodeficiencies (Bloom syndrome, Wiskott-

Table 13-4. CLASSIFICATION OF THE NON-HODGKIN'S LYMPHOMAS BY THE WORKING FORMULATION

Subtype	Frequency (%)	Growth Pattern	Median Age	Potentially Curable with Chemotherapy?
Low Grade				
A. Small lymphocytic	4	Diffuse	61	Unproved
B. Follicular small cleaved cell	23	Follicular	54	Unproved
C. Follicular mixed cell	8	Follicular	56	Controversial
Intermediate Grade				
D. Follicular large cell	4	Follicular	55	Controversial
E. Diffuse small cleaved cell	7	Diffuse	58	Controversial
F. Diffuse mixed cell	7	Diffuse	58	Yes
G. Diffuse large cell	20	Diffuse	57	Yes
High grade				
H. Immunoblastic	8	Diffuse	51	Yes
I. Lymphoblastic	4	Diffuse	17	Yes
J. Small noncleaved cell	5	Diffuse	30	Yes

From Armitage JO. Treatment of non-Hodgkin's lymphoma. N Engl J Med 328:1023–1030, 1993.

Aldrich syndrome, or common variable immunodeficiency), AIDS, organ transplantation, and autoimmune disease (Sjögren syndrome, systemic lupus erythematosus [SLE], or rheumatoid arthritis).

Viruses may play a role in the pathogenesis of at least some of these lesions. For example, Epstein-Barr virus (EBV) has been implicated, but not proven, to be an etiopathogenic agent in Burkitt's lymphoma (see p. 436), a type of high-grade, small, noncleaved B-cell lymphoma. A blood-borne human retrovirus called HTLV-1 has been shown to cause an aggressive form of peripheral T-cell lymphoma among certain populations in the Caribbean, central Africa, and southwestern Japan.

Clinical and Radiographic Features

Non-Hodgkin's lymphoma occurs primarily in adults, although children may be affected, particularly by the more aggressive intermediate- and high-grade lymphomas. The condition most commonly presents in the lymph nodes, but so-called extranodal lymphomas are also found. With a nodal presentation, the patient usually is aware of a nontender mass that has been slowly enlarging for months. The lesion typically involves a local lymph node collection, such as the cervical, axillary, or inguinal nodes; one or two freely movable nodules are noticed initially. As the malignancy progresses, the nodes become more numerous and are fixed to adjacent structures or matted together (Fig. 13–16). Gradually, other lymph node groups are involved by the process, and invasion of adjoining normal tissues occurs.

In the oral cavity, lymphoma usually presents as extranodal disease. Although the oral lesions of lymphoma are often a component of more widely disseminated disease, at times the lymphoma begins in the oral tissues and has not spread to other sites. The malignancy may develop in the oral soft tissues or centrally within the jaws. Soft tissue lesions appear as nontender, diffuse swellings; they most commonly affect the buccal vestibule, gingiva, or posterior hard palate (Fig. 13–17). Such swellings characteristically have a boggy consistency. The lesion may appear erythematous or purplish, and it may or may not be ulcerated. Patients who wear a denture that involves the lesional site often complain that their denture does not fit because it is "too tight."

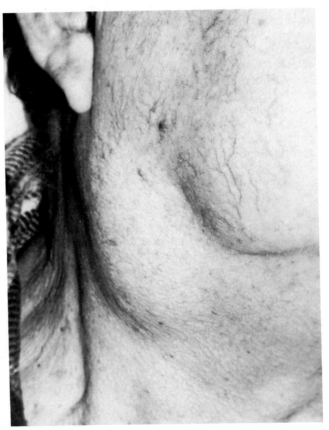

FIGURE 13–16. **Non-Hodgkin's lymphoma.** The matted, nontender lymph node enlargement in the lateral cervical region represents a common presentation of lymphoma.

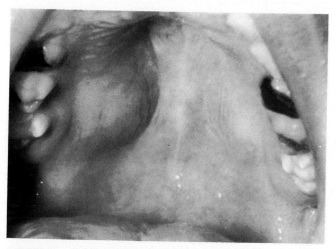

FIGURE 13–17. **Non-Hodgkin's lymphoma.** One of the frequent locations of extranodal lymphoma in the head and neck area is the palate, where the tumor presents as a nontender, boggy swelling. This case is unusual because it affects an 8-year-old child.

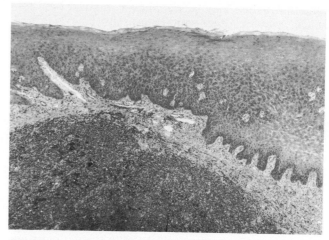

FIGURE 13–19. **Non-Hodgkin's lymphoma.** This low-power photomicrograph shows a diffuse infiltration of the subepithelial connective tissue by lymphoma.

Lymphoma of bone may present with vague pain or discomfort, which might be mistaken for a toothache. The patient may complain of paresthesia, particularly with a mandibular lesion. Radiographs usually show an ill-defined or ragged radiolucency. If it is untreated, the process typically causes expansion of the bone, which eventually perforates the cortical plate and produces a soft tissue swelling (Fig. 13–18). Such lesions have been mistaken for a dental abscess, although a significant amount of pain is not present in most cases.

Clinical staging to determine the extent to which the disease has spread is an important factor in assessing the prognosis for a particular patient. The staging evaluation should include a history, physical examination, complete blood count, liver function studies, routine chest radiographs, CT scans of the pelvic and abdominal regions, lymphangiography, and bone marrow biopsy. The stag-

ing system for Hodgkin's disease (see Table 13–3) has been widely adopted for use with the non-Hodgkin's lymphomas.

Histopathologic Features

Non-Hodgkin's lymphomas are histopathologically characterized by a proliferation of lymphocytic-appearing cells that may show varying degrees of differentiation, depending on the type of lymphoma. Low-grade lesions consist of well-differentiated small lymphocytes. High-grade lesions tend to be composed of less differentiated cells. All lymphomas grow as infiltrative, broad sheets of relatively uniform neoplastic cells, which show little or no evidence of lesional tissue necrosis (Figs. 13–19 and 13–20). In some lesions, particularly those of B-lymphocyte origin, a vague semblance of germinal

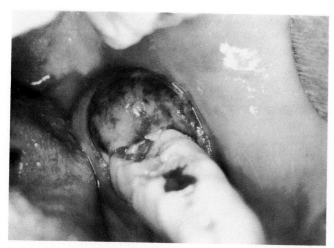

FIGURE 13–18. **Non-Hodgkin's lymphoma.** The ulcerated mass of the retromolar region represents extranodal lymphoma, which originated in bone and now involves the oral soft tissue.

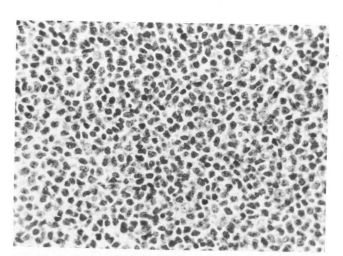

FIGURE 13–20. **Non-Hodgkin's lymphoma.** This high-power photomicrograph shows lesional cells of lymphoma, consisting of a uniform population of dark, round, poorly differentiated cells of the lymphocytic series with minimal cytoplasm.

center formation may be seen, i.e., a "nodular" or "follicular" pattern. Other lymphomas show no evidence of such differentiation, and this pattern is termed "diffuse." If the lymphoma arises in a lymph node, the tumor destroys the normal architecture of the node. An extranodal lymphoma destroys the normal adjacent host tissue by infiltrating throughout the area.

Treatment and Prognosis

The treatment of a patient with non-Hodgkin's lymphoma consists of radiation therapy and/or chemotherapy, depending on the stage and grade of the lymphoma. Surgical management is not usually indicated.

Low-grade lymphomas are perhaps the most controversial in terms of treatment. Some authorities recommend no particular treatment because these tumors are slow-growing and tend to recur despite chemotherapy. Given the fact that low-grade lymphomas arise in older adults and the median survival without treatment is 8 to 10 years, many clinicians opt for a "watch and wait" strategy, treating the patient only if symptoms occur.

For the *intermediate-grade* and *high-grade* lymphomas, the treatment depends not only on the grade of the lesion but also on the stage of the disease. If the tumor is localized, radiation therapy alone may be used. If the tumor is in a more advanced stage, then radiation plus chemotherapy or chemotherapy alone usually is implemented. Multiagent chemotherapy is used routinely, and new combinations are being evaluated continuously. Unfortunately, although the response rate of many lesions is good and much progress has been made in this area, the cure rate is not high. For intermediate-grade lesions, a failure rate of 30 to 50 percent can be expected. High-grade lymphomas are associated with a 60 percent mortality rate at 5 years after diagnosis and treatment.

MYCOSIS FUNGOIDES (Cutaneous T-Cell Lymphoma)

From its name, one might think that **mycosis fungoides** is a fungal infection. The early dermatologists who first recognized mycosis fungoides knew that this was not the case; however, they still thought the disease resembled a fungal condition. Thus this term has persisted. This condition in fact represents a lymphoma that is derived from T lymphocytes, specifically the T-helper (CD4+) lymphocyte. Mycosis fungoides is a relatively rare malignancy; only about 400 new cases are diagnosed in the United States annually. This condition exhibits a peculiar property called *epidermotropism*, i.e., a propensity to invade the epidermis of the skin. Oral involvement, although infrequent, may also be present.

Clinical Features

Mycosis fungoides is a condition that usually affects middle-aged adult men; there is a 2:1 male-to-female ratio and a mean age at diagnosis of 55 to 60 years. The disease progresses through three stages, usually over the course of several years.

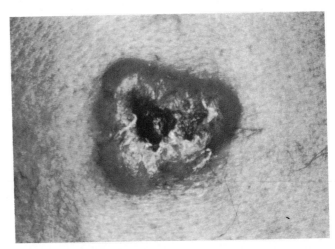

FIGURE 13–21. **Mycosis fungoides.** In the tumor stage of the disease, patients with mycosis fungoides have ulcerated nodules of the skin. (Damm DD, et al. Mycosis fungoides: Initial diagnosis via palatal biopsy with discussion of diagnostic advantages of plastic embedding. Oral Surg Oral Med Oral Pathol 58:413–419, 1984.)

The first stage, known as the *eczematous* (*erythematous*) stage, is often mistaken for psoriasis of the skin because of the well-demarcated, scaly, erythematous patches that characterize these lesions. Patients may complain of pruritus. With time, the erythematous patches evolve into slightly elevated, red lesions (*plaque stage*). These plaques tend to grow and become distinct papules and nodules. At this time, the disease has entered the *tumor stage* (Fig. 13–21). Visceral involvement is also seen at this point.

Approximately 25 cases of mycosis fungoides with oral involvement have been reported. The most commonly affected sites are the gingiva, hard and soft palates, and tongue (Fig. 13–22). The buccal mucosa, tonsils, lips, sinuses, and nasopharynx may also be affected. The oral lesions present as erythematous, indurated plaques or

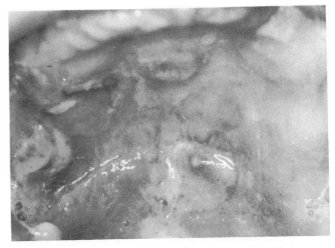

FIGURE 13–22. **Mycosis fungoides.** The ulcerated palatal lesions represent a rare example of oral mucosal involvement by mycosis fungoides.

nodules that are typically ulcerated. Generally, these lesions appear late in the course of the disease and develop after the cutaneous lesions.

Sézary syndrome is an aggressive expression of mycosis fungoides that essentially represents a dermatopathic T-cell leukemia. The patient has a generalized exfoliative erythroderma as well as lymphadenopathy, hepatomegaly, and splenomegaly. The lungs, kidneys, and central nervous system can also be involved. This condition follows a fulminant course and typically results in the patient's death within a short period of time; the median survival is 2 to 3 years.

Histopathologic Features

Eczematous Stage

The early stages of mycosis fungoides may be difficult to diagnose histopathologically because of the subtle changes that characterize the initial lesions. A psoriasiform pattern of epithelial alteration is seen, with parakeratin production and elongation of the epithelial rete ridges. Scattered, slightly atypical lymphocytic cells may be seen in the connective tissue papillae, but such features are often mistaken for an inflammatory process.

Plaque Stage

With the development of the plaque stage, a more readily identifiable microscopic pattern emerges. Examination of the surface epithelium reveals infiltration by atypical lymphocytic cells, which are sometimes referred to as "mycosis cells" or "Sézary cells" (Fig. 13–23). The lesional cells have an extremely unusual nucleus because of the marked infolding of the nuclear membrane, which results in what is termed a "cerebriform nucleus." This feature can best be appreciated when viewed in special semithin, plastic-embedded microscopic sections. These atypical lymphocytes classically form small intraepithelial aggregates termed "Pautrier's microabscesses" (Fig. 13–24). A mixed infiltrate of eosinophils, histiocytes,

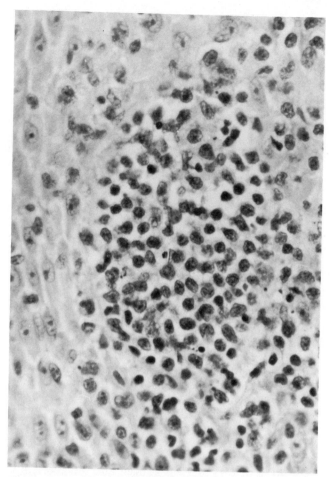

FIGURE 13–24. **Mycosis fungoides.** This high-power photomicrograph reveals the atypical, malignant lymphoid cells of mycosis fungoides forming a Pautrier's microabscess within the epithelium.

and plasma cells may be observed in the subepithelial connective tissue.

Tumor Stage

As the condition progresses to the tumor stage, the diffuse infiltration of the dermis and epidermis by atypical lymphocytic cells makes it easier to identify as a malignant process. Other types of lymphoma would enter into the histopathologic differential diagnosis.

Electron microscopic studies showing convoluted nuclei and immunohistochemical studies demonstrating a T-helper phenotype would help to establish the diagnosis of mycosis fungoides. Examination of the peripheral blood of a patient with Sézary syndrome shows circulating atypical lymphoid cells.

Treatment and Prognosis

Topical nitrogen mustard, electron beam therapy, or photochemotherapy (**PUVA** [8-methoxyPsoralen + UltraViolet A]) are effective in controlling mycosis fungoides during the early stages. Ultimately, the topical forms of therapy fail, and aggressive chemotherapy is necessary, particularly if there is visceral involvement. If

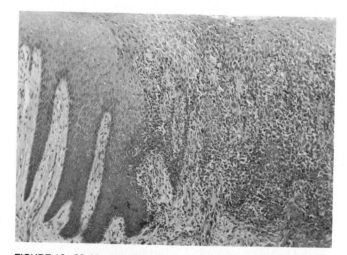

FIGURE 13–23. **Mycosis fungoides.** This low-power photomicrograph of an oral lesion of mycosis fungoides shows infiltration of the epithelium by the malignant infiltrate (*right*). Note normal adjacent epithelium (*left*).

Sézary syndrome develops, extracorporeal photopheresis or chemotherapy is used as a treatment modality. Extracorporeal photopheresis involves the ingestion of the photoactive drug 8-methoxypsoralen, followed by the removal of a portion of the patient's blood and a separation of red and white blood cells. The red blood cells are returned to the patient immediately. The white blood cells are irradiated outside the body (extracorporeal) with UV-A. These altered white cells are then infused back into the patient. Their altered state may help generate an immunologic response to the patient's own abnormal lymphocytes.

Although the prognosis for patients with mycosis fungoides is poor, the disease is usually slowly progressive. As a result, there is a median survival time of 8 to 10 years. Once the disease progresses beyond the cutaneous involvement, the course becomes much worse. The patient usually dies of organ failure or sepsis within 1 year.

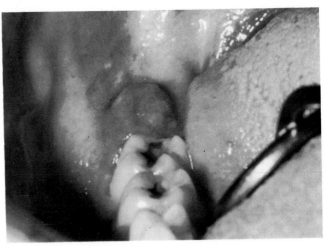

FIGURE 13–25. **Burkitt's lymphoma.** This patient had documented American Burkitt's lymphoma involving the abdominal region. The retromolar swelling represents oral involvement with the malignancy.

BURKITT'S LYMPHOMA

Burkitt's lymphoma is a malignancy of B-lymphocyte origin that represents an undifferentiated lymphoma. It was named after the missionary doctor, Denis Burkitt, who first documented the process. In the original report, this type of lymphoma was described in young African children, and it seemed to have a predilection for the jaws. Subsequently, the tumor was postulated to be related pathogenetically to Epstein-Barr virus (EBV) because more than 90 percent of the tumor cells show expression of EBV nuclear antigen and the affected patients have elevated antibody titers to EBV. Characteristic cytogenetic chromosomal translocations, which may also be responsible for neoplastic transformation, have also been described.

Tumors with a similar histomorphology, commonly referred to as **American Burkitt's lymphoma**, have been observed in other countries where the neoplasm is usually first detected as an abdominal mass. Some HIV-related lymphomas may also have the microscopic features of Burkitt's lymphoma.

Clinical and Radiographic Features

As many as 50 to 70 percent of the cases of the African form of Burkitt's lymphoma present in the jaws. The malignancy usually affects children (peak prevalence, about 7 years of age) who live in Central Africa, where this tumor is endemic. The posterior segments of the jaws are more commonly affected, and the maxilla is involved more commonly than the mandible (a 2:1 ratio). Sometimes all four quadrants of the jaws show tumor involvement.

The tendency for jaw involvement seems to be age-related; nearly 90 percent of 3-year-old patients have jaw lesions in contrast to only 25 percent of patients older than age 15. American Burkitt's lymphoma tends to affect patients over a greater age range than is noted for the African tumor. Although the abdominal region is usually affected, jaw lesions have been reported in American Burkitt's lymphoma (Fig. 13–25).

The growth of the tumor mass may produce facial swelling and proptosis. Pain, tenderness, and paresthesia are usually minimal, although marked tooth mobility may be present because of the aggressive destruction of the alveolar bone.

The radiographic features are consistent with a malignant process and include a radiolucent destruction of the bone with ragged, ill-defined margins. This process may begin as several smaller sites, which eventually enlarge and coalesce. Patchy loss of the lamina dura has been mentioned as an early sign of Burkitt's lymphoma.

Histopathologic Features

Burkitt's lymphoma histopathologically represents an undifferentiated, small, noncleaved B-cell lymphoma. The lesional tissue invades as broad sheets of tumor cells and exhibits round nuclei with several prominent nucleoli and numerous mitoses. A classic "starry-sky" pattern is associated with the lesional tissue, a phenomenon that is caused by the presence of macrophages within the tumor tissue (Fig. 13–26). These macrophages have abundant cytoplasm, which microscopically appears less intensely stained in comparison with the surrounding process. Thus these cells tend to stand out as "stars" set against the "night sky" of deeply hyperchromatic neoplastic lymphoid cells (Fig. 13–27).

Treatment and Prognosis

Burkitt's lymphoma is an aggressive malignancy that usually results in the death of the patient within 4 to 6 months after diagnosis if it is not treated. Treatment generally consists of an intensive chemotherapeutic regimen, which emphasizes the use of high doses of cyclophosphamide. More than 90 percent of the patients respond to this treatment. Unfortunately, most experience recurrences and ultimately die of their disease.

The prognosis for Burkitt's lymphoma in the past was poor, with a median survival time of only 10½ months.

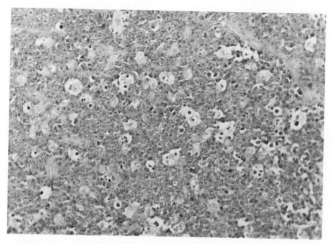

FIGURE 13-26. **Burkitt's lymphoma.** This low-power photomicrograph shows the classic "starry-sky" appearance, a pattern due to interspersed histiocytic cells with abundant cytoplasm ("stars") set against a background of malignant, darkly staining lymphoma cells ("night sky").

More recent trials with more intensive, multiagent chemotherapeutic protocols show a 68 percent remission rate after 38 months of follow-up.

MULTIPLE MYELOMA

Multiple myeloma is a relatively rare malignancy of plasma cell origin that often appears to have a multicentric origin within bone. The cause of the condition is unknown, although sometimes a plasmacytoma (see p. 438) may evolve into multiple myeloma. This disease makes up about 1 percent of all malignancies and 10 to 15 percent of hematologic malignancies. If metastatic disease is excluded, multiple myeloma accounts for nearly 50 percent of all malignancies that involve the bone. More than 12,000 cases are diagnosed annually in the United States.

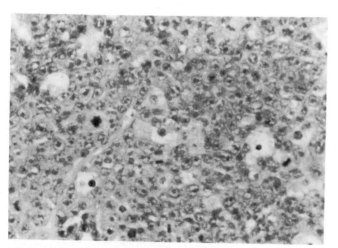

FIGURE 13-27. **Burkitt's lymphoma.** This high-power photomicrograph demonstrates the undifferentiated, small, dark lesional cells with occasional histiocytes.

The abnormal plasma cells that compose this tumor are typically monoclonal. The abnormal cells probably arose from a single malignant precursor that has undergone uncontrolled mitotic division and has spread throughout the body. Because the neoplasm has developed from a single cell, all the daughter cells that compose the lesional tissue have the same genetic make-up and produce the same proteins. These proteins are the immunoglobulin components that the plasma cell would normally produce, although in the case of this malignant tumor the immunoglobulins are not normal or functional. The signs and symptoms of this disease result from the uncontrolled proliferation of the tumor cells and the uncontrolled manufacture of their protein products.

Clinical and Radiographic Features

Multiple myeloma is typically a disease of older men. The median age at diagnosis is 70 years, and it rarely presents before age 40. A male-to-female ratio of 2:1 is seen; for reasons that are not understood, the disease occurs twice as frequently in blacks as whites.

Bone pain is the most characteristic presenting symptom. Some patients present with pathologic fractures caused by tumor destruction of bone. They may also present with fatigue as a consequence of myelophthisic anemia. Petechial hemorrhages of the skin and oral mucosa may be seen if platelet production has been affected. Fever may be present as a result of neutropenia with increased susceptibility to infection. Metastatic calcifications may involve the soft tissues and are thought to be due to hypercalcemia secondary to tumor-related osteolysis.

Radiographically, multiple well-defined, "punched-out" radiolucencies or ragged radiolucent lesions may be seen in multiple myeloma (Fig. 13-28). These may be especially evident on a skull film. Although any bone may be affected, the jaws have been reported to be involved in as many as 30 percent of cases. The radiolucent areas of the bone contain the abnormal plasma cell proliferations that characterize multiple myeloma.

Renal failure may be a presenting sign in these patients because the kidneys become overburdened with the excess circulating light chain proteins of the tumor cells. These light chain products, which are found in the urine of 30 to 50 percent of patients with multiple myeloma, are called *Bence Jones proteins*, after the British physician who first described them in detail.

Some patients with multiple myeloma show deposition of amyloid (see p. 599) in various soft tissues of the body, and this may be the initial manifestation of the disease. Amyloid deposits are due to the accumulation of the abnormal light chain proteins. Sites that are classically affected include the oral mucosa, particularly the tongue. The tongue may show diffuse enlargement and firmness or may have more of a nodular appearance. Sometimes the nodules are ulcerated. Another area that is commonly affected is the periorbital skin, with the amyloid deposits appearing as waxy, firm, plaque-like lesions.

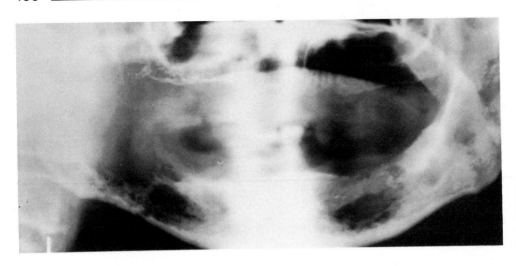

FIGURE 13–28. **Multiple myeloma.** Multiple myeloma affecting the mandible, in this case producing several radiolucencies with rather ragged, ill-defined margins. (Courtesy of Dr. Joseph Finelli.)

Histopathologic Features

Histopathologic examination of the lesional tissue in multiple myeloma shows diffuse, monotonous sheets of neoplastic, variably differentiated, plasmacytoid cells that invade and replace the normal host tissue (Fig. 13–29). Mitotic activity may be seen with some frequency. Occasionally, deposition of amyloid may be observed in association with the neoplastic cells. Like other types of amyloid, this material appears homogeneous, eosinophilic, and relatively acellular. It stains metachromatically with crystal violet and shows an affinity for Congo red, demonstrating apple-green birefringence on viewing with polarized light. A biopsy specimen of bone marrow from a patient with multiple myeloma should show at least 10 percent atypical plasma cells making up the marrow cell population.

Although the histopathologic and radiographic findings strongly suggest a diagnosis of multiple myeloma, serum or urine protein immunoelectrophoresis should be performed as an additional parameter to establish the diagnosis. The serum and urine protein immunoelectrophoresis should show the presence of myeloma protein (M-protein), which represents the massive overproduction of one abnormal immunoglobulin by the neoplastic clone of plasma cells. This monoclonal protein consists of two heavy chain polypeptides of the same immunoglobulin (Ig) class (IgA, IgG, IgM, IgD, or IgE) and two light chain polypeptides of the same class (*kappa* or *lambda*).

Treatment and Prognosis

The treatment of multiple myeloma consists of chemotherapy. An alkylating agent, such as melphalan or cyclophosphamide, is often used in conjunction with prednisone.

The prognosis is considered poor. A median survival time of about 30 to 36 months can be expected after the onset of symptoms. In the past, a 10 percent 5-year survival rate was typical; the prognosis today has not improved dramatically. Most hematology and oncology centers report a 5-year survival rate of 25 percent.

PLASMACYTOMA

The **plasmacytoma** is a unifocal, monoclonal, neoplastic proliferation of plasma cells that usually arises within bone. Occasionally, it is seen in soft tissue. In the latter case, the term **extramedullary plasmacytoma** is used. Some investigators believe that this lesion represents the least aggressive part of a spectrum of plasma cell neoplasms that extends to **multiple myeloma**. The plasmacytoma is therefore important because it may ultimately give rise to the more serious problem of multiple myeloma.

Clinical and Radiographic Features

The plasmacytoma usually is detected in an adult man with an average age of 55 years. The male-to-female ratio is 3:1. Most of the lesions present centrally within a bone, and the spine is the most commonly involved site. About one third of the cases are reported in that location. The initial symptoms often relate to swelling or bone

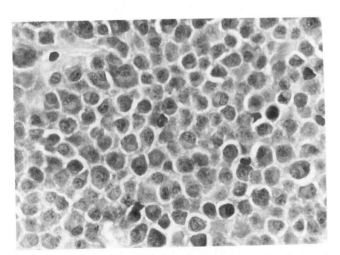

FIGURE 13–29. **Multiple myeloma.** This high-power photomicrograph reveals sheets of monotonous, malignant, plasmacytoid cells with eccentric nuclei and stippled nuclear chromatin.

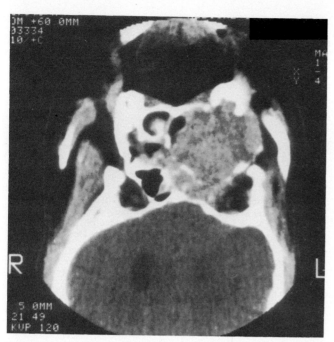

FIGURE 13–30. **Plasmacytoma.** This CT scan depicts a solitary plasmacytoma involving the left maxillary sinus and nasal cavity.

pain; occasionally, however, this lesion is detected on routine radiographic examination. The extramedullary plasmacytoma appears as a relatively nondescript, well-circumscribed, nontender soft tissue mass. In the head and neck, such lesions have been reported in the tonsillar region, the maxillary sinus, and the parotid gland.

Radiographically, the lesion may be seen as a well-defined, unilocular radiolucency with no evidence of sclerotic borders, or as a ragged radiolucency similar to the appearance of multiple myeloma (Fig. 13–30). No other lesions should be identifiable by a skeletal survey or careful physical examination, however.

Histopathologic Features

The histopathologic features of the plasmacytoma are identical to those of multiple myeloma. Sheets of plasma cells show varying degrees of differentiation. Immuno-histochemical studies demonstrate that these plasma cells are monoclonal. As many as 25 to 50 percent of these patients also show a monoclonal gammopathy on evaluation by serum protein immunoelectrophoresis. Unlike multiple myeloma, however, no evidence of plasma cell infiltration should be seen by a random bone marrow biopsy, and the patient should not show signs of anemia, hypercalcemia, or renal failure.

Treatment and Prognosis

Plasmacytomas are usually treated with radiation therapy, typically given as 4000 cGy to the tumor site. A few lesions have been surgically excised with good results, although this is not the preferred treatment in most instances. Unfortunately, when these patients are observed on a long-term basis, most will eventually develop multi-

ple myeloma. About 25 percent show evidence of disseminated disease within 2 to 3 years. However, one third of patients with solitary plasmacytomas will not have symptoms of multiple myeloma for as long as 10 years.

MIDLINE LETHAL GRANULOMA
(Malignant Granuloma; Idiopathic Midline Destructive Disease; Stewart's Granuloma; Midline Nonhealing Malignant Granuloma; Polymorphic Reticulosis; Midline Malignant Reticulosis; Lymphomatoid Granulomatosis; Pseudolymphoma; Angiocentric Immunoproliferative Lesion; T-Cell Lymphoma of Palatal Midline)

Midline lethal granuloma is a rare process that is characterized clinically by aggressive, non-relenting destruction of the midline structures of the palate and nasal fossa. The controversial nature of this process can readily be appreciated by the wide variety of terms by which it has been called.

Even today, a consensus may be difficult to reach with respect to what this process really represents, although most investigators believe that it probably should be classified with the T-cell lymphomas. Even though midline lethal granuloma often does not have the classic histopathologic features of lymphoma microscopically, it behaves in a malignant fashion and seems to respond to the same treatments to which lymphomas respond. Furthermore, recent immunologic and molecular genetic studies have shown features that are consistent with lymphoma.

Clinical Features

Midline lethal granuloma typically presents in adults. The initial signs and symptoms may be localized to the nasal region and include nasal stuffiness or epistaxis. Pain may accompany the nasal symptoms, or the lesion may be localized to the hard palatal region. Swelling of the soft palate or posterior hard palate may precede the formation of a deep, necrotic ulceration, which usually occupies a midline position. This ulceration enlarges and destroys the palatal tissues, which typically creates an oronasal fistula (Fig. 13–31). Secondary infection may complicate the course of the disease, and life-threatening hemorrhage is a potential problem in some instances.

Histopathologic Features

Histopathologic examination of midline lethal granuloma shows a mixed infiltrate of a variety of inflammatory cells, often arranged around blood vessels ("angiocentric") (Fig. 13–32). The lesional process appears to invade and destroy the normal tissue in the area. Necrosis is often present in some areas of the lesion. Large, angular, lymphocytic cells with an atypical appearance

radiation therapy, a feature that is similar to that of T-cell lymphomas of other sites. Approximately 4500 cGy is required to control the disease, and most patients show no evidence of recurrence or dissemination of the lesion.

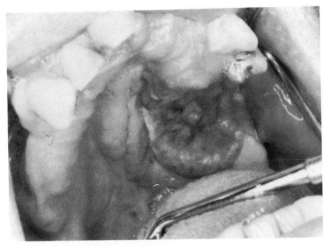

FIGURE 13–31. **Midline lethal granuloma.** The ulcerated palatal lesion represents polymorphic reticulosis, one of several lesions that may present as midline lethal granuloma. (Courtesy of Dr. Dick Lee.)

are usually identified as a component of the inflammatory infiltrate. Immunohistochemical evaluation of this infiltrate often shows a monoclonal T-lymphocyte proliferation. Molecular genetic studies may show gene rearrangements of the T-lymphocyte receptor consistent with a lymphoreticular malignancy.

Treatment and Prognosis

Without treatment, midline lethal granuloma is a relentlessly progressive, highly destructive process that ultimately leads to the patient's death by secondary infection, massive hemorrhage, or infiltration of vital structures in the area. The condition usually responds to

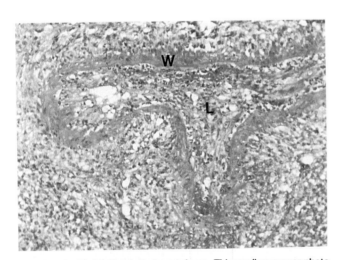

FIGURE 13–32. **Midline lethal granuloma.** This medium-power photomicrograph of polymorphic reticulosis shows atypical lymphoid cells infiltrating the wall (W) and filling the lumen (L) of a blood vessel. Such a pattern is termed "angiocentric" (meaning "around blood vessels"). This feature is characteristic of lesions categorized as midline lethal granuloma.

REFERENCES

Lymphoid Hyperplasia

Bradley G, et al. Benign lymphoid hyperplasia of the palate. J Oral Pathol 16:18–26, 1987.
Davila MA, Thompson SH. Reactive lymphoid hyperplasia of the hard palate. J Oral Maxillofac Surg 46:1103–1105, 1988.
Harsany DL, Ross J, Fee WE. Follicular lymphoid hyperplasia of the hard palate simulating lymphoma. Otolaryngol Head Neck Surg 88:349–356, 1980.
Napier SS, Newlands C. Benign lymphoid hyperplasia of the palate: Report of two cases and immunohistochemical profile. J Oral Pathol Med 19:221–225, 1990.
Wright J, Dunsworth A. Follicular lymphoid hyperplasia of the hard palate: A benign lymphoproliferative process. Oral Surg Oral Med Oral Pathol 55:162–168, 1983.

Hemophilia

Green JB. Hereditary and acquired coagulation factor abnormalities: A primary care primer. Postgrad Med 76:118–127, 1984.
Kitchens CS. Approach to the bleeding patient. Hematol Oncol Clin North Am 6:983–989, 1992.
Lusher JM, et al. Recombinant factor VIII for the treatment of previously untreated patients with hemophilia A. N Engl J Med 328:453–459, 1993.
Lusher JM, Warrier I. Hemophilia A. Hematol Oncol Clin North Am 6:1021–1033, 1992.
Stevens R. Haemophilia and haemorrhagic disorders. Practitioner 237:350–354, 1993.

Anemia

Beddall A. Anaemias. Practitioner 234:713–715, 1990.
Brown RG. Determining the cause of anemia: General approach, with emphasis on microcytic hypochromic anemias. Postgrad Med 89:161–170, 1991.
Hoggarth K. Macrocytic anaemias. Practitioner 237:331–335, 1993.
Hoggarth K. Microcytic anaemias. Practitioner 237:338–341, 1993.
Welborn JL, Meyers FJ. A three-point approach to anemia. Postgrad Med 89:179–186, 1991.

Sickle Cell Anemia

Darbyshire P. Sickle cell disease in the UK. Practitioner 234:722–726, 1990.
Fuller J. Sickle cell disease and thalassaemia. Practitioner 237:344–349, 1993.
Kan YW. Development of DNA analysis for human diseases. JAMA 267:1532–1536, 1992.
Lubin BH, Witkowska E, Kleman K. Laboratory diagnosis of hemoglobinopathies. Clin Biochem 24:363–374, 1991.
Sansevere JJ, Milles M. Management of the oral and maxillofacial surgery patient with sickle cell disease and related hemoglobinopathies. J Oral Maxillofac Surg 51:912–916, 1993.
Steingart R. Management of patients with sickle cell disease. Med Clin North Am 76:669–682, 1992.
Wang W, et al. Medical management and prevention guidelines for children with sickle cell disease. J Tenn Med Assoc 85:209–214, 1992.
Ware RE, Filston HC. Surgical management of children with hemoglobinopathies. Surg Clin North Am 72:1223–1236, 1992.

Thalassemia

Cannell H. The development of oral and facial signs in beta-thalassaemia major. Br Dent J 164:50–51, 1988.

Evans DIK. Bone marrow transplantation for thalassemia major. J Clin Pathol 45:553–555, 1992.

Giardina PJ, Hilgartner MW. Update on thalassemia. Pediatr Rev 13:55–63, 1992.

Lucarelli G, et al. Marrow transplantation in patients with thalassemia responsive to iron chelation therapy. N Engl J Med 329:840–844, 1993.

Piomelli S, Loew T. Management of thalassemia major (Cooley's anemia). Hematol Oncol Clin North Am 5:557–569, 1991.

Riggs DR. The thalassaemia syndromes. Q Rev Med 86:559–564, 1993.

Aplastic Anemia

Frickhofen N, Liu JM, Young NS. Etiologic mechanisms of hematopoietic failure. Am J Pediatr Hematol Oncol 12:385–395, 1990.

Hibbs J, et al. Aplastic anemia and viral hepatitis: Non-A, non-B, non-C? JAMA 267:2051–2054, 1992.

Luker J, Scully C, Oakhill A. Gingival swelling as a manifestation of aplastic anemia. Oral Surg Oral Med Oral Pathol 71:55–56, 1991.

Malkin D, Koren G, Saunders EF. Drug-induced aplastic anemia: Pathogenesis and clinical aspects. Am J Pediatr Hematol Oncol 12:402–410, 1990.

Nissen C, Gratwohl A, Speck B. Management of aplastic anemia. Eur J Haematol 46:193–197, 1991.

Schrezenmeier H, Raghavachar A, Heimpel H. Granulocyte-macrophage colony-stimulating factor in the sera of patients with aplastic anemia. Clin Invest 71:102–108, 1993.

Socie G, et al. Malignant tumors occurring after treatment of aplastic anemia. N Engl J Med 329:1152–1157, 1993.

Stewart FM. Hypoplastic/aplastic anemia: Role of bone marrow transplantation. Med Clin North Am 76:683–697, 1992.

Neutropenia

Boxer LA, Hutchinson R, Emerson S. Recombinant human granulocyte-colony-stimulating factor in the treatment of patients with neutropenia. Clin Immunol Immunopathol 62:S39–S46, 1992.

Agranulocytosis

Bergman OJ. Oral infections in haematological patients. Dan Med Bull 39:15–29, 1992.

Glasser L, Duncan BR, Corrigan JJ. Measurement of serum granulocyte-colony-stimulating factor in a patient with congenital agranulocytosis (Kostmann's syndrome). Am J Dis Child 145:925–928, 1991.

Kuipers EJ, et al. Sulfasalazine induced agranulocytosis treated with granulocyte-macrophage colony stimulating factor. J Rheumatol 19:621–622, 1992.

Pisciotta AV. Drug-induced agranulocytosis: Peripheral destruction of polymorphonuclear leukocytes and their marrow precursors. Blood Rev 4:226–237, 1990.

Salama A, Mueller-Eckhardt C. Immune-mediated blood cell dyscrasias related to drugs. Semin Hematol 29:54–63, 1992.

Cyclic Neutropenia

Boxer LA, Hutchinson R, Emerson S. Recombinant human granulocyte-colony-stimulating factor in the treatment of patients with neutropenia. Clin Immunol Immunopathol 62:S39–S46, 1992.

Dale DC, Hammond WP. Cyclic neutropenia: A clinical review. Blood Rev 2:178–185, 1988.

Rylander H, Ericsson I. Manifestations and treatment of periodontal disease in a patient suffering from cyclic neutropenia. J Clin Periodontol 8:77–87, 1981.

Thrombocytopenia

Palmer RL. Laboratory diagnosis of bleeding disorders: Basic screening tests. Postgrad Med 76:137–148, 1984.

Salama A, Mueller-Eckhardt C. Immune-mediated blood cell dyscrasias related to drugs. Semin Hematol 29:54–63, 1992.

Taylor RE, Blatt PM. Clinical evaluation of the patient with bruising and bleeding. J Am Acad Dermatol 4:348–368, 1981.

Thompson CC, et al. Purpuric oral and cutaneous lesions in a case of drug-induced thrombocytopenia. J Am Dent Assoc 105:465–467, 1982.

Polycythemia Vera

Boughton B. Polycythaemia. Practitioner 234:728–730, 1990.

de Wolf JTM, Vellenga E, Halie MR. Polycythaemia vera. Neth J Med 41:295–304, 1992.

Messinezy M, Pearson T. Polycythaemias. Practitioner 237:355–357, 1993.

Murphy S. Polycythemia vera. Dis Mon 38:153–212, 1992.

Rosenthal DS. Clinical aspects of chronic myeloproliferative diseases. Am J Med Sci 304:109–124, 1992.

Leukemia

Barrett AP. Gingival lesions in leukemia: A classification. J Periodontol 55:585–588, 1984.

Champlin R, Golde DW. The leukemias. *In*: Harrison's Principles of Internal Medicine, 12th ed. Edited by Wilson JD, et al. New York, McGraw-Hill, 1991, pp 1552–1563.

Cheson BD. Chronic lymphocytic leukemia and hairy-cell leukemia. Curr Opin Oncol 3:54–62, 1991.

Chessells JM. Treatment of childhood acute lymphoblastic leukaemia: Present issues and future projects. Blood Rev 6:193–203, 1992.

Hollsberg P, Hafler DA. Pathogenesis of diseases induced by human lymphotropic virus type 1 infection. N Engl J Med 328:1173–1182, 1993.

Karmiris TD, Lister TA, Rohatiner AZ. Chronic lymphocytic leukaemia. Br J Hosp Med 46:379–385, 1991.

Marks DI, et al. Allogeneic bone marrow transplantation for chronic myeloid leukemia using sibling and volunteer unrelated donors: A comparison of complications in the first 2 years. Ann Intern Med 119:207–214, 1993.

Peterson DE, Gerad H, Williams LT. An unusual instance of leukemic infiltrate: Diagnosis and management of periapical tooth involvement. Cancer 51:1716–1719, 1983.

Rivera GK, et al. Treatment of acute lymphoblastic leukemia—30 years' experience at St. Jude Children's Research Hospital. N Engl J Med 329:1289–1295, 1993.

Hodgkin's Disease

Anastasi J, Bitter MA, Vardiman JW. The histopathologic diagnosis and subclassification of Hodgkin's disease. Hematol Oncol Clin North Am 3:187–204, 1989.

Butler JJ. The histologic diagnosis of Hodgkin's disease. Semin Diagn Pathol 9:252–256, 1992.

DeVita VT, Hubbard SM. Drug therapy: Hodgkin's disease. N Engl J Med 328:560–565, 1993.

Harris NL. The relationship between Hodgkin's disease and non-Hodgkin's lymphoma. Semin Diagn Pathol 9:304–310, 1992.

Mooreier JA, Williams SF, Golomb HM. The staging of Hodgkin's disease. Hematol Oncol Clin North Am 3:237–251, 1989.

Poppema S. Lymphocyte-predominance Hodgkin's disease. Semin Diagn Pathol 9:257–264, 1992.

Weinshel EL, Peterson BA. Hodgkin's disease. CA Cancer J Clin 43:327–346, 1993.

Non-Hodgkin's Lymphoma

Armitage JO. Drug therapy: Treatment of non-Hodgkin's lymphoma. N Engl J Med 328:1023–1030, 1993.

Freedman AS, Nadler LM. Immunologic markers in non-Hodgkin's lymphoma. Hematol Oncol Clin North Am 5:871–889, 1991.

Garson OM, Lukeis RE. Cytogenetics of malignant lymphoma. J Histotechnol 15:253–261, 1992.

Handlers JP, et al. Extranodal lymphoma: Part I. A morphologic and immunoperoxidase study of 34 cases. Oral Surg Oral Med Oral Pathol 61:362–367, 1986.

Howell RE, et al. Extranodal oral lymphoma: Part II. Relationships between clinical features and the Lukes-Collins classification of 34 cases. Oral Surg Oral Med Oral Pathol 64:597–602, 1987.

Jacobs C, Weiss L, Hoppe RT. The management of extranodal head and neck lymphomas. Arch Otolaryngol Head Neck Surg 112:654–658, 1986.

Leong AS-Y. Malignant lymphoma: Nomenclature, recently recognized subtypes, and current concepts. J Histotechnol 15:175–184, 1992.

Newell GR, et al. Incidence of lymphoma in the US classified by the working formulation. Cancer 59:857–861, 1987.

Ostrowski ML, et al. Malignant lymphoma of bone. Cancer 58:2646–2655, 1986.

Takahashi H, Tsuda N, Tezuda F. Immunophenotypic analysis of extranodal non-Hodgkin's lymphomas in the oral cavity. Pathol Res Pract 189:300–311, 1993.

Tomich CE, Shafer WG. Lymphoproliferative disease of the hard palate: A clinicopathologic entity. Oral Surg Oral Med Oral Pathol 39:754–768, 1975.

Vose JM, et al. The therapy of non-Hodgkin's lymphomas. Hematol Oncol Clin North Am 5:845–852, 1991.

Wallace C, Ramsay AD, Quiney RE. Non-Hodgkin's extranodal lymphoma: A clinico-pathological study of 24 cases involving head and neck sites. J Laryngol Otol 102:914–922, 1988.

White L, Siegel SE, Quah TC. Non-Hodgkin's lymphomas in children: I. Patterns of disease and classification. Crit Rev Oncol Hematol 13:55–71, 1992.

Mycosis Fungoides

Abel EA, Wood GS, Hoppe RT. Mycosis fungoides: Clinical and histologic features, staging, evaluation, and approach to treatment. CA Cancer J Clin 43:93–115, 1993.

Damm DD, et al. Mycosis fungoides: Initial diagnosis via palatal biopsy with discussion of diagnostic advantages of plastic embedding. Oral Surg Oral Med Oral Pathol 58:413–419, 1984.

Evans GE, Dalziel KL. Mycosis fungoides with oral involvement: A case report and literature review. Int J Oral Maxillofac Surg 16:634–637, 1987.

Hoppe RT, Wood GS, Abel EA. Mycosis fungoides and the Sézary syndrome: Pathology, staging, and treatment. Curr Probl Cancer 14:297–361, 1990.

Sirois DA, et al. Oral manifestations of cutaneous T-cell lymphoma: A report of eight cases. Oral Surg Oral Med Oral Pathol 75:700–705, 1993.

Wright JM, Balciunas BA, Muus JH. Mycosis fungoides with oral manifestations: Report of a case and review of the literature. Oral Surg Oral Med Oral Pathol 51:24–31, 1981.

Zic J, et al. Extracorporeal photopheresis for the treatment of cutaneous T-cell lymphoma. J Am Acad Dermatol 27:729–736, 1992.

Burkitt's Lymphoma

Jacobs P. The malignant lymphomas in Africa. Hematol Oncol Clin North Am 5:953–982, 1991.

Pavlova Z, et al. Small noncleaved follicular center cell lymphoma: Burkitt's and non-Burkitt's variants in the US: II. Pathologic and immunologic features. Cancer 59:1892–1902, 1987.

White L, Siegel SE, Quah TC. Non-Hodgkin's lymphomas in children. Crit Rev Oncol Hematol 13:73–89, 1992.

Yih WY, et al. African Burkitt's lymphoma: Case report and light and electron microscopic findings. Oral Surg Oral Med Oral Pathol 70:760–764, 1990.

Young L, Rowe M. Epstein-Barr virus, lymphomas and Hodgkin's disease. Semin Cancer Biol 3:273–284, 1992.

Multiple Myeloma

Baldini L, et al. No correlation between response and survival in patients with multiple myeloma treated with vincristine, melphalan, cyclophosphamide, and prednisone. Cancer 68:62–67, 1991.

Cherng NC, et al. Prognostic factors in multiple myeloma. Cancer 67:3150–3156, 1991.

Dimopoulos MA, et al. Risk of disease progression in asymptomatic multiple myeloma. Am J Med 94:57–61, 1993.

Greipp PR. Advances in the diagnosis and management of myeloma. Semin Hematol 29(suppl 2):24–45, 1992.

Kyle RA. Diagnostic criteria of multiple myeloma. Hematol Oncol Clin North Am 6:347–358, 1992.

Niesvizky R, Siegel D, Michaeli J. Biology and treatment of multiple myeloma. Blood Rev 7:24–33, 1993.

Riedel DA, Pottern LM. The epidemiology of multiple myeloma. Hematol Oncol Clin North Am 6:225–247, 1992.

Plasmacytoma

Dimopoulos MA, et al. Solitary plasmacytoma of bone and asymptomatic multiple myeloma. Hematol Oncol Clin North Am 6:359–369, 1992.

Gonzalez J, et al. Plasma-cell tumors of the condyle. Br J Oral Maxillofac Surg 29:274–276, 1991.

Meis JM, et al. Solitary plasmacytomas of bone and extramedullary plasmacytomas: A clinicopathologic and immunohistochemical study. Cancer 59:1475–1485, 1987.

Rothfield RE, Johnson JT, Stavrides A. Extramedullary plasmacytoma of the parotid. Head Neck 12:352–354, 1990.

Midline Lethal Granuloma

Batsakis JG, Luna MA. Midfacial necrotizing lesions. Semin Diagn Pathol 4:90–116, 1987.

Gaulard P, et al. Lethal midline granuloma (polymorphic reticulosis) and lymphomatoid granulomatosis. Cancer 62:705–710, 1988.

Harabuchi Y, et al. Lethal midline granuloma (peripheral T-cell lymphoma) after lymphomatoid papulosis. Cancer 70:835–839, 1992.

Lippman SM, et al. Lethal midline granuloma with a novel T-cell phenotype as found in peripheral T-cell lymphoma. Cancer 59:936–939, 1987.

Nadimi H, et al. T-cell lymphoma of palatal midline. Report of 2 cases. Int J Oral Maxillofac Surg 17:377–381, 1988.

Sirois DA, et al. Oral manifestations of cutaneous T-cell lymphoma: A report of eight cases. Oral Surg Oral Med Oral Pathol 75:700–705, 1993.

14

Bone Pathology

Charles A. Waldron

OSTEOGENESIS IMPERFECTA

Osteogenesis imperfecta comprises a heterogeneous group of heritable connective tissue disorders characterized by bone fragility. Some affected individuals also have blue sclera, opalescent dentin, hearing loss, long bone and spine deformities, and joint hyperextensibility. Osteogenesis imperfecta is the most common type of inherited bone disease. Both autosomal dominant and recessive hereditary patterns occur, and many cases are sporadic. The severity of the disease varies widely, even in affected members of a single family.

Clinical and Radiographic Features

Four major types of osteogenesis imperfecta are recognized, each having several subtypes.

Type I Osteogenesis Imperfecta

Type I is the most common form. It shows an autosomal dominant inheritance pattern. Affected patients have mild to moderately severe bone fragility. Fractures are present at birth in about 10 percent of cases, but there is great variability in frequency and age of onset of fractures. Hearing loss commonly develops before age 30, and most older patients have hearing deficits. Some affected patients have normal teeth, but others show opalescent dentin. (See **dentinogenesis imperfecta**, p. 84.)

Type II Osteogenesis Imperfecta

Type II patients have extreme bone fragility and frequent fractures, which may occur during delivery. Many patients are stillborn, and 90 percent die before 4 weeks of age. Blue sclerae are present (Fig. 14–1; see Color Figure 89). Both autosomal recessive and dominant patterns may occur, and many cases appear to be sporadic. Tooth anomalies (dentinogenesis imperfecta) may be present.

Type III Osteogenesis Imperfecta

Type III is associated with moderately severe to severe bone fragility. The sclerae are blue in infants, but the blue color fades as the child grows older. Fractures may be present at birth, but there is a low mortality in infancy. The mortality rate is higher in older children. Death usually results from cardiopulmonary complications caused by kyphoscoliosis. Some patients have opalescent dentin, whereas others have normal teeth. Both autosomal dominant and recessive hereditary patterns are noted.

Type IV Osteogenesis Imperfecta

Type IV appears to be inherited as an autosomal dominant trait. Patients have mild to moderately severe bone fragility. The sclera may be pale blue in early childhood, but the blue color fades later in life. Fractures are present at birth in about 50 percent of these patients. The frequency of fractures decreases after puberty, and some individuals never experience bone fracture at any time. Some of these patients have opalescent dentin; others have normal teeth.

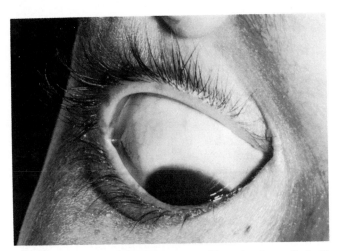

FIGURE 14–1. **Osteogenesis imperfecta.** Blue sclera in a patient with osteogenesis imperfecta. See Color Plates.

Histopathologic Features

Osteogenesis imperfecta is a generalized disease of connective tissue with abnormalities in collagen synthesis. The bone abnormalities are due to defective osteoblasts, and the mass of cortical and cancellous bone is greatly reduced. Cortical bone is very scant. Osteoblasts are present, but bone matrix production is markedly reduced. The bone architecture remains immature throughout life, and there is a failure of woven bone to become transformed to lamellar bone. Woven bone may usually be seen in adult patients. The bone fractures heal quickly with abundant callus formation. The dental defects in osteogenesis imperfecta are described on p. 84.

Treatment and Prognosis

There is no treatment for osteogenesis imperfecta. Management of the fractures may be a major problem. Patients with opalescent dentin usually show severe attrition of their teeth, leading to tooth loss. Extensive restorative procedures with full crown coverage are sometimes performed to preserve the dentition and provide good aesthetics.

The prognosis varies from relatively good to very poor. Some patients have little to no disability, whereas others have severe crippling as a result of the fractures. In severe forms, death occurs *in utero*, during delivery, or early in childhood.

OSTEOPETROSIS (Albers-Schönberg Disease; Marble Bone Disease)

Osteopetrosis is a rare hereditary skeletal disorder characterized by a marked increase in bone density resulting from a defect in bone remodeling. The clinical severity of the disease varies widely. Two distinct hereditary patterns occur.

The severe *infantile* form of osteopetrosis is transmitted as an autosomal recessive trait. It is usually discovered within the first few months of life. In addition to exhibiting widespread osteosclerosis, these patients also have hematologic and neurologic manifestations. Most affected individuals die before age 20 as a result of anemia or infection. The anemia is the result of a decrease in the hematopoietic marrow compartment, which becomes filled with bone.

The more common *adult* form of osteopetrosis is transmitted as an autosomal dominant trait. This form may be relatively mild. In some instances, it is only detected when radiographs are made for some other purpose.

Clinical and Radiographic Features

Infantile Osteopetrosis

The initial signs of infantile osteopetrosis are often normocytic anemia and hepatosplenomegaly resulting from compensatory extramedullary hematopoiesis. Increased susceptibility to infection is common as a result of granulocytopenia. Facial deformity develops in many of the children, manifesting as a broad face, hypertelorism, snub nose, and frontal bossing. Tooth eruption is almost always delayed. Failure of resorption and remodeling of the skull bones produces narrowings of the various skull foramina that press on the various cranial nerves and result in optic nerve atrophy and blindness, deafness, and facial paralysis. In spite of the dense bone, pathologic fractures are common. Osteomyelitis of the jaws is a common complication of tooth extraction (Fig. 14–2).

Radiographically, there is a widespread increase in skeletal density with defects in metaphyseal remodeling. The radiographic distinction between cortical and cancellous bone is lost (Fig. 14–3).

Adult Osteopetrosis

The autosomal dominant form of osteopetrosis is a milder disease that is usually detected at a later age than the autosomal recessive type. The disease probably begins asymptomatically in early life and progressively

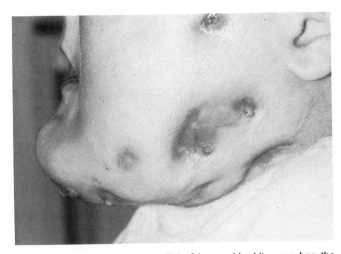

FIGURE 14–2. **Osteopetrosis.** This 24-year-old white man has the infantile form of osteopetrosis. He has suffered from mandibular osteomyelitis, and multiple draining fistulae are present on his face. (Courtesy of Dr. Dan Sarasin.)

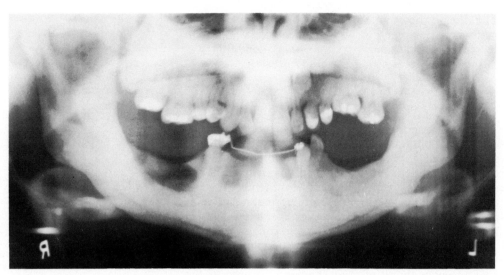

FIGURE 14-3. **Osteopetrosis.** Extensive mandibular involvement is apparent in this radiograph of a 31-year-old woman. She had been diagnosed as having osteopetrosis as a child. There is a history of multiple fractures and osteomyelitis of the jaws. (Courtesy of Dr. Dan Sarasin.)

involves more bone. It is usually not life-threatening, and may be detected only when radiographs are taken for some other purpose. The patients do not have anemia or hepatosplenomegaly; blindness and deafness do not usually develop. Long-bone fractures after minor trauma are not common. When the mandible is involved, however, fracture and osteomyelitis after tooth extraction are significant complications.

The radiographic appearance of adult osteopetrosis is similar to that of the infantile form, although defects in metaphyseal remodeling are not prominent.

Histopathologic Features

The basic defect in osteopetrosis is failure of normal osteoclast function. The number of osteoclasts present is often increased; however, because of their failure to function normally, bone is not resorbed. On microscopic examination, the osteoclasts may appear atypical. Defective osteoclastic bone resorption, combined with continued bone formation and endochondral ossification, results in the marked increase of the calcified skeletal tissue.

Several patterns of abnormal endosteal bone formation have been described. These include:

- Tortuous lamellar trabeculae replacing the cancellous portion of the bone
- Globular amorphous bone deposition in the marrow spaces (Fig. 14-4)
- Osteophytic bone formation

Numerous osteoclasts may be seen, but there is no evidence that they function because Howship's lacunae are not visible.

Treatment and Prognosis

There is no specific therapy for osteopetrosis. Treatment consists of supportive measures, such as transfusions and antibiotics for the complications.

The prognosis for the severe recessive (infantile) form of the disease is very poor. Death usually results from anemia or infection, usually before age 20. Supportive therapy directed toward control of the hematologic problems and control of infections is required. A milder form of autosomal recessive osteopetrosis is recognized, and the outlook is better for this type.

The prognosis for the autosomal dominant (adult) form is variable, although better. The frequency of osteomyelitis and jaw fracture after extraction is a major problem, and efforts should be directed to prevent the necessity for tooth extraction. Measures include frequent prophylaxis, good home care, and topical fluorides.

CLEIDOCRANIAL DYSPLASIA

The bone defects in patients with **cleidocranial dysplasia** chiefly involve the skull and clavicles, although a wide variety of anomalies may be found in other bones.

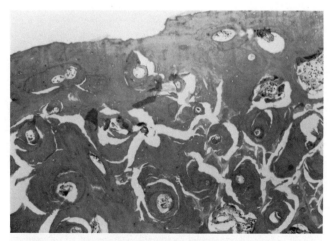

FIGURE 14-4. **Osteopetrosis.** Low-power photomicrograph showing nodules of dense, sclerotic bone that are replacing the cancellous bone.

The disease shows an autosomal dominant inheritance pattern, but as many as 40 percent of cases appear to represent spontaneous mutations. This condition was formerly known as **cleidocranial dysostosis**.

Clinical and Radiographic Features

The appearance of the patient affected by cleidocranial dysplasia is often diagnostic. The patients tend to be of short stature and have large heads with pronounced frontal and parietal bossing. Ocular hypertelorism is frequently present. The mid-facial skeleton tends to be hypoplastic, and this—combined with normal mandibular growth—results in a relative prognathism. The nose is often broad at the base with a depressed nasal bridge.

The patient's neck appears long; the shoulders are narrow and show marked drooping. The patients show an unusual mobility of their shoulders because of the absence or hypoplasia of the clavicles. In some instances, the patient can approximate the shoulders in front of the chest (Fig. 14–5). Although the clavicular defects result in variations of the muscles related to the clavicles, function is remarkably good.

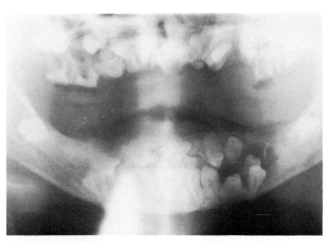

FIGURE 14–6. **Cleidocranial dysplasia.** Panoramic radiograph showing multiple unerupted teeth. (Courtesy of Dr. John R. Cramer.)

The patients often have a narrow high-arched palate, and there is an increased prevalence of cleft palate. Prolonged retention of deciduous teeth and delay or complete failure of eruption of permanent teeth are characteristic findings.

On skull radiographs, the sutures and fontanels show delayed closure or may remain open throughout the patient's life. Secondary centers of ossification appear in the suture lines, and many wormian bones may be seen. The clavicles may be totally absent, either unilaterally or bilaterally, in about 10 percent of all cases. More commonly, the clavicles show varying degrees of hypoplasia and malformation.

Jaw radiographs usually show many unerupted permanent teeth. Supernumerary teeth are often present, frequently with distorted crown and root shapes (Fig. 14–6).

Histopathologic Features

The reason for failure of permanent tooth eruption in patients with cleidocranial dysplasia is not well understood. Microscopic study of unerupted permanent teeth shows that these teeth lack secondary cementum.

Treatment and Prognosis

There is no treatment for the skull, clavicular, and other bone anomalies associated with cleidocranial dysplasia. Most patients function well without any significant problems. It is not unusual for an affected individual to be unaware of the disease until some professional calls it to his or her attention.

Treatment of the dental problems associated with the disease, however, may be a major problem. Extraction of the retained deciduous teeth does not promote eruption of unerupted permanent teeth. Surgical exposure of unerupted teeth, combined with orthodontic therapy, has been successful in some cases. Other authors advocate early surgical exposure of unerupted teeth to stimulate root formation and eruption. Some patients may require orthognathic surgery and prostheses.

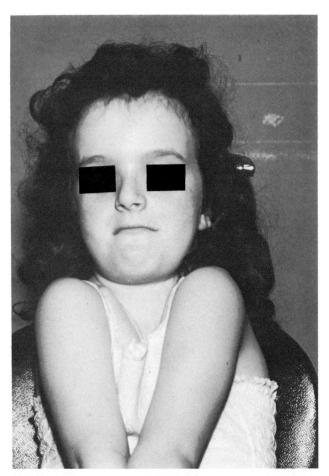

FIGURE 14–5. **Cleidocranial dysplasia.** The patient can almost approximate her shoulders in front of her chest. (Courtesy of Dr. William Bruce.)

FOCAL OSTEOPOROTIC MARROW DEFECT

The **focal osteoporotic marrow defect** does not represent a pathologic process, but its radiographic features may be confused with a variety of pathoses. The pathogenesis of this condition is unknown. Various theories include:

- Aberrant bone regeneration following tooth extraction
- Persistence of fetal marrow
- Marrow hyperplasia in response to increased demand for erythrocytes

Clinical and Radiographic Features

The focal osteoporotic marrow defect is invariably asymptomatic and is detected as an incidental finding on a radiographic examination. The area presents as a radiolucent lesion, varying in size from several millimeters to several centimeters in diameter. The borders of the radiolucency are ill defined. The radiolucency typically shows fine central trabeculations that may be seen on a high-detail periapical radiograph (Fig. 14–7). More than 75 percent of all cases are discovered in adult women. About 70 percent occur in the posterior mandible, most often in edentulous areas. No expansion of the jaw is noted clinically.

Histopathologic Features

Microscopically, the defects contain cellular hematopoietic marrow. Lymphoid aggregates may be present. Bone trabeculae included in the biopsy specimen show no evidence of abnormal osteoblastic or osteoclastic activity (Fig. 14–8).

Treatment and Prognosis

The radiographic findings, while often suggestive of the diagnosis, are not specific and may simulate those of

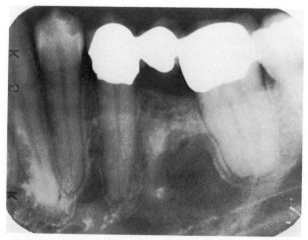

FIGURE 14–7. **Focal osteoporotic marrow defect.** The periapical film shows a radiolucent area containing fine trabeculations. (Courtesy of Dr. Ed McGaha.)

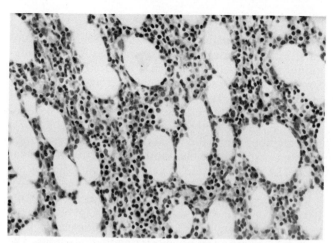

FIGURE 14–8. **Focal osteoporotic marrow defect.** Photomicrograph of a biopsy specimen of a lesion similar to that shown in Figure 14–7. The hematopoietic marrow is normal.

a variety of other diseases. Incisional biopsy, therefore, is often necessary to establish the diagnosis.

Once the diagnosis is established, no further treatment is needed. The prognosis is excellent, and no association between focal osteoporotic marrow defects and anemia or other hematologic disorders has been established.

IDIOPATHIC OSTEOSCLEROSIS (Dense Bone Island)

Asymptomatic, uniformly radiopaque foci composed of dense bone are not uncommonly noted on review of dental radiographs. Some of these radiopaque foci occur in the periapical areas of teeth with nonvital pulps and are believed to represent a response to a low-grade inflammatory stimulus. These lesions are often designated as **condensing osteitis** or **focal chronic sclerosing osteomyelitis** (see p. 117). The areas may persist in the bone after extraction of the tooth.

In addition, similar-appearing areas that cannot be attributed to inflammatory, dysplastic, or neoplastic causes are commonly encountered. Several studies involving large numbers of patients suggest that these opaque foci may be present in as much as 5 percent of the population. A number of terms, such as "bone whorl," "bone scar," "enostosis," "focal periapical osteopetrosis," and "dense bone island," have been used to designate these lesions. **Idiopathic osteosclerosis** is suggested as an adequate designation for these lesions. These sclerotic areas are not restricted to the jaws, and radiologically similar lesions may be found in other bones.

Because past studies did not distinguish the idiopathic lesions from those of inflammatory origin, a confusion in terminology has resulted. More recently, most investigators have advocated that the idiopathic lesions be classified separately from those of inflammatory etiology.

Clinical and Radiographic Features

Although idiopathic osteosclerosis may be encountered in patients over a wide age range, it is most commonly seen in people between 20 and 40 years of age. Some reports have shown a female predilection, whereas others have not. The condition seems to be somewhat more prevalent in black persons. Idiopathic osteosclerosis is invariably asymptomatic and is detected during a radiographic examination. About 90 percent of examples are seen in the mandible, most often in the first molar area. The second premolar and second molar areas are also common sites. In most cases, only one focus of sclerotic bone is present. A small number of patients have two or even three separate areas of involvement.

Radiographically, the lesions are characterized by a well-defined, rounded, or elliptical radiodense mass. The lesions vary from 3 mm to more than 2.0 cm in greatest extent. The radiodense area is not surrounded by a radiolucent rim. Most examples of idiopathic osteosclerosis are associated with a root apex. In a lesser number of cases, the sclerotic area may extend into or be located only in the inter-radicular area (Fig. 14–9). In about 20 percent of cases, the sclerotic area is located in the jaw, with no apparent relationship to a tooth. Root resorption, usually involving the roots of first molar teeth, has been noted in about 10 percent of cases.

Histopathologic Features

Because idiopathic osteosclerosis is seldom subjected to biopsy, few microscopic studies have been reported. Studies have shown that the lesion consists of dense lamellar bone with scant fibro-fatty marrow. Inflammatory cells are inconspicuous or totally absent.

Diagnosis

A diagnosis of idiopathic osteosclerosis may usually be made with confidence on the basis of history, clinical features, and radiographic findings. Differentiation from condensing osteitis may be difficult, but in the absence of a deep restoration or caries, a periapical radiodense area associated with a vital tooth is likely to represent idiopathic osteosclerosis.

Treatment and Prognosis

No treatment is indicated for idiopathic osteosclerosis, and there is little or no tendency for the lesions to progress or change. Serial radiographic study in some cases has shown that the lesions often develop during the teen years, and once the lesion is fully mature, little to no change occurs. Some lesions, however, may disappear in the older patient.

MASSIVE OSTEOLYSIS (Gorham's Disease; Vanishing Bone Disease; Phantom Bone Disease)

Massive osteolysis is a rare disease that is characterized by spontaneous and usually progressive destruction of one or more bones. The destroyed bone does not regenerate or repair itself, and it is replaced by dense fibrous tissue.

The cause of massive osteolysis is unknown. There is no evidence of any underlying metabolic or endocrine imbalance. Many investigators believe that massive osteolysis is related to hemangioma of bone. Lesions have occurred in almost any bone or combination of bones. The maxillofacial bones, particularly the mandible, are among the most commonly affected sites. The mandible and maxilla are often simultaneously involved.

Clinical and Radiographic Features

Most cases of massive osteolysis occur in children and adults under age 40. The disease is somewhat more common in males than females. About 50 percent of all patients report an episode of trauma prior to the diagnosis, but this is often trivial in nature. The onset of the disease is often insidious, and pain is seldom a feature unless pathologic fracture develops.

Radiographically, the earliest changes consist of intramedullary radiolucent foci of varying size and indistinct margins. These coalesce to become larger and involve the cortical bone. Eventually, large portions of the involved bone disappear. In the end stage, the involved bone is completely missing (Fig. 14–10).

Laboratory Findings

The results of laboratory studies generally are completely within normal limits.

Histopathologic Features

The microscopic findings in massive osteolysis contrast sharply with the striking clinical and radiologic findings. In the early stages of disease, specimens removed from the radiolucent defects consist of a nonspecific vas-

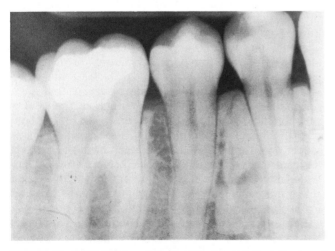

FIGURE 14–9. **Idiopathic osteosclerosis.** An asymptomatic area of bone sclerosis is present in the inter-radicular area between vital mandibular premolar teeth.

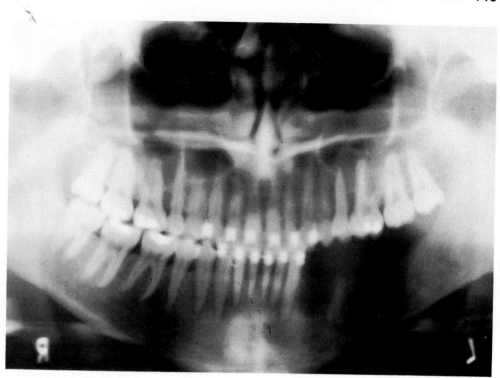

FIGURE 14–10. **Massive osteolysis.** Panographic film showing extensive bone loss and a pathologic fracture of the left mandible in a 24-year-old woman. This process was first noted as a presumed periapical cyst or granuloma and progressed to the extent shown over an 8-month period. (Courtesy of Dr. John R. Cramer.)

cular fibrous connective tissue containing foci of lymphocytes and plasma cells. A slight to moderate vascular proliferation is present. This is characterized by thin-walled channels that may be capillary or cavernous in nature (Fig. 14–11). Osteoclastic reaction in the adjacent bone fragments is usually not conspicuous.

In the later stages, tissue from the area of bone loss is more collagenized. Evidence of repair by new bone formation is not seen.

Treatment and Prognosis

The clinical course of massive osteolysis is variable and impossible to predict. In most cases, bone destruction progresses over months to a few years and results in the total loss of the affected bone or bones. Some patients, however, experience a spontaneous arrest of the process without complete loss of the affected bone. The prognosis varies from slight to severe disability. Mortality from massive osteolysis is relatively uncommon and is usually the result of severe chest cage involvement or destruction of vertebral bodies with spinal cord compression.

Treatment is not particularly satisfactory. Insertion of prostheses and radiation therapy have each been employed with variable but limited success. Bone grafting has been used in many cases, but the success rate is poor because the graft may also undergo osteolysis. The results of therapy are difficult to evaluate because the disease may spontaneously arrest in some patients.

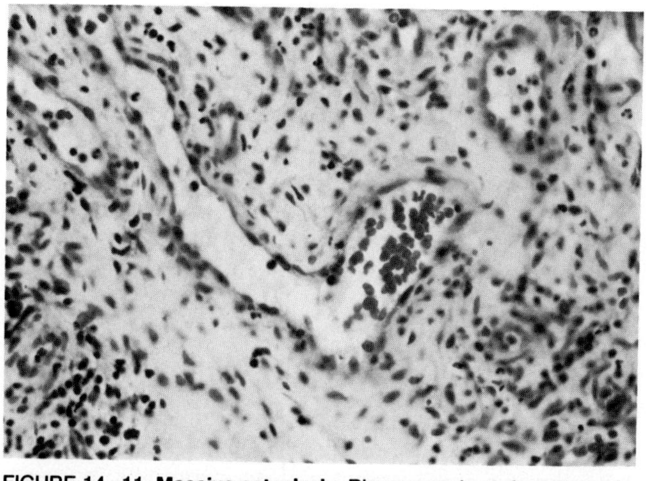

PAGET'S DISEASE OF BONE (Osteitis Deformans)

Paget's disease of bone is characterized by abnormal and anarchic resorption and deposition of bone, resulting in distortion and weakening of the affected bones. The disease principally affects older people and is rarely encountered in patients younger than 40 years of age. Paget's disease is relatively common, although there is a marked geographic variance in its prevalence. It is more common in Britain than in the United States. The frequency of the disease varies in areas of the same country. Paget's disease is rare in Africa and Asia. Some studies show that 2 to 4 percent of residents of certain geographic locations have radiographic evidence of Paget's disease.

The cause of Paget's disease is unknown. Inflammatory, genetic, and endocrine factors may be contributing

FIGURE 14–11. **Massive osteolysis.** Biopsy specimen from the same patient shown in Figure 14–10. The loose, highly vascular connective tissue shows a diffuse infiltrate of lymphocytes and plasma cells.

agents. The possibility that the disease is the result of a slow virus infection has received considerable attention in recent years, but a viral cause remains unproven.

Clinical and Radiographic Features

Most cases of Paget's disease are *polyostotic* (more than one bone is affected). The disease, however, may be *monostotic* (limited to one bone). Men are affected about twice as often as women, and whites are affected more than blacks. Symptoms vary, and some patients may remain relatively asymptomatic. Bone pain, which may be quite severe, is a common complaint.

The bones affected by Paget's disease become thickened, enlarged, and weakened. The lumbar vertebrae, pelvis, skull, and femur are the most commonly affected bones. Jaw involvement is present in 10 to 15 percent of cases. As a result of weakening by the disease process, weight-bearing bones often show bowing deformity, resulting in what is described as a simian ("monkey-like") stance. Skull involvement generally leads to a progressive increase in the circumference of the head.

Maxillary involvement, which is far more common than mandibular involvement, results in enlargement of the middle third of the face. In extreme cases, the enlargement results in a "lion-like" facial deformity (*leontiasis ossea*). The alveolar ridges tend to become grossly enlarged, and the enlargement is usually symmetric. If the patient is dentulous, the enlargement causes spacing of the teeth. Edentulous patients may complain that their dentures no longer fit because of the alveolar enlargement.

Radiographically, the early stages of Paget's disease reveal a decreased radiodensity of the bone and alteration of the trabecular pattern. Particularly in the skull, large circumscribed areas of radiolucency may be present (*osteoporosis circumscripta*).

During the osteoblastic phases of the disease, patchy areas of sclerotic bone are formed. These tend to become confluent. The patchy sclerotic areas are often described as having a "cotton wool" appearance (Figs. 14–12 and

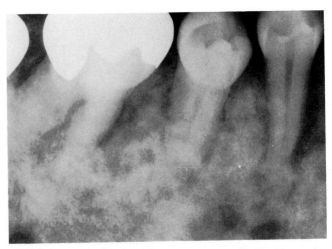

FIGURE 14–13. **Paget's disease.** Periapical film showing the "cotton wool" appearance of the bone.

14–13). On radiographic examination, the teeth often demonstrate extensive hypercementosis.

Radiographic findings of Paget's disease closely resemble those of cemento-osseous dysplasia (see p. 464). Patients with presumed cemento-osseous dysplasia who demonstrate clinical expansion of the jaws should be evaluated further to rule out Paget's disease.

Laboratory Findings

Patients with Paget's disease show marked elevations in serum alkaline phosphatase levels but usually have normal blood calcium and phosphorus levels. Urinary hydroxyproline levels may also be markedly elevated.

Histopathologic Features

Microscopic examination shows an apparent uncontrolled alternating resorption and formation of bone. In the active resorptive stages, numerous osteoclasts surround bone trabeculae, which show evidence of resorptive activity. Simultaneously, osteoblastic activity is seen with formation of osteoid rims around bone trabeculae. The marrow is replaced by a vascular fibrous connective tissue (Fig. 14–14). A characteristic microscopic feature is the presence of basophilic reversal lines in the bone. These lines indicate the junction between alternating resorptive and formative phases of the bone and result in a "jigsaw puzzle," or mosaic, appearance of the bone (Fig. 14–15). In the less active phases, large masses of dense bone showing prominent reversal lines are present.

Treatment and Prognosis

Although Paget's disease is chronic and slowly progressive, it is seldom the cause of death. In patients with more limited involvement and no symptoms, no treatment is required. Bone pain, the most common symptom, may often be controlled by aspirin or other analge-

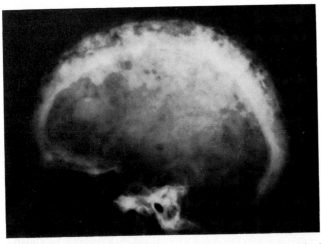

FIGURE 14–12. **Paget's disease.** Lateral skull film shows marked enlargement of the cranium with new bone formation above the outer table of the skull and a patchy, dense, "cotton wool" appearance. (Courtesy of Dr. Reg Munden.)

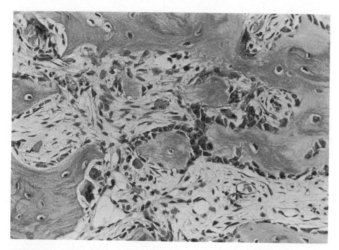

FIGURE 14–14. **Paget's disease.** Prominent osteoblastic and osteoclastic activity surround the bone trabeculae.

sics. Neurologic complications, such as deafness or visual disturbances, may result from bony encroachment on cranial nerves passing through skull foramina. Use of parathyroid hormone antagonists, such as calcitonin and biphosphonates, can reduce bone turnover and improve the biochemical abnormalities.

Dental complications include difficulties in extraction of grossly hypercementosed teeth. Edentulous patients may require new and larger dentures periodically to compensate for progressive enlargement of the alveolar processes.

Development of a malignant bone tumor, usually an osteosarcoma, is a recognized complication of Paget's disease. Osteosarcoma in adults over the age of 40 is quite uncommon in individuals who do not have Paget's disease. The frequency of bone sarcoma complicating Paget's disease ranges from 0.9 to 13 percent in various studies. The true frequency is probably in the range of 1 percent or less. Most of the osteosarcomas develop in the pelvis and long bones of the lower extremities. The skull and jaws are very rare sites for sarcomas associated with

Paget's disease. Benign and malignant giant cell tumors (see p. 455) may also develop in bones affected by Paget's disease. Most of these occur in the craniofacial skeleton.

LANGERHANS CELL DISEASE
(Histiocytosis X; Idiopathic Histiocytosis; Eosinophilic Granuloma; Langerhans Cell Granuloma)

The term **histiocytosis X** was introduced as a collective designation for a spectrum of clinicopathologic disorders characterized by proliferation of histiocyte-like cells that are accompanied by varying numbers of eosinophilic leukocytes, lymphocytes, plasma cells, and multinucleated giant cells. There is general agreement that the distinctive histiocytic cells present in this lesion are Langerhans cells, and many believe that the condition is best designated as **Langerhans cell disease** or **Langerhans cell granuloma**. Langerhans cells are dendritic mononuclear cells normally found in the epidermis, mucosa, lymph nodes, and bone marrow. These cells process and present antigens to T lymphocytes. Langerhans cell disease is considered to be a non-neoplastic condition, but the cause is obscure.

Clinical and Radiographic Features

The clinicopathologic spectrum traditionally considered under the designation of histiocytosis X includes:

1. Solitary or multiple bone lesions without visceral involvement — **eosinophilic granuloma of bone**.
2. A chronic disseminated disease involving bone and skin and viscera (**Hand-Schüller-Christian disease**).
3. An acute disseminated disease with prominent cutaneous, visceral, and bone marrow involvement occurring mainly in infants (**Letterer-Siwe disease**).

It is difficult to categorize many patients into one of these classic designations because of overlapping clinical features. The often cited Hand-Schüller-Christian triad — bone lesions, exophthalmos, and diabetes insipidus — is present in only a few patients with chronic disseminated disease. It is widely believed that the traditional designations of Hand-Schüller-Christian and Letterer-Siwe disease serve no useful purpose and should be discontinued. The acute disseminated form of the disease remains controversial. Many investigators believe that the designation of Letterer-Siwe disease in the past included obscure infections, immunodeficiency syndromes, and malignant histiocytic lesions.

Although Langerhans cell disease may be encountered in patients over a wide age range, more than 50 percent of all cases are seen in patients under age 10. There is a definite male predilection. Bone lesions, either solitary or multiple, are the most common clinical presentation. Lesions may be found in almost any bone, but the skull, ribs, vertebrae, and mandible are among the most frequent sites. Children younger than age 10 most often have skull and femoral lesions; patients over age 20 more often have lesions in the ribs, shoulder girdle, and man-

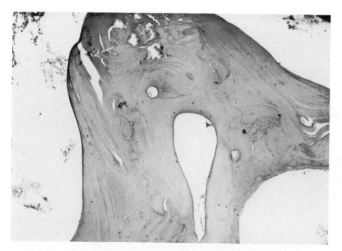

FIGURE 14–15. **Paget's disease.** Prominent reversal lines are present in the bone in this inactive stage of the disease.

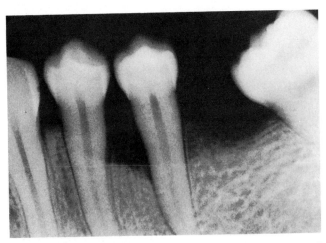

FIGURE 14–16. **Langerhans cell disease.** Periapical radiograph showing bone loss between the premolar teeth; this is suggestive of periodontitis.

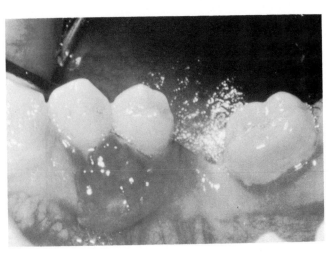

FIGURE 14–17. **Langerhans cell disease.** Clinical photograph of the same patient shown in Figure 14–16. Note the soft tissue changes.

dible. Patients with solitary or multiple bone lesions may have lymphadenopathy but usually do not have significant visceral involvement.

The jaws are affected in 10 to 20 percent of all cases. Bone lesions are often accompanied by dull pain and tenderness. Bone involvement in the mandible most often occurs in the posterior areas. The alveolar bone is often affected, resulting in bone destruction and loosening of the teeth, which clinically resembles severe destructive periodontitis (Fig. 14–16). This is usually accompanied by mucosal involvement, which appears as an ulcerative lesion or a proliferative gingival mass (Fig. 14–17). Lesions also occur within the body of the man-

dible and maxilla. These may occur over the periapical area of a tooth and simulate a periapical granuloma or periapical cyst.

Radiographically, the lesions often appear as sharply punched-out radiolucencies, but other examples reveal an ill-defined radiolucency. Extensive alveolar involvement causes the teeth to appear as if they are "floating in air" (Fig. 14–18).

Histopathologic Features

The bone lesions in patients with Langerhans cell disease show a diffuse infiltration of large, pale-staining

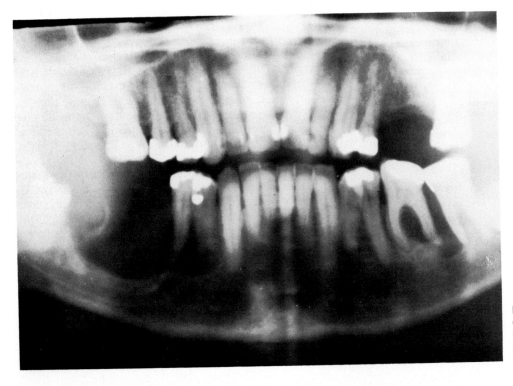

FIGURE 14–18. **Langerhans cell disease.** Severe bone loss in the mandibular molar regions. The left mandibular molar appears to be "floating in air."

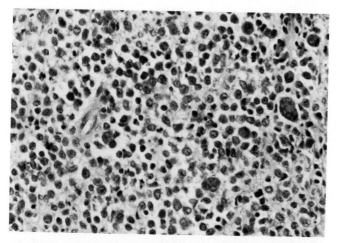

FIGURE 14–19. **Langerhans cell disease.** There is a diffuse infiltrate of pale-staining Langerhans cells with focal accumulations of darker-staining eosinophils. Several multinucleated giant cells are also present.

mononuclear cells. These cells have indistinct cytoplasmic borders and rounded or indented vesicular nuclei. Varying numbers of eosinophils may be interspersed among the histiocyte-like cells. Plasma cells, lymphocytes, and multinucleated giant cells may also be seen as well as areas of necrosis and hemorrhage (Fig. 14–19).

Some pathologists require the identification of Langerhans cells to confirm the diagnosis. Electron microscopy or immunohistochemical procedures are necessary because Langerhans cells cannot be differentiated from other histiocytes by routine histologic staining. Ultrastructurally, Langerhans cells contain rod-shaped cytoplasmic structures known as *Birbeck granules,* which differentiate them from other mononuclear phagocytes (Fig. 14–20).

Immunohistochemical studies are also helpful in confirming the presence of Langerhans cells. Langerhans cells stain positively for S-100 protein. They also show binding for peanut agglutinin (PNA).

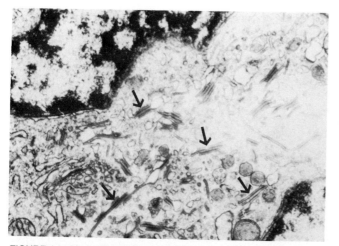

FIGURE 14–20. **Langerhans cell disease.** Electron micrograph showing rod-shaped Birbeck bodies (*black arrows*) in the cytoplasm of a Langerhans cell. (Courtesy of Dr. Richard Wesley.)

Treatment and Prognosis

Accessible bone lesions, such as those in the maxilla and mandible, are usually treated by curettage. Low doses of radiation are often employed for less accessible bone lesions.

The prognosis for bone lesions in the absence of significant visceral involvement is generally good, although progression or dissemination of the disease may occur. If a patient has not experienced recurrence or progression of the disease by 1 year after treatment, he or she is considered cured.

Chronic disseminated disease is often associated with considerable morbidity, but few patients die as a result of the disease. The acute disseminated form of the disease seen in infants and young children is associated with a poor prognosis and is often fatal. Treatment consists of use of multiple chemotherapeutic agents. The prognosis is poorer for patients in whom the first sign of the disease develops at a very young age and somewhat better for patients who are older at the time of onset.

CENTRAL GIANT CELL GRANULOMA
(Giant Cell Lesion; Giant Cell Tumor)

The giant cell granuloma is widely considered to be a non-neoplastic lesion. Although formerly designated as "giant cell reparative granuloma," there is little evidence that the lesion represents a reparative response. Some lesions demonstrate aggressive behavior similar to that of a neoplasm. The term "reparative" has been dropped by most oral and maxillofacial pathologists; today these lesions are designated as "giant cell granuloma" or by the more noncommittal term, **giant cell lesion.** Whether or not "true" **giant cell tumors** occur in the jaws is uncertain and controversial. This topic is discussed later.

Clinical and Radiographic Features

Giant cell granulomas may be encountered in patients ranging from 2 to 80 years of age, although more than 60 percent of all cases present before age 30. There is a distinct gender predilection, with 65 percent of cases occurring in females. About 70 percent of cases occur in the mandible. Lesions are more common in the anterior portions of the jaws, and mandibular lesions frequently cross the midline.

Most giant cell lesions of the jaws are asymptomatic and first come to attention during a routine radiographic examination or as a result of painless expansion of the affected bone. A minority of cases, however, may be associated with pain, paresthesia, or perforation of the cortical bone plate, resulting in ulceration of the mucosal surface by the underlying lesion (Fig. 14–21).

On the basis of the clinical and radiologic features, several groups of investigators have suggested that central giant cell lesions of the jaws may be divided into two categories:

1. *Non-aggressive* lesions, which make up most cases, present with few or no symptoms, demonstrate slow

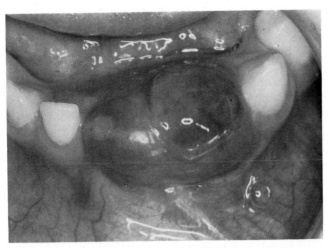

FIGURE 14-21. **Central giant cell granuloma.** A bluish-purple mass is present on the anterior alveolar ridge of this 4-year-old white boy.

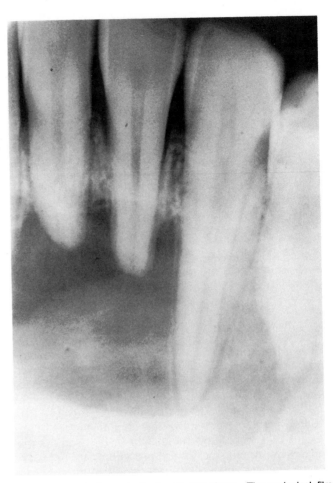

FIGURE 14-23. **Central giant cell granuloma.** The periapical film shows a radiolucent area in the anterior mandible. The incisors show apical root resorption. (Courtesy of Dr. Mark Bowden.)

growth, and do not show cortical perforation or root resorption of teeth involved in the lesion.

2. *Aggressive* lesions are characterized by pain, rapid growth, cortical perforation, and root resorption. They show a marked tendency to recur after treatment compared with the non-aggressive types.

Radiographically, central giant cell lesions present as radiolucent defects, which may be unilocular or multilocular. The defect is usually well delineated, but the margins are generally non-corticated. The lesion may vary from a 5- × 5-mm incidental radiographic finding to a destructive lesion greater than 10 cm in size. The radiographic findings are not specifically diagnostic. Small unilocular lesions may be confused with periapical granulomas or cysts (Figs. 14-22 to 14-25). Multilocular giant cell lesions cannot be radiographically distinguished from ameloblastomas or other multilocular lesions.

Histopathologic Features

Giant cell lesions of the jaw show a variety of features. Common to all is the presence of few to many multinucleated giant cells in a background of ovoid to spindle-shaped mesenchymal cells (Figs. 14-26*A, B*). The giant

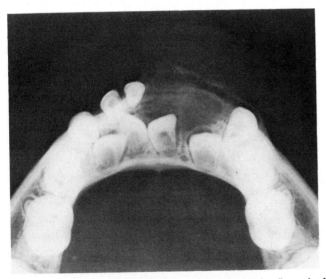

FIGURE 14-22. **Central giant cell granuloma.** Occlusal radiograph of the same patient shown in Figure 14-21. There is an ill-defined radiolucent lesion with cortical expansion.

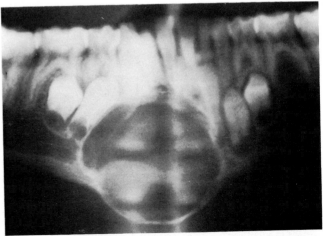

FIGURE 14-24. **Central giant cell granuloma.** Panoramic radiograph showing a large, expansile radiolucent lesion in the anterior mandible. (Courtesy of Dr. Gregory R. Erena.)

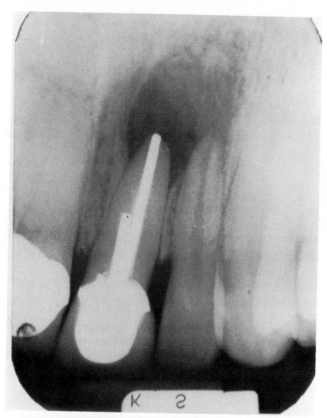

FIGURE 14–25. **Central giant cell granuloma.** The periapical radiograph shows a radiolucent area involving the periapical area of an endodontically treated tooth. This was preoperatively considered to represent a periapical granuloma or periapical cyst.

In some cases, the stroma is loosely arranged and edematous; in other cases, it may be quite cellular. Areas of erythrocyte extravasation and hemosiderin deposition may be prominent. Some lesions show considerable fibrosis of the stroma. Foci of osteoid and newly formed bone may be present within the lesion. The histopathologic findings closely resemble, and may be identical with, those seen in cherubism (see p. 456) and in the brown tumor of hyperparathyroidism (see p. 612).

Treatment and Prognosis

Central giant cell lesions of the jaws are usually treated by curettage. In reports of large series of cases, recurrence rates range from 11 to 50 percent or greater. Most studies indicate a recurrence rate of about 15 to 20 percent. Those lesions considered on clinical and radiologic grounds to be potentially aggressive show a higher frequency of recurrence. Recurrent lesions often respond to further curettage, although with some aggressive lesions more radical surgery is required for cure.

The long-term prognosis, however, is good, and metastases do not develop. Correlation of the histopathologic features with clinical behavior remains debatable, but lesions showing large, uniformly distributed giant cells and a predominantly cellular stroma appear more likely to be clinically aggressive with a greater tendency to recur.

cells may be focally aggregated in the lesional tissue or may be diffusely present throughout the lesion. These cells may vary considerably in size and shape from case to case. Some are small and irregular in shape and contain only a few nuclei. In other cases, the giant cells are large and round and contain 20 or more nuclei. There is evidence that these giant cells represent osteoclasts.

Giant Cell Tumor

The question of whether "true" **giant cell tumors**, which most often occur in the epiphyses of long tubular bones, occur in the jaws has been argued for many years and is still unresolved. Although most central giant cell lesions can be distinguished histopathologically from the long bone tumors, a small number of jaw lesions are microscopically indistinguishable from the typical giant cell tumor of long bone (Figs. 14–27A, B). In spite of the histopathologic similarity, these jaw lesions appear to

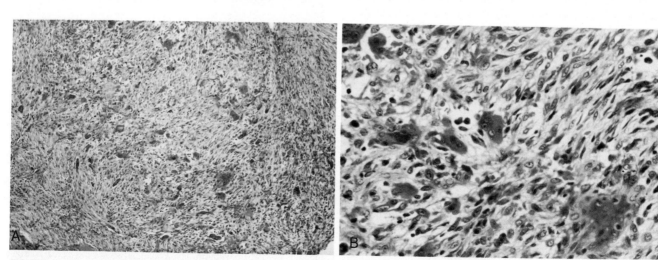

FIGURE 14–26. **Central giant cell granuloma.** A, Spindle-shaped mesenchymal cells with focal aggregates of small multinucleated giant cells. B, Higher magnification showing cellular details.

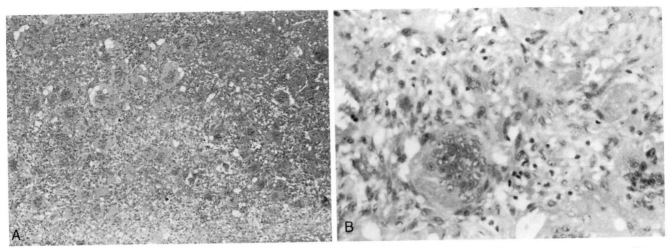

FIGURE 14–27. **Central giant cell granuloma.** *A*, Photomicrograph of a clinically aggressive and recurrent giant cell lesion of the maxilla in a 28-year-old white woman. Large giant cells are evenly distributed in a cellular mesenchymal tissue. *B*, Higher magnification of the same case showing the large giant cells and cellular mesenchymal tissue. The histopathologic features are identical with those of a giant cell tumor of long bone.

have a biologically different behavior from long bone lesions, which have higher recurrence rates after curettage and show malignant change in up to 10 percent of cases. One case of metastasis from a mandibular tumor, however, has been reported. It has been suggested that giant cell granulomas of the jaws and giant cell tumors of the extragnathic skeleton are not distinct and separate entities but rather represent a continuum of a single disease process modified by the age of the patient, their location, and possibly other factors that are not yet clearly understood.

CHERUBISM

Cherubism is a rare developmental jaw condition. The name "cherubism" was applied because the characteristic bilateral posterior mandibular swellings seen in affected patients result in a facial appearance similar to that of the plump-cheeked little angels (cherubs) depicted in Renaissance paintings. Although cherubism has also been called "familial fibrous dysplasia," this term should be avoided because this condition has no relationship to fibrous dysplasia of bone (see p. 461). There is an autosomal dominant pattern of inheritance, and pedigrees showing involvement through three or more generations have been reported. In a number of cases, however, no family history can be obtained, and these presumably represent spontaneous mutations.

Clinical and Radiographic Features

The lesions of cherubism occur in children, with some examples being manifested as early as 1 year of age. The mean age for detection is 7 years, but milder cases may not be detected until the patient reaches 10 to 12 years of age. A painless, bilateral expansion of the posterior mandible is the common early manifestation. The lesions tend to involve the mandibular angles and ascending rami. The bony expansion tends to be bilaterally sym-

metric and imparts the "chubby" facial appearance (Fig. 14–28). In severe cases, most of the mandible is involved. Milder maxillary involvement occurs in the tuberosity areas; in severe cases, the entire maxilla can be involved.

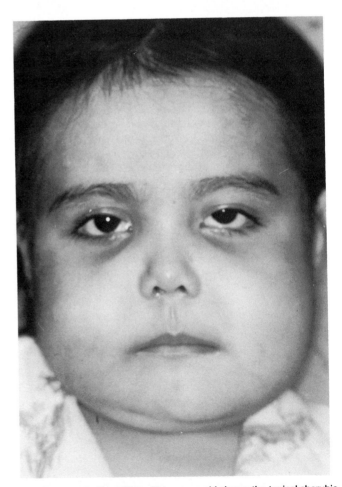

FIGURE 14–28. **Cherubism.** This young girl shows the typical cherubic facies resulting from bilateral expansile mandibular and maxillary lesions. (Courtesy of Dr. Román Carlos.)

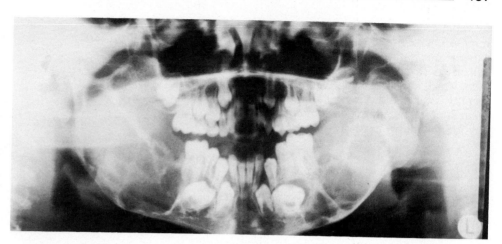

FIGURE 14–29. **Cherubism.** Panoramic radiograph showing large multilocular lesions involving the posterior body and ascending rami of the right and left mandibles. (Courtesy of Dr. Tom Brock.)

Extensive maxillary involvement causes stretching of the skin of the upper face to expose the sclerae. This results in an "eyes upturned to heaven" appearance. Extensive bone involvement causes a marked widening and distortion of the alveoli. Developing teeth are often displaced and fail to erupt. The extent of facial deformity, however, is variable and some patients show only minimal bone expansion and mild facial deformity. Although there have been rare reports of unilateral cherubism, it is difficult to accept these as examples of this disease unless there is a strong family history.

Radiographically, the lesions are typically multilocular, expansile radiolucencies (Fig. 14–29). The appearance is virtually diagnostic as a result of their bilateral location. Less commonly, the lesions present as unilocular radiolucencies. These may be associated with unerupted teeth and simulate the appearance of a dentigerous cyst.

No unusual biochemical findings have been reported in patients with cherubism. In rare instances, extragnathic bone lesions have been noted. Most of these have been isolated, incidental findings, and their nature and relationship to cherubism are uncertain.

An association between cherubism and Noonan-like syndrome has been reported. Noonan syndrome is a complex condition characterized by short stature, unusual facies, cardiac defects, and mental retardation. It is inherited as an autosomal dominant trait but may occur sporadically. The association between these two rare inherited diseases suggests that they are independent diseases that may be transmitted by genes closely linked on the same chromosome.

Histopathologic Features

The microscopic findings of cherubism are essentially similar to those of the isolated giant cell granulomas; however, the stroma in cherubism often tends to be more loosely arranged than that seen in giant cell granulomas. The microscopic features seldom permit a specific diagnosis of cherubism in the absence of clinical and radiologic information. The lesional tissue consists of vascular fibrous tissue containing variable numbers of multinucleated giant cells. The giant cells tend to be small and are usually focally aggregated (Fig. 14–30). Foci of

extravasated blood are commonly present. Some cases of cherubism reveal eosinophilic cuff-like deposits surrounding small blood vessels throughout the lesion. This feature appears to be specific for cherubism; however, these deposits are not present in many cases, so that their absence does not exclude a diagnosis of cherubism. In older, resolving lesions of cherubism, the tissue becomes more fibrous, the number of giant cells decreases, and new bone formation is seen.

Treatment and Prognosis

The prognosis in any given case is unpredictable. In some instances, the lesions tend to show varying degrees of remission and involution after puberty, although some degree of facial deformity may persist. However, cases demonstrating active disease persisting into adult life have been reported.

The question of whether to actively treat or simply observe a patient with cherubism is difficult. Excellent results have been obtained in some cases by early surgical intervention with curettage of the lesions. Conversely, early surgical intervention has sometimes been followed

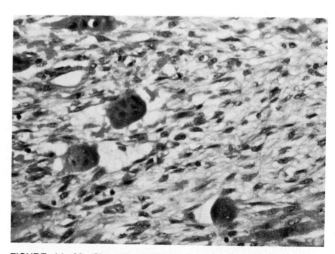

FIGURE 14–30. **Cherubism.** Photomicrograph showing loosely arranged fibrous stroma containing scattered, small giant cells.

by rapid regrowth of the lesions and worsening deformity. A course limited only to observation may result in extreme and sometimes grotesque facial deformity with associated psychologic problems and functional deformity, which may necessitate extensive surgery. Radiation therapy is contraindicated because of the risk of development of post-irradiation bone sarcoma. The optimal therapy for cherubism has not been determined.

SIMPLE BONE CYST (Traumatic Bone Cyst; Hemorrhagic Bone Cyst; Solitary Bone Cyst; Idiopathic Bone Cavity)

The **simple bone cyst** is undoubtedly more common in the jaws than the literature would indicate. The cause and pathogenesis are uncertain and controversial. Several theories have been proposed, but none of them explains all of the clinical and pathologic features of this disease.

The *trauma-hemorrhage theory* has many advocates, as evidenced by the widely used designation **traumatic bone cyst**. This theory suggests that trauma to the bone that is insufficient to cause a fracture results in an intraosseous hematoma. If the hematoma does not undergo organization and repair, it may liquefy, resulting in a cystic defect. Although the trauma-hemorrhage theory appears to be widely held in the dental literature, it has little support in the orthopedic literature to explain similar cysts most commonly found in the proximal diaphysis of the femur and tibia in young patients.

Similar simple cysts may be associated with lesions of cemento-osseous dysplasia and other fibro-osseous tumors. These are discussed later (see p. 466).

Clinical and Radiographic Features

Most simple bone cysts of the jaws are encountered in patients between 10 and 20 years of age. The lesion is rare in children under age 5 and is seldom seen in patients over age 35. Simple bone cysts of the jaws are essentially restricted to the mandible, although there have been reports of the lesion in the maxilla. Bilateral simple bone cysts of the mandible are occasionally encountered. About 60 percent of cases occur in males.

The simple bone cyst usually produces no symptoms and is discovered only when radiographs are taken for some other reason. About 20 percent of patients, however, have a painless swelling of the affected area. Pain and paresthesia may be noted in a few cases. Some patients may recall an episode of trauma to the affected area, but this anecdotal information is of uncertain significance and has not been subjected to detailed, controlled analysis. Although any area of the mandible may be involved, simple cysts are more common in the premolar and molar areas. Extensive lesions involving a substantial portion of the body and ascending ramus may be encountered.

Radiographically, the lesion presents as a well-delineated radiolucent defect. In some areas, the margins of the defect are sharply defined; in other areas, the margins

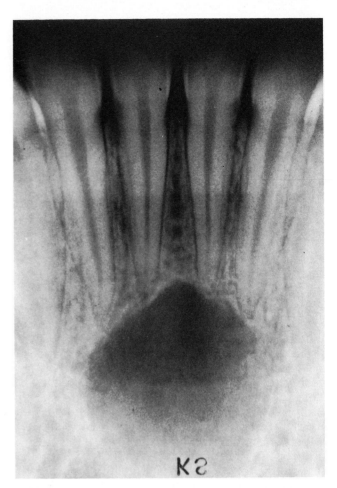

FIGURE 14–31. **Simple bone cyst.** Periapical radiograph showing a radiolucent area in the apical region of the anterior mandible. The incisor teeth responded normally to vitality testing, and no restorations are present.

are ill defined. The defect may range from 1 to 10 cm in diameter. When several teeth are involved in the lesion, the radiolucent defect often shows dome-like projections that scallop upward between the roots. This feature is highly suggestive but not diagnostic of a simple bone cyst (Figs. 14–31 and 14–32). Teeth that appear to be involved in the lesion are generally vital and do not show root resorption. When mandibular expansion is present, an occlusal radiograph may reveal that the cortical bone is reduced to a thin shell and no cortical bone reaction is seen.

Diagnosis

The radiologic features of the simple bone cyst, while often suggestive of the diagnosis, are not diagnostic and may be confused with a wide variety of odontogenic and non-odontogenic radiolucent jaw lesions. Surgical exploration is necessary to establish the diagnosis.

Because little to no tissue is obtained at the time of surgery, the diagnosis of simple bone cyst is based primarily on the clinical and radiographic features together with the surgical findings. In about one third of cases, the

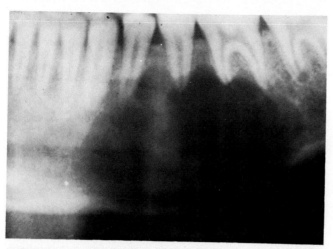

FIGURE 14–32. **Simple bone cyst.** Panoramic film showing a large simple bone cyst of the mandible in a 12-year-old girl. The scalloping superior aspect of the cyst between the roots of the teeth is highly suggestive of, but not diagnostic for, a simple bone cyst. (Courtesy of Dr. Lon Doles.)

lytic defect will be found to be an empty cavity with smooth, shiny bony walls. In about two thirds of cases, the cavity will contain small amounts of serosanguineous fluid. The mandibular neurovascular bundle may be seen lying free in the cavity.

Histopathologic Features

Histopathologic study is usually limited to the bone "window," which is removed to obtain access to the lesion. This shows a thin membrane of vascular connective tissue, fibrin, erythrocytes, and occasional giant cells on the bone surface next to the cavity (Fig. 14–33). A well-developed fibrous cyst wall is not present, and there is never any evidence of an epithelial lining. The bony surface next to the cavity often shows resorptive areas (Howship's lacunae) indicative of past osteoclastic activity.

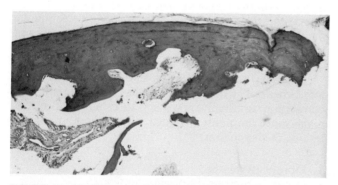

FIGURE 14–33. **Simple bone cyst.** Photomicrograph of the bony "window" removed during surgical exploration of a lesion similar to that shown in Figure 14–32. The cortical bone adjacent to the cyst cavity (*bottom*) shows evidence of osteoclastic resorption. A thin, vascular connective tissue membrane is adjacent to the bone.

Treatment and Prognosis

Surgical exploration to establish the diagnosis is usually the curative therapy. After surgical exploration with or without curettage of the bony walls, obliteration of the defect by new bone formation is generally rapid. Even large defects may show normal radiographic findings within 6 months after exploration. Recurrence or persistence of the lesion is most unusual, and the prognosis is excellent. The chief problem associated with simple bone cysts relates to clinical and radiologic misdiagnosis as some other radiolucent pathosis leading to unnecessarily extensive surgery, such as extraction of teeth or even local resection of the area.

Although the bone walls of the cavity at surgical exploration appear smooth and shiny, it is wise to curette them and submit the small amount of tissue obtained for microscopic examination to rule out more serious diseases. Rarely, a lesion considered to be a simple bone cyst at surgical exploration will prove to be a thin-walled cystic ameloblastoma or an odontogenic keratocyst after microscopic study.

ANEURYSMAL BONE CYST

Aneurysmal bone cysts are most commonly located in the shaft of a long bone or in the vertebral column in patients younger than age 30. The lesion is uncommon in the jaws, with fewer than 50 examples having been reported.

The cause and pathogenesis of the aneurysmal bone cyst are poorly understood, and there is controversy as to whether the lesion arises *de novo* or represents the result of some form of vascular "accident" in a pre-existing lesion. Some authors have presented large series of cases involving the extragnathic skeleton and claim that none of their cases has shown evidence of a pre-existing lesion. Others have reported similar large series and contend that a pre-existing lesion may be evident in one third of cases. Aneurysmal bone cyst–like areas may also develop in malignant bone tumors, such as osteosarcoma. It is likely that the aneurysmal bone cyst may occur as a primary lesion or may result from development of a dilated vascular bed in a pre-existing intrabony lesion.

Clinical and Radiographic Features

Most aneurysmal bone cysts of the jaws have occurred in patients younger than age 20. There is a slight female predilection. The mandible is more often involved than the maxilla, and the lesions occur mostly in the molar regions. The lesion is most often associated with an obvious facial swelling that has usually developed rapidly. Pain is often reported.

Radiographic study shows a unilocular or multilocular radiolucent lesion often associated with marked cortical expansion and thinning (Fig. 14–34). This is frequently described as a ballooning or "blow-out" distention of the contour of the affected bone. At the time of surgery, intact periosteum and a thin shell of bone are found covering the lesion. When the periosteum and bony shell

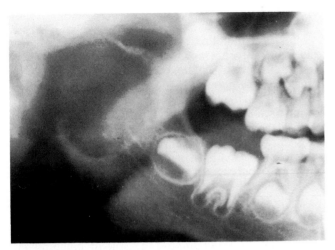

FIGURE 14-34. **Aneurysmal bone cyst.** A large multilocular radiolucent lesion involves most of the ascending ramus in a 5-year-old white boy. (Courtesy of Dr. Samuel McKenna.)

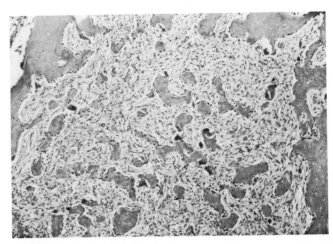

FIGURE 14-36. **Aneurysmal bone cyst.** Photomicrograph of solid areas in the lesion. The histopathologic features resemble those of an ossifying fibroma.

are removed, dark venous blood frequently wells up and the bleeding may be difficult to control. The appearance at surgery has been likened to that of a "blood-soaked sponge."

Histopathologic Features

Microscopically, the aneurysmal bone cyst is characterized by spaces of varying size, filled with unclotted blood surrounded by fibroblastic tissue containing multinucleated giant cells and trabeculae of osteoid and woven bone. The blood-filled spaces are not lined by endothelium (Fig. 14-35). In some cases, the lesion may contain larger solid areas that resemble giant cell granuloma, fibrous dysplasia, ossifying fibroma, or other jaw tumors (Fig. 14-36).

Treatment and Prognosis

Aneurysmal bone cysts of the jaws are usually treated by curettage. Recurrence rates as high as 50 percent have been reported. This may be related to the difficulty in curetting large, vascular lesions. Significant blood loss at surgery, however, is seldom a problem. The long-term prognosis appears favorable, although more extensive surgical resection, supplemented with cryosurgery, may be required to control recurrent lesions.

FIBRO-OSSEOUS LESIONS OF THE JAWS

Fibro-osseous lesions comprise a diverse group of processes that are characterized by replacement of normal bone by a fibrous tissue containing a newly formed mineralized product. The designation "fibro-osseous lesion" is not a specific diagnosis and describes only a process. Fibro-osseous lesions of the jaws include developmental (hamartomatous) lesions, reactive or dysplastic processes, and neoplasms.

The pathologic features on a biopsy specimen may be very similar in lesions of diverse etiology, behavior, and prognosis. Clinical, radiologic, and histopathologic correlation is usually necessary to establish a specific diagnosis. Commonly included among the fibro-osseous lesions of the jaws are:

1. Fibrous dysplasia
2. Cemento-osseous dysplasia
   a. Periapical cemento-osseous dysplasia
   b. Focal cemento-osseous dysplasia
   c. Florid cemento-osseous dysplasia
3. Ossifying (cemento-ossifying) fibroma

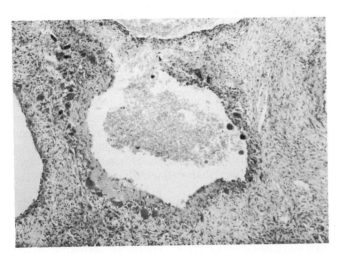

FIGURE 14-35. **Aneurysmal bone cyst.** Photomicrograph showing large, blood-filled spaces surrounded by fibroblastic connective tissue. Numerous multinucleated giant cells are adjacent to the vascular spaces.

FIBROUS DYSPLASIA

Fibrous dysplasia of bone is considered to represent a developmental tumor-like lesion. Most cases represent *monostotic* disease (limited to a single bone). This type accounts for about 80 to 85 percent of all cases of fibrous dysplasia.

Polyostotic fibrous dysplasia (affecting several to many bones) is relatively uncommon. In extreme cases, three fourths of the entire skeleton may be involved. This form of polyostotic fibrous dysplasia is sometimes termed the **Jaffe type.**

About 3 percent of patients with polyostotic fibrous dysplasia also have multiple areas of cutaneous pigmentation and autonomous hyperfunction of one or more of the endocrine glands. This is known as the **McCune-Albright syndrome.**

The skull and jaws are commonly involved in all three forms of the disease.

Clinical and Radiographic Features

Monostotic Fibrous Dysplasia of the Jaws

The jaws are among the most commonly affected sites in patients with **monostotic fibrous dysplasia.** The disease usually becomes manifest during the first or second decade of life, but milder examples may escape detection until later. Males and females are affected with about equal frequency. A painless swelling of the affected area is the most common feature (Fig. 14–37). Growth is generally slow, and the patient or parents are often unable to recall when the lesion was first noted. Occasionally, however, the growth may be fairly rapid. The maxilla is involved more often than the mandible.

Although mandibular lesions are truly monostotic, maxillary lesions often involve adjacent bones, such as the zygoma, sphenoid, and occiput, and are not strictly monostotic. The designation of **craniofacial fibrous dysplasia** is appropriate for these lesions. Teeth involved in the lesion usually remain firm but may be displaced by the bony mass.

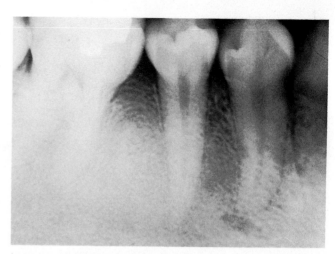

FIGURE 14–38. **Fibrous dysplasia.** Periapical radiograph showing a diffuse "ground glass" radiographic appearance.

The chief radiologic feature is a fine "ground glass" opacification that results from superimposition of a myriad of poorly calcified bone trabeculae arranged in a disorganized pattern. Radiographically, the lesions of fibrous dysplasia are not well defined and the margins blend imperceptibly into the adjacent normal bone so that the limits of the lesion may be difficult to define (Figs. 14–38 and 14–39). In the earlier stages, the lesion may be largely radiolucent or mottled. When the maxilla is involved, the lesional tissue commonly fills and obliterates the maxillary sinus. Lateral skull films in cases with maxillary involvement may show increased density of the base of the skull involving the occiput, sphenoid, roof of the orbit, and frontal bones. This is said to be the most characteristic radiographic feature of fibrous dysplasia of the skull.

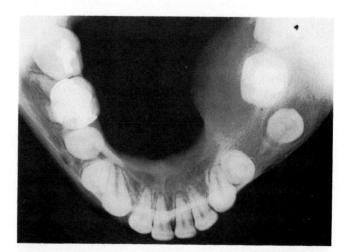

FIGURE 14–39. **Fibrous dysplasia.** Occlusal radiograph showing localized expansion of the mandible and the "ground glass" radiographic appearance. The margins of the lesion are not well defined and blend into the adjacent bone. (From Waldron CA, Giansanti JS. Benign fibro-osseous lesions of the jaws: A clinical-radiologic-histologic review of 65 cases. Part I. Fibrous dysplasia of the jaws. Oral Surg Oral Med Oral Pathol 35:190–201, 1973.)

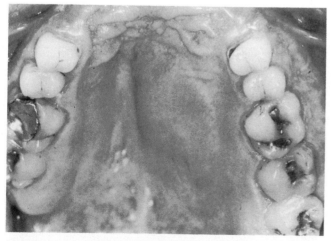

FIGURE 14–37. **Fibrous dysplasia.** Clinical photograph showing the typical unilateral maxillary enlargement in a patient with fibrous dysplasia.

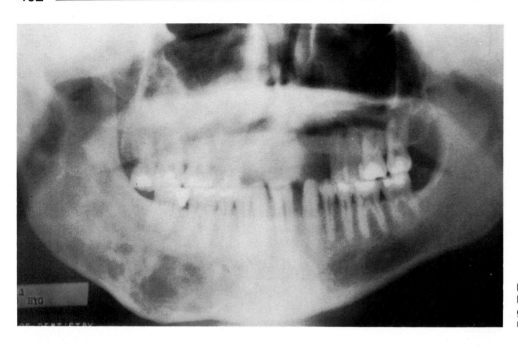

FIGURE 14–40. **Polyostotic fibrous dysplasia.** Panoramic radiograph showing involvement of the right maxilla and mandible.

Polyostotic Fibrous Dysplasia and McCune-Albright Syndrome

Although the skull and jaws may be affected with resultant facial asymmetry, the clinical picture in patients with **polyostotic fibrous dysplasia** is usually dominated by symptoms related to the long bone lesions (Fig. 14–40). Pathologic fracture with resulting pain and deformity is very common. Leg length discrepancy is very common as a result of involvement of the upper portion of the femur ("hockey stick" deformity).

Patients with the **McCune-Albright syndrome** have *café au lait* (coffee with milk) pigmentation, which consists of well-defined, generally unilateral tan macules on the trunk and thighs. These pigmented lesions may be congenital, and oral mucosal pigmented macules may be present. The margins of the *café au lait* spots are typically very irregular, resembling a map of the coastline of Maine (Fig. 14–41). This is in contrast to the *café au lait* spots of neurofibromatosis (see p. 381), which have smooth borders (like the coast of California).

Sexual precocity is the most common endocrine manifestation of the syndrome, particularly in females. Menstrual bleeding may occur during the first few months of life. Breast development and pubic hair may be apparent within the first few years of life in affected girls.

Histopathologic Features

The typical microscopic findings of fibrous dysplasia show irregularly shaped trabeculae of immature (woven) bone in a cellular, loosely arranged fibrous stroma. The bone trabeculae are not connected to each other. They often assume curvilinear shapes, which have been likened to Chinese script writing. The bone trabeculae are considered to arise by metaplasia and are not surrounded by osteoid seams or plump appositional osteoblasts (Fig. 14–42). The lesional bone fuses directly to normal bone at the periphery of the lesion, so that no capsule or line of

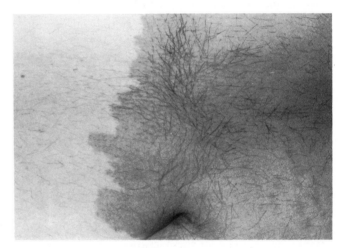

FIGURE 14–41. **Polyostotic fibrous dysplasia.** McCune-Albright syndrome: *Café au lait* pigmentation of the abdomen. This is the same patient as shown in Figures 14–37 and 14–40.

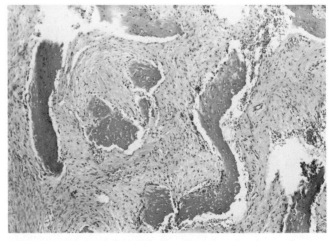

FIGURE 14–42. **Fibrous dysplasia.** Irregularly shaped trabeculae of woven bone in a fibrous stroma.

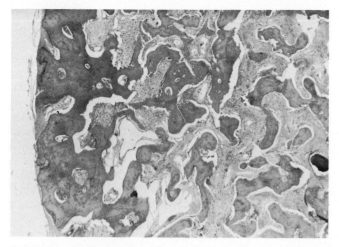

FIGURE 14–43. **Fibrous dysplasia.** The lesional bone is fused to the overlying cortical bone on the left side.

demarcation is present (Fig. 14–43). Although fibrous dysplasia of the long bones does not undergo maturation, jaw and skull lesions tend to be more ossified than their counterparts in the rest of the skeleton. This is particularly true in specimens from older patients (Figs. 14–44*A, B*).

Serial biopsy specimens in some cases have shown that histopathologically classic fibrous dysplasia of the jaws may undergo progressive maturation to a lesion consisting of lamellar bone in a moderately cellular connective tissue stroma. The bone trabeculae in these mature lesions tend to run parallel to one another (Fig. 14–45).

Treatment and Prognosis

Clinical management of fibrous dysplasia of the jaws may present a major problem. Although smaller lesions,

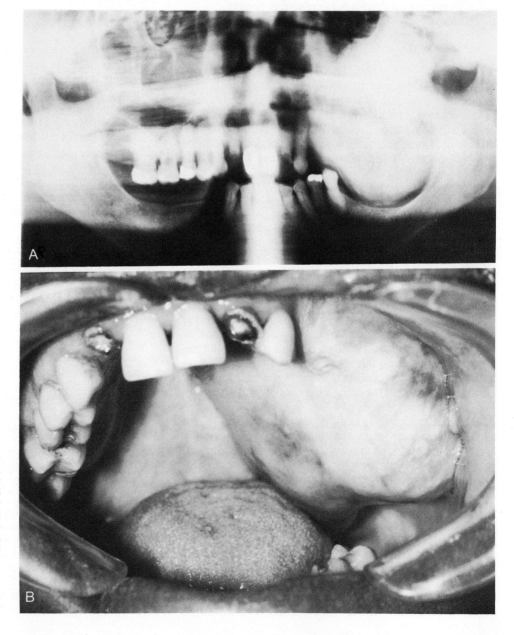

FIGURE 14–44. **Fibrous dysplasia.** *A*, Panoramic radiograph of a "mature" lesion of fibrous dysplasia of the left posterior maxilla and maxillary sinus. The patient, a 45-year-old woman, was known to have a lesion in this area for more than 20 years. (Courtesy of Dr. Richard Brock.) *B*, Clinical photograph of the same patient shown in *A*. Note prominent unilateral maxillary enlargement.

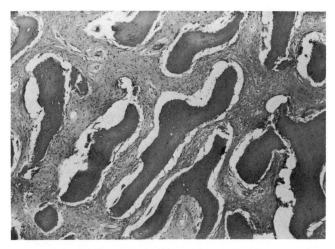

FIGURE 14–45. **Fibrous dysplasia.** This specimen is from a "shave-down" procedure performed on the same patient depicted in Figure 14–44. Trabeculae of mature lamellar bone showing a parallel arrangement are present in a fibrous stroma. This is characteristic of the mature fibrous dysplasia lesions in the craniofacial skeleton.

particularly in the mandible, may be completely surgically resected without too much difficulty, the diffuse nature and large size of many lesions, particularly those of the maxilla, preclude removal without extensive surgery. In many cases, the disease tends to stabilize and essentially stops enlarging when skeletal maturation is reached. Some lesions, however, continue to grow, although generally slowly, in adult patients.

Some patients with minimal cosmetic or functional deformity may not require or desire surgical treatment. Cosmetic deformity with associated psychologic problems or functional deformity may dictate surgical intervention in the younger patient. Such a procedure usually entails surgical reduction of the lesion to an acceptable contour without attempts to remove the entire lesion. The cosmetic result is usually good, but regrowth of the lesion occurs over time.

The prevalence of regrowth after surgical reduction is difficult to determine, but it has been estimated that between 25 and 50 percent of patients show some regrowth after surgical shave-down of the lesion. The regrowth is more common in younger patients, and many surgeons believe that surgical intervention should be delayed for as long as possible.

Malignant change, usually development of an osteosarcoma, has been rarely associated with fibrous dysplasia. Most examples have been found in patients who had received radiation therapy for fibrous dysplasia, but a few examples of spontaneous sarcomatous changes have been reported. Radiation therapy for fibrous dysplasia is contraindicated because it carries the risk for development of post-irradiation bone sarcoma.

CEMENTO-OSSEOUS DYSPLASIAS

Cemento-osseous dysplasias occur in the tooth-bearing areas of the jaws and are probably the most common types of fibro-osseous lesions encountered in clinical practice. Microscopically, they consist of fibrous tissue, bone, and cementum-like calcifications. The pathologic features may be similar to those of fibrous dysplasia and ossifying fibroma. However, these lesions do not appear to be developmental in nature, such as fibrous dysplasia, nor do they show the characteristics of neoplasia, such as ossifying fibroma. The pathogenesis of the cemento-osseous dysplasias is unknown, but they appear to represent some form of reactive or dysplastic process.

On the basis of their clinical and radiologic features, it is convenient to separate the cemento-osseous dysplasias into three groups: *periapical, focal,* and *florid.* It is likely, however, that these categories represent only variants of the same pathologic process.

Periapical Cemento-osseous Dysplasia
(Periapical Cemental Dysplasia; Periapical Cementoma)

Clinical and Radiographic Features

Periapical cemento-osseous dysplasia predominantly involves the lower anterior periapical region. Occasionally, however, it appears in other periapical areas. Solitary lesions may occur, but multiple lesions are present more frequently. There is a marked predilection for female patients (14:1) and for blacks; the reasons for the gender and racial predilection are unclear. Most people are between ages 30 and 50 when the lesions are first detected. Teeth associated with the lesions are almost invariably vital and seldom have restorations.

Periapical cemento-osseous dysplasia is an asymptomatic condition that is discovered when radiographs are taken for other purposes. Early lesions present as circumscribed areas of radiolucency involving the apical area of a tooth. At this stage, the lesion cannot be radiographically differentiated from a periapical granuloma or periapical cyst (Fig. 14–46).

Serial radiographic studies reveal that the lesions tend to "mature" over time to have a mixed radiolucent and radiopaque appearance. In the end stage, the lesions show a circumscribed dense calcification surrounded by a narrow radiolucent rim (Fig. 14–47). Individual lesions seldom exceed 1.0 cm in diameter. Each lesion is self-limiting and does not expand the cortex. Progressive growth seldom, if ever, occurs.

Histopathologic Features

In the early (radiolucent) stages, the lesion consists of a fibroblastic proliferation that may contain small foci of osteoid formation. There is no evidence of inflammation.

In the later stages, the lesion shows progressive deposition of bone or cementum-like material. In the end stage, the lesion consists of a dense mineralized mass.

Treatment and Prognosis

Patients with periapical cemento-osseous dysplasia do not require treatment. In the typical case (i.e., a black

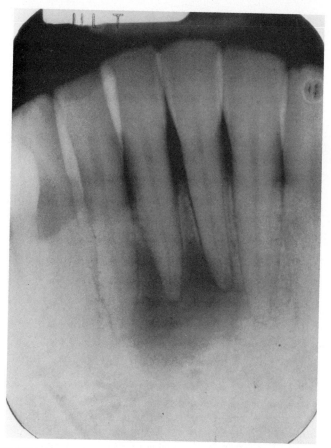

FIGURE 14–46. **Periapical cemento-osseous dysplasia.** Periapical radiograph showing a radiolucent lesion in the apical area of the mandibular central incisors. The teeth are vital, and no restorations are present. This early stage of periapical cemento-osseous dysplasia could be mistaken for chronic inflammatory periapical pathosis.

female with multiple lesions involving vital lower incisor teeth), biopsy is not indicated. Solitary lesions in a less typical clinical presentation may indicate the need for a biopsy, but if the lesion is in a periapical location and the involved tooth responds to vitality testing, the lesion most probably represents periapical cemento-osseous dysplasia. The major concern is the failure to recognize the nature of the lesion, which may result in unnecessary endodontic treatment or extractions on the assumption that the lesion represents inflammatory periapical pathosis.

Focal Cemento-osseous Dysplasia

Focal cemento-osseous dysplasia is a benign cemento-osseous lesion that occupies a portion of the spectrum between the periapical and florid cemento-osseous dysplasias. These lesions show histopathologic features similar to the periapical and florid dysplasias, but they do not have the same characteristic clinical-radiologic presentations. Although focal cemento-osseous dysplasia has received scant attention in the literature, it is likely the most common fibro-osseous lesion encountered in the oral pathology laboratory.

Clinical and Radiographic Features

About 80 percent of cases of focal cemento-osseous dysplasia occur in females, with the greatest prevalence in the fourth and fifth decades of life. The lesions are found more often in whites. This is in contrast to the marked predominance of the periapical and florid cemento-osseous dysplasias in blacks. Focal cemento-osseous dysplasia may occur in any area of the jaws, but the posterior mandible is the predominant site. The disease is almost invariably asymptomatic and is detected only on a radiographic examination. Most lesions are smaller than 1.5 cm in diameter.

Radiographically, the lesion varies from completely radiolucent to densely radiopaque. Most commonly, however, there is a mixed radiolucent and radiopaque pattern (Figs. 14–48*A*, *B*). The lesion tends to be well defined, but the borders are usually slightly irregular. Lesions may occur in dentulous as well as edentulous areas. Many examples occur in extraction sites. Usually, the patient has only one lesion.

Histopathologic Features

On surgical exploration, the tissue occupying the bony defect consists of easily fragmented gritty tissue, which

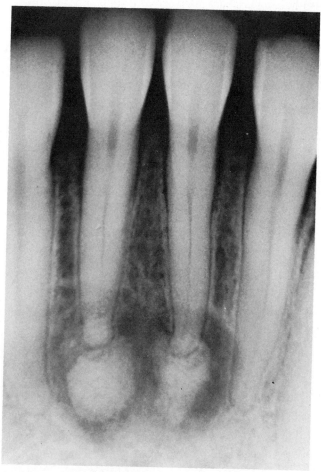

FIGURE 14–47. **Periapical cemento-osseous dysplasia.** Periapical radiograph showing a more advanced stage of the disease.

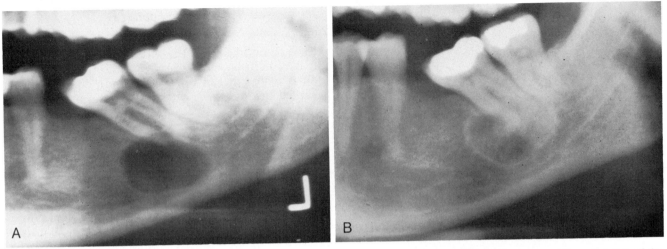

FIGURE 14–48. **Focal cemento-osseous dysplasia.** *A*, A radiolucent area involves the edentulous first molar area and the apical area of the second molar. *B*, Radiograph of the same patient taken 9 years later showing a mixed radiolucent-radiopaque pattern.

can be curetted from the defect, often with some difficulty. Microscopically, the tissue consists of fragments of cellular mesenchymal tissue composed of spindle-shaped fibroblasts and collagen fibers with numerous small blood vessels. Trabeculae of woven bone and cementum-like material are interspersed throughout the fibrous framework. Areas of fresh surgical hemorrhage are frequently present. Inflammatory cells are usually not visible (Fig. 14–49*A*).

Treatment and Prognosis

In patients with focal cemento-osseous dysplasia, the lesion is often only partially removed at biopsy and follow-up study often shows little or no tendency for progression and enlargement of the lesion. The prognosis is

excellent. Once the diagnosis has been established by biopsy, only periodic observation is required. Simple bone cysts (see p. 458) may develop within an area of focal cemento-osseous dysplasia, and this may cause enlargement of the area (Fig. 14–49*B*). In such instances, surgical exploration is necessary to establish the diagnosis and the lesion is usually subjected to curettage. In a few instances, a patient with focal cemento-osseous dysplasia has additional lesions and the condition has progressed to a point where it may be considered to represent florid cemento-osseous dysplasia.

Differentiation of focal cemento-osseous dysplasia from ossifying (cemento-ossifying) fibroma can be difficult. Many lesions that have been diagnosed as ossifying fibroma in the past are better considered to represent focal cemento-osseous dysplasia. The findings at surgery

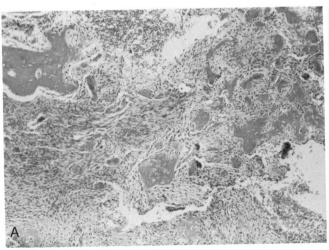
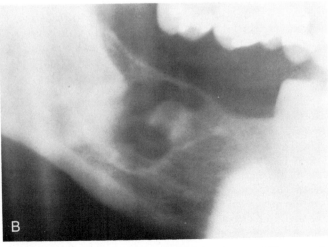

FIGURE 14–49. **Focal cemento-osseous dysplasia.** *A*, Biopsy specimen showing trabeculae of bone and cementum-like material in a vascular fibrous stroma. *B*, The radiolucent area adjacent to the calcified structure represents a simple bone cyst arising in a focal cemento-osseous dysplasia. (Courtesy of Dr. H. T. Daniel.)

are very helpful in distinguishing between these two lesions. Focal cemento-osseous dysplasia does not separate cleanly from the bone and is removed by curettage in fragments. In contrast, ossifying fibromas tend to separate cleanly from the bone in one or several large masses.

Florid Cemento-osseous Dysplasia

Florid cemento-osseous dysplasia clearly appears to be a form of bone and cemental dysplasia that is limited to the jaws. Patients do not have laboratory or radiologic evidence of bone disease in other parts of the skeleton. Secondary infection, usually as the result of exposure of the abnormal calcified material to the oral cavity, often results in a low-grade osteomyelitis. Many cases formerly reported as **chronic sclerosing osteomyelitis** or **sclerosing osteitis** appear to represent florid cemento-osseous dysplasia with secondary infections.

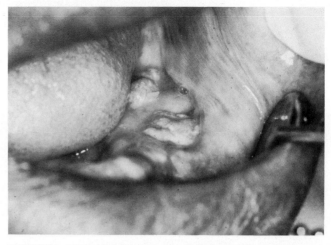

FIGURE 14–50. **Florid cemento-osseous dysplasia.** Yellowish, avascular cementum-like material is beginning to exfoliate through the oral mucosa.

Clinical and Radiographic Features

This distinctive form of cemento-osseous dysplasia shows a striking predilection to involve adult black women (in some series, more than 90 percent of patients). The reason for this racial and gender predilection is unknown. A familial tendency has been reported in some cases, but most examples appear to represent isolated instances.

The lesions show a marked tendency for bilateral and often quite symmetric involvement, and it is not unusual to encounter extensive involvement of all four posterior quadrants. The disease may be completely asymptomatic and in such cases is discovered only when radiographs are taken for some other purpose. In other instances, the patient may complain of dull pain, and an alveolar mucosal fistula may be present. In some cases, yellowish, avascular bone-like material is exposed to the oral cavity through a mucosal defect (Fig. 14–50). One or more of the involved areas of the jaws may demonstrate some degree of expansion.

Radiographically, the most typical lesions are highly radiodense and lobular in configuration. These dense lobular areas are often interspersed with less well-defined mixed radiolucent and radiopaque alterations in the radiographic pattern (Figs. 14–51 and 14–52). Serial radiographic study has shown that the mixed radiolucent and radiopaque areas tend to become more heavily calcified with time.

Both dentulous and edentulous areas may be affected, and involvement appears to be unrelated to the presence or absence of teeth. The lower anterior teeth, if present, often show the radiographic features associated with periapical cemento-osseous dysplasia. More sharply defined radiolucent areas, which on surgical exploration prove to be simple bone cysts (see p. 458), may be intermixed with

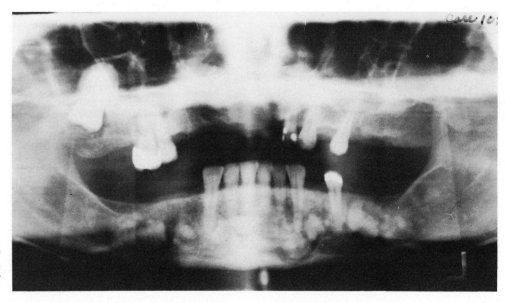

FIGURE 14–51. **Florid cemento-osseous dysplasia.** Multiple, mixed radiolucent/radiopaque lesions involve the mandible.

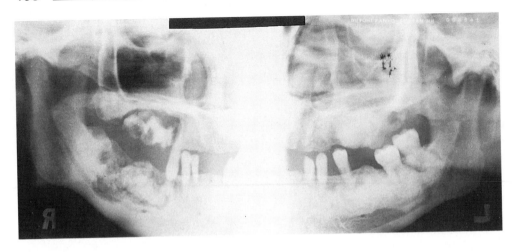

FIGURE 14–52. Florid cemento-osseous dysplasia. Densely sclerotic lesions involve the four posterior quadrants. The mass in the upper right quadrant is exposed to the mouth and is sequestrating.

the other lesional elements. The cysts may be single or multiple, and in some cases represent a sizable portion of the lesion. These cysts often do not heal as rapidly as the cysts in a younger patient who does not have cemento-osseous dysplasia. In some cases, the cysts persist or enlarge after surgical intervention; when they fill in, the bone retains an abnormal radiographic appearance.

Histopathologic Features

Microscopically, the lesions show a fibroblastic proliferation associated with irregular trabeculae of woven bone and cementum-like material. The densely sclerotic lobular masses are composed of sheets or fused globules of relatively acellular material, which is interpreted by most pathologists to represent cementum (Fig. 14–53). Varying numbers of inflammatory cells may be present in biopsy specimens from symptomatic patients. The simple bone cysts associated with florid cemento-osseous dysplasia show a thin lining of loosely arranged fibrous connective tissue.

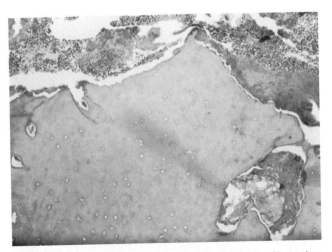

FIGURE 14–53. Florid cemento-osseous dysplasia. Photomicrograph of sequestrum from patient shown in Figure 14–52. The necrotic dense cementum-like material is surfaced by bacterial colonies and inflammatory cells.

Treatment and Prognosis

Management of florid cemento-osseous dysplasia may be difficult and not very satisfactory. The disease may persist for indefinite periods of time without causing any symptoms. For the asymptomatic patient, the best management consists of regular recall examinations with prophylaxis and reinforcement of good home hygiene care to control periodontal disease and prevent tooth loss. Because the onset of symptoms is usually associated with exposure of the sclerotic masses to the oral cavity, biopsy or elective extraction of teeth should be avoided. In other instances, symptoms begin after exposure of the sclerotic masses to the oral cavity as a result of progressive alveolar atrophy under a denture. Affected patients should be encouraged to retain their teeth to prevent development of symptoms later.

Management of the symptomatic patient is more difficult. At this stage, there is an inflammatory component to the disease and the process is basically a chronic osteomyelitis involving dysplastic bone and cementum. Antibiotics may be indicated but may not be effective. Sequestration of the sclerotic cementum-like masses occurs slowly and is followed by healing. Saucerization of dead bone and cementum may speed healing.

FAMILIAL GIGANTIFORM CEMENTOMA

The term **gigantiform cementoma** is used as a synonym for florid cemento-osseous dysplasia in the 1992 World Health Organization (WHO) classification, and a few cases of typical florid cemento-osseous dysplasia have been reported under this designation. A rare familial form of the disease, however, has also has been designated as **familial gigantiform cementoma**. Patients have significantly different clinical features from those affected by typical florid cemento-osseous dysplasia. This suggests that familial gigantiform cementoma may deserve separate classification.

Familial gigantiform cementoma appears to be an autosomal dominant inherited condition showing variable phenotypic expression. In one report, 16 members of a family were affected for more than five generations. In contrast to the marked black female predominance in typical florid cemento-osseous dysplasia, familial gigantiform cementomas occur almost exclusively in whites. Males are affected as commonly as females.

Clinical and Radiographic Findings

In contrast to the usual findings in typical florid cemento-osseous dysplasia, familial gigantiform cementoma is often clinically and radiographically manifest during the first and second decades of life. The lesions characteristically show relatively rapid growth, resulting in prominent facial deformity.

Histopathologic Features

Histopathologically, familial gigantiform cementoma shows the same spectrum of changes seen in florid cemento-osseous dysplasia, and the two cannot be distinguished microscopically.

Treatment and Prognosis

Attempts to improve aesthetics by shave-down surgical procedures have not been successful because the dysplastic tissue rapidly regrows. The condition is not life-threatening, but facial asymmetry may continue to present problems.

OSSIFYING FIBROMA (Cementifying Fibroma; Cemento-ossifying Fibroma)

The **ossifying fibroma** is a well-demarcated and occasionally encapsulated neoplasm composed of fibrous tissue that contains varying amounts of calcified tissue resembling bone, cementum, or both. Formerly, many investigators separately classified **cementifying fibromas**, which were considered to be *odontogenic* tumors, from **ossifying fibromas**, which were believed to be tumors of *osteogenic* origin. Today, however, it is agreed that these are one and the same lesion and are best classified as osteogenic neoplasms.

Although some of these tumors contain only cementum-like calcifications and others show only bony material, admixtures of the two types of calcifications are commonly seen in a single lesion. This has led to the widely used designation of **cemento-ossifying fibroma**. Whether or not the amorphous calcifications truly represent cementum is not certain because such structures may be encountered in fibro-osseous skull lesions located some distance from the teeth as well as in lesions of the extragnathic skeleton.

The designations ossifying fibroma, cemento-ossifying fibroma, and cementifying fibroma are all appropriate for this tumor; ossifying fibroma is the personal choice of this author.

Clinical and Radiographic Features

Ossifying fibromas occur over a wide age range, but the greatest number of cases are encountered during the

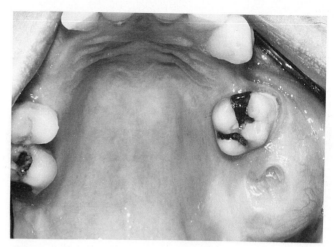

FIGURE 14–54. **Ossifying fibroma.** Expansion of the left posterior maxilla caused by a large ossifying fibroma.

third and fourth decades of life. There is a definite female predilection, with female-to-male ratios as high as 5:1 being reported in some series of cases. The mandible is involved far more often than the maxilla, and some reports indicate 90 percent of all cases are located in the mandible. The mandibular premolar-molar area is the most common site.

Small lesions seldom cause any symptoms and are detected only on radiographic examination. Larger tumors result in a painless swelling of the involved bone (Fig. 14–54); they may cause obvious facial asymmetry, which on occasion reaches grotesque size. Pain and paresthesia are rarely associated with an ossifying fibroma.

Radiographically, the lesion most often is well defined and unilocular (Fig. 14–55). Some examples show a sclerotic border. Depending on the amount of calcified material produced in the tumor, it may appear as completely radiolucent; more often it shows varying degrees of radiopacity (Fig. 14–56). Some lesions may be largely

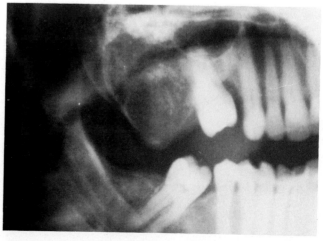

FIGURE 14–55. **Ossifying fibroma.** Radiograph of the same patient shown in Figure 14–54. Note the well-defined unilocular radiolucent lesion containing radiopaque calcifications.

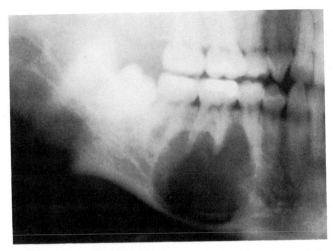

FIGURE 14-56. **Ossifying fibroma.** A large ossifying fibroma of the mandible presenting as a well-demarcated radiolucent lesion.

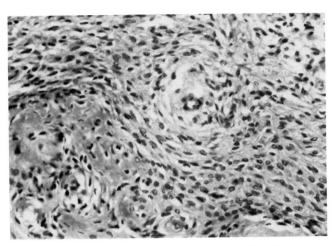

FIGURE 14-58. **Ossifying fibroma.** This cellular fibroblastic tumor shows early osteoid formation that is present in the lower left.

radiopaque with a radiolucent periphery. Root divergence or resorption of roots of teeth associated with the tumor may be noted, but these findings are not common. Large ossifying fibromas of the mandible often demonstrate a characteristic "downward bowing" of the inferior cortex of the mandible.

Histopathologic Features

At surgical exploration, the lesion is well demarcated from the surrounding bone, thus permitting relatively easy separation of the tumor from its bony bed. A few ossifying fibromas will grossly and microscopically show a fibrous capsule surrounding the tumor (Fig. 14-57). Most are not encapsulated but are grossly and microscopically well demarcated from the surrounding bone.

On microscopic study, the tumor is composed of fibrous tissue of varying degrees of cellularity containing calcified material. This may be in the form of trabeculae of osteoid and bone or basophilic ovoid calcifications that resemble cementum-like material. Admixtures of the two types of calcifications are commonly seen (Figs. 14-58 and 14-59).

Treatment and Prognosis

The circumscribed nature of the ossifying fibroma generally permits enucleation of the tumor with relative ease. Some examples, however, which have grown large and destroyed considerable bone, may necessitate surgical resection and bone grafting. The prognosis, however, is very good, and recurrence after removal of the tumor is rarely encountered. There is no evidence that ossifying fibromas ever undergo malignant change.

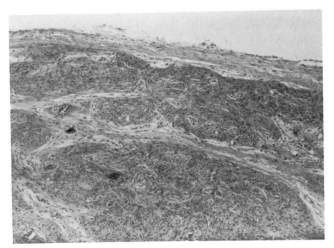

FIGURE 14-57. **Ossifying fibroma.** This low-magnification photomicrograph shows a well-developed fibrous capsule surrounding the tumor.

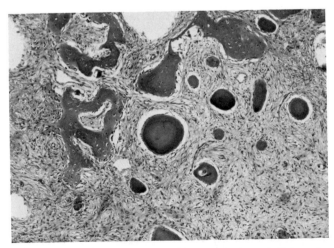

FIGURE 14-59. **Ossifying fibroma.** This tumor shows both bone trabeculae and acellular droplets of cementum-like material in a moderately cellular fibrous stroma.

JUVENILE OSSIFYING FIBROMA
(Juvenile Active Ossifying Fibroma; Juvenile Aggressive Ossifying Fibroma)

The **juvenile ossifying fibroma** is a controversial lesion that has been distinguished from the larger group of ossifying fibromas on the basis of the age of the patients, most common sites of involvement, and clinical behavior. Juvenile ossifying fibromas are uncommon lesions compared with the usual ossifying fibromas previously described. Unfortunately, the histopathologic criteria for differentiating juvenile ossifying fibromas from other ossifying fibromas are neither well defined nor generally accepted. Some have suggested that juvenile ossifying fibromas are basically a type of osteoblastoma occurring in the facial bones.

Clinical and Radiographic Features

Juvenile ossifying fibromas are most commonly seen in patients younger than age 15, although similar lesions may be seen in older patients. The orbital and frontal bones and paranasal sinuses are more common sites than the jaws for these lesions. The maxilla is considerably more commonly involved than the mandible. Some tumors demonstrate rapid growth. Lesions involving the sinuses and orbital bones may cause exophthalmos and proptosis. Nasal obstruction may also develop.

The radiographic features are variable and depend on the tumor's location and the amount of calcified tissue being produced. Varying degrees of lucency and opacity may be present. The juvenile ossifying fibroma tends to be radiographically fairly well demarcated, but it may demonstrate invasion and erosion of the surrounding bone (Fig. 14–60).

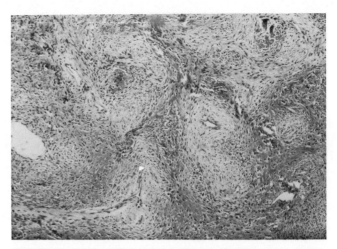

FIGURE 14–61. **Juvenile ossifying fibroma.** Small strands of immature osteoid are present in a cellular fibrous stroma.

Histopathologic Features

The histopathologic features ascribed to the juvenile ossifying fibroma by different investigators are variable. The tumor stroma consists of a cell-rich proliferation of spindle-shaped and polyhedral cells with scant collagen formation. Small strands of immature cellular osteoid form within the lesion. Maturation of the lesion results in the formation of more typical trabeculae of woven bone (Fig. 14–61). Clusters of multinucleated giant cells may also be present. Other investigators believe that the formation of small spherical ossicles surrounded by osteoid rims is the characteristic microscopic feature (Fig. 14–62).

Treatment and Prognosis

The clinical management and prognosis of the juvenile ossifying fibroma are uncertain. Some lesions may re-

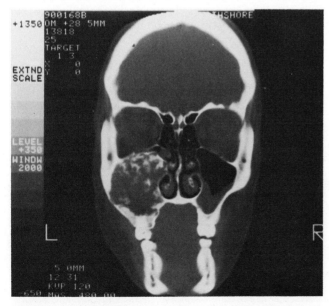

FIGURE 14–60. **Juvenile ossifying fibroma.** Computed tomography scan showing a large tumor involving the left maxilla and maxillary sinus of a 12-year-old girl. Clinically, the tumor was growing rapidly.

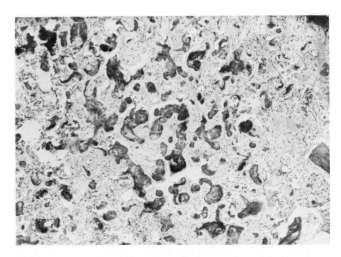

FIGURE 14–62. **Juvenile ossifying fibroma.** Small spherical ossicles are present in a cellular fibroblastic stroma. This pattern is considered by some to be the most characteristic for the juvenile active ossifying fibroma.

main for long periods of time, causing only minimal symptoms. Other lesions, particularly in young children, may demonstrate rapid growth and aggressive local behavior.

For smaller lesions, complete local excision or thorough curettage appears adequate. For some rapidly growing lesions, wider resection may be required.

In contrast to the negligible recurrence rate seen in the common types of ossifying fibromas, recurrence rates of 30 to 58 percent have been reported for juvenile ossifying fibromas.

OSTEOMA

Osteomas are benign tumors composed of mature compact or cancellous bone. Osteomas are essentially restricted to the craniofacial skeleton and are rarely, if ever, diagnosed in other bones. There is some question as to whether osteomas represent true neoplasms, and not all lesions designated as an "osteoma" may represent a single entity. Some likely represent the end stage of an injury or inflammatory process or the end stage of a hamartomatous process, such as fibrous dysplasia. The common palatal and mandibular tori and buccal exostoses (see pp. 17–20) are not considered to represent osteomas, although they are histopathologically identical to osteomas. Because many osteomas are small, asymptomatic lesions, there is little reliable information as to their true frequency.

Clinical and Radiographic Features

Osteomas of the jaws may arise on the surface of the bone, as a polypoid or sessile mass (**periosteal osteoma**), or they may be located in the medullary bone (**endosteal osteoma**). Most jaw osteomas are detected in young adults and are generally asymptomatic, solitary lesions. There is little valid information as to whether there is any gender predilection.

Periosteal osteomas present as slowly growing masses on the surface of the mandible or maxilla. Some types may reach a large size, resulting in facial deformity.

An osteoma involving the mandibular condyle may cause a slowly progressing shift in the patient's occlusion, with deviation of the midline of the chin toward the unaffected side. These condylar lesions are considered by some to represent osteomas; others designate them as hyperostoses.

Small endosteal osteomas are asymptomatic, but large lesions cause a slowly progressive enlargement of the affected area.

Osteomas arising in the paranasal sinuses may cause such symptoms as sinusitis, headache, or ophthalmologic manifestations.

Radiographically, osteomas present as circumscribed sclerotic masses. Periosteal osteomas may show a uniform sclerotic pattern or may demonstrate a sclerotic periphery with a central trabecular pattern (Fig. 14–63). Smaller endosteal osteomas are difficult, if not impossible, to differentiate from foci of sclerotic bone representing the end stage of an inflammatory process (condens-

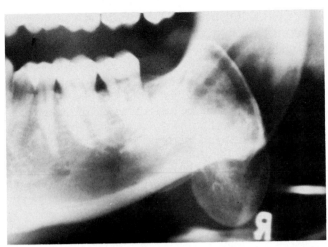

FIGURE 14–63. **Osteoma**. The radiograph shows a pedunculated cancellous osteoma arising from the lingual surface of the mandible near the crest of the alveolar ridge.

ing osteitis, focal chronic sclerosing osteomyelitis) or from nonpathologic foci of sclerotic bone (idiopathic osteosclerosis). Osteomas may also be radiographically confused with complex odontomas.

Histopathologic Features

Compact osteomas are composed of normal-appearing dense bone showing minimal marrow tissue (Fig. 14–64). **Cancellous** osteomas are composed of trabeculae of bone and fibro-fatty marrow. Osteoblastic activity may be fairly prominent.

Treatment and Prognosis

Larger osteomas causing symptoms or cosmetic deformity are treated by conservative surgical excision. Small, asymptomatic osteomas, particularly those located endosteally, probably do not need to be treated but should

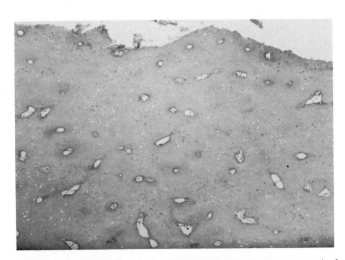

FIGURE 14–64. **Osteoma**. This compact osteoma is composed of dense bone with only minimal marrow elements.

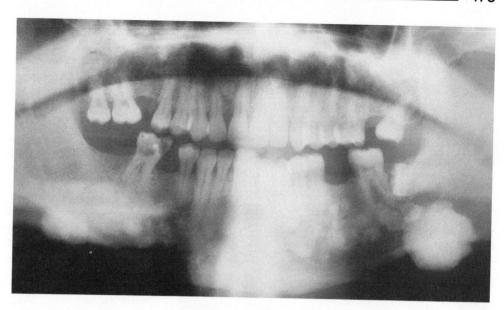

FIGURE 14–65. **Gardner syndrome.** Panoramic radiograph showing multiple osteomas of the mandible.

be observed periodically. The lesion is completely benign, and patients do not experience malignant change or recurrences after excision.

GARDNER SYNDROME

Gardner syndrome is a rare disorder that is inherited as an autosomal dominant trait. It is considered to be part of a spectrum of diseases characterized by familial colorectal polyposis. The chief manifestations of Gardner syndrome include multiple adenomatous polyps of the colon and rectum, multiple osteomas, cutaneous epidermoid cysts, and fibromas. The presence of multiple osteomas of the facial bones is an important early marker for this syndrome. Such patients and other family members should be evaluated for other manifestations.

Clinical and Radiographic Features

Osteomas may occur in any bone as a component of Gardner syndrome, but they are particularly common in the jaws, frontal bones, and frontal and ethmoid sinuses. They often occur in the region of the mandibular angles, where they may cause prominent facial deformity (Fig. 14–65). The osteomas often are noted during puberty and precede the development of, or any symptomatology from, the bowel polyps (Fig. 14–66). Most patients also show one or several epidermoid cysts of the skin (Fig. 14–67).

Radiographically, the jaw osteomas show features similar to the previously described solitary osteomas. Multiple odontomas, supernumerary teeth, and impacted teeth are also seen in patients with Gardner syndrome, but the reported prevalence varies.

Histopathologic Features

Histopathologically, the osteomas generally are of the compact type. An individual lesion cannot be microscopically differentiated from a solitary osteoma.

Treatment and Prognosis

The major problem for patients with Gardner syndrome is the high rate of malignant transformation of bowel polyps into invasive adenocarcinoma. By age 30, about 50 percent of patients with Gardner syndrome will develop colorectal carcinoma. The frequency of malignant change approaches 100 percent in older patients.

Prophylactic colectomy is usually recommended. Removal of jaw osteomas and epidermoid cysts for cosmetic reasons may sometimes be indicated, but the long-term prognosis depends on the behavior of the bowel adenocarcinomas.

OSTEOID OSTEOMA AND OSTEOBLASTOMA

Osteoid osteoma and **osteoblastoma** are closely related benign bone tumors. There is general agreement that the

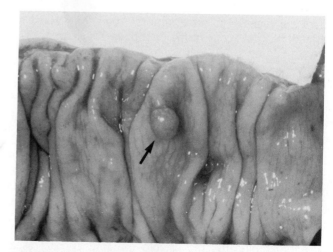

FIGURE 14–66. **Gardner syndrome.** A segment of resected large bowel showing polyp formation (*arrow*).

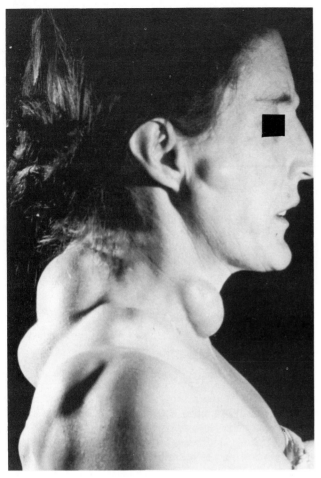

FIGURE 14–67. **Gardner syndrome.** This patient has multiple, large epidermoid cysts. (Courtesy of Dr. William Welton.)

histopathologic features of these two lesions are identical, and they are distinguished from one another only by site of occurrence, size of the lesion, and symptomatology. However, there are many cases with overlapping features, which makes differentiation difficult. Some authors prefer to classify all of these lesions as osteoblastomas. They are uncommon lesions, accounting for less than 1 percent of all bone tumors. About 15 percent of osteoblastomas occur in the craniofacial skeleton.

Clinical and Radiographic Features

Osteoid osteomas and osteoblastomas may occur over a wide age range, but 85 percent of cases occur before age 30. They are twice as common in males as in females.

Osteoid Osteoma

Tumors considered to be typical osteoid osteomas occur most often in the femur, tibia, and phalanges. They are very rare in the jaws. Pain is the most common presenting symptom. It is usually nocturnal in nature and is alleviated by salicylates.

Radiographically, the osteoid osteoma appears as a well-circumscribed radiolucent defect, usually less than 1 cm in diameter, with a surrounding zone of sclerosis of varying thickness. The sclerotic zone is reactive in nature and is not part of the tumor. To be classified as an osteoid osteoma, the radiolucent zone should never be more than 2 cm in diameter. A small radiopaque nidus may be present, resulting in a "target"-like appearance radiographically (Fig. 14–68).

Osteoblastoma

Conventional osteoblastomas are most often located in the vertebral column. Other common sites include the femur, tibia, fibula, and mandible, but virtually any bone may be affected. Jaw osteoblastomas are twice as common in the mandible as the maxilla. Osteoblastomas are larger than osteoid osteomas and are not less than 2 cm in diameter. Most examples are between 2 and 4 cm, but they may be as large as 10 cm. Pain is also a common presenting feature, but it is less often nocturnal in character. In contrast to the typical osteoid osteoma, the osteoblastoma is not as well relieved by aspirin.

Radiographically, the osteoblastoma may appear as a well-defined or ill-defined radiolucent lesion. Reactive sclerosis surrounding the lesion is not a constant feature. Some lesions show a patchy area of calcification within the radiolucent area, and some may demonstrate considerable calcification (Figs. 14–69 and 14–70).

Histopathologic Features

Although some pathologists claim subtle microscopic differences between osteoid osteoma and osteoblastoma, most consider that the pathologic changes are identical in the two lesions. These consist of anastomosing osteoid trabeculae in a cellular fibrovascular stroma. The osteoid trabeculae, which often appear basophilic, are surrounded by prominent osteoblasts. Osteoclasts are usually present and may be numerous. Varying degrees of mineralization of the osteoid trabeculae are present. Some examples may show prominent cement lines in the mineralized component. The rich cellularity of the lesion

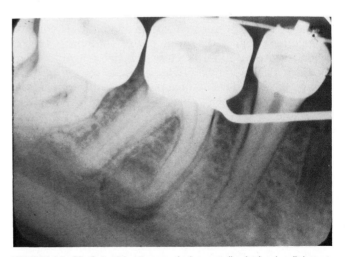

FIGURE 14–68. **Osteoid osteoma.** A circumscribed mixed radiolucent-radiopaque lesion near the apex of mesial root of mandibular first molar. The patient had dull, nocturnal pain that was relieved by aspirin. (Courtesy of Dr. Ellen Eisenberg.)

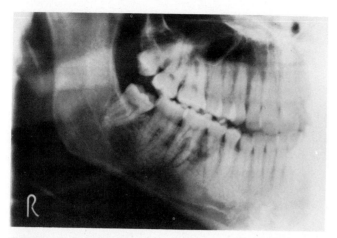

FIGURE 14–69. **Osteoblastoma.** Panoramic radiograph showing an ill-defined radiolucent-radiopaque lesion in the molar-premolar area of a 29-year-old woman. (Courtesy of Dr. John Kalmar.)

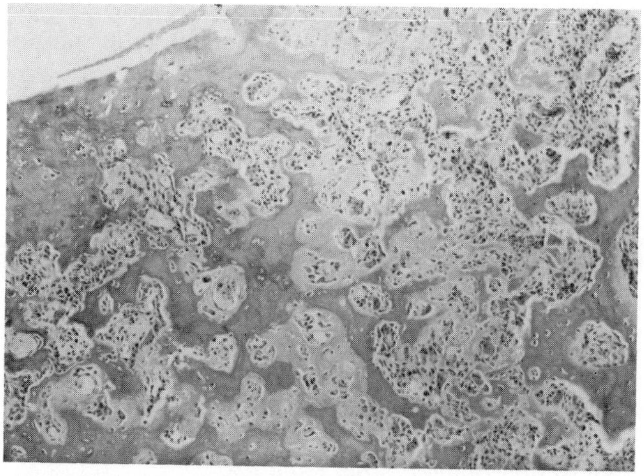

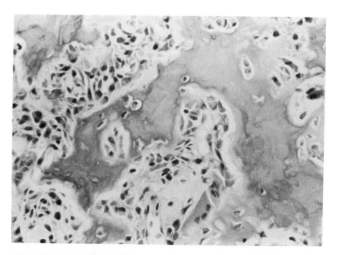

FIGURE 14–71. **Osteoblastoma.** Anastomosing osteoid trabeculae are surrounded by prominent osteoblasts.

may lead to an erroneous diagnosis of osteosarcoma (Figs. 14–71 and 14–72).

Differentiation between some osteoblastomas and low-grade osteosarcomas may be very difficult. Some low-grade osteosarcomas may closely resemble the microscopic appearance of osteoblastomas, and some lesions may have microscopic features intermediate between osteoblastoma and osteosarcoma.

Treatment and Prognosis

Most cases of osteoid osteoma and osteoblastoma are treated by local excision or curettage. The prognosis is good, and some lesions will regress even after incomplete excision. A small number of lesions will recur, and in

rare instances an osteoblastoma may undergo transformation into an osteosarcoma.

Aggressive Osteoblastomas

A small group of osteoblastomas ("**aggressive**" **osteoblastomas**) are characterized by more atypical histopathologic features and locally aggressive behavior. These tumors occur more often in older patients, most being over 30 years of age. A variety of bones, including the mandible, may be involved. Pain is a common symptom and may be severe.

Radiographically, these lesions show the features of conventional osteoblastomas but tend to be larger.

Microscopically, aggressive osteoblastomas are characterized by the presence of large (epithelioid) osteoblasts with increased mitotic activity, and non-trabecular sheets or lace-like areas of osteoid production.

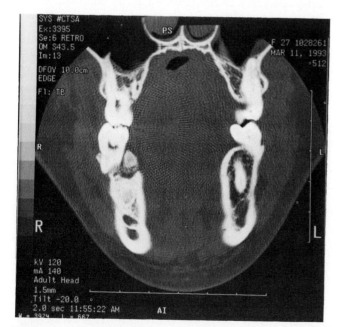

FIGURE 14–70. **Osteoblastoma.** Computed tomography scan of the same patient shown in Figure 14–69. Note the destruction of the lingual cortex in the right molar area. (Courtesy of Dr. John Kalmar.)

FIGURE 14–72. **Osteoblastoma.** Higher magnification of Figure 14–71 showing prominent osteoblastic rimming around mineralized osteoid trabeculae.

Although about 50 percent of these aggressive osteoblastomas will recur, metastasis or death from the tumor has not been reported.

CEMENTOBLASTOMA (TRUE CEMENTOMA)

Although most oral and maxillofacial pathologists consider the **cementoblastoma** to be a benign odontogenic tumor, its close relationship to osteoblastoma warrants its inclusion in this chapter. A number of noted authorities in orthopedic pathology consider cementoblastoma and osteoblastoma to be identical lesions and prefer to designate them as osteoblastomas.

Clinical and Radiographic Features

Most cementoblastomas occur in the mandibular molar region. They occur predominantly in patients under age 25. There does not appear to be any significant gender predilection. Cementoblastomas are slowly growing lesions and may eventually cause localized expansion of the affected area. Pain may or may not be associated with the lesion.

The radiographic findings are distinctive and essentially diagnostic. These show a calcified mass that is intimately associated with the root or roots of a tooth. Most reported cases have been associated with the mandibular permanent first molar tooth (Figs. 14–73 and 14–74). Rarely, a deciduous tooth has been involved. The outline of the root or roots of the involved tooth is usually obscured as a result of root resorption and fusion of the tumor with the tooth. The calcified mass is usually surrounded by a radiolucent rim of uniform width.

Histopathologic Features

The bulk of the cementoblastoma is composed of sheets or thick trabeculae of mineralized material with

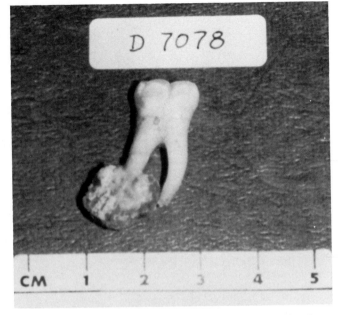

FIGURE 14–74. **Cementoblastoma.** Surgical specimen showing a mass attached to a mandibular molar root. (Courtesy of Dr. John Wright.)

irregularly placed lacunae and prominent basophilic reversal lines. Cellular fibrovascular tissue is present between the mineralized trabeculae. Multinucleated giant cells are often present, and the mineralized trabeculae are often lined by prominent blast-like cells (Fig. 14–75). The periphery of the lesion, corresponding to the radiolucent zone seen on the radiograph, is composed of uncalcified matrix, which is often arranged in radiating columns (Fig. 14–76). Unless the clinical and radiographic features are appreciated, a small peripheral biopsy specimen of the mass might be confused with a low-grade osteoblastic osteosarcoma.

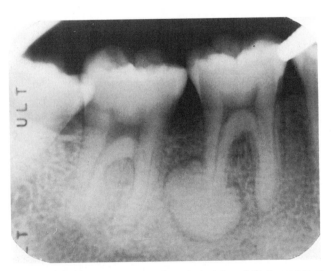

FIGURE 14–73. **Cementoblastoma.** A densely calcified mass is attached to the distal root of the first molar. The root is partially resorbed. (Courtesy of Dr. John Wright.)

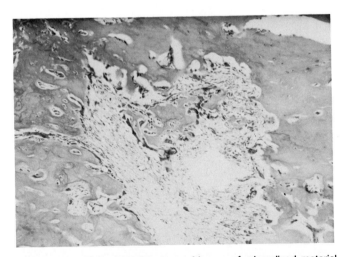

FIGURE 14–75. **Cementoblastoma.** Masses of mineralized material showing prominent reversal lines. Blast cells are present at the margins of the mineralized material. The soft tissue component is composed of loose vascular fibrous tissue. This microscopic field cannot be distinguished from that seen in an osteoblastoma.

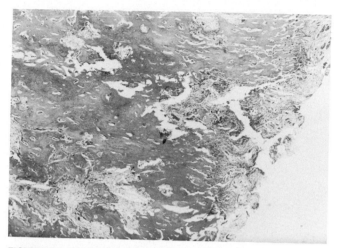

FIGURE 14–76. **Cementoblastoma.** Poorly mineralized tissue at the periphery of a cementoblastoma is arranged in radiating parallel columns.

The major differential diagnostic problem relates to differentiation of cementoblastoma from osteoblastoma. The histopathologic features of the two may be quite similar in some microscopic fields, and in some instances it might be argued that the lesion in question was an osteoblastoma that had grown to envelop the roots of a tooth rather than a neoplasm originating from cementoblasts on a root surface. Cementoblastomas and osteoblastomas should be considered closely related lesions.

Treatment and Prognosis

Treatment of a cementoblastoma usually consists of surgical extraction of the tooth together with the attached calcified mass. Surgical excision of the mass with root amputation and endodontic treatment of the involved tooth may be considered.

The prognosis is excellent, and recurrence of the tumor after its total removal does not occur. Progressive growth of the tumor after extraction of the involved tooth and incomplete removal of the mass has been documented.

CHONDROMA

Chondromas are benign tumors composed of mature hyaline cartilage. They are one of the more common bone tumors and are most often located in the short tubular bones of the hands and feet. Chondromas have rarely been reported in the jaws. Most examples have been found in the anterior maxilla of adult patients.

Histopathologic Features

The microscopic distinction between a benign chondroma and a low-grade chondrosarcoma is very difficult (see p. 485 for a discussion of chondromatous neoplasms of the jaws). Many experienced pathologists believe that a diagnosis of chondroma for a jaw tumor should be regarded with considerable suspicion because most of these lesions eventually prove to be chondrosarcomas.

Treatment and Prognosis

It is wise to consider any lesion diagnosed as chondroma of the jaws to represent a potential chondrosarcoma. Treatment is directed toward total surgical removal of the tumor.

CHONDROMYXOID FIBROMA

The **chondromyxoid fibroma** is an uncommon benign neoplasm accounting for less than 1 percent of all primary bone tumors. It is most commonly located in the metaphyseal region of the long bones. Chondromyxoid fibromas rarely involve the jaws.

Clinical and Radiographic Features

Chondromyxoid fibromas of the jaws have been encountered in patients ranging in age from 10 to 67 years. Most often, patients under age 25 are affected. There is no gender predilection. Of the 16 reported cases in the jaws, 14 have involved the mandible. Initial symptoms commonly include pain or expansion of the involved area. Some cases have been asymptomatic, being detected only on a radiographic examination.

Radiographically, the lesion presents as a circumscribed radiolucent defect with sclerotic or scalloped margins. Calcifications are sometimes present within the lesion.

Histopathologic Features

The tumor consists of lobulated areas of spindle-shaped or stellate cells and abundant myxoid or chondroid intercellular substance. The lobules are characteristically separated by zones of a more cellular tissue composed of spindle-shaped or round cells with varying numbers of multinucleated cells (Fig. 14–77).

Large, pleomorphic cells that may cause confusion with chondrosarcoma may be seen. Focal areas of calcification and spicules of residual bone may also be present within the tumor.

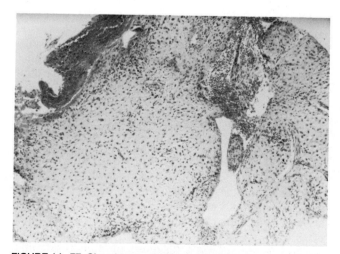

FIGURE 14–77. **Chondromyxoid fibroma.** Lobulated masses of immature cartilage and stellate myxoid cells.

Treatment and Prognosis

Although the chondromyxoid fibroma is a benign tumor, approximately 25 percent of cases in the long bones recur after curettage. Some orthopedic surgeons recommend block excision as the initial treatment. Chondromyxoid fibromas of the jaws have generally been treated by curettage, and recurrence has been reported in only one case.

Differential diagnosis between a chondromyxoid fibroma and chondrosarcoma may be difficult. Examples of both underdiagnosis and overdiagnosis, with resultant improper treatment, have been noted.

SYNOVIAL CHONDROMATOSIS
(Chondrometaplasia)

Synovial chondromatosis is a rare, benign, non-neoplastic arthropathy characterized by the metaplastic development of cartilaginous nodules within the synovial membrane. The cause is unknown. The disease most commonly affects large joints, such as the knee, elbow, hip, and shoulder. About 50 cases involving the temporomandibular joint have been reported. The disease is usually limited to one joint.

Clinical and Radiographic Features

Synovial chondromatosis of the temporomandibular joint is usually diagnosed in middle-aged patients with an average age of 47 years. In contrast to the findings in other joints, there is a predilection for females. Periarticular swelling, pain, crepitus, and limitation of joint motion are usually present. These features are common to a number of pathoses involving the temporomandibular joint and are not diagnostic for synovial chondromatosis. In rare instances, the disease may produce no symptoms.

Radiographically, the most common feature is the presence of loose bodies in the joint. These consist of rounded, irregularly shaped, and variably sized radiopaque structures in the region of the joint. Other features include irregularity of the joint space, widened joint space, and irregularity of the condylar head.

These findings, however, are not diagnostic of synovial chondromatosis and may be seen in other degenerative joint diseases. The absence of loose bodies does not preclude a diagnosis of synovial chondromatosis. Computed tomography (CT) scans and magnetic resonance imaging (MRI) have been advocated as more specific diagnostic imaging procedures.

Histopathologic Features

Nodules of cartilage are present within the synovium and lie loose in the joint space. As many as 100 nodules may be present. These cartilaginous nodules often become calcified and may ossify. The cartilage may appear atypical with hyperchromatic and binucleated chondrocytes (Fig. 14–78). In another clinical situation, these features would suggest a diagnosis of chondrosarcoma, but these changes are not considered significant in synovial chondromatosis.

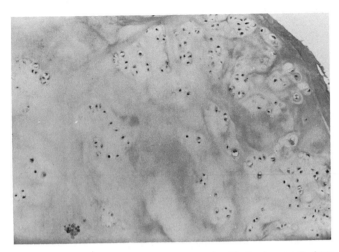

FIGURE 14–78. **Synovial chondromatosis.** Photomicrograph from one of many nodules removed at the time of synovectomy. The cartilage shows some degree of atypia, and in a different clinical setting this histopathology could be interpreted to represent a low-grade chondrosarcoma.

Treatment and Prognosis

For patients with synovial chondromatosis, the involved synovium and all loose bodies are surgically removed. Some surgeons advocate total synovectomy to prevent recurrence. Meniscectomy may be necessary if the disc cannot be repaired. A few cases of erosion of the glenoid fossa and cranial extension of the process have been reported.

The prognosis is good, with a low frequency of recurrence after surgical excision. Malignant transformation of synovial chondromatosis of the temporomandibular joint has not been noted. Most patients experience improved joint function and pain relief after surgery.

HEMANGIOMA OF BONE

Central **hemangiomas** are uncommon intrabony lesions that are composed of capillary, cavernous, or venous blood vessels. Some of them appear to represent tumor-like malformations (*hamartomas*), some appear to be traumatic in origin, and others are regarded as true neoplasms. The skull, vertebrae, and jaws are the most common sites.

Clinical and Radiographic Features

Hemangiomas of the jaws are most often noted in patients between 10 and 20 years of age. They are considerably more common in females than males and occur twice as often in the mandible as the maxilla. The lesion may be totally asymptomatic, but most examples are associated with pain and swelling. Mobility of teeth or bleeding from the gingival sulcus may occur. A bruit or pulsation may be apparent on auscultation and palpation.

The radiographic appearance is variable. Most commonly, the lesion shows a multilocular radiolucent defect. The individual lobules may be small (honeycomb

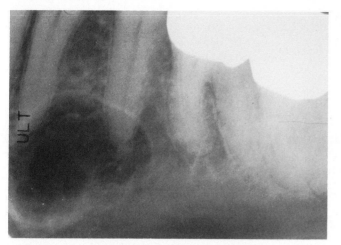

FIGURE 14–79. **Hemangioma.** Mandibular hemangioma presenting as a circumscribed radiolucency containing fine trabeculations.

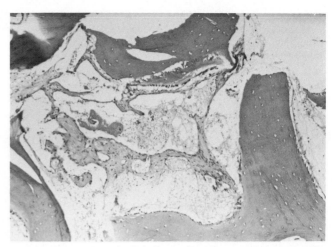

FIGURE 14–81. **Hemangioma.** Biopsy specimen from the same patient shown in Figure 14–80. Multiple vascular spaces lined by endothelial cells occupy the marrow spaces between the bone trabeculae.

appearance) or large (soap bubble appearance). In other cases, the hemangioma may present as an ill-defined radiolucent area or a well-defined, cyst-like radiolucency (Fig. 14–79). Resorption of the roots of teeth involved in the lesion is common. Large lesions may cause cortical expansion, and occasionally a "sunburst" radiographic pattern is produced (Fig. 14–80).

Histopathologic Features

Hemangiomas are composed of a fibrous connective tissue stroma supporting numerous vascular channels lined with a single layer of endothelial cells (Fig. 14–81). The lesion may be of the cavernous type, showing larger vascular spaces, or of the capillary type. An admixture of the two types is frequently encountered.

Treatment and Prognosis

Hemangiomas of the jaws are potentially dangerous lesions because of the risk of severe bleeding, which may occur spontaneously or during surgical manipulation.

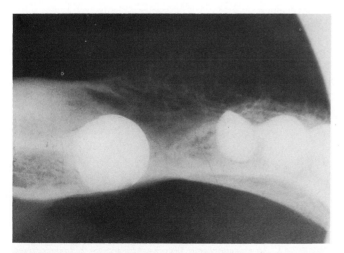

FIGURE 14–80. **Hemangioma.** Occlusal radiograph demonstrating cortical destruction and a "sunburst" periosteal reaction resembling osteosarcoma.

Needle aspiration of any undiagnosed intrabony lesion prior to biopsy is a wise precaution to rule out the possibility of a hemangioma. Severe and even fatal hemorrhages have occurred after incisional biopsy or extraction of teeth involved in a hemangioma.

Hemangiomas of the jaws may be successfully treated with a variety of methods. The selection of therapy is influenced by the size and location of the lesion and by the blood supply to the tumor, as determined by angiographic study. Effective control or total elimination of hemangiomas of the jaws has been obtained by surgical resection or curettage, cryotherapy, radiation, or injections of sclerosing solutions. Presurgical embolization can effectively reduce bleeding during surgery.

If complications due to hemorrhage are avoided, the prognosis is good.

Arteriovenous Aneurysm of Bone

Some authorities regard the **arteriovenous aneurysm of bone** as a distinct entity; others include it under the general heading of "intrabony hemangioma." Arteriovenous aneurysms represent direct communication between an artery and vein, with the blood flow bypassing the capillary circulation. Arteriovenous aneurysms may be congenital in nature or acquired as a result of trauma, usually a fracture. Lesions considered by some to represent arteriovenous aneurysms of the mandible have presented with progressive swelling, pulsation, and often discoloration of the facial skin overlying the mandible.

Radiographs may reveal irregular lytic destruction of the bone (Figs. 14–82 and 14–83). Histopathologically, the lesion consists of multiple large communicating arterial and venous vessels. Most reported cases have been treated with surgical resection.

Other Vascular Tumors Involving Bone

Vascular tumors generally considered to be of low-grade or high-grade malignancy also may involve the

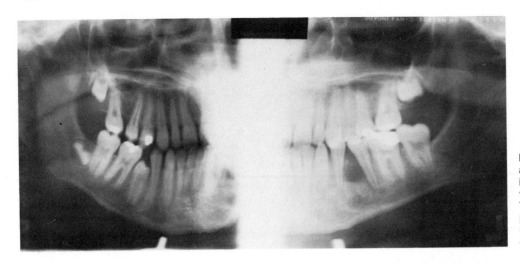

FIGURE 14–82. **Arteriovenous aneurysm.** Panoramic film showing a radiolucent lesion between the left mandibular premolar roots. This was believed to be a lateral periodontal cyst, but pulsation was noted on palpation of the area. (Courtesy of Dr. H. W. Allsup.)

skeleton. The jaws are rarely the site for tumors of this type, but examples have been reported. The terminology for these lesions is controversial and confusing. Terms such as **angiosarcoma, hemangioendothelioma, malignant hemangioendothelioma, epithelioid hemangioendothelioma,** and **histiocytoid hemangioma** have been used to designate members of this group. These tumors show a marked tendency for multicentric skeletal involvement. Some types are highly malignant; others, although locally aggressive, are essentially benign.

DESMOPLASTIC FIBROMA

The **desmoplastic fibroma** of bone is a rare tumor that appears to be the osseous counterpart of soft tissue fibromatosis (desmoid tumor; see p. 369). Although the metaphyseal regions of the humerus and tibia are the sites of slightly more than 50 percent of all cases, the mandible is the fourth most commonly affected bone.

Clinical and Radiographic Features

Most examples of desmoplastic fibroma of bone are discovered in patients younger than 30 years of age. There is no sex predilection. Of the reported cases involving the jaws, 90 percent have occurred in the mandible, most often in the molar–angle–ascending ramus area. The mean age for patients with jaw desmoplastic fibromas is 15.7 years.

A painless swelling of the affected area is the most common initial complaint.

Radiographically, the lesion presents as a unilocular or occasionally multilocular radiolucent area. The margins may be well defined or ill defined (Fig. 14–84). The bone is expanded, and the cortex is thinned; however, cortical reaction is not present. If the lesion erodes through the cortex, an accompanying soft tissue mass will be present. When this occurs, it may be difficult to determine whether the lesion is a desmoplastic fibroma of bone with soft tissue extension or a soft tissue fibromatosis with secondary extension into bone. The roots of teeth involved in the lesion often show resorption.

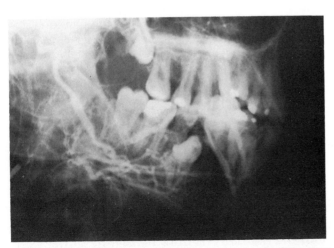

FIGURE 14–83. **Arteriovenous aneurysm.** Lateral jaw film of the same patient (shown in Figure 14–82) after angiography. The radiopaque dye fills the radiolucent defect that was noted on the conventional film.

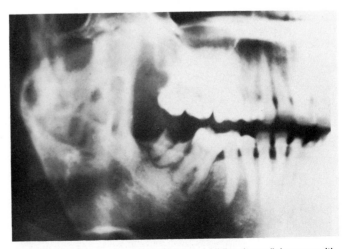

FIGURE 14–84. **Desmoplastic fibroma.** Multilocular radiolucency with poorly defined margins in the ascending ramus of a middle-aged woman.

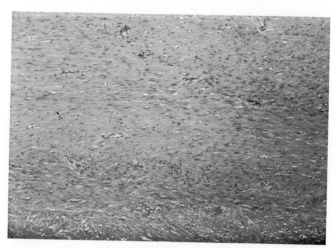

FIGURE 14–85. **Desmoplastic fibroma.** The tumor is composed of bundles of uniform spindle-shaped fibroblasts with abundant collagen.

Histopathologic Findings

The tumor is composed of small elongated fibroblasts and abundant collagen fibers (Fig. 14–85). The degree of cellularity may vary from area to area in a given lesion, and the cellular areas may show plumper fibroblasts and less collagen. The fibroblasts are not atypical, however, and mitoses are essentially absent. Bone spicules may be present at the interface between the tumor and adjacent bone but are never an integral part of the lesion.

Treatment and Prognosis

Although the desmoplastic fibroma is considered to be a benign tumor, it often behaves in a locally aggressive fashion, with extensive bone destruction and soft tissue extension, so that radical surgery may be required to control the disease. Initial curettage appears to be the most common treatment for desmoplastic fibromas of the jaws. Tumor recurrence, however, develops in about 30 percent of cases. Large lesions with soft tissue extension or recurrent lesions may need to be resected. Although metastases do not occur and the long-term prognosis is good, the lesion may be associated with considerable morbidity.

It may be very difficult to distinguish desmoplastic fibroma of bone from well-differentiated fibrosarcoma. Some authorities suggest that all desmoplastic fibromas of bone be considered potentially malignant.

FIBROSARCOMA OF BONE

Fibrosarcoma of bone is a malignant fibroblastic tumor that shows varying degrees of collagen production without formation of tumor bone, osteoid, or cartilage in the primary tumor or any metastatic site. Fibrosarcomas of bone may arise in the medullary portion of a bone or in a periosteal location. The tumor may arise as a "primary" lesion or "secondary" to a variety of benign bone lesions or after irradiation of a bone.

Fibrosarcoma of bone is one of the least common types of primary bone sarcomas. In recent years, the criteria for diagnosis of fibrosarcoma of both soft tissue and bone have been considerably refined and the diagnosis of fibrosarcoma is less commonly made today than in the past. Many tumors formerly classified as fibrosarcoma are now considered to be malignant fibrous histiocytoma or some other type of neoplasm.

Clinical and Radiographic Features

Fibrosarcomas of bone may be encountered in patients over a wide age range. The average age is 40 years. There is no gender predilection. The tumor most commonly occurs in the long tubular bones, particularly the femur and humerus. About 15 percent of cases occur in the craniofacial bones, and the mandible is the predominant site. Fibrosarcomas arising in the medullary portion of a bone are about twice as common as those arising in the periosteal region. Pain, swelling, paresthesia, and loosening of teeth are often associated with fibrosarcomas of the jaws.

Radiographically, fibrosarcomas of bone present as lytic, destructive lesions. In patients with relatively slow-growing tumors, the radiolucent area may be fairly well defined, suggesting a benign process. Films of more rapidly growing tumors show a radiolucent lesion with ill-defined margins (Fig. 14–86).

Histopathologic Features

Fibrosarcomas of bone show the same histopathologic features as fibrosarcomas of soft tissue (see p. 401). Low-grade tumors are characterized by abundant intercellular collagen with a herringbone pattern. The tumor cells are relatively uniform, and mitoses are not prominent (Fig. 14–87). High-grade tumors show cellular pleomorphism, increased mitotic activity, loss of the herringbone pattern, and less collagen formation.

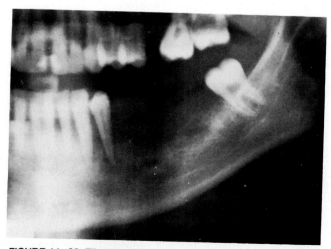

FIGURE 14–86. **Fibrosarcoma.** The panoramic film shows an irregular lytic destructive lesion associated with a soft tissue density on the superior aspect of the edentulous alveolar ridge.

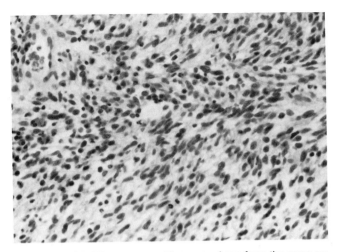

FIGURE 14–87. **Fibrosarcoma.** Biopsy specimen from the same patient shown in Figure 14–86. Note the interlacing bundles of hyperchromatic spindle-shaped cells. Mitoses are not prominent, and little collagen is being formed.

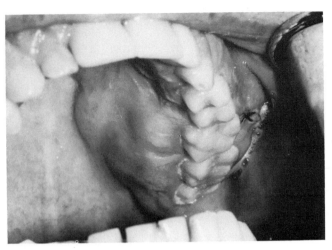

FIGURE 14–88. **Osteosarcoma.** This patient shows a firm, painful swelling of the left maxilla of recent onset.

Treatment and Prognosis

Fibrosarcoma of bone is treated with radical resection. The efficacy of chemotherapy is not well established. The prognosis for tumors originating in the medullary portion of the bone is poorer than for those arising in a periosteal position. There are few valid data on patient survival from fibrosarcomas of the jaws. The overall reported survival rate for fibrosarcoma of bone varies from 40 to 50 percent in various studies.

OSTEOSARCOMA (Osteogenic Sarcoma)

Osteosarcoma is the most common type of primary malignant tumor of bone. The distal femur and proximal tibia are the most frequent sites for this tumor, although about 7 percent of all osteosarcomas occur in the jaws.

Clinical and Radiographic Features

Osteosarcomas of the jaws have been diagnosed in patients ranging from young children to the elderly, and they most often occur in the third and fourth decades of life. The mean age for patients with osteosarcoma of the jaw is about 33 years, which is 10 to 15 years older than the mean age for osteosarcomas of the long bones. Osteosarcomas of the jaws are somewhat more common in males than in females. The maxilla and mandible are involved with about equal frequency.

Swelling and pain are the most common symptoms (Fig. 14–88). Loosening of teeth, paresthesia, and nasal obstruction (in the case of maxillary tumors) may also be noted. Some patients report symptoms for relatively long periods prior to diagnosis, which indicates that some osteosarcomas of the jaws grow rather slowly. In one study of 66 patients, the average duration of signs and symptoms prior to diagnosis was 3.9 months, with a range of 1 to 240 months.

The radiographic findings vary from dense sclerosis, to a mixed sclerotic and radiolucent lesion, to an entirely radiolucent process (Fig. 14–89). The peripheral border of the lesion is usually ill defined and indistinct, making it difficult to determine the extent of the tumor radiographically. In some cases, an extensive osteosarcoma may show only minimal and subtle radiographic change with only slight variation in the trabecular pattern. There is often resorption of the roots of teeth involved by the tumor. This feature is often described as "spiking" resorption as a result of the tapered narrowing of the root. The "classic" sunburst or sun-ray appearance caused by osteophytic bone production on the surface of the lesion is noted in about 25 percent of jaw osteosarcomas. This is often best appreciated on an occlusal projection (Fig. 14–90).

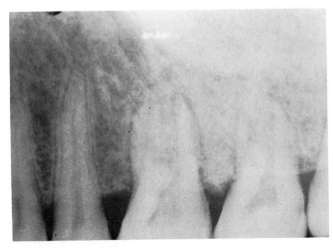

FIGURE 14–89. **Osteosarcoma.** Periapical radiograph from the same patient shown in Figure 14–88. Note the irregular, dense sclerotic change in the bone pattern.

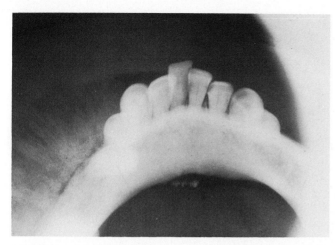

FIGURE 14-90. **Osteosarcoma.** Occlusal radiograph demonstrating prominent exophytic tumor bone production on the buccal surface of the mandible, resulting in the "sunburst" pattern. (Courtesy of Dr. Lewis Gilbert.)

An important early radiographic change in patients with osteosarcoma consists of a symmetric widening of the periodontal ligament space around a tooth or several teeth. This is the result of tumor infiltration along the periodontal ligament space (Figs. 14-91*A*, *B*). Widening

of the periodontal ligament space is not specific for osteosarcoma and may be seen associated with other malignancies. This radiographic finding, when accompanied by pain or discomfort and other minimal radiographic changes, may be of great importance in the early diagnosis of jaw osteosarcomas.

Histopathologic Features

Osteosarcomas of the jaws display considerable histopathologic variability. The essential microscopic criterion is the direct production of osteoid by malignant mesenchymal cells (Figs. 14-92*A*, *B*). In addition to osteoid, the cells of the tumor may produce chondroid material and fibrous connective tissue. The tumor cells may vary from relatively uniform round or spindle-shaped cells to highly pleomorphic cells with bizarre nuclear and cytoplasmic shapes. The amount of matrix material produced in the tumor may vary considerably. In some instances, osteoid production may be very minimal and difficult to demonstrate (Fig. 14-93). Most osteosarcomas of the jaws tend to be better differentiated than osteosarcomas of the extragnathic skeleton.

Depending on the relative amounts of osteoid, cartilage, or collagen fibers produced by the tumor, many

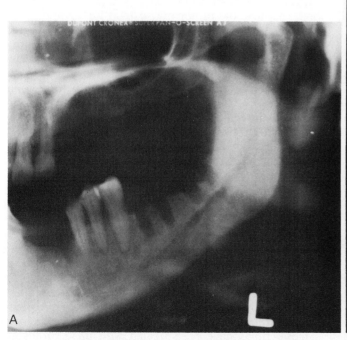

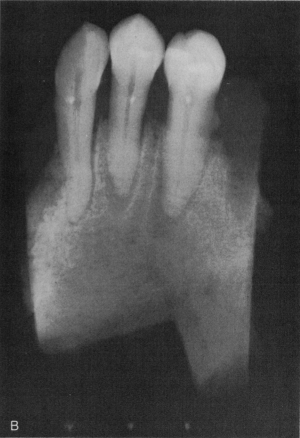

FIGURE 14-91. **Osteosarcoma.** *A,* Lateral jaw radiograph of a 50-year-old woman. A large osteosarcoma of the left mandible extends from the incisor region to the condyle. Two molar teeth had been recently extracted, and the patient had been treated for presumed osteomyelitis for a month. Periodontal ligament widening is noted in the apical area of the premolar teeth. *B,* Radiograph of a portion of the resection specimen from the same patient. Widening of the periodontal ligament space is well demonstrated. Microscopically, this was due to infiltration of osteosarcoma into the periodontal ligament space.

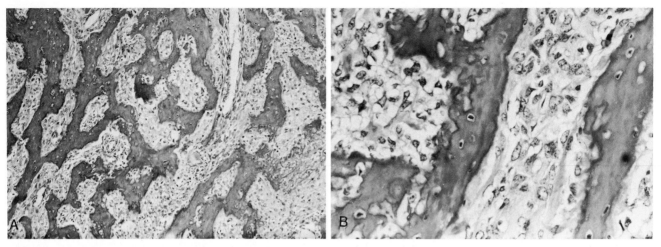

FIGURE 14-92. Osteosarcoma. *A*, Trabeculae of osteoid and bone are being produced by the malignant cells. *B*, Higher magnification shows cellular details.

pathologists subclassify osteosarcomas into the following types:

- Osteoblastic
- Chondroblastic
- Fibroblastic

These histopathologic subtypes, however, do not have any great bearing on the prognosis.

Chondroblastic osteosarcomas constitute a substantial proportion of all osteosarcomas of the jaws. Some examples may be composed almost entirely of malignant cartilage growing in lobules with only small foci of direct osteoid production by tumor cells being identified. Such lesions, however, should be classified as osteosarcomas rather than chondrosarcomas.

Low-grade, well-differentiated osteosarcomas may show only minimal cellular atypia of the stromal cells and abundant bone formation. On microscopic examina-

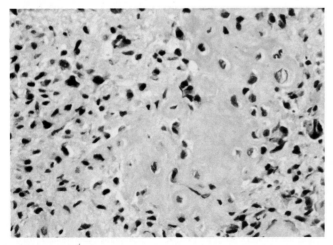

FIGURE 14-93. Osteosarcoma. Malignant mesenchymal cells with a focus of osteoid production. Only small amounts of osteoid were present in this tumor.

tion, these lesions may be difficult to differentiate from benign bone lesions, such as fibrous dysplasia or ossifying fibroma.

A rare form of osteosarcoma has been designated as **small cell osteosarcoma**. The tumor cells resemble those of Ewing's sarcoma, but the small round cells produce osteoid. This type of osteosarcoma is most common in young patients. Examples have occurred in the jaws.

Treatment and Prognosis

Radical surgical excision has been the most common treatment for osteosarcoma of the jaws. This may be supplemented with chemotherapy, radiation therapy, or both. Because the tumor may extend for some distance beyond the apparent clinical and radiologic margins, local recurrence after surgery is a major problem. In one reported series of 66 patients, there was a local recurrence rate of 70 percent that was attributed to inadequate initial surgery. Local uncontrolled disease is more often the cause of death for patients with jaw osteosarcoma than are the effects of distant metastases. Most deaths from uncontrolled local disease occur within 2 years of the initial treatment.

Jaw osteosarcomas have a lesser tendency to metastasize than do osteosarcomas of long bones. Although regional lymph nodes may be involved, metastases most often involve the lungs and brain. The prevalence of metastases reported from jaw osteosarcomas ranges from 6 to 50 percent in different series. Some major cancer centers advocate preoperative chemotherapy for osteosarcoma. This is followed by radical surgical excision with careful pathologic examination of the specimen to evaluate chemotherapy effects on the tumor. Depending on the results, further chemotherapy or radiation may then be employed. Limited numbers of patients with jaw osteosarcomas have been treated with these protocols, and superior results have been claimed compared with surgical treatment alone.

The prognosis, however, remains serious. Various studies indicate a 30 to 50 percent survival rate. Survival rates of up to 80 percent have been reported for patients receiving initial radical surgery.

Peripheral (Juxtacortical) Osteosarcoma

In contrast to the usual forms of osteosarcoma, which arise in the medullary portion of the bone, several varieties originate on the surface of the bone and initially grow outward from the bone surface. The terminology used for these lesions by different authors is somewhat confusing. These **peripheral (juxtacortical) osteosarcomas** usually occur in the long bones, but a few examples involving the jaws have been reported.

The **parosteal** type of osteosarcoma is characterized by a high degree of structural differentiation, and the bland histopathologic appearance may lead to a benign diagnosis. This lesion, however, tends to recur with less than *en bloc* or radical surgery and may eventually develop into a higher-grade osteosarcoma.

The **periosteal** form of osteosarcoma is a histopathologically higher grade of tumor with a prominent cartilaginous component.

Peripheral osteosarcomas are associated with a considerably better prognosis than the conventional intramedullary tumors. Because few cases of juxtacortical osteosarcomas have been reported in the jaws, there is little valid information as to the biologic behavior of this lesion. In all likelihood, however, the prognosis is as good as for the juxtacortical lesions of long bones.

Post-irradiation Bone Sarcoma

Sarcoma arising in a bone that has been previously subjected to radiation therapy is a well-recognized phenomenon. The jaws are closely situated to tissues that commonly receive therapeutic radiation and are a common site for post-irradiation bone sarcomas. Post-irradiation sarcomas may develop as early as 3 years after radiation, but the average latent period is about 14 years. The frequency of development of sarcoma is related to radiation dosage. Post-irradiation sarcoma develops in about 0.2 percent of patients receiving 7000 rad (cGy); there is no increased prevalence of sarcoma for those receiving less than 1000 rad.

Osteosarcoma is the most common type of post-irradiation sarcoma, accounting for 50 percent of all cases. About 40 percent of post-irradiation sarcomas are **fibrosarcomas,** with **chondrosarcomas** and other histologic types making up the rest. Post-irradiation bone sarcomas have no distinctive histopathologic features that allow them to be distinguished from other bone sarcomas of the same type that arise *de novo.*

The prognosis for post-irradiation sarcomas is about the same as for *de novo* tumors of the same type.

CHONDROSARCOMA

Chondrosarcoma is a malignant tumor characterized by the formation of cartilage, but not bone, by the tumor cells. Chondrosarcomas compose about 10 percent of all primary tumors of the skeleton but are considered by most authorities to involve the jaws only rarely; probably less than 1 percent of all chondrosarcomas arise in the head and neck area. Some institutions report a somewhat greater frequency of chondrosarcomas in the jaws. This is probably due to differing criteria used by the pathologists for distinguishing chondrogenic osteosarcomas from chondrosarcomas.

Clinical and Radiographic Findings

Chondrosarcomas of the jaws occur in patients over a wide age range. The average age is 33 years. The tumor is slightly more prevalent in males than in females. A painless mass or swelling is the most common presenting sign. This may be associated with separation or loosening of teeth. Pain is less often associated with chondrosarcomas than with osteosarcomas and is reported in less than 50 percent of patients with chondrosarcomas of the jaws. The maxilla and mandible are involved with about equal frequency. The tumor is encountered in all areas of the jaws. Maxillary tumors may cause nasal obstruction or epistaxis.

Radiologically, the tumor usually shows features suggestive of a malignancy, consisting of a radiolucent process with poorly defined borders. The radiolucent area often contains scattered and variable amounts of radiopaque foci, which are caused by calcification or ossification of the cartilage matrix (Fig. 14–94). Some chondrosarcomas show extensive calcification and radiologically present as a densely calcified mass with irregular peripheral margins. Penetration of the cortex can result in a sunburst pattern similar to that seen in some osteosarcomas.

Chondrosarcomas often demonstrate extensive infiltration between the osseous trabeculae of the pre-existing bone without causing appreciable resorption. In such cases, the extent of the tumor is difficult to determine by radiographic examination. Root resorption or symmetric widening of the periodontal ligament space about teeth

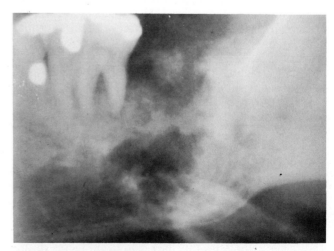

FIGURE 14–94. **Chondrosarcoma.** Ill-defined radiolucent lesion of posterior mandible containing radiopaque foci. (Courtesy of Dr. Ben B. Henry.)

involved in the tumor may also be noted. Chondrosarcomas may grow in a lobular pattern with minimal or no foci of calcification. In such instances, the lesion can present as a multilocular radiolucency and mimic a benign process.

Histopathologic Features

Chondrosarcomas are composed of cartilage showing varying degrees of maturation and cellularity. In most cases, typical lacunar formation within the chondroid matrix is visible, although this feature may be scarce in poorly differentiated tumors. The tumor often shows a lobular growth pattern, with tumor lobules separated by thin fibrous connective tissue septa. The central areas of the lobules demonstrate the greatest degree of maturation. The peripheral areas consist of immature cartilage and mesenchymal tissue consisting of round or spindle-shaped cells. Calcification or ossification may occur within the chondroid matrix. Neoplastic cartilage may be replaced by bone in a manner similar to normal endochondral ossification.

Chondrosarcomas may be divided into three histopathologic grades of malignancy. This grading system correlates well with the rate of tumor growth and prognosis for chondrosarcomas of the extragnathic skeleton. Grading has not been widely applied to jaw chondrosarcomas because of their rarity.

Grades

Grade I chondrosarcomas closely mimic the appearance of a **chondroma,** composed of chondroid matrix and chondroblasts that show only subtle variation from the appearance of normal cartilage. The distinction between benign and well-differentiated malignant cartilaginous tumors is notoriously difficult. Many believe that a tumor should be considered malignant when large, plump chondroblasts and binucleated chondrocytes are present, even in only scattered microscopic fields. Calcification or ossification of the cartilaginous matrix is often prominent, and mitoses are rare.

Grade II chondrosarcomas show a greater proportion of moderately sized nuclei and increased cellularity, particularly about the periphery of the lobules. The cartilaginous matrix tends to be more myxoid with a less prominent hyaline matrix. The mitotic rate, however, is low (Fig. 14–95).

Grade III chondrosarcomas are highly cellular and may show a prominent spindle cell proliferation. Mitoses may be prominent. Easily recognizable cartilaginous matrix containing cells within lacunae may be scarce.

Chondrosarcomas of the jaws are predominantly of the histopathologic grades I and II. Grade III tumors are very uncommon.

Variants

Several uncommon microscopic variants of chondrosarcoma are also recognized.

The **clear cell chondrosarcoma** shows cells with abundant clear cytoplasm; this may lead to problems in differentiation from a metastatic clear cell carcinoma. The

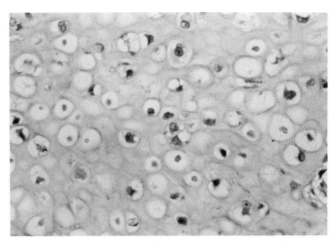

FIGURE 14–95. **Chondrosarcoma.** This grade II chondrosarcoma shows a variation in size of chondrocyte nuclei. Occasional double nuclei are seen in the lacunae.

clear cell chondrosarcoma is considered to be a low-grade lesion.

Dedifferentiated chondrosarcoma is a high-grade malignancy that shows an admixture of well-differentiated chondrosarcoma and a malignant mesenchymal tumor resembling fibrosarcoma. If these variants occur in the jaws, they are exceedingly rare.

Treatment and Prognosis

Radical surgical excision has been the most widely advocated treatment for chondrosarcomas of the jaws. Chondrosarcomas are not very radiosensitive, and the response to chemotherapy is less than that noted for osteosarcomas.

The prognosis is poorer than that for osteosarcomas of the jaws. This contrasts with the better prognosis for chondrosarcomas than osteosarcomas in extragnathic sites. Chondrosarcomas of the jaws do not tend to metastasize. Most treatment failures are due to local recurrence.

Mesenchymal Chondrosarcoma

The **mesenchymal chondrosarcoma,** an uncommon and distinctive tumor of bone and soft tissue, shows a biphasic histopathologic pattern. About one third to one fourth of all examples arise in the soft tissues rather than in bone.

Clinical and Radiographic Features

The mesenchymal chondrosarcoma is most often seen in patients between 10 and 30 years of age but may be encountered at any age. Between one fourth and one third of all cases occur in the craniofacial region, and the jaws are fairly common sites for this tumor.

Swelling and pain, often of fairly short duration, are the most common symptoms. Radiographically, the

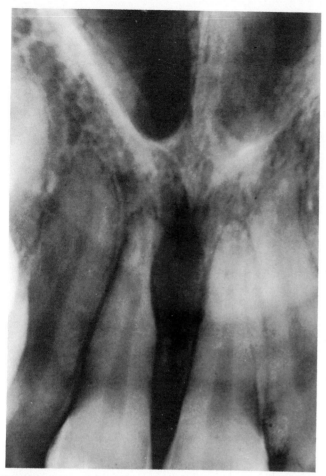

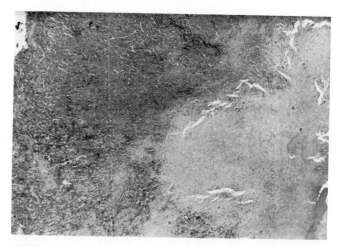

FIGURE 14–97. **Mesenchymal chondrosarcoma.** Photomicrograph from the same lesion shown in Figure 14–96. The pale-staining area (*right*) is composed of cartilage showing only minimal cytologic atypia. The darker-staining mass (*left*) is composed of undifferentiated malignant cells.

Treatment and Prognosis

Surgical resection is the treatment of choice. This may be combined with chemotherapy. Mesenchymal chondrosarcomas are highly malignant tumors, although the clinical course in a given case may be variable. In some patients, lymphatic and hematogenous metastases develop rapidly; in others, there may be long symptom-free periods after surgery. However, about 70 percent of patients eventually die from their tumor.

EWING'S SARCOMA

Ewing's sarcoma is a distinctive primary malignant tumor of bone of uncertain histogenesis. Ewing's sarcomas constitute 6 to 10 percent of all primary malignant

FIGURE 14–96. **Mesenchymal chondrosarcoma.** Periapical radiograph showing a radiolucent lesion between the roots of the central incisors in a 29-year-old woman. The roots of the incisors show resorption. At surgery, the lesion was considerably larger than indicated on the radiograph. (Courtesy of Dr. Gary Baker.)

tumor demonstrates a circumscribed radiolucency with infiltrative margins. Stippled calcification may be present within the radiolucent area (Fig. 14–96).

Histopathologic Features

Microscopically, the mesenchymal chondrosarcoma reveals sheets or patternless masses of small, undifferentiated spindle or round cells surrounding discrete nodules of cartilage (Fig. 14–97). The chondroid tissue is well differentiated, and its degree of cellularity and atypia may vary from that of a benign chondroma to a low-grade chondrosarcoma. The non-cartilaginous component of the tumor is difficult to differentiate from, and may be confused with, a variety of small cell tumors of bone, such as Ewing's sarcoma, malignant lymphoma, and metastatic small cell carcinoma (Fig. 14–98). In some cases, a prominent, branching vascular pattern is present in the soft tissue component of a mesenchymal chondrosarcoma. In the absence of cartilaginous foci, the tumor may be misdiagnosed as a hemangiopericytoma.

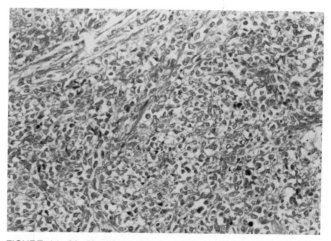

FIGURE 14–98. **Mesenchymal chondrosarcoma.** Higher magnification of the same lesion depicted in Fig. 14–97 showing undifferentiated malignant cells forming the soft tissue component of this tumor.

bone tumors. The femur and pelvic bones are the site of nearly 50 percent of all cases. Jaw involvement is uncommon; less than 3 percent of all Ewing's sarcomas originate in the gnathic bones.

The cell of origin for Ewing's sarcoma has been controversial for many years. Endothelial cells, hematopoietic cells, and primitive mesenchymal cells have been suggested as the possible progenitor cells. Many investigators now believe that Ewing's sarcoma is of neuroectodermal derivation. Tumors indistinguishable from Ewing's sarcoma of bone are occasionally located in the soft tissues without any evidence of bone involvement.

Clinical and Radiographic Features

Ewing's sarcoma is primarily a disease of children and adolescents. About 80 percent of all cases occur in the first and second decades of life. The tumor is very rare in patients younger than 5 or older than 30 years of age. Ewing's sarcoma is predominantly seen in whites; blacks and Asians are not commonly affected. More than 60 percent of cases occur in males.

Pain, often associated with swelling, is the most common symptom. It is usually intermittent and varies from dull to severe. Fever, leukocytosis, and an elevated erythrocyte sedimentation rate may also be present and may lead to an erroneous diagnosis of osteomyelitis. The tumor commonly penetrates the cortex, resulting in a soft tissue mass overlying the affected area of the bone (Fig. 14–99). Jaw involvement is more common in the mandible than the maxilla. Paresthesia and loosening of teeth are common findings in Ewing's sarcomas of the jaws.

Radiographically, there is irregular lytic bone destruction with ill-defined margins (Fig. 14–100). Cortical destruction or expansion may or may not be present. The characteristic "onion-skin" periosteal reaction, commonly observed in Ewing's sarcoma of long bones, is seldom seen in jaw lesions.

Histopathologic Features

Ewing's sarcoma is composed of small round cells with well-delineated nuclear outlines and ill-defined cellular borders (Fig. 14–101). The tumor cells are often arranged in broad sheets without any distinct pattern. In some cases, variable-sized nests of tumor cells are separated by fibrovascular septa, creating a lobular pattern. Large areas of necrosis and hemorrhage are commonly present. Ewing's sarcomas are not as morphologically homogeneous as was once believed. Some examples contain foci or may be mostly composed of larger cells. These are designated as **large cell (atypical) Ewing's sarcomas.**

About 75 percent of cases contain glycogen granules in the cytoplasm of the tumor cells. This is a helpful diagnostic feature, but it is not specific because glycogen can also be demonstrated in some other primitive tumors. About 25 percent of well-documented Ewing's tumors do not show glycogen.

Diagnosis of Ewing's sarcoma may be very difficult. The tumor must be differentiated from other primitive

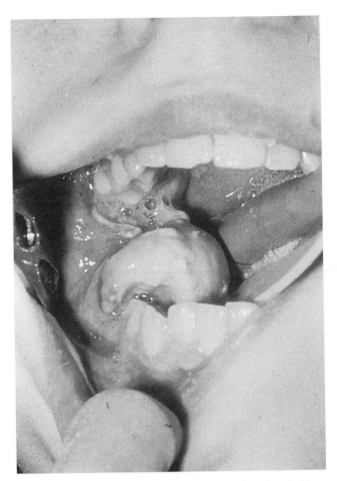

FIGURE 14–99. **Ewing's sarcoma.** A rapidly growing, ulcerated tumor of the right posterior mandible. (Courtesy of Dr. George Blozis.)

small cell tumors involving bone and soft tissues in young patients. These include metastatic neuroblastoma, malignant lymphoma, small cell osteosarcoma, embryonal rhabdomyosarcoma, and the primitive neuroectodermal tumor. Metastatic small cell carcinoma must

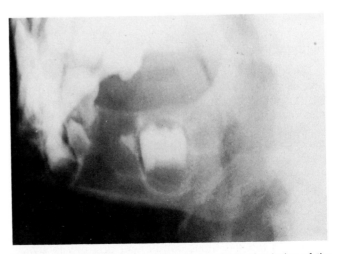

FIGURE 14–100. **Ewing's sarcoma.** Lytic destructive lesion of the mandible in a 4-year-old boy. The developing premolars have been displaced by the tumor, and the developing second premolar is partially resorbed by the tumor.

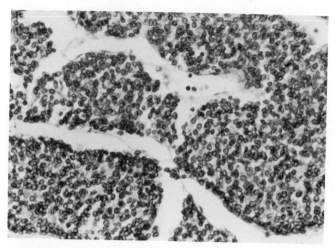

FIGURE 14–101. **Ewing's sarcoma.** Broad sheets of small round cells with well-defined nuclear outlines and ill-defined cytoplasmic borders.

also be considered in the differential diagnosis of a suspected Ewing's sarcoma in an older patient. A battery of immunohistochemical stains and electron microscopy may be required for confirmation of the diagnosis of Ewing's sarcoma in some cases.

Treatment and Prognosis

The prognosis for patients with Ewing's sarcoma has improved dramatically in recent years. Formerly, less than 5 percent of patients survived more than 5 years. Current treatment, consisting of combined surgery, radiotherapy, and multidrug chemotherapy, has led to 40 to 80 percent survival rates.

Ewing's sarcomas frequently metastasize to the lungs, liver, lymph nodes, and other bones. The anatomic location of the tumor is a critical factor in prognosis. Pelvic lesions are associated with the poorest prognosis. Distal lesions have a better prognosis than those in a proximal location. With modern therapy, patients with Ewing's sarcoma of the jaws probably have an improved prognosis; however, there is a scarcity of good information because of the small number of cases.

METASTATIC TUMORS TO THE JAWS

Metastatic carcinoma is the most common form of cancer involving bone. Autopsy studies have shown that more than two thirds of breast carcinomas, one half of all prostate carcinomas, and one third of all lung and kidney carcinomas spread to one or more bones before a patient dies.

Although metastatic lesions may be observed in any bone, the vertebrae, ribs, pelvis, and skull are the most frequent sites for metastasis. The jaws are usually considered to be uncommon sites for metastasis but may be involved more often than generally appreciated. One population-based study has shown that almost 4 percent of upper aerodigestive tract carcinomas in the study group represented metastatic disease from a primary tumor arising outside of the upper aerodigestive tract. In

about 50 percent of the cases, the metastatic lesion was the first evidence of malignancy.

A study of carcinomas arising in various extraoral sites demonstrated that 10 (16 percent) of 62 autopsied cases of carcinoma showed histopathologic evidence of metastasis to the mandible, even though radiographic study of the mandibles removed at autopsy in these cases failed to show evidence of metastatic disease. Metastasis to the maxilla is uncommon, and more than 80 percent of reported metastases to the jaws have occurred in the mandible. Although bone metastasis may arise from primary carcinomas of any anatomic site, carcinomas of the breast, lung, thyroid, prostate, and kidney give rise to the majority of bone metastases. Metastatic spread of a carcinoma to the jaws occurs by the hematogenous route. Sarcomas arising in soft tissues or other bones may metastasize to the jaws, but this is very rare.

Clinical and Radiographic Features

Most patients with metastatic carcinoma are older. This finding is a reflection of the greater incidence of carcinoma in the elderly. Metastatic involvement of the jaws presents with a wide variety of symptoms. In some instances, the patient may be completely asymptomatic, and the diagnosis of metastatic carcinoma occurs only after microscopic study of a lesion noted on radiographic examination. More commonly, however, the patient may experience pain, swelling, loosening of teeth, a mass, or paresthesia. These symptoms, however, are not specific for metastatic disease and are often associated with primary inflammatory or neoplastic diseases of the jaws. Of particular interest are those cases in which diagnosis of a jaw metastasis is the first indication that the patient has a primary malignancy in some other anatomic site. Detection of the occult primary tumor may be difficult, requiring extensive evaluation.

Radiographically, metastatic deposits in the jaws usually present as radiolucent defects. The defect may be well circumscribed, resembling a cyst, or it may be ill defined with a "moth-eaten" appearance (Fig. 14–102).

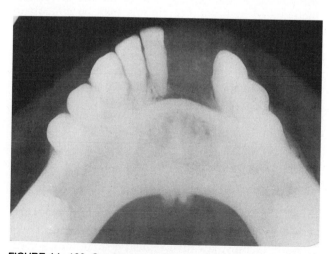

FIGURE 14–102. **Carcinoma metastatic to the jaws.** Occlusal radiograph showing a destructive radiolucent area in the anterior mandible of a 60-year-old woman. This proved to be a metastasis from a carcinoma of the large bowel.

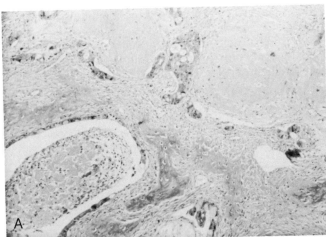
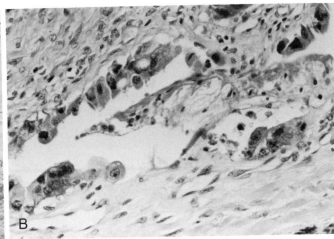

FIGURE 14–103. **Metastatic carcinoma.** *A,* Biopsy specimen from the same patient shown in Figure 14–102. Islands of adenocarcinoma are present in a fibrous stroma. The histopathologic pattern suggests that the tumor arose in the gastrointestinal tract. *B,* Higher magnification of the same metastatic tumor. Some of the tumor cells contain mucin.

Involvement of the alveolus may clinically and radiographically resemble periodontal disease. Some carcinomas, particularly from the prostate and breast, may stimulate new bone formation in the metastatic site, resulting in radiopaque or mixed radiolucent and radiopaque lesions.

Histopathologic Features

The microscopic appearance of metastatic carcinoma in bone varies. In some instances, the metastatic tumor is well differentiated and closely resembles a carcinoma of a specific site, such as the kidney, colon, or thyroid. In such instances, the pathologist can say with reasonable certainty that a given metastatic tumor comes from a specific primary site (Figs. 14–103*A, B*). More often, however, metastatic carcinomas are poorly differentiated and histopathologic study of the metastatic deposit gives little clue as to the primary site of the tumor. Poorly differentiated metastatic carcinoma may be difficult to differentiate from anaplastic small cell sarcomas, malignant lymphomas, and malignant melanoma. Immunohistochemical staining is usually necessary in such cases to establish the diagnosis. Although the diagnosis of metastatic carcinoma can usually be determined by microscopic examination, the final diagnosis depends mostly on a careful medical history and complete physical examination with appropriate laboratory studies.

Treatment and Prognosis

The prognosis for metastatic carcinoma of the jaws is poor, because by definition osseous metastasis automatically places the patient in Stage IV disease. Although a solitary metastatic focus may be treated by excision or radiation therapy, jaw involvement is often only a component of widely disseminated disease. Five-year survival after detection of metastatic carcinoma involving the jaws is exceedingly rare, and most patients do not survive more than a year.

REFERENCES

Osteogenesis Imperfecta

Gorlin RJ, Cohen MM Jr, Levin LS. The osteogenesis imperfectas. *In*: Syndromes of the Head and Neck, 3rd ed. New York, Oxford Press, 1990, pp 155–166.

Levin LS, et al. Dentinogenesis imperfecta in the Brandywine isolate (DI Type III): Clinical, radiologic and scanning electron microscopic studies of the dentition. Oral Surg Oral Med Oral Pathol 56:267–274, 1983.

Osteopetrosis

Steiner M, Gould AR, Means WR. Osteomyelitis of the mandible associated with osteopetrosis. J Oral Maxillofac Surg 41:395–405, 1983.

Younai F, Eisenbud L, Sciubba JJ. Osteopetrosis: A case report including gross and microscopic findings in the mandible at autopsy. Oral Surg Oral Med Oral Pathol 65:214–221, 1988.

Cleidocranial Dysplasia

Farrar EL, van Sickels JE. Early surgical management of cleidocranial dysplasia: A preliminary report. J Oral Maxillofac Surg 41:527–529, 1983.

Gorlin RJ, Cohen MM Jr, Levin LS. Cleidocranial dysplasia. *In*: Syndromes of the Head and Neck, 3rd ed. New York, Oxford Press, 1990, pp 249–253.

Trimble LD, West RA, McNeil RW. Cleidocranial dysplasia: Comprehensive treatment of the dentofacial abnormalities. J Am Dent Assoc 105:661–666, 1982.

Focal Osteoporotic Marrow Defect

Barker BF, Jensen JL, Howell FV. Focal osteoporotic marrow defects of the jaws. Oral Surg Oral Med Oral Pathol 38:404–413, 1974.

Crawford BE, Weathers DR. Osteoporotic marrow defects of the jaws. J Oral Surg 28:600–603, 1970.

Idiopathic Osteosclerosis

Geist JR, Katz JO. The frequency and distribution of idiopathic osteosclerosis. Oral Surg Oral Med Oral Pathol 69:388–393, 1990.

McDonnell D. Dense bone island: A review of 107 patients. Oral Surg Oral Med Oral Pathol 76:124–128, 1993.

Massive Osteolysis

Frederiksen NL, et al. Massive osteolysis of the maxillofacial skeleton: A clinical, radiographic, histologic and ultrastructural study. Oral Surg Oral Med Oral Pathol 55:470–480, 1983.

Heffez L, et al. Perspective of massive osteolysis: Report of a case and review of the literature. Oral Surg Oral Med Oral Pathol 55:331–343, 1983.

Paget's Disease

Carrillo R, et al. Benign fibro-osseous lesions in Paget's disease of the jaws. Oral Surg Oral Med Oral Pathol 71:588–592, 1991.

Smith J, Eveson J. Paget's disease of bone with particular reference to dentistry. J Oral Pathol 10:233–247, 1981.

Tillman H. Paget's disease of bone: A clinical, radiographic and histopathologic study of 24 cases involving the jaws. Oral Surg Oral Med Oral Pathol 15:1225–1234, 1962.

Langerhans Cell Disease

Dagenais M, Pharoah MJ, Sikorski PA. The radiographic characteristics of histiocytosis X: A study of 29 cases that involve the jaws. Oral Surg Oral Med Oral Pathol 74:230–236, 1992.

Hartman KH. A review of 114 cases of histiocytosis X. Oral Surg Oral Med Oral Pathol 49:38–54, 1980.

Pringle GA, et al. Langerhans cell histiocytosis in association with periapical granulomas and cysts. Oral Surg Oral Med Oral Pathol 74:186–192, 1992.

Sedano HO, et al. Histiocytosis X: Clinical, radiologic and histologic findings with special attention to oral manifestations. Oral Surg Oral Med Oral Pathol 27:760–771, 1969.

Central Giant Cell Granuloma

Abrams B, Shear MA. A histologic comparison of the giant cells in central giant cell granuloma and the giant cell tumor of long bone. J Oral Pathol 3:217–223, 1974.

Auclair PL, et al. A clinical and histomorphologic comparison of the central giant cell granuloma and the giant cell tumor. Oral Surg Oral Med Oral Pathol 66:197–208, 1988.

Ficarra G, Kaban LB, Hansen LS. Giant cell lesions of the jaws: A clinicopathologic and cytometric study. Oral Surg Oral Med Oral Pathol 64:44–49, 1987.

Whitaker SB, Waldron CA. Central giant cell lesions of the jaws: A clinical, radiologic and histopathologic study. Oral Surg Oral Med Oral Pathol 75:199–208, 1993.

Cherubism

Dunlap C, et al. The Noonan syndrome/cherubism association. Oral Surg Oral Med Oral Pathol 67:698–705, 1989.

Hamner JE, Ketcham AS. Cherubism: An analysis of treatment. Cancer 23:1133–1143, 1969.

Peters WJN. Cherubism: A study of twenty cases from one family. Oral Surg Oral Med Oral Pathol 47:307–311, 1979.

Simple Bone Cyst

Howe GL. Haemorrhagic cysts of the mandible: I. Br J Oral Surg 3:77–91, 1965.

Kaugars GE, Cale AE. Traumatic bone cyst. Oral Surg Oral Med Oral Pathol 63:318–324, 1987.

Saito Y, et al. Simple bone cyst: A clinical and histopathologic study of fifteen cases. Oral Surg Oral Med Oral Pathol 74:487–491, 1992.

Sapp JP, Stark ML. Self-healing traumatic bone cysts. Oral Surg Oral Med Oral Pathol 69:597–602, 1990.

Aneurysmal Bone Cyst

Struthers PJ, Shear M. Aneurysmal bone cyst of the jaws. I: Clinicopathologic features. Int J Oral Surg 13:85–91, 1984.

Struthers PJ, Shear M. Aneurysmal bone cyst of the jaws. II: Pathogenesis. Int J Oral Surg 13:92–100, 1984.

Toljanic JS, et al. Aneurysmal bone cyst of the jaws: A case study and review of the literature. Oral Surg Oral Med Oral Pathol 64:72–77, 1987.

Fibro-osseous Lesions—General Aspects and Classification

Eversole LS, Sabes WR, Rovin S. Fibrous dysplasia: A nosologic problem in the diagnosis of fibro-osseous lesions of the jaws. J Oral Pathol 1:189–220, 1972.

Hamner JE, Scofield HH, Cornyn J. Benign fibro-osseous lesions of periodontal membrane origin. Cancer 22:861–878, 1968.

Sissons HA, Steiner GC, Dorfman HD. Calcified spherules in fibro-osseous lesions of bone. Arch Pathol Lab Med 117:284–290, 1993.

Waldron CA. Fibro-osseous lesions of the jaws. J Oral Maxillofac Surg 51:828–835, 1993.

Fibrous Dysplasia

Gorlin RJ, Cohen MM Jr, Levin LS. McCune-Albright syndrome. *In*: Syndromes of the Head and Neck, 3rd ed. New York, Oxford Press, 1990, pp 273–277.

Harris WH, Dudley HR Jr, Barry RJ. The natural history of fibrous dysplasia. J Bone Joint Surg 44A:207–233, 1962.

Slow IN, Stern D, Friedman EW. Osteogenic sarcoma arising in pre-existing fibrous dysplasia. J Oral Surg 29:126–129, 1971.

Waldron CA, Giansanti JS. Benign fibro-osseous lesions of the jaws, part I: Fibrous dysplasia of the jaws. Oral Surg Oral Med Oral Pathol 35:190–201, 1973.

Cemento-osseous Dysplasias

Cannon JS, Keller EE, Dahlin DC. Gigantiform cementoma: Report of two cases (mother and son). J Oral Surg 38:65–70, 1980.

Higuchi Y, Nakamura N, Tashiro H. Clinicopathologic study of cemento-osseous dysplasia producing cysts of the mandible. Oral Surg Oral Med Oral Pathol 65:339–342, 1988.

Melrose RJ, Abrams AM, Mills BG. Florid osseous dysplasia. Oral Surg Oral Med Oral Pathol 41:62–82, 1976.

Robinson HBG. Osseous dysplasia: Reaction of bone to injury. J Oral Surg 14:3–14, 1956.

Schneider LC, Mesa ML. Differences between florid osseous dysplasia and diffuse sclerosing osteomyelitis. Oral Surg Oral Med Oral Pathol 70:308–312, 1990.

Waldron CA. Fibro-osseous lesions of the jaws. J Oral Maxillofac Surg 43:249–262, 1985.

Young SK, et al. Familial gigantiform cementoma: Classification and presentation of a large pedigree. Oral Surg Oral Med Oral Pathol 68:740–747, 1989.

Zegarelli EV, et al. The cementoma—a study of 230 patients with cementomas. Oral Surg Oral Med Oral Pathol 17:219–224, 1964.

Fibro-osseous Neoplasms—Ossifying Fibroma and Juvenile Ossifying Fibroma

Eversole LR, Leider AS, Nelson K. Ossifying fibroma: A clinicopathologic study of 64 cases. Oral Surg Oral Med Oral Pathol 60:505–511, 1985.

Johnson LC, et al. Juvenile active ossifying fibroma: Its nature, dynamics and origin. Acta Otolaryngol Suppl (Stockh) 488:1–40, 1991.

Makek MS. So-called "fibro-osseous lesions" of tumorous origin: Biology confronts terminology. J Craniomaxillofac Surg 15:154–168, 1987.

Margo C, et al. Psammomatoid (juvenile) ossifying fibroma of the orbit. Ophthalmology 92:150–159, 1985.

Slootweg PJ, Muller H. Juvenile ossifying fibroma: Report of 4 cases. J Craniomaxillofac Surg 18:125–129, 1990.

Waldron CA, Giansanti JS. Benign fibro-osseous lesions of the jaws, part II: Benign fibro-osseous lesions of periodontal ligament origin. Oral Surg Oral Med Oral Pathol 35:340–350, 1973.

Osteoma

Cutilli BJ, Quinn PD. Traumatically induced peripheral osteoma: Report of case. Oral Surg Oral Med Oral Pathol 73:667–669, 1992.

Richards HE, et al. Large peripheral osteoma arising from the genial tubercle area. Oral Surg Oral Med Oral Pathol 61:268–271, 1986.

Schneider LC, Dolinski HB, Grodjesk JE. Solitary peripheral osteoma of the jaws: Report of a case and review of the literature. Oral Surg Oral Med Oral Pathol 38:452–455, 1980.

Gardner Syndrome

Haggitt RC, Reid BJ. Hereditary gastrointestinal polyposis syndromes. Am J Surg Pathol 10:871–893, 1986.

Ida M, Nakamura T, Utsunomiya J. Osteomatous changes and tooth abnormalities found in the jaws of patients with adenomatosis coli. Oral Surg Oral Med Oral Pathol 52:2–11, 1981.

Sondergaard J, et al. Dental anomalies in familial adenomatous polyposis. Acta Odontol Scand 45:61–63, 1987.

Osteoblastoma

Dorfman HD, Weiss SW. Borderline osteoblastic tumors: Problems in differential diagnosis of aggressive osteoblastoma and low grade osteosarcoma. Semin Diagn Pathol 1:215–245, 1984.

Eisenbud L, Kahn L, Friedman E. Benign osteoblastoma of the mandible: Fifteen year follow-up showing spontaneous regression after biopsy. J Oral Maxillofac Surg 45:53–57, 1987.

Smith RA, et al. Comparison of osteoblastoma in gnathic and extragnathic sites. Oral Surg Oral Med Oral Pathol 54:285–298, 1982.

Weinberg S, Katsikeris N, Pharoah M. Osteoblastoma of the mandibular condyle: Review of the literature and report of a case. J Oral Maxillofac Surg 45:350–355, 1987.

Cementoblastoma (True Cementoma)

Abrams AM, Kirby JW, Melrose RJ. Cementoblastoma. Oral Surg Oral Med Oral Pathol 38:394–403, 1974.

Dahlin DC, Unni KK. Bone Tumors: General Aspects and Data on 8542 Cases, 4th ed. Springfield, Ill, Charles C Thomas, 1986, pp 114–115.

Jelic JS, et al. Benign cementoblastoma: Report of an unusual case and analysis of 14 additional cases. J Oral Maxillofac Surg 51:1033–1037, 1993.

Monks FT, Bradley JC, Turner EP. Central osteoblastoma or cementoblastoma? A case report and 12 year review. Br J Oral Surg 19:29–37, 1981.

Slootweg PJ. Cementoblastoma and osteoblastoma: A comparison of histologic features. J Oral Pathol Med 21:385–389, 1992.

Chondroma

Hyams VJ, Batsakis JG, Michaels L. Tumors of the Upper Respiratory Tract and Ear. Atlas of Tumor Pathology, 2nd Series, Fascicle 25. Washington, DC, Armed Forces Institute of Pathology, 1988, pp 163–164.

Chondromyxoid Fibroma

Damm DD, et al. Chondromyxoid fibroma of the maxilla: Electron microscopic findings and review of the literature. Oral Surg Oral Med Oral Pathol 59:176–183, 1985.

Müller S, Whitaker SB, Weathers DR. Chondromyxoid fibroma of the mandible: Diagnostic image cytometry findings and review of the literature. Oral Surg Oral Med Oral Pathol 73:465–468, 1992.

Synovial Chondromatosis

Deahl ST, Ruprecht A. Asymptomatic, radiographically detected chondrometaplasia in the temporomandibular joint. Oral Surg Oral Med Oral Pathol 72:371–374, 1991.

Lustman J, Zeltzer R. Synovial chondromatosis of the temporomandibular joint: Review of the literature and case report. Int J Oral Maxillofac Surg 18:90–94, 1989.

Quinn PD, Stanton DC, Foote JW. Synovial chondromatosis with cranial extension. Oral Surg Oral Med Oral Pathol 73:398–402, 1992.

Hemangioma and Other Vascular Tumors

Bonel K, Sindet-Pederson S. Central hemangioma of the mandible. Oral Surg Oral Med Oral Pathol 75:565–570, 1993.

Freedman PD, Kerpel SM. Epithelioid angiosarcoma of the maxilla: A case report and review of the literature. Oral Surg Oral Med Oral Pathol 74:319–325, 1992.

Greene LA, et al. Capillary hemangioma of the maxilla: A report of two cases in which angiography and embolization were used. Oral Surg Oral Med Oral Pathol 70:268–273, 1990.

Lund BA, Dahlin DC. Hemangiomas of the maxilla and mandible. J Oral Surg 22:234–242, 1964.

Desmoplastic Fibroma

Bertoni F, et al. Desmoplastic fibroma of the jaw: The experience of the Institute Beretta. Oral Surg Oral Med Oral Pathol 61:179–184, 1986.

Freedman PD, et al. Desmoplastic fibroma (fibromatosis) of the jawbones: Report of a case and review of the literature. Oral Surg Oral Med Oral Pathol 46:386–395, 1978.

Fibrosarcoma

Dahlin DC, Ivins JC. Fibrosarcoma of bone: A study of 114 cases. Cancer 23:35–41, 1969.

Van Blarcom CW, Masson JK, Dahlin DC. Fibrosarcoma of the mandible. Oral Surg Oral Med Oral Pathol 32:428–439, 1969.

Osteosarcoma

Bras JM, Donner R, van der Kwast WAM. Juxtacortical osteogenic sarcoma. Oral Surg Oral Med Oral Pathol 50:535–544, 1980.

Clark JJ, et al. Osteosarcoma of the jaws. Cancer 51:2311–2316, 1983.

Garrington GE, et al. Osteosarcoma of the jaws: Analysis of 56 cases. Cancer 20:377–391, 1967.

Huvos AG, et al. Postradiation sarcoma of bone and soft tissues: A clinicopathologic study of 66 patients. Cancer 55:1244–1255, 1985.

Martin SE, et al. Small cell osteosarcoma. Cancer 50:990–996, 1982.

Rosen G, et al. Preoperative chemotherapy for osteogenic sarcoma: Selection of postoperative chemotherapy based upon the response of the primary tumor to preoperative chemotherapy. Cancer 49:1221–1230, 1982

Slootweg PJ, Müller H. Osteosarcoma of the jawbones. J Maxillofac Surg 13:158–166, 1985.

Unni KK, et al. Intraosseous well-differentiated osteosarcoma. Cancer 40:1337–1347, 1977.

Zarbo RJ, Regezi JA, Baker SR. Periosteal osteogenic sarcoma of the mandible. Oral Surg Oral Med Oral Pathol 57:643–647, 1984.

Chondrosarcoma

Christensen RE Jr. Mesenchymal chondrosarcoma of the jaws. Oral Surg Oral Med Oral Pathol 54:197–206, 1982.

Finn DG, Goepfert H, Batsakis JG. Chondrosarcoma of the head and neck. Laryngoscope 94:1539–1544, 1984.

Garrington GE, Collett WK. Chondrosarcoma. I: A selected literature review. J Oral Pathol 17:1–11, 1988.

Garrington GE, Collett WK. Chondrosarcoma. II: Chondrosarcoma of the jaws: Analysis of 37 cases. J Oral Pathol 17:12–20, 1988.

Ewing's Sarcoma

Arafat A, Ellis G, Adrian JC. Ewing's sarcoma of the jaws. Oral Surg Oral Med Oral Pathol 55:589–596, 1983.

Dehner LP. Primitive neuroectodermal tumor and Ewing's sarcoma. Am J Surg Pathol 17:1–13, 1993.

Kissane JM, et al. Ewing's sarcoma of bone: Clinicopathologic aspects of 303 cases from the intergroup Ewing's sarcoma study. Hum Pathol 14:773–779, 1983.

Tumors Metastatic to the Jaws

Bouquot JE, Weiland LH, Kurland LT. Metastasis to and from the upper aero-digestive tract in the population of Rochester, Minnesota, 1935–1984. Head Neck 11:212–218, 1989.

Clausen F, Poulson H. Metastatic carcinoma of the jaws. Acta Pathol Microbiol Scand 57:361–374, 1963.

Hashimoto N, et al. Pathologic characteristics of metastatic carcinoma in the human mandible. J Oral Pathol 16:362–367, 1987.

O'Carroll MK, Krolls SO, Mosca NG. Metastatic carcinoma to the mandible: Report of two cases. Oral Surg Oral Med Oral Pathol 76:368–374, 1993.

Zachariades N. Neoplasms metastatic to the mouth, jaws and surrounding tissues. J Craniomaxillofac Surg 17:283–290, 1989.

15

Odontogenic Cysts and Tumors

Charles A. Waldron

Odontogenic cysts and tumors constitute an important aspect of oral and maxillofacial pathology. Odontogenic cysts are encountered relatively commonly in dental practice. Odontogenic tumors, by contrast, are uncommon lesions. Even in the specialized oral and maxillofacial pathology laboratory, less than 1 percent of all specimens received are odontogenic tumors.

Odontogenic Cysts

With rare exceptions, epithelium-lined cysts in bone are seen only in the jaws. Other than a few cysts that may result from the inclusion of epithelium along embryonic lines of fusion, most jaw cysts are lined by epithelium that is derived from odontogenic epithelium. These are referred to as **odontogenic cysts**. (*Non-odontogenic* jaw cysts are discussed in Chapter 1.)

Odontogenic cysts are subclassified as developmental or inflammatory in origin. *Developmental cysts* are of unknown etiology but they do not appear to be the result of an inflammatory reaction. *Inflammatory cysts* are the result of inflammation. Table 15–1 presents categories of odontogenic cysts based on the widely accepted 1992 World Health Organization (WHO) classification. (Inflammatory odontogenic cysts are discussed in Chapter 3.)

DENTIGEROUS CYST (Follicular Cyst)

The **dentigerous cyst** is defined as a cyst that originates by the separation of the follicle from around the crown of an unerupted tooth. This is the most common type of developmental odontogenic cyst, making up about 20 percent of all epithelium-lined cysts of the jaws. The dentigerous cyst encloses the crown of an unerupted tooth and is attached to the tooth at the cemento-enamel junction (Fig. 15–1). The pathogenesis of this cyst, however, is unknown. Some dentigerous cysts may develop earlier in odontogenesis by degeneration of the stellate reticulum of the enamel organ. In such cases, the involved tooth shows enamel hypoplasia. However, the crowns of the teeth involved in most dentigerous cysts are fully formed, which suggests that the cyst develops by accumulation of fluid between the reduced enamel epithelium and the crown.

Clinical and Radiographic Features

Although dentigerous cysts may involve any unerupted tooth, most often they involve mandibular third molars. Maxillary canines are the second most commonly involved teeth. Dentigerous cysts rarely involve unerupted deciduous teeth. They are occasionally associated with supernumerary teeth or odontomas.

Although dentigerous cysts may be encountered in patients over a wide age range, they are most frequently discovered in patients between 10 and 30 years of age. There is a slight male predilection, and the prevalence is higher for whites than for blacks. Small dentigerous cysts

Table 15–1. CLASSIFICATION OF ODONTOGENIC CYSTS

A. Developmental
 1. Dentigerous cyst
 2. Eruption cyst
 3. Odontogenic keratocyst
 4. Gingival (alveolar) cyst of the newborn
 5. Gingival cyst of the adult
 6. Lateral periodontal cyst
 7. Calcifying odontogenic cyst*
 8. Glandular odontogenic cyst

B. Inflammatory
 1. Radicular cyst
 2. Residual radicular cyst
 3. Paradental cyst

*The term "calcifying odontogenic cyst" includes both non-neoplastic cysts and true neoplasms. Although the calcifying odontogenic cyst is included with odontogenic tumors in the 1992 WHO classification, we discuss it with the odontogenic cysts in this chapter.

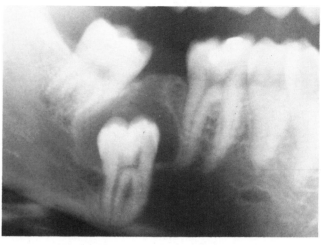

FIGURE 15–2. **Dentigerous cyst**. Central type showing the crown projecting into the cystic cavity. (Courtesy of Dr. Stephen E. Irwin.)

are usually completely asymptomatic and are discovered only on a routine radiographic examination or when films are taken to determine the reason for the failure of a tooth to erupt. Dentigerous cysts can grow to a considerable size, and large cysts may be associated with a painless expansion of the bone in the involved area. Extensive lesions may result in facial asymmetry. Large dentigerous cysts are uncommon, and most lesions that are considered to be large dentigerous cysts on radiographic examination will prove to be odontogenic keratocysts or ameloblastomas. Dentigerous cysts may become infected, presumably by the hematogenous route, and be associated with pain and swelling. Infection may also involve a dentigerous cyst that is associated with a partially erupted tooth or by extension from a periapical or periodontal lesion that affects an adjacent tooth.

Radiographically, the dentigerous cyst typically shows a unilocular radiolucent area that is associated with the crown of an unerupted tooth. The radiolucency usually has a well-defined and often sclerotic border, but an infected cyst may show ill-defined borders. A large dentigerous cyst may give the impression of a multilocular process because of the persistence of bone trabeculae within the radiolucency. Dentigerous cysts, however, are grossly and histopathologically unilocular processes and probably never are truly multilocular lesions.

The cyst-crown relationship shows several radiographic variations. In the *central* variety, which is the most common, the cyst surrounds the crown of the tooth and the crown projects into the cyst (Fig. 15–2). The *lateral* variety is usually associated with mesioangular impacted mandibular third molars that are partially erupted. The cyst grows laterally along the root surface and partially surrounds the crown (Fig. 15–3). In the *circumferential* variant, the cyst surrounds the crown and extends for some distance along the root so that a signifi-

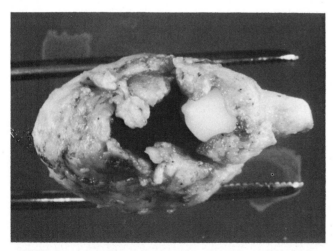

FIGURE 15–1. **Dentigerous cyst**. Gross specimen of a dentigerous cyst involving a maxillary canine tooth. The cyst has been cut open to show the cyst-crown relationship.

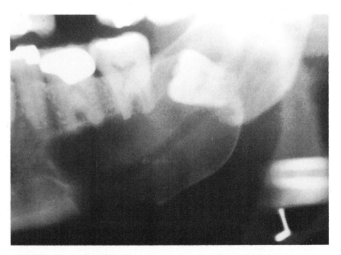

FIGURE 15–3. **Dentigerous cyst**. Lateral variety showing a large cyst along the mesial root of the unerupted molar. This cyst exhibited mucous cell prosoplasia. (Courtesy of Dr. John R. Cramer.)

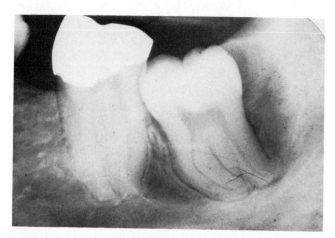

FIGURE 15–4. **Dentigerous cyst**. Circumferential variety showing cyst extension along the mesial and distal roots of the unerupted tooth. (Courtesy of Dr. Richard Marks.)

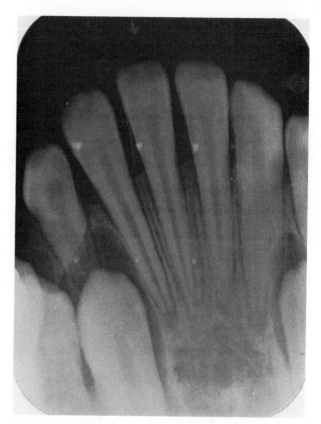

FIGURE 15–5. **Dentigerous cyst or enlarged follicle.** Radiolucent lesion involving the crown of an unerupted mandibular canine. Distinction between a dentigerous cyst and an enlarged follicle for a lesion of this size by radiographic and even histopathologic means is difficult, if not impossible.

cant portion of the root appears to lie within the cyst (Fig. 15–4). Rarely, a third molar may be displaced to the lower border of the mandible or higher up into the ascending ramus. Maxillary anterior teeth may be displaced into the floor of the nose, and other maxillary teeth may be moved through the maxillary sinus to the floor of the orbit. Dentigerous cysts may displace the involved tooth for a considerable distance.

In about 50 percent of cases, dentigerous cysts in contact with adjacent erupted teeth cause root resorption of these teeth. This is a considerably higher rate than the frequency of root resorption associated with other odontogenic cysts. This may be related to the dental follicle's role in the resorption of deciduous roots.

Radiographic distinction between a small dentigerous cyst and an enlarged follicle about the crown of an unerupted tooth is difficult and may be largely an academic exercise (Fig. 15–5). For the lesion to be considered a dentigerous cyst, some investigators believe that the radiolucent area should be at least 3 to 4 mm in diameter. Radiographic findings are not diagnostic for a dentigerous cyst, however, because odontogenic keratocysts, unilocular ameloblastomas, and many other odontogenic and non-odontogenic tumors may have radiographic features that are essentially identical to those of a dentigerous cyst.

Histopathologic Features

The histopathologic findings of dentigerous cysts vary, depending on whether the cyst is inflamed or not inflamed. In the *non-inflamed* dentigerous cyst, the fibrous connective tissue wall is loosely arranged and contains considerable glycosaminoglycan ground substance. Small islands or cords of inactive-appearing odontogenic epithelial rests may be present in the fibrous wall. The epithelial lining consists of two to four layers of cuboidal epithelial cells, and the epithelium–connective tissue interface is flat (Fig. 15–6).

In the fairly common *inflamed* dentigerous cyst, the fibrous wall is more collagenized, with a variable infiltra-

tion of chronic inflammatory cells. The epithelial lining may show varying amounts of hyperplasia with the development of rete ridges and squamous features (Fig. 15–7). A keratinized surface is sometimes seen. These changes must be differentiated from those observed in the odontogenic keratocyst. Focal areas of mucous cells may be found in the epithelial lining of dentigerous cysts.

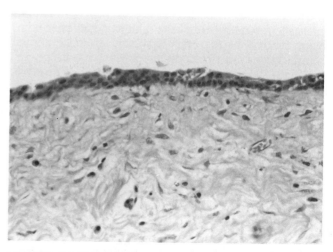

FIGURE 15–6. **Dentigerous cyst**. This non-inflamed dentigerous cyst shows a thin, non-keratinized epithelial lining.

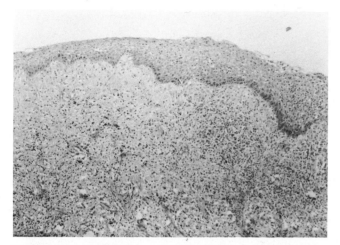

FIGURE 15–7. **Dentigerous cyst**. This inflamed dentigerous cyst shows a thicker epithelial lining with rete ridges. The fibrous cyst capsule shows a diffuse chronic inflammatory infiltrate.

Rarely, ciliated epithelial cells are present. Small nests of sebaceous cells may rarely be noted within the fibrous cyst wall. These mucous, ciliated, and sebaceous elements are believed to represent the multipotentiality of the odontogenic epithelial lining in a dentigerous cyst. Gross examination of the wall of a dentigerous cyst may reveal one or several areas of nodular thickening on the luminal surface. These areas must be examined microscopically to rule out the presence of early neoplastic change.

Treatment and Prognosis

The usual treatment for a dentigerous cyst is careful enucleation of the cyst together with removal of the unerupted tooth. If eruption of the involved tooth is considered feasible, the tooth may be left in place after partial removal of the cyst wall. Patients may need orthodontic treatment to assist eruption. Large dentigerous cysts may also be treated by marsupialization. This permits decompression of the cyst, with a resulting reduction in the size of the bone defect. The cyst can then be excised at a later date with a less extensive surgical procedure.

The prognosis associated with most dentigerous cysts is excellent, and recurrence is seldom noted after complete removal of the cyst. However, several potential complications must be considered. Much has been written about the possibility that the lining of a dentigerous cyst might undergo neoplastic transformation to an **ameloblastoma**. Although this undoubtedly occasionally occurs, the frequency of such neoplastic transformation is low. Rarely, a **squamous cell carcinoma** may arise in the lining of a dentigerous cyst (see p. 510). It is likely that some **intraosseous mucoepidermoid carcinomas** (see p. 351) develop from mucous cells in the lining of a dentigerous cyst.

ERUPTION CYST (Eruption Hematoma)

The **eruption cyst** is the soft tissue analogue of the dentigerous cyst. The cyst develops as a result of separa-

tion of the dental follicle from around the crown of an erupting tooth that is within the soft tissues overlying the alveolar bone.

Clinical Features

The eruption cyst is a soft, often translucent swelling in the gingival mucosa overlying the crown of an erupting deciduous or permanent tooth. Most examples are seen in children younger than age 10. Although the cyst may occur with any erupting tooth, the lesion is most commonly seen in the mandibular molar region. Surface trauma may result in a considerable amount of blood in the cystic fluid, which imparts a purplish or brown color. Such lesions are sometimes referred to as **eruption hematomas** (Fig. 15–8; see Color Figure 90).

Histopathologic Features

Intact eruption cysts are seldom submitted to the oral and maxillofacial pathology laboratory, and most examples consist of the excised roof of the cyst, which has been removed to facilitate tooth eruption. These show surface oral epithelium on the superior aspect. The underlying lamina propria shows a variable inflammatory cell infiltrate. The deep portion of the specimen, which represents the roof of the cyst, shows a thin layer of non-keratinizing squamous epithelium (Fig. 15–9).

Treatment and Prognosis

Treatment may not be required because the cyst usually ruptures spontaneously, permitting the tooth to erupt. If this does not occur, simple excision of the roof of the cyst generally permits speedy eruption of the tooth.

PRIMORDIAL CYST

The concept and meaning of the term **primordial cyst** continue to be controversial and confusing. In the older classification of cysts widely used in the United States,

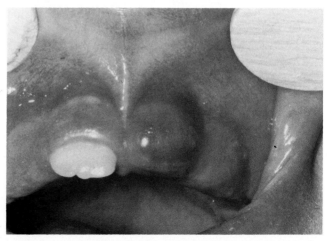

FIGURE 15–8. **Eruption cyst.** This soft gingival swelling contains considerable blood and can also be designated as an eruption hematoma.

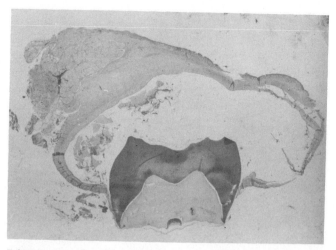

FIGURE 15–9. **Eruption cyst.** The cyst is attached to the molar tooth at the cemento-enamel junction. Intact oral mucosa is present superior to the cyst.

the primordial cyst was considered to originate from cystic degeneration of the enamel organ epithelium before the development of dental hard tissue. Therefore, the primordial cyst occurs in place of a tooth.

In the mid-1950s, oral pathologists in Europe introduced the term **odontogenic keratocyst** to denote a cyst with specific histopathologic features and clinical behavior, which was believed to arise from the dental lamina (i.e., the dental primordium). This concept was subsequently widely accepted, and the terms **odontogenic keratocyst** and **primordial cyst** were used synonymously. The 1972 WHO classification used the designation primordial cyst as the preferred term for this lesion. The 1992 WHO classification, however, lists odontogenic keratocyst as the preferred designation.

Whether there is a primordial cyst that is not microscopically an odontogenic keratocyst is still unsettled. Many believe that all primordial cysts are odontogenic keratocysts, although some recognize the existence of a primordial cyst that does not have the histopathologic features of the odontogenic keratocyst. If such a lesion exists, it must be exceedingly uncommon. Reference to this lesion is almost nonexistent in the current literature, and there are no reported series that include a significant number of cases. In the present author's experience, a cyst considered to represent a primordial cyst clinically, in the older meaning of the term, almost always is an odontogenic keratocyst after microscopic study (Fig. 15–10).

ODONTOGENIC KERATOCYST

The **odontogenic keratocyst** is a distinctive form of developmental odontogenic cyst that deserves special consideration because of its specific histopathologic features and clinical behavior. There is general agreement that the odontogenic keratocyst arises from cell rests of the dental lamina. This cyst shows a different growth mechanism and biologic behavior from the more com-

mon dentigerous cyst and radicular cyst. Most authors believe that dentigerous and radicular cysts continue to enlarge as a result of increased osmotic pressure within the lumen of the cyst. This mechanism does not appear to hold true for odontogenic keratocysts, and their growth may be related to unknown factors inherent in the epithelium itself or enzymatic activity in the fibrous wall. Several investigators suggest that odontogenic keratocysts be regarded as benign cystic neoplasms rather than cysts. Although there are wide variations in the reported frequency of odontogenic keratocysts compared with that of other types of odontogenic cysts, several studies that include large series of cysts indicate that odontogenic keratocysts make up 10 to 12 percent of all developmental odontogenic cysts.

Clinical and Radiographic Features

Odontogenic keratocysts may be found in patients who range in age from infancy to old age, but about 60 percent of all cases are diagnosed in people between 10 and 40 years of age. There is a definite male predilection. The mandible is involved in 60 to 80 percent of cases, with a marked tendency to involve the posterior body and ascending ramus.

Small odontogenic keratocysts are usually asymptomatic and are discovered only during the course of a radiographic examination. Larger odontogenic keratocysts may be associated with pain, swelling, or drainage. Extremely large cysts, however, may cause no symptoms.

Odontogenic keratocysts tend to grow in an anteroposterior direction within the medullary cavity of the bone without causing obvious bone expansion. This feature may be useful in differential clinical and radiologic diagnosis because dentigerous and radicular cysts of comparable size are usually associated with bony expansion. Multiple odontogenic keratocysts may be present, and such patients should be evaluated for other manifestations of the **nevoid basal cell carcinoma (Gorlin) syndrome.**

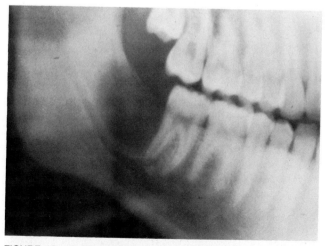

FIGURE 15–10. **Primordial cyst.** This patient gave no history of extraction of the third molar. A cyst is located in the third molar area. The cyst was excised, and pathologic examination revealed an odontogenic keratocyst.

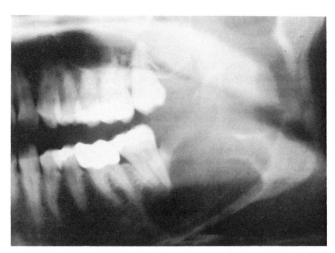

FIGURE 15–11. **Odontogenic keratocyst.** Large, multilocular cyst involving most of the ascending ramus. (Courtesy of Dr. S. C. Roddy.)

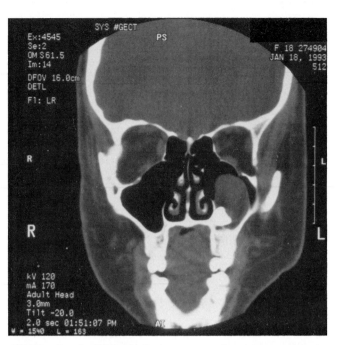

FIGURE 15–13. **Odontogenic keratocyst.** Computed tomography scan showing a large cyst involving the crown of an unerupted maxillary third molar. The cyst largely fills the maxillary sinus. (Courtesy of Dr. E. B. Bass.)

Odontogenic keratocysts demonstrate a well-defined radiolucent area with smooth and often corticated margins. Large lesions, particularly in the posterior body and ascending ramus of the mandible, may appear multilocular (Fig. 15–11). An unerupted tooth is involved in the lesion in 25 to 40 percent of cases; in such instances, the radiographic features suggest the diagnosis of dentigerous (follicular) cyst (Figs. 15–12 and 15–13). In these cases, the cyst has presumably arisen from dental lamina rests in the vicinity of an unerupted tooth and has grown to envelop the unerupted tooth. Resorption of the roots of erupted teeth adjacent to odontogenic keratocysts is less common than that noted with dentigerous and radicular cysts.

The diagnosis of odontogenic keratocyst is based on the histopathologic features. The radiographic findings, although often highly suggestive, are not diagnostic. The radiographic findings in an odontogenic keratocyst may simulate those of a dentigerous cyst, a radicular cyst, a residual cyst, a lateral periodontal cyst, or a so-called globulomaxillary cyst (Fig. 15–14).

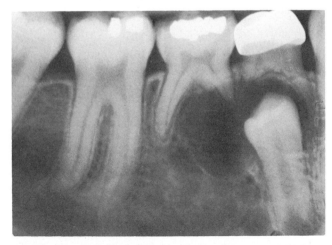

FIGURE 15–12. **Odontogenic keratocyst.** This cyst involves the crown of an unerupted premolar. Radiographically, this lesion cannot be differentiated from a dentigerous cyst.

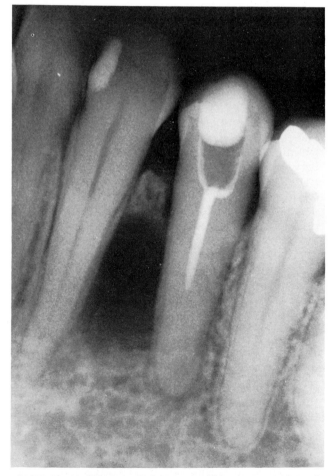

FIGURE 15–14. **Odontogenic keratocyst.** This cyst cannot be radiographically differentiated from a lateral periodontal cyst. (Courtesy of Dr. Keith Lemmerman.)

Histopathologic Features

The odontogenic keratocyst typically shows a thin, friable wall, which is often difficult to enucleate from the bone in one piece. The cystic lumen may contain a clear liquid that is similar to a transudate of serum, or it may be filled with a cheesy material, which on microscopic examination consists of keratinaceous debris. Microscopically, the thin fibrous wall is essentially devoid of any inflammatory infiltrate. The epithelial lining is composed of a uniform layer of stratified squamous epithelium, usually six to eight cells in thickness. The epithelium–connective tissue interface is usually flat, and rete ridge formation is inconspicuous. Detachment of portions of the cyst-lining epithelium from the fibrous wall is commonly observed (Fig. 15–15). The luminal surface shows flattened parakeratotic epithelial cells, which present a wavy or corrugated appearance (Fig. 15–16). The basal epithelial layer is composed of a palisaded layer of cuboidal or columnar epithelial cells, which are often hyperchromatic. Small satellite cysts, cords, or islands of odontogenic epithelium may be seen within the fibrous wall. These structures have been present in 7 to 26 percent of cases in various reported series.

In the presence of inflammatory changes, the typical features of the odontogenic keratocyst may be altered. The parakeratinized luminal surface may disappear, and the epithelium may proliferate to form rete ridges with the loss of the characteristic palisaded basal layer (Fig. 15–17). Areas of the epithelial surface may develop an orthokeratinized surface. When these changes involve most of the cyst lining, the diagnosis of odontogenic keratocyst cannot be confirmed unless other sections show the typical features described earlier.

Some investigators recognize a microscopic orthokeratotic variant and include this lesion as a subtype of the odontogenic keratocyst. However, the clinical and histopathologic features and the clinical behavior of orthokeratotic cysts differ markedly from those of the typical odontogenic (parakeratinized) cysts described previously.

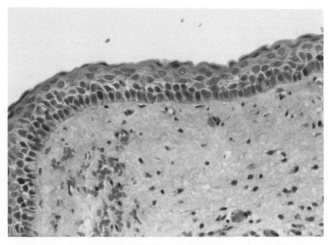

FIGURE 15–16. **Odontogenic keratocyst.** Higher magnification of an odontogenic keratocyst. The basal epithelial layer is composed of hyperchromatic, columnar cells. The thin epithelial lining shows a parakeratinized surface with "wavy" or corrugated appearance.

We believe that it is more logical to discuss these orthokeratinizing cysts separately.

Treatment and Prognosis

Although the presence of an odontogenic keratocyst may be suspected on clinical or radiologic grounds, histopathologic confirmation is required for the diagnosis. Consequently, most odontogenic keratocysts are treated similarly to other odontogenic cysts, that is, by enucleation and curettage. Complete removal of the cyst in one piece is often difficult because of the thin, friable nature of the cyst wall. In contrast to other odontogenic cysts, odontogenic keratocysts often tend to recur after treatment. Whether this is due to fragments of the original cyst that were not removed at the time of the operation or to a "new" cyst that has developed from dental lamina rests in the general area of the original cyst cannot be determined with certainty.

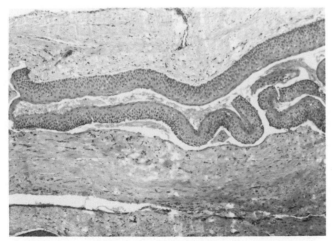

FIGURE 15–15. **Odontogenic keratocyst.** A thin parakeratotic epithelial lining is visible. A portion of the lining has become detached from the fibrous capsule. This is often seen in sections of odontogenic keratocysts.

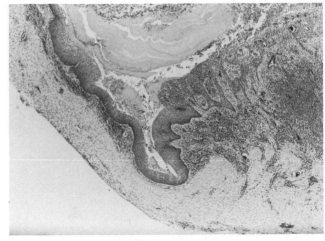

FIGURE 15–17. **Odontogenic keratocyst.** The cyst lining has undergone alteration with the formation of rete ridges in the area of severe inflammation on the right. The epithelial lining on the left retains the features of an odontogenic keratocyst.

The reported frequency of recurrence in various studies ranges from 5 to 62 percent. This wide variation may be related to the total number of cases studied, the length of follow-up periods, and the inclusion or exclusion of orthokeratinized cysts in the study group. Several reports that include large numbers of cases indicate a recurrence rate of approximately 30 percent. Recurrence is encountered more often in mandibular odontogenic keratocysts, particularly those in the posterior body and ascending ramus. Multiple recurrences are not unusual. Some surgeons advocate the use of chemical cautery agents after enucleation of a keratocyst or peripheral ostectomy with a bone bur to reduce the frequency of recurrence. Although many odontogenic keratocysts recur within 5 years of the original surgery, a significant number of recurrences may not be manifested until 10 or more years after the original surgical procedure. Long-term clinical and radiologic follow-up, therefore, is necessary.

Other than the tendency for recurrences, the overall prognosis for odontogenic keratocysts is good. Occasionally, a locally aggressive odontogenic keratocyst cannot be controlled without local resection and bone grafting. A few examples of carcinoma arising in an odontogenic keratocyst have been reported, but the propensity for an odontogenic keratocyst to undergo malignant alteration is no greater and is possibly less than that for other types of odontogenic cysts. Patients with odontogenic keratocysts should be evaluated for manifestations of the nevoid basal cell carcinoma syndrome (see p. 501).

ORTHOKERATINIZED ODONTOGENIC CYSTS

The designation **orthokeratinized odontogenic cyst** does not denote a specific clinical type of odontogenic cyst but refers only to an odontogenic cyst that microscopically has an orthokeratinized epithelial lining.

Some investigators suggest that these orthokeratinized cysts are a variant of the **odontogenic keratocyst** and designate them as **odontogenic keratocysts–orthokeratotic variant**. This designation, however, is confusing because these cysts show little if any of the histopathologic features of the odontogenic keratocyst and their clinical behavior differs from that of the typical odontogenic keratocyst.

Clinical and Radiographic Features

Orthokeratinized odontogenic cysts have no clinical or radiologic features that differentiate them from the other inflammatory or developmental odontogenic cysts described previously. Most cases are encountered in a lesion that appears clinically and radiologically to represent a dentigerous cyst; they most often involve an unerupted mandibular third molar tooth (Fig. 15–18). Similar histopathologic changes are occasionally noted in longstanding radicular cysts or residual cysts.

Histopathologic Features

The cyst lining is composed of stratified squamous epithelium, which shows an orthokeratotic surface of

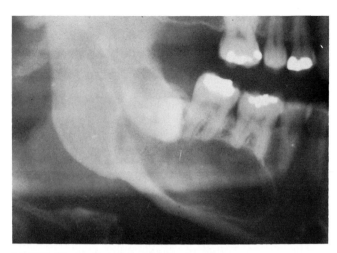

FIGURE 15–18. **Orthokeratinized odontogenic cyst.** A large dentigerous cyst involving a horizontally impacted lower third molar. On microscopic examination, this was an orthokeratinized odontogenic cyst. (Courtesy of Dr. Carroll Gallagher.)

varying thickness. Keratohyalin granules may be prominent in the superficial epithelial layer subjacent to the orthokeratin. The epithelial lining may be relatively thin, and a prominent palisaded basal layer, characteristic of the odontogenic keratocyst, is not present (Fig. 15–19).

Treatment and Prognosis

Enucleation with curettage is the usual treatment for orthokeratinized odontogenic cysts. Recurrence has rarely been noted, and the reported frequency is less than 2 percent, which is in marked contrast with the 30 percent or higher recurrence rate associated with odontogenic keratocysts. It has been suggested that cysts with an orthokeratinized surface may be at slightly greater risk for malignant transformation, but evidence for this is scant.

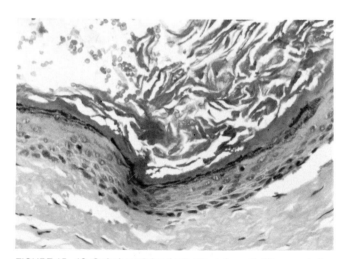

FIGURE 15–19. **Orthokeratinized odontogenic cyst.** Microscopic features showing a thin epithelial lining. The basal epithelial layer does not demonstrate palisading. Prominent keratohyalin granules are present beneath the orthokeratotic surface. Flakes of orthokeratin are present in the lumen.

Orthokeratinized cysts have not been associated with nevoid basal cell carcinoma syndrome.

NEVOID BASAL CELL CARCINOMA SYNDROME (Gorlin Syndrome)

Nevoid basal cell carcinoma syndrome is inherited as an autosomal dominant trait with a high penetrance and variable expressivity. The chief components are multiple basal cell carcinomas of the skin, jaw cysts, rib anomalies, vertebral anomalies, and intracranial calcification. Many other anomalies have been reported in these patients and probably also represent manifestations of the syndrome.

Clinical and Radiographic Features

There is great variability in the expressivity of nevoid basal cell carcinoma syndrome, and no single component is present in all patients. The patient often has a characteristic facies, with frontal and temporoparietal bossing, which results in an increased cranial circumference. The eyes may appear widely separated, and 40 percent of patients have true ocular hypertelorism. Mild mandibular prognathism is also commonly present (Fig. 15–20).

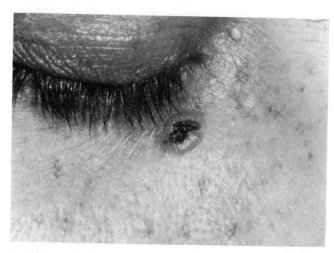

FIGURE 15–21. **Nevoid basal cell carcinoma syndrome.** An ulcerating basal cell carcinoma is present on the upper face.

Skin tumors are a major component of the syndrome. They usually appear at puberty or in the second and third decades of life but can first appear in young children. The tumors may vary from flesh-colored papules to ulcerating plaques. They are often present on non–sun-exposed skin but are most commonly located in the mid-face area (Fig. 15–21). The number of skin tumors may vary from only a few to many hundreds. Palmar and plantar pits are present in about 60 percent of patients. These punctate lesions represent a localized retardation of the maturation of basal epithelial cells. Basal cell carcinomas may develop at the base of the pits (Fig. 15–22).

Skeletal anomalies are present in 60 to 75 percent of patients with this syndrome. The most common anomaly is a bifid rib or splayed ribs. This anomaly may involve several ribs and may be bilateral. Kyphoscoliosis has been observed in about 50 percent of patients, and a number of other anomalies, such as spina bifida occulta and shortened metacarpals, seem to occur with unusual frequency in these patients. A distinctive lamellar calcification of the falx cerebri, noted on an anteroposterior skull radiograph, is a common finding and is present in most affected patients (Fig. 15–23).

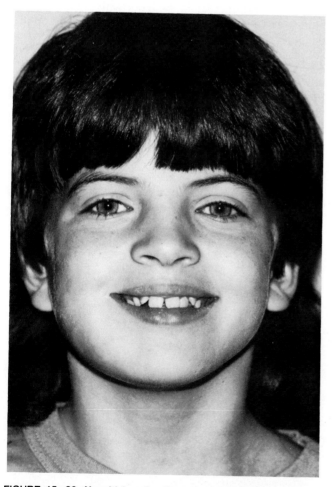

FIGURE 15–20. **Nevoid basal cell carcinoma syndrome.** This 11-year-old girl shows hypertelorism and mandibular swelling. (Courtesy of Dr. Richard DeChamplain.)

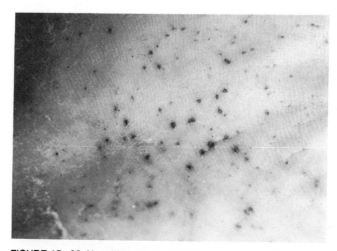

FIGURE 15–22. **Nevoid basal cell carcinoma syndrome.** Plantar pits.

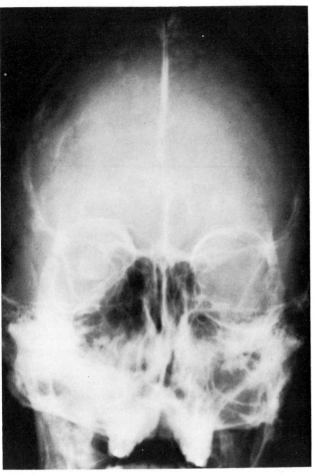

FIGURE 15–23. **Nevoid basal cell carcinoma syndrome.** Anteroposterior skull film showing calcification of the falx cerebri.

Ovarian fibromas and medulloblastomas occur with increased frequency in affected patients. Hyporesponsiveness to parathyroid hormone has also been reported to be a manifestation of this syndrome, but this has been recently questioned.

Jaw cysts are one of the most constant features of the syndrome and are present in at least 75 percent of the patients. The cysts are **odontogenic keratocysts**, although there are some differences between the cysts in patients with nevoid basal cell carcinoma syndrome and in those with isolated keratocysts. The cysts are frequently multiple; some patients have had as many as ten separate cysts. The patient's age when the first keratocyst is removed is significantly younger in those affected by this syndrome than in those with isolated keratocysts. For most patients with this syndrome, their first keratocyst is removed before age 19. About one third of patients with nevoid basal cell carcinoma syndrome have only a solitary cyst at the time of the initial presentation, but in most cases additional cysts will develop over periods ranging from 1 to 20 years.

Radiographically, the cysts in patients with nevoid basal cell carcinoma syndrome do not differ significantly from isolated keratocysts. The cysts in patients with this syndrome are often associated with the crowns of unerupted teeth; on radiographs they may mimic dentigerous cysts (Fig. 15–24).

Histopathologic Features

The cysts in the nevoid basal cell carcinoma syndrome histopathologically are invariably odontogenic keratocysts. The keratocysts in patients with this syndrome tend to have more satellite cysts, solid islands of epithelial proliferation, and odontogenic epithelial rests within the fibrous capsule than do isolated keratocysts (Fig. 15–25). These features, however, are not diagnostic for nevoid basal cell carcinoma syndrome because they may be seen in isolated keratocysts. The basal cell tumors of the skin exhibit a wide spectrum of histopathologic findings that range from benign adnexal basal cell lesions to aggressive, ulcerating basal cell carcinomas.

Treatment and Prognosis

Most of the anomalies in nevoid basal cell carcinoma syndrome are minor and usually not life-threatening.

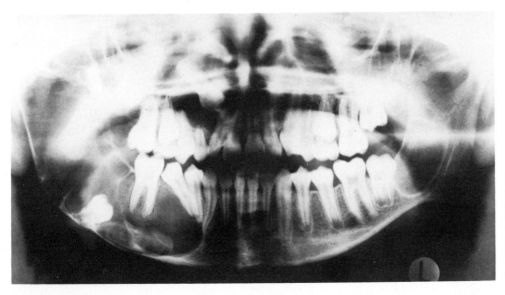

FIGURE 15–24. **Nevoid basal cell carcinoma syndrome.** Large cysts are present in the right and left mandibular molar regions together with a smaller cyst involving the right maxillary canine in the same patient shown in Figure 15–20. (Courtesy of Dr. Richard DeChamplain.)

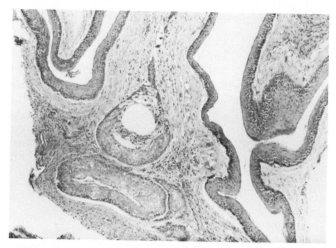

FIGURE 15-25. **Nevoid basal cell carcinoma syndrome.** The large cyst cavity shows a lining typical for an odontogenic keratocyst. Small satellite cysts and solid epithelial islands are present in the fibrous capsule.

The prognosis generally depends on the behavior of the skin tumors. In a few cases, aggressive basal cell carcinomas have caused the death of the patient as a result of tumor invasion of the brain or other vital structures (Fig. 15-26). The jaw cysts are treated by enucleation, but in many patients additional cysts will continue to develop. Varying degrees of jaw deformity may result from the operations for multiple cysts. Infection of the cysts in patients with this syndrome is also relatively common. Genetic counseling may be helpful.

GINGIVAL (ALVEOLAR) CYST OF THE NEWBORN

Gingival cysts of the newborn are small, superficial, keratin-filled cysts that are found on the alveolar mucosa

of infants. These cysts arise from remnants of the dental lamina. They are fairly common lesions, but because they disappear spontaneously by rupture into the oral cavity, the lesion is seldom noticed or sampled for biopsy. Similar inclusion cysts (e.g., **Epstein's pearls** and **Bohn's nodules**) are also found in the midline of the palate or laterally on the hard and soft palate (see p. 23).

Clinical Features

Gingival cysts of the newborn appear as small, usually multiple whitish papules on the mucosa overlying the alveolar processes of neonates (Fig. 15-27). The individual cysts are usually smaller than 2 mm in diameter. The maxillary alveolus is more commonly involved than the mandibular.

Histopathologic Features

Examination of an intact gingival cyst of the newborn shows a thin, flattened epithelial lining with a parakeratotic surface. The lumen contains keratinaceous debris.

Treatment and Prognosis

Treatment is not indicated for gingival cysts of the newborn because the lesions spontaneously involute as a result of the rupture of the cysts and resultant contact with the oral mucosal surface.

GINGIVAL CYST OF THE ADULT

The **gingival cyst of the adult** is an uncommon lesion. It is considered to represent the soft tissue counterpart of the **lateral periodontal cyst** (see next topic), being derived from rests of the dental lamina. The diagnosis of gingival cyst of the adult should be restricted to lesions with the same histopathologic features as those of the lateral periodontal cyst.

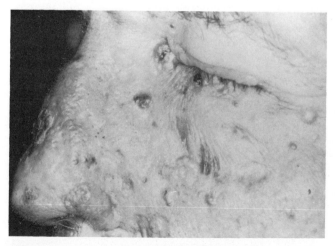

FIGURE 15-26. **Nevoid basal cell carcinoma syndrome.** This 52-year-old man had more than 100 basal cell carcinomas removed from his face over a 30-year period. Several basal cell carcinomas are present in this photograph. The lesion at the inner canthus of the eye was deeply invasive and was eventually fatal as a result of brain invasion.

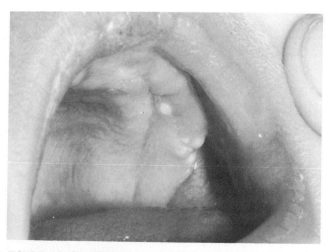

FIGURE 15-27. **Gingival cyst of the newborn.** Multiple whitish papules on the alveolar ridge of a newborn infant.

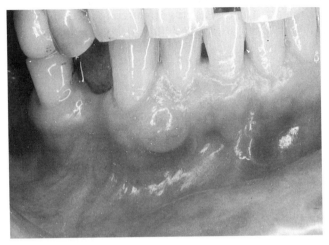

FIGURE 15-28. **Gingival cyst of the adult.** Tense, fluid-filled swelling on the facial gingiva.

Clinical Features

Like the lateral periodontal cyst, the gingival cyst of the adult shows a striking predilection to occur in the mandibular canine-premolar area (60 to 75 percent of cases). Gingival cysts of the adult are most commonly found in patients in the fifth and sixth decades of life. They are almost invariably located on the facial gingiva or alveolar mucosa. Maxillary gingival cysts are usually found in the incisor, canine, and premolar areas.

Clinically, the cysts appear as painless, dome-like swellings, usually less than 0.5 cm in diameter, although rarely they may be somewhat larger (Fig. 15-28; see Color Figure 91). They are often bluish or bluish-gray. In some instances, the cyst may cause a superficial "cupping-out" of the alveolar bone, which is usually not detected on a radiograph but is apparent when the cyst is excised. If more bone is missing, one could argue that the lesion may be a lateral periodontal cyst that has eroded the cortical bone rather than a gingival cyst that originated in the mucosa.

Histopathologic Features

In most cases, the histopathologic features of the gingival cyst of the adult are similar to those of the lateral periodontal cyst, consisting of a thin, flattened epithelial lining with or without focal plaques and isolated nests that contain clear cells (Fig. 15-29A, B). Some cysts of the gingiva show a thin layer of keratinized or non-keratinized squamous epithelium. Such cysts are also classified as gingival cysts by those who take a less restrictive view of the definition of the gingival cyst of the adult; however, these lesions probably represent epidermal inclusion cysts or peripheral odontogenic keratocysts.

Treatment and Prognosis

The gingival cyst of the adult responds well to simple surgical excision. The prognosis is excellent.

LATERAL PERIODONTAL CYST

The **lateral periodontal cyst** is a rare type of developmental odontogenic cyst that accounts for less than 2 percent of all epithelium-lined jaw cysts. The diagnosis of lateral periodontal cyst should be reserved for a cyst that occurs in the lateral periodontal region in which an inflammatory origin (see lateral radicular cyst, p. 105) or a diagnosis of odontogenic keratocyst has been excluded by clinical and histopathologic means.

The histogenesis of the lateral periodontal cyst is uncertain, but the lesion is believed to result from a proliferation of rests of the dental lamina. Others say that the lateral periodontal cyst may arise from the proliferation of the reduced enamel epithelium along the lateral root surface.

Clinical and Radiographic Features

The lateral periodontal cyst is most often an asymptomatic lesion that is detected only during a radiographic

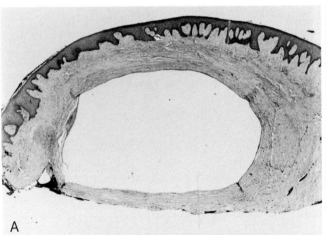

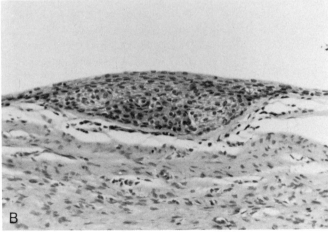

FIGURE 15-29. **Gingival cyst of the adult.** *A*, Cystic lesion with a thin epithelial lining in the gingival lamina propria. *B*, Higher magnification showing focal epithelial thickening (plaque) in the epithelial lining.

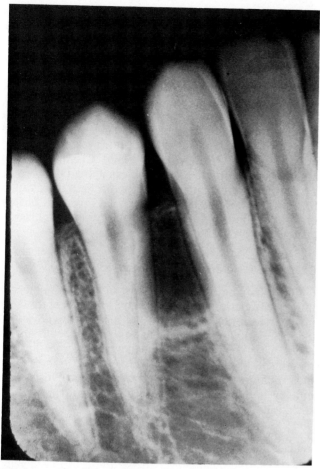

FIGURE 15–30. **Lateral periodontal cyst.** Radiolucent lesion between the roots of a vital mandibular canine and first premolar.

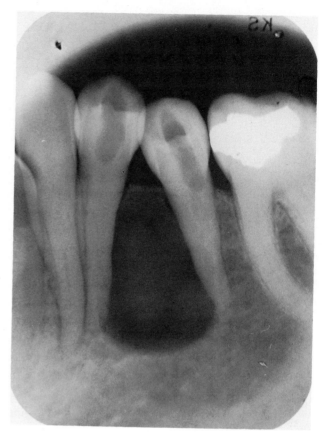

FIGURE 15–31. **Lateral periodontal cyst.** A larger lesion causing root divergence.

examination. It is usually encountered in patients older than age 30, and there is a male predilection. At least 65 percent of cases occur in the mandibular canine-premolar area. The less common maxillary examples are usually seen in the lateral incisor region.

Radiographically, the cyst presents as a well-circumscribed radiolucent area located laterally to the root(s) of vital teeth. Most such cysts are less than 1.0 cm in greatest diameter (Figs. 15–30 and 15–31).

Occasionally, the cyst may have a multilocular appearance. These lesions have been termed **botryoid odontogenic cysts**. Grossly and microscopically, they show a "grape-like" cluster of small individual cysts (Fig. 15–32). These lesions are generally considered to represent a variant of the lateral periodontal cyst, possibly the result of cystic degeneration and subsequent fusion of adjacent foci of dental lamina rests. The botryoid type may also appear unilocular on the radiograph but microscopically shows the clustering of multiple cysts.

The radiologic features of the lateral periodontal cyst are not diagnostic; an odontogenic keratocyst that develops between the roots of adjacent teeth may show identical radiographic findings. An inflammatory radicular cyst that occurs laterally to a root in relation to an accessory foramen or a cyst that arises from periodontal

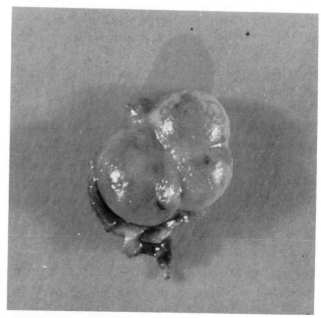

FIGURE 15–32. **Lateral periodontal cyst.** Gross specimen of a botryoid variant. Microscopically, three separate cysts formed this "grape-like" cluster.

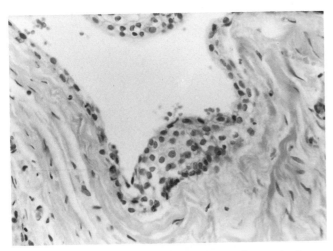

FIGURE 15–33. **Lateral periodontal cyst.** Photomicrograph of a portion of the cyst wall showing a thin lining of cuboidal epithelium. A localized thickened plaque containing clear cells is present.

inflammation may also simulate a lateral periodontal cyst radiographically (see p. 106). In one study of 46 cases of cystic lesions in the lateral periodontal region, only 13 met the histopathologic criteria for the lateral periodontal cyst. Eight were odontogenic keratocysts, 20 were inflammatory cysts, and five were of undetermined origin.

Histopathologic Features

The lateral periodontal cyst has a thin, generally non-inflamed, fibrous wall lined by a thin layer of squamous epithelium. The epithelial cells are often cuboidal. Foci of glycogen-rich clear cells may be interspersed among the lining epithelial cells. Some cysts show thickening of the lining epithelium, which is chiefly composed of clear cells (Fig. 15–33). Clear cell epithelial rests are sometimes seen within the fibrous wall.

Treatment and Prognosis

Conservative enucleation of the lateral periodontal cyst is the treatment of choice. This can usually be accomplished without damage to the adjacent teeth. Recurrence is unusual, although it has been reported with the botryoid variant. An exceedingly rare case of squamous cell carcinoma, which apparently originated in a lateral periodontal cyst, has also been reported.

CALCIFYING ODONTOGENIC CYST
(Gorlin Cyst)

The **calcifying odontogenic cyst** is an uncommon lesion that demonstrates considerable histopathologic diversity and variable clinical behavior. Although it is widely considered to represent a cyst, some investigators prefer to classify it as a neoplasm. Some calcifying odontogenic cysts appear to represent non-neoplastic cysts;

other members of this group, variously designated as **dentinogenic ghost cell tumors, epithelial odontogenic ghost cell tumors,** or **ghost cell tumors,** have no cystic features, may be infiltrative or even malignant, and are regarded as neoplasms.

In addition, the calcifying odontogenic cyst may be associated with other recognized odontogenic tumors, most commonly **odontomas.** However, **adenomatoid odontogenic tumors** and **ameloblastomas** have also been associated with calcifying odontogenic cysts. The revised World Health Organization (WHO) Classification of Odontogenic Tumors groups the calcifying odontogenic cyst with all its variants as an odontogenic tumor rather than an odontogenic cyst, although it admits that further experience may provide more reliable criteria for classification of the variants.

Clinical and Radiographic Features

The calcifying odontogenic cyst is predominantly an intraosseous lesion, although 13 to 21 percent of the cysts in reported series appeared as peripheral (extraosseous) lesions. Both the intraosseous and extraosseous forms occur with about equal frequency in the maxilla and mandible. About 65 percent of cases are found in the incisor-canine areas. Patients may range in age from infancy to elderly. The mean age is 33 years, and most cases are diagnosed in the second and third decades of life. Calcifying odontogenic cysts that are associated with odontomas tend to occur in younger patients, with a mean age of 17 years. The rare neoplastic variants of the calcifying odontogenic cyst appear to occur in older patients; because of the paucity of reported cases, however, this may not be significant.

Extraosseous calcifying odontogenic cysts present as localized sessile or pedunculated gingival masses with no distinctive clinical features. They can resemble common gingival fibromas, gingival cysts, or peripheral giant cell granulomas.

The central calcifying odontogenic cyst usually presents as a unilocular, well-defined radiolucency, although the lesion may occasionally appear multilocular. Radiopaque structures within the lesion, either irregular calcifications or tooth-like densities, are present in about 50 percent of cases (Fig. 15–34). In approximately one third of cases, the radiolucent lesion is associated with an unerupted tooth, most often a canine (Fig. 15–35). Most calcifying odontogenic cysts are between 2.0 and 4.0 cm in greatest diameter, but lesions as large as 12.0 cm have been noted. Root resorption or divergence of adjacent teeth is seen with some frequency (Fig. 15–36).

Histopathologic Features

The cystic (non-neoplastic) forms comprise 86 to 98 percent of all calcifying odontogenic cysts in various reported series. These may occur both intraosseously and extraosseously. Most commonly, a well-defined cystic lesion is found with a fibrous capsule and a lining of odontogenic epithelium of four to ten cells in thickness. The basal cells of the epithelial lining may be cuboidal or columnar and are similar to ameloblasts. The overlying

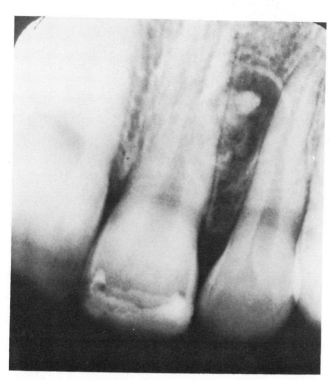

FIGURE 15–34. **Calcifying odontogenic cyst.** Maxillary radiolucent lesion containing calcified structures.

layer of loosely arranged epithelium may resemble the stellate reticulum of an ameloblastoma.

The most characteristic histopathologic feature of the calcifying odontogenic cyst is the presence of variable numbers of *ghost cells* within the epithelial component. These eosinophilic ghost cells are altered epithelial cells that are characterized by the loss of nuclei with preservation of the basic cell outline (Fig. 15–37).

The nature of the ghost cell change is controversial. Some believe that this change represents coagulative necrosis; others contend it is a form of normal or aberrant keratinization of odontogenic epithelium. Masses of ghost cells may fuse to form large sheets of amorphous,

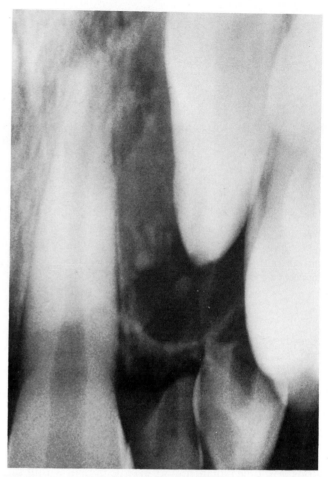

FIGURE 15–35. **Calcifying odontogenic cyst.** Radiolucent lesion associated with an unerupted maxillary canine. Fine calcifications are present in the lesion. (Courtesy of Dr. Bob M. Crider.)

acellular material. Calcification within the ghost cells is common. This first appears as fine basophilic granules within the ghost cells. The granules may increase in size and number to form extensive masses of calcified material. Areas of an eosinophilic matrix material that are

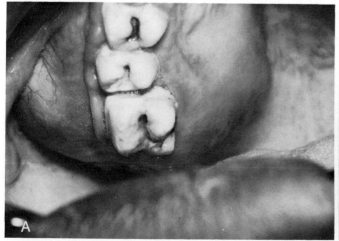

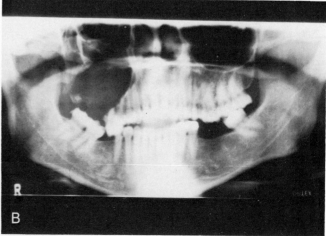

FIGURE 15–36. **Calcifying odontogenic cyst.** *A*, Expansion of the posterior maxillary alveolus caused by a large calcifying odontogenic cyst. *B*, Panoramic radiograph of the same patient shown in *A*. Note the large radiolucent area in the posterior maxilla. A small calcified structure is seen in the lower portion of the cyst. (*A* and *B*, Courtesy of Dr. Tom Brock.)

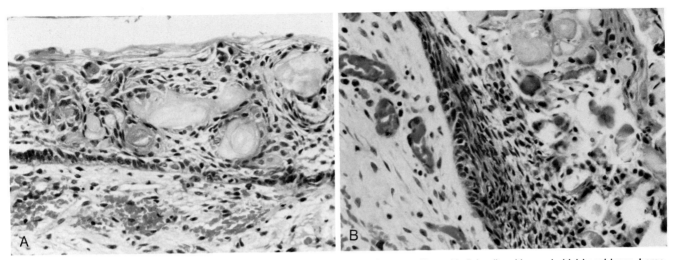

FIGURE 15–37. **Calcifying odontogenic cyst.** *A,* The cyst lining shows ameloblastoma-like epithelial cells with a cuboidal basal layer. Large eosinophilic ghost cells are present within the epithelial lining. *B,* Calcifications are present in the ghost cells.

considered to represent dysplastic dentin (dentinoid) may also be present adjacent to the epithelial component. This is widely believed to be the result of an inductive effect by the odontogenic epithelium on the adjacent mesenchymal tissue (Fig. 15–38).

Several variants of the cystic type of calcifying odontogenic cyst are seen. In some cases, the epithelial lining proliferates into the lumen so that the lumen is largely filled with masses of ghost cells and dystrophic calcifications. Multiple daughter cysts may be present within the fibrous wall, and a foreign-body reaction to herniated ghost cells may be conspicuous.

In another variant, unifocal or multifocal epithelial proliferation of the cyst lining into the lumen may resemble ameloblastoma. These proliferations are intermixed with varying numbers of ghost cells. These epithelial proliferations superficially resemble, but do not meet the strict histopathologic criteria for, ameloblastoma.

About 20 percent of cystic calcifying odontogenic cysts are associated with **odontomas**. This variant is usually a unicystic lesion that shows the features of calcifying odontogenic cyst together with those of a small complex or compound odontoma.

Neoplastic (solid) calcifying odontogenic cysts are uncommon, accounting for 2 to 16 percent of all calcifying odontogenic cysts in reported series. These may occur intraosseously or extraosseously.

The *extraosseous* forms of the solid variant appear to be the most common. These show varying-sized islands of odontogenic epithelium in a fibrous stroma. The epithelial islands show peripheral palisaded columnar cells and central stellate reticulum, which resemble ameloblastoma. Nests of ghost cells, however, are present within the epithelium, and juxtaepithelial dentinoid is commonly present. These features differentiate this lesion from the peripheral ameloblastoma.

The rare *intraosseous* variant is a solid tumor that consists of ameloblastoma-like strands and islands of odontogenic epithelium in a mature fibrous connective tissue stroma. Variable numbers of ghost cells and juxtaepithelial dentinoid are present.

A small number of aggressive or malignant epithelial odontogenic ghost cell tumors have been reported. These lesions have cellular pleomorphism and mitotic activity with invasion of the surrounding tissues (Fig. 15–39*A,* *B*).

Treatment and Prognosis

The prognosis for a patient with cystic calcifying odontogenic cyst is good; only a few recurrences after simple enucleation have been reported. The prognosis for those with the neoplastic types is less certain because of the rarity of this lesion. The peripheral neoplastic calcifying odontogenic cyst appears to be associated with the same prognosis as that for a peripheral ameloblastoma, with minimal chance of recurrence after simple surgical excision.

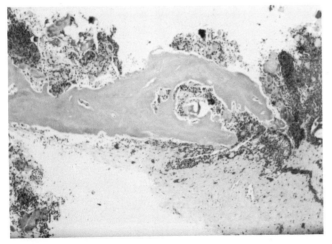

FIGURE 15–38. **Calcifying odontogenic cyst.** Eosinophilic matrix material (dentinoid) is present adjacent to the epithelial lining.

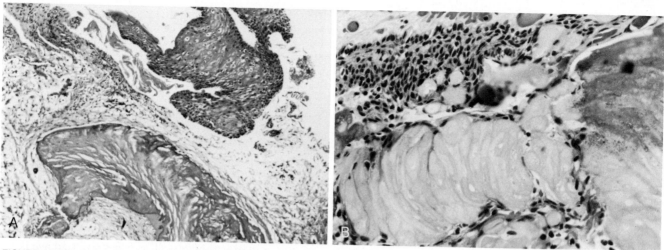

FIGURE 15–39. **Calcifying odontogenic cyst–epithelial odontogenic ghost cell tumor.** *A,* A mass of calcified ghost cells is present (*bottom*). The proliferating epithelium (*top*) shows epithelial atypia. This lesion was interpreted as a squamous carcinoma arising in a calcifying odontogenic cyst. *B,* Higher magnification from another portion of the same specimen showing ghost cells, early calcification, and hyperchromatic, atypical epithelial cells.

The outlook for the aggressive intraosseous epithelial odontogenic ghost cell tumors is less certain because of the few known cases. Two reported patients died as a result of invasion of vital structures or presumed metastasis. When a calcifying odontogenic cyst is associated with some other recognized odontogenic tumor, such as an ameloblastoma, the treatment and prognosis are likely to be the same as for the associated tumor.

GLANDULAR ODONTOGENIC CYST

In rare instances, jaw cysts are encountered that microscopically do not fit into established classifications. Terms such as **mucoepidermoid odontogenic cyst** and **sialo-odontogenic cyst** have been used to designate one such lesion. The term **glandular odontogenic cyst** has been proposed as the most appropriate designation for this lesion because of its glandular differentiation. Although this cyst clearly appears to be of odontogenic origin, its pathogenesis is unknown.

Clinical and Radiographic Features

The paucity of reported cases of glandular odontogenic cysts precludes any reliable data as to age or sex predilection or the most common location. Most reported examples have been located in the mandible of adults. Smaller glandular odontogenic cysts are asymptomatic, although larger cysts may cause bony expansion.

Radiographically, the lesion may appear as a unilocular or, more commonly, a multilocular radiolucency. The margins of the radiolucency are usually well defined with a sclerotic rim (Fig. 15–40).

Histopathologic Features

The glandular odontogenic cyst is lined by squamous epithelium of varying thickness. The interface between

the epithelium and the fibrous connective tissue wall is generally flat. The fibrous cyst wall is usually devoid of any inflammatory cell infiltrate. The superficial epithelial cells that line the cyst cavity tend to be cuboidal and have an irregular and sometimes papillary surface. Cilia

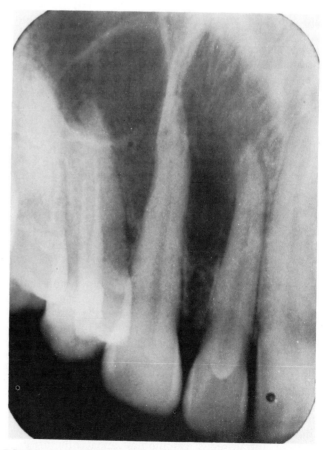

FIGURE 15–40. **Glandular odontogenic cyst.** Multilocular radiolucent lesion in the anterior maxilla. (Courtesy of Dr. Ed Marshall.)

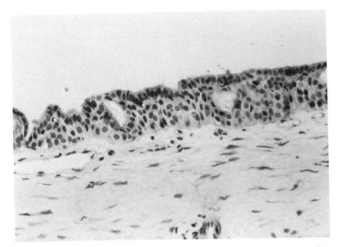

FIGURE 15–41. **Glandular odontogenic cyst.** Multiple cyst-like spaces lined by cuboidal epithelium are present within the epithelial lining. The superficial epithelial cells of the cyst lining are cuboidal, and a few show cilia.

may occasionally be noted. Pools of mucicarminophilic material are often present within the epithelium. These pools are usually lined with cuboidal cells (Fig. 15–41). Mucous cells may or may not be present within the epithelium. In focal areas, the epithelial lining cells may form spherical nodules, similar to those seen in lateral periodontal cysts. There is some histopathologic overlap between the features of the glandular odontogenic cyst and those of some intraosseous, low-grade, predominantly cystic mucoepidermoid carcinomas (see p. 351). In selected microscopic fields, the microscopic features may be identical. Examination of multiple sections, however, usually permits the differentiation of these lesions.

Treatment and Prognosis

In some cases of glandular odontogenic cyst, recurrence has been noted after curettage, but the number of reported cases is too small to draw reliable conclusions as to the behavior of these cysts. It appears, however, that the overall prognosis is good.

CARCINOMA ARISING IN ODONTOGENIC CYSTS

Carcinoma arising within bone is a rare lesion that is essentially limited to the jaws. Because the putative source of the epithelium giving rise to the carcinoma is odontogenic, these intraosseous jaw carcinomas are collectively known as **odontogenic carcinomas**. Odontogenic carcinomas may arise in an ameloblastoma, rarely from other odontogenic tumors, *de novo* (without evidence of a pre-existing lesion), or from the epithelial lining of odontogenic cysts. Some intraosseous mucoepidermoid carcinomas (see p. 351) may also arise from mucous cells lining a dentigerous cyst.

Most intraosseous carcinomas apparently arise in odontogenic cysts. Although there are probably fewer than 100 well-documented cases in the literature, carcinomatous transformation of the lining of an odontogenic cyst may be more common than is generally appreciated. Several studies have shown that 1 to 2 percent of all oral cavity carcinomas seen in some oral and maxillofacial pathology services may originate from odontogenic cysts. The pathogenesis of carcinomas arising in odontogenic cysts is unknown. Occasionally, areas within the lining of odontogenic cysts histopathologically demonstrate varying degrees of epithelial dysplasia, and such changes likely give rise to the carcinoma (Fig. 15–42).

Clinical and Radiographic Features

Although carcinomas arising in cysts may be seen in patients over a wide age range, they are most often encountered in older patients. The mean reported age is 59 years. This lesion is about twice as common in men as in women. Pain and swelling are the most common complaints. However, many patients have no symptoms, and the diagnosis of carcinoma is made only after microscopic examination of a presumed odontogenic cyst.

Radiographic findings may mimic those of any odontogenic cyst, although the margins of the radiolucent defect are usually irregular and "ragged." A lesion considered to be a **residual periapical cyst** is apparently the most common type associated with carcinomatous transformation. In about 25 percent of reported cases, the carcinoma appeared to have arisen in a **dentigerous cyst** (Fig. 15–43). A few examples of carcinoma arising in an **odontogenic keratocyst** have also been documented (Fig. 15–44); in one patient, the carcinoma appeared to originate in a **lateral periodontal cyst**.

Histopathologic Features

Most carcinomas arising in cysts have histopathologically been well-differentiated **squamous cell carcinomas**. It is sometimes possible to identify a transition from a normal-appearing cyst lining to invasive squamous cell carcinoma (Figs. 15–45 and 15–46).

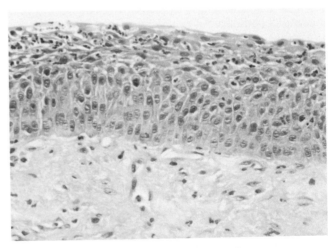

FIGURE 15–42. **Epithelial dysplasia in a dentigerous cyst.** This was an incidental finding in histopathologic study of an otherwise typical dentigerous cyst in a middle-aged man.

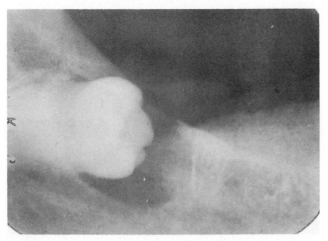

FIGURE 15–43. **Carcinoma arising in a dentigerous cyst.** Radiolucent lesion surrounding the crown of an impacted third molar in a 56-year-old white woman. This was clinically considered to be a dentigerous cyst. (Courtesy of Dr. Richard Ziegler.)

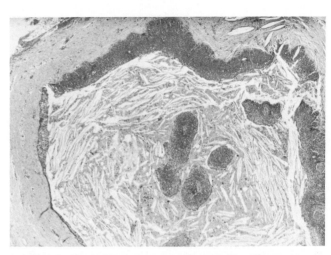

FIGURE 15–45. **Carcinoma arising in a cyst.** Low-power view of a dentigerous cyst from a 53-year-old man. A thin, benign stratified epithelial lining is present (*lower left*). This merges into the thicker, more darkly staining lining, which is microscopically carcinoma *in situ*. Invasive carcinoma was found in other portions of the specimen.

Treatment and Prognosis

The treatment of patients with carcinomas arising in cysts has varied from local block excision to radical resection, with or without radiation or adjunctive chemotherapy. The prognosis is difficult to evaluate because most reports consist of isolated cases; often, the follow-up is inadequate. Several larger studies indicate an approximate 50 percent 5-year survival rate after treatment. Metastases to regional lymph nodes have been demonstrated in a few cases.

Before a given lesion can be accepted as an example of primary intraosseous carcinoma, the possibility that the tumor represents metastatic spread from an intraoral or extraoral site must be ruled out by appropriate studies.

Odontogenic Tumors

Odontogenic tumors comprise a complex group of lesions of diverse histopathologic types and clinical behavior. Some of these lesions are true neoplasms and may rarely exhibit malignant behavior. Others may represent tumor-like malformations (hamartomas).

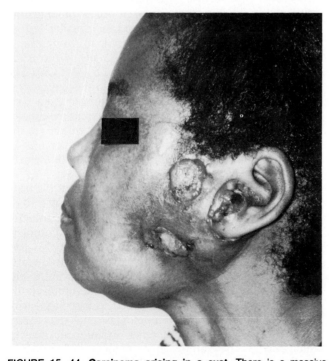

FIGURE 15–44. **Carcinoma arising in a cyst.** There is a massive carcinoma of the mandible with extension into the parotid gland, the face, and the base of the brain. Nineteen years previously, a large odontogenic keratocyst with areas of epithelial dysplasia had been removed from the ascending ramus. The patient had suffered multiple recurrences with eventual change into invasive carcinoma.

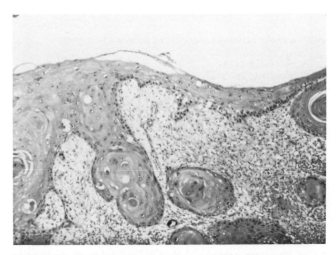

FIGURE 15–46. **Carcinoma arising in a cyst.** Well-differentiated squamous cell carcinoma arising in a large residual cyst of the mandible.

Odontogenic tumors, like normal odontogenesis, demonstrate varying inductive interactions between odontogenic epithelium and odontogenic ectomesenchyme (mesodermal elements). Some odontogenic tumors are composed only of odontogenic epithelium without any participation of odontogenic ectomesenchyme.

Others, sometimes referred to as **mixed odontogenic tumors**, are composed of odontogenic epithelium and ectomesenchymal elements. Dental hard tissue may or may not be formed in these lesions.

A third group of odontogenic tumors are composed principally of odontogenic ectomesenchyme. Odontogenic epithelium may be included within these lesions, but it does not play any essential role in their pathogenesis.

Table 15–2 presents categories of odontogenic tumors based on the 1992 World Health Organization (WHO) classification.

Tumors of Odontogenic Epithelium Without Odontogenic Ectomesenchyme

Epithelial odontogenic tumors are composed of odontogenic epithelium without participation of odontogenic ectomesenchyme. Four different tumors are included in the group; ameloblastoma is the most important and common of them.

AMELOBLASTOMA

The **ameloblastoma** is the most common clinically significant odontogenic tumor. Its relative frequency equals the combined frequency of all other odontogenic tumors,

---

Table 15–2. CLASSIFICATION OF ODONTOGENIC TUMORS

A. Tumors of odontogenic epithelium without odontogenic ectomesenchyme
  1. Ameloblastoma
  2. Calcifying epithelial odontogenic tumor
  3. Squamous odontogenic tumor
  4. Clear cell odontogenic tumor

B. Tumors of odontogenic epithelium with odontogenic ectomesenchyme, with or without dental hard tissue formation
  1. Ameloblastic fibroma
  2. Ameloblastic fibro-odontoma
  3. Tumors of odontoameloblastoma
  4. Adenomatoid odontogenic tumor
  5. Complex odontoma
  6. Compound odontoma

C. Tumors of odontogenic ectomesenchyme with or without included odontogenic epithelium
  1. Odontogenic fibroma
  2. Myxoma
  3. Cementoblastoma

---

excluding odontomas. Ameloblastomas are tumors of odontogenic epithelial origin. Theoretically, they may arise from cell rests of the enamel organ, from a developing enamel organ, from the epithelial lining of an odontogenic cyst, or from the basal cells of the oral mucosa. Ameloblastomas are slow-growing, locally invasive tumors that run a benign course in most cases.

Ameloblastomas occur in three different clinicoradiologic situations, which deserve separate consideration because of differing therapeutic considerations and prognosis. These are:

1. Conventional solid or multicystic (about 86 percent of all cases).
2. Unicystic (about 13 percent of all cases).
3. Peripheral (extraosseous) (about 1 percent of all cases).

Conventional Solid or Multicystic Intraosseous Ameloblastoma

Clinical and Radiographic Features

Conventional solid or multicystic intraosseous ameloblastoma is encountered in patients over a wide age range. It is rare in children younger than age 10 and relatively uncommon in the 10- to 19-year-old group. The tumor shows an approximately equal prevalence in the third to seventh decades of life. There is no significant gender predilection. Some studies indicate a greater frequency in blacks; others show no racial predilection. The tumor is often asymptomatic, and smaller lesions are detected only during a radiographic examination. A painless swelling or expansion of the jaw is the usual clinical presentation (Figs. 15–47 to 15–49A, B). The lesion may grow slowly to massive or grotesque proportions. Pain and paresthesia are uncommon, even with large tumors. About 85 percent of conventional ameloblastomas occur in the mandible, most often in the molar–ascending ramus area. About 15 percent of ameloblastomas occur in the maxilla, usually in the posterior regions.

The most typical radiographic feature is that of a multilocular radiolucent lesion. The lesion is often described as having a "soap bubble" appearance when the radiolucent loculations are large and as being "honeycombed" when the loculations are small (Figs. 15–50 to 15–53). Buccal and lingual cortical expansion is frequently present. Resorption of the roots of teeth adjacent to the tumor is common. In many cases, an unerupted tooth, most often a mandibular third molar, is associated with the radiolucent defect. Solid ameloblastomas may radiographically present as unilocular radiolucent defects, which may resemble almost any type of cystic lesion. The margins of these radiolucent lesions, however, often show irregular scalloping. Although the radiographic features, particularly of the typical multilocular defect, may be highly suggestive of ameloblastoma, a variety of odontogenic and non-odontogenic lesions may show similar radiographic features.

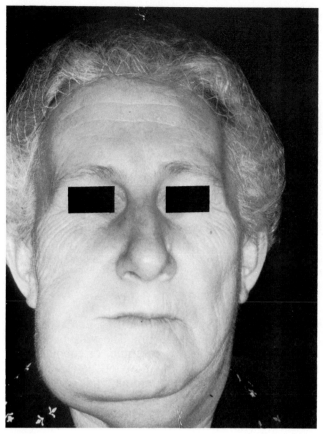

FIGURE 15-47. **Ameloblastoma.** Facial asymmetry caused by a large mandibular ameloblastoma of 10 years' duration.

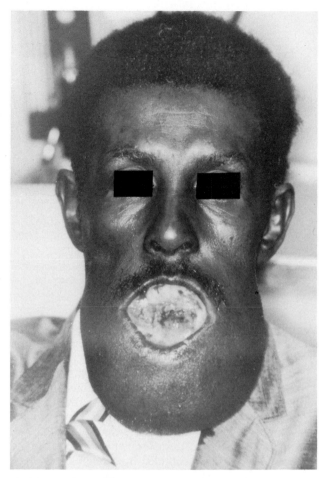

FIGURE 15-48. **Ameloblastoma.** Massive tumor of the anterior mandible. (Courtesy of Dr. Ronald Baughman.)

Histopathologic Features

Conventional solid or multicystic intraosseous ameloblastomas show a remarkable tendency to undergo cystic change; grossly, most tumors have varying combinations of cystic and solid features. The cysts may be seen only at the microscopic level or may be present as multiple large cysts that include most of the tumor. Several microscopic subtypes of conventional ameloblastomas

are recognized, but these microscopic patterns generally have little bearing on the behavior of the tumor. Large tumors often show a combination of microscopic patterns.

The *follicular* and *plexiform* patterns are the most

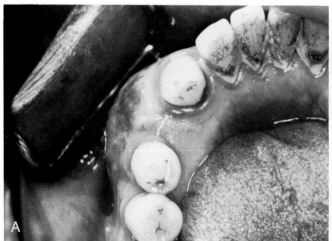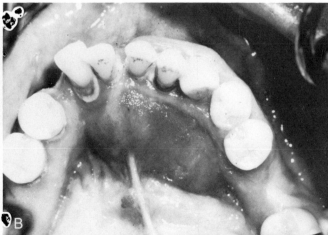

FIGURE 15-49. **Ameloblastoma.** *A,* Localized enlargement of the mandible caused by an ameloblastoma. *B,* Prominent expansion of the lingual alveolus caused by a large ameloblastoma of the mandibular symphysis. The radiograph of the patient is shown in Figure 15-53.

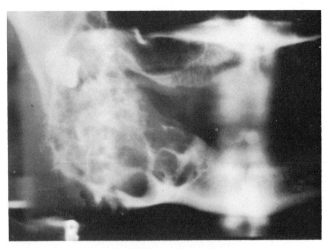

FIGURE 15–50. **Ameloblastoma.** Large multilocular lesion involving the mandibular angle and ascending ramus. The large loculations show the "soap bubble" appearance. An unerupted third molar has been displaced high into the ramus.

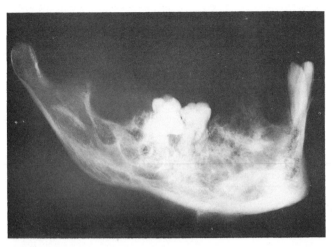

FIGURE 15–52. **Ameloblastoma.** Radiograph of a hemimandibulectomy specimen. The tumor extends from the coronoid notch to the midline area.

common. Less common histopathologic patterns include the *acanthomatous, granular cell, desmoplastic,* and *basal cell* types.

Follicular Pattern. The follicular histopathologic pattern is the most common and recognizable. Islands of epithelium resemble enamel organ epithelium in a mature fibrous connective tissue stroma. The epithelial nests consist of a core of loosely arranged angular cells resembling the stellate reticulum of an enamel organ. This central core is surrounded by a single layer of tall columnar ameloblast-like cells. The nuclei of these cells are located at the opposite pole to the basement membrane (*reversed polarity*). In other areas, the peripheral cells may be more cuboidal and resemble basal cells. Cyst formation is common and may vary from microcysts, which form within the epithelial islands, to large macroscopic cysts, which may be several or more centimeters in diameter (Figs. 15–54 and 15–55*A, B*).

Plexiform Pattern. The plexiform type of ameloblas-

toma consists of long, anastomosing cords or larger sheets of odontogenic epithelium. The cords or sheets of epithelium are bounded by columnar or cuboidal ameloblast-like cells surrounding more loosely arranged epithelial cells. The supporting stroma tends to be loosely arranged and vascular. Cyst formation is relatively uncommon in this variety. When it occurs, it is more often associated with stromal degeneration rather than cystic change within the epithelium (Fig. 15–56).

Acanthomatous Pattern. When extensive squamous metaplasia, often associated with keratin formation, occurs in the central portions of the epithelial islands of a follicular ameloblastoma, the term **acanthomatous ameloblastoma** is sometimes applied. This change does not indicate a more aggressive course for the lesion; histopathologically, however, such a lesion may be confused with squamous cell carcinoma or squamous odontogenic tumor (Fig. 15–57).

Granular Cell Pattern. Ameloblastomas may some-

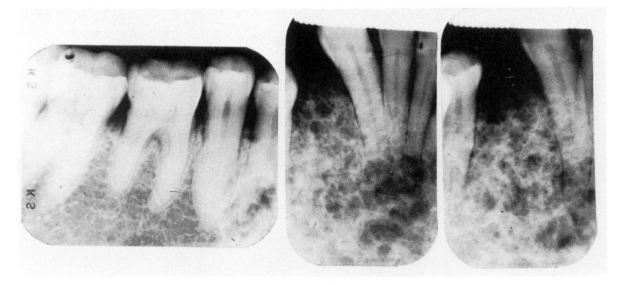

FIGURE 15–51. **Ameloblastoma.** Periapical films showing the "honeycombed" appearance. (Courtesy of Dr. John Hann.)

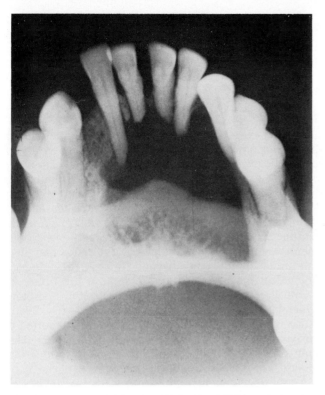

FIGURE 15–53. **Ameloblastoma.** Unilocular radiolucent lesion associated with root resorption of the anterior teeth. (Courtesy of Dr. Richard Brock.)

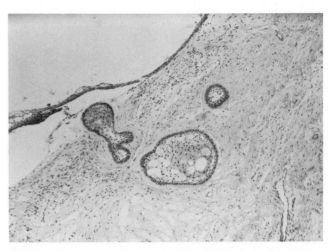

FIGURE 15–54. **Ameloblastoma, follicular pattern.** Three small follicular islands are present in a fibrous stroma. A portion of a large cyst is present in the upper half of the photograph. The epithelial lining of the large cyst is flattened as a result of cyst pressure and does not show the typical microscopic features of ameloblastoma.

times show transformation of groups of epithelial cells to granular cells. These cells have abundant cytoplasm filled with eosinophilic granules. The nature of this granular change is unknown. The eosinophilic cytoplasmic granules resemble lysosomes at the ultrastructural and histochemical levels. Although it was originally considered to represent an aging or degenerative change in longstanding lesions, this variant has been seen in young patients

and in clinically aggressive tumors. When this granular cell change is extensive in an ameloblastoma, the designation of **granular cell ameloblastoma** is appropriate (Fig. 15–58).

Desmoplastic Pattern. The desmoplastic variant of ameloblastoma has been recently recognized. This type contains small islands and cords of odontogenic epithelium in a densely collagenized stroma. Peripheral columnar ameloblast-like cells are inconspicuous about the epithelial islands (Fig. 15–59*A, B*). This variant has a marked predilection to occur in the anterior regions of the jaws, particularly the maxilla. Radiographically, this type seldom suggests the diagnosis of ameloblastoma and usually resembles a fibro-osseous lesion because of its mixed radiolucent and radiopaque appearance (Fig. 15–60).

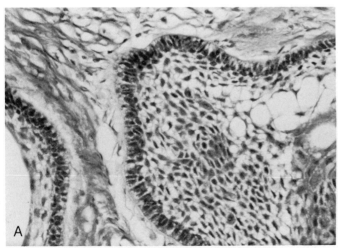

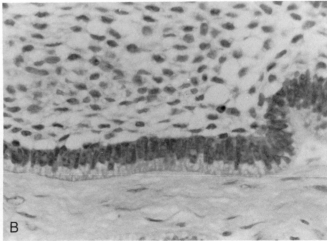

FIGURE 15–55. **Ameloblastoma, follicular pattern.** *A*, The columnar peripheral cells resemble ameloblasts with reverse polarity of their nuclei. The central portions of the islands show loosely arranged epithelial cells resembling the stellate reticulum of the enamel organ. Early microcyst formation is seen. *B*, Higher magnification showing reverse polarity and basal cytoplasmic vacuolization of the peripheral cells.

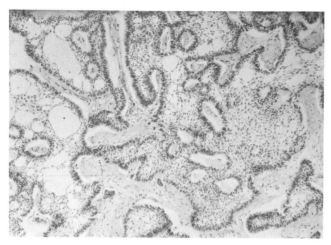

FIGURE 15–56. **Ameloblastoma, plexiform pattern.** Large anastomosing sheets of epithelium bounded by columnar ameloblast-like cells.

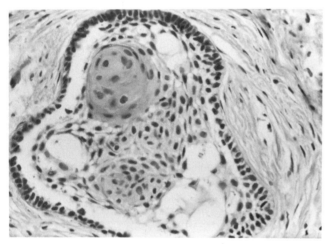

FIGURE 15–57. **Ameloblastoma, acanthomatous pattern.** A focus of squamous metaplasia with keratin formation is present in this tumor island.

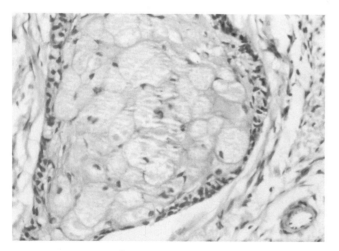

FIGURE 15–58. **Ameloblastoma, granular cell variant.** The central portion of this follicular nest is filled with large eosinophilic granular cells. The cuboidal peripheral cells retain their ameloblastic features.

Basaloid Pattern. The basaloid variant of ameloblastoma is the least common type. These lesions are composed of nests of uniform basaloid cells. No stellate reticulum is present in the central portions of the nests. The peripheral cells about the nests tend to be cuboidal rather than columnar (Fig. 15–61).

Treatment and Prognosis

Patients with conventional solid or multicystic intraosseous ameloblastomas have been treated by a variety of means. These range from simple enucleation and curettage to *en bloc* resection. The optimal method of treatment has been the subject of controversy for many years. The conventional ameloblastoma tends to infiltrate between intact cancellous bone trabeculae at the periphery of the lesion before bone resorption becomes radiographically evident. Therefore, the actual margin of the tumor often extends beyond its apparent radiologic or clinical margin. Attempts to remove the tumor by curettage leave small islands of tumor within the bone, which later manifest as recurrences (Fig. 15–62). Recurrence rates of 55 to 90 percent have been reported in various studies after curettage. Recurrence often takes many years to become clinically manifest, and 5-year disease-free periods do not indicate a cure.

Marginal resection is the most widely used treatment, but recurrence rates of up to 15 percent have been reported after marginal or block resection. Many surgeons advocate that the margin of the resection should be at least 1.0 cm past the radiographic limits of the tumor. Ameloblastomas of the posterior maxilla are particularly dangerous because of the difficulty of obtaining an adequate surgical margin around the tumor. Radiation therapy has seldom been used for ameloblastomas, although some studies suggest that the tumor may be radiosensitive.

The conventional ameloblastoma is a persistent, infiltrative neoplasm that may kill the patient by progressive spread to involve vital structures. Most of these tumors, however, are not life-threatening lesions. Rarely, an ameloblastoma exhibits frank malignant behavior. These are discussed separately.

Unicystic Ameloblastoma

The **unicystic ameloblastoma** deserves separate consideration on the basis of its clinical, radiologic, and pathologic features and its response to treatment. Unicystic ameloblastomas account for 10 to 15 percent of all intraosseous ameloblastomas in various studies. Whether the unicystic ameloblastoma originates *de novo* as a neoplasm or whether it is the result of neoplastic transformation of non-neoplastic cyst epithelium has been long debated. Both mechanisms probably occur, but proof of which is involved in an individual patient is virtually impossible to obtain.

Clinical and Radiographic Features

Unicystic ameloblastomas are most often seen in younger patients, with about 50 percent of all such

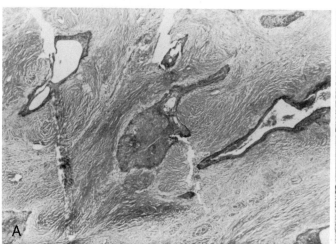

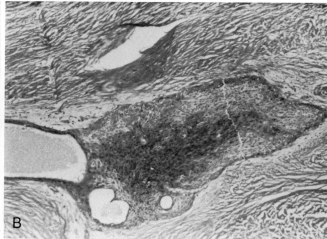

FIGURE 15-59. **Ameloblastoma, desmoplastic variant.** A, Small nests of tumor cells are present in an abundant, densely collagenized stroma. B, Higher magnification showing lack of columnar cells at the periphery of the tumor islands. The central epithelial cells are spindle-shaped.

tumors diagnosed during the second decade of life. The average age in one large series was 23 years. More than 90 percent of unicystic ameloblastomas are found in the mandible, usually in the posterior regions. The lesion is often asymptomatic, although large lesions may cause a painless swelling of the jaws.

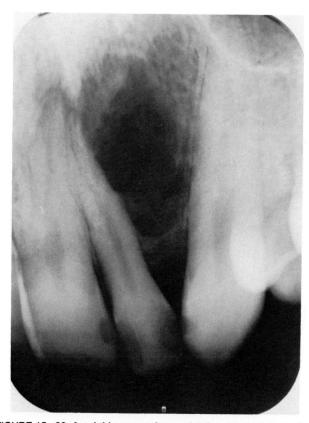

FIGURE 15-60. **Ameloblastoma, desmoplastic variant.** Periapical radiograph showing an ill-defined mixed radiolucent/radiopaque lesion. (From Waldron CA. The importance of histologic study of the various radiolucent areas of the jaws. Oral Surg Oral Med Oral Pathol 12:19-30, 1959.)

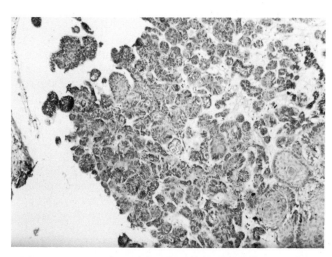

FIGURE 15-61. **Ameloblastoma, basal cell variant.** The tumor is composed of nests of basaloid-appearing cells bounded by cuboidal cells.

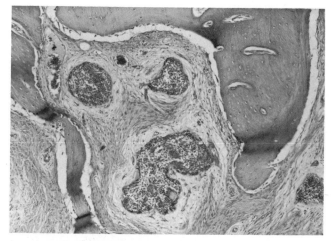

FIGURE 15-62. **Ameloblastoma.** Follicular islands infiltrating marrow spaces between cancellous bone trabeculae.

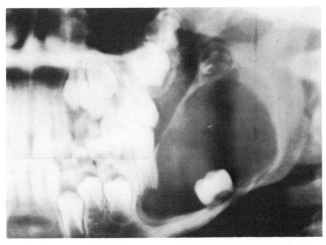

FIGURE 15-63. **Unicystic ameloblastoma.** A large radiolucency in a 7-year-old boy with displacement of the developing second molar to the inferior border of the mandible. This was believed to be a large dentigerous cyst. (Courtesy of Dr. Larry Chewning.)

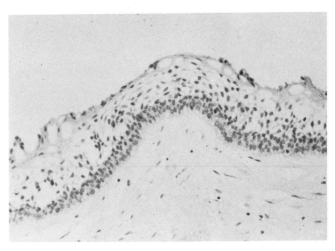

FIGURE 15-65. **Unicystic ameloblastoma, luminal type.** The cyst is lined with ameloblastic epithelium showing a hyperchromatic, polarized basal layer. The overlying epithelial cells are loosely cohesive and resemble stellate reticulum.

In many patients, this lesion typically appears as a circumscribed radiolucency that surrounds the crown of an unerupted mandibular third molar (Fig. 15-63). Other tumors simply appear as sharply defined radiolucent areas. These are usually considered to be a primordial, radicular, or residual cyst, depending on the relationship of the lesion to teeth in the area. (Fig. 15-64). In some instances, the radiolucent area may have scalloped margins but is still a unicystic ameloblastoma.

The surgical findings may also suggest that the lesion in question is a cyst, and the diagnosis of ameloblastoma is made only after microscopic study of the specimen.

Histopathologic Features

Three histopathologic variants of unicystic ameloblastoma may be seen. In the first type (**luminal ameloblastoma**), the tumor is confined to the luminal surface of the cyst. The lesion consists of a fibrous cyst wall with a lining that consists totally or partially of ameloblastic epithelium. This demonstrates a basal layer of columnar or cuboidal cells with hyperchromatic nuclei that show reverse polarity and basilar cytoplasmic vacuolization. The overlying epithelial cells are loosely cohesive and resemble stellate reticulum. This finding does not seem to be related to inflammatory edema (Fig. 15-65).

In the second microscopic variant, one or more nodules of ameloblastoma project from the cystic lining into the lumen of the cyst. This type is called an **intraluminal ameloblastoma**. These nodules may be relatively small or largely fill the cystic lumen. In some cases, the nodule of tumor that projects into the lumen demonstrates an edematous, plexiform pattern that resembles the plexiform pattern seen in conventional ameloblastomas. These lesions are sometimes referred to as **plexiform unicystic ameloblastomas**. The intraluminal cellular proliferation does not always meet the strict histopathologic criteria for ameloblastoma, but more typical ameloblastoma is usually found in other parts of the specimen (Fig. 15-66A, B).

In the third variant, known as **mural ameloblastoma**, the fibrous wall of the cyst is infiltrated by typical follicular or plexiform ameloblastoma. The extent and depth of the ameloblastic infiltration may vary considerably, and multiple sections through many levels of the specimen are needed to determine the extent of the tumor (Fig. 15-67).

Treatment and Prognosis

The clinical and radiologic findings in most cases of unicystic ameloblastoma suggest that the lesion is an odontogenic cyst. These tumors are usually treated as cysts by enucleation. The diagnosis of ameloblastoma is made only after microscopic examination of the presumed cyst. If the ameloblastic elements are confined to the lumen of the cyst with or without intraluminal tumor

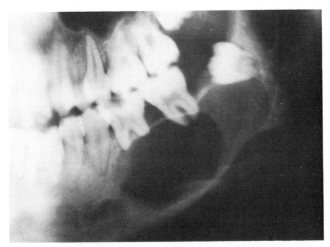

FIGURE 15-64. **Unicystic ameloblastoma.** Large unicystic lesion showing root resorption of the first and second molar teeth.

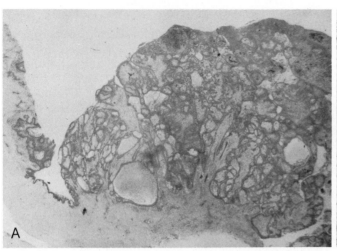
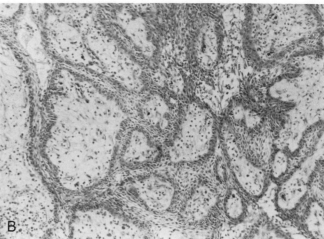

FIGURE 15–66. **Unicystic ameloblastoma, intraluminal plexiform type.** *A,* Photomicrograph of the intraluminal mass arising from the cyst wall in the same patient shown in Figure 15–63. *B,* Higher magnification of the intraluminal mass.

extension, the cyst enucleation has probably been adequate treatment. The patient, however, should be kept under long-term follow-up. If the specimen shows extension of the tumor into the fibrous cyst wall for any appreciable distance, subsequent management of the patient is more controversial. Some surgeons believe that local resection of the area is indicated as a prophylactic measure; others prefer to keep the patient under close radiographic observation and delay further treatment until there is evidence of recurrence.

Recurrence rates of 10 to 20 percent have been reported after enucleation and curettage of unicystic ameloblastomas. This is considerably less than the 50 to 90 percent recurrence rates noted after curettage of conventional solid and multicystic intraosseous ameloblastomas.

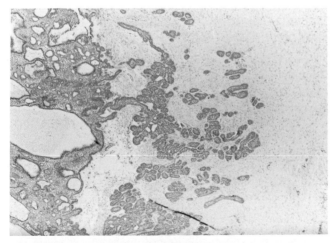

FIGURE 15–67. **Unicystic ameloblastoma, mural type.** Islands of follicular ameloblastoma are infiltrating into the fibrous cyst capsule. A plexiform intraluminal projection is seen (*left*).

Peripheral (Extraosseous) Ameloblastoma

The **peripheral ameloblastoma** is uncommon and accounts for about 1 percent of all ameloblastomas. This tumor probably arises from odontogenic epithelial rests beneath the oral mucosa or from the basal epithelial cells of the surface epithelium. Histopathologically, these lesions have the same features as the intraosseous form of the tumor.

Clinical Features

The peripheral ameloblastoma usually presents as a painless, non-ulcerated sessile or pedunculated gingival or alveolar mucosal lesion. The clinical features are nonspecific, and most lesions are clinically considered to represent some form of fibroma. Most examples are smaller than 1.5 cm, but larger lesions have been reported (Fig. 15–68). The tumor has been found in patients over a wide age range, but most are seen in middle-aged patients.

Peripheral ameloblastomas are most commonly found on the posterior gingival and alveolar mucosa, and they are somewhat more common in mandibular than in maxillary areas. In a few cases, the superficial alveolar bone becomes slightly eroded, but significant bone involvement does not occur. A few examples of a microscopically identical lesion have been reported in the buccal mucosa at some distance from the alveolar or gingival soft tissues.

Histopathologic Features

Peripheral ameloblastomas have islands of ameloblastic epithelium that occupy the lamina propria underneath the surface epithelium. The proliferating epithelium may show any of the features described for the

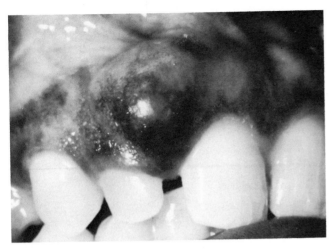

FIGURE 15-68. **Peripheral ameloblastoma.** Sessile gingival mass. (Courtesy of Dr. Dean K. White.)

intraosseous ameloblastoma; plexiform or follicular patterns are the most common. Connection of the tumor with the basal layer of the surface epithelium is seen in about 50 percent of cases. Whether this represents origin of the tumor from the basal layer of the epithelium or merging of the tumor into the surface epithelium has not been ascertained (Fig. 15-69).

Basal call carcinomas of the oral mucosa have been reported, but most authors consider them to represent peripheral ameloblastomas. A **peripheral odontogenic fibroma** may be confused microscopically with a peripheral ameloblastoma, particularly if a prominent epithelial component is present in the former. The presence of dysplastic dentin or cementum-like elements in the peripheral odontogenic fibroma and the lack of peripheral columnar differentiation and reverse polarization of the epithelium should serve to distinguish the two lesions.

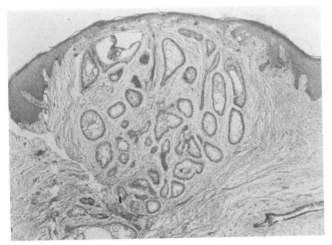

FIGURE 15-69. **Peripheral ameloblastoma.** This small lesion is composed of follicular ameloblastoma occupying the gingival lamina propria. The tumor is not connected to the overlying atrophic surface epithelium, and no bone involvement is present.

Treatment and Prognosis

Unlike the intraosseous ameloblastoma, the peripheral ameloblastoma shows an innocuous clinical behavior. Patients respond well to local surgical excision. Although local recurrence has been noted in about 25 percent of cases, further local excision almost always results in a cure. Several examples of malignant change in a peripheral ameloblastoma have been reported, but this is rare.

MALIGNANT AMELOBLASTOMA AND AMELOBLASTIC CARCINOMA

Rarely, an ameloblastoma exhibits frank malignant behavior with development of metastases. The frequency of malignant behavior in ameloblastomas is difficult to determine but probably occurs in far less than 1 percent of all ameloblastomas.

The terminology for these lesions is somewhat controversial. We believe that the term **malignant ameloblastoma** should refer to a tumor that shows the histopathologic features of ameloblastoma, both in the primary tumor and in the metastatic deposits. The term **ameloblastic carcinoma** should be reserved for an ameloblastoma that has cytologic features of malignancy in the primary tumor, in a recurrence, or in any metastatic deposit. These lesions may follow a markedly aggressive local course, but metastases do not necessarily occur.

Clinical and Radiographic Features

Malignant ameloblastomas have been observed in patients who range in age from 4 to 75 years (mean age, 30 years). In patients with documented metastases, the interval between the initial treatment of the ameloblastoma and first evidence of metastasis varies from 1 to 30 years. In nearly one third of cases, metastases do not become apparent until 10 years after treatment of the primary tumor.

Metastases from ameloblastomas are most often found in the lungs. These have sometimes been regarded as "aspiration" or "implant" metastases. However, the peripheral location of some metastatic deposits in the lung suggests that aspiration cannot explain many lung deposits, which must have occurred by blood or lymphatic routes (Fig. 15-70).

Cervical lymph nodes are the second most common site for metastasis of an ameloblastoma. Spread to vertebrae, other bones, and viscera has also occasionally been confirmed.

The radiologic findings of malignant ameloblastomas may be essentially the same as those in typical non-metastasizing ameloblastomas. Ameloblastic carcinomas are often more aggressive lesions with ill-defined margins and cortical destruction (Fig. 15-71A, B).

Histopathologic Features

With malignant ameloblastomas, the primary jaw tumor and the metastatic deposits show no microscopic features that differ from those of ameloblastomas with a

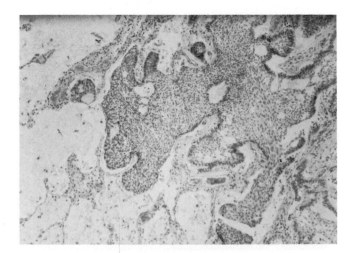

FIGURE 15-70. **Malignant ameloblastoma.** Metastatic deposit in the lung of a 61-year-old man. The metastatic tumor deposit is cytologically benign. Pulmonary alveoli are present (*lower left*).

completely benign local course. With ameloblastic carcinomas, the metastatic deposits or primary tumor shows the microscopic pattern of ameloblastoma in addition to cytologic features of malignancy. These include an increased nuclear/cytoplasmic ratio, nuclear hyperchromatism, and the presence of mitoses. Necrosis in tumor islands and areas of dystrophic calcification may also be present (Fig. 15-72*A*, *B*).

Treatment and Prognosis

The prognosis of patients with malignant ameloblastomas appears to be poor, but the paucity of documented cases with long-term follow-up does not permit accurate assumptions to be made. About 50 percent of the patients with documented metastases and long-term follow-up have died. Lesions designated as ameloblastic carcinoma have demonstrated a uniformly aggressive clinical course with perforation of the cortical plates of

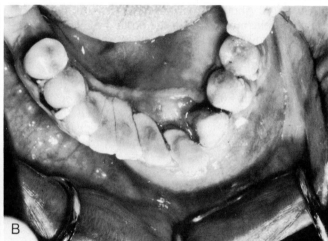

FIGURE 15-71. **Ameloblastic carcinoma.** *A*, Panoramic radiograph of a rapidly growing destructive lesion of the mandible. (From Neville BW, Damm DD, White DK, Waldron CA. Color Atlas of Clinical Oral Pathology. Philadelphia, Lea & Febiger, 1991.) *B*, Clinical photograph of the same patient shown in *A*. There is prominent labial expansion of the mandible in the incisor-premolar area.

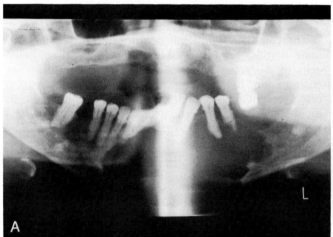

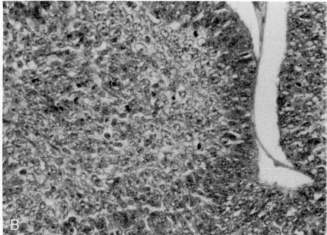

FIGURE 15-72. **Ameloblastic carcinoma.** *A*, The tumor from the same patient depicted in Figure 15-71 is highly cellular. It shows the pattern of a plexiform ameloblastoma with peripheral columnar cells. Cytologic epithelial dysplasia is present. *B*, Higher magnification showing cytologic atypia and mitoses.

the jaw and extension of the tumor into adjacent soft tissues.

CALCIFYING EPITHELIAL ODONTOGENIC TUMOR (Pindborg Tumor)

The **calcifying epithelial odontogenic tumor**, also widely known as the **Pindborg tumor**, is an uncommon lesion that accounts for fewer than 1 percent of all odontogenic tumors. Although the tumor is clearly of odontogenic origin, its histogenesis is uncertain. The tumor cells bear a close morphologic resemblance to the cells of the stratum intermedium of the enamel organ.

Clinical and Radiographic Features

Although the calcifying epithelial odontogenic tumor has been found in patients over a wide age range and in many parts of the jaw, it is most often encountered in patients between 30 and 50 years of age. There is no sex predilection. About 75 percent of all cases are found in the mandible, most often in the posterior areas. A painless, slow-growing swelling is the most common presenting sign.

Radiographically, the tumor shows a unilocular or, more often, a multilocular radiolucent defect (Fig. 15–73). The margins of the lytic defect are often scalloped. The lesion may be entirely radiolucent, but the defect frequently contains calcified structures of varying size and density (Fig. 15–74). The tumor is frequently associated with an impacted tooth, most often a mandibular third molar. Calcifications within the tumor are often most prominent around the crown of the impacted tooth (Fig. 15–75).

A few cases of peripheral (extraosseous) calcifying epithelial odontogenic tumors have been reported. These present as nonspecific, sessile gingival masses, most often on the anterior gingiva. Some of these have been associated with cup-like erosion of the underlying bone.

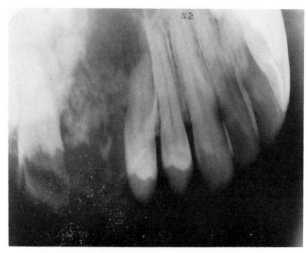

FIGURE 15–74. **Calcifying epithelial odontogenic tumor.** Radiolucent maxillary lesion containing larger calcifications. (From Gnepp DR. Pathology of the Head and Neck. New York, Churchill Livingstone, 1988.)

Histopathologic Features

The calcifying epithelial odontogenic tumor has discrete islands, strands, or sheets of polyhedral epithelial cells in a fibrous stroma. Large areas of amorphous, eosinophilic, hyalinized extracellular material are also often present. The cellular outlines of the epithelial cells are distinct, and intercellular bridges may be noted. The nuclei show considerable variation, and giant nuclei may be seen (Fig. 15–76). Some tumors show considerable nuclear pleomorphism, but this feature is not considered to indicate malignancy. The tumor islands frequently enclose masses of hyaline (amyloid-like) material; this results in a cribriform appearance (Fig. 15–77). The calcifications, which are a distinctive feature of the tumor, develop within the amyloid-like material and form concentric rings (Liesegang ring calcifications). These tend to fuse together and form large, complex masses (Fig. 15–78).

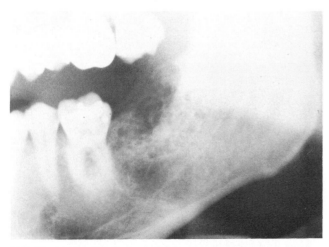

FIGURE 15–73. **Calcifying epithelial odontogenic tumor.** "Honeycombed" multilocular radiolucency containing fine calcifications.

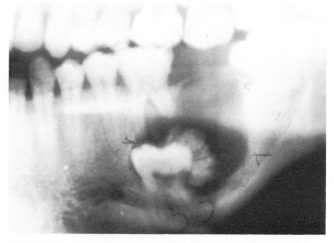

FIGURE 15–75. **Calcifying epithelial odontogenic tumor.** Prominent calcification around the crown of an impacted second molar that is involved in the tumor. (Courtesy of Dr. Harold Peacock.)

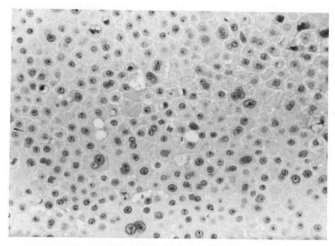

FIGURE 15-76. Calcifying epithelial odontogenic tumor. Sheets of polyhedral epithelial cells showing intercellular bridging. Giant nuclei and multinucleated cells are present.

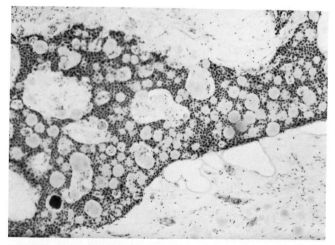

FIGURE 15-77. Calcifying epithelial odontogenic tumor. The tumor cells surround islands of amyloid-like material, giving a cribriform appearance. Calcification in an island of amyloid is present (*lower left*).

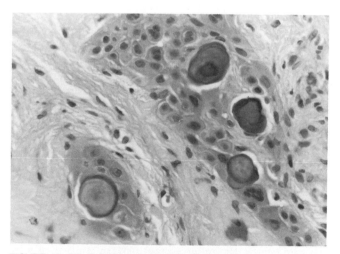

FIGURE 15-78. Calcifying epithelial odontogenic tumor. Liesegang ring calcifications forming within tumor cell islands.

Several microscopic variations may be encountered. Some tumors consist of large sheets of epithelial cells with minimal production of amyloid-like material and calcifications. Others show large diffuse masses of amyloid-like material that contain only small nests or islands of epithelium. A clear cell variant has also been described, in which clear cells constitute a significant portion of the epithelial component.

The amyloid-like material in the Pindborg tumor has been extensively investigated by histochemical, immunologic, and biochemical methods and by electron microscopy. Its precise nature, however, is still uncertain. This material generally stains for amyloid (i.e., positive staining results with Congo red or thioflavine T). The material appears closely related to some form of amyloid and may represent degradation of the lamina densa material that is produced by the epithelial cells.

Treatment and Prognosis

Although it was originally believed that the calcifying epithelial odontogenic tumor had about the same biologic behavior as the ameloblastoma, accumulating experience indicates that it tends to be less aggressive. Conservative local resection to include a narrow rim of surrounding bone appears to be the treatment of choice. A recurrence rate of about 15 percent has been reported; tumors treated by curettage have the highest frequency of recurrence. The overall prognosis appears good, although a single case with regional lymph node metastasis was reported.

SQUAMOUS ODONTOGENIC TUMOR

Squamous odontogenic tumor is a rare benign odontogenic neoplasm that was first described in 1975 and is now recognized as a distinct entity. Fewer than 30 examples have been reported at the time of this writing. Before 1975, this lesion was probably believed to represent an atypical acanthomatous ameloblastoma or even a squamous cell carcinoma. The squamous odontogenic tumor is presumed to arise from neoplastic transformation of the epithelial rests of Malassez. The tumor appears to originate within the periodontal ligament that is associated with the lateral root surface of an erupted tooth.

Clinical and Radiographic Features

Squamous odontogenic tumors have been found in patients whose ages ranged from 11 to 67 years (average age, 37). They are randomly distributed throughout the alveolar processes of the maxilla and mandible, with no site of predilection. A few patients have had multiple squamous odontogenic tumors that involved several quadrants of the mouth. There is no apparent sex predilection. A painless or mildly painful gingival swelling, often associated with mobility of the associated teeth, is the most common complaint. About 25 percent of reported patients have had no symptoms, and their lesions were detected during a radiographic examination.

The radiographic findings are not specific or diagnostic

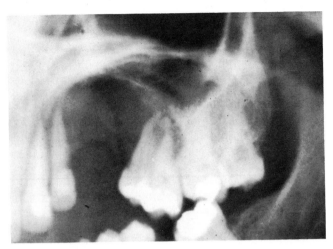

FIGURE 15–79. **Squamous odontogenic tumor.** Lucent defect extending along the roots of the lateral incisor and first premolar teeth. (Courtesy of Dr. Ed McGaha.)

and consist of a triangular radiolucent defect lateral to the root or roots of the teeth (Fig. 15–79). In some instances, this suggests vertical periodontal bone loss. The radiolucent area may be somewhat ill defined or may show a well-defined, sclerotic margin. Most examples are relatively small lesions that seldom exceed 1.5 cm in greatest diameter.

Histopathologic Features

The microscopic findings of squamous odontogenic tumor are distinctive and consist of varying-shaped islands of bland-appearing squamous epithelium in a mature fibrous connective tissue stroma. The peripheral cells of the epithelial islands do not show the characteristic polarization seen in ameloblastomas (Fig. 15–80). Microcystic vacuolization and individual cell keratinization within the epithelial islands are common features. Small microcysts are sometimes present within the epithelial islands. Laminated calcified bodies and globular

eosinophilic structures, which do not stain for amyloid, are present within the epithelium in some cases. The former probably represents dystrophic calcifications; the nature of the latter is unknown.

Islands of epithelium that closely resemble those of the squamous odontogenic tumor have been observed within the fibrous walls of dentigerous and radicular cysts. These have been designated as squamous odontogenic tumor–like proliferations in odontogenic cysts. These islands do not appear to have any significance relative to the behavior of the cyst, and evaluation of the clinical, radiologic, and histopathologic features should permit differentiation from a squamous odontogenic tumor.

In published reports, some squamous odontogenic tumors have been initially misdiagnosed as ameloblastomas, with resulting unnecessarily radical surgery.

Treatment and Prognosis

Conservative local excision or curettage appears to be effective for patients with squamous odontogenic tumors, and most reported cases have not recurred after local excision. A few instances of recurrence have been reported, but these have responded well to further local excision. Maxillary squamous odontogenic tumors, may be somewhat more aggressive than mandibular lesions, with a greater tendency to invade adjacent structures. This may be due to the porous, spongy nature of the maxillary bone.

CLEAR CELL ODONTOGENIC TUMOR
(Clear Cell Odontogenic Carcinoma)

Clear cell odontogenic tumor is a rare jaw tumor that was first described in 1985. To date, only a small number of cases have been documented. The tumor appears to be of odontogenic origin, but its histogenesis is uncertain. Histochemical and ultrastructural studies show that the clear cells, which are the prominent feature of this neoplasm, have similarities to glycogen-rich presecretory ameloblasts.

Clinical and Radiographic Features

Because of the paucity of reported cases, there is little valid clinical information regarding the clear cell odontogenic tumor. Most cases are diagnosed in patients older than age 50, and both the mandible and maxilla have been involved. Some patients complain of pain and bony swelling; others are relatively symptom-free.

Radiologically, the lesions appear as unilocular or multilocular radiolucencies. The margins of the radiolucency are often somewhat ill defined or irregular (Fig. 15–81).

Histopathologic Features

Several histopathologic patterns or combinations of patterns may be seen in the clear cell odontogenic tumor. In some cases, the predominant pattern consists of varying-sized nests of epithelial cells with a clear or faintly

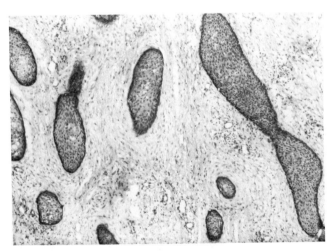

FIGURE 15–80. **Squamous odontogenic tumor.** Islands of bland-appearing epithelium in a fibrous stroma.

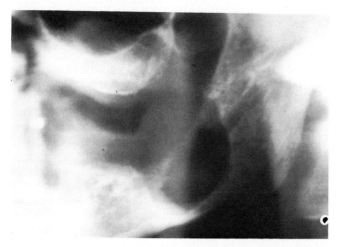

FIGURE 15–81. **Clear cell odontogenic tumor.** Unilocular radiolucent defect.

eosinophilic cytoplasm. The clear cell nests are separated by thin strands of hyalinized connective tissue (Fig. 15–82A, B). The peripheral cells of the clear cell islands may demonstrate palisading. In other instances, the dominant pattern consists of cords or small islands of hyperchromatic basaloid epithelial cells in a fibrous stroma. The epithelial islands or cords contain varying numbers of clear cells.

The clear cells contain small amounts of glycogen, but mucin stains are negative. In some cases, islands more typical of ameloblastoma are interspersed among the other tumor elements. Clear cell odontogenic tumors may be difficult to differentiate from intraosseous mucoepidermoid carcinomas with a prominent clear cell component. A clear cell variant of the calcifying epithelial odontogenic tumor may also present problems in the differential diagnosis. A metastatic clear cell neoplasm, such as a renal cell carcinoma, must also be ruled out before the diagnosis of clear cell odontogenic tumor can be established.

Treatment and Prognosis

Clear cell odontogenic tumors largely demonstrate an aggressive clinical course, with invasion of contiguous structures and a tendency to recur. Most patients require fairly radical surgery. Pulmonary or lymphatic metastases may occur. Clear cell odontogenic tumors should be regarded as potentially malignant or malignant neoplasms, and the designation **clear cell odontogenic carcinoma** is preferred by some investigators.

Tumors of Odontogenic Epithelium with Odontogenic Ectomesenchyme

A group of mixed odontogenic tumors, composed of proliferating odontogenic epithelium in a cellular ectomesenchyme resembling the dental papilla, poses problems in classification. Some of these lesions show varying degrees of inductive effect by the epithelium on the mesenchyme, leading to the formation of varying amounts of enamel and dentin. Some of these lesions (the common odontomas) are clearly non-neoplastic developmental anomalies; others appear to be true neoplasms. The nature of others is uncertain.

The histopathologic findings alone cannot distinguish between the neoplastic lesions and the developmental anomalies. Clinical and radiologic features are of considerable assistance in making this distinction.

AMELOBLASTIC FIBROMA

The **ameloblastic fibroma** is considered to be a true mixed tumor in which the epithelial and mesenchymal tissues are both neoplastic. It is an uncommon tumor, but the data are difficult to evaluate because some lesions diagnosed as ameloblastic fibromas may only represent the early developing stage of an odontoma.

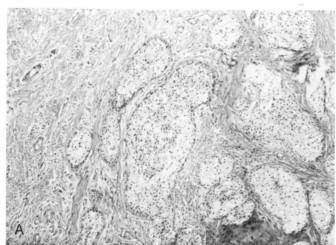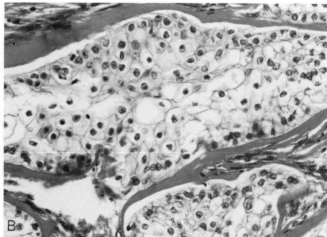

FIGURE 15–82. **Clear cell odontogenic tumor.** *A*, Nests of clear epithelial cells in a fibrous stroma. *B*, Higher magnification showing tumor islands surrounded by hyalinized connective tissue. Some tumor cells have a clear cytoplasm; others have a faintly granular cytoplasm.

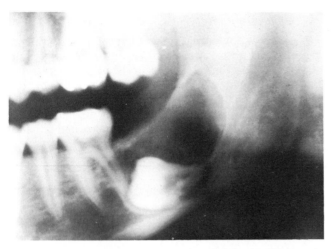

FIGURE 15–83. **Ameloblastic fibroma.** Well-defined radiolucent defect containing an unerupted second molar. (Courtesy of Dr. Robert Lauer.)

Clinical and Radiographic Features

Ameloblastic fibromas tend to occur in younger patients; most lesions are diagnosed in the first two decades of life. This lesion, however, is occasionally encountered in middle-aged patients. The tumor is slightly more common in males than in females. Small ameloblastic fibromas are asymptomatic; larger tumors are associated with swelling of the jaws. The posterior mandible is the most common site; about 70 percent of all cases are located in this area.

Radiographically, either a unilocular or multilocular radiolucent lesion is seen. The margins of the defect tend to be well defined, and they may be sclerotic. An unerupted tooth is associated with the lesion in about 50 percent of cases (Fig. 15–83). The ameloblastic fibroma may grow to a large size, and cases that involve a considerable portion of the body and ascending ramus of the mandible have been reported.

Histopathologic Features

The ameloblastic fibroma presents as a solid, soft tissue mass with a smooth outer surface. A definite capsule may or may not be present. Microscopically, the tumor is composed of a cell-rich mesenchymal tissue resembling the primitive dental papilla admixed with proliferating odontogenic epithelium. The latter may have one of two patterns, both of which are usually present in any given case. The most common epithelial pattern consists of long, narrow cords of odontogenic epithelium, often in an anastomosing arrangement. These cords are usually only two cells in thickness and are composed of cuboidal or columnar cells (Fig. 15–84A, B). In the other pattern, the epithelial cells form small, discrete islands that resemble the follicular stage of the developing enamel organ. These show peripheral columnar cells, which surround a mass of loosely arranged epithelial cells that resemble stellate reticulum. In contrast to the follicular type of ameloblastoma, these follicular islands in the ameloblastic fibroma seldom demonstrate microcyst formation.

The mesenchymal portion of the ameloblastic fibroma consists of plump stellate and ovoid cells in a loose matrix, which closely resembles the developing dental papilla. Collagen formation is generally inconspicuous. Juxtaepithelial hyalinization of the mesenchymal portion of the tumor is sometimes seen.

Treatment and Prognosis

It was formerly believed that the ameloblastic fibroma was an innocuous lesion that seldom, if ever, recurred after simple local excision or curettage. More recent reports, however, indicate a substantial risk of recurrence after conservative local excision. Some of this problem may be related to the probable inclusion of some small lesions that were probably developing odontomas among the neoplastic ameloblastic fibromas. About 20 percent of ameloblastic fibromas may recur after conservative

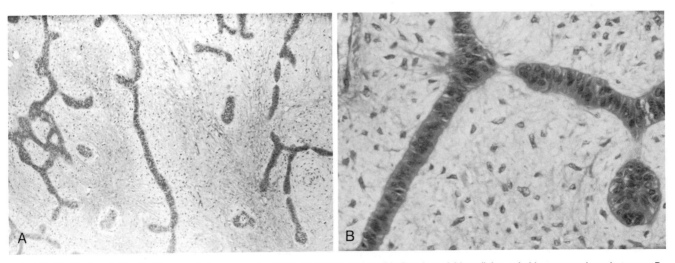

FIGURE 15–84. **Ameloblastic fibroma.** *A,* Long, narrow cords of odontogenic epithelium in a richly cellular, primitive mesenchymal stroma. *B,* Higher magnification showing the plump, stellate-shaped mesenchymal cells in a loose matrix.

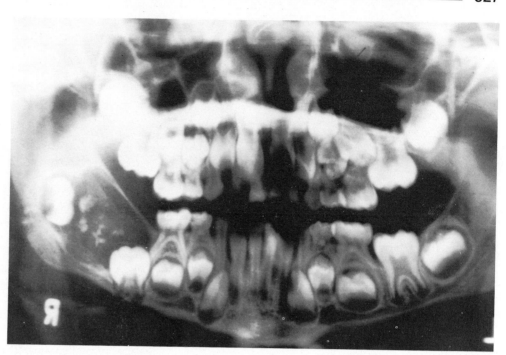

FIGURE 15–85. **Ameloblastic fibro-odontoma.** Radiolucent defect in the ramus containing small calcifications having the radiodensity of tooth structure.

removal, and some surgeons recommend a more aggressive surgical excision. Approximately 50 percent of the cases of the rare ameloblastic fibrosarcoma develop as a recurrence of an ameloblastic fibroma.

AMELOBLASTIC FIBRO-ODONTOMA

The **ameloblastic fibro-odontoma** is defined as a tumor with the general features of an ameloblastic fibroma but that also contains enamel and dentin. Some investigators believe that the ameloblastic fibro-odontoma is only a stage in the development of an odontoma and do not consider it to be a separate entity. In some cases, however, the tumor can undergo progressive growth, which causes considerable deformity and bone destruction. Such lesions appear to be true neoplasms, and it is likely that some lesions diagnosed as ameloblastic fibro-odontomas are neoplastic. Others may only represent a stage in the development of an odontoma. However, differentiation of these entities cannot be made on histopathologic grounds alone.

Clinical and Radiographic Features

The ameloblastic fibro-odontoma is usually encountered in children with an average age of 10 years. It is rarely encountered in adults. In contrast to the **ameloblastic fibroma**, ameloblastic fibro-odontomas occur with about equal frequency in the maxilla and mandible. There is no significant gender predilection. The lesion is commonly asymptomatic and is discovered when radiographs are taken to determine the reason for failure of a tooth to erupt. Large examples may be associated with a painless swelling of the affected bone.

Radiographically, the tumor shows a well-circumscribed unilocular or, rarely, multilocular radiolucent defect that contains a variable amount of calcified material with the radiodensity of tooth structure. The calcified material within the lesion may appear as multiple, small radiopacities or as a solid conglomerate mass (Fig. 15–85). In most instances, an unerupted tooth is present at the margin of the lesion, or the crown of the unerupted tooth may be included within the defect. Some ameloblastic fibro-odontomas contain only a minimal amount of calcifying enamel and dentin matrix and appear radiographically as radiolucent lesions (Fig. 15–86). These cannot be differentiated from the wide variety of unilocular radiolucencies that may involve the jaws. At the other extreme, some ameloblastic fibro-odontomas appear as largely calcified masses with only a narrow rim of radiolucency about the periphery of the lesion.

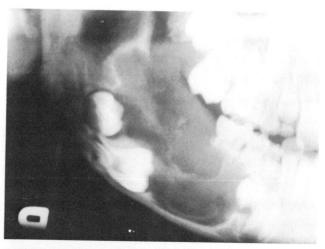

FIGURE 15–86. **Ameloblastic fibro-odontoma.** Radiolucent defect involving several unerupted teeth. Little calcified material is present in the radiolucent defect.

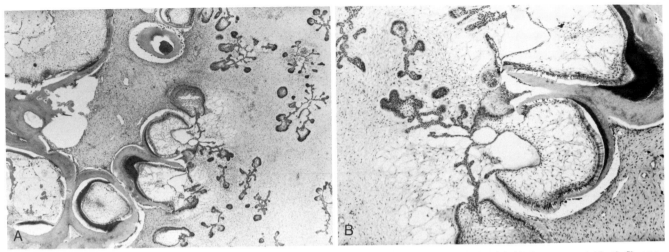

FIGURE 15–87. **Ameloblastic fibro-odontoma.** A, The soft tissue component of the tumor (*right*) is indistinguishable from an ameloblastic fibroma. Developing rudimentary tooth-like structures are shown (*left*). B, Higher magnification showing enamel matrix and dentin formation in the tumor.

Histopathologic Features

The soft tissue component of ameloblastic fibro-odontomas is microscopically identical to the **ameloblastic fibroma** and has narrow cords and small islands of odontogenic epithelium in a loose primitive-appearing connective tissue that resembles the dental papilla. The calcifying element consists of foci of enamel and dentin matrix formation in close relationship to the epithelial structures (Fig. 15–87*A*, *B*). The more calcified lesions show mature dental structures in the form of rudimentary small teeth or conglomerate masses of enamel and dentin. A similar tumor in which the calcifying component consists only of dentin matrix and dentinoid material has been designated by some as **ameloblastic fibro-dentinoma**. It is questionable whether this lesion represents a separate entity, and it is probably best considered as only a variant of the ameloblastic fibro-odontoma.

Treatment and Prognosis

A patient with an ameloblastic fibro-odontoma is generally treated by conservative curettage, and the lesion usually separates easily from its bony bed. The tumor is well circumscribed and does not invade the surrounding bone.

The prognosis is excellent, and recurrence after conservative removal is unusual. Development of an ameloblastic fibrosarcoma after curettage of an ameloblastic fibro-odontoma has been reported, but this is exceedingly rare.

AMELOBLASTIC FIBROSARCOMA
(Ameloblastic Sarcoma)

The rare **ameloblastic fibrosarcoma** is considered to be the malignant counterpart of the **ameloblastic fibroma**, in which the mesenchymal portion of the lesion shows features of malignancy. The tumor may apparently arise *de novo*, although in somewhat more than 50 percent of known cases, the malignant lesion represents a recurrence of a tumor previously diagnosed as an ameloblastic fibroma or an **ameloblastic fibro-odontoma**.

Clinical and Radiographic Features

Ameloblastic fibrosarcomas occur about twice as often in males as in females. The lesion tends to occur in younger patients (mean reported age, 26 years). Although either the maxilla or mandible may be involved, about 75 percent of cases have occurred in the mandible. Pain and swelling associated with rapid clinical growth are the common complaints.

Radiographically, the ameloblastic fibrosarcoma shows an ill-defined destructive radiolucent lesion that suggests a malignant process (Fig. 15–88*A*, *B*).

Histopathologic Features

Ameloblastic fibrosarcomas contain an epithelial component similar to that seen in the ameloblastic fibroma, although it is frequently less prominent than that present in the typical ameloblastic fibroma. The epithelial component appears histopathologically benign and does not demonstrate any cytologic atypia. The mesenchymal portion of the tumor, however, is highly cellular and shows hyperchromatic and often bizarre pleomorphic cells (Fig. 15–89). Mitoses are usually prominent. In some cases with multiple recurrences, the epithelial component becomes progressively less conspicuous so that the tumor eventually shows only a poorly differentiated fibrosarcoma.

In a few instances, dysplastic dentin or small amounts of enamel may be formed. Such lesions have been called **ameloblastic dentinosarcomas** or **ameloblastic fibro-odontosarcomas** by some. This additional subclassification, however, appears unnecessary.

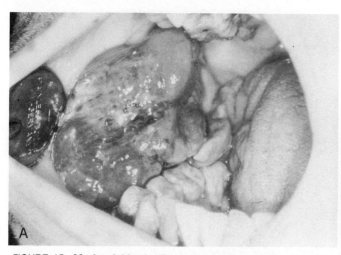
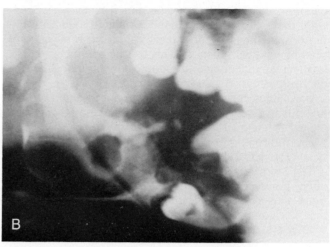

FIGURE 15-88. **Ameloblastic fibrosarcoma.** *A*, A 21-year-old white woman complained of facial asymmetry and recent increase in size of a mandibular mass that had been present for some years. *B*, Radiograph of the same patient shown in *A*. Note the lytic destruction of the posterior mandible. (*A* and *B*, Courtesy of Dr. Sam McKenna.)

Treatment and Prognosis

Once the diagnosis of ameloblastic fibrosarcoma has been confirmed, radical surgical excision appears to be the treatment of choice. Curettage or local excision is usually followed by rapid local recurrence. The tumor is locally aggressive and infiltrates adjacent bone and soft tissues.

The long-term prognosis is difficult to ascertain because of the few reported cases with adequate follow-up. Most deaths have resulted from uncontrolled local disease, but both regional and distant metastases have occurred.

ADENOMATOID ODONTOGENIC TUMOR

The **adenomatoid odontogenic tumor** represents 3 to 7 percent of all odontogenic tumors. Although this lesion

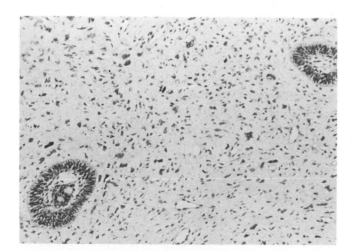

FIGURE 15-89. **Ameloblastic fibrosarcoma.** The cellular mesenchymal tissue shows hyperchromatism and atypical cells. Two small islands of benign-appearing odontogenic epithelium are present.

was formerly considered to be a variant of the ameloblastoma and was designated as "adenoameloblastoma," its clinical features and biologic behavior indicate that it is a separate entity. There is good evidence that the tumor cells are derived from enamel organ epithelium.

Although the adenomatoid odontogenic tumor is often classified as an epithelial odontogenic tumor, the fact that some of these lesions also produce dentinoid material—and rarely enamel matrix—suggests it is more logical to consider it an epithelial tumor with an inductive effect on the odontogenic ectomesenchyme.

Clinical and Radiographic Features

Adenomatoid odontogenic tumors are largely limited to younger patients, and two thirds of all cases are diagnosed when patients are 10 to 19 years of age. This tumor is definitely uncommon in a patient older than age 30. It has a striking tendency to occur in the anterior portions of the jaws and is found twice as often in the maxilla as in the mandible. Females are affected about twice as often as males.

Most adenomatoid odontogenic tumors are relatively small. They seldom exceed 3.0 cm in greatest diameter, although a few large lesions have been reported. Peripheral (extraosseous) forms of the tumor are also encountered but are rare. These usually present as small, sessile masses on the facial gingiva of the maxilla. Clinically, these lesions cannot be differentiated from the common gingival fibrous lesions.

Adenomatoid odontogenic tumors are frequently asymptomatic and are discovered during the course of a radiographic examination or when films are made to determine why a tooth has not erupted. Larger lesions cause a painless expansion of the bone.

In about 75 percent of cases, the tumor presents as a circumscribed, radiolucent area that involves the crown of an unerupted tooth, most often a canine. This follicular type of adenomatoid odontogenic tumor may be impossible to differentiate radiographically from the more common dentigerous cyst. The radiolucency associated with the follicular type of adenomatoid odontogenic tumor sometimes extends apically along the root past the cemento-enamel junction. This feature may help to distinguish an adenomatoid odontogenic tumor from a dentigerous cyst (Fig. 15–90).

Less often the adenomatoid odontogenic tumor presents as a well-delineated radiolucent lesion that is not related to an unerupted tooth and is often located between the roots of several erupted teeth (extrafollicular type) (Fig. 15–91).

The lesion may appear completely radiolucent; more often, however, it contains fine ("snowflake") calcifications. This feature is helpful in differentiating the adenomatoid odontogenic tumor from a dentigerous or other type of cyst.

Histopathologic Features

The adenomatoid odontogenic tumor is a well-defined lesion that is usually surrounded by a thick, fibrous capsule. When the lesion is bisected, the central portion of the tumor may be essentially solid or may show varying degrees of cystic change.

Microscopically, the tumor is composed of spindle-shaped epithelial cells that form sheets, strands, or whorled masses of cells in a scant fibrous stroma. The epithelial cells may form rosette-like structures about a central space, which may be empty or contain small amounts of eosinophilic material. This material may stain for amyloid.

The tubular or duct-like structures, which are the characteristic feature of the adenomatoid odontogenic tumor, may be prominent, scanty, or even absent in a given lesion. These consist of a central space surrounded by a layer of columnar or cuboidal epithelial cells. The nuclei of these cells tend to be polarized away from the central space. The mechanism of formation of these tubular structures is not entirely clear but is likely due to

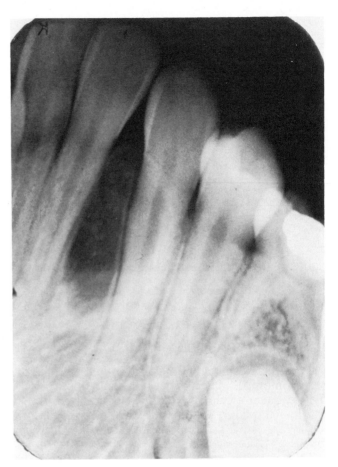

FIGURE 15–91. **Adenomatoid odontogenic tumor, extrafollicular type.** A small radiolucency is present between the roots of the lateral incisor and canine. (Courtesy of Dr. Ramesh Narang.)

the secretory activity of the tumor cells, which appear to be preameloblasts. In any event, these structures are not true ducts, and no glandular elements are present in the tumor (Fig. 15–92).

Small foci of calcification may also be scattered throughout the tumor. These have been interpreted as abortive enamel formation. Some adenomatoid odontogenic tumors contain larger areas of matrix material or calcification. This material has been interpreted as dentinoid or cementum.

Some lesions also have another pattern, particularly at the periphery of the tumor adjacent to the capsule. This consists of narrow, often anastomosing cords of epithelium in an eosinophilic, loosely arranged matrix.

The histopathologic features of this lesion are distinctive and should not be confused with any other odontogenic tumor. The chief problem relates to mistaking this tumor for an ameloblastoma by a pathologist who is not familiar with this lesion. This error can lead to unnecessarily radical surgery.

Treatment and Prognosis

The adenomatoid odontogenic tumor is completely benign; because of its capsule, it enucleates easily from the bone. Aggressive behavior has not been documented, and recurrence after enucleation seldom, if ever, occurs.

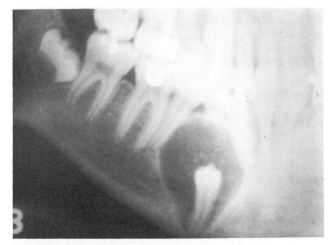

FIGURE 15–90. **Adenomatoid odontogenic tumor, follicular type.** Radiolucent lesion involving an unerupted mandibular first premolar. Fine "snowflake" calcifications are present in the radiolucent area. In contrast to the usual dentigerous cyst, the radiolucency extends almost to the apex of the tooth. (Courtesy of Dr. Tony Traynham.)

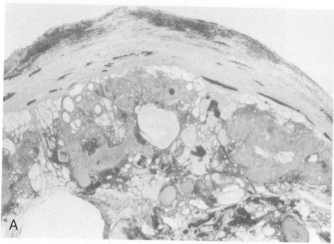
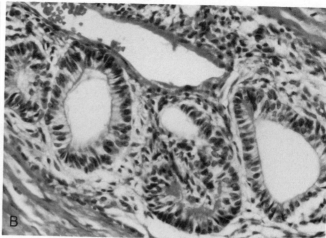

FIGURE 15–92. Adenomatoid odontogenic tumor. *A,* Low-power view demonstrating a thick capsule surrounding the tumor. *B,* Higher magnification showing the duct-like epithelial structures. The nuclei of the columnar cells are polarized away from the central spaces.

ODONTOAMELOBLASTOMA

The **odontoameloblastoma** is an extremely rare odontogenic tumor that contains an ameloblastomatous component together with odontoma-like elements. This tumor was formerly called **ameloblastic odontoma** and was confused with the more common lesion currently designated as **ameloblastic fibro-odontoma**. The former deserves special classification, and the term odontoameloblastoma is the preferred designation.

Clinical and Radiographic Features

Because of the rarity of odontoameloblastomas, little reliable information is available. The lesion appears to occur more often in the mandible of younger patients. Pain, delayed eruption of teeth, and expansion of the affected bone may be noted.

Radiographically, the tumor shows a radiolucent, destructive process that contains calcified structures. These have the radiodensity of tooth structure and may resemble miniature teeth or occur as larger masses of calcified material similar to a complex odontoma.

Histopathologic Features

The histopathologic features of the odontoameloblastoma are complex. The proliferating epithelial portion of the tumor has features of an **ameloblastoma**, most often of the plexiform or follicular pattern. The ameloblastic component is intermingled with immature or more mature dental tissue in the form of developing rudimentary teeth, which is similar to the appearance of a **compound odontoma,** or conglomerate masses of enamel, dentin, and cementum, as seen in a **complex odontoma.**

Treatment and Prognosis

Multiple recurrences of odontoameloblastomas have been reported after local curettage, and it appears that this tumor has the same biologic potential as the ameloblastoma. It is probably wise to treat a patient with this lesion in the same manner as one with an ameloblastoma. However, there are no valid data on the long-term prognosis.

ODONTOMA

Odontomas are the most common types of odontogenic tumors. Their prevalence exceeds that of all other odontogenic tumors combined. Odontomas are considered to be developmental anomalies (**hamartomas**) rather than true neoplasms. When fully developed, odontomas consist chiefly of enamel and dentin with variable amounts of pulp and cementum. In their earlier developmental stages, varying amounts of proliferating odontogenic epithelium and mesenchyme are present.

Odontomas are further subdivided into compound and complex types. The **compound odontoma** is composed of multiple, small tooth-like structures. The **complex odontoma** consists of a conglomerate mass of enamel and dentin, which bears no anatomic resemblance to a tooth. Compound and complex odontomas occur with about equal frequency. Some odontomas, however, show features of both types.

Clinical and Radiographic Features

Most odontomas are detected during the first two decades of life, and the mean age at the time of diagnosis is 14 years. Most odontomas are completely asymptomatic, being discovered on a routine radiographic examination or when films are taken to determine the reason for failure of a tooth to erupt. Most odontomas are relatively small and seldom exceed the size of a tooth in the area where they are located. However, large odontomas up to 6 cm or more in diameter are occasionally seen. These large odontomas can cause expansion of the jaw.

Odontomas occur somewhat more frequently in the

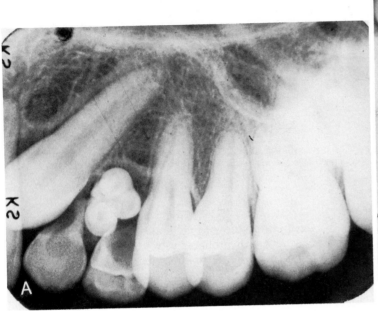

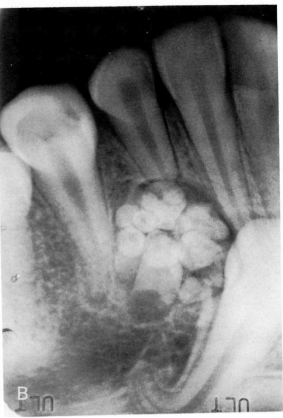

FIGURE 15–93. **Compound odontomas.** In both *A* and *B*, a group of tooth-like structures is preventing the eruption of a permanent tooth. (*A*, Courtesy of Dr. Robert J. Powers. *B*, Courtesy of Dr. Brent Bernard.)

maxilla than in the mandible. Although compound and complex odontomas may be found in any site, the compound type is more often seen in the anterior maxilla; complex odontomas occur more often in the molar regions of either jaw.

Radiographically, the **compound odontoma** presents as a collection of tooth-like structures of varying size and shape surrounded by a narrow radiolucent zone (Fig. 15–93*A*, *B*). The **complex odontoma** presents as a calcified mass with the radiodensity of tooth structure, which

is also surrounded by a narrow radiolucent rim. An unerupted tooth is frequently associated with the odontoma, and the odontoma prevents eruption of the tooth (Fig. 15–94). Some small odontomas are present between the roots of erupted teeth and are not associated with disturbance in eruption. The radiographic findings are usually diagnostic, and the compound odontoma is seldom confused with any other lesion. A developing odontoma may show little evidence of calcification and appear as a circumscribed radiolucent lesion. A complex

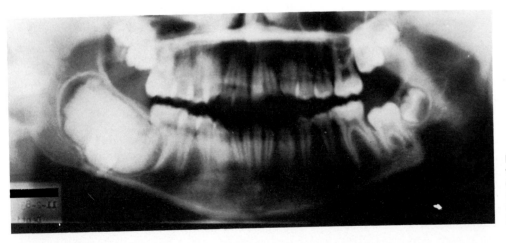

FIGURE 15–94. **Complex odontoma.** A large radiopaque mass is overlying the crown of the mandibular right second molar, which has been displaced to the inferior border of the mandible.

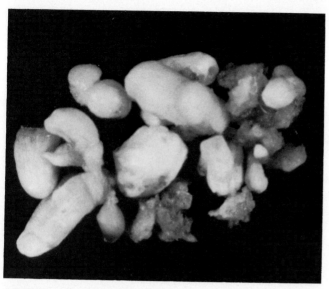

FIGURE 15–95. **Compound odontoma.** Surgical specimen consisting of more than 20 malformed tooth-like structures.

odontoma, however, may be radiographically confused with an osteoma or some other highly calcified bone lesion.

Histopathologic Features

The compound odontoma consists of multiple structures resembling small, single-rooted teeth, contained in a loose fibrous matrix (Fig. 15–95). The mature enamel caps of the tooth-like structures are lost during decalcification for preparation of the microscopic section, but varying amounts of enamel matrix are often present. Pulp tissue may be seen in the coronal and root portions of the tooth-like structures. In patients with developing odontomas, structures that resemble tooth germs are present.

Complex odontomas consist largely of mature tubular dentin. This dentin encloses clefts or hollow circular structures that contained the mature enamel that was removed during decalcification. The spaces may contain small amounts of enamel matrix or immature enamel (Fig. 15–96). Small islands of eosinophilic-staining epithelial ghost cells are present in about 20 percent of complex odontomas. These may represent remnants of odontogenic epithelium that have undergone keratinization and cell death from the local anoxia. A thin layer of cementum is often present about the periphery of the mass. Occasionally, a dentigerous cyst may arise from the epithelial lining of the fibrous capsule of a complex odontoma.

Treatment and Prognosis

Odontomas are treated by simple local excision, and the prognosis is excellent.

Tumors of Odontogenic Ectomesenchyme with or without Included Odontogenic Epithelium

These odontogenic tumors are composed of **odontogenic ectomesenchyme**. Odontogenic epithelium may or may not be included in the tumor, but the epithelial elements do not appear to play any active role in the lesion.

ODONTOGENIC FIBROMA

The **odontogenic fibroma** is an uncommon and somewhat controversial lesion. Fewer than 50 examples have been reported.

Clinical and Radiographic Features

Odontogenic fibromas have been reported in patients whose ages ranged from 9 to 80 years (mean age, 40 years). There is a marked female predilection: 7.4 to 1. About 60 percent of reported cases have occurred in the maxilla; most maxillary lesions are located anterior to the first molar tooth. In the mandible, however, about 50 percent of the tumors are located posterior to the first molar. An unerupted third molar has been associated with a few mandibular odontogenic fibromas. Smaller odontogenic fibromas are usually completely asymptomatic; larger lesions may be associated with localized bony expansion or loosening of teeth.

Radiographically, smaller odontogenic fibromas tend to be well-defined, unilocular, radiolucent lesions often associated with the apical area of erupted teeth (Fig. 15–97). Larger lesions tend to be multilocular radiolucencies. Many lesions have a sclerotic border. Root resorption of associated teeth is common, and lesions located between the teeth may result in root divergence.

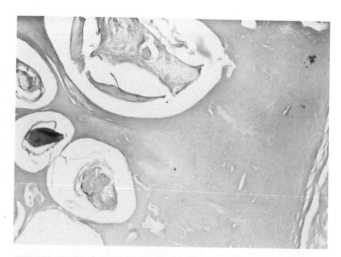

FIGURE 15–96. **Complex odontoma.** This decalcified section is largely composed of mature dentin. The hollow circular areas contain remnants of enamel matrix. The mature enamel was removed during decalcification.

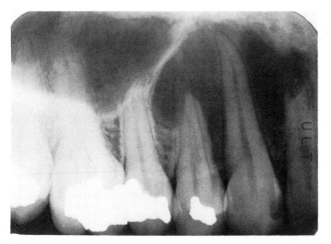

FIGURE 15-97. **Odontogenic fibroma.** Apical radiolucent lesion in the incisor-premolar area. (Courtesy of Dr. Robert Provencher Jr.)

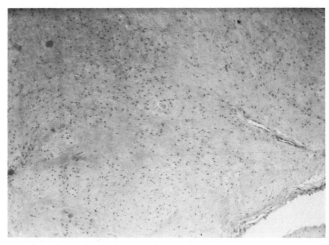

FIGURE 15-98. **Odontogenic fibroma, simple type.** Fibroblasts arranged in a whorled pattern with fine collagen fibrils. No epithelial rests were found on multiple sections from this tumor.

Histopathologic Features

The odontogenic fibroma shows considerable histopathologic diversity; this has led some authors to describe two separate types. The **simple odontogenic fibroma** is composed of stellate fibroblasts, often arranged in a whorled pattern with fine collagen fibrils and considerable ground substance (Fig. 15-98). Small foci of odontogenic epithelial rests may or may not be present. Occasional foci of dystrophic calcification may be present.

The so-called **WHO** (World Health Organization) **odontogenic fibroma** has a more complex pattern, which often consists of a fairly cellular fibrous connective tissue with collagen fibers arranged in interlacing bundles. Odontogenic epithelium in the form of long strands or isolated nests is present throughout the lesion and may be a prominent component (Fig. 15-99A, B). The fibrous component may vary from myxoid to densely hyalinized. Calcifications composed of cementum-like material or dentinoid are present in some cases.

In a few cases, a central odontogenic fibroma has been associated with a **giant cell granuloma**-like response. It seems unlikely that this represents a "collision" tumor with synchronous occurrence of an odontogenic fibroma and a giant cell granuloma. It is more likely that the odontogenic fibroma somehow induced the giant cell response in these patients.

The more cellular collagenized odontogenic fibroma needs to be differentiated from a desmoplastic fibroma. The desmoplastic fibroma, however, does not contain an epithelial component. Formerly, some oral and maxillofacial pathologists designated solid fibrous masses that were almost always associated with the crown of an unerupted tooth as odontogenic fibromas. Most oral and

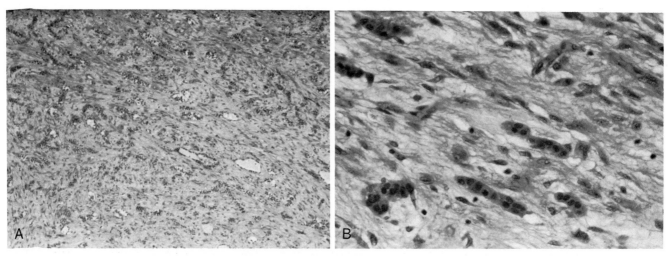

FIGURE 15-99. **Odontogenic fibroma, World Health Organization (WHO) type.** A, A cellular fibroblastic lesion containing narrow cords of odontogenic epithelium. B, Higher magnification shows the epithelial strands and cellular fibroblastic tissue.

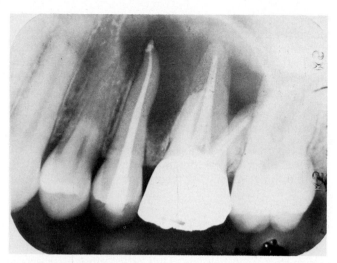

FIGURE 15–100. **Granular cell odontogenic fibroma.** Radiolucent lesion involving the apical area of endodontically treated maxillary teeth. (Courtesy of Dr. Steve Ferry.)

maxillofacial pathologists today consider such lesions to represent only hyperplastic dental follicles, and these should not be considered to be neoplasms.

Treatment and Prognosis

Odontogenic fibromas are usually treated by enucleation and curettage. Although the tumor does not have a definite capsule, it appears to have a limited growth potential, particularly in the anterior regions of the jaws. Although a few recurrences have been documented, the prognosis is very good.

GRANULAR CELL ODONTOGENIC FIBROMA (Granular Cell Odontogenic Tumor)

The rare **granular cell odontogenic fibroma** was first described as a "granular cell ameloblastic fibroma."

However, it is probably more appropriate to designate it as a granular cell odontogenic fibroma or by the noncommittal term **granular cell odontogenic tumor**. Only 14 documented cases have been reported.

Clinical and Radiographic Features

With only one exception, all patients with granular cell odontogenic fibromas have been older than 40 years of age. The tumor occurs in the maxilla and mandible and most often in the molar regions. Some lesions are completely asymptomatic; others present as a painless, localized expansion of the affected area.

Radiographically, the lesion presents as a well-demarcated radiolucent area, which may show small calcifications (Fig. 15–100).

Histopathologic Features

The granular cell odontogenic fibroma is composed of large eosinophilic granular cells, which closely resemble the granular cells seen in the soft tissue granular cell tumor (see p. 387) or the granular cells seen in the granular cell variant of the ameloblastoma (see p. 514). Narrow cords or small islands of odontogenic epithelium are scattered among the granular cells. Small cementum-like or dystrophic calcifications have been seen in some lesions associated with the granular cells (Fig. 15–101).

The nature of the granular cells is controversial. Ultrastructural studies reveal the features of mesenchymal cells. Immunohistochemically, the granular cells in the granular cell odontogenic fibroma are S-100 negative, in contrast to the positive S-100 staining in the granular cell tumor.

Treatment and Prognosis

The granular cell odontogenic fibroma appears to be completely benign and responds well to curettage. No recurrences have been reported.

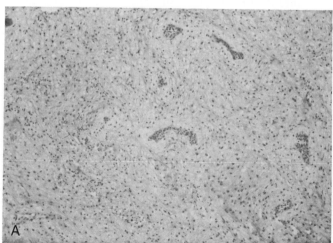
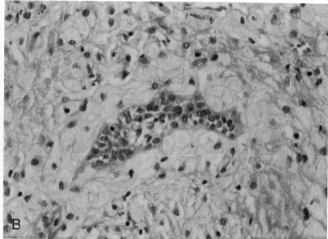

FIGURE 15–101. **Granular cell odontogenic fibroma.** *A*, Sheets of large granular mesenchymal cells and small nests of odontogenic epithelium. *B*, Higher magnification shows details of granular cells and epithelial islands.

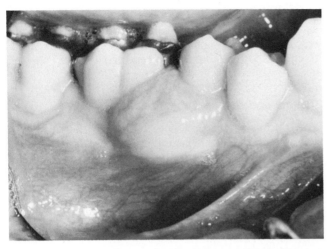

FIGURE 15-102. **Peripheral odontogenic fibroma.** This sessile gingival mass cannot be clinically distinguished from the common peripheral ossifying fibroma. (Courtesy of Dr. Jerry Stovall.)

PERIPHERAL ODONTOGENIC FIBROMA

The relatively rare **peripheral odontogenic fibroma** is considered to represent the soft tissue counterpart of the **central (intraosseous) odontogenic fibroma**. In the past, clinically and histopathologically similar lesions have been designated by some as **odontogenic epithelial hamartoma** or as **peripheral fibro-ameloblastic dentinoma**. It is likely that all of these terms refer to the same lesion, and peripheral odontogenic fibroma seems to be the most appropriate designation. Although this uncommon gingival lesion is occasionally encountered in the oral and maxillofacial pathology laboratory, there are few published reports analyzing large numbers of cases.

Clinical and Radiographic Features

The peripheral odontogenic fibroma appears as a firm, slow-growing, and usually sessile gingival mass, covered by normal-appearing mucosa (Fig. 15-102). Clinically, the peripheral odontogenic fibroma cannot be distinguished from the much more common fibrous gingival lesions (see Chapter 12). The lesion is most often encountered on the facial gingiva of the mandible. It usually varies between 1.5 and 3.5 cm in diameter and may cause displacement of the teeth. Peripheral odontogenic fibromas have been recorded in patients over a wide age range.

Radiographic studies demonstrate a soft tissue mass, which in some cases has shown areas of calcification. The lesion, however, does not involve the underlying bone.

Histopathologic Features

The peripheral odontogenic fibroma shows similar histopathologic features to the central odontogenic fibroma (WHO type). The tumor consists of interwoven strands of cellular fibrous connective tissue, which may be interspersed with areas of less cellular, myxoid connective tissue. Islands or strands of odontogenic epithelium are scattered throughout the connective tissue. These may be prominent or scarce. The epithelial cells may show vacuolization. Dysplastic dentin, amorphous ovoid cementum-like calcifications, and trabeculae of osteoid may also be present.

Treatment and Prognosis

The peripheral odontogenic fibroma is treated by local surgical excision. The prognosis is excellent, and there is little to no tendency for recurrence.

MYXOMA

Myxomas of the jaws are believed to arise from odontogenic ectomesenchyme. They bear a close microscopic resemblance to the mesenchymal portion of a developing tooth. Formerly, some investigators made a distinction between **odontogenic myxomas** (derived from odontogenic mesenchyme) and **osteogenic myxomas** (presumably derived from primitive bone tissue). However, most authorities in orthopedic pathologic practice do not recognize myxomas in the extragnathic skeleton, and all myxomas of the jaws are currently considered to be of odontogenic origin.

Clinical and Radiographic Features

Myxomas are predominantly found in young adults but may occur over a wide age group. The average age for patients with myxomas is 25 to 30 years. There is no sex predilection. The tumor may be found in almost any area of the jaws, and the mandible is slightly more commonly involved than the maxilla. Smaller lesions may be asymptomatic and are discovered only during a radiographic examination. Larger lesions are often associated with a painless expansion of the involved bone. In some instances, clinical growth of the tumor may be rapid; this is probably related to the accumulation of myxoid ground substance in the tumor.

Radiographically, the myxoma presents as a unilocular or multilocular radiolucent defect. The margins of the defect are often irregular or scalloped. The radiolucent defect may contain thin trabeculae of residual bone, which are often arranged at right angles to one another (Fig. 15-103). Large myxomas of the mandible may show a "soap bubble" radiolucent pattern, which is indistinguishable from that seen in ameloblastomas (Fig. 15-104).

Histopathologic Features

At the time of surgery or gross examination of the specimen, the gelatinous, loose structure of the myxoma is obvious. Microscopically, the tumor is composed of loosely arranged stellate, spindle-shaped, and round cells in an abundant, loose myxoid stroma that contains only a few collagen fibrils (Fig. 15-105A, B). Histochemical study shows that the ground substance is acid mucopolysaccharide, chiefly hyaluronic acid and chondroitin sul-

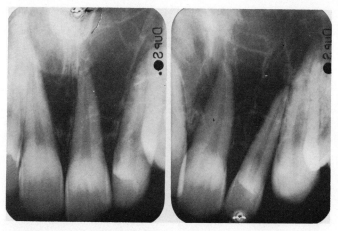

FIGURE 15–103. **Myxoma.** Radiolucent lesion of anterior maxilla showing fine residual bone trabeculae arranged at right angles to one another ("stepladder" pattern).

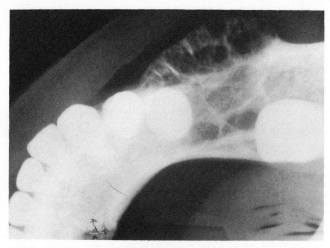

FIGURE 15–104. **Myxoma.** Occlusal view of a large myxoma showing buccal expansion and "soap bubble" radiolucency similar to that seen in an ameloblastoma. (Courtesy of Dr. Mike Rohrer.)

fate. Small islands of inactive-appearing odontogenic epithelial rests may be scattered throughout the myxoid ground substance. These epithelial rests are not required for the diagnosis and are not obvious in most cases. In some patients, the tumor may have a greater tendency to form collagen fibers; such lesions are sometimes designated as **fibro-myxomas** or **myxofibromas**. There is no evidence that these more collagenized forms deserve separate consideration, and they are considered only variants of the myxoma.

A myxoma may be microscopically confused with other myxoid jaw neoplasms, such as the rare chondromyxoid fibroma (see p. 477). Myxoid change in an enlarged dental follicle or the dental papilla of a developing tooth may be microscopically similar to a myxoma. Evaluation of the clinical and radiologic features, however, will prevent overdiagnosis of these lesions as myxomas.

Treatment and Prognosis

Small myxomas are generally treated by curettage. For larger lesions, more extensive resection may be required. Myxomas are not encapsulated and tend to infiltrate the surrounding bone. Complete removal of the tumor by curettage is often difficult to accomplish. Recurrence rates of up to 25 percent have been reported in various studies. In most instances, this probably relates to incomplete removal of the original lesion. In spite of local recurrences, the overall prognosis is good, and metastases do not occur.

In rare cases, the myxoma microscopically shows marked cellularity and cellular atypism. These lesions have been designated by some as **myxosarcomas**. They appear to have a more aggressive local course than do the usual myxomas, but distant metastases have not been reported.

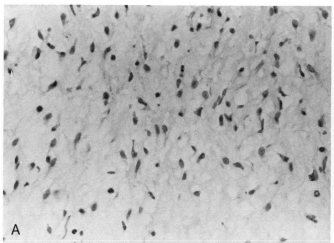

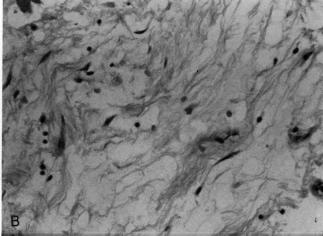

FIGURE 15–105. **Myxoma.** *A*, Stellate cells in a loose, myxoid matrix. *B*, Higher magnification shows stellate-shaped cells and fine collagen fibrils.

CEMENTOBLASTOMA (True Cementoma)

Many oral and maxillofacial pathologists consider the **cementoblastoma** to represent an odontogenic tumor. However, many pathologists have pointed out that the histopathologic features of cementoblastomas of the jaws are identical to those of a bone tumor, **osteoblastoma**, seen both in the jaws and extragnathic skeleton. Cementoblastomas are discussed together with osteoblastomas in Chapter 14 (see p. 476).

REFERENCES

Odontogenic Cysts and Tumors—General References and Classification

Kramer IRH, Pindborg JJ, Shear M. Histological Typing of Odontogenic Tumors, 2nd ed. Berlin, Springer-Verlag, 1992.

Shear M. Cysts of the Oral Regions, 2nd ed. Bristol, Wright PSG, 1983.

Dentigerous Cyst

Al-Talabani NG, Smith CJ. Experimental dentigerous cysts and enamel hypoplasia: Their possible significance in explaining the pathogenesis of human dentigerous cysts. J Oral Pathol 9:82–91, 1980.

Gorlin RJ. Potentialities of oral epithelium manifest by mandibular dentigerous cysts. Oral Surg Oral Med Oral Pathol 10:271–284, 1957.

Kusukawa J, et al. Dentigerous cyst associated with a deciduous tooth: A case report. Oral Surg Oral Med Oral Pathol 73:415–418, 1992.

Lustmann L, Bodner L. Dentigerous cysts associated with supernumerary teeth. Int J Oral Maxillofac Surg 17:100–102, 1988.

McMillan MD, Smillie AC. Ameloblastomas associated with dentigerous cysts. Oral Surg Oral Med Oral Pathol 51:489–496, 1981.

Norris LH, Papageorge MB. Multiple dentigerous cysts of the maxilla and mandible: Report of a case. J Oral Maxillofac Surg 45:694–697, 1987.

Shear M. Cysts of the jaws: Recent advances. J Oral Pathol 14:43–59, 1985.

Skouteris CA. Fiberoptic endoscopy of a marsupialized dentigerous cyst. J Oral Maxillofac Surg 46:74–77, 1988.

Eruption Cyst

Clark CA. A survey of eruption cysts in the newborn. Oral Surg Oral Med Oral Pathol 15:917, 1962.

Seward MH. Eruption cyst: An analysis of its clinical features. J Oral Surg 31:31–35, 1973.

Primordial Cyst

Brannon RB. The odontogenic keratocyst—a clinicopathologic study of 312 cases: Part I: Clinical features. Oral Surg Oral Med Oral Pathol 42:54–72, 1976

Odontogenic Keratocyst

Ahlfors E, Larsson A, Sjögren S. The odontogenic keratocyst: A benign cystic tumor? J Oral Maxillofac Surg 42:10–19, 1984.

Brannon RB. The odontogenic keratocyst—a clinicopathologic study of 312 cases: Part I: Clinical features. Oral Surg Oral Med Oral Pathol 42:54–72, 1976.

Brannon RB. The odontogenic keratocyst—a clinicopathologic study of 312 cases: Part II: Histologic features. Oral Surg Oral Med Oral Pathol 43:233–255, 1977.

Browne RM. The odontogenic keratocyst—histological features and their correlation with clinical behavior. Br Dent J 131:249–259, 1971.

Forssell K, Forssell H, Kahnberg K-E. Recurrence of keratocysts: A long-term follow-up study. Int J Oral Maxillofac Surg 17:25–28, 1988.

Orthokeratinized Odontogenic Cysts

Crowley TE, Kaugars GE, Gunsolley JC. Odontogenic keratocysts: A clinical and histologic comparison of the parakeratin and orthokeratin variants. J Oral Maxillofac Surg 50:22–26, 1992.

Vuhahula E, et al. Jaw cysts with orthokeratinization: Analysis of 12 cases. J Oral Pathol Med 22:35–40, 1993.

Wright JM. The odontogenic keratocyst: Orthokeratinized variant. Oral Surg Oral Med Oral Pathol 51:609–618, 1981.

Nevoid Basal Cell Carcinoma Syndrome

Gorlin RJ. Nevoid basal cell carcinoma syndrome. Medicine 66:98–113, 1987.

Gorlin RJ, et al. The multiple basal cell nevi syndrome: An analysis of a syndrome consisting of multiple nevoid basal cell carcinomas, jaw cysts, skeletal anomalies, medulloblastoma and hyporesponsiveness to parathormone. Cancer 18:89–103, 1965.

Gorlin RJ, Goltz R. Multiple nevoid basal cell epithelioma, jaw cysts and bifid rib syndrome. N Engl J Med 262:908–914, 1960.

Woolgar JA, Rippin JW, Browne RM: The odontogenic keratocyst and its occurrence in the nevoid basal cell carcinoma syndrome. Oral Surg Oral Med Oral Pathol 64:727–730, 1987.

Woolgar JA, Rippin JW, Browne RM: A comparative histologic study of odontogenic keratocysts in basal cell nevus syndrome and non-syndrome patients. J Oral Pathol 16:75–80, 1987.

Gingival Cyst of the Newborn

Cataldo E, Berkman M. Cysts of the oral mucosa in newborns. Am J Dis Child 116:44–48, 1968.

Gingival Cyst of the Adult

Buchner A, Hansen LS. The histomorphologic spectrum of the gingival cyst in the adult. Oral Surg Oral Med Oral Pathol 48:532–539, 1979.

Lateral Periodontal Cyst

Altini M, Shear M. The lateral periodontal cyst: An update. J Oral Pathol Med 21:245–250, 1992.

Fantasia JE. Lateral periodontal cyst. An analysis of forty-six cases. Oral Surg Oral Med Oral Pathol 48:237–243, 1979.

Greer RO, Johnson M. Botryoid odontogenic cyst: Clinicopathologic analysis of ten cases with three recurrences. J Oral Maxillofac Surg 46:574–579, 1988.

Wysocki GP, et al. Histogenesis of the lateral periodontal cyst and the gingival cyst of the adult. Oral Surg Oral Med Oral Pathol 50:327–334, 1980.

Calcifying Odontogenic Cyst

Buchner A. The central (intraosseous) calcifying odontogenic cyst: An analysis of 215 cases. J Oral Maxillofac Surg 49:330–339, 1991.

Buchner A, et al. Peripheral (extraosseous) calcifying odontogenic cysts: A review of forty-five cases. Oral Surg Oral Med Oral Pathol 72:65–70, 1991.

Ellis GL, Shmookler BM. Aggressive (malignant?) epithelial odontogenic ghost cell tumor. Oral Surg Oral Med Oral Pathol 61:471–478, 1986.

Hong SP, Ellis GL, Hartman KS. Calcifying odontogenic cyst: A review of ninety-two cases with reevaluation of their nature as cysts or neoplasms, the nature of the ghost cells and subclassification. Oral Surg Oral Med Oral Pathol 72:56–64, 1991.

Praetorius F, et al. Calcifying odontogenic cyst. Range, variations and neoplastic potential. Acta Odontol Scand 39:227–240, 1981.

Tajima Y, et al. Ameloblastoma arising in calcifying odontogenic cyst. Oral Surg Oral Med Oral Pathol 74:776–779, 1992.

Glandular Odontogenic Cyst

Ficarra G, Chou L, Panzoni E. Glandular odontogenic cyst (sialo-odontogenic cyst): A case report. Int J Oral Maxillofac Surg 19:331–333, 1990.

Gardner DG, et al. The glandular odontogenic cyst: An apparent entity. J Oral Pathol 17:359–366, 1988.

Patron M, Colmenero C, Larrouri J. Glandular odontogenic cyst: Clinicopathologic analysis of three cases. Oral Surg Oral Med Oral Pathol 72:71–74, 1991.

Carcinoma Arising in Odontogenic Cysts

Eversole LR, Sabes WR, Rovin S. Aggressive growth and neoplastic potential of odontogenic cysts. Cancer 35:270–282, 1975.

Müller S, Waldron CA. Primary intraosseous carcinoma: Report of two cases. Int J Oral Maxillofac Surg 20:362–365, 1991.

Stoelinga PJ, Bronkhorst FB. The incidence, multiple presentation and recurrence of aggressive cysts of the jaws. J Craniomaxillofac Surg 16:184–195, 1988.

van der Waal I, et al. Squamous cell carcinoma arising in the lining of odontogenic cysts. Int J Oral Surg 14:146–152, 1985.

Waldron CA, Mustoe TA. Primary intraosseous carcinoma of the mandible with probable origin in an odontogenic cyst. Oral Surg Oral Med Oral Pathol 67:716–724, 1989.

Ameloblastoma

Eversole LR, Leider AS, Hansen LS. Ameloblastomas with pronounced desmoplasia. J Oral Maxillofac Surg 42:735–740, 1984.

Gardner DG, Pecak AMJ. The treatment of ameloblastoma based on pathologic and anatomic principles. Cancer 46:2514–2519, 1980.

Hartman KS. Granular cell ameloblastoma. Oral Surg Oral Med Oral Pathol 38:241–253, 1974.

Leider AS, Eversole LR, Barkin ME. Cystic ameloblastoma: A clinicopathologic analysis. Oral Surg Oral Med Oral Pathol 60:624–630, 1985.

Mehlisch DR, Dahlin DC, Masson JK. Ameloblastoma: A clinicopathologic study. J Oral Surg 30:9–22, 1972.

Müller H, Slootweg PJ. The ameloblastoma: The controversial approach to therapy. J Maxillofac Surg 13:79–84, 1984.

Philipsen HP, Ormiston IW, Reichart PA. The desmo- and osteoplastic ameloblastoma: Histologic variant or clinicopathologic entity? Int J Oral Maxillofac Surg 21:352–357, 1992.

Small IA, Waldron CA. Ameloblastoma of the jaws. Oral Surg Oral Med Oral Pathol 8:281–297, 1955.

Waldron CA, El-Mofty S. A histopathologic study of 116 ameloblastomas with special reference to the desmoplastic variant. Oral Surg Oral Med Oral Pathol 63:441–451, 1987.

Unicystic Ameloblastoma

Ackerman GL, Altini M, Shear M. The unicystic ameloblastoma: A clinicopathologic study of 57 cases. J Oral Pathol 17:541–546, 1988.

Gardner DG, Corio RL. The relationship of plexiform unicystic ameloblastoma to conventional ameloblastoma. Oral Surg Oral Med Oral Pathol 56:54–60, 1983.

Robinson L, Martinez MG: Unicystic ameloblastoma: A prognostically distinct entity. Cancer 40:2278–2285, 1977.

Vickers RA, Gorlin RJ. Ameloblastoma: Delineation of early histopathologic features of neoplasia. Cancer 26:699–710, 1970.

Peripheral (Extraosseous) Ameloblastoma

Baden E, Doyle JL, Petriella V. Malignant transformation of peripheral ameloblastoma. Oral Surg Oral Med Oral Pathol 75:214–219, 1993.

Gardner DG. Peripheral ameloblastoma: A study of 21 cases including 5 reported as basal cell carcinoma of the gingiva. Cancer 39:1625–1633, 1977.

Woo SB, et al. Peripheral ameloblastoma of the buccal mucosa: Case report and review of the English language literature. Oral Surg Oral Med Oral Pathol 63:73–84, 1987.

Malignant Ameloblastoma and Ameloblastic Carcinoma

Corio RL, et al. Ameloblastic carcinoma: A clinicopathologic assessment of eight cases. Oral Surg Oral Med Oral Pathol 64:570–576, 1987.

Eliasson A, Moser RJ III, Tenholder MF. Diagnosis and treatment of metastatic ameloblastoma. South Med J 82:1165–1168, 1989.

Ikumera K, et al. Ameloblastoma of the mandible with metastasis to lungs and lymph nodes. Cancer 29:930–940, 1972.

Slootweg PJ, Müller H. Malignant ameloblastoma or ameloblastic carcinoma. Oral Surg Oral Med Oral Pathol 57:168–176, 1984.

Calcifying Epithelial Odontogenic Tumor

Basu MK, et al. Calcifying epithelial odontogenic tumor: A case showing features of malignancy. J Oral Pathol 13:310–319, 1984.

Chaudhry AP, et al. Calcifying epithelial odontogenic tumor: A histochemical and ultrastructural study. Cancer 30:519–529, 1972.

Franklin CD, et al. An investigation into the origin and nature of "amyloid" in a calcifying epithelial odontogenic tumor. J Oral Pathol 10:417–429, 1981.

Franklin CD, Pindborg JJ. The calcifying epithelial odontogenic tumor: A review and analysis of 113 cases. Oral Surg Oral Med Oral Pathol 42:753–765, 1976.

Krolls SO, Pindborg JJ. Calcifying epithelial odontogenic tumor: A survey of 23 cases and discussion of histomorphologic variations. Arch Pathol Lab Med 98:206–210, 1974.

Pindborg JJ. A calcifying epithelial odontogenic tumor. Cancer 11:838–843, 1958.

Squamous Odontogenic Tumor

Baden E, et al. Squamous odontogenic tumor: Report of three cases including the first extraosseous case. Oral Surg Oral Med Oral Pathol 75:733–738, 1993.

Goldblatt LI, Brannon RB, Ellis GL. Squamous odontogenic tumor: Report of five cases and review of the literature. Oral Surg Oral Med Oral Pathol 54:187–196, 1982.

Mills WP, et al. Squamous odontogenic tumor: Report of a case with lesions in three quadrants. Oral Surg Oral Med Oral Pathol 61:557–563, 1986.

Pullon PA, et al. Squamous odontogenic tumor: Report of six cases of a previously undescribed lesion. Oral Surg Oral Med Oral Pathol 40:616–630, 1975.

Wright JM. Squamous odontogenic tumor-like proliferations in odontogenic cysts. Oral Surg Oral Med Oral Pathol 47:354–358, 1979.

Clear Cell Odontogenic Tumor

Bang G, et al. Clear cell odontogenic carcinoma: Report of three cases and lymph node metastasis. J Oral Pathol Med 18:113–118, 1989.

Fan J, et al. Clear cell odontogenic carcinoma: A case report with massive invasion of neighboring organs and lymph node metastasis. Oral Surg Oral Med Oral Pathol 74:768–775, 1992.

Hansen LS, et al. Clear cell odontogenic tumor—a new histologic variant with aggressive potential. Head Neck Surg 8:115–123, 1985.

Waldron CA, Small IA, Silverman H. Clear cell ameloblastoma—an odontogenic carcinoma. J Oral Maxillofac Surg 43:709–717, 1985.

Mixed Odontogenic Tumors

Gardner DG. The mixed odontogenic tumors. Oral Surg Oral Med Oral Pathol 58:166–168, 1984.

Hansen LS, Ficarra G. Mixed odontogenic tumors: An analysis of 23 new cases. Head Neck Surg 10:330–343, 1988.

Slootweg PJ. An analysis of the interrelationship of the mixed odontogenic tumors—ameloblastic fibroma, ameloblastic fibro-odontoma and the odontomas. Oral Surg Oral Med Oral Pathol 51:266–276, 1981.

Ameloblastic Fibroma

Sawyer DR, Nwoku AL, Mosadomi A. Recurrent ameloblastic fibroma: Report of 2 cases. Oral Surg Oral Med Oral Pathol 53:19–24, 1982.

Trodahl JN. Ameloblastic fibroma: A survey of cases from the Armed Forces Institute of Pathology. Oral Surg Oral Med Oral Pathol 33:547–558, 1972.

Zallen RD, Preskar MH, McClary SA. Ameloblastic fibroma. J Oral Maxillofac Surg 40:513–517, 1982.

Ameloblastic Fibro-Odontoma

Miller AS, et al. Ameloblastic fibro-odontoma. Oral Surg Oral Med Oral Pathol 41:354–365, 1976.

Slootweg PJ. Epithelio-mesenchymal morphology in ameloblastic fibro-odontoma: A light and electron microscopic study. J Oral Pathol 9:29–40, 1980.

Van Wyk CW, Van der Vyrer PC. Ameloblastic fibroma with dentinoid formation/immature dentinoma: A microscopic and ultrastructural study of the epithelial-connective tissue interface. J Oral Pathol 12:37–46, 1983.

Ameloblastic Fibrosarcoma

Altini M, et al. Ameloblastic sarcoma of the mandible. J Oral Maxillofac Surg 43:789–794, 1985.

Chomette G, et al. Ameloblastic fibrosarcoma of the jaws—report of three cases. Pathol Res Pract 178:40–47, 1983.

Leider AS, Nelson JF, Trodahl JN. Ameloblastic fibrosarcoma of the jaws. Oral Surg Oral Med Oral Pathol 33:559–569, 1972.

Wood RM, et al. Ameloblastic fibrosarcoma. Oral Surg Oral Med Oral Pathol 66:74–77, 1988.

Adenomatoid Odontogenic Tumor

Courtney RM, Kerr DA. The odontogenic adenomatoid tumor: A comprehensive review of 21 cases. Oral Surg Oral Med Oral Pathol 39:424–435, 1975.

Giansanti JS, Someren A, Waldron CA. Odontogenic adenomatoid tumor (adenoameloblastoma). Oral Surg Oral Med Oral Pathol 30:69–86, 1970.

Philipsen HP, et al. Adenomatoid odontogenic tumor: Biologic profile on 499 cases. J Oral Pathol Med 20:149–158, 1991.

Poulson TC, Greer RO. Adenomatoid odontogenic tumor: Clinicopathologic and ultrastructural concepts. J Oral Maxillofac Surg 41:818–824, 1983.

Odontoameloblastoma

LaBriola JP, et al. Odontoameloblastoma. J Oral Surg 38:139–143, 1980.

Odontoma

Budnick SD. Compound and complex odontomas. Oral Surg Oral Med Oral Pathol 42:501–506, 1976.

Sapp JP, Gardner DG. An ultrastructural study of the calcifications in calcifying odontogenic cysts and odontomas. Oral Surg Oral Med Oral Pathol 44:754–766, 1977.

Sedano HO, Pindborg JJ. Ghost cell epithelium in odontomas. J Oral Pathol 4:27–30, 1975.

Odontogenic Fibroma

Allen CM, Hammond HL, Stimson PG. Central odontogenic fibroma WHO type: A report of 3 cases with an unusual associated giant cell reaction. Oral Surg Oral Med Oral Pathol 73:62–66, 1992.

Gardner DG. The central odontogenic fibroma: An attempt at clarification. Oral Surg Oral Med Oral Pathol 50:425–432, 1980.

Handlers JP, et al. Central odontogenic fibroma: Clinicopathologic features of 19 cases and review of the literature. J Oral Maxillofac Surg 49:46–54, 1991.

Slootweg PJ, Müller H. Central fibroma of the jaw: Odontogenic or desmoplastic. Oral Surg Oral Med Oral Pathol 56:61–70, 1983.

Granular Cell Odontogenic Fibroma

Vincent SD, et al. Central granular cell odontogenic fibroma. Oral Surg Oral Med Oral Pathol 63:715–721, 1987.

Waldron CA, Thompson CW, Conner WA. Granular cell ameloblastic fibroma. Oral Surg Oral Med Oral Pathol 16:1202–1213, 1963.

White DK, et al. Central granular cell tumor of the jaws (the so-called granular cell ameloblastic fibroma). Oral Surg Oral Med Oral Pathol 45:396–405, 1978.

Peripheral Odontogenic Fibroma

Baden E, Moskow BS, Moskow R. Odontogenic epithelial hamartoma. J Oral Surg 26:702–714, 1968.

Buchner A. Peripheral odontogenic fibroma. J Craniomaxillofac Surg 17:134–138, 1989.

Buchner A, Ficarra G, Hansen LS. Peripheral odontogenic fibroma. Oral Surg Oral Med Oral Pathol 64:432–438, 1987.

Slabbert H, Altini M. Peripheral odontogenic fibroma: A clinicopathologic study. Oral Surg Oral Med Oral Pathol 72:86–90, 1991.

Myxoma

Barros RE, Dominguez PV, Cabrini RL. Myxoma of the jaws. Oral Surg Oral Med Oral Pathol 27:225–236, 1969.

Goldblatt LI. Ultrastructural study of an odontogenic myxoma. Oral Surg Oral Med Oral Pathol 42:206–220, 1976.

Gosh BC, et al. Myxoma of the jaw bones. Cancer 31:237–240, 1973.

Lamberg MA, et al. A case of malignant myxoma (myxosarcoma) of the maxilla. Scand J Dent Res 92:352–357, 1984.

White DK, et al. Odontogenic myxoma: A clinical and ultrastructural study. Oral Surg Oral Med Oral Pathol 39:901–917, 1975.

Zimmerman DC, Dahlin DC. Myxomatous tumors of the jaws. Oral Surg Oral Med Oral Pathol 11:1069–1080, 1958.

16

Dermatologic Diseases

ECTODERMAL DYSPLASIA

Ectodermal dysplasia represents a group of inherited conditions in which two or more ectodermally derived anatomic structures fail to develop. Thus, depending on the type of ectodermal dysplasia, hypoplasia or aplasia of tissues, such as skin, hair, nails, teeth, or sweat glands, may be seen. The various types of this disorder may be inherited in any one of several genetic patterns, including autosomal dominant, autosomal recessive, and X-linked. Even though by some accounts 121 different subtypes of ectodermal dysplasia can be defined, these disorders are considered to be relatively rare, with an estimated frequency of 1 case occurring in every 10,000 to 100,000 births.

Clinical Features

Perhaps the best known of the ectodermal dysplasia syndromes is **hypohidrotic ectodermal dysplasia**. In most instances, this disorder seems to show an X-linked inheritance pattern; therefore, a male predominance is usually seen. Affected individuals typically display heat intolerance because of a reduced number of sweat glands.

Sometimes the diagnosis is made during infancy because the baby appears to have a fever of undetermined origin; however, the infant simply cannot regulate body temperature appropriately because of the decreased number of sweat glands. Uncommonly, death results from the markedly elevated body temperature. Sometimes, as a diagnostic aid, a special impression can be made of the patient's fingertips and then examined microscopically in order to count the density of the sweat glands. Such findings should be interpreted in conjunction with appropriate age-matched controls.

Other signs of this disorder include fine, sparse blonde hair, including a reduced density of eyebrow and eyelash hair (Fig. 16-1). The periocular skin may show a fine wrinkling with hyperpigmentation (Fig. 16-2), and mid-face hypoplasia is frequently observed, often resulting in protuberant lips. Because the salivary glands are ectodermally derived, patients may exhibit varying degrees of xerostomia. The nails may also appear dystrophic and brittle.

The teeth are usually markedly reduced in number (**oligodontia** or **hypodontia**), and their crown shapes are characteristically abnormal (Fig. 16-3). The incisor crowns usually appear tapered, conical, or pointed, and the molar crowns are reduced in diameter.

Female patients may show partial expression of the abnormal gene; that is, their teeth may be reduced in number or may have mild structural changes. This incomplete presentation can be explained by the _Lyon hypothesis,_ with half of the female patient's X chromosomes expressing the normal gene and the other half expressing the defective gene.

Histopathologic Features

Histopathologic examination of the skin from a patient with hypohidrotic ectodermal dysplasia shows a decreased number of sweat glands and hair follicles.

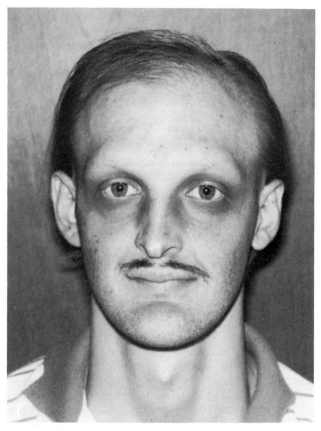

FIGURE 16-1. **Ectodermal dysplasia**. The sparse hair, periocular hyperpigmentation, and mild midfacial hypoplasia are characteristic features evident in this affected patient.

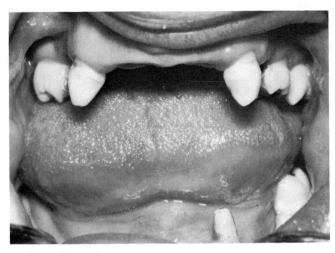

FIGURE 16-3. **Ectodermal dysplasia**. Oligodontia and conical crown forms are typical oral manifestations. (Courtesy of Dr. Charles Hook and Dr. Bob Gellin.)

Those adnexal structures that are present are hypoplastic and malformed.

Treatment and Prognosis

Management of hypohidrotic ectodermal dysplasia warrants genetic counseling for the parents and the pa-

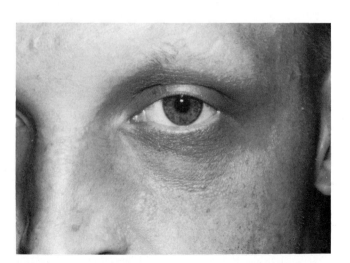

FIGURE 16-2. **Ectodermal dysplasia**. Closer view of the same patient depicted in Figure 16-1. Fine periocular wrinkling as well as sparse eyelash and eyebrow hair can be observed.

tient. The dental problems are best managed by prosthetic replacement of the dentition with complete dentures, overdentures, or fixed appliances, depending on the number and location of the remaining teeth. Endosseous dental implants may be considered for facilitating prosthetic management in patients older than 12 years of age.

WHITE SPONGE NEVUS (Cannon's Disease; Familial White Folded Dysplasia)

White sponge nevus is a relatively rare genodermatosis (a genetically determined skin disorder) that is inherited as an autosomal dominant trait displaying a high degree of penetrance and variable expressivity. Patients usually have the lesions at birth or in early childhood, but sometimes the condition develops during adolescence.

Clinical Features

The lesions of white sponge nevus appear as symmetric, thickened, white, corrugated or velvety, diffuse plaques that primarily affect the buccal mucosa bilaterally (Fig. 16-4). Other common intraoral sites of involvement include the ventral tongue, labial mucosa, soft palate, alveolar mucosa, and floor of the mouth, although the extent of involvement can vary. Extraoral mucosal sites appear to be less commonly affected, such as the nasal, esophageal, laryngeal, and anogenital mucosa. Patients are usually asymptomatic.

Histopathologic Features

The microscopic features of white sponge nevus are characteristic but not necessarily pathognomonic. Prominent hyperparakeratosis and marked acanthosis with clearing of the cytoplasm of the cells in the spinous layer are common features (Figs. 16-5 and 16-6); however,

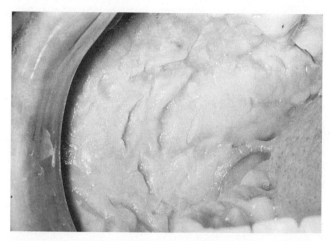

FIGURE 16-4. **White sponge nevus.** Diffuse, thickened white plaques of the buccal mucosa.

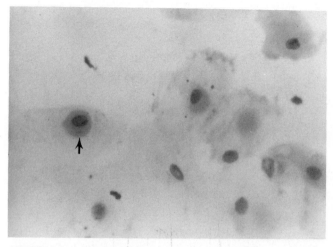

FIGURE 16-7. **White sponge nevus.** This high-power photomicrograph of a Papanicolaou-stained cytologic preparation shows the pathognomonic perinuclear condensation of keratin tonofilaments (*arrow*).

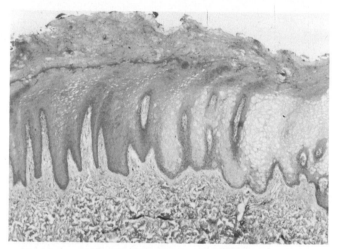

FIGURE 16-5. **White sponge nevus.** This low-power photomicrograph shows prominent parakeratosis as well as marked thickening (acanthosis) and vacuolation of the spinous cell layer.

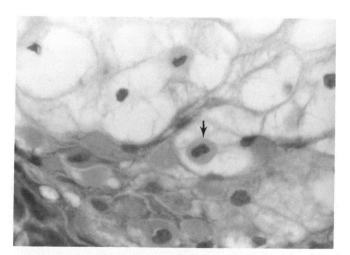

FIGURE 16-6. **White sponge nevus.** This high-power photomicrograph shows vacuolation of the cytoplasm of the cells of the spinous layer, with no evidence of epithelial atypia. Perinuclear condensation of keratin tonofilaments can also be observed in some cells (*arrow*).

similar microscopic findings may be associated with leukoedema and hereditary benign intraepithelial dyskeratosis. In some instances, an eosinophilic condensation is noted in the perinuclear region of the cells in the superficial layers of the epithelium, a feature that is unique to white sponge nevus. Ultrastructurally, this condensed material can be identified as tangled masses of keratin tonofilaments.

Exfoliative cytologic studies may provide more definitive diagnostic information. A cytologic preparation stained with the Papanicolaou method often shows the eosinophilic perinuclear condensation of the epithelial cell cytoplasm to a greater extent than does the histopathologic section (Fig. 16-7).

Treatment and Prognosis

Because this is a benign condition, no treatment is necessary. The prognosis is good.

HEREDITARY BENIGN INTRAEPITHELIAL DYSKERATOSIS
(Witkop-Von Sallmann Syndrome)

Hereditary benign intraepithelial dyskeratosis (HBID) is a rare genodermatosis primarily affecting descendants of a triracial isolate (Native American, African-American, and white) of people who originally lived in North Carolina. The condition is inherited as an autosomal dominant trait.

Clinical Features

The lesions of HBID usually appear during childhood, in most instances affecting the oral and conjunctival mucosa. The oral lesions appear similar to those of white sponge nevus, with both conditions showing thick, corrugated white plaques involving the buccal and labial

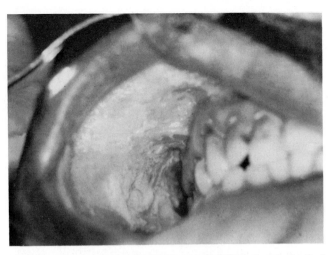

FIGURE 16-8. **Hereditary benign intraepithelial dyskeratosis.** Oral lesions appear as corrugated white plaques of the buccal and labial mucosa. (Courtesy of Dr. Carl Witkop.)

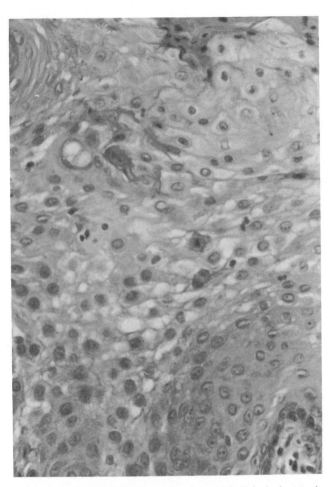

FIGURE 16-10. **Hereditary benign intraepithelial dyskeratosis.** Marked thickening and vacuolation of the spinous layer of the epithelium is noted in this medium-power photomicrograph.

mucosa (Fig. 16-8). Milder cases may exhibit the opalescent appearance of leukoedema. Other oral mucosal sites, such as the floor of the mouth and lateral tongue, may also be affected. These oral lesions may exhibit a superimposed candidal infection as well.

The most interesting feature of HBID is the ocular lesions, which begin to develop very early in life. These appear as thick, opaque, gelatinous plaques affecting the bulbar conjunctiva adjacent to the cornea (Fig. 16-9) and sometimes involving the cornea itself. When the lesions are active, patients may experience tearing, photophobia, and itching of the eyes. In many patients, the plaques are most prominent in the spring and tend to regress during the summer or autumn. Sometimes blindness may result from the induction of vascularity of the cornea secondary to the shedding process.

Histopathologic Features

The histopathologic features of HBID include prominent parakeratin production in addition to marked acanthosis. A peculiar dyskeratotic process, similar to that of Darier's disease, is scattered throughout the upper spinous layer of the surface oral epithelium (Fig. 16-10). With this dyskeratotic process, an epithelial cell appears to be surrounded or engulfed by an adjacent epithelial cell, resulting in the so-called "cell-within-a-cell" phenomenon.

Treatment and Prognosis

Because HBID is a benign condition, no treatment is generally required or indicated for the oral lesions. If superimposed candidiasis develops, an antifungal medication can be used. Patients with symptomatic ocular lesions should be referred to an ophthalmologist. Typically, the plaques that obscure vision must be surgically excised. This procedure, however, is recognized as a temporary measure because ultimately the lesions often recur.

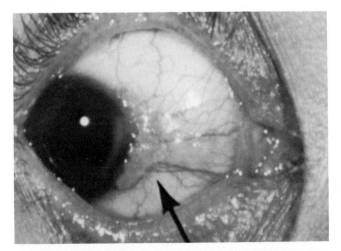

FIGURE 16-9. **Hereditary benign intraepithelial dyskeratosis.** Ocular lesions appear as gelatinous plaques (*arrow*) of the bulbar conjunctivae. (Courtesy of Dr. Carl Witkop.)

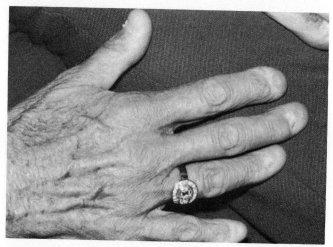

FIGURE 16–11. **Pachyonychia congenita**. Loss of fingernails. (Courtesy of Dr. John Lenox.)

PACHYONYCHIA CONGENITA
(Jadassohn-Lewandowsky Syndrome)

Pachyonychia congenita is a rare genodermatosis that is usually inherited as an autosomal dominant trait. The nails are dramatically affected in most patients, but oral lesions are also seen in a significant number. Fewer than 200 cases have been reported.

Clinical Features

Virtually all patients with pachyonychia congenita exhibit characteristic nail changes either at birth or in the early neonatal period. The free margins of the nails are lifted up because of an accumulation of keratinaceous material in the nail beds. This results in a pinched, tubular configuration. Ultimately, nail loss may occur (Fig. 16–11).

Other skin changes that may occur include marked hyperkeratosis of the palmar and plantar surfaces, producing thick, callous-like lesions (Fig. 16–12). Hyperhidrosis of the palms and soles is also commonly present. The rest of the skin shows punctate papules, representing an abnormal accumulation of keratin in the hair follicles. One disabling feature of the syndrome is that painful blisters form on the soles of the feet when the patient walks for a few minutes during warm weather.

The oral lesions consist of thickened white plaques that involve the lateral margins and dorsal surface of the tongue. Other oral mucosal regions that are frequently exposed to mild trauma, such as the palate, buccal mucosa, and alveolar mucosa, may also be affected (Fig. 16–13). Neonatal teeth have been reported in some of these patients. Hoarseness and dyspnea have been described in some patients as a result of laryngeal mucosal involvement.

Histopathologic Features

Microscopic examination of lesional oral mucosa shows marked hyperparakeratosis and acanthosis with perinuclear clearing of the epithelial cells.

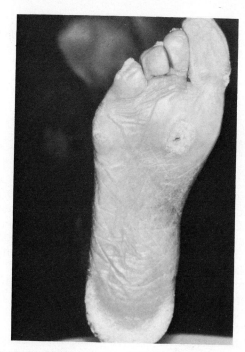

FIGURE 16–12. **Pachyonychia congenita**. The soles of the feet of affected patients typically show marked callus-like thickenings. (Courtesy of Dr. Lou Young.)

Treatment and Prognosis

Because the oral lesions of pachyonychia congenita show no apparent tendency for malignant transformation, no treatment is required. The nails are often lost or may need to be surgically removed because of the deformity. Patients should receive genetic counseling.

DYSKERATOSIS CONGENITA

Dyskeratosis congenita is a rare genodermatosis that is thought to be inherited as an X-linked recessive trait

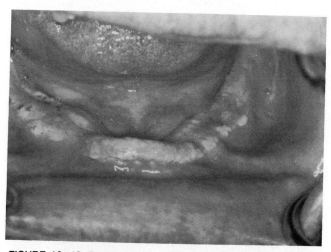

FIGURE 16–13. **Pachyonychia congenita**. Although tongue lesions are more common in patients with pachyonychia congenita, other oral mucosal sites exposed to minor trauma, such as the alveolar mucosa, may develop thickened white patches. (Courtesy of Dr. John Lenox.)

because of its striking male predilection. Some studies suggest that the condition shows genetic heterogeneity, with autosomal dominant and autosomal recessive forms being reported. The clinician should be aware of the condition because the oral lesions may undergo malignant transformation, and patients are susceptible to aplastic anemia.

Clinical Features

Dyskeratosis congenita usually becomes evident during the first 10 years of life. A reticular pattern of skin hyperpigmentation develops, affecting the upper chest and neck. In addition, abnormal, dysplastic changes of the nails are evident at this time (Fig. 16–14).

Intraorally, the tongue and buccal mucosa develop bullae; these are followed by erosions and, eventually, leukoplakic lesions (Fig. 16–15). The leukoplakic lesions are considered to be premalignant, and approximately one third of them become malignant in a 10- to 30-year period. Rapidly progressive periodontal disease has been reported sporadically.

Thrombocytopenia is usually the first hematologic problem that develops, typically during the second decade of life, followed by anemia. Ultimately, **aplastic anemia** develops in approximately 45 percent of these patients (see p. 422). Mild to moderate mental retardation may also be present. Generally, the autosomal recessive and X-linked recessive forms show a more severe pattern of disease expression.

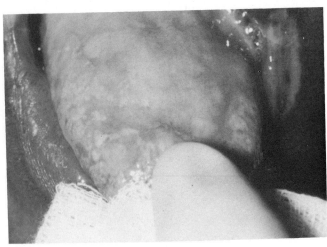

FIGURE 16–15. **Dyskeratosis congenita**. Atrophy and hyperkeratosis of the dorsal tongue mucosa are visible.

Histopathologic Features

Biopsy specimens of the early oral mucosal lesions show hyperorthokeratosis with epithelial atrophy. As the lesions progress, epithelial dysplasia develops until frank squamous cell carcinoma evolves.

Treatment and Prognosis

The discomfort of the oral lesions is managed symptomatically, and careful periodic oral mucosal examinations are performed to check for evidence of malignant transformation. Routine medical evaluation is warranted to monitor the patient for the development of aplastic anemia.

As a result of these potentially life-threatening complications, the prognosis is guarded. The average life span for the more severely affected patients is 32 years of age. The parents and the patient should also receive genetic counseling.

XERODERMA PIGMENTOSUM

Xeroderma pigmentosum is a rare genodermatosis in which numerous cutaneous malignancies develop at a very early age. The condition is inherited as an autosomal recessive trait and is caused by one of several defects in the excision repair and/or postreplication repair mechanism of DNA. As a result of the inability of the epithelial cells to repair ultraviolet light-induced damage, mutations in the epithelial cells occur, leading to the development of skin cancer.

Clinical Features

During the first few years of life, patients affected by xeroderma pigmentosum show a markedly increased tendency to sunburn. Skin changes, such as atrophy, freckled pigmentation, and patchy depigmentation, soon follow (Fig. 16–16). In early childhood, **actinic keratoses**

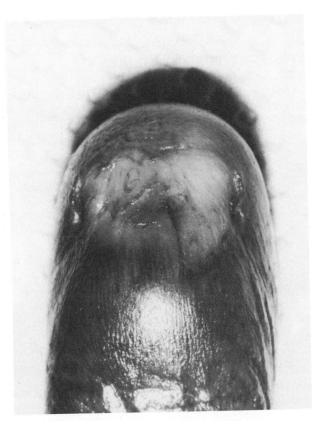

FIGURE 16–14. **Dyskeratosis congenita**. Dysplastic nail changes.

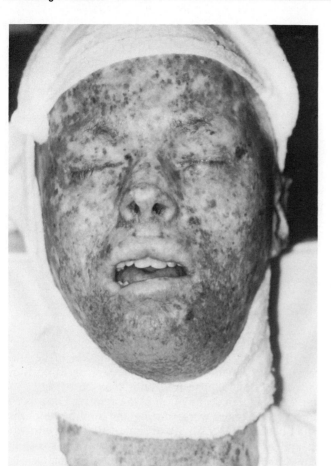

FIGURE 16-16. **Xeroderma pigmentosum**. The atrophic changes and pigmentation disturbances shown are characteristic of xeroderma pigmentosum.

begin developing, a process that normally does not take place before 40 years of age. These lesions quickly progress to **squamous cell carcinoma**, with **basal cell carcinomas** also appearing, so that in most patients a non-melanoma skin cancer develops during the first decade of life. **Melanoma** develops in about 5 percent of patients with xeroderma pigmentosum, but it evolves at a slightly later time. As a consequence of sun exposure, the head and neck region is the site most frequently affected by these cutaneous malignancies. Neurologic manifestations include subnormal intelligence in 80 percent of affected individuals.

Oral manifestations, which often occur before 20 years of age, include development of **squamous cell carcinoma** of the lower lip and the tip of the tongue. This latter site is most unusual for oral cancer, and its involvement is again undoubtedly related to the increased sun exposure, however minimal, which this area receives in contrast to the rest of the oral mucosa.

The diagnosis of xeroderma pigmentosum is usually made when the patient is evaluated for the cutaneous lesions, because it is highly unusual for a very young person to have skin cancer. Because xeroderma pigmentosum is an autosomal recessive trait, a family history of the disorder is not likely to be present, but the possibility of a consanguineous relationship of the affected child's parents should be investigated.

Histopathologic Features

The histopathologic features of xeroderma pigmentosum are relatively nonspecific, in that the cutaneous premalignant lesions and malignancies that occur are microscopically indistinguishable from those observed in unaffected patients.

Treatment and Prognosis

Treatment of xeroderma pigmentosum is challenging because in most instances significant sun damage has already occurred by the time of diagnosis. Patients are advised to avoid sunlight and unfiltered fluorescent light and to wear appropriate protective clothing and sunscreens if they cannot avoid sun exposure. A dermatologist should evaluate the patient every 3 months to monitor the development of cutaneous lesions.

Actinic keratoses may be treated by topical chemotherapeutic agents, such as 5-fluorouracil. Non-melanoma skin cancers should be excised conservatively, preferably with microscopically controlled excision (Mohs surgery) in order to preserve as much normal tissue as possible. Patients should also receive genetic counseling because a high number of consanguineous marriages have been reported in some series.

The prognosis is still poor. Most patients die 30 years earlier than the normal population, either directly from cutaneous malignancy or from complications associated with the treatment of the cancer.

INCONTINENTIA PIGMENTI (Bloch-Sulzberger Syndrome)

Incontinentia pigmenti is a relatively rare inherited disorder, with approximately 800 cases reported worldwide. It typically evolves in several stages, primarily affecting the skin, eyes, and central nervous system as well as oral structures. There is a marked female predilection, with a 37:1 female-to-male ratio reported. The condition is thought to be inherited as an X-linked dominant trait, with the single unpaired gene on the X chromosome being lethal for most males. Recent studies suggest that affected patients show chromosomal instability, which may lead to a small increased risk of childhood malignancy.

Clinical Features

The clinical manifestations of incontinentia pigmenti usually begin in the first few weeks of infancy. There are four stages:

1. *Vesicular stage.* Vesiculobullous lesions appear on the skin of the trunk and limbs. Spontaneous resolution occurs within 4 months.
2. *Verrucous stage.* Verrucous cutaneous plaques de-

velop, affecting the limbs. These clear by 6 months of age, evolving into the third stage.

3. *Hyperpigmentation stage.* Macular, brown skin lesions appear, characterized by a strange swirling pattern.
4. *Atrophy and depigmentation stage.* Atrophy and depigmentation of the skin ultimately occur.

Central nervous system abnormalities occur in 30 to 50 percent of affected patients. The most common problems are mental retardation, seizure disorders, and motor difficulties. Ocular problems (e.g., strabismus, cataracts, and optic atrophy) may also be identified in approximately 30 percent of these patients.

The oral manifestations of incontinentia pigmenti, noted in 60 to 80 percent of the cases, include *oligodontia (hypodontia),* delayed eruption, and hypoplasia of the teeth. The teeth are small and cone-shaped; both the primary and permanent dentitions are affected.

Histopathologic Features

The microscopic findings in incontinentia pigmenti vary, depending on when a biopsy of the skin lesions is performed.

In the initial *vesicular* stage, intraepithelial clefts filled with eosinophils are observed. During the *verrucous* stage, hyperkeratosis, acanthosis, and papillomatosis are noted. The *hyperpigmentation* stage shows numerous melanin-containing macrophages (melanin "incontinence") in the subepithelial connective tissue, the feature from which the disorder derives its name.

Treatment and Prognosis

Treatment of incontinentia pigmenti is directed toward the various abnormalities. Dental management includes appropriate prosthodontic and restorative care, although this is sometimes difficult if central nervous system problems are severe.

DARIER'S DISEASE (Keratosis Follicularis; Dyskeratosis Follicularis; Darier-White Disease)

Darier's disease is an uncommon genodermatosis with rather striking skin involvement and relatively subtle oral mucosal lesions. The condition is inherited as an autosomal dominant trait having a high degree of penetrance and variable expressivity. Although the precise defect is unknown, the adherence mechanism between surface squamous epithelial cells appears to be abnormal. Estimates of the prevalence of Darier's disease in northern European populations range from 1 in 36,000 to 1 in 100,000.

Clinical Features

Patients with Darier's disease have numerous erythematous, often pruritic, papules on the skin of the

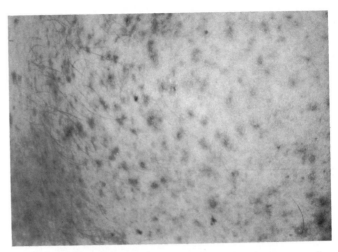

FIGURE 16–17. **Darier's disease**. Erythematous cutaneous papules on the chest.

trunk and the scalp that develop during the second decade of life (Fig. 16–17). An accumulation of keratin, producing a rough texture, may be seen in association with the lesions, and a foul odor may be present as a result of bacterial degradation of the keratin. The process generally becomes worse during the summer months, either because of sensitivity of some patients to ultraviolet light or because increased heat results in sweating, which induces more epithelial clefting. The palms and soles often exhibit pits and keratoses. The nails show longitudinal lines, ridges, or painful splits.

The oral lesions are typically asymptomatic and are discovered on routine examination. The frequency of occurrence of oral lesions ranges from 15 to 50 percent. They consist of multiple, normal-colored or white, flat-topped papules that, if numerous enough to be confluent, result in a cobblestone mucosal appearance (Fig. 16–18). These lesions affect the hard palate and alveolar mucosa primarily, although the buccal mucosa or tongue may occasionally be involved. If the palatal lesions are prominent, the condition may resemble inflammatory papillary hyperplasia or nicotine stomatitis. Some patients with this condition also experience recurrent obstructive parotid swelling.

Histopathologic Features

Microscopic examination of the cutaneous or mucosal lesions shows a dyskeratotic process characterized by a central keratin plug that overlies epithelium exhibiting a suprabasilar cleft (Fig. 16–19). This intraepithelial clefting phenomenon, also known as *acantholysis,* is not unique to Darier's disease and may be seen in conditions such as pemphigus vulgaris (see p. 559). In addition, the epithelial rete ridges associated with the lesions appear narrow, elongated, and "test tube"–shaped. Closer inspection of the epithelium reveals varying numbers of two types of dyskeratotic cells, called *corps ronds* (round bodies) or grains (because they resemble cereal grains) (Fig. 16–20).

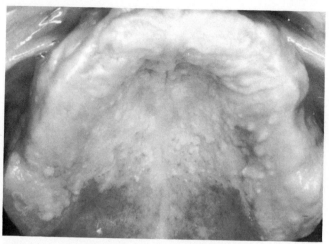

FIGURE 16-18. **Darier's disease**. The oral mucosa may show multiple white papules. (Courtesy of Dr. George Blozis.)

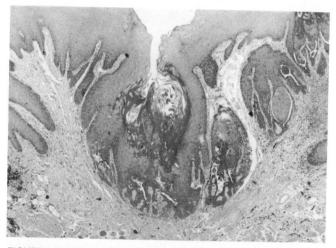

FIGURE 16-19. **Darier's disease**. Low-power photomicrograph showing a thick keratin plug, intraepithelial clefting, and elongated rete ridges.

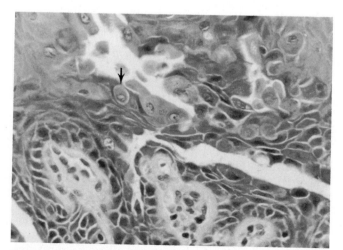

FIGURE 16-20. **Darier's disease**. High-power photomicrograph showing characteristic dyskeratotic cells (*arrow*).

Treatment and Prognosis

Treatment of Darier's disease depends on the severity of involvement. Photosensitive patients should use a sunscreen, and all patients should minimize unnecessary exposure to hot environments. For relatively mild cases, keratolytic agents may be the only treatment required. For more severely affected patients, systemic retinoids are often beneficial, but the side effects of such medications have to be carefully monitored by the physician. Although the condition is not premalignant or otherwise life-threatening, genetic counseling is appropriate.

WARTY DYSKERATOMA (Isolated Darier's Disease; Isolated Dyskeratosis Follicularis; Focal Acantholytic Dyskeratosis)

The **warty dyskeratoma** is a distinctly uncommon solitary lesion that can occur on skin or oral mucosa. It is histopathologically identical to Darier's disease. For this reason, the lesion has been termed **isolated Darier's disease**. The lesion is not otherwise related to Darier's disease, however, and its cause remains unknown.

Clinical Features

The cutaneous warty dyskeratoma typically presents as a solitary, asymptomatic, umbilicated papule on the skin of the head or neck of an older adult. The intraoral lesion also develops in patients older than age 40, and a slight male predilection has been identified. The intraoral warty dyskeratoma appears as a pink or white, umbilicated papule located on the keratinized mucosa, especially the hard palate and the alveolar ridge. A warty or roughened surface is noted in some lesions. Most warty dyskeratomas are smaller than 0.5 cm in diameter and produce no symptoms.

Histopathologic Features

Histopathologically, the warty dyskeratoma appears very similar to **keratosis follicularis**. Both conditions display dyskeratosis and a suprabasilar cleft. The warty dyskeratoma is a solitary lesion, however, and the formation of *corps ronds* and grains is not a prominent feature.

Treatment and Prognosis

Treatment of the warty dyskeratoma consists of conservative excision. The prognosis is excellent; these lesions have not been reported to recur, and they have no apparent malignant potential. Careful histopathologic evaluation of the tissue should be performed because some epithelial dysplasias may show a marked lack of cellular cohesiveness, resulting in an acantholytic appearance microscopically.

PEUTZ-JEGHERS SYNDROME

Peutz-Jeghers syndrome is a relatively rare but well-recognized condition. It is characterized by freckle-like lesions of the hands, perioral skin, and oral mucosa in conjunction with intestinal polyposis. The syndrome is generally inherited as an autosomal dominant trait, although 35 percent of cases represent new mutations.

Clinical Features

The skin lesions of Peutz-Jeghers syndrome usually develop early in childhood and involve the periorificial areas (mouth, nose, anus, genital region). The skin of the extremities is affected in about 50 percent of patients (Fig. 16–21). The lesions resemble freckles, but they do not wax and wane with sun exposure, as true freckles do.

The intestinal polyps, generally considered to be hamartomatous growths, are scattered throughout the mucus-producing areas of the gastrointestinal tract. The jejunum and ileum are most commonly affected. Patients often have problems with intestinal obstruction because of intussusception ("telescoping" of a proximal segment of the bowel into a distal portion), a problem that usually becomes evident during the third decade of life. Most of these episodes are self-correcting, but surgical intervention is sometimes necessary in order to prevent ischemic necrosis of the bowel with subsequent peritonitis. Gastrointestinal adenocarcinoma develops in 2 to 3 percent of affected patients, although the polyps themselves do not appear to be premalignant. Other tumors are also seen with increased frequency, affecting the pancreas, breast, and ovary.

The oral lesions essentially represent an extension of the perioral freckling. These 1- to 4-mm blue-gray macules affect the vermilion zone, labial and buccal mucosa, and tongue primarily and are seen in more than 90 percent of these patients (Fig. 16–22; see Color Figure 92). The number of lesions and the extent of involvement can vary markedly from patient to patient.

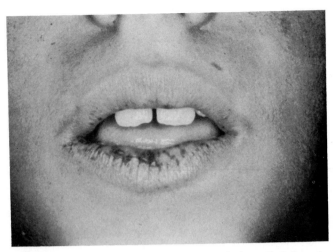

FIGURE 16–22. **Peutz-Jeghers syndrome.** Oral manifestations include multiple, dark, freckle-like lesions of the lips. See Color Plates. (Courtesy of Dr. Ahmed Uthman.)

Histopathologic Features

The gastrointestinal polyps of Peutz-Jeghers syndrome histopathologically represent benign overgrowths of intestinal glandular epithelium supported by a core of smooth muscle. Epithelial atypia is not usually a prominent feature, unlike the polyps of Gardner syndrome (see p. 473).

Microscopic evaluation of the pigmented cutaneous lesions shows slight acanthosis of the epithelium with elongation of the rete ridges. No apparent increase in melanocyte number is detected by electron microscopy, but the dendritic processes of the melanocytes are elongated. Furthermore, the melanin pigment appears to be retained in the melanocytes rather than being transferred to adjacent keratinocytes.

Treatment and Prognosis

Patients with Peutz-Jeghers syndrome should be monitored for development of intussusception or tumor formation. Genetic counseling is also appropriate.

HEREDITARY HEMORRHAGIC TELANGIECTASIA (Osler-Weber-Rendu Syndrome)

Hereditary hemorrhagic telangiectasia (HHT) is an uncommon mucocutaneous disorder that is inherited as an autosomal dominant trait. Numerous vascular hamartomas develop, affecting the skin and mucosa; however, other vascular problems, such as arteriovenous fistulas, may also be seen. The clinician should be familiar with HHT because the oral lesions are often the most dramatic and most easily identified component of this syndrome.

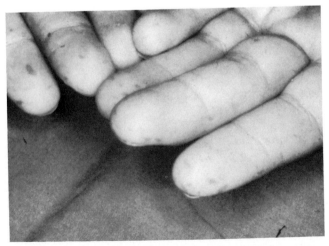

FIGURE 16–21. **Peutz-Jeghers syndrome.** Cutaneous lesions appear as brown, macular, freckle-like areas, often concentrated around the mouth or on the hands. (Courtesy of Dr. Ahmed Uthman.)

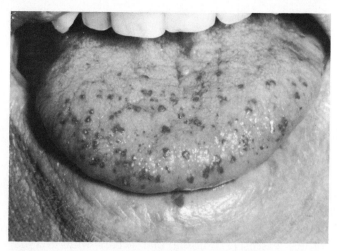

FIGURE 16-23. **Hereditary hemorrhagic telangiectasia**. The tongue of this patient shows multiple red papules, which represent superficial collections of dilated capillary spaces. See Color Plates.

Clinical Features

Patients with HHT are often diagnosed initially because of frequent episodes of epistaxis. On further examination, the nasal and oropharyngeal mucosae exhibit numerous scattered red papules, 1 to 2 mm in size, which blanch when diascopy is used. This blanching indicates that the red color is due to blood contained within blood vessels, in this case, small collections of dilated capillaries (*telangiectasias*) that are close to the surface of the mucosa. These telangiectatic vessels are most frequently found on the vermilion zone of the lips, tongue, and buccal mucosa, although any oral mucosal site may be affected (Figs. 16-23 [see Color Figure 93] and 16-24).

In many patients, telangiectasias are seen on the hands and feet. The lesions are often distributed throughout the gastrointestinal mucosa as well as the genitourinary mucosa and the conjunctival mucosa. The gastrointestinal telangiectasias have a tendency to rupture, which may cause significant blood loss. Chronic iron-deficiency ane-

mia is often a problem for such individuals. Significantly, arteriovenous fistulas may develop in the lungs, liver, and brain. The brain lesions seem to predispose these patients to the development of brain abscesses.

In some instances, CREST syndrome (see p. 586) must be considered in the differential diagnosis. In these cases, serologic studies for anti-centromere autoantibodies often help to distinguish between the two conditions because these antibodies would be present only in CREST syndrome.

Histopathologic Features

If one of the telangiectasias is submitted for biopsy, the microscopic features essentially show a superficially located collection of thin-walled vascular spaces that contain erythrocytes (Fig. 16-25).

Treatment and Prognosis

For mild cases of HHT, no treatment may be required. Moderate cases may be managed by selective cryosurgery or electrocautery of the most bothersome of the telangiectatic vessels. More severely affected patients, particularly those troubled by repeated episodes of epistaxis, may require a surgical procedure of the nasal septum (septal dermoplasty). The involved nasal mucosa is removed and replaced by a skin graft.

Estrogen therapy may benefit some patients, and iron replacement therapy is indicated for the iron-deficient patient. Occasionally, blood transfusions may be necessary to compensate for blood loss.

From a dental standpoint, some authors recommend the use of prophylactic antibiotics prior to dental procedures that might cause bacteremia in patients with HHT. The antibiotics are advocated because of the 1 percent prevalence of brain abscesses in these patients. It is believed that antibiotic coverage, similar to that for endocarditis prophylaxis, may prevent this serious complication.

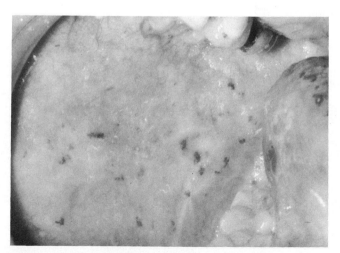

FIGURE 16-24. **Hereditary hemorrhagic telangiectasia**. Red macules similar to the tongue lesions are observed on the buccal mucosa.

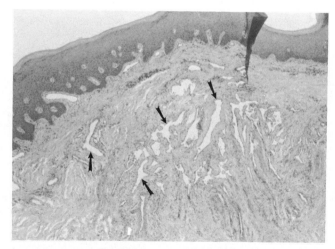

FIGURE 16-25. **Hereditary hemorrhagic telangiectasia**. This low-power photomicrograph shows multiple dilated vascular spaces (*arrows*) located immediately subjacent to the epithelium.

The prognosis is generally good, although a 1 to 2 percent mortality rate is reported from complications related to blood loss. For patients with brain abscesses, the mortality rate is 10 percent, even with early diagnosis and appropriate therapy.

EHLERS-DANLOS SYNDROMES

The **Ehlers-Danlos syndromes**, a group of inherited connective tissue disorders, are relatively heterogeneous. At least ten types have been defined. The patient presents with problems that are usually attributed to the production of abnormal collagen, the protein that is the main structural component of the connective tissue. Because the production of collagen necessitates many biochemical steps that are controlled by several genes, the potential exists for any one of these genes to mutate, producing selective defects in collagen synthesis. The various forms of abnormal collagen result in many overlapping clinical features for each of the types of the Ehlers-Danlos syndrome (Table 16–1). The discussion here will concentrate on the most common and significant forms of this group of conditions.

Patients typically exhibit such clinical findings as hypermobility of the joints, easy bruisability, and marked elasticity of the skin. Some patients have worked in circus sideshows as the "Indian rubber man" or the "contortionist" as a result of their pronounced joint mobility and ability to stretch the skin.

Clinical Features

The pattern of inheritance and the clinical manifestations vary with the type of Ehlers-Danlos syndrome being examined. About 80 percent of patients have either the **type I (severe)** or **type II (mild)** form. Both types are inherited as autosomal dominant traits. Hyperelasticity of the skin (Fig. 16–26) as well as cutaneous fragility can be observed. An unusual healing response that often occurs with relatively minor injury to the skin is termed *papyraceous scarring* because it resembles crumpled cigarette paper (Fig. 16–27).

Patients with **type III** Ehlers-Danlos syndrome exhibit remarkable joint hypermobility but no evidence of scarring.

Type IV is also known as the *ecchymotic* type because of the extensive bruising that occurs with everyday trauma. There may be a dominant or recessive inheritance pattern, and the patient may be mistaken for a victim of child abuse. The life expectancy of type IV patients is often greatly reduced because of the tendency for aortic aneurysm formation and rupture.

Type VIII Ehlers-Danlos syndrome was originally reported as having dental manifestations as one of its hallmark features, with patients showing marked periodontal disease activity at a relatively early age. More recent studies suggest that these patients may be best classified as having type IV, however, because (1) type IV patients have increased periodontal disease activity and (2) types IV and VIII patients have decreased amounts of a specific form of collagen (type III collagen).

Table 16–1. EHLERS-DANLOS (ED) SYNDROMES

Type	Clinical Features	Inheritance	Defect
I: Gravis (severe)	Hyperextensible skin, easy bruising, hypermobile joints, papyraceous scarring of skin	AD	Not known
II: Mitis (mild)	Similar to ED type I, but less severe	AD	Not known
III: Familial hypermobility	Soft skin, no scarring, marked joint hyperextensibility	AD	Not known
IV: Arterial	Severe bruising, arterial and uterine rupture	AD, AR	Abnormal type III collagen
V: X-linked	Very rare; similar to ED type II	XLR	Not known
VI: Ocular	Ocular fragility, hyperextensible skin, hypermobile joints, scoliosis	AR	Lysyl hydroxylase deficiency
VII: Arthrochalasis multiplex congenita	Congenital hip dislocation, joint hypermobility, normal scarring, mandibular hypoplasia	AD	Structural defect in collagen molecule
VIII: Periodontal	Rapidly progressive periodontitis, otherwise similar to ED type IV	AD	Not known
IX: (Vacant)	(Formerly, occipital horn syndrome)		
X: FIbronectin	Similar to ED types II and III	AR	Defect in fibronectin

AD, autosomal dominant; AR, autosomal recessive; XLR, X-linked recessive.

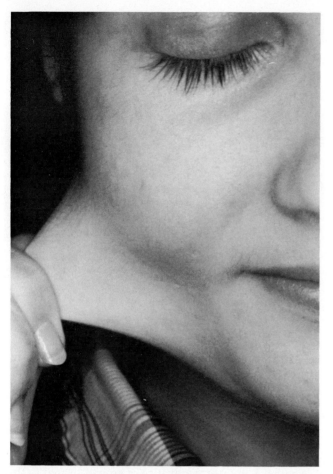

FIGURE 16–26. **Ehlers-Danlos syndrome**. The hyperelasticity of the skin is evident in this patient affected by type II (mild) Ehlers-Danlos syndrome.

mal life span, although affected women may have problems with placental tearing and hemorrhage during gestation.

Accurate diagnosis is important because it impacts heavily on the prognosis. Similarly, because the various types of this syndrome show a variety of inheritance patterns, an accurate diagnosis is required so that appropriate genetic counseling can be provided.

TUBEROUS SCLEROSIS

Tuberous sclerosis is an uncommon syndrome that is classically characterized by mental retardation, seizure disorders, and angiofibromas of the skin. The condition can be inherited as an autosomal dominant trait, but more than 50 percent of the cases appear to represent new mutations. There is a wide range of clinical severity, and more than one gene may be responsible for this disease. Milder forms may be difficult to diagnose.

The prevalence is between 1 in 10,000 and 1 in 23,000 in the general population, although in some long-term care facilities tuberous sclerosis accounts for as high as 1 percent of the mentally retarded patients.

Clinical Features

Several clinical features characterize tuberous sclerosis. The first of these, **facial angiofibromas**, used to be called "adenoma sebaceum." Because these lesions are neither

The oral manifestations of Ehlers-Danlos syndrome include the ability of 50 percent of these patients to touch the tip of their nose with their tongue *(Gorlin sign)*, a feat that can be achieved by less than 10 percent of normal people. Some authors have noted easy bruising and bleeding during minor manipulations of the oral mucosa; others state that oral mucosal friability is present. A tendency for recurrent subluxation of the temporomandibular joint has also been reported.

Most patients with Ehlers-Danlos syndrome have normal teeth. A variety of dental abnormalities have been described, including malformed, stunted tooth roots, large pulp stones, and hypoplastic enamel. These findings, however, have not been consistently correlated with any particular type of the syndrome.

Treatment and Prognosis

The prognosis for the patient with Ehlers-Danlos syndrome depends on the type. Some forms, such as the ecchymotic type, can be very serious, with sudden death occurring from rupture of the aorta secondary to the weakened, abnormal collagen that constitutes the vessel wall. The mild type is generally compatible with a nor-

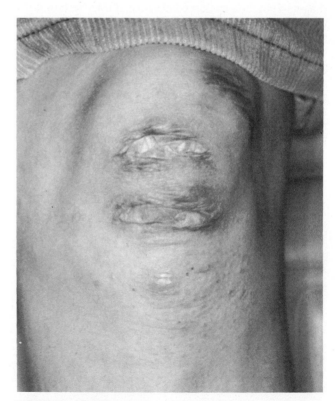

FIGURE 16–27. **Ehlers-Danlos syndrome**. Scarring that resembles crumpled cigarette paper (papyraceous scarring) is associated with minimal trauma in patients with Ehlers-Danlos syndromes. These lesions involve the skin of the knee.

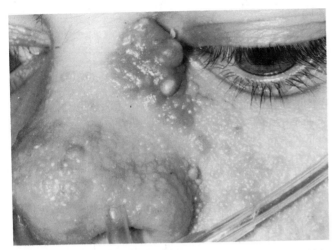

FIGURE 16–28. **Tuberous sclerosis.** Patients typically have multiple papular facial lesions that microscopically are angiofibromas.

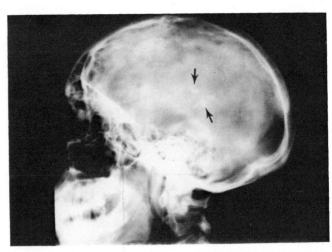

FIGURE 16–30. **Tuberous sclerosis.** Patchy calcifications (*arrows*) associated with intracranial hamartoma formation are seen on this lateral skull radiograph. (Courtesy of Dr. Reg Munden.)

adenomas nor sebaceous, the use of that term should be discontinued. Facial angiofibromas present as multiple, smooth-surfaced papules and occur primarily in the nasolabial fold area (Fig. 16–28). Similar lesions, called **ungual fibromas**, are seen around or under the margins of the nails (Fig. 16–29).

Two other characteristic skin lesions are connective tissue hamartomas called **shagreen patches** and ovoid areas of hypopigmentation called **ash-leaf spots.** The shagreen patches, so named because of their resemblance to sharkskin-derived shagreen cloth, affect the skin of the trunk. The ash-leaf spots may appear on any cutaneous surface and may be best visualized using ultraviolet (Wood's lamp) illumination.

Central nervous system manifestations include seizure disorders in nearly 90 percent of affected patients and mental retardation in 33 to 60 percent. In addition, hamartomatous proliferations in the central nervous system develop into the potato-like growths ("tubers") seen

at autopsy, from which the term tuberous sclerosis is derived (Fig. 16–30).

A relatively rare tumor of the heart muscle, called **cardiac rhabdomyoma**, is also typically associated with this syndrome. This lesion, which probably represents a hamartoma rather than a true neoplasm, occurs in approximately 30 percent of affected patients. Problems with myocardial function often develop as a result of this process.

Another hamartomatous type of growth related to this disorder is the **angiomyolipoma.** This is a benign neoplasm composed of vascular smooth muscle and adipose tissue and occurs primarily in the kidney.

Oral manifestations of tuberous sclerosis include developmental pitting of the enamel on the facial aspect of the anterior permanent dentition in 50 to 100 percent of patients. Multiple fibrous papules affect 11 to 56 percent of patients. The fibrous papules are seen predominantly on the anterior gingival mucosa (Fig. 16–31), although the lips, buccal mucosa, palate, and tongue may be involved. Diffuse fibrous gingival enlargement is reported in affected patients who are not taking phenytoin; however, most cases of gingival hyperplasia in these individuals are probably related to medication taken to control seizures.

The diagnosis of tuberous sclerosis can be based on the finding of one primary criterion, such as:

- Facial angiofibromas
- Ungual fibromas
- Central nervous system hamartomas

The presence of two secondary criteria may also confirm the diagnosis. These include:

- Infantile seizure disorder
- Ash-leaf hypopigmented areas
- Shagreen patch
- Cardiac rhabdomyoma
- A first-degree relative affected by the syndrome

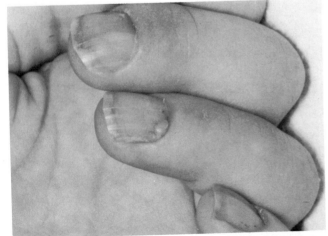

FIGURE 16–29. **Tuberous sclerosis.** Examination of the fingers often shows periungual fibromas.

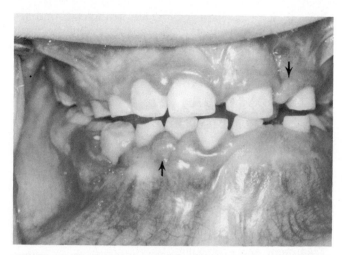

FIGURE 16–31. **Tuberous sclerosis**. Patients often exhibit gingival hyperplasia, which may be secondary to phenytoin medications used to control seizures in some cases. Fibrous papules of the gingiva (*arrows*) may also be present.

Histopathologic Features

Microscopic examination of the fibrous papules of the oral mucosa or the enlarged gingivae shows a nonspecific fibrous hyperplasia. The angiofibroma of the skin is a benign aggregation of delicate fibrous connective tissue characterized by plump, uniformly spaced fibroblasts with numerous interspersed thin-walled vascular channels.

Treatment and Prognosis

For patients with tuberous sclerosis, most of the treatment is directed toward the management of the seizure disorder with anticonvulsant agents. Mentally retarded patients may have problems with oral hygiene procedures, and poor oral hygiene contributes to phenytoin-induced gingival hyperplasia. Patients affected by this condition have a slightly reduced life span compared with the general population, with death usually related to central nervous system or kidney disease.

MULTIPLE HAMARTOMA SYNDROME
(Cowden Syndrome)

Multiple hamartoma syndrome is a rare condition that has important implications for the affected patient, because malignancies, in addition to the benign hamartomatous growths, develop in a high percentage of these individuals. Usually, the syndrome is inherited as an autosomal dominant trait showing a high degree of penetrance and a range of expressivity.

Clinical Features

Cutaneous manifestations are present in most patients with multiple hamartoma syndrome, usually developing during the second decade of life. Some skin lesions present as multiple, small papules primarily on the facial skin, especially around the mouth, nose, and ears (Fig. 16–32). Most are less than 1 mm in size.

Microscopically, most of these papules represent hair follicle hamartomas called **trichilemmomas**. Other common skin lesions are the **acral keratosis**, a warty-appearing growth that develops on the dorsal surface of the hand, and **palmoplantar keratosis**, a prominent callus-like lesion on the palms or soles. Cutaneous **hemangiomas, xanthomas,** and **lipomas** have also been described.

Other problems can appear in these patients as well. Thyroid disease usually presents as either a goiter or thyroid adenoma.

In women, fibrocystic disease of the breast is frequently observed. Unfortunately, breast cancer occurs with a relatively high frequency (30 to 50 percent) in these patients. The mean age is 40 years, which is much younger than usual.

In the gastrointestinal tract, multiple benign hamartomatous polyps may be present.

In addition, several types of benign and malignant tumors may develop in association with the female genitourinary tract more frequently than in the normal population.

The oral lesions vary in severity from patient to patient and usually consist of multiple papules affecting the gingivae, dorsal tongue, and buccal mucosa (Figs. 16–33 to 16–35). These lesions have been reported in more than 80 percent of affected patients and generally produce no symptoms. Other possible oral findings include a high-arched palate, periodontitis, and extensive dental caries, although it is unclear whether the latter two conditions are significantly related to the syndrome.

Histopathologic Features

The histopathologic features of the oral lesions are rather nonspecific, essentially representing fibroepithelial hyperplasia. Other lesions associated with this syndrome

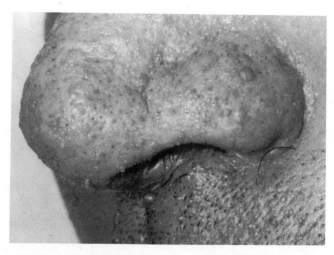

FIGURE 16–32. **Multiple hamartoma syndrome**. These tiny cutaneous facial papules represent the hair follicle hamartomas called trichilemmomas.

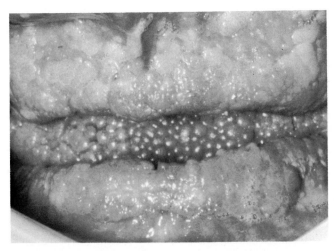

FIGURE 16–33. **Multiple hamartoma syndrome.** Multiple, irregular fibroepithelial papules involve the tongue (*center*) and alveolar ridge mucosa.

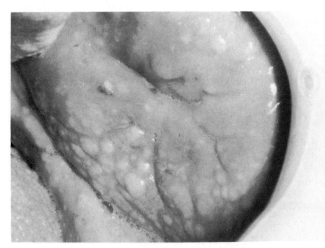

FIGURE 16–34. **Multiple hamartoma syndrome.** Oral lesions may present as papules on the buccal mucosa as well.

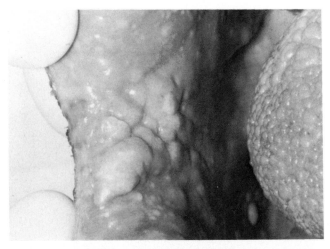

FIGURE 16–35. **Multiple hamartoma syndrome.** The oral lesions show a marked range of expression, as evidenced by the cobblestone-like texture of the contralateral buccal mucosa of the same patient depicted in Figure 16–34.

have their own characteristic histopathologic findings, depending on the hamartomatous or neoplastic tissue origin.

Diagnosis

The diagnosis is based on the finding of two of the following three signs:

- Multiple facial trichilemmomas
- Multiple oral papules
- Acral keratoses

A positive family history is also helpful in confirming the diagnosis.

Treatment and Prognosis

Treatment of multiple hamartoma syndrome is controversial. Although most of the tumors that develop are benign, the prevalence of malignancy is higher than in the general population. Some investigators recommend bilateral prophylactic mastectomies as early as the third decade of life for female patients because of the associated increased risk of breast cancer.

EPIDERMOLYSIS BULLOSA

The term **epidermolysis bullosa** describes a heterogeneous group of inherited blistering mucocutaneous disorders. Each has a specific defect in the attachment mechanisms of the epithelial cells, either to each other or to the underlying connective tissue. At least 25 different forms have been identified. Depending on the defective mechanism of cellular cohesion, there are three broad categories:

- Simplex
- Junctional
- Dystrophic

Each category consists of several forms of the disorder. A variety of inheritance patterns may be seen, depending on the particular form. The degree of severity can range from relatively mild, annoying forms, such as the **simplex** types, through a spectrum that includes severe, fatal disease. For example, many cases of **junctional** epidermolysis bullosa result in death at birth because of the significant sloughing of the skin during passage through the birth canal.

A few representative examples of the types of epidermolysis bullosa are summarized in Table 16–2. Because oral lesions are most commonly observed in the dystrophic forms, our discussion centers on these. Dental abnormalities, such as anodontia, enamel hypoplasia, neonatal teeth, and severe dental caries, have been variably associated with several of the different types of epidermolysis bullosa. A disorder termed **epidermolysis bullosa acquisita** is mentioned because of the similarity of its name; however, this appears to be an unrelated condition, having an autoimmune, rather than genetic, etiology (see p. 565).

Table 16–2. EXAMPLES OF EPIDERMOLYSIS BULLOSA (EB)

Form	Inheritance	Clinical Features	Defect
EB simplex	AD	Blistering of the hands and feet; mucosal involvement uncommon; blisters heal without scarring; prognosis usually good	Keratin gene defects
Junctional EB, generalized gravis variant	AR	Severe blistering at birth; granulation tissue around the mouth; oral erosions common; pitted enamel hypoplasia; often fatal (previously called EB letalis)	Defects of hemi-desmosomes
Dominant, dystrophic EB, Pasini type	AD	Generalized blistering, white papules	Defect in type VII collagen
Dominant, dystrophic EB, Cockayne-Touraine type	AD	Extremities primarily affected	Defect in type VII collagen
Recessive, dystrophic EB, generalized gravis type	AR	Severe mucosal involvement; mitten-like scarring; deformities of hands and feet; patients usually do not survive past early adulthood	Defect in type VII collagen
Recessive, dystrophic EB, inverse type	AR	Involvement of groin and axilla; severe oral and esophageal lesions	Defect in type VII collagen

AD, autosomal dominant; AR, autosomal recessive.

Clinical Features

Dominant Type

The **dystrophic** forms of epidermolysis bullosa that are inherited in an autosomal dominant fashion are not usually life-threatening, although they may certainly be disfiguring and pose many problems. The initial lesions are vesicles or bullae, which are seen early in life and develop on areas exposed to low-grade, chronic trauma, such as the knuckles or knees. The bullae rupture, resulting in erosions or ulcerations that ultimately heal with scarring. In the process, appendages such as fingernails may be lost (Fig. 16–36).

The oral manifestations are typically mild, with some gingival erythema and tenderness. Gingival recession and reduction in the depth of the buccal vestibule may be observed (Fig. 16–37).

Recessive Type

Generalized recessive dystrophic epidermolysis bullosa represents one of the more debilitating forms of the disease. Vesicles and bullae form with even the most minor trauma. Secondary infections are often a problem because of the large surface areas that may be involved. If the patient manages to survive into the second decade, hand function is often greatly diminished because of the

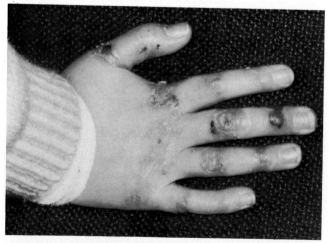

FIGURE 16–36. **Epidermolysis bullosa.** A young girl, affected by the dominant dystrophic form of epidermolysis bullosa, shows the characteristic hemorrhagic bullae, scarring, and erosion associated with minimal trauma to the hands.

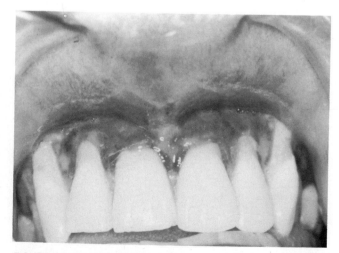

FIGURE 16–37. **Epidermolysis bullosa.** A teen-aged boy, affected by dominant dystrophic epidermolysis bullosa, shows a reduced depth of the labial vestibule caused by repeated mucosal tearing and healing with scarring.

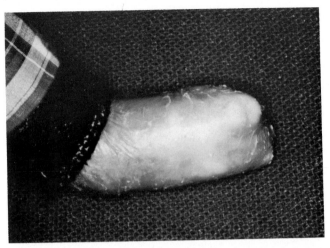

FIGURE 16–38. **Epidermolysis bullosa**. A 19-year-old man, affected by recessive dystrophic epidermolysis bullosa, shows the typical mitten-like deformity of the hand caused by scarring of the tissue following damage associated with normal activity.

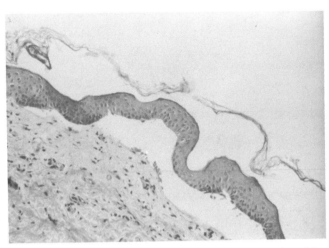

FIGURE 16–40. **Epidermolysis bullosa**. Complete separation of the epithelium from the connective tissue is seen in this photomicrograph of a tissue section obtained from a patient affected by a junctional form of epidermolysis bullosa.

repeated episodes of cutaneous breakdown and healing with scarring, resulting in fusion of the fingers into a mitten-like deformity (Fig. 16–38).

The oral problems are no less severe. Bulla and vesicle formation is induced by virtually any food having some degree of texture. Even with a soft diet, the repeated cycles of scarring often result in **microstomia** (Fig. 16–39), and similar mucosal injury and scarring may cause severe stricture of the esophagus. Because a soft diet is usually highly cariogenic, carious destruction of the dentition at an early age is common.

Histopathologic Features

The histopathologic features of epidermolysis bullosa vary with the type being examined. The **simplex** form shows intraepithelial clefting by light microscopy. **Junctional** and **dystrophic** forms show subepithelial clefting (Fig. 16–40). Electron microscopic examination reveals clefting at the level of the lamina lucida of the basement membrane in the **junctional** forms and below the lamina densa of the basement membrane in the **dystrophic** forms. Immunohistochemical evaluation of perilesional tissue may help to identify specific defects in order to further classify and subtype the condition.

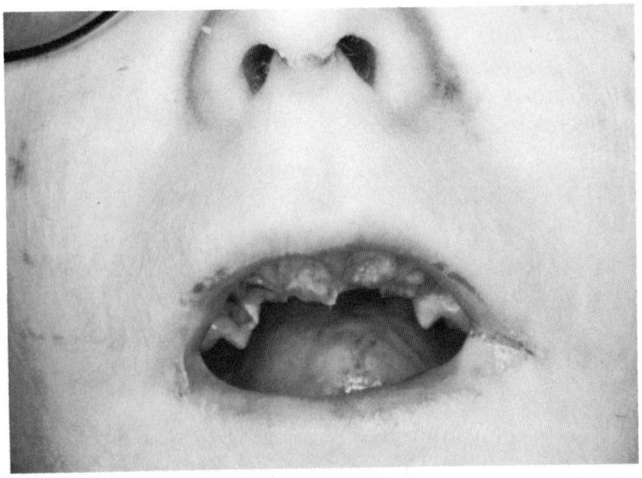

Treatment and Prognosis

Treatment of epidermolysis bullosa varies with the type. For milder cases, no treatment other than local wound care may be needed. Sterile drainage of larger blisters and the use of topical antibiotics are often indicated in these situations. For the more severe cases, intensive management with oral antibiotics may be necessary if cellulitis develops; despite intensive medical care, some patients die as a result of infectious complications.

The "mitten deformity" of the hands, seen in the recessive dystrophic form, can be corrected with plastic surgery, but the problem usually recurs after a period of time. With esophageal involvement, dysphagia may be a significant problem, resulting in malnutrition and weight loss. Placement of a gastrostomy tube may be necessary at times. Patients with the **dystrophic** forms are also predisposed to development of cutaneous **squamous cell carcinoma**.

Management of the oral manifestations also depends on the type of the disease. For patients who are susceptible to mucosal bulla formation, dental manipulation should be kept to a minimum. To achieve this, topical fluoride solutions should be administered daily to prevent dental caries. A soft diet that is as non-cariogenic as possible, as well as atraumatic oral hygiene procedures, should be encouraged.

Unfortunately, because of the genetic nature of the disease, no cure exists.

FIGURE 16–39. **Epidermolysis bullosa**. Same patient as depicted in Figure 16–38. Microstomia has been caused by repeated trauma and healing with scarring. Note the severe dental caries activity associated with a soft cariogenic diet.

PEMPHIGUS

The condition known as **pemphigus** represents four related diseases of an autoimmune etiology:

- Pemphigus vulgaris
- Pemphigus vegetans
- Pemphigus erythematosus
- Pemphigus foliaceus

Only the first two of these affect the oral mucosa with any degree of frequency. Because **pemphigus vegetans** itself is rare, the discussion is limited to **pemphigus vulgaris.**

Pemphigus vulgaris is the most common of these disorders (*vulgaris* is Latin for "common"). Even so, it is not seen very often. The estimated incidence is 1 to 5 cases per million people diagnosed each year in the general population. Nevertheless, pemphigus vulgaris is an important condition because, if untreated, it often results in the patient's death. Furthermore, the oral lesions are often the first sign of the disease, and they are the most difficult to resolve with therapy. This has prompted the description of the oral lesions as "the first to show, and the last to go."

The blistering that typifies this disease is due to an abnormal production, for unknown reasons, of autoantibodies directed against an epidermal cell surface glycoprotein, which is a component of *desmosomes* (structures that essentially bind epithelial cells to each other). As a result of this immunologic attack on the desmosomes, a split develops within the epithelium, causing a blister to form.

Occasionally, a pemphigus-like oral and cutaneous eruption may occur in patients taking certain medications, such as penicillamine, or in patients suffering from malignancy, especially lymphoreticular malignancies (so-called **paraneoplastic pemphigus**; see p. 561). Similarly, a variety of other conditions may produce chronic vesiculoulcerative lesions of the oral mucosa, and these often need to be considered in the differential diagnosis (Table 16–3).

Clinical Features

The initial manifestations of pemphigus vulgaris often involve the oral mucosa, typically in adults. The average age at diagnosis is 50 years, although rare cases may be seen in childhood. No sex predilection is observed, and the condition seems to be more common in Jews.

Patients usually complain of oral soreness, and examination shows superficial, ragged erosions and ulcerations distributed haphazardly on the oral mucosa (Figs. 16–41 to 16–43; see Color Figure 94). Such lesions may affect virtually any oral mucosal location, although the palate, labial mucosa, buccal mucosa, ventral tongue, and gingivae are often involved. Patients rarely report vesicle or bulla formation intraorally, and such lesions can seldom be identified by the examining clinician, probably because of the thin, friable roof of the lesions. Nearly 50 percent of the patients have oral mucosal lesions prior to the onset of cutaneous lesions, sometimes by as much as a year or more. Eventually, however, nearly all patients have intraoral involvement. The skin lesions appear as flaccid vesicles and bullae (Fig. 16–44) that rupture

Table 16–3. CHRONIC VESICULOULCERATIVE DISEASES

Condition	Mean Age	Sex Predilection	Clinical Features	Histopathologic Features	Direct Immunofluorescence	Indirect Immunofluorescence
Pemphigus vulgaris	4th to 6th decade	Equal	Vesicles, erosions, and ulcerations on any oral mucosal or skin surface	Intraepithelial clefting	Positive intercellular	Positive
Paraneoplastic pemphigus	6th or 7th decade	Equal	Vesicles, erosions, and ulcerations on any mucosal or skin surface	Subepithelial and intraepithelial clefting	Positive, intercellular, and basement membrane zone	Positive (rat bladder)
Cicatricial pemphigoid	6th or 7th decade	Female	Primarily mucosal lesions	Subepithelial clefting	Positive, basement membrane zone	Negative
Bullous pemphigoid	7th or 8th decade	Equal	Primarily skin lesions	Subepithelial clefting	Positive, basement membrane zone	Positive
Erythema multiforme	3rd or 4th decade	Male	Skin and mucosa involved; "target lesions" on skin	Subepithelial edema and perivascular inflammation	Nondiagnostic	Negative
Lichen planus	5th or 6th decade	Female	Oral and/or skin lesions; may or may not be erosive.	Hyperkeratosis, saw-toothed rete ridges, band-like infiltrate of lymphocytes	Fibrinogen, basement membrane zone	Negative

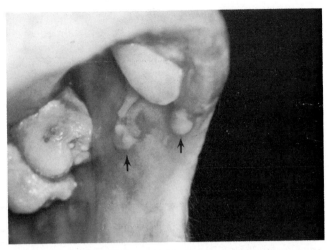

FIGURE 16–41. **Pemphigus vulgaris**. The oral lesions appear as diffusely distributed, irregular ulcerations (*arrows*), in this case involving the anterior buccal mucosa.

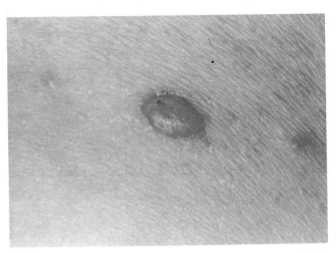

FIGURE 16–44. **Pemphigus vulgaris**. This flaccid cutaneous bulla is characteristic of skin involvement.

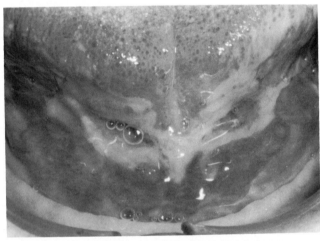

FIGURE 16–42. **Pemphigus vulgaris**. Large, irregularly shaped ulcerations involving the floor of the mouth and ventral tongue. See Color Plates.

quickly, usually within hours to a few days, leaving an erythematous, denuded surface.

Without proper treatment, the oral and cutaneous lesions tend to persist and progressively involve more surface area. A characteristic feature of pemphigus vulgaris is that a bulla can be induced on normal-appearing skin if firm lateral pressure is exerted. This is called a *positive Nikolsky sign*.

Histopathologic Features

Biopsy specimens of perilesional tissue show characteristic intraepithelial separation, which occurs just above the basal cell layer of the epithelium (Fig. 16–45). Sometimes the entire superficial layers of the epithelium are stripped away, leaving only the basal cells, which have been described as resembling a "row of tombstones." The cells of the spinous layer of the surface epithelium typically appear to fall apart, a feature that

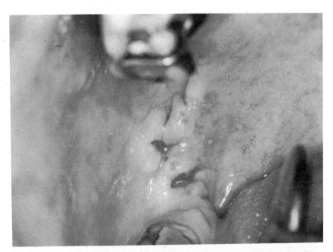

FIGURE 16–43. **Pemphigus vulgaris**. The patient, with a known diagnosis of pemphigus vulgaris, had been treated with immunosuppressive therapy. The oral erosions shown here were the only persistent manifestation of her disease.

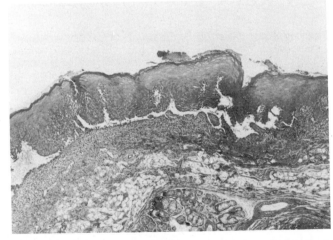

FIGURE 16–45. **Pemphigus vulgaris**. Low-power photomicrograph of perilesional mucosa affected by pemphigus vulgaris. An intraepithelial cleft is located just above the basal cell layer.

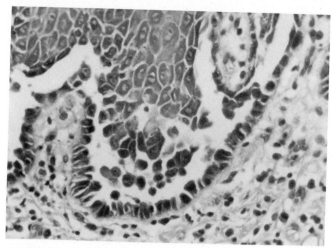

FIGURE 16-46. **Pemphigus vulgaris**. High-power photomicrograph showing rounded, acantholytic epithelial cells sitting within the intraepithelial cleft.

has been termed *acantholysis*, and the loose cells tend to assume a rounded shape (Fig. 16-46). This feature of pemphigus vulgaris can be used in making a diagnosis based on the identification of these rounded cells ("Tzanck cells") in an exfoliative cytologic preparation. A mild to moderate chronic inflammatory cell infiltrate is usually seen in the underlying connective tissue.

The diagnosis of pemphigus vulgaris should be confirmed by direct immunofluorescence examination of fresh perilesional tissue or tissue submitted in Michel's solution. With this procedure, antibodies (usually IgG or IgM) and complement components (usually C3) can be demonstrated in the intercellular spaces between the epithelial cells (Fig. 16-47) in almost all patients with this disease. Indirect immunofluorescence is also typically positive in 80 to 90 percent of cases, demonstrating the presence of circulating autoantibodies in the patient's serum.

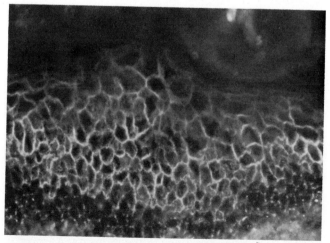

FIGURE 16-47. **Pemphigus vulgaris**. Photomicrograph depicting the direct immunofluorescence pattern of pemphigus vulgaris. Immunoreactants are deposited in the intercellular areas between the surface epithelial cells. (Courtesy of Dr. Ronald Grimwood.)

It is critical that perilesional tissue be obtained for both light microscopy and direct immunofluorescence in order to maximize the probability of a diagnostic sample. If ulcerated mucosa is submitted for testing, the results are often inconclusive because of either a lack of an intact epithelium–connective tissue interface or a great deal of nonspecific inflammation.

Treatment and Prognosis

A diagnosis of pemphigus vulgaris should be made as early in its course as possible because control is generally easier to achieve. Treatment consists primarily of systemic corticosteroids (usually prednisone), often in combination with other immunosuppressive drugs (so-called "steroid-sparing" agents), such as azathioprine. The potential side effects associated with the long-term use of systemic corticosteroids are significant and include:

- Diabetes mellitus
- Adrenal suppression
- Weight gain
- Osteoporosis
- Peptic ulcers
- Severe mood swings
- Increased susceptibility to a wide range of infections

Thus, ideally the patient should be managed by a physician with expertise in immunosuppressive therapy. The most common approach is to attempt to maintain the patient on as low a dose of corticosteroids as is necessary to control the condition. Often the success of therapy can be monitored by measuring the titers of circulating autoantibodies using indirect immunofluorescence, since disease activity often correlates with the abnormal antibody levels. Pemphigus rarely undergoes complete resolution, although remissions and exacerbations are common.

Prior to the development of corticosteroid therapy, as many as 60 to 80 percent of these patients died, primarily as a result of infections and electrolyte imbalances. Even today, the mortality rate associated with pemphigus vulgaris is in the range of 5 to 10 percent, usually because of the complications of long-term systemic corticosteroid use.

PARANEOPLASTIC PEMPHIGUS
(Neoplasia-Induced Pemphigus)

Paraneoplastic pemphigus is a recently described vesiculobullous disorder that affects patients who have a neoplasm, usually **lymphoma** or **chronic lymphocytic leukemia**. It is thought that a cross-reactivity develops between antibodies produced in response to the tumor and antigens associated with the desmosomal complex and the basement membrane zone of the epithelium. A variety of different antibodies that attack these epithelial adherence structures are produced, resulting in an array of clinical features, histopathologic findings, and immunopathologic findings that may be perplexing if the clinician is unfamiliar with this disease process.

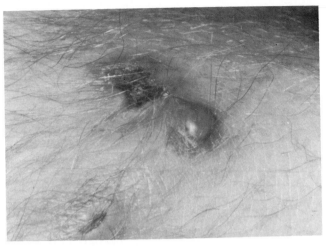

FIGURE 16-48. **Paraneoplastic pemphigus**. The bulla and crusted ulcerations on this patient's arm are representative of the polymorphous cutaneous lesions.

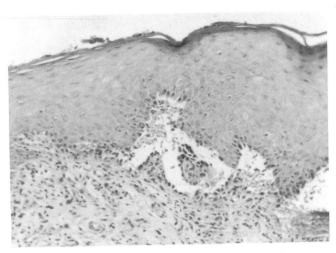

FIGURE 16-50. **Paraneoplastic pemphigus**. This medium-power photomicrograph shows both intraepithelial and subepithelial clefting.

Clinical Features

Patients typically have a history of a malignant lymphoreticular neoplasm. The neoplastic disease may or may not be under control at the time of onset of the paraneoplastic condition. Signs and symptoms of paraneoplastic pemphigus usually begin suddenly and may appear polymorphous. In some instances, multiple vesiculobullous lesions affect the skin (Fig. 16-48) and oral mucosa. In other instances, the cutaneous lesions appear more papular and pruritic, similar to cutaneous lichen planus. The lips often show hemorrhagic crusting similar to that of erythema multiforme. The oral mucosa shows multiple areas of erythema and diffuse, irregular ulceration (Fig. 16-49), affecting virtually any oral mucosal surface. If the lesions remain untreated, they persist and worsen.

Other mucosal surfaces are also commonly affected, particularly the conjunctival mucosa. In this area, a cicatrizing (scarring) conjunctivitis develops, similar to that seen with cicatricial pemphigoid. The vaginal mucosa as well as the mucosa of the respiratory tract may be involved.

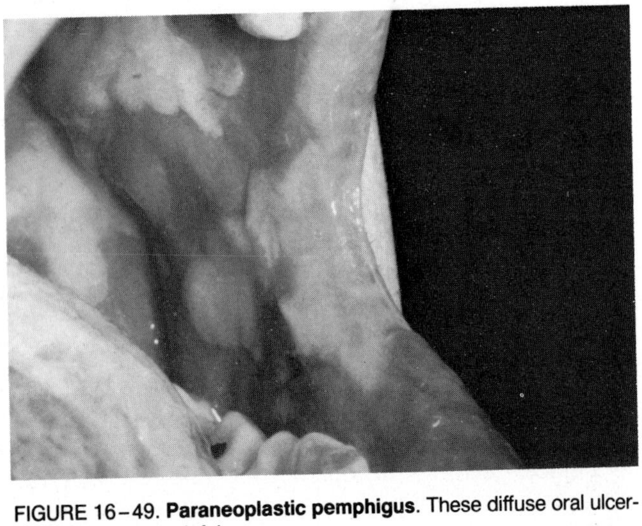

Histopathologic Features

The features of paraneoplastic pemphigus on light microscopy may be as diverse as the clinical features. In most cases, a lichenoid mucositis is seen, usually with subepithelial clefting (like pemphigoid) or intraepithelial clefting (like pemphigus) (Fig. 16-50).

Direct immunofluorescence studies may show either a weakly positive deposition of immunoreactants (IgG and complement) in the intercellular zones of the epithelium and/or a linear deposition of immunoreactants at the basement membrane zone. Indirect immunofluorescence should be conducted using a transitional type of epithelium (such as rat urinary bladder mucosa) as the substrate. This shows a highly specific pattern of antibody localization to the intercellular areas of the epithelium.

Treatment and Prognosis

Paraneoplastic pemphigus is a very serious condition with a high morbidity and mortality rate. Treatment essentially consists of systemic immunosuppressive agents, particularly prednisone and azathioprine. Unfortunately, although the immunosuppressive therapy often manages to control the autoimmune disease, this immunosuppression often seems to trigger a reactivation of the malignant neoplasm. Thus, a high mortality rate is seen, with patients either succumbing to complications of the vesiculobullous lesions or to the progression of malignant disease. Occasionally, long-term survivors are reported, but these seem to be in the minority. As more of these patients are identified, therapeutic strategies can be better evaluated and modified for optimal care in the future.

FIGURE 16-49. **Paraneoplastic pemphigus**. These diffuse oral ulcerations are quite painful.

CICATRICIAL PEMPHIGOID (Benign Mucous Membrane Pemphigoid; Mucous Membrane Pemphigoid)

Cicatricial pemphigoid is a chronic, blistering, mucocutaneous autoimmune disease in which tissue-bound autoantibodies are directed against one or more components of the basement membrane. Some investigators suggest that this condition may have a heterogeneous etiology. The precise incidence is unknown, but most authors believe that it is at least twice as common as pemphigus vulgaris.

The term *pemphigoid* is used because clinically it often appears similar (the meaning of the "*-oid*" suffix) to **pemphigus**. The prognosis and microscopic features of pemphigoid, however, are very different.

The term *cicatricial* is derived from the word *cicatrix*, meaning "scar." When the conjunctival mucosa is affected, the scarring that results is the most significant aspect of this disorder because it invariably results in blindness unless the condition is recognized and treated. Interestingly, the oral lesions often do not exhibit this tendency for scar formation.

Clinical Features

Cicatricial pemphigoid usually affects older adults, with an average age of 60 years at the onset of disease. Females are affected more frequently than males by a 2:1 ratio. Oral lesions are seen in most patients, but other sites, such as conjunctival, nasal, esophageal, laryngeal, and vaginal mucosa as well as the skin (Fig. 16–51) may be involved.

The oral lesions begin as either vesicles or bullae that may occasionally be identified clinically (Fig. 16–52; see Color Figure 95). In patients with pemphigus, however, such blisters are rarely seen. The most likely explanation for this difference is that the pemphigoid blister forms in a subepithelial location, producing a thicker, stronger

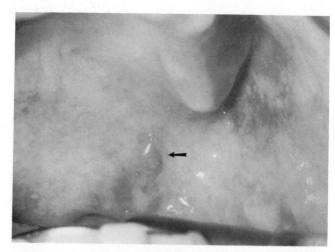

FIGURE 16–52. Cicatricial pemphigoid. One or more intraoral vesicles, as seen on the soft palate (*arrow*), may be detected in patients with cicatricial pemphigoid. Usually, ulcerations of the oral mucosa are also present. See Color Plates.

roof than the intraepithelial, acantholytic pemphigus blister. Eventually, the oral blisters rupture, leaving large, superficial, ulcerated, and denuded areas of mucosa (Fig. 16–53; see Color Figure 96). The ulcerated lesions are usually painful and persist for weeks to months if untreated.

Often this process is seen diffusely throughout the mouth, but it may be limited to certain areas, especially the gingiva (Fig. 16–54). Gingival involvement produces a clinical reaction pattern termed **desquamative gingivitis** (see p. 128). This pattern may also be seen in other conditions, such as **erosive lichen planus** or, much less frequently, **pemphigus vulgaris**.

The most significant complication of cicatricial pemphigoid, however, is ocular involvement. This occurs in approximately 25 percent of patients with oral lesions. One eye may be affected before the other. The earliest

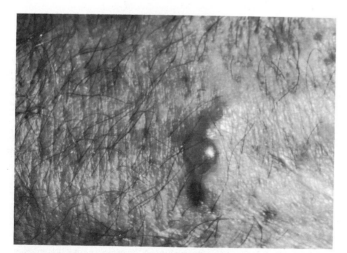

FIGURE 16–51. Cicatricial pemphigoid. Although cutaneous lesions are not common, tense bullae such as these may develop on the skin of 20 percent of affected patients. (Courtesy of Dr. Charles Camisa.)

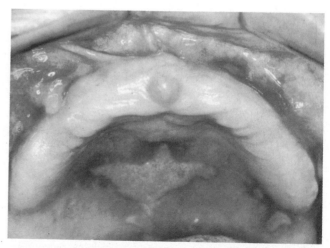

FIGURE 16–53. Cicatricial pemphigoid. Large, irregular oral ulcerations characterize the lesions after the initial bullae rupture. See Color Plates.

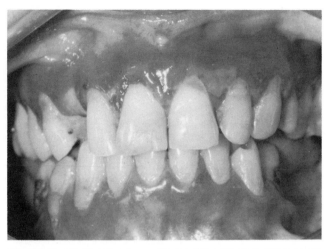

FIGURE 16-54. **Cicatricial pemphigoid**. Often the gingival tissues are the only affected site, resulting in a clinical pattern known as desquamative gingivitis. Such a pattern may also be seen with lichen planus and pemphigus vulgaris.

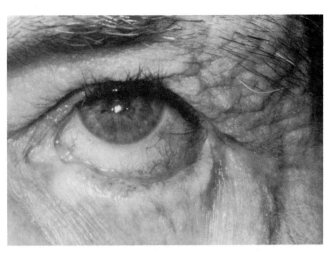

FIGURE 16-56. **Cicatricial pemphigoid**. The disease has caused the upper eyelid of this patient to turn inward (entropion), resulting in the eyelashes rubbing against the eye itself (trichiasis). Also note the obliteration of the lower fornix of the eye.

change is subconjunctival fibrosis, which usually can be detected by an ophthalmologist using slit-lamp examination. As the disease progresses, the conjunctiva becomes inflamed and eroded. Attempts at healing lead to scarring between the bulbar (lining the globe of the eye) and palpebral (lining the inner surface of the eyelid) conjunctiva. Adhesions called *symblepharons* result (Fig. 16-55). Without treatment the inflammatory changes become more severe, although conjunctival vesicle formation is rarely seen (Fig. 16-56). Scarring can ultimately cause the eyelids to turn inward *(entropion)*. This causes the eyelashes to rub against the cornea and globe *(trichiasis)* (Fig. 16-57; see Color Figure 97). The scarring closes off the openings of the lacrimal glands as well, and with the loss of tears, the eye becomes extremely dry.

The cornea then produces keratin as a protective mechanism; however, keratin is an opaque material, and blindness ensues. End-stage ocular involvement may also be characterized by adhesions between the upper and lower eyelids themselves (Fig. 16-58).

Other mucosal sites may also be involved and cause considerable difficulty for the patient. In female patients, the vaginal mucosal lesions may cause considerable pain during attempts at intercourse *(dyspareunia)*.

Laryngeal lesions, which are fairly uncommon, may be especially significant because of the possibility of airway obstruction by the bullae that are formed. Patients who present with a sudden change in vocalization or who have difficulty breathing should undergo examination with laryngoscopy.

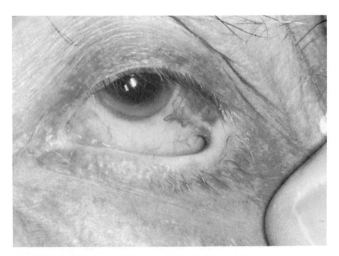

FIGURE 16-55. **Cicatricial pemphigoid**. Although the earliest ocular changes are difficult to identify, patients with ocular involvement may show adhesions (symblepharons) between the bulbar and palpebral conjunctivae before severe ocular damage occurs.

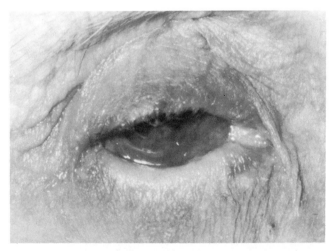

FIGURE 16-57. **Cicatricial pemphigoid**. A patient with ocular involvement shows severe conjunctival inflammation. The lower eyelashes were removed by an ophthalmologist because of trichiasis associated with entropion. See Color Plates.

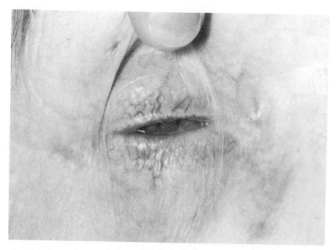

FIGURE 16–58. **Cicatricial pemphigoid.** In this patient, the ocular involvement has resulted in nearly complete scarring between the conjunctival mucosa and the eyelids themselves, producing blindness.

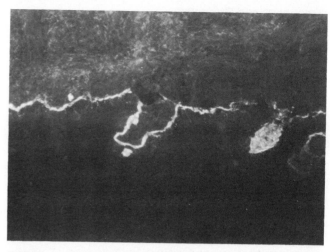

FIGURE 16–60. **Cicatricial pemphigoid.** Direct immunofluorescence studies show a deposition of immunoreactants at the basement membrane zone of the epithelium. (Courtesy of Dr. Ronald Grimwood.)

Histopathologic Features

Biopsy of perilesional mucosa shows a split between the surface epithelium and the underlying connective tissue (Fig. 16–59). A mild chronic inflammatory cell infiltrate is present in the superficial submucosa.

Direct immunofluorescence studies of perilesional mucosa show a continuous linear band of immunoreactants at the basement membrane zone in nearly 90 percent of affected patients (Fig. 16–60). The immune deposits consist primarily of IgG and C3, although IgA and IgM may also be identified. These immunoreactants may play a role in the pathogenesis of the subepithelial vesicle formation by weakening the attachment of the basement membrane.

Indirect immunofluorescence is positive in only 5 percent of these patients, indicating a relatively consistent lack of circulating autoantibodies.

For an accurate diagnosis, perilesional tissue—rather than the ulcerated lesion itself—should be obtained.

Often the epithelium in the area of the lesion is so loosely adherent that it strips off as the clinician attempts to perform the biopsy. Such tissue is not usually adequate for diagnostic purposes because an intact epithelium-connective tissue interface is no longer present (although some investigators have shown positive immunofluorescence with this tissue).

Other relatively rare conditions can mimic pemphigoid histopathologically. These include **linear IgA disease** and **epidermolysis bullosa acquisita**.

Linear IgA Disease

Linear IgA disease, as the name indicates, is characterized by the linear deposition of IgA along the basement membrane zone; thus, this disease can be distinguished from cicatricial pemphigoid on an immunopathologic basis.

Epidermolysis Bullosa Acquisita

Epidermolysis bullosa acquisita is an immunologically mediated condition characterized by autoantibodies directed against type VII collagen, the principal component of the anchoring fibrils. The anchoring fibrils play an important role in bonding the epithelium to the underlying connective tissue. As a result, their immunologic destruction results in the formation of bullous lesions of the skin and mucosa with minimal trauma.

Oral lesions are present in nearly 50 percent of the cases, although such lesions have not been reported in the absence of cutaneous lesions. In order to distinguish epidermolysis bullosa acquisita from other immunobullous diseases with subepithelial clefting, a special technique is performed. A sample of the patient's perilesional skin is incubated in a concentrated salt solution; this causes the epithelium to separate from the connective tissue, forming an artificially induced bulla. Immunohistochemical evaluation shows deposition of IgG autoantibodies on the floor of the bulla. This finding is in contrast to that of cicatricial pemphigoid, in which the autoantibodies are localized to the roof of the induced blister.

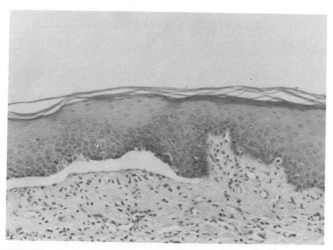

FIGURE 16–59. **Cicatricial pemphigoid.** Low-power photomicrograph of perilesional tissue shows characteristic subepithelial clefting.

Treatment and Prognosis

Once the diagnosis of cicatricial pemphigoid has been established by light microscopy and direct immunofluorescence, the patient should be referred to an ophthalmologist who is familiar with the ocular lesions of this condition for a baseline examination of the conjunctivae. This should be done whether or not the patient is experiencing ocular complaints.

Topical Agents

If only oral lesions are present, sometimes the disease can be controlled with application of one of the more potent topical corticosteroids to the lesions several times each day. Once control is achieved, the applications can be discontinued, although the lesions are certain to flare up again. Sometimes alternate-day application prevents such exacerbations of disease activity.

Patients with only gingival lesions may also benefit from good oral hygiene measures, which can help to decrease the severity of the lesions and reduce the amount of topical corticosteroids required. As an additional aid in treating gingival lesions, a flexible mouth guard may be fabricated to use as a carrier for the corticosteroid medication.

Systemic Agents

If topical corticosteroids are unsuccessful, systemic corticosteroids plus other immunosuppressive agents (particularly cyclophosphamide) may be used if the patient has no medical contraindications. This type of aggressive treatment is absolutely indicated in the presence of advancing ocular disease. Attempts at surgical correction of the symblepharons must be done when the disease is under control or quiescent; otherwise, the manipulation often induces an acute flare of the ocular lesions.

An alternative systemic therapy that may produce fewer serious side effects is the use of dapsone, a sulfa drug derivative. Some centers report good results with dapsone, but others observe that a minority of patients respond adequately. Contraindications to its use include glucose-6-phosphate dehydrogenase deficiency or allergy to sulfa drugs.

BULLOUS PEMPHIGOID

Bullous pemphigoid is an autoimmune condition characterized by the production of autoantibodies directed against a component of the basement membrane. In many respects, bullous pemphigoid resembles **cicatricial pemphigoid**, but most investigators note that there are enough differences to consider these diseases as distinct but related entities. One significant difference is that the clinical course in patients with bullous pemphigoid is usually limited, whereas the course in patients with cicatricial pemphigoid is usually protracted and progressive.

Clinical Features

Bullous pemphigoid typically develops in older people; most patients are between 60 and 80 years of age. No sex or racial predilection is seen. Pruritus may be an early

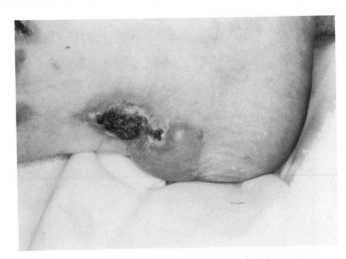

FIGURE 16–61. **Bullous pemphigoid**. The vesiculobullous cutaneous lesions eventually rupture, leaving hemorrhagic crusted areas.

symptom. This is followed by the development of multiple, tense bullae on either normal or erythematous skin (Fig. 16–61). These lesions eventually rupture after several days, causing a superficial crust to form. Eventually, healing takes place without scarring.

Oral mucosal involvement is uncommon, although the reported prevalence in several series of cases has ranged from 8 to 39 percent. Referral bias may explain the discrepancy in prevalence rates. The oral lesions, like the skin lesions, begin as bullae, but they tend to rupture sooner, probably as a result of the constant low-grade trauma to which the oral mucosa is subjected. Large, shallow ulcerations with smooth, distinct margins are present after the bullae rupture (Fig. 16–62).

Histopathologic Features

Microscopic examination of tissue obtained from the perilesional margin of a bulla shows separation of the epithelium from the connective tissue at the basement

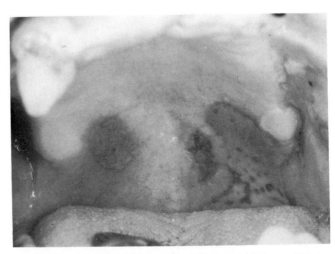

FIGURE 16–62. **Bullous pemphigoid**. These oral lesions appear as large, shallow ulcerations involving the soft palate.

membrane zone, resulting in a subepithelial separation. Modest numbers of both acute and chronic inflammatory cells are typically seen in the lesional area, and the presence of eosinophils within the bulla itself is characteristic.

Direct immunofluorescence studies show a continuous linear band of immunoreactants, usually IgG and C3, localized to the basement membrane zone in 90 to 100 percent of affected patients. These antibodies may bind to a protein associated with *hemidesmosomes*, structures that bind the basal cell layer of the epithelium to the basement membrane and the underlying connective tissue. This protein has been designated as *bullous pemphigoid antigen*, and immunoelectron microscopy has demonstrated its localization to the upper portion of the lamina lucida of the basement membrane.

In addition to the tissue-bound autoantibodies, 40 to 70 percent of the patients also have circulating autoantibodies in the serum, producing an indirect immunofluorescent pattern that is identical to that of the direct immunofluorescence. Unlike pemphigus vulgaris, the antibody titers seen in bullous pemphigoid do not appear to correlate with disease activity.

Treatment and Prognosis

Management of the patient with bullous pemphigoid consists of systemic immunosuppressive therapy. Moderate daily doses of systemic prednisone usually control the condition, after which alternate-day therapy may be given to reduce the risk of corticosteroid complications. If the lesions do not respond to prednisone alone, another immunosuppressive agent, such as azathioprine or methotrexate, may be added to the regimen. Dapsone, a sulfa derivative, may also be used as an alternative therapeutic agent.

The prognosis is good, with many patients experiencing spontaneous remission after 2 to 3 years. The condition is rarely fatal.

ERYTHEMA MULTIFORME

Erythema multiforme is a blistering, ulcerative mucocutaneous condition of uncertain etiopathogenesis. This is probably an immunologically mediated process, although the cause is poorly understood. In about 50 percent of the cases, one can identify either a preceding infection, such as *Herpes simplex* or *Mycoplasma pneumoniae*, or exposure to any one of a variety of drugs and medications, particularly antibiotics or analgesics. These agents may trigger the immunologic derangement that produces the disease. Sophisticated techniques in molecular biology have demonstrated the presence of *Herpes simplex* DNA in patients with recurrent erythema multiforme, thus supporting the concept of an immunologic precipitating event. Interestingly, direct and indirect immunofluorescence studies are nonspecific and are not really very useful diagnostically except to rule out other vesiculobullous diseases.

Clinical Features

Erythema multiforme usually has an acute onset and may present with a wide spectrum of clinical disease. On the mild end of the spectrum, ulcerations develop, affecting the oral mucosa primarily. In its most severe form, diffuse sloughing and ulceration of the entire skin and mucosal surfaces may be seen (**toxic epidermal necrolysis,** or **Lyell's disease**).

Patients are usually young adults in their 20s or 30s. Men are affected more frequently than women.

Prodromal symptoms include fever, malaise, headache, cough, and sore throat, occurring approximately 1 week prior to onset. Although the disease is self-limiting, usually lasting 2 to 6 weeks, about 20 percent of patients experience recurrent episodes, usually in the spring and autumn.

Erythematous skin lesions develop in about 50 percent of cases. A variety of appearances (*multiforme* = many forms) may be present. Typically, early lesions are flat, round, and dusky-red, appearing on the extremities. These become slightly elevated and may evolve into bullae with necrotic centers. Sometimes particular skin lesions develop that are highly characteristic for the disease. These lesions present as concentric circular erythematous rings resembling a target or bull's-eye *(target lesions)* (Fig. 16–63; see Color Figure 98).

The oral lesions begin as erythematous patches that undergo epithelial necrosis and evolve into large, shallow erosions and ulcerations with irregular borders (Fig. 16–64). Hemorrhagic crusting of the vermilion zone of the lips is common (Fig. 16–65; see Color Figure 99). These oral lesions, like the skin lesions, emerge quickly and are uncomfortable. Sometimes patients are dehydrated because they are unable to ingest liquids as a result of mouth pain. The ulcerations often have a diffuse distribution. The lips, labial mucosa, buccal mucosa, tongue, floor of the mouth, and soft palate are the most common sites of involvement. Usually, the gingivae and hard palate are relatively spared.

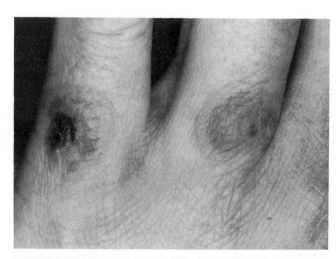

FIGURE 16–63. **Erythema multiforme.** The concentric erythematous pattern of the cutaneous lesions on the fingers resembles a target or bull's-eye. See Color Plates.

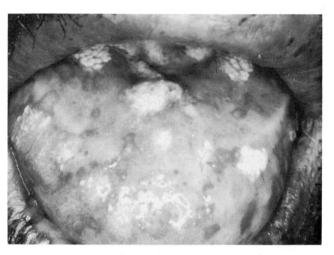

FIGURE 16–64. **Erythema multiforme**. Diffuse ulcerations and erosions involving the dorsal surface of this patient's tongue.

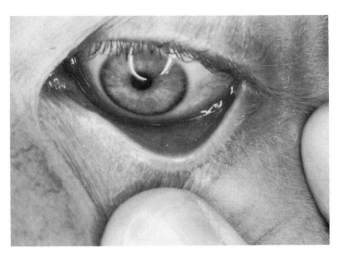

FIGURE 16–66. **Stevens-Johnson syndrome**. With erythema multiforme major (Stevens-Johnson syndrome), other mucosal surfaces may show involvement, such as the severe conjunctivitis depicted in this photograph. See Color Plates.

Erythema Multiforme Major

A more severe form of the disease, known as **erythema multiforme major** or **Stevens-Johnson syndrome**, is usually triggered by a drug rather than infection. For such a diagnosis to be made, the ocular (Fig. 16–66; see Color Figure 100) and genital (Fig. 16–67) mucosae should be affected in conjunction with the oral and skin lesions. With severe ocular involvement, scarring (symblepharon formation) may occur, similar to that in cicatricial pemphigoid (see p. 563).

Toxic Epidermal Necrolysis

Many dermatologists consider **toxic epidermal necrolysis** to represent the most severe form of erythema multiforme. It is almost always triggered by drug exposure. There is diffuse sloughing of a significant proportion of the skin and mucosal surfaces, appearing as if the patient had been badly scalded (Figs. 16–68 and 16–69). In contrast to erythema multiforme major, toxic epidermal

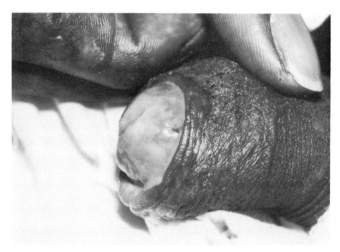

FIGURE 16–67. **Stevens-Johnson syndrome**. Genital ulcerations, demonstrated in this patient by the involvement of the glans penis, may also be a component.

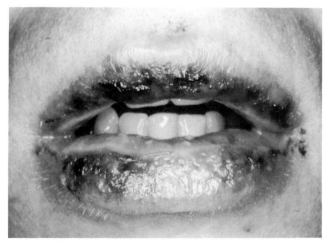

FIGURE 16–65. **Erythema multiforme**. Ulceration of the labial mucosa with hemorrhagic crusting of the vermilion zone of the lips. See Color Plates.

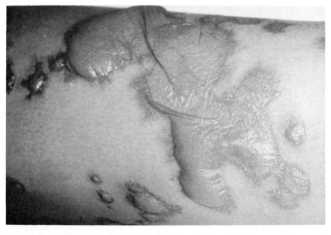

FIGURE 16–68. **Toxic epidermal necrolysis**. This severe form of erythema multiforme exhibits diffuse bullous skin lesions. (Courtesy of Dr. Peter Larsen.)

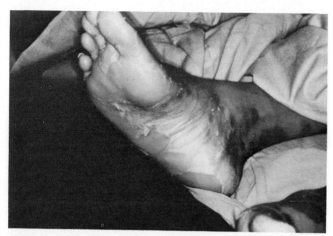

FIGURE 16-69. **Toxic epidermal necrolysis.** The desquamation of the skin of the foot is characteristic of the diffuse sloughing cutaneous lesions. (Courtesy of Dr. Peter Larsen.)

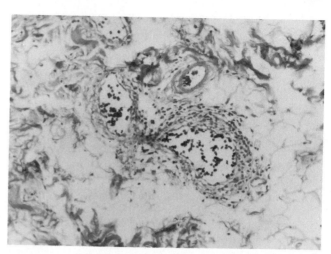

FIGURE 16-71. **Erythema multiforme.** This medium-power photomicrograph shows the perivascular inflammatory infiltrate, typically seen in erythema multiforme.

necrolysis tends to occur in older people. A female predilection is observed. If the patient survives, the cutaneous process resolves in 2 to 4 weeks; however, oral lesions may take longer to heal, and significant residual ocular damage is evident in half the patients. These more severe presentations of erythema multiforme are rare. Erythema multiforme major occurs at an average rate of five cases per million population per year, and toxic epidermal necrolysis occurs at a rate of about one case per million per year.

Histopathologic Features

Histopathologic examination of the perilesional mucosa in erythema multiforme reveals a pattern that is characteristic but not pathognomonic. Subepithelial vesiculation is usually seen in association with necrotic basal keratinocytes (Fig. 16-70). A mixed inflammatory infiltrate is present, consisting of lymphocytes, neutrophils, and often eosinophils. Sometimes these cells are arranged in a perivascular orientation (Fig. 16-71). Because the immunopathologic features are also nonspe-

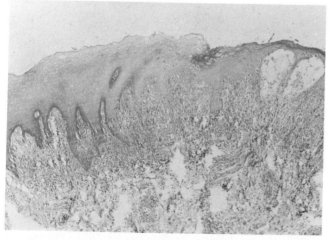

FIGURE 16-70. **Erythema multiforme.** This low-power photomicrograph shows subepithelial edema and inflammation, features that are characteristic, but not pathognomonic, of erythema multiforme.

cific, the diagnosis is often based on the clinical presentation and the exclusion of other vesiculobullous disorders.

Treatment and Prognosis

Management of erythema multiforme, particularly the minor and major forms, includes the use of systemic corticosteroids, especially in the early stages of the disease. Sometimes oral lesions in patients with the minor form of the condition may be managed effectively with topical corticosteroid syrups or elixirs.

If the patient is dehydrated as a result of an inability to eat because of oral pain, intravenous rehydration may be necessary along with topical anesthetic agents to decrease discomfort.

If recurrent episodes of erythema multiforme are a problem, an initiating factor, such as recurrent herpesvirus infection or drug exposure, should be sought. If disease is triggered by *H. simplex,* continuous oral acyclovir therapy can prevent recurrences.

Generally, erythema multiforme is not life-threatening except in its most severe forms. The mortality rate in patients with toxic epidermal necrolysis is approximately 34 percent; the rate in those with Stevens-Johnson syndrome is 2 to 10 percent. Corticosteroids should probably be avoided in the management of toxic epidermal necrolysis because some investigators have found that such drugs may be detrimental. Because the lesions of toxic epidermal necrolysis are analogous to those suffered by burn patients, management of these patients in the burn unit of the hospital is often successful.

ERYTHEMA MIGRANS (Geographic Tongue; Benign Migratory Glossitis; Wandering Rash of the Tongue; Erythema Areata Migrans; Stomatitis Areata Migrans)

Erythema migrans is a common benign condition that primarily affects the tongue. It is often detected on routine examination of the oral mucosa. The lesion occurs in 1 to 3 percent of the population. Females are affected more frequently than males by a 2:1 ratio. Patients may occasionally consult a health care professional if they happen to notice the unusual appearance of their tongue or if the lingual mucosa becomes sensitive to hot or spicy foods as a result of the process.

Even though erythema migrans has been documented for many years, the etiopathogenesis is still unknown. Some investigators have suggested that erythema migrans occurs with increased frequency in atopic individuals, thus raising the possibility that it represents a type of hypersensitivity to an environmental factor. In addition, it has recently been reported that the lesions of erythema migrans in a female patient seemed to wax and wane predictably with oral contraceptive therapy, suggesting that hormonal factors may be relevant.

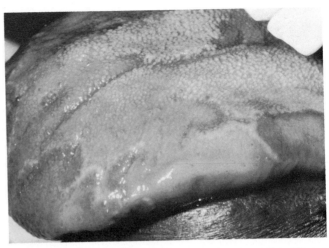

FIGURE 16–73. **Erythema migrans**. Lingual mucosa of a different patient than the one in Figure 16–72. The lateral distribution of the lesions is shown.

Clinical Features

The characteristic lesions of erythema migrans are seen on the anterior two thirds of the dorsal tongue mucosa. They present as multiple, well-demarcated zones of erythema (Figs. 16–72 and 16–73; see Color Figure 101), concentrated at the tip and lateral borders of the tongue. This erythema is due to atrophy of the filiform papillae, and these atrophic areas are typically surrounded at least partially by a slightly elevated, yellowish-white, serpentine border (Fig. 16–74; see Color Figure 102). The patient who is aware of the process is often able to describe the lesions as appearing quickly in one area, healing within a few days or weeks, then developing in a totally different area. Frequently, the lesion begins as a small white patch, which then develops a central erythematous atrophic zone and enlarges centrifugally. Often patients with **fissured tongue** (see p. 11) are affected with erythema migrans as well. Some patients may have only a solitary lesion, but this is uncommon. The lesions are usually asymptomatic, although a burn-

ing sensation or sensitivity to hot or spicy foods may be noted when the lesions are active. Only rarely is the burning sensation more constant and severe.

Very infrequently, erythema migrans may occur on oral mucosal sites other than the tongue. In these instances, the tongue is almost always affected; however, other lesions develop on the buccal mucosa, the labial mucosa and, less frequently, the soft palate (Fig. 16–75). These lesions typically produce no symptoms, and they can be identified by their yellowish-white serpentine border, which surrounds an erythematous zone. These features should prevent confusion with such conditions as candidiasis or erythroplakia.

Histopathologic Features

If a biopsy specimen of the peripheral region of erythema migrans is examined, a characteristic histopatho-

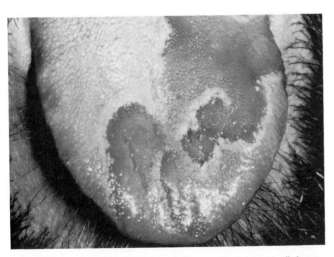

FIGURE 16–72. **Erythema migrans**. The erythematous, well-demarcated areas of papillary atrophy are characteristic of erythema migrans affecting the tongue (benign migratory glossitis). Note the asymmetric distribution and the tendency to involve the lateral aspects of the tongue. See Color Plates.

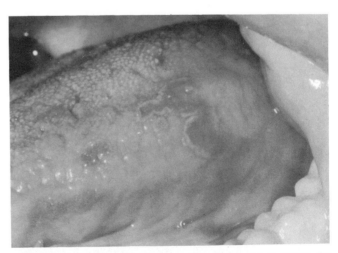

FIGURE 16–74. **Erythema migrans**. This photograph illustrates the slightly elevated, yellowish-white, scalloped margin that is characteristically associated with the periphery of the erythematous, atrophic regions. See Color Plates.

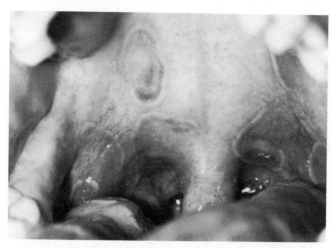

FIGURE 16-75. **Erythema migrans.** Lesions may infrequently be found on other oral mucosal sites. These palatal lesions show well-demarcated erythematous areas surrounded by a white border, similar to the process involving the tongue.

logic pattern is observed. Hyperparakeratosis, spongiosis, acanthosis, and elongation of the epithelial rete ridges are seen (Fig. 16-76). In addition, collections of neutrophils *(Munro abscesses)* are observed within the epithelium (Fig. 16-77); lymphocytes and neutrophils involve the submucosa. The intense neutrophilic infiltrate may be responsible for the destruction of the superficial portion of the epithelium, thus producing an atrophic, reddened mucosa as the lesion progresses. Because these histopathologic features are reminiscent of **psoriasis,** this is called a *psoriasiform mucositis.* In one case-control study of psoriatic patients, erythema migrans occurred at a rate of about 10 percent; only 2.5 percent of an age-matched and sex-matched population were affected. Whether these findings mean that erythema migrans represents oral psoriasis or that psoriatics are just more susceptible to erythema migrans is open to debate.

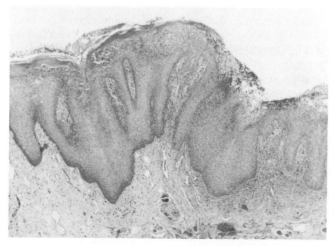

FIGURE 16-76. **Erythema migrans.** This low-power photomicrograph shows the elongation of the rete ridges with parakeratosis and underlying inflammation. Such features are also common in psoriasis, which explains why this is known as a "psoriasiform" mucositis.

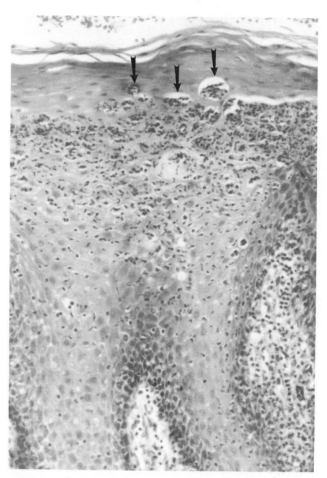

FIGURE 16-77. **Erythema migrans.** This high-power photomicrograph shows collections of neutrophils in the superficial spinous layer of the epithelium *(arrows).*

Treatment and Prognosis

Generally, no treatment is indicated for patients with erythema migrans. Reassuring the patient that the condition is completely benign is often all that is necessary. Infrequently, patients may complain of tenderness or a burning sensation that is so severe that it disrupts their lifestyle. In such cases, topical corticosteroids, such as fluocinonide gel, may provide relief when it is applied as a thin film several times a day to the lesional areas. One uncontrolled study has recently suggested that zinc supplementation is effective for symptomatic erythema migrans.

REITER'S SYNDROME

Reiter's syndrome is an uncommon disease that most likely represents an immunologically mediated condition. Current evidence suggests that the disorder may be triggered by any one of several infectious agents in a genetically susceptible person. A classic triad of signs has been described:

- Nongonococcal urethritis
- Arthritis
- Conjunctivitis

However, most patients do not exhibit all three of these signs.

It is interesting that Reiter's syndrome has been reported with some frequency in patients infected with the human immunodeficiency virus (HIV).

Clinical Features

Reiter's syndrome is particularly prevalent in young adult men. According to most series, there is a male-to-female ratio of 9:1. The majority (60 to 90 percent) of these patients are positive for HLA-B27, a haplotype present in only 4 to 8 percent of the population. The syndrome usually develops 1 to 4 weeks after an episode of dysentery or venereal disease.

Urethritis is often the first sign and is seen in both affected males and females. Females may also have an inflammation of the uterine cervix. Conjunctivitis usually appears concurrently with the urethritis, and after several days, arthritis ensues. The arthritis usually affects the joints of the lower extremities. Skin lesions often take the form of a characteristic lesion of the glans penis (**balanitis circinata**). These lesions develop in about one third of patients with Reiter's syndrome, and they appear as well-circumscribed erythematous erosions with a scalloped, whitish linear boundary.

The oral lesions, which occur in slightly less than 20 percent of patients with this disorder, are described in various ways. Some reports mention painless erythematous papules distributed on the buccal mucosa and palate; other reports suggest that oral involvement includes shallow, painless ulcers that affect the tongue, buccal mucosa, palate, and gingiva. Some authors have even implied that **geographic tongue** may be a component of Reiter's syndrome, probably because geographic tongue bears a superficial resemblance to the lesions of balanitis circinata.

The American Rheumatism Association has defined Reiter's syndrome on the basis of the clinical findings of a peripheral arthritis that lasts longer than 1 month in conjunction with urethritis, cervicitis, or both.

Histopathologic Features

The histopathologic findings of the cutaneous lesions in patients with Reiter's syndrome are frequently similar to those found in patients with **psoriasis**, particularly with respect to the presence of microabscesses within the superficial layers of the surface epithelium. Other features in common with psoriasis include hyperparakeratosis with elongated, thin rete ridges.

Treatment and Prognosis

Some patients with Reiter's syndrome experience spontaneous resolution of their disease, but many others have chronic symptoms that may wax and wane. Treatment may not be necessary for the milder cases. For symptomatic patients, particularly those with urethritis, a course of doxycycline or minocycline may be helpful. Nonsteroidal anti-inflammatory agents are initially used for managing arthritis, and sulfasalazine may be helpful

in resolving cases that do not respond. Immunosuppressive agents, such as azathioprine and methotrexate, are reserved for the most resistant cases if they are not associated with HIV infection.

Physical therapy probably helps to reduce joint fibrosis associated with arthritis. About 10 to 25 percent of patients with this disorder have severe disability, usually from arthritis.

LICHEN PLANUS

Lichen planus is a relatively common, chronic dermatologic disease that often affects the oral mucosa. The strange name of the condition was provided by the British physician Erasmus Wilson, who first described it in 1869. Lichens are primitive plants composed of symbiotic algae and fungi. The term *planus* is Latin for "flat." Wilson probably thought that the skin lesions looked similar enough to the lichens growing on rocks to merit this designation. Even though the term lichen planus suggests a flat, fungal condition, current evidence indicates that this is an immunologically mediated mucocutaneous disorder.

A variety of medications may induce lesions that appear clinically identical to the idiopathic form of the condition; however, the term **lichenoid mucositis** (or **lichenoid dermatitis,** depending on the site involved) is probably a better name for the drug-related alterations.

The relationship of stress or anxiety to the development of lichen planus is controversial, and most cited cases appear to be anecdotal. One study attempted to use psychologic questionnaires to resolve this question. Patients with oral lichen planus had no greater degree of stress in their lives than did age-matched and sex-matched controls. It might be that stress has no bearing on the pathogenesis of lichen planus; however, an alternative explanation might be that those patients who have lichen planus simply respond in this fashion to levels of stress that do not induce lesions in other people.

Clinical Features

Most patients who present with lichen planus are middle-aged adults. It is rare for children to be affected. Women predominate in most series of cases, usually by a 3:2 ratio over men. Approximately 1 percent of the population may have cutaneous lichen planus. The prevalence of oral lichen planus is between 0.1 and 2.2 percent.

The skin lesions of lichen planus have been classically described as purple, pruritic, polygonal papules (Fig. 16-78; see Color Figure 103). These usually affect the flexor surfaces of the extremities. Excoriations may not be visible, despite the fact that the lesions itch, because it hurts the patient when he or she scratches them.

Careful examination of the surface of the skin papules reveals a fine, lace-like network of white lines (*Wickham's striae*). Other sites of extraoral involvement include the glans penis, the vulvar mucosa, and the nails (Fig. 16-79).

There are essentially two forms of oral lesions: reticular and erosive.

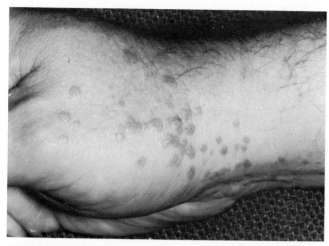

FIGURE 16-78. **Lichen planus**. The cutaneous lesions on the wrist appear as purple, polygonal papules. Careful examination shows a network of fine white lines (Wickham's striae) on the surface of the papules. See Color Plates.

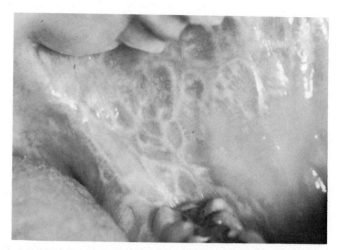

FIGURE 16-80. **Lichen planus**. The interlacing white lines are typical of reticular lichen planus involving the posterior buccal mucosa, the most common site of oral involvement. (Courtesy of Dr. William Bruce.)

Reticular Lichen Planus

Reticular lichen planus is much more common than the erosive form, but the erosive form predominates in several studies. This is probably due to referral bias, since the erosive form is symptomatic. The reticular form usually causes no symptoms and involves the posterior buccal mucosa bilaterally. Other oral mucosal surfaces may also be involved concurrently, such as the lateral and dorsal tongue, the gingivae, and the palate.

Reticular lichen planus is thus named because of its characteristic pattern of interlacing white lines (also referred to as *Wickham's striae*) (Figs. 16-80 and 16-81); however, the white lesions may present as papules in some instances. These lesions are typically not static, but wax and wane over weeks or months (Figs. 16-82 and 16-83). The reticular pattern may not be as evident in some sites, such as the dorsal tongue, where the lesions present more as keratotic plaques with atrophy of the papillae (Fig. 16-84).

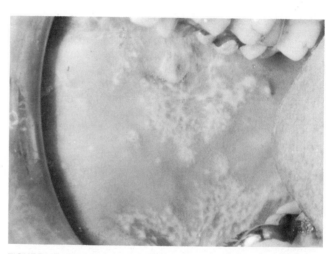

FIGURE 16-81. **Lichen planus**. The patient is affected by oral lichen planus in its reticular form. The white interlacing striae are present on the buccal mucosa, but the pattern differs markedly from that of the lesions depicted in Figure 16-80.

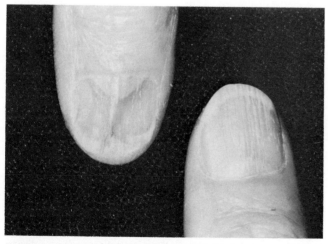

FIGURE 16-79. **Lichen planus**. Dysplastic appearance of the fingernails.

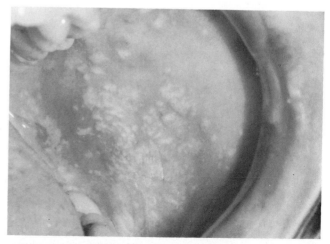

FIGURE 16-82. **Lichen planus**. A more papular form of reticular lichen planus involving the buccal mucosa.

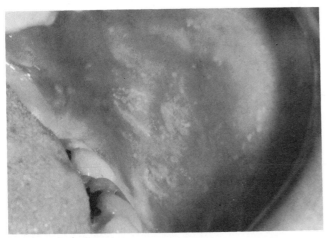

FIGURE 16-83. **Lichen planus**. Same patient as depicted in Figure 16-82. The oral lesions have waned with no treatment. Of course, in a few more weeks, these lesions may return to their original degree of severity.

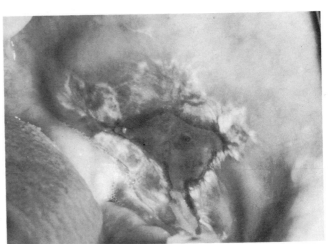

FIGURE 16-85. **Lichen planus**. Ulceration of the buccal mucosa shows peripheral radiating keratotic striae, characteristic of oral erosive lichen planus. See Color Plates.

Erosive Lichen Planus

Erosive lichen planus, although not as common as the reticular form, is more significant for the patient because the lesions are usually symptomatic. Clinically, there are atrophic, erythematous areas with central ulceration of varying degrees. The periphery of the atrophic regions is usually bordered by fine, white radiating striae (Figs. 16-85 [see Color Figure 104] to 16-87). Sometimes the atrophy and ulceration are confined to the gingival mucosa, producing the reaction pattern called **desquamative gingivitis** (see p. 128) (Fig. 16-88; see Color Figure 105). In such cases, biopsy specimens should be obtained for light microscopic and immunofluorescent studies of perilesional tissue, since cicatricial pemphigoid (see p. 563) and pemphigus vulgaris (see p. 559) may present in a similar fashion.

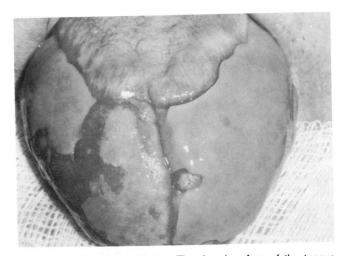

FIGURE 16-86. **Lichen planus**. The dorsal surface of the tongue shows extensive ulceration caused by erosive lichen planus. Note the fine white streaks at the periphery of the ulcerations.

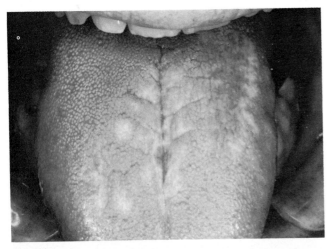

FIGURE 16-84. **Lichen planus**. With involvement of the dorsal tongue by reticular lichen planus, the characteristic interlacing striae seen in the buccal mucosal lesions are usually not present. Instead, smooth, white plaques are typically observed replacing the normal papillary surface of the tongue.

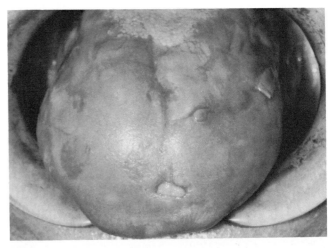

FIGURE 16-87. **Lichen planus**. Same patient as depicted in Figure 16-86 after systemic corticosteroid therapy. Much of the mucosa has re-epithelialized, with only focal ulcerations remaining.

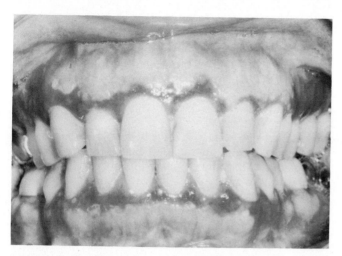

FIGURE 16–88. **Lichen planus**. Erosive lichen planus often presents as a desquamative gingivitis, producing gingival erythema and tenderness. See Color Plates.

If the erosive component is severe, epithelial separation may occur. This results in the relatively rare presentation of **bullous lichen planus**.

Histopathologic Features

The histopathologic features of lichen planus are characteristic but may not be specific; this is because other conditions, such as **lichenoid drug reactions**, may also show a similar histopathologic pattern. Varying degrees of orthokeratosis and parakeratosis may be present on the surface of the epithelium, depending on whether the biopsy specimen is taken from an erosive or reticular lesion.

The thickness of the spinous layer can also vary. The rete ridges may be absent or hyperplastic, but they classically have a pointed or "saw-toothed" shape (Fig. 16–89).

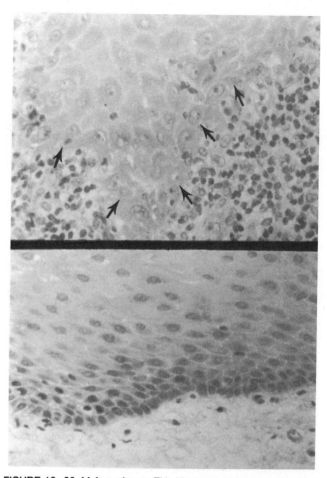

FIGURE 16–90. **Lichen planus**. This high-power photomicrograph of lichen planus (*top*) shows degeneration of the basal cell layer of the epithelium (*arrows*) compared with normal oral mucosa (*bottom*).

Destruction of the basal cell layer of the epithelium *(hydropic degeneration)* is also evident. This is accompanied by an intense, band-like infiltrate of predominantly T lymphocytes immediately subjacent to the epithelium (Fig. 16–90). Degenerating keratinocytes may be seen in the area of the epithelium–connective tissue interface and have been termed *colloid, cytoid, hyaline,* or *Civatte bodies*. No significant degree of epithelial atypia is expected in oral lichen planus, although lesions having a superimposed candidal infection may appear worrisome. These should be re-evaluated histopathologically after the candidal infection is treated.

The immunopathologic features of lichen planus are nonspecific. Most lesions show the deposition of a shaggy band of fibrinogen at the basement membrane zone

Diagnosis

The diagnosis of **reticular lichen planus** can often be made on the basis of the clinical findings alone. The interlacing white striae presenting bilaterally on the posterior buccal mucosa are virtually pathognomonic. Difficulties in diagnosis may arise if candidiasis is superimposed on the lesions because the organism may disturb

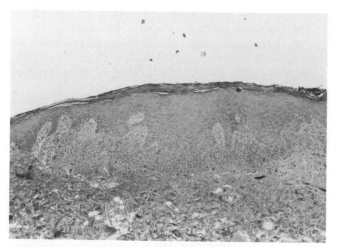

FIGURE 16–89. **Lichen planus**. This low-power photomicrograph of an oral lesion shows hyperkeratosis, saw-toothed rete ridges, and a band-like infiltrate of lymphocytes immediately subjacent to the epithelium.

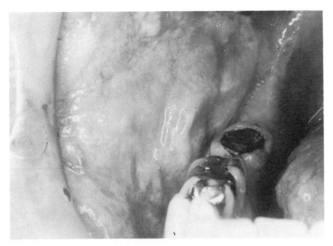

FIGURE 16-91. **Lichen planus**. These relatively nondescript white lesions affected the buccal mucosa of a patient who had complained of a burning sensation. Histopathologic evaluation of the lesion showed a lichenoid mucositis with superimposed candidiasis. See Color Plates.

the characteristic reticular pattern of the lichen planus (Figs. 16-91 and 16-92; see Color Figures 106 and 107).

Erosive lichen planus is sometimes more challenging than the reticular form to diagnose simply on the basis of its clinical features. If the typical radiating white striae and erythematous, atrophic mucosa are present at the periphery of well-demarcated ulcerations on the posterior buccal mucosa, the diagnosis can sometimes be rendered without the support of histopathologic findings. However, a biopsy is often necessary to rule out other vesiculoerosive diseases, such as lupus erythematosus or the recently described entity chronic ulcerative stomatitis.

Chronic ulcerative stomatitis usually affects adult women. It may appear as desquamative gingivitis or as ulcerations of the tongue or buccal mucosa. In many instances, the histopathologic features are similar to

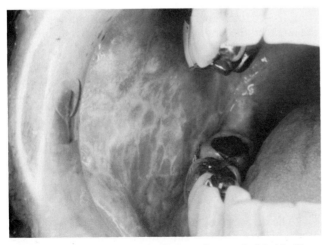

FIGURE 16-92. **Lichen planus**. Same patient as depicted in Figure 16-91 two weeks following antifungal therapy. Once the mucosal reaction to the candidal organism has been eliminated, the characteristic white striae of reticular lichen planus can be identified. See Color Plates.

those of lichen planus. A characteristic immunopathologic pattern, however, consists of autoantibodies directed against the nuclei of stratified squamous epithelial cells. Both direct and indirect immunofluorescence studies are positive for these antibodies. Unlike the lesions of erosive lichen planus, the lesions associated with chronic ulcerative stomatitis are less responsive to topical or systemic corticosteroid therapy.

Specimens of isolated erosive lichenoid lesions, particularly those of the soft palate, the lateral-ventral tongue, or the floor of the mouth, should be obtained for biopsy to rule out premalignant changes or malignancy. Another condition that may mimic an isolated lesion of lichen planus, both clinically and histopathologically, is a **lichenoid reaction to dental amalgam** (see p. 252).

Treatment and Prognosis

Reticular lichen planus typically produces no symptoms, and no treatment is needed. Occasionally, affected patients may have a superimposed candidiasis, in which case they may complain of a burning sensation of the oral mucosa. Antifungal therapy is necessary in such a case. Some investigators recommend annual re-evaluation of the reticular lesions of oral lichen planus.

Erosive lichen planus is often bothersome because of the open sores in the mouth. Because it is an immunologically mediated condition, corticosteroids are recommended. The lesions respond to systemic corticosteroids, but such drastic therapy is usually not necessary. A topical corticosteroid, such as fluocinonide gel, applied several times per day to the most symptomatic areas is usually sufficient to induce healing. The patient should be warned, however, that the condition will undoubtedly flare up again, in which case the corticosteroids should be reapplied. In addition, the possibility of iatrogenic candidiasis associated with corticosteroid use should be monitored (Figs. 16-93 to 16-95). Some investigators suggest that patients with oral erosive lichen planus be evaluated every 3 months, particularly if the lesions are not typical.

The question of the malignant potential of lichen planus, particularly the erosive form, is yet to be resolved. Most cases of reported malignant transformation are rather poorly documented. Some of these reported cases may not have been true lichen planus, but rather may have actually been dysplastic leukoplakias with a secondary lichenoid inflammatory infiltrate that mimicked lichen planus ("lichenoid dysplasia"). In addition, the argument can be made that because both lichen planus and squamous cell carcinoma are not rare, some people may have both problems simultaneously, and the two processes may be unrelated to one another. Conversely, some investigators say that the atrophic epithelium of lichen planus may be more susceptible to the action of carcinogens, resulting in an increased risk of malignant transformation. If the potential for malignant transformation exists, it appears to be small and generally confined to patients with the erosive form of lichen planus.

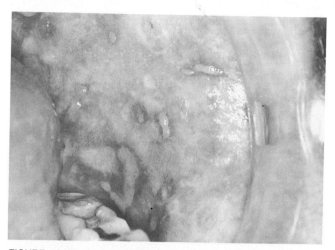

FIGURE 16–93. **Lichen planus**. This patient presented with erosive lichen planus affecting the buccal mucosa and was treated with topical corticosteroids.

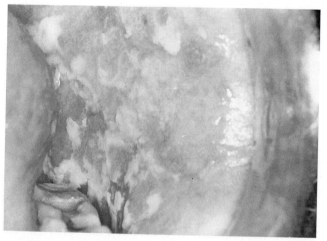

FIGURE 16–94. **Lichen planus**. Same patient as depicted in Figure 16–93. The creamy-white plaques of pseudomembranous candidiasis have developed as a result of the corticosteroid therapy.

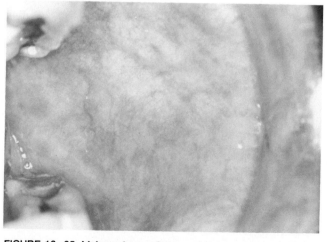

FIGURE 16–95. **Lichen planus**. Same patient as depicted in Figures 16–93 and 16–94 after antifungal therapy. At this point, the patient was asymptomatic.

GRAFT-VERSUS-HOST DISEASE

Graft-versus-host disease (GVHD) occurs in recipients of allogeneic bone marrow transplants. Such transplantations are performed at major medical centers to treat life-threatening diseases of the blood or bone marrow, such as leukemia, aplastic anemia, or disseminated metastatic disease. Cytotoxic drugs, radiation or both may be used to destroy the malignant cells, but in the process the normal hematopoietic cells of the patient are destroyed. To provide the patient with an immune system, an HLA-matched donor must be found. Bone marrow from the donor is transfused into the patient, whose own hematopoietic and immune cells have been destroyed. These transfused hematopoietic cells make their way to the recipient's bone marrow and begin to re-establish normal function.

Unfortunately, the HLA match is not always exact, and despite the use of immunomodulating and immunosuppressive drugs, such as cyclosporine and prednisone, the engrafted cells often recognize that they are not in their own environment. When this happens, these cells start attacking what they perceive as a foreign body. The result of this attack is known as graft-versus-host disease, and it can be quite devastating to the patient.

Clinical Features

The systemic signs of GVHD are varied, depending on the organ system involved and whether the problem is acute or chronic.

Acute GVHD is typically observed within the first few weeks after a bone marrow transplantation (by definition, within 100 days after the procedure). The disease affects about 50 percent of bone marrow transplant patients. The skin lesions that develop may range from a mild rash to a diffuse severe sloughing that resembles toxic epidermal necrolysis (see p. 568). These signs may be accompanied by diarrhea, nausea, vomiting, abdominal pain, and liver dysfunction.

Chronic GVHD may represent a continuation of a previously diagnosed case of acute GVHD, or it may develop later than 100 days after bone marrow transplantation, sometimes not appearing for several years after the procedure. Chronic GVHD can be expected to develop in 25 to 45 percent of bone marrow transplant recipients. The condition often mimics any one of a variety of autoimmune conditions, such as systemic lupus erythematosus, Sjögren's syndrome, or primary biliary cirrhosis. Skin involvement, which is the most common manifestation, may resemble lichen planus or even systemic sclerosis.

The oral mucosal manifestations of GVHD can also vary, depending on the duration and severity of the attack and the targeted oral tissues. Of patients with acute GVHD, 33 to 75 percent will have oral involvement; of patients with chronic GVHD, 80 percent or more will have oral lesions. In most patients with oral GVHD, there is a fine, reticular network of white striae that resembles oral lichen planus, although a more diffuse pattern of pinpoint white papules has also been described (Figs. 16–96 and 16–97). The tongue, the labial mucosa,

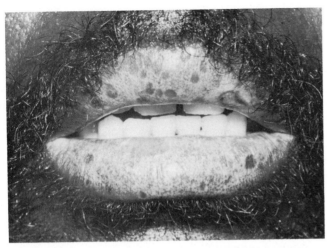

FIGURE 16-96. **Graft-versus-host disease.** Confluent, interlacing white linear lesions of the vermilion zone superficially resemble oral lichen planus.

and the buccal mucosa are the oral mucosal sites most frequently involved. Patients often complain of a burning sensation of the oral mucosa, and care must be taken not to overlook possible candidiasis. Atrophy of the oral mucosa may be present, and this can contribute to the mucosal discomfort. Ulcerations that are related to the chemotherapeutic conditioning and neutropenic state of the patient often develop during the first 2 weeks after bone marrow transplantation. Ulcers that persist longer than 2 weeks may represent acute GVHD, and these should be differentiated from intraoral herpesvirus infection or bacterial infection.

Xerostomia is also a common complaint. If the patient is not taking drugs that dry the mouth, it is likely that the immunologic response is destroying the salivary gland tissue. Other evidence of salivary gland involvement includes the development of mucoceles, particularly on the soft palate.

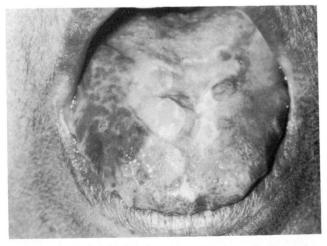

FIGURE 16-97. **Graft-versus-host disease.** Involvement of the tongue showing erosions and ulcerations that resemble erosive lichen planus.

Histopathologic Features

The histopathologic features of GVHD resemble those of oral lichen planus to a certain degree. Both lesions display hyperorthokeratosis; short, pointed rete ridges; and degeneration of the basal cell layer. The inflammatory response in GVHD is usually not as intense as in lichen planus. With advanced cases, an abnormal deposition of collagen is present, similar to the pattern in systemic sclerosis. Minor salivary gland tissue usually shows periductal inflammation in the early stages, with gradual acinar destruction and extensive fibrosis appearing later.

Diagnosis

The diagnosis of GVHD may be difficult because of the varied clinical manifestations. Such a diagnosis is of great clinical significance to the patient because complications of the condition and its treatment may be lethal. Although the diagnosis of GVHD is based on the clinical and histopathologic findings, each patient may present with a different constellation of signs and symptoms. Oral lesions appear to have value as a highly predictive index of the presence of GVHD.

Treatment and Prognosis

The primary strategy for dealing with GVHD is to reduce or prevent its occurrence. Careful tissue histocompatibility matching is performed, and the patient is given prophylactic therapy with immunomodulatory and immunosuppressive agents, such as cyclosporine and prednisone. The addition of the immunosuppressive drug methotrexate to this regimen has reduced the prevalence of acute GVHD even further. If GVHD develops, the doses of these drugs may be increased or similar pharmacologic agents may be added. The drug thalidomide has shown some promise for cases of chronic GVHD that have been resistant to standard therapy.

Topical corticosteroids may facilitate the healing of focal oral ulcerations associated with GVHD. Topical anesthetic agents are prescribed to provide patient comfort while the lesions are present. The use of **P**soralen and **U**ltraviolet **A** (PUVA) therapy has recently been shown to improve the cutaneous and oral lesions of patients with the lichenoid form of GVHD. If significant xerostomia is present in a dentulous patient, topical fluorides should be used daily to prevent xerostomia-related caries.

In general, some degree of GVHD is expected in most allogeneic bone marrow transplant recipients. The prognosis depends on the extent to which the condition progresses and whether or not it can be controlled. The significance of this complication is reflected in the survival of 55 percent of patients with relatively mild GVHD compared with 15 percent of patients with severe GVHD.

PSORIASIS

Psoriasis is a common chronic skin disease affecting 1 to 2 percent of people in the United States. According to some estimates, 150,000 new cases of psoriasis are diagnosed each year in the United States.

Psoriasis is characterized by an increased proliferative activity of the cutaneous keratinocytes. The etiopathogenesis of this increased proliferation is poorly understood but probably results from an abnormal production of cytokines. Genetic factors seem to play a role, since as many as one third of these patients have affected relatives. And yet, if one twin in a set of identical twins has psoriasis, there is only a 35 percent chance that the other twin will have it. This suggests that genetic factors are not entirely responsible for the condition and that one or more unidentified environmental agents must influence its pathogenesis.

Clinical Features

Psoriasis often has its onset during the second decade of life and tends to persist for years, with periods of exacerbation and quiescence. Patients often report that the lesions improve during the summer and worsen during the winter, an observation that may be related to lesional exposure to ultraviolet light. The lesions appear in certain favored locations, such as the scalp, elbows, and knees. The classic description is a well-demarcated, erythematous plaque with a silvery scale on its surface (Fig. 16–98; see Color Figure 108). The lesions are typically asymptomatic, but occasionally an affected patient complains of itching. An unfortunate complication affecting approximately 4 percent of these patients is **psoriatic arthritis**, which may involve the temporomandibular joint.

Oral lesions may occur in patients with psoriasis, but they are distinctly uncommon. Because descriptions of these lesions have ranged from white plaques to red plaques to ulcerations, it is difficult to determine the true nature of intraoral psoriasis (Fig. 16–99). To render a diagnosis of intraoral psoriasis, some investigators say that the activity of the oral lesions should parallel that of the cutaneous lesions. Some authors refer to **erythema**

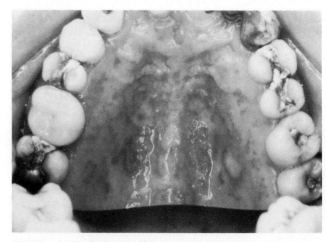

FIGURE 16–99. **Psoriasis.** This is an example of the relatively rare involvement of the oral mucosa by psoriasis. The erythematous linear patches tended to flare with the patient's cutaneous lesions. (Courtesy of Dr. George Blozis.)

migrans (see p. 569) as "intraoral psoriasis," and the prevalence of erythema migrans in psoriatic patients appears to be slightly greater than that seen in the rest of the population. It is difficult, however, to prove a direct correlation of that common mucosal alteration with psoriasis.

Histopathologic Features

Microscopically, psoriasis shows a characteristic pattern. The surface epithelium shows marked parakeratin production, and the epithelial rete ridges are elongated (Fig. 16–100). The connective tissue papillae, which contain dilated capillaries, approach close to the epithelial surface, and a perivascular chronic inflammatory cell infiltrate is present. In addition, collections of neutrophils *(Munro abscesses),* are seen within the parakeratin layer.

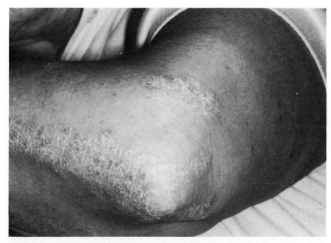

FIGURE 16–98. **Psoriasis.** Characteristic cutaneous lesions on the skin of the elbow. Note the erythematous plaques surmounted by silvery keratotic scales. See Color Plates.

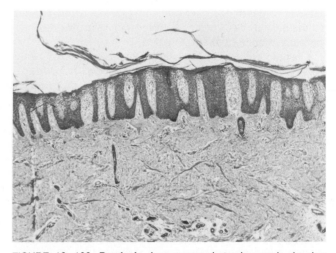

FIGURE 16–100. **Psoriasis.** Low-power photomicrograph showing elongation of the rete ridges, parakeratosis, and inflammation of the papillary dermis.

With respect to oral lesions, good correlation with skin disease activity should be seen in addition to the characteristic histopathology, since other intraoral lesions, such as erythema migrans and oral mucosal cinnamon reaction (see p. 251), exhibit a psoriasiform microscopic appearance.

Treatment and Prognosis

The treatment of psoriasis depends on the severity of the disease activity. For mild lesions, no treatment may be necessary.

For moderate involvement, topical therapeutic agents, such as corticosteroids, coal tar derivatives, and keratolytic agents, may be used. Exposure to ultraviolet radiation may also be helpful for mild to moderate disease.

For severe cases, PUVA (**P**soralen and **U**ltraviolet **A**) therapy may be needed. Methotrexate or, more recently, cyclosporine may also be used as systemic treatments for severe disease.

Although the mortality rate is not increased in patients with psoriasis, the condition often persists for years despite therapy. Some studies have shown a modest increase in the risk for cutaneous squamous cell carcinoma in psoriasis patients, possibly related to their PUVA or methotrexate therapy.

LUPUS ERYTHEMATOSUS

Lupus erythematosus (LE) is a classic example of an immunologically mediated condition. It may present in any one of several clinicopathologic forms.

Systemic lupus erythematosus (SLE) is a serious multisystem disease with a variety of cutaneous and oral manifestations. There is an increase in the activity of the humoral limb (B lymphocytes) of the immune system in conjunction with abnormal function of the T lymphocytes. Although genetic factors probably play a role in the pathogenesis of SLE, the precise cause is unknown. Undoubtedly, an interplay between genetic and environmental factors occurs, for if SLE develops in one monozygotic (identical) twin, the other twin has a 32 percent chance of having SLE as well. In contrast, if one dizygotic (fraternal) twin has SLE, the other twin has only a 6 percent chance of being affected.

Chronic cutaneous lupus erythematosus (CCLE) may represent a different, but related, process. It primarily affects the skin and oral mucosa, and the prognosis is good.

Subacute cutaneous lupus erythematosus is a third form of the disease, which has clinical features intermediate between those of SLE and CCLE.

Clinical Features

Systemic Lupus Erythematosus

Systemic lupus erythematosus can be a very difficult disease to diagnose in its early stages because it often presents in a nonspecific, vague fashion, frequently with periods of remission or disease inactivity. Women are affected nearly eight to ten times more frequently than

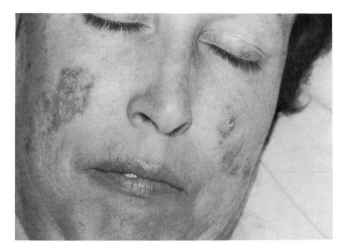

FIGURE 16–101. **Systemic lupus erythematosus**. The erythematous patches seen in the malar regions are a characteristic sign.

men. The average age at diagnosis is 31 years. Common findings include fever, weight loss, arthritis, and general malaise. In 40 to 50 percent of affected patients, a characteristic rash, having the pattern of a butterfly, develops over the malar area and nose (Fig. 16–101). Sunlight often makes the lesions worse.

The kidneys are affected in approximately 40 to 50 percent of SLE patients. This complication may ultimately lead to kidney failure and thus is typically the most significant aspect of the disease.

Cardiac involvement is also common. At autopsy nearly 50 percent of SLE patients display warty vegetations affecting the heart valves (*Libman-Sacks endocarditis*). Its significance is debatable, although some patients may develop a superimposed subacute bacterial endocarditis on these otherwise sterile outgrowths of fibrinoid material and connective tissue cells.

The oral lesions of SLE develop in 5 to 25 percent of these patients, although some studies indicate a prevalence as high as 40 percent. The lesions usually affect the palate, buccal mucosa, and gingivae. Sometimes they appear as lichenoid areas, but they may also look nonspecific or even somewhat granulomatous (Fig. 16–102).

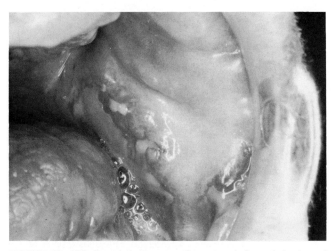

FIGURE 16–102. **Systemic lupus erythematosus**. Irregularly shaped ulcerations of the buccal mucosa.

Table 16–4. CLINICAL DIAGNOSTIC CRITERIA OF SYSTEMIC LUPUS ERYTHEMATOSUS

According to the American Rheumatism Association criteria, a diagnosis of systemic lupus erythematosus can be made if a patient has two abnormal immunologic findings in addition to at least two of the following clinical findings. The findings indented to the right under one heading are counted only as one abnormality.

Finding	Affected Patients (%)
Nonerosive polyarthritis	60%
Malar rash	50
Discoid rash	15
Photosensitivity	40
Oral ulcers	40
Hematologic abnormalities	
Anemia of chronic disease	70
Hemolytic anemia	10
Leukopenia (<4000/mm³)	65
Lymphopenia (<1500/mm³)	50
Thrombocytopenia (<100,000/mm³)	15
Neurologic symptoms	
Psychosis	10
Seizures	20
Cardiopulmonary	
Pleurisy	50
Pericarditis	30
Myocarditis	10
Renal	
Proteinuria >500 mg/24 hr	50
Cellular casts	50
Nephrotic syndrome	25
Renal failure	5%–10%

Adapted from Braunwald E. Harrison's Principles of Internal Medicine, 12th ed. New York, McGraw-Hill, 1991, p 1434.

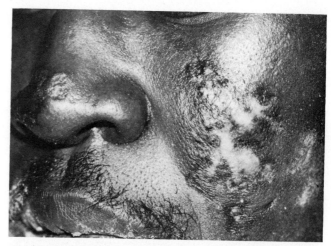

FIGURE 16–103. **Chronic cutaneous lupus erythematosus**. The skin lesions are characterized by scaling, atrophy, and pigmentary disturbances, which are most evident on sun-exposed skin.

Varying degrees of ulceration, pain, erythema, and hyperkeratosis may be present.

Confirming the diagnosis of SLE can often be difficult, particularly in the early stages. Criteria for making the diagnosis of SLE have been established by the American Rheumatism Association, and these include both clinical and laboratory findings (see Table 16–4).

Chronic Cutaneous Lupus Erythematosus

Patients with chronic cutaneous lupus erythematosus (CCLE) usually have few or no systemic signs or symptoms, with lesions being limited to skin or mucosal surfaces. The skin lesions of CCLE are known as **discoid lupus erythematosus**. They begin as scaly, erythematous patches that are frequently distributed on sun-exposed skin, especially in the head and neck area (Fig. 16–103). Patients may indicate that the lesions are exacerbated by sun exposure. With time, the lesions may heal spontaneously in one area, only to appear in another area. The healing process usually results in cutaneous atrophy with scarring and hypopigmentation or hyperpigmentation of the resolving lesion.

In most cases, the oral manifestations of CCLE essentially appear clinically identical to the lesions of erosive lichen planus. Unlike the oral lesions of lichen planus, however, the oral lesions of CCLE rarely occur in the absence of skin lesions. An ulcerated or atrophic, erythematous central zone, surrounded by white, fine, radiating striae, characterizes the oral lesion of CCLE (Figs.

16–104 [see Color Fig. 109] and 16–105). Sometimes the erythematous, atrophic central region of a lesion may show a fine stippling of white dots. As with erosive lichen planus, the ulcerative and atrophic oral lesions of CCLE may be painful, especially when exposed to acidic or salty foods.

Subacute Cutaneous Lupus Erythematosus

Patients with subacute cutaneous lupus erythematosus have clinical manifestations intermediate between those of SLE and CCLE. The skin lesions are the most prominent feature of this variation. They are characterized by photosensitivity and are therefore generally present in sun-exposed areas. These lesions do not show the induration and scarring seen with the skin lesions of CCLE. Usually, the renal or neurologic abnormalities associated with SLE are not present either, with most patients having arthritis or musculoskeletal problems.

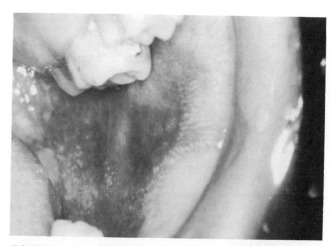

FIGURE 16–104. **Chronic cutaneous lupus erythematosus**. Erythematous zones of the buccal mucosa are surrounded by radiating keratotic striae. These features are similar to those of erosive lichen planus. See Color Plates.

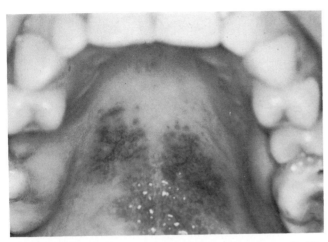

FIGURE 16–105. **Chronic cutaneous lupus erythematosus**. Oral involvement may also include relatively nondescript erythematous patches, such as this one in the palate.

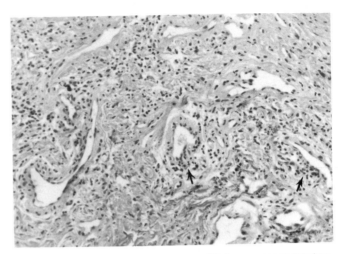

FIGURE 16–107. **Lupus erythematosus**. Medium-power photomicrograph showing the perivascular chronic inflammatory cell infiltrate (*arrows*).

Histopathologic Features

The histopathologic features of the skin and oral lesions of the various forms of lupus erythematosus show some features in common but are different enough to warrant separate discussions.

The skin lesions of chronic cutaneous lupus erythematosus are characterized by hyperkeratosis, often displaying keratin packed into the openings of hair follicles ("follicular plugging"). In all forms of lupus erythematosus, degeneration of the basal cell layer is frequently observed, and the underlying connective tissue supports patchy to dense aggregates of chronic inflammatory cells (Fig. 16–106). In the deeper connective tissue, the inflammatory infiltrate often surrounds the small blood vessels (Fig. 16–107).

The oral lesions demonstrate hyperkeratosis, alternating atrophy and thickening of the spinous cell layer, degeneration of the basal cell layer, and subepithelial lymphocytic infiltration. These features may also be seen in oral lichen planus; however, the two conditions can usually be distinguished by the presence in LE of patchy

deposits of a periodic acid–Schiff (PAS)–positive material in the basement membrane zone, subepithelial edema (sometimes to the point of vesicle formation), and a more diffuse, deep inflammatory infiltrate, often in a perivascular orientation.

Diagnosis

In addition to the clinical and microscopic features, a number of additional immunologic studies may be helpful in making the diagnosis of lupus erythematosus.

Direct immunofluorescence testing of lesional tissue shows deposition of one or more immunoreactants (usually IgM, IgG, or C3) in a shaggy or granular band at the basement membrane zone. In addition, direct immunofluorescence testing of clinically normal skin of SLE patients often shows a similar deposition of IgG, IgM, or complement components. This finding is known as a *positive lupus band test*.

Evaluation of serum obtained from a patient with systemic lupus erythematosus shows various immunologic abnormalities. Approximately 95 percent of these patients have antibodies directed against multiple nuclear antigens (antinuclear antibodies [ANAs]). Although this is a nonspecific finding that may be seen in other autoimmune diseases as well as in otherwise healthy elderly individuals, it is nevertheless useful as a screening study. Furthermore, if results are negative on multiple occasions, the diagnosis of SLE should probably be doubted. Antibodies directed against double-stranded DNA are noted in 70 percent of patients with SLE, and these are more specific for the disease. Another 30 percent of patients show antibodies directed against Sm, a protein that is complexed with small nuclear RNA. This finding is very specific for SLE.

A summary of selected immunologic findings in lupus erythematosus is shown in Table 16–5.

Treatment and Prognosis

Patients with SLE should avoid excessive exposure to sunlight because ultraviolet light may precipitate disease

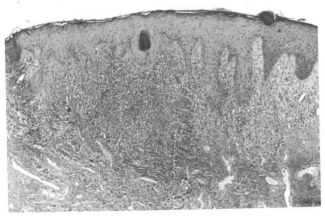

FIGURE 16–106. **Lupus erythematosus**. Low-power photomicrograph showing the lichenoid reaction with follicular plugging, characteristic of chronic cutaneous lupus erythematosus.

Table 16–5. SELECTED ABNORMAL IMMUNOLOGIC FINDINGS IN LUPUS ERYTHEMATOSUS

Finding	Frequency		Significance
Direct immunofluorescence, lesional skin	CCLE:	90%	May help distinguish among the various types of lupus erythematosus
	SLE:	95%	
Direct immunofluorescence, normal skin	CCLE:	0%	"Lupus band test"
	SLE:	25–60%	
Antinuclear antibodies	CCLE:	0–10%	Very sensitive for SLE, however not very specific; not useful for CCLE diagnosis.
	SLE:	95%	
Anti–double-stranded DNA antibodies	CCLE:	0%	Specific for SLE; may indicate disease activity or kidney involvement
	SLE:	70–80%	
Anti-Sm antibodies	CCLE:	0%	Specific for SLE
	SLE:	10–30%	

CCLE, chronic cutaneous lupus erythematosus; SLE, systemic lupus erythematosus.

activity. For acute episodes, systemic corticosteroids are generally indicated and these may be combined with other immunosuppressive agents. At times, antimalarial drugs may be effective, although they are usually more effective for CCLE or subacute cutaneous LE. If oral lesions are present, they typically respond to the systemic therapy.

As with SLE patients, patients with CCLE should avoid excessive sunlight exposure. Because most of the manifestations of CCLE are cutaneous, topical corticosteroids are often reasonably effective. For cases that are resistant to topical therapy, systemic antimalarial drugs may produce a response. Topical corticosteroids are also helpful in treating the oral lesions of CCLE.

The prognosis for the patient with SLE is variable. For patients undergoing treatment today, the 5-year survival rate is approximately 95 percent; however, by 15 years, the survival rate falls to 75 percent. Ultimately, the prognosis depends on which organs are affected and how frequently the disease is reactivated. The most common cause of death is renal failure due to kidney involvement. For reasons that are poorly understood, the prognosis is worse for men than for women.

The prognosis for patients with CCLE is considerably better than that for patients with SLE, although transformation to SLE may be seen in approximately 5 percent of CCLE patients. Usually, CCLE remains confined to the skin, but it may persist and be quite a nuisance. For about 50 percent of CCLE patients, the problem eventually resolves after several years.

SYSTEMIC SCLEROSIS (Scleroderma; Hide-Bound Disease)

Systemic sclerosis is a relatively rare condition that probably has an immunologically mediated pathogenesis. For reasons that are not understood, dense collagen is deposited in the tissues of the body in extraordinary amounts. Although its most dramatic effects are seen in association with the skin, the disease is often quite serious, with most organs of the body affected.

Clinical and Radiographic Features

Systemic sclerosis affects approximately 19 persons per million population each year. Women have the condition three times more frequently than men do. Most patients are adults. The onset of the disease is often insidious, with the cutaneous changes often responsible for bringing the problem to the patient's attention.

Often one of the first signs of the disease is *Raynaud's phenomenon*, a vasoconstrictive event triggered by emotional distress or exposure to cold. Raynaud's phenomenon (see **CREST syndrome,** p. 586) is not specific for systemic sclerosis, however, because it may be present in other immunologically mediated diseases and in otherwise healthy people. Resorption of the terminal phalanges *(acro-osteolysis)* and flexion contractures produce shortened, claw-like fingers (Fig. 16–108). The vascular events and the abnormal collagen deposition contribute to the production of ulcerations on the fingertips (Fig. 16–109).

The skin develops a diffuse, hard texture (*sclero* = hard; *derma* = skin), and its surface is usually smooth.

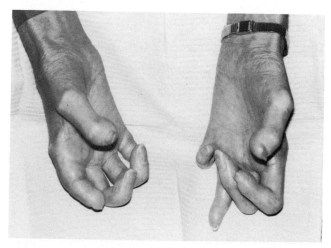

FIGURE 16–108. **Systemic sclerosis.** The tense, shiny appearance of the skin is evident. Note that the fingers are fixed in a claw-like position, with some showing shortening as a result of acro-osteolysis.

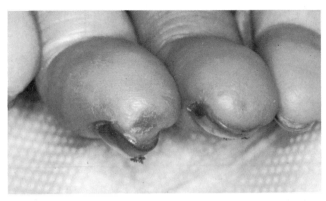

FIGURE 16–109. **Systemic sclerosis.** Ulcerations of the fingertips.

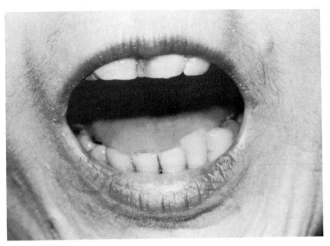

FIGURE 16–111. **Systemic sclerosis.** Same patient as depicted in Figure 16–110. Because of the associated microstomia, this is the patient's maximal opening.

Involvement of the facial skin by the subcutaneous collagen deposition results in the characteristic smooth, taut, "mask-like" facies (Fig. 16–110). Similarly, the nasal alae become atrophied, resulting in a pinched appearance to the nose, called a "mouse facies."

Involvement of other organs may be more subtle at first, but the results are more serious. Fibrosis of the lungs, heart, kidneys, and gastrointestinal tract leads to

organ failure. Pulmonary fibrosis is particularly significant, leading to pulmonary hypertension and heart failure, a primary cause of death for these patients.

The oral manifestations occur in varying degrees. *Microstomia* often develops as a result of the collagen deposition in the perioral tissues. This causes a limitation of opening the mouth in nearly 70 percent of these patients (Fig. 16–111). Characteristic furrows radiating from the mouth produce a "purse-string" appearance. Loss of attached gingival mucosa and multiple areas of gingival recession may occur in some patients. Dysphagia often develops as a result of deposition of collagen in the lingual and esophageal submucosa, producing a firm, hypomobile tongue and an inelastic esophagus, thus hindering swallowing.

On dental radiographs, diffuse widening of the periodontal ligament space is often present throughout the dentition. The extent of the widening may vary, with some examples being subtle and others quite dramatic (Fig. 16–112). Varying degrees of resorption of the poste-

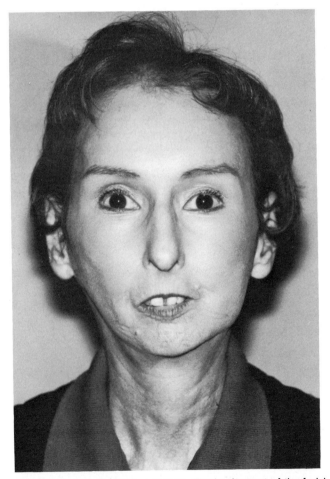

FIGURE 16–110. **Systemic sclerosis.** The involvement of the facial skin with abnormal collagen deposition produces a mask-like facies. Note the loss of the alae of the nose.

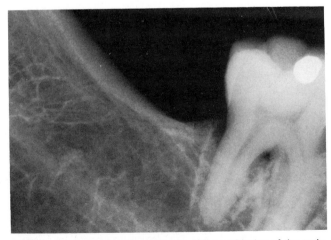

FIGURE 16–112. **Systemic sclerosis.** Diffuse widening of the periodontal ligament space is often identified on evaluation of periapical radiographs.

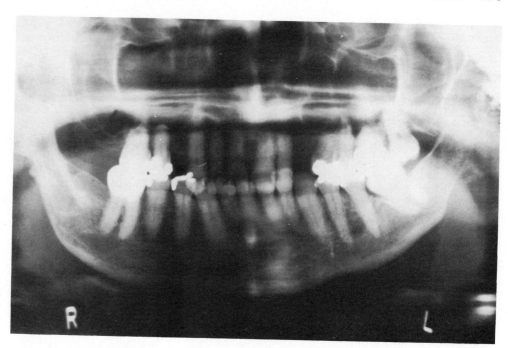

FIGURE 16–113. **Systemic sclerosis**. Panoramic radiographic evaluation may show a characteristic resorption of the ramus, coronoid process, or condyle.

rior ramus of the mandible, the coronoid process, and the condyle may be detected on panoramic radiographs, affecting approximately 20 percent of patients (Fig. 16–113). In theory, these areas are resorbed because of the increased pressure associated with the abnormal collagen production.

A mild variant of this condition, called **localized scleroderma**, usually affects only a solitary patch of skin. Because these lesions often look like scars, the name *coup de sabre* ("strike of the sword") is used to describe them (Fig. 16–114; see Color Figure 110). This problem is primarily cosmetic and, unlike systemic sclerosis, it is rarely life-threatening.

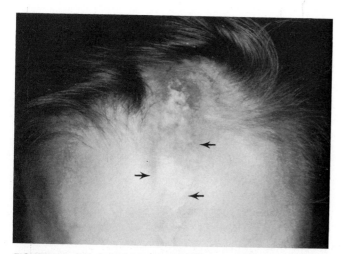

FIGURE 16–114. **Localized scleroderma**. The cutaneous alteration on the patient's forehead (*arrows*) represents a limited form of scleroderma called *coup de sabre* because the lesion resembles a scar that might result from a cut with a sword. See Color Plates.

Histopathologic Features

Microscopic examination of tissue involved by systemic sclerosis shows diffuse deposition of dense collagen within and around the normal structures (Fig. 16–115). This abnormal collagen replaces and destroys the normal tissue, causing the loss of normal tissue function.

Diagnosis

During the early phases, it may be difficult to make a diagnosis of systemic sclerosis. Generally, the clinical signs of stiffened skin texture along with the development of Raynaud's phenomenon are suggestive of the diagnosis. A skin biopsy may be supportive of the diagnosis if abundant collagen deposition is observed microscopically.

Laboratory studies may be helpful to the diagnostic process if anti-centromere antibodies or anti-Scl 70 (topoisomerase I) is detected. Anti-Scl 70 antibodies are seen more often with systemic sclerosis; anti-centromere antibodies are usually associated with more limited forms of scleroderma or **CREST syndrome** (see next topic).

Treatment and Prognosis

The management of systemic sclerosis is difficult. Systemic medications, such as D-penicillamine, are prescribed in an attempt to inhibit collagen production. Surprisingly, corticosteroids are of little benefit. Extracorporeal photochemotherapy has shown some beneficial effect on the skin lesions; however, no improvement of the pulmonary function tests is observed.

Other management strategies are directed at controlling symptoms. Such techniques as esophageal dilation

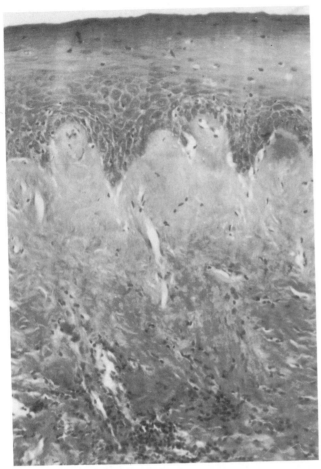

FIGURE 16–115. **Systemic sclerosis**. Medium-power photomicrograph of an oral biopsy specimen. Diffuse deposition of collagen is apparent throughout the lamina propria.

are used, for example, to temporarily correct the esophageal dysfunction and dysphagia. Nifedipine helps to increase peripheral blood flow and reduce the symptoms of Raynaud's phenomenon.

From a dental standpoint, problems may develop for patients who wear prostheses because of the microstomia and inelasticity of the mouth. For the same reasons, patients may also have problems with maintaining good oral hygiene and they have a decreased ability to manipulate a toothbrush as a result of sclerotic changes in the fingers and hands. Infrequently, the resorption of the mandible may become so great as to cause a pathologic fracture.

The prognosis is poor, although the outlook is better for patients with limited cutaneous involvement than for those with diffuse involvement. In one large study, it was shown that approximately 80 percent of patients will survive 2 years following diagnosis, but survival drops off with time. Only 50 percent will survive 8 years, and the survival rate drops to 30 percent at 12 years.

CREST SYNDROME (Acrosclerosis)

CREST syndrome is an uncommon condition that may be a relatively mild variant of systemic sclerosis.

The term CREST is an acronym for **C**alcinosis cutis, **R**aynaud's phenomenon, **E**sophageal dysfunction, **S**clerodactyly, and **T**elangiectasia.

Clinical Features

As with **systemic sclerosis**, most patients with CREST syndrome are women in the sixth or seventh decade of life. The characteristic signs may not appear synchronously but instead may develop sequentially over a period of months to years.

Calcinosis cutis occurs in the form of movable, nontender, subcutaneous nodules, 0.5 to 2.0 cm in size, which are usually multiple (Fig. 16–116).

Raynaud's phenomenon may be observed when a person's hands or feet are exposed to cold temperatures. The initial clinical sign is a dramatic blanching of the digits, which appear dead-white in color as a result of severe vasospasm. A few minutes later, the affected extremity takes on a bluish color because of venous stasis. After warming, increased blood flow results in a dusky-red hue with the return of hyperemic blood flow. This may be accompanied by varying degrees of throbbing pain.

Esophageal dysfunction, caused by abnormal collagen deposition in the esophageal submucosa, may not be noticeable in the early phases of CREST syndrome. Often the subtle initial signs of this problem must be demonstrated by barium swallow radiologic studies.

The **sclerodactyly** of CREST syndrome is rather remarkable. The fingers become stiff, and the skin takes on a smooth, shiny appearance. Often the fingers undergo permanent flexure, resulting in a characteristic "claw" deformity (Fig. 16–117). As with **systemic sclerosis**, this change is due to abnormal deposition of collagen within the dermis in these areas.

The **telangiectasias** in this syndrome are similar to those seen in hereditary hemorrhagic telangiectasia (see p. 550). As with that condition, significant bleeding from the superficial dilated capillaries may occur. The facial skin and the vermilion zone of the lips are commonly affected (Fig. 16–118; see Color Figure 111).

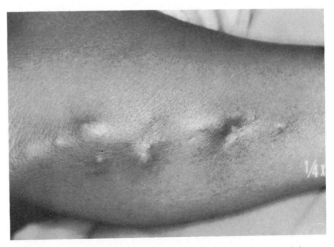

FIGURE 16–116. **CREST syndrome**. The subcutaneous nodules on this patient's arm represent deposition of calcium salts (calcinosis cutis). (Courtesy of Dr. Román Carlos.)

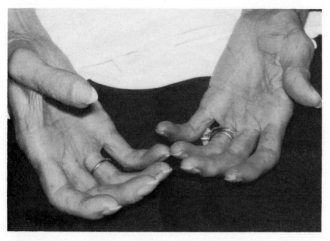

FIGURE 16–117. **CREST syndrome.** Claw-like deformity affecting the hands (sclerodactyly).

Diagnosis

Sometimes **hereditary hemorrhagic telangiectasia** may be considered in the differential diagnosis if the history is unclear and the other signs of CREST are not yet evident. In these cases, laboratory studies directed at identi-

fying anti-centromere antibodies may be useful, since this test is relatively specific for CREST.

Histopathologic Features

The histopathologic findings in CREST syndrome are similar, although milder, to those seen in systemic sclerosis. Superficial dilated capillaries are observed if a telangiectatic vessel is included in the biopsy specimen.

Treatment and Prognosis

The treatment of patients with CREST syndrome is essentially the same as that of those with systemic sclerosis. Because CREST syndrome usually is not as severe, the treatment does not have to be as aggressive. The prognosis is much better than that for systemic sclerosis.

ACANTHOSIS NIGRICANS

Acanthosis nigricans is an acquired dermatologic problem characterized by the development of a velvety, brownish alteration of the skin. In some instances, this unusual condition develops in conjunction with gastrointestinal cancer and is termed **malignant acanthosis nigricans**. The cutaneous lesion itself is benign, yet it is significant because it represents a cutaneous marker for internal malignancy. The etiology of malignant acanthosis nigricans is unknown, although a cytokine-like peptide capable of affecting the epidermal cells may be produced by the malignancy.

Most cases, estimated to affect as many as 5 percent of adults, are not associated with a malignancy and are termed **benign acanthosis nigricans**. A clinically similar form, **pseudo–acanthosis nigricans**, may occur in some obese people. Some benign forms of acanthosis nigricans may be inherited or may occur in association with various endocrinopathies, such as diabetes mellitus, Addison's disease, hypothyroidism, and acromegaly. Furthermore, benign acanthosis nigricans may occur with certain syndromes (e.g., Crouzon syndrome) or drug ingestion (oral contraceptives, corticosteroids). These forms of the condition are typically associated with resistance of their tissues to the effects of insulin, similar to the insulin resistance seen in non–insulin-dependent diabetes mellitus. Even though the affected individuals may not have overt diabetes mellitus, they often show increased levels of insulin or an abnormal response to exogenously administered insulin.

Clinical Features

The malignant form of acanthosis nigricans develops in association with an internal malignancy, particularly adenocarcinoma of the gastrointestinal tract. Approximately 20 percent of the cases of malignant acanthosis nigricans are identified before the malignancy is found, but most appear at about the same time as discovery of the gastrointestinal tumor or thereafter.

Both forms of acanthosis nigricans affect the flexural areas of the skin predominantly, appearing as finely pap-

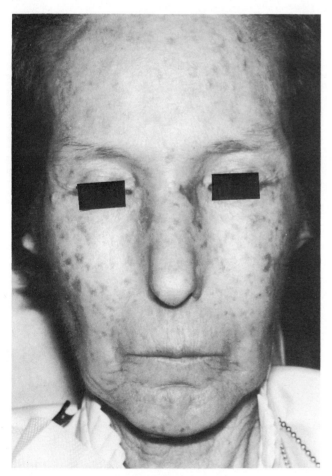

FIGURE 16–118. **CREST syndrome.** The patient shows numerous red facial macules representing telangiectatic blood vessels. See Color Plates.

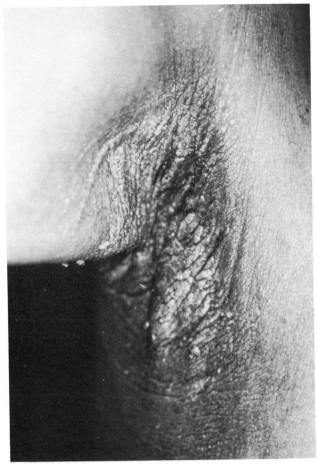

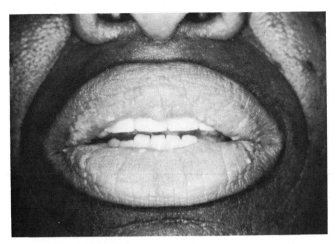

FIGURE 16-120. **Acanthosis nigricans**. The vermilion zone of the lips are affected. (Courtesy of Dr. George Blozis.)

FIGURE 16-119. **Acanthosis nigricans**. The lesions are characterized by numerous fine, almost velvety, confluent papules. The lesions most often affect the flexural areas, such as the axilla depicted in this photograph. (From Hall JM, Moreland A, Cox GJ, Wade TR. Oral acanthosis nigricans: Report of a case and comparison of oral and cutaneous pathology. Am J Dermatopathol 10:68-73, 1988.)

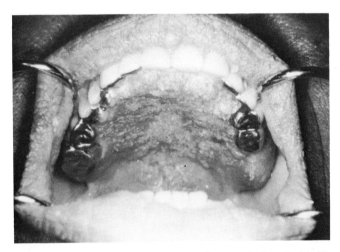

FIGURE 16-121. **Acanthosis nigricans**. Same patient as depicted in Figure 16-120. Note involvement of the palatal mucosa. (Courtesy of Dr. George Blozis.)

illary, hyperkeratotic, brownish patches that are usually asymptomatic (Fig. 16-119). The texture of the lesions has been variably described as either velvety or leathery.

Oral lesions of acanthosis nigricans have also been reported, and may occur in 25 to 50 percent of affected patients, especially those with the malignant form. These lesions appear as diffuse, finely papillary areas of mucosal alteration that most often involve the tongue or lips, particularly the upper lip (Figs. 16-120 and 16-121). The buccal mucosa may also be affected. The brownish pigmentation associated with the cutaneous lesions is usually not seen in oral acanthosis nigricans.

Histopathologic Features

The histopathologic features of the various forms of acanthosis nigricans are essentially identical. The epidermis exhibits hyperorthokeratosis and papillomatosis. Usually, some degree of increased melanin deposition is noted, but the extent of *acanthosis* (thickening of the spinous layer) is really rather mild. The oral lesions have much more acanthosis, but show minimal increased melanin pigmentation (Fig. 16-122).

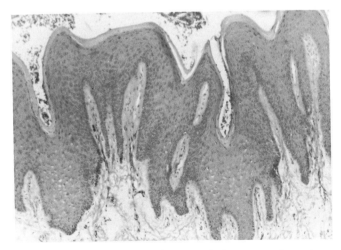

FIGURE 16-122. **Acanthosis nigricans**. Medium-power photomicrograph of an oral lesion showing papillomatosis, mild hyperkeratosis, and acanthosis of the epithelium.

Treatment and Prognosis

Although acanthosis nigricans itself is a harmless process, the patient should be evaluated to ascertain which form of the disease is present. Identification and treatment of the underlying malignancy obviously are important for patients with the malignant type; unfortunately the prognosis for these individuals is very poor. Interestingly, malignant acanthosis nigricans may resolve when the cancer is treated. Keratolytic agents may improve the appearance of the benign forms.

REFERENCES

Ectodermal Dysplasia

Anton-Lamprecht I, Schieiermacher E, Wolf M. Autosomal recessive anhidrotic ectodermal dysplasia: Report of a case and discrimination of diagnostic features. Birth Defects 24:183–195, 1988.

Berg D, et al. Sweating in ectodermal dysplasia syndromes. Arch Dermatol 126:1075–1079, 1990.

Farrington FH. The team approach to the management of ectodermal dysplasias. Birth Defects 24:237–242, 1988.

Jorgenson RJ, et al. A population study on the density of palmar sweat pores. Birth Defects 24:51–63, 1988.

Levin LS. Dental and oral abnormalities in selected ectodermal dysplasia syndromes. Birth Defects 24:205–227, 1988.

Nowak AJ. Dental treatment for patients with ectodermal dysplasias. Birth Defects 24:243–252, 1988.

Siegel MB, Potsic WP. Ectodermal dysplasia: The otolaryngologic manifestations and management. Int J Pediatr Otorhinolaryngol 19:265–271, 1990.

White Sponge Nevus

Cox MF, et al. Human papillomavirus type 16 DNA in oral white sponge nevus. Oral Surg Oral Med Oral Pathol 73:476–478, 1992.

Jorgenson RJ, Levin LS. White sponge nevus. Arch Dermatol 117:73–76, 1981.

Krajewska IA, Moore L, Brown JH. White sponge nevus presenting in the esophagus—case report and literature review. Pathology 24:112–115, 1992.

Miller CS, Craig RM. White corrugated mucosa. J Am Dent Assoc 117:345–346, 1988.

Morris R, et al. White sponge nevus: Diagnosis by light microscopic and ultrastructural cytology. Acta Cytol 32:357–361, 1988.

Nichols GE, et al. White sponge nevus. Obstet Gynecol 76:545–548, 1990.

Hereditary Benign Intraepithelial Dyskeratosis

Reed JW, Cashwell LF, Klintworth GK. Corneal manifestations of hereditary benign intraepithelial dyskeratosis. Arch Ophthalmol 97:297–300, 1979.

Sadeghi EM, Witkop CJ. The presence of *Candida albicans* in hereditary benign intraepithelial dyskeratosis: An ultrastructural observation. Oral Surg Oral Med Oral Pathol 48:342–346, 1979.

Pachyonychia Congenita

Stieglitz JB, Centerwall WR. Pachyonychia congenita (Jadassohn-Lewandowsky syndrome): A seventeen member, four-generation pedigree with unusual respiratory and dental involvement. Am J Med Genet 14:21–28, 1983.

Dyskeratosis Congenita

Davidson HR, Connor JM. Dyskeratosis congenita. J Med Genet 25:843–846, 1988.

Drachtman RA, Alter BP. Dyskeratosis congenita: Clinical and genetic heterogeneity: Report of a new case and review of the literature. Am J Pediatr Hematol Oncol 14:297–304, 1992.

Kawaguchi K, et al. Dyskeratosis congenita (Zinsser-Cole-Engman syndrome): An autopsy case presenting with rectal carcinoma, noncirrhotic portal hypertension, and *Pneumocystis carinii* pneumonia. Virchows Arch A Pathol Anat Histopathol 417:247–253, 1990.

Loh HS, Koh ML, Giam YC. Dyskeratosis congenita in two male cousins. Br J Oral Maxillofac Surg 25:492–499, 1987.

Ogden GR, Conner E, Chisholm DM. Dyskeratosis congenita: Report of a case and review of the literature. Oral Surg Oral Med Oral Pathol 65:586–591, 1988.

Ogden GR, et al. Cytokeratin profiles in dyskeratosis congenita: An immunocytochemical investigation of lingual hyperkeratosis. J Oral Pathol Med 21:353–357, 1992.

Ogden GR, Lane DP, Chisholm DM. p53 expression in dyskeratosis congenita: A marker for oral premalignancy? J Clin Pathol 46:169–170, 1993.

Putterman C, et al. Treatment of the hematological manifestations of dyskeratosis congenita. Ann Hematol 66:209–212, 1993.

Yavazyilmaz E, et al. Oral-dental findings in dyskeratosis congenita. J Oral Pathol Med 21:280–284, 1992.

Xeroderma Pigmentosum

Khatri ML, Shafi M, Mashina A. Xeroderma pigmentosum: A clinical study of 24 Libyan cases. J Am Acad Dermatol 26:75–78, 1992.

Kraemer KH, Lee MM, Scotto J. Xeroderma pigmentosum: Cutaneous, ocular, and neurologic abnormalities in 830 published cases. Arch Dermatol 123:241–250, 1987.

Osguthorpe JD, Lang P. Management of xeroderma pigmentosum. Arch Otolaryngol Head Neck Surg 113:292–294, 1987.

Patton LL, Valdez IH. Xeroderma pigmentosum: Review and report of a case. Oral Surg Oral Med Oral Pathol 71:297–300, 1991.

Shumrick KA, Coldiron B. Genetic syndromes associated with skin cancer. Otolaryngol Clin North Am 26:117–137, 1993.

Incontinentia Pigmenti

Emery MM, et al. Incontinentia pigmenti: Transmission from father to daughter. J Am Acad Dermatol 29:368–372, 1993.

Landy SJ, Donnai D. Incontinentia pigmenti (Bloch-Sulzberger syndrome). J Med Genet 30:53–59, 1993.

Milam PE, Griffin TJ, Shapiro RD. A dentofacial deformity associated with incontinentia pigmenti: Report of a case. Oral Surg Oral Med Oral Pathol 70:420–424, 1990.

Vogt J, Matheson J. Incontinentia pigmenti (Bloch-Sulzberger syndrome): A case report. Oral Surg Oral Med Oral Pathol 71:454–456, 1991.

Wiss K. Neurocutaneous disorders: Tuberous sclerosis, incontinentia pigmenti, and hypomelanosis of Ito. Semin Neurol 12:364–373, 1992.

Darier's Disease

Berg D, Bassett AS. Darier's disease: Current understanding of pathogenesis and future role of genetic studies. Int J Dermatol 32:397–400, 1993.

Burge SM, Wilkinson JD. Darier-White disease: A review of the clinical features in 163 patients. J Am Acad Dermatol 27:40–50, 1992.

Ferris T, Lamey P-J, Rennie JS. Darier's disease: Oral features and genetic aspects. Br Dent J 168:71–73, 1990.

Macleod RI, Munro CS. The incidence and distribution of oral lesions in patients with Darier's disease. Br Dent J 171:133–136, 1991.

Munro CS. The phenotype of Darier's disease: Penetrance and expressivity in adults and children. Br J Dermatol 127:126–130, 1992.

Warty Dyskeratoma

Chau MNY, Radden BG. Oral warty dyskeratoma. J Oral Pathol 13:546–556, 1984.

Kaugars GE, Lieb RJ, Abbey LM. Focal oral warty dyskeratoma. Int J Dermatol 23:123–130, 1984.

Laskaris G, Sklavounou A. Warty dyskeratoma of the oral mucosa. Br J Oral Maxillofac Surg 23:371–375, 1985.

Mesa ML, et al. Oral warty dyskeratoma. Cutis 33:293–296, 1984.

Peutz-Jeghers Syndrome

Buck JL, et al. Peutz-Jeghers syndrome. Radiographics 12:365–378, 1992.

Hizawa K, et al. Cancer in Peutz-Jeghers syndrome. Cancer 72:2777–2781, 1993.

Rodu B, Martinez MG. Peutz-Jeghers syndrome and cancer. Oral Surg Oral Med Oral Pathol 58:584–588, 1984.

Uno A, Hori Y. Disturbance of melanosome transfer in pigmented macules of Peutz-Jeghers syndrome. *In*: Brown Melanoderma. Edited by Fitzpatrick TB, et al. Tokyo, University of Tokyo Press, 1986, pp 173–178.

Hereditary Hemorrhagic Telangiectasia

Bevelaqua FA, et al. Osler-Weber-Rendu disease: Diagnosis and management of spontaneous hemothorax during pregnancy. N Y State J Med 92:551–552, 1992.

Braverman IM, Keh A, Jacobson BS. Ultrastructure and three-dimensional organization of the telangiectases of hereditary hemorrhagic telangiectasia. J Invest Dermatol 95:422–427, 1990.

Goldberg SH, Bullock JD. Hereditary hemorrhagic telangiectasia. Ophthal Plast Reconstr Surg 6:136–138, 1990.

Peery WH. Clinical spectrum of hereditary hemorrhagic telangiectasia (Osler-Weber-Rendu disease). Am J Med 82:989–997, 1987.

Reilly PJ, Nostrant TT. Clinical manifestations of hereditary hemorrhagic telangiectasia. Am J Gastroenterol 79:363–367, 1984.

Swanson DL, Dahl MV. Embolic abscesses in hereditary hemorrhagic telangiectasia. J Am Acad Dermatol 24:580–583, 1991.

Ehlers-Danlos Syndromes

Dyne KM, et al. Ehlers-Danlos syndrome type VIII: Biochemical, stereological and immunocytochemical studies on dermis from a child with clinical signs of Ehlers-Danlos syndrome and a family history of premature loss of permanent teeth. Br J Dermatol 128:458–463, 1993.

Fridrich KL, et al. Dental implications in Ehlers-Danlos syndrome: A case report. Oral Surg Oral Med Oral Pathol 69:431–435, 1990.

Hartsfield JK, Kousseff BG. Phenotypic overlap of Ehlers-Danlos syndrome types IV and VIII. Am J Med Genet 37:465–470, 1990.

Hoff M. Dental manifestations in Ehlers-Danlos syndrome: Report of a case. Oral Surg Oral Med Oral Pathol 44:864–871, 1977.

Nelson DL, King RA. Ehlers-Danlos syndrome type VIII. J Am Acad Dermatol 5:297–303, 1981.

Ooshima T, et al. Oral manifestations of Ehlers-Danlos syndrome type VII: Histological examination of a primary tooth. Pediatr Dent 12:102–106, 1990.

Pope FM. Ehlers-Danlos syndrome. Baillieres Clin Rheumatol 5:321–349, 1991.

Pope FM, et al. Ehlers Danlos syndrome type I with novel dental features. J Oral Pathol Med 21:418–421, 1992.

Sacks H, Zelig D, Schabes G. Recurrent temporomandibular joint subluxation and facial ecchymosis leading to diagnosis of Ehlers-Danlos syndrome: Report of surgical management and review of the literature. J Oral Maxillofac Surg 48:641–647, 1990.

Sakala EP, Harding MD. Ehlers-Danlos syndrome type III and pregnancy: A case report. J Reprod Med 36:622–624, 1991.

Tuberous Sclerosis

Fitzpatrick TB. History and significance of white macules, earliest visible sign of tuberous sclerosis. Ann N Y Acad Sci 615:26–35, 1991.

Haines JL, et al. Genetic heterogeneity in tuberous sclerosis: Study of a large collaborative dataset. Ann N Y Acad Sci 615:256–264, 1991.

Houser OW, Shepherd CW, Gomez MR. Imaging of intracranial tuberous sclerosis. Ann N Y Acad Sci 615:81–93, 1991.

Lygidakis NA, Lindenbaum RH. Oral fibromatosis in tuberous sclerosis. Oral Surg Oral Med Oral Pathol 68:725–728, 1989.

Mlynarczyk G. Enamel pitting: A common symptom of tuberous sclerosis. Oral Surg Oral Med Oral Pathol 71:63–67, 1991.

Northrup H. Tuberous sclerosis complex: Genetic aspects. J Dermatol 19:914–919, 1992.

Osborne JP, Fryer A, Webb D. Epidemiology of tuberous sclerosis. Ann N Y Acad Sci 615:125–127, 1991.

Sampson JR, et al. Pitted enamel hypoplasia in tuberous sclerosis. Clin Genet 42:50–52, 1992.

Shepherd CW, Gomez MR. Mortality in the Mayo Clinic tuberous sclerosis complex study. Ann N Y Acad Sci 615:375–377, 1991.

Stirrups DR, Inglis J. Tuberous sclerosis with nonhydantoin gingival hyperplasia: Report of a case. Oral Surg Oral Med Oral Pathol 49:211–213, 1980.

Thomas D, et al. Tuberous sclerosis with gingival overgrowth. J Periodontol 63:713–717, 1992.

Tillman HH, De Caro F. Tuberous sclerosis. Oral Surg Oral Med Oral Pathol 71:301–302, 1991.

Multiple Hamartoma Syndrome

Albrecht S, et al. Cowden syndrome and Lhermitte-Duclos disease. Cancer 70:869–876, 1992.

Bagan JV, Penarrocha M, Vera-Sempere F. Cowden syndrome: Clinical and pathological considerations in two new cases. J Oral Maxillofac Surg 47:291–294, 1989.

Devlin MF, Barrie R, Ward-Booth RP. Cowden's disease: A rare but important manifestation of oral papillomatosis. Br J Oral Maxillofac Surg 30:335–336, 1992.

Poole S, Fenske NA. Cutaneous markers of internal malignancy, I: Malignant involvement of the skin and the genodermatoses. J Am Acad Dermatol 28:1–13, 1993.

Shapiro SD, Lambert WC, Schwartz RA. Cowden's disease: A marker for malignancy. Int J Dermatol 27:232–237, 1988.

Swart JGN, Lekkas C, Allard RHB. Oral manifestations in Cowden's syndrome. Oral Surg Oral Med Oral Pathol 59:264–268, 1985.

Takenoshita Y, et al. Oral and facial lesions in Cowden's disease: Report of two cases and a review of the literature. J Oral Maxillofac Surg 51:682–687, 1993.

Williard W, et al. Cowden's disease: A case report with analyses at the molecular level. Cancer 69:2969–2974, 1992.

Epidermolysis Bullosa

Fine J-D, et al. Revised clinical and laboratory criteria for subtypes of inherited epidermolysis bullosa. J Am Acad Dermatol 24:119–135, 1991.

Haber RM, et al. Hereditary epidermolysis bullosa. J Am Acad Dermatol 13:252–278, 1985.

Hochberg MS, Vazquez-Santiago IA, Sher M. Epidermolysis bullosa: A case report. Oral Surg Oral Med Oral Pathol 75:54–57, 1993.

Kero M, Niemi K-M. Epidermolysis bullosa. Int J Dermatol 25:75–82, 1986.

Lin AN, Carter DM. Epidermolysis bullosa. Annu Rev Med 44:189–199, 1993.

McGrath JA, et al. Mitten deformity in severe generalized recessive dystrophic epidermolysis bullosa: Histological, immunofluorescence, and ultrastructural study. J Cutan Pathol 19:385–389, 1992.

McGrath JA, et al. Structural variations in anchoring fibrils in dystrophic epidermolysis bullosa: Correlation with Type VII collagen expression. J Invest Dermatol 100:366–372, 1993.

Nowak AJ. Oropharyngeal lesions and their management in epidermolysis bullosa. Arch Dermatol 124:724–745, 1988.

Pearson RW. Clinicopathologic types of epidermolysis bullosa and their nondermatological complications. Arch Dermatol 124:718–725, 1988.

Schaffer SR. Head and neck manifestations of epidermolysis bullosa. Clin Pediatr (Phila) 31:81–88, 1992.

Uitto J, Christiano AM. Inherited epidermolysis bullosa: Clinical features, molecular genetics, and pathoetiologic mechanisms. Dermatol Clin 11:549–563, 1993.

Wright JT. Comprehensive dental care and general anesthetic management of hereditary epidermolysis bullosa: A review of fourteen cases. Oral Surg Oral Med Oral Pathol 70:573–578, 1990.

Wright JT, Fine J-D, Johnson LB. Oral soft tissues in hereditary epidermolysis bullosa. Oral Surg Oral Med Oral Pathol 71:440–446, 1991.

Pemphigus

Becker BA, Gaspari AA. Pemphigus vulgaris and vegetans. Dermatol Clin 11:429–452, 1993.

Calvanico NJ, Robledo MA, Diaz LA. Immunopathology of pemphigus. J Autoimmun 4:3–16, 1991.

Eisenberg E, et al. Pemphigus-like mucosal lesions: A side effect of penicillamine therapy. Oral Surg Oral Med Oral Pathol 51:409–414, 1981.

Korman NJ. Pemphigus. Dermatol Clin 8:689–700, 1990.

Korman NJ. Pemphigus. J Am Acad Dermatol 18:1219–1238, 1988.

Lamey P-J, et al. Oral presentation of pemphigus vulgaris and its response to systemic steroid therapy. Oral Surg Oral Med Oral Pathol 74:54–57, 1992.

Laskaris G, Stoufi E. Oral pemphigus vulgaris in a 6-year-old girl. Oral Surg Oral Med Oral Pathol 69:609–613, 1990.

Mutasim DF, Pelc NJ, Anhalt GJ. Drug-induced pemphigus. Dermatol Clin 11:463–471, 1993.

Paterson AJ, et al. Pemphigus vulgaris precipitated by glibenclamide therapy. J Oral Pathol Med 22:92–95, 1993.

Ruocco V, Sacerdoti G. Pemphigus and bullous pemphigoid due to drugs. Int J Dermatol 30:307–312, 1991.

Stanley JR. Cell adhesion molecules as targets of autoantibodies in pemphigus and pemphigoid, bullous diseases due to defective epidermal cell adhesion. Adv Immunol 53:291–325, 1993.

Paraneoplastic Pemphigus

Anhalt GJ, et al. Paraneoplastic pemphigus: An autoimmune mucocutaneous disease associated with neoplasia. N Engl J Med 323:1729–1735, 1990.

Camisa C, Helm TN. Paraneoplastic pemphigus is a distinct neoplasia-induced autoimmune disease. Arch Dermatol 129:883–886, 1993.

Camisa C, et al. Paraneoplastic pemphigus: A report of three cases including one long-term survivor. J Am Acad Dermatol 27:547–553, 1992.

Helm TN, et al. Paraneoplastic pemphigus: A distinct autoimmune vesiculobullous disorder associated with neoplasia. Oral Surg Oral Med Oral Pathol 75:209–213, 1993.

Horn TD, Anhalt GJ. Histologic features of paraneoplastic pemphigus. Arch Dermatol 128:1091–1095, 1992.

Liu AY, et al. Indirect immunofluorescence on rat bladder transitional epithelium: A test with high specificity for paraneoplastic pemphigus. J Am Acad Dermatol 28:696–699, 1993.

Meyers SJ, et al. Conjunctival involvement in paraneoplastic pemphigus. Am J Ophthalmol 114:621–624, 1992.

Mutasim DF, Pelc NJ, Anhalt GJ. Paraneoplastic pemphigus. Dermatol Clin 11:473–481, 1993.

Rybojad M, et al. Paraneoplastic pemphigus in a child with a T-cell lymphoblastic lymphoma. Br J Dermatol 128:418–422, 1993.

Cicatricial Pemphigoid

Ahmed AR, Kurgis BS, Rogers RS. Cicatricial pemphigoid. J Am Acad Dermatol 24:987–1001, 1991.

Camisa C, Meisler DM. Immunobullous diseases with ocular involvement. Dermatol Clin 10:555–570, 1992.

Chan LS, et al. Immune-mediated subepithelial blistering diseases of mucous membranes. Arch Dermatol 129:448–455, 1993.

Fern AI, et al. Dapsone therapy for the acute inflammatory phase of ocular pemphigoid. Br J Ophthalmol 76:332–335, 1992.

Gammon WR. Epidermolysis bullosa acquisita: A disease of autoimmunity to type VII collagen. J Autoimmun 4:59–71, 1991.

Hanson RD, Olsen KD, Rogers RS. Upper aerodigestive tract manifestations of cicatricial pemphigoid. Ann Otol Rhinol Laryngol 97:493–499, 1988.

Lamey P-J, et al. Mucous membrane pemphigoid: Treatment experience at two institutions. Oral Surg Oral Med Oral Pathol 74:50–53, 1992.

Laskaris G, Angelopoulos A. Cicatricial pemphigoid: Direct and indirect immunofluorescent studies. Oral Surg Oral Med Oral Pathol 51:48–54, 1981.

Matsumura Y, et al. Epidermolysis bullosa acquisita (EBA) with nonclassical distribution of eruptions. J Dermatol 20:159–163, 1993.

Mondino BJ. Cicatricial pemphigoid and erythema multiforme. Ophthalmology 97:939–952, 1990.

Mutasim DF, Pelc NJ, Anhalt GJ. Cicatricial pemphigoid. Dermatol Clin 11:499–510, 1993.

Niimi Y, Zhu X-J, Bystryn J-C. Identification of cicatricial pemphigoid antigens. Arch Dermatol 128:54–57, 1992.

Siegel MA, Anhalt GJ. Direct immunofluorescence of detached gingival epithelium for diagnosis of cicatricial pemphigoid: Report of five cases. Oral Surg Oral Med Oral Pathol 75:296–302, 1993.

Thuong-Nguyen V, et al. Inhibition of neutrophil adherence to antibody by dapsone: A possible therapeutic mechanism of dapsone in the treatment of IgA dermatoses. J Invest Dermatol 100:349–355, 1993.

Vincent SD, Lilly GE, Baker KA. Clinical, historic, and therapeutic features of cicatricial pemphigoid: A literature review and open therapeutic trial with corticosteroids. Oral Surg Oral Med Oral Pathol 76:453–459, 1993.

Williams DM, et al. Benign mucous membrane (cicatricial) pemphigoid revisited: A clinical and immunological reappraisal. Br Dent J 157:313–316, 1984.

Bullous Pemphigoid

Anhalt GJ. Pemphigoid: Bullous and cicatricial. Dermatol Clin 8:701–716, 1990.

Anhalt GJ, Morrison LH. Bullous and cicatricial pemphigoid. J Autoimmun 4:17–35, 1991.

Korman NJ. Bullous pemphigoid. Dermatol Clin 11:483–498, 1993.

Vassileva S. Immunofluorescence in dermatology. Int J Dermatol 32:153–161, 1993.

Venning VA, et al. Mucosal involvement in bullous and cicatricial pemphigoid: A clinical and immunopathological study. Br J Dermatol 118:7–15, 1988.

Williams DM. Vesiculo-bullous mucocutaneous disease: Benign mucous membrane and bullous pemphigoid. J Oral Pathol Med 19:16–23, 1990.

Erythema Multiforme

Aslanzadeh J, et al. Detection of HSV-specific DNA in biopsy tissue of patients with erythema multiforme by polymerase chain reaction. Br J Dermatol 126:19–23, 1992.

Barone CM, et al. Treatment of toxic epidermal necrolysis and Stevens-Johnson syndrome in children. J Oral Maxillofac Surg 51:264–268, 1993.

Bastuji-Garin S, et al. Clinical classification of cases of toxic epidermal necrolysis, Stevens-Johnson syndrome, and erythema multiforme. Arch Dermatol 129:92–96, 1993.

Hurwitz S. Erythema multiforme: A review of its characteristics, diagnostic criteria, and management. Pediatr Rev 11:217–222, 1990.

Lozada-Nur F, Cram D, Gorsky M. Clinical response to levamisole in thirty-nine patients with erythema multiforme: An open prospective study. Oral Surg Oral Med Oral Pathol 74:294–298, 1992.

Lyell A. Toxic epidermal necrolysis: An eruption resembling scalding of the skin. Br J Dermatol 68:355–361, 1956.

Parsons JM. Toxic epidermal necrolysis. Int J Dermatol 31:749–768, 1992.

Roujeau J-C, et al. Toxic epidermal necrolysis (Lyell syndrome). J Am Acad Dermatol 23:1039–1058, 1990.

Schofield JK, Tatnall FM, Leigh IM. Recurrent erythema multiforme: Clinical features and treatment in a large series of patients. Br J Dermatol 128:542–545, 1993.

Schopf E, et al. Toxic epidermal necrolysis and Stevens-Johnson syndrome: An epidemiologic study from West Germany. Arch Dermatol 127:839–842, 1991.

Stampien TM, Schwartz RA. Erythema multiforme. Am Fam Physician 46:1171–1176, 1992.

Wilkins J, Morrison L, White CR. Oculocutaneous manifestations of the erythema multiforme/Stevens-Johnson syndrome/toxic epidermal necrolysis spectrum. Dermatol Clin 10:571–582, 1992.

Erythema Migrans

Espelid M, et al. Geographic stomatitis: Report of 6 cases. J Oral Pathol Med 20:425–428, 1991.

Gibson J, et al. Geographic tongue: The clinical response to zinc supplementation. J Trace Elem Exp Med 3:203–208, 1990.

Marks R, Radden BG. Geographic tongue: A clinico-pathological review. Australas J Dermatol 22:75–79, 1981.

Sigal MJ, Mock D. Symptomatic benign migratory glossitis: Report of two cases and literature review. Pediatr Dent 14:392–396, 1992.

Waltimo J. Geographic tongue during a year of oral contraceptive cycles. Br Dent J 171:94–96, 1991.

Reiter's Syndrome

Edwards L, Hansen RC. Reiter's syndrome of the vulva. Arch Dermatol 128:811–814, 1992.

Keat A, Rowe I. Reiter's syndrome and associated arthritides. Rheum Dis Clin North Am 17:25–42, 1991.

Rothe MJ, Kerdel FA. Reiter syndrome. Int J Dermatol 30:173–180, 1991.

Lichen Planus

Beutner EH, et al. Ten cases of chronic ulcerative stomatitis with stratified epithelium-specific antinuclear antibody. J Am Acad Dermatol 24:781–782, 1991.

Borghelli RF, et al. Oral lichen planus in patients with diabetes: An epidemiologic study. Oral Surg Oral Med Oral Pathol 75:498–500, 1993.

Boyd AS, Nelder KH. Lichen planus. J Am Acad Dermatol 25:593–619, 1991.

Brown RS, et al. A retrospective evaluation of 193 patients with oral lichen planus. J Oral Pathol Med 22:69–72, 1993.

Camisa C. Lichen planus and related conditions. Adv Dermatol 2:47–70, 1987.

Eisen D. The therapy of oral lichen planus. Crit Rev Oral Biol Med 4:141–158, 1993.

Eisenberg E. Lichen planus and oral cancer: Is there a connection between the two? J Am Dent Assoc 123:104–108, 1992.

Firth NA, et al. Assessment of the value of immunofluorescence microscopy in the diagnosis of oral mucosal lichen planus. J Oral Pathol Med 19:295–297, 1990.

Halevy S, Shai A. Lichenoid drug eruptions. J Am Acad Dermatol 29:249–255, 1993.

Holmstrup P, et al. Malignant development of lichen planus-affected oral mucosa. J Oral Pathol 17:219–225, 1988.

Jaremko WM, et al. Chronic ulcerative stomatitis associated with a specific immunologic marker. J Am Acad Dermatol 22:215–220, 1990.

Jungell P. Oral lichen planus: A review. Int J Oral Maxillofac Surg 20:129–135, 1991.

Scully C, El-Kom M. Lichen planus: Review and update on pathogenesis. J Oral Pathol 14:431–458, 1985.

Silverman S. Lichen planus. Curr Opin Dent 1:769–772, 1991.

Silverman S, et al. A prospective study of findings and management in 214 patients with oral lichen planus. Oral Surg Oral Med Oral Pathol 72:665–670, 1991.

Thorn JJ, et al. Course of various clinical forms of oral lichen planus: A prospective follow-up study of 611 patients. J Oral Pathol 17:213–218, 1988.

Voute ABE, et al. Possible premalignant character of oral lichen planus. J Oral Pathol Med 21:326–329, 1992.

Voute ABE, et al. Fluocinonide in an adhesive base for treatment of oral lichen planus: A double-blind, placebo-controlled clinical study. Oral Surg Oral Med Oral Pathol 75:181–185, 1993.

Walsh LJ, et al. Immunopathogenesis of oral lichen planus. J Oral Pathol Med 19:389–396, 1990.

Graft-versus-Host Disease

Barrett AP, Bilous AM. Oral patterns of acute and chronic graft-v-host disease. Arch Dermatol 120:1461–1465, 1984.

Carl W, Higby DJ. Oral manifestations of bone marrow transplantation. Am J Clin Oncol 8:81–87, 1985.

Chao NJ, et al. Cyclosporine, methotrexate, and prednisone compared with cyclosporine and prednisone for prophylaxis of acute graft-versus-host disease. N Engl J Med 329:1225–1230, 1993.

Chosidow O, et al. Sclerodermatous chronic graft-versus-host disease. J Am Acad Dermatol 26:49–55, 1992.

Jampel RCM, et al. PUVA therapy for chronic cutaneous graft-vs-host disease. Arch Dermatol 127:1673–1678, 1991.

Kernan NA, et al. Analysis of 462 transplantations from unrelated donors facilitated by the National Marrow Donor Program. N Engl J Med 328:593–602, 1993.

Rodu B, Gockerman JP. Oral manifestations of the chronic graft-v-host reaction. JAMA 249:504–507, 1983.

Schubert MM, et al. Oral manifestations of chronic graft-v-host disease. Arch Intern Med 144:1591–1595, 1984.

Schubert MM, Sullivan KM. Recognition, incidence and management of oral graft-versus-host disease. NCI Monogr 9:135–143, 1990.

Schubert MM, et al. Clinical assessment scale for the rating of oral mucosal changes associated with bone marrow transplantation: Development of an oral mucositis index. Cancer 69:2469–2477, 1992.

Tanaka K, et al. A clinical review: Cutaneous manifestations of acute and chronic graft-versus-host disease following bone marrow transplantation. J Dermatol 18:11–17, 1991.

Vogelsang GB. Acute and chronic graft-versus-host disease. Curr Opin Oncol 5:276–281, 1993.

Woo S-B, et al. A longitudinal study of oral ulcerative mucositis in bone marrow transplant recipients. Cancer 72:1612–1617, 1993.

Psoriasis

Bhate SM, et al. Prevalence of skin and other cancers in patients with psoriasis. Clin Exp Dermatol 18:401–404, 1993.

Duffy DL, Spelman LS, Martin NG. Psoriasis in Australian twins. J Am Acad Dermatol 29:428–434, 1993.

Eastman JR, Goldblatt LI. Psoriasis: Palatal manifestations and physiologic considerations. J Periodontol 54:736–739, 1983.

Khandke L, et al. Cyclosporine in psoriasis treatment. Arch Dermatol 127:1172–1179, 1991.

Morris LF, et al. Oral lesions in patients with psoriasis: A controlled study. Cutis 49:339–344, 1992.

Sklavounou A, Laskaris G. Oral psoriasis: Report of a case and review of the literature. Dermatologica 180:157–159, 1990.

Stern RS, Laird N. The carcinogenic risk of treatments for severe psoriasis. Cancer 73:2759–2764, 1994.

Yamada J, Amar S, Petrungaro P. Psoriasis-associated periodontitis: A case report. J Periodontol 63:854–857, 1992.

Lupus Erythematosus

Burge SM, et al. Mucosal involvement in systemic and chronic cutaneous lupus erythematosus. Br J Dermatol 121:727–741, 1989.

Callen JP. Mucocutaneous changes in patients with lupus erythematosus: The relationship of these lesions to systemic disease. Rheum Dis Clin North Am 14:79–97, 1988.

Cervera R, et al. Systemic lupus erythematosus: Clinical and immunologic patterns of disease expression in a cohort of 1,000 patients. Medicine (Baltimore) 72:113–124, 1993.

David-Bajar KM, et al. Clinical, histologic, and immunofluorescent distinctions between subacute cutaneous lupus erythematosus and discoid lupus erythematosus. J Invest Dermatol 99:251–257, 1992.

Lahita RG. Overview of lupus erythematosus. Clin Dermatol 10:389–392, 1993.

Rhodus NL, Johnson DK. The prevalence of oral manifestations of systemic lupus erythematosus. Quintessence Int 21:461–465, 1990.

Steinberg AD, Klinman DM. Pathogenesis of systemic lupus erythematosus. Rheum Dis Clin North Am 14:25–41, 1988.

Velthuis PJ, et al. Direct immunofluorescence patterns in clinically healthy skin of patients with collagen diseases. Clin Dermatol 10:423–430, 1993.

Systemic Sclerosis

Asboe-Hansen G. Scleroderma. J Am Acad Dermatol 17:102–108, 1987.

Black CM. The aetiopathogenesis of systemic sclerosis. J Intern Med 234:3–8, 1993.

Clements P. Clinical aspects of localized and systemic sclerosis. Curr Opin Rheumatol 4:843–850, 1992.

Eversole LR, Jacobsen PL, Stone CE. Oral and gingival changes in systemic sclerosis (scleroderma). J Periodontol 55:175–178, 1984.

Jablonska S, et al. Clinical relevance of immunologic findings in scleroderma. Clin Dermatol 10:407–421, 1993.

Marmary Y, Glaiss R, Pisanty S. Scleroderma: Oral manifestations. Oral Surg Oral Med Oral Pathol 52:32–37, 1981.

Müller-Ladner U, Benning K, Lang B. Current therapy of systemic sclerosis (scleroderma). Clin Investig 71:257–263, 1993.

Naylor WP. Oral management of the scleroderma patient. J Am Dent Assoc 105:814–817, 1982.

Perez MI, Kohn SR. Systemic sclerosis. J Am Acad Dermatol 28:525–547, 1993.

Rook AH, et al. Treatment of systemic sclerosis with extracorporeal photochemotherapy: Results of a multicenter trial. Arch Dermatol 128:337–346, 1992.

Steen VD, Medsger TA. Epidemiology and natural history of systemic sclerosis. Rheum Dis Clin North Am 16:1–10, 1990.

Wigley FM. Treatment of systemic sclerosis. Curr Opin Rheumatol 4:878–886, 1992.

CREST Syndrome

Paley M, McLoughlin P. Oral problems associated with CREST syndrome: A case report. Br Dent J 175:295–296, 1993.

Ueda M, et al. Prominent telangiectasia associated with marked bleeding in CREST syndrome. J Dermatol 20:180–184, 1993.

Acanthosis Nigricans

Flier JS. Metabolic importance of acanthosis nigricans. Arch Dermatol 121:193–194, 1985.

Hall JM, et al. Oral acanthosis nigricans: Report of a case and comparison of oral and cutaneous pathology. Am J Dermatopathol 10:68–73, 1988.

Mostofi RS, Hayden NP, Soltani K. Oral malignant acanthosis nigricans. Oral Surg Oral Med Oral Pathol 56:372–374, 1983.

Rogers DL. Acanthosis nigricans. Semin Dermatol 10:160–163, 1991.

Schwartz RA. Acanthosis nigricans. J Am Acad Dermatol 31:1–19, 1994.

Tasjian D, Jarratt M. Familial acanthosis nigricans. Arch Dermatol 120:1351–1354, 1984.

17

Oral Manifestations of Systemic Disease

MUCOPOLYSACCHARIDOSIS

The **mucopolysaccharidoses** are a heterogeneous group of metabolic disorders that are usually inherited in an autosomal recessive fashion. These disorders are all characterized by the lack of any one of several normal enzymes needed to process the important intercellular substances known as glycosaminoglycans. These materials used to be known as mucopolysaccharides, thus the term mucopolysaccharidosis. Examples of glycosaminoglycans include:

- Heparan sulfate
- Dermatan sulfate
- Keratan sulfate
- Chondroitin sulfate

The type of mucopolysaccharidosis that is seen clinically depends on which of these substrates lacks its particular enzyme.

Clinical and Radiographic Features

The clinical features of the mucopolysaccharidoses vary, depending on the particular syndrome that is examined (Table 17–1). Furthermore, affected patients with a particular type of this disorder often exhibit a wide range of severity of involvement. Most types of mucopolysaccharidoses display some degree of mental retardation. Often, the facial features of affected patients are somewhat coarse, with heavy brow ridges (Fig. 17–1), and there are other skeletal changes, such as stiff joints. Cloudy degeneration of the corneas, a problem that frequently leads to blindness, is seen in several forms of mucopolysaccharidosis.

The oral manifestations vary according to the particular type of mucopolysaccharidosis. Most types show some degree of macroglossia. Gingival hyperplasia may be present, particularly in the anterior regions, as a result of the drying and irritating effects of mouth breathing. The dental changes include thin enamel with pointed cusps on the posterior teeth, although this seems to be a feature unique to mucopolysaccharidosis type IV-A. Other dental manifestations include numerous impacted teeth with prominent follicular spaces (Fig. 17–2), possibly caused by the accumulation of glycosaminoglycans in the follicular connective tissue. Some investigators have reported the occurrence of multiple impacted teeth that are congregated in a single large follicle, forming a rosette-like pattern radiographically.

Treatment and Prognosis

There is no satisfactory systemic treatment of the mucopolysaccharidoses at this time, although the possibility of enzyme replacement has generated a great deal of interest. This could be accomplished either by infusing the missing enzyme itself or by introducing genetically corrected host cells or transplanted normal cells into the affected patient. Limited success has been achieved with allogeneic bone marrow transplantation in humans.

Management of the dental problems of these patients

Table 17–1. FEATURES OF SELECTED MUCOPOLYSACCHARIDOSIS SYNDROMES

Type	Eponym	Inheritance	Enzyme Deficiency	Stored Substrate	Clinical Features
I-H	Hurler	AR	Alpha-L-iduronidase	HS and DS	Presents in infancy, cloudy corneas, growth retardation, reduced intelligence, coronary artery disease, rarely live 10 years
I-S	Scheie	AR	Alpha-L-iduronidase	HS and DS	Onset in late childhood, cloudy corneas, normal intelligence, aortic regurgitation, survive to adulthood
II	Hunter	X-linked R	Iduronate-2-sulfatase	HS and DS	Presents at 1–2 years of age, clear corneas, reduced intelligence, growth retardation, stiff joints
III-A	Sanfilippo-A	AR	Sulfamidase	HS	Presents at 4–6 years of age, clear corneas, reduced intelligence, mild skeletal changes, death in adolescence
III-B	Sanfilippo-B	AR	Alpha-N-acetylglucosaminidase	HS	Generally same as Sanfilippo A
IV-A	Morquio-A	AR	Galactose-6-sulfatase	KS, CS, GalNAc6S	Presents at 1–2 years of age, cloudy corneas, normal intelligence, lax joints, may survive to middle age
IV-B	Morquio-B	AR	Beta-D-galactosidase	KS	Generally similar to Morquio A
VI	Maroteaux-Lamy	AR	N-acetylgalactos-amine-4-sulfatase	DS, CS, GalNAc4S, GalNAc4, 6diS	Presents at 2–6 years of age, cloudy corneas, normal intelligence, growth retardation, stiff joints, may survive to adulthood

AR, autosomal recessive; DS, dermatan sulfate; KS, keratan sulfate; CS, chondroitin sulfate; HS, heparan sulfate; GalNAc, N-acetylgalactosamine; S, sulfate; diS, disulfate.

is essentially no different than that of any other patient. Several factors may have to be taken into account, however, such as:

- The degree of mental retardation (if any)
- The presence or absence of a seizure disorder
- The degree of joint stiffening
- The extent of other related medical problems

Depending on which of these factors is present and the extent of involvement, dental care may warrant sedation, hospitalization, or general anesthesia of the patient for optimal results.

LIPID RETICULOENDOTHELIOSES

The **lipid reticuloendothelioses** are a relatively rare group of inherited disorders. These include the conditions known as:

- Gaucher disease
- Niemann-Pick disease
- Tay-Sachs disease

These conditions are seen with increased frequency in patients with Ashkenazi Jewish heritage. Affected patients lack certain enzymes necessary for processing specific lipids, and this results in an accumulation of the lipids within a variety of cells. Because of this accumulation, it appears that cells may be attempting to store these substances; therefore, the term "storage disease" has been commonly used for these disorders.

In **Gaucher disease** (the most common of the reticuloendothelioses), a lack of glucocerebrosidase results in the accumulation of glucosylceramide, particularly within the lysosomes of cells of the macrophage/monocyte lineage.

Niemann-Pick disease is characterized by a deficiency of acid sphingomyelinase, resulting in the accumulation of sphingomyelin, also within the lysosomes of macrophages.

Tay-Sachs disease is caused by a lack of hexosaminidase A, which results in the accumulation of a ganglioside, principally within the lysosomes of neurons.

All these disorders are inherited as autosomal recessive traits. When the genetic mutation known to cause Gaucher disease was evaluated for the Ashkenazi Jewish population, a gene frequency of 0.032 was found. Most of the persons identified as having the gene, however, were heterozygous and, therefore, asymptomatic.

Clinical and Radiographic Features

Gaucher Disease

The clinical features of Gaucher disease are generally due to the effects of the abnormal storage of glucosylcer-

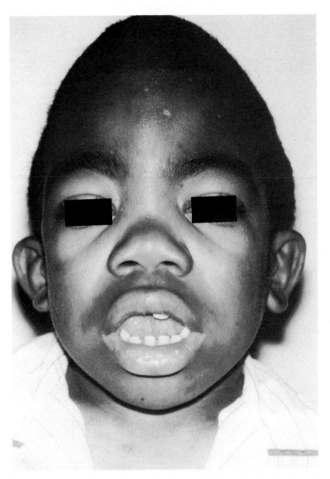

FIGURE 17–1. **Mucopolysaccharidosis**. This patient, affected by Hunter's syndrome, exhibits the characteristic facial features of this disorder.

amide. Macrophages laden with this glucocerebroside are typically rendered relatively nonfunctional, and they tend to accumulate within the bone marrow of the affected patient. This accumulation displaces the normal hematopoietic cells and produces anemia and thrombocytopenia. In addition, these patients are susceptible to bone infarctions. The resulting bone pain is often the presenting complaint. Characteristic "Erlenmeyer flask" deformities of the long bones, particularly of the femur, are often identified. Accumulations of the macrophages in the spleen and liver result in visceral enlargement. Many affected patients show a significant degree of growth retardation. Neurologic deterioration may also occur in a few patients. Jaw lesions typically present as ill-defined radiolucencies that usually affect the mandible without causing devitalization of the teeth or resorption of the lamina dura.

Niemann-Pick Disease

Niemann-Pick disease occurs as several different types, each associated with a different clinical expression and prognosis. Generally, two subgroups are identified: the neuronopathic and the visceral.

The *neuronopathic* type is characterized by psychomotor retardation, dementia, spasticity, hepatosplenomegaly, and death during the first or second decade of life. The *visceral* type is primarily characterized by hepatosplenomegaly, sometimes with pulmonary involvement, but patients normally survive into adulthood.

Tay-Sachs Disease

Tay-Sachs disease may have a wide clinical range because the condition is genetically heterogeneous. Some forms are mild, with patients surviving into adulthood.

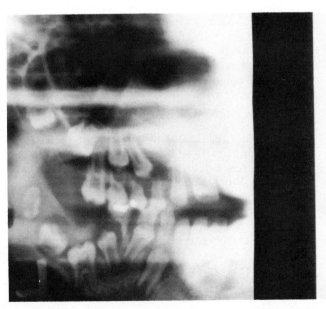
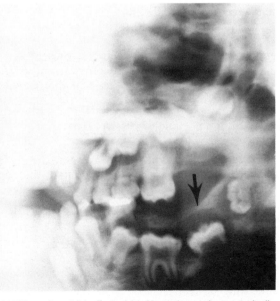

FIGURE 17–2. **Mucopolysaccharidosis**. Radiographic examination of the dentition of a child affected by Hunter's syndrome typically shows radiolucencies (*arrow*) associated with the crowns of unerupted teeth.

In the severe infantile form, however, rapidly progressive neuronal degeneration develops shortly after birth. Signs and symptoms include blindness, developmental retardation, and intractable seizures. Death usually occurs by 3 to 5 years of age.

Histopathologic Features

Histopathologic examination of an osseous lesion of Gaucher disease shows sheets of macrophages exhibiting abundant bluish cytoplasm, which has a fine texture resembling "wrinkled silk." In Niemann-Pick disease, the characteristic cell seen on examination of a bone marrow aspirate is the "sea-blue" histiocyte.

Treatment and Prognosis

Gaucher Disease

For patients with a mild expression of Gaucher disease, no treatment may be necessary. Recent reports have shown some success with enzyme replacement therapy when a macrophage-targeted glucocerebrosidase was used. After 9 to 12 months of therapy, patients tend to exhibit improvement in the status of their anemia, a decrease in plasma glucocerebroside levels, a decrease in hepatosplenomegaly, and perhaps slight resolution of the radiographic changes. Children treated with this regimen may show significant gain in height. Bone marrow transplantation has also been attempted; however, the problems inherent in graft-versus-host disease are still present with that form of therapy. A case-control study showed that adults with Gaucher disease have an increased risk for hematologic malignancies, particularly lymphoma and multiple myeloma.

Niemann-Pick and Tay-Sachs Disease

Niemann-Pick disease and the infantile form of Tay-Sachs disease are associated with a poor prognosis. Genetic counseling should be provided for affected families. Molecular markers of these disorders have been developed to identify carriers. Such identification allows earlier intervention in terms of counseling.

LIPOID PROTEINOSIS (Hyalinosis Cutis et Mucosae; Urbach-Wiethe Syndrome)

A rare condition, **lipoid proteinosis** is inherited as an autosomal recessive trait. It is characterized by the deposition of a waxy material in the dermis and submucosal connective tissue of affected patients. Lipoid proteinosis was originally described in 1929, and more than 300 patients, most of whom are of European background, have been reported to date. The precise nature of the biochemical defect associated with this disease is still controversial and essentially unknown, although some investigators claim that it is a lysosomal storage disease.

Clinical Features

The laryngeal mucosa and vocal cords are usually the sites that are initially affected by lipoid proteinosis. Therefore, the first sign of the disease may be:

- An inability of the infant to make a crying sound
- A hoarse cry in infancy
- The development of a hoarse voice during early childhood

The vocal cords become thickened as the accumulation of an amorphous material begins to affect the laryngeal mucosa. This infiltrative mucosal process may also involve the pharynx, esophagus, tonsils, vulva, and rectum. Skin lesions also develop early in life, appearing as thickened, yellowish, waxy areas that often affect the face, particularly the lips and the margins of the eyelids. Some lesions may begin as dark-crusted vesicles, which heal as atrophic hyperpigmented patches.

Eventually, most patients exhibit a thickened, furrowed appearance of the skin. Other areas of the skin that may be involved include the neck, palms, axillae, elbows, scrotum, knees, and digits. In those areas subjected to chronic trauma, a hyperkeratotic, verrucous surface often develops. In addition to the cutaneous manifestations, intracranial calcifications have been identified in approximately 70 percent of affected patients. These lesions are usually asymptomatic, although a few patients have been reported to have a seizure disorder.

The oral mucosal abnormalities typically become evident in the second decade of life. The tongue, labial mucosa, and buccal mucosa become nodular, diffusely enlarged, and thickened because of infiltration with waxy, yellow-white plaques and nodules. The dorsal tongue papillae are eventually destroyed, and the tongue develops a smooth surface. The accumulation of the amorphous material within the tongue may result in its being bound to the floor of the mouth. Therefore, the patient may not be able to protrude the tongue.

Histopathologic Features

A biopsy specimen of an early lesion of lipoid proteinosis typically reveals the deposition of a lamellar material around the blood vessels, nerves, hair follicles, and sweat glands. This material stains positively with the periodic acid–Schiff method and is not digested by diastase. The location of this material and its staining properties suggest a basement membrane origin.

Biopsy specimens of a lesion in its later stages usually show not only the lamellar material but also deposition of an amorphous substance within the dermal connective tissue (Fig. 17–3).

Treatment and Prognosis

Generally, no specific treatment is available for lipoid proteinosis other than genetic counseling. In rare instances, the infiltration of the laryngeal mucosa may produce difficult breathing for some infants, in which case debulking of the mucosal lesions may be necessary. Most patients with lipoid proteinosis have a normal life span. Certainly, however, the vocal hoarseness and the appearance of the skin may influence the quality of life for affected patients.

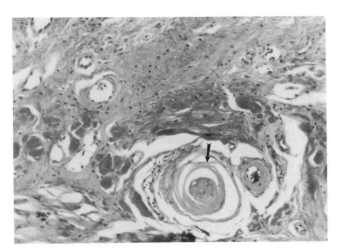

FIGURE 17–3. **Lipoid proteinosis**. This medium-power photomicrograph shows the deposition of a lamellar, acellular material (*arrow*).

JAUNDICE (Icterus)

Jaundice is a condition characterized by excess bilirubin in the blood stream. The bilirubin accumulates in the tissues, which results in a yellowish discoloration of the skin and mucosa. To understand jaundice, it is important to know something about the metabolism of bilirubin. Most bilirubin is derived from the breakdown of hemoglobin, the oxygen-carrying pigment of erythrocytes. The average life span of an erythrocyte in the circulation is 120 days. After this time, it undergoes physiologic breakdown. The hemoglobin is degraded and processed by the cells of the reticuloendothelial system, and bilirubin is liberated into the blood stream in an unconjugated state. In the liver, bilirubin is taken up by the hepatocytes and conjugated with glucuronic acid, which produces conjugated bilirubin, a soluble product that can be excreted in the bile.

There are numerous causes for increased serum levels of bilirubin; some are physiologic, and many are pathologic. Therefore, the presence of jaundice is not a specific sign and generally necessitates physical examination and laboratory studies to determine the precise cause. The basic disturbances associated with increased bilirubin levels include an increased production of bilirubin. This occurs when the red blood cells are being broken down at such a rapid rate that the liver cannot keep pace with processing. This breakdown is seen in such conditions as **autoimmune hemolytic anemia** or **sickle cell anemia**.

In addition, the liver may not be functioning correctly, resulting in decreased uptake of the bilirubin from the circulation or decreased conjugation of bilirubin in the liver cells. Jaundice is frequently present at birth as a result of the low level of activity of the enzyme system that conjugates bilirubin. Defects in this enzyme system may also be seen with certain inherited problems. Because most of these examples of jaundice occur with impaired processing of bilirubin, laboratory studies usually show unconjugated bilirubin in the serum.

The presence of conjugated bilirubinemia in jaundice can usually be explained by the reduced excretion of bilirubin into the bile ducts. This can be due to swelling of the hepatocytes (resulting in an occlusion of the bile canaliculi) or hepatocyte necrosis with disruption of the bile canaliculi and liberation of conjugated bilirubin. Thus, liver function may be disturbed because of any one of a variety of infections (e.g., viruses) or toxins (e.g., alcohol). Occlusion of the bile duct from gallstones, stricture, or cancer can also force conjugated bilirubin into the blood stream.

Clinical Features

The patient affected by jaundice exhibits a diffuse, uniform, yellowish discoloration of the skin and mucosa. The color varies in intensity, depending on the serum level of bilirubin. The sclera of the eye is often the first site at which the yellow color is noted (Fig. 17–4; see Color Figure 112). The yellow discoloration caused by hypercarotenemia (caused by excess ingestion of carotene, a vitamin A precursor found in yellow vegetables and fruits) may be confused with jaundice, but the sclera is not involved in that condition.

Other signs and symptoms associated with jaundice vary with the underlying cause of the hyperbilirubinemia. For example, patients with viral hepatitis usually have a fever, abdominal pain, anorexia, and fatigue. The patient who presents with jaundice typically requires a complete medical evaluation to determine the precise cause of the condition so that proper therapy can be instituted.

Treatment and Prognosis

The treatment and prognosis of the patient with jaundice vary with the cause. The jaundice that is commonly noted at birth resolves spontaneously, although if the infant is placed under special lights the clearing will occur more quickly because conjugation of the bilirubin molecule is triggered by exposure to blue light. If the episode of jaundice is due to significant liver damage, as may be seen with viral hepatitis B or hepatotoxic chemi-

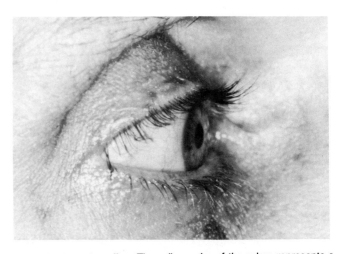

FIGURE 17–4. **Jaundice**. The yellow color of the sclera represents a common finding. See Color Plates.

cal injury, the prognosis will vary, depending on the extent of liver damage. The prognosis for patients with jaundice secondary to liver damage associated with metastatic malignancy is poor.

AMYLOIDOSIS

Amyloidosis represents a heterogeneous group of conditions characterized by the deposition of an extracellular proteinaceous material called *amyloid*. The term amyloid was coined by Virchow in the mid-19th century because he believed it to be a starch-like material (*amyl* = starch; *oid* = resembling).

Amyloidosis can produce a variety of effects, depending on the organ of involvement and the extent to which the amyloid is deposited. With limited cutaneous forms of amyloidosis, virtually no impact on survival is seen. With some forms of systemic amyloidosis, however, death may occur within a few years of the diagnosis as a result of cardiac or renal failure. Furthermore, the presence of amyloid may be associated with other problems, such as multiple myeloma or chronic infections. Although amyloid may have several sources, all types of amyloid have the common feature of a beta-pleated sheet molecular configuration, which is seen with x-ray diffraction crystallographic analysis. Because of this similarity of molecular structure, the different types of amyloid have similar staining patterns with special stains.

Clinical Features

Several classifications of amyloidosis have been proposed in the past decade, each evolving as our knowledge of this unusual condition increases. None of the classifications is completely satisfactory. In this discussion, we attempt to be as concise and direct as possible.

Essentially, amyloidosis may be divided into *organ-limited* and *systemic* forms.

Organ-Limited Amyloidosis

Although organ-limited amyloidosis may occur in a variety of organs, it has rarely been reported in the oral soft tissues. An example of a limited form of amyloidosis is the amyloid nodule, which appears as a solitary, otherwise asymptomatic, submucosal deposit. Most of the organ-limited forms of amyloidosis consist of aggregates of immunoglobulin light chains and are not associated with any systemic alteration.

Systemic Amyloidosis

Systemic amyloidosis may occur in several forms:

- Primary
- Myeloma-associated
- Secondary
- Hemodialysis-associated
- Heredofamilial

Primary and Myeloma-Associated Amyloidosis. The primary and myeloma-associated forms of amyloidosis usually affect older adults (average age 65 years), and a

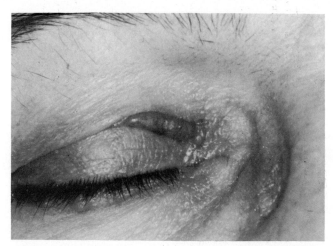

FIGURE 17–5. **Amyloidosis**. This patient exhibits a firm, waxy nodular lesion in the periocular region, a finding characteristic for this condition. See Color Plates.

slight male predilection is present. The initial signs and symptoms may be nonspecific, often resulting in a delayed diagnosis. Fatigue, weight loss, paresthesia, hoarseness, edema, and orthostatic hypotension are among the first indications of this disease process. Eventually, carpal tunnel syndrome, mucocutaneous lesions, hepatomegaly, and macroglossia develop as a result of the deposition of the amyloid protein. The skin lesions appear as smooth-surfaced, firm, waxy papules and plaques. These most commonly affect the eyelid region (Fig. 17–5; see Color Figure 113), the retroauricular region, the neck, and the lips. The lesions are often associated with petechiae and ecchymoses. Macroglossia has been reported in 12 to 40 percent of these patients and may appear as diffuse or nodular enlargement of the tongue (Fig. 17–6; see Color Figure 114). Sometimes oral amyloid nodules show ulceration and submucosal hemorrhage overlying the lesions. Infrequently, patients may complain of dry

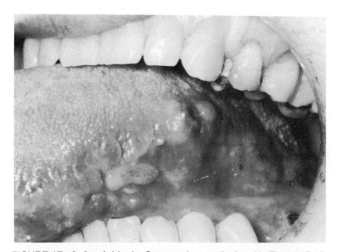

FIGURE 17–6. **Amyloidosis**. Same patient as depicted in Figure 17–5. Note amyloid nodules of lateral tongue, some of which are ulcerated. The patient's amyloidosis was due to previously undiagnosed multiple myeloma. See Color Plates.

eyes or dry mouth, which is secondary to amyloid infiltration and destruction of the lacrimal and salivary glands. When significant blood vessel infiltration has occurred, claudication of the jaw musculature may be noticed.

Secondary Amyloidosis. Secondary amyloidosis is so named because it characteristically develops as a result of a chronic inflammatory process, such as long-standing osteomyelitis, tuberculosis, or sarcoidosis. The heart is usually not affected as in other forms of amyloidosis. Liver, kidney, spleen, and adrenal involvement are typical, however.

Hemodialysis-Associated Amyloidosis. Patients who have undergone long-term renal dialysis also are susceptible to amyloidosis, although in this case the amyloid protein has been identified as beta-2 microglobulin. This normally occurring protein is not removed by the dialysis procedure, and it accumulates in the plasma. Eventually, it forms deposits, particularly in the bones and joints. Often, carpal tunnel syndrome as well as cervical spine pain and dysfunction occur. Tongue involvement has been reported.

Heredofamilial Amyloidosis. Heredofamilial amyloidosis is an uncommon but significant form of the disease. Several kindreds have been identified in Swedish, Portuguese, and Japanese populations, and most are inherited as autosomal dominant traits. An autosomal recessive form, known as **familial Mediterranean fever**, has also been described. Most of these conditions present as polyneuropathies, although other manifestations, such as cardiomyopathy, cardiac arrhythmias, congestive heart failure, and renal failure eventually develop as the amyloid deposition continues.

Histopathologic Features

Biopsy of rectal mucosa has classically been used to confirm a diagnosis of amyloidosis. Up to 80 percent of such biopsy specimens yield positive findings. Alternative tissue sources, however, are the gingiva and labial salivary gland. Histopathologic examination of gingival tissue that has been affected by amyloidosis shows extracellular deposition in the submucosal connective tissue of an amorphous, eosinophilic material, which may be arranged in a perivascular orientation or may be diffusely present throughout the tissue (Fig. 17–7). Labial salivary gland tissue shows deposition of amyloid in a periductal or perivascular location in more than 80 percent of the cases.

A standard means of identifying amyloid uses the dye Congo red, which displays an affinity for the abnormal protein. In tissue sections stained with Congo red, the amyloid appears red. When the tissue is viewed with polarized light, it exhibits an apple-green birefringence. Microscopic sections stained with crystal violet reveal a characteristic metachromasia; this normally purple dye appears more reddish when it reacts with amyloid. Staining with thioflavine T, a fluorescent dye, also gives positive results if amyloid is present. Ultrastructurally, amyloid is seen as a collection of 7.5- to 10-nm diameter, nonbranching, linear fibrils.

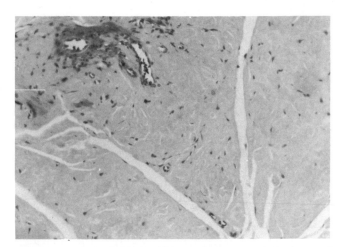

FIGURE 17–7. **Amyloidosis**. This medium-power photomicrograph shows the eosinophilic, acellular deposits that are characteristic of amyloid deposition.

Diagnosis

Once the histopathologic diagnosis of amyloidosis has been made, the patient must be evaluated medically to determine the type of amyloidosis that is present. This often entails a workup that includes serum electrophoresis to determine whether a monoclonal gammopathy exists so that multiple myeloma can be ruled out. Family history and physical examination findings are also important.

Treatment and Prognosis

In most instances, no effective therapy is available for amyloidosis. Selected forms of amyloidosis may respond to treatment, or at least their progression may be slowed, depending on the underlying cause. In cases of secondary amyloidosis associated with an infectious agent, treatment of the infection and reduction of the inflammation often result in clinical improvement. Renal transplantation may arrest the progression of the bone lesions in hemodialysis-associated amyloidosis, but this procedure apparently does not reverse the process. Familial Mediterranean fever may respond to systemic colchicine therapy. Treatment trials with colchicine, prednisone, and melphalan are being examined for their efficacy in managing other forms of amyloidosis, although in most instances the prognosis is guarded to poor. Most patients die of cardiac failure, arrhythmia, or renal disease within a few years after the diagnosis.

VITAMIN DEFICIENCY

In the United States today, significant vitamin deficiencies are not common. Patients with malabsorption syndromes or eating disorders, persons who follow fad diets, and alcoholics are the groups most commonly affected.

Vitamin A (retinol) is essential for the maintenance of

vision, and it also plays a role in growth and tissue differentiation. Vitamin A can be obtained directly from dietary sources, such as organ meats or milk, or the body can synthesize it from beta-carotene, which is abundant in red and yellow vegetables.

Vitamin B_1 (thiamin) acts as a coenzyme for several metabolic reactions and probably maintains the proper functioning of neurons. Thiamin is found in many animal and vegetable food sources.

Vitamin B_2 (riboflavin) is necessary for cellular oxidation-reduction reactions. Foods that contain significant amounts of riboflavin include milk, green vegetables, meat (especially liver), fish, and eggs.

Vitamin B_3 (niacin) acts as a coenzyme for oxidation-reduction reactions. Rich sources include food from animal sources, especially lean meat and liver, and peanuts, yeast, and cereal bran or germ.

Vitamin B_6 (pyridoxine) serves as a cofactor associated with enzymes that participate in amino acid synthesis. It is found in many animal and vegetable food sources.

Vitamin C (ascorbic acid) is necessary for the proper synthesis of collagen. This vitamin is present in a wide variety of vegetables and fruits, although it is particularly abundant in citrus fruits.

Vitamin D, which is now considered to be a hormone, can be synthesized in adequate amounts within the epidermis if the skin is exposed to a moderate degree of sunlight. Most milk and processed cereal is fortified with vitamin D in the United States today, however. Appropriate levels of vitamin D and its active metabolites are necessary for calcium absorption from the gut.

Vitamin E (alpha-tocopherol) is a fat-soluble vitamin that is widely stored throughout the body. It probably functions as an antioxidant. Vegetable oil and fresh greens and vegetables are good sources of vitamin E.

Vitamin K is a fat-soluble vitamin found in a wide variety of green vegetables; it is also produced by intestinal bacteria. This vitamin is necessary for the proper synthesis of various proteins, including the clotting factors II, VII, IX, and X.

Clinical Features

Vitamin A

A severe deficiency of vitamin A during infancy may result in blindness. The early changes associated with a lack of this vitamin later in life include an inability of the eye to adapt to reduced light conditions (night blindness). With more severe, prolonged deficiency, dryness of the skin and conjunctiva develop, and the ocular changes may progress to ulceration of the cornea, leading to blindness.

Thiamin

A deficiency of thiamin results in a condition called **beriberi**, a problem that is relatively uncommon except in alcoholics or other individuals who do not receive a balanced diet. The condition became prevalent in southeast Asia when the practice of removing the outer husks of the rice grain by machine was introduced. Because

these outer husks contained nearly all of the thiamin, people who subsisted on the "polished" rice became deficient in this vitamin. The disorder is manifested by cardiovascular problems (such as peripheral vasodilation, heart failure, and edema) as well as neurologic problems (including peripheral neuropathy and Wernicke's encephalopathy). Patients with Wernicke's encephalopathy experience vomiting, nystagmus, and progressive mental deterioration, which may lead to coma and death.

Riboflavin

A diet that is chronically deficient in riboflavin causes a number of oral alterations, including glossitis, angular cheilitis, sore throat, and swelling and erythema of the oral mucosa. A normocytic, normochromic anemia may be present, and seborrheic dermatitis may affect the skin.

Niacin

A deficiency of niacin causes a condition known as **pellagra**, which may occur in populations that use corn as a principal component of their diets. Pellagra was once common in the southeastern United States and may still be seen in some parts of the world. The classic systemic signs and symptoms include the triad of dermatitis, dementia, and diarrhea. The dermatitis is distributed symmetrically; sun-exposed areas, such as the face, neck, and forearms, are affected most severely. The oral manifestations have been described as stomatitis and glossitis, with the tongue appearing red, smooth, and raw. Without correction of the niacin deficiency, the disease may evolve and persist over a period of years, eventually leading to death.

Pyridoxine

A deficiency of pyridoxine is unusual because of its widespread occurrence in a variety of foods. A number of drugs, such as the antituberculosis drug isoniazid, act as pyridoxine antagonists, and patients who receive these medications may therefore have a deficiency state. Because the vitamin plays a role in neuronal function, patients may show weakness, dizziness, or seizure disorders. Cheilitis and glossitis, reported in people with pellagra, are also reported in patients with pyridoxine deficiency.

Vitamin C

A deficiency of vitamin C is known as **scurvy**, and its occurrence in the United States is usually limited to people whose diets lack fresh fruits and vegetables. Commonly affected groups include inner-city infants (whose diets often consist entirely of milk) and elderly edentulous men, particularly those who live alone.

The clinical signs of scurvy are typically related to inadequate collagen synthesis. For example, weakened vascular walls may result in widespread petechial hemorrhage and ecchymosis. Similarly, wound healing is delayed, and recently healed wounds may break down. In childhood, painful subperiosteal hemorrhages may occur.

The oral manifestations are well documented and in-

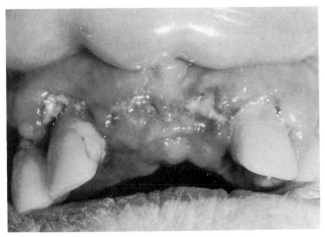

FIGURE 17–8. **Scurvy.** The gingival inflammation and ulceration (*scorbutic gingivitis*) are due to severe vitamin C deficiency.

clude generalized gingival swelling with spontaneous hemorrhage, ulceration, tooth mobility, and increased severity of periodontal infection and periodontal bone loss. The gingival lesions have been termed **scorbutic gingivitis** (Fig. 17–8). If untreated, scurvy may ultimately lead to death, often as a result of intracranial hemorrhage.

Vitamin D

A deficiency of vitamin D during infancy results in a condition called **rickets**; adults who are deficient in this vitamin develop **osteomalacia**. With the vitamin D supplementation of milk and cereal, rickets is a relatively uncommon disease today in the United States. In past centuries, however, rickets was often seen, particularly in the temperate zones of the world, which often do not receive adequate sunlight to ensure physiologic levels of vitamin D.

Clinical manifestations of rickets include irritability, growth retardation, and prominence of the costochondral junctions ("rachitic rosary"). As the child ages and begins to put weight on the long bones of the legs, significant bowing results because of the poor mineralization of the skeleton.

A similar pattern of poorly mineralized bone is seen in osteomalacia in adults. Bone normally undergoes continuous remodeling and turnover, and the osteoid that is produced during this process does not have sufficient calcium to mineralize completely. Thus a weak, fragile bone structure results. Patients affected by osteomalacia frequently complain of diffuse skeletal pain, and their bones are susceptible to fracture with relatively minor injury.

Vitamin E

A deficiency of vitamin E is rare and occurs primarily in children who suffer from chronic cholestatic liver disease. These patients have severe malabsorption of all fat-soluble vitamins, but particularly vitamin E. Multiple neurologic signs develop as a result of abnormalities in the central and peripheral nervous system.

Vitamin K

A deficiency of vitamin K may be seen in patients with malabsorption syndromes or in those whose intestinal microflora has been eliminated by long-term, broad-spectrum antibiotic use. Oral anticoagulants in the dicumarol family also inhibit the normal enzymatic activity of vitamin K. A deficiency or inhibition of synthesis of vitamin K leads to a coagulopathy because of the inadequate synthesis of prothrombin and other clotting factors. Intraorally, this coagulopathy is most often manifested by gingival bleeding. If uncorrected, death may result from uncontrolled systemic hemorrhage.

Treatment and Prognosis

Replacement therapy is indicated for vitamin deficiencies. However, such deficiencies are uncommon, except for the situations described earlier. In fact, vitamin excess is perhaps more likely to be encountered in the United States today because so many people self-medicate with unnecessary and potentially harmful vitamin supplements. For example, excess vitamin A may cause abdominal pain, vomiting, headache, joint pain, and exostoses whereas excess vitamin C may induce the formation of kidney stones in some individuals.

IRON-DEFICIENCY ANEMIA

Iron-deficiency anemia is the most common cause of anemia in the United States and throughout the world. This form of anemia develops when the amount of iron available to the body cannot keep pace with the need for iron in the production of red blood cells. This type of anemia develops under four conditions:

1. Excessive blood loss.
2. Increased demands for red blood cells.
3. Decreased intake of iron.
4. Decreased absorption of iron.

It is estimated that 20 percent of women of childbearing age in the United States are iron-deficient as a result of the chronic blood loss associated with excessive menstrual flow (*menorrhagia*). Similarly, 2 percent of adult men are iron-deficient because of chronic blood loss, usually associated with gastrointestinal disease, such as peptic ulcer disease, diverticulosis, hiatal hernia, or malignancy.

An increased demand for erythrocyte production occurs during childhood growth spurts and during pregnancy. A decreased intake of iron may be seen during infancy when the diet consists of relatively iron-poor foods, such as cereals and milk. Likewise, the diets of elderly people may be deficient if their dental condition prohibits them from eating the proper foods or if they cannot afford iron-rich foods, such as meats and vegetables.

Decreased absorption is a much less common problem; however, it can be seen in patients who have had a complete gastrectomy or who have **celiac sprue**, a condition that results in severe chronic diarrhea because of sensitivity to the plant protein gluten.

Clinical Features

Patients with iron-deficiency anemia that is severe enough to cause symptoms may complain of fatigue, easy tiring, palpitations, lightheadedness, and lack of energy.

Oral manifestations include angular cheilitis and atrophic glossitis or generalized oral mucosal atrophy. The glossitis has been described as a diffuse or patchy atrophy of the dorsal tongue papillae, often accompanied by tenderness or a burning sensation. Such findings are also evident in oral candidiasis, and some investigators have suggested that iron deficiency predisposes the patient to candidal infection, which results in the changes seen at the corners of the mouth and on the tongue. Such lesions are rarely seen in the United States, perhaps because the anemia is usually detected relatively early before the oral mucosal changes have had a chance to develop.

Laboratory Findings

The diagnosis should be established by means of a complete blood count with red blood cell indices because many other conditions, such as hypothyroidism, other anemias, or chronic depression, may elicit similar systemic clinical complaints. The laboratory evaluation characteristically shows hypochromic microcytic red blood cells in addition to reduced numbers of erythrocytes.

Treatment and Prognosis

Therapy for most cases of iron-deficiency anemia consists of dietary iron supplementation by means of oral ferrous sulfate. For patients with malabsorption problems, parenteral iron may be given periodically. The response to therapy is usually prompt, with red cell parameters returning to normal within 1 to 2 months. The underlying cause of the anemia should be identified so that it may be addressed, if feasible.

PLUMMER-VINSON SYNDROME
(Paterson-Kelly Syndrome; Sideropenic Dysphagia)

Plummer-Vinson syndrome is a rare condition characterized by iron-deficiency anemia, seen in conjunction with glossitis and dysphagia. Its incidence in developed countries has been declining, probably as a result of the improved nutritional status of the populations. The condition is significant in that it has been associated with a high frequency of both oral and esophageal squamous cell carcinoma and is therefore considered a premalignant process.

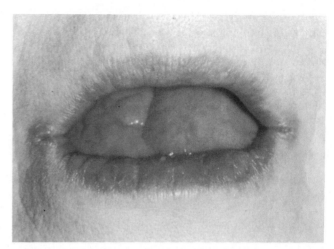

FIGURE 17–9. **Plummer-Vinson syndrome**. Patients often show angular cheilitis.

Clinical and Radiographic Features

Most reported patients with Plummer-Vinson syndrome have been Scandinavian or northern European women between 30 and 50 years of age. Patients typically complain of a burning sensation associated with the tongue and oral mucosa. Sometimes this discomfort is so severe that dentures cannot be worn. Angular cheilitis is often present and may be severe (Fig. 17–9). Marked atrophy of the lingual papillae, which produces a smooth, red appearance of the dorsal tongue, is seen clinically (Fig. 17–10; see Color Figure 115).

Patients also frequently complain of difficulty in swallowing (*dysphagia*) or pain on swallowing. An evaluation with endoscopy or esophageal barium contrast radiographic studies usually shows the presence of abnormal bands of tissue in the esophagus, called *esoph-*

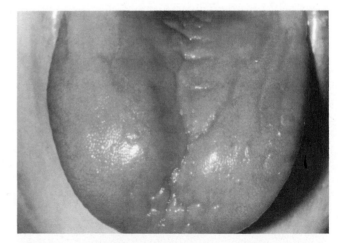

FIGURE 17–10. **Plummer-Vinson syndrome**. The diffuse papillary atrophy of the dorsal tongue is characteristic of the oral changes. See Color Plates. (From Neville BW, Damm DD, White DK, Waldron CA. Color Atlas of Clinical Oral Pathology. Philadelphia, Lea & Febiger, 1991, p 319.)

ageal webs. Another sign is an alteration of the growth pattern of the nails, which results in a spoon-shaped configuration (*koilonychia*). The nails may also be brittle.

Symptoms of anemia may prompt patients with Plummer-Vinson syndrome to seek medical care. Fatigue, shortness of breath, and weakness are characteristic symptoms.

Laboratory Findings

Hematologic studies show a hypochromic microcytic anemia that is consistent with an iron-deficiency anemia.

Histopathologic Features

A biopsy specimen of involved mucosa from a patient with Plummer-Vinson syndrome typically shows epithelial atrophy with varying degrees of submucosal chronic inflammation. In advanced cases, evidence of epithelial atypia or dysplasia may be seen.

Treatment and Prognosis

Treatment of Plummer-Vinson syndrome is primarily directed at correcting the iron-deficiency anemia by means of dietary iron supplementation. This therapy usually resolves the anemia, relieves the glossodynia, and may reduce the severity of the esophageal symptoms. Occasionally, esophageal dilation is necessary to help improve the symptoms of dysphagia. Patients with Plummer-Vinson syndrome should be evaluated periodically for oral, hypopharyngeal, and esophageal cancer because a 5 to 50 percent prevalence of upper aerodigestive tract malignancy has been reported in affected persons.

PERNICIOUS ANEMIA

Pernicious anemia is an uncommon condition that occurs with greatest frequency among elderly patients of northern European heritage. The disease is a megaloblastic anemia caused by poor absorption of cobalamin (vitamin B$_{12}$, extrinsic factor). Intrinsic factor, which is produced by the parietal cells of the stomach lining, is needed for vitamin B$_{12}$ absorption. Normally, when cobalamin is ingested, it binds to intrinsic factor in the duodenum. Because the lining cells of the intestine can only take up the cobalamin–intrinsic factor complex, the vitamin cannot be absorbed unless both components are present.

In the case of pernicious anemia, most patients appear to lack intrinsic factor, probably because of an autoimmune destruction of the parietal cells of the stomach, and this results in decreased absorption of cobalamin. A decreased ability to absorb cobalamin may also occur following gastrointestinal bypass operations.

Because cobalamin is necessary for normal nucleic acid synthesis, anything that disrupts the absorption of the vitamin causes problems, especially for cells that are multiplying rapidly and therefore synthesizing large amounts of nucleic acids. The cells that are the most mitotically active are affected to the greatest degree, especially the hematopoietic cells and the gastrointestinal lining epithelial cells.

Clinical Features

With respect to systemic complaints, patients with pernicious anemia often report fatigue, weakness, shortness of breath, headache, and feeling faint. Such symptoms are associated with most anemias and probably reflect the reduced oxygen-carrying capacity of the blood. In addition, many patients report paresthesia, tingling, or numbness of the extremities. Difficulty in walking and diminished vibratory and positional sense may be present.

Oral symptoms often consist of a burning sensation of the tongue, lips, buccal mucosa, or other mucosal sites. The clinical examination may show focal patchy areas of oral mucosal erythema and atrophy (Figs. 17–11 and 17–12; see Color Figures 116 and 117), or the process may be more diffuse, depending on the severity and

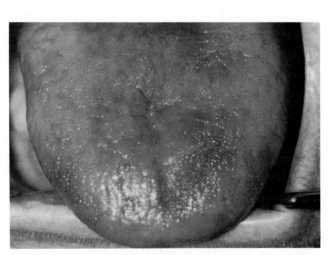

FIGURE 17–11. **Pernicious anemia**. The dorsal tongue shows erythema and atrophy. See Color Plates.

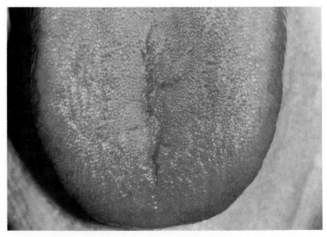

FIGURE 17–12. **Pernicious anemia**. Same patient as depicted in Figure 17–11. After therapy with vitamin B$_{12}$, the mucosal alteration resolved. See Color Plates.

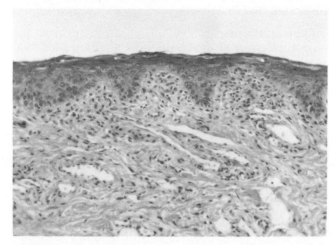

FIGURE 17–13. **Pernicious anemia**. This medium-power photomicrograph shows epithelial atrophy and atypia with chronic inflammation of the underlying connective tissue. These features are characteristic of a megaloblastic anemia, such as pernicious anemia.

duration of the condition. The tongue may be affected in as many as 50 to 60 percent of patients with pernicious anemia, but it may not show as much involvement as other areas of the oral mucosa in some instances. The atrophy and erythema may be easier to appreciate on the dorsal tongue than at other sites, however.

Histopathologic Features

Histopathologic examination of an erythematous portion of the oral mucosa shows marked epithelial atrophy with loss of rete ridges, an increased nuclear-to-cytoplasmic ratio, and prominent nucleoli (Fig. 17–13). This pattern can be misinterpreted as epithelial dysplasia at times, although the nuclei in pernicious anemia typically are pale-staining and show peripheral chromatin clumping. A patchy diffuse chronic inflammatory cell infiltrate is usually noted in the underlying connective tissue.

Laboratory Findings

Hematologic evaluation shows a macrocytic anemia, and serum cobalamin levels are reduced. The Schilling test is used to determine the pathogenesis of the cobalamin deficiency by comparing absorption and excretion rates of radiolabeled cobalamin.

Treatment and Prognosis

Once the diagnosis of pernicious anemia is established, treatment consists of monthly intramuscular injections of cyanocobalamin. The condition responds rapidly once therapy is initiated, with reports of clearing of oral lesions within 5 days. One study has confirmed that there is an increased risk of malignancy, particularly gastric carcinoma, a complication that affects between 1 and 2 percent of this population.

PITUITARY DWARFISM

Pituitary dwarfism is a relatively rare condition that results from either the diminished production of growth hormone by the anterior pituitary gland or a reduced capacity of the tissues to respond to growth hormone. Affected patients are typically much shorter than normal, although their body proportions are generally appropriate.

Several conditions may cause short stature, and a careful evaluation of the patient must be performed to rule out other possible causes, such as: (1) intrinsic defects in the patient's tissues (including certain skeletal dysplasias, chromosomal abnormalities, or idiopathic short stature) or (2) alterations in the environment of the growing tissues (such as malnutrition, hypothyroidism, or diabetes mellitus). If a lack of growth hormone is detected, the cause should be determined. Sometimes the fault lies with the pituitary gland itself (e.g., aplasia or hypoplasia). In other instances, the problem may be related to destruction of the pituitary or hypothalamus by tumors, therapeutic radiation, or infection.

If the hypothalamus is affected, a deficiency in growth hormone–releasing hormone, which is produced by the hypothalamus, results in a deficiency of growth hormone. Often deficiencies in other hormones, such as thyroid hormone and cortisol, are also detected in patients with primary pituitary or hypothalamic disorders.

Some patients exhibit normal or even elevated levels of growth hormone, yet still show little evidence of growth. These individuals usually have inherited an autosomal recessive trait, resulting in abnormal and reduced growth hormone receptors on the patients' cells. Thus, normal growth cannot proceed.

Clinical Features

Perhaps the most striking feature of pituitary dwarfism is the remarkably short stature of the affected patient. Sometimes this is not noticed until the early years of childhood, but a review of the patient's growth history should show a consistent pattern of failure to achieve the minimal height on the standard growth chart. Often the patient's height may be as much as three standard deviations below normal for a given age. Unlike the body proportions in many of the dysmorphic syndromes and skeletal dysplasias, the body proportions of patients affected by a lack of growth hormone are usually normal. One possible exception is the size of the skull, which is usually within normal limits. Because the facial skeleton does not keep pace with the skull, however, the face of an affected patient may appear smaller than it should be. Mental status is generally within normal limits.

The maxilla and mandible of affected patients are smaller than normal, and the teeth show a delayed pattern of eruption. The delay ranges from 1 to 3 years for teeth that normally erupt during the first decade of life and from 3 to 10 years for teeth that normally erupt in the second decade of life. Often the shedding of deciduous teeth is delayed by several years, and the development of the roots of the permanent teeth also appears to be delayed. A lack of development of the third molars seems to be a common finding. The size of the teeth is usually reduced in proportion to the other anatomic structures.

Laboratory Findings

Radioimmunoassay for human growth hormone shows levels that are markedly below normal.

Treatment and Prognosis

Replacement therapy with human growth hormone is the treatment of choice for patients with pituitary dwarfism if the disorder is detected prior to closure of the epiphyseal growth plates. In the past, growth hormone was extracted from cadaveric pituitary glands; today, genetically engineered human growth hormone is produced with recombinant DNA technology. For patients with a growth hormone deficiency caused by a hypothalamic defect, treatment with growth hormone–releasing hormone is appropriate. If patients are identified and treated at an early age, they can be expected to achieve a relatively normal height. For patients who lack growth hormone receptors, no treatment is available.

GIGANTISM

Gigantism is a rare condition caused by an increased production of growth hormone, usually related to a functional pituitary adenoma. The increased production of growth hormone takes place before closure of the epiphyseal plates, and the affected person grows at a much more rapid pace, becoming abnormally tall. Although the average height of the population of the United States has been gradually increasing during the past several decades, individuals who exceed the mean height by more than three standard deviations may be considered candidates for endocrinologic evaluation.

Clinical and Radiographic Features

Patients with gigantism usually show markedly accelerated growth during childhood, irrespective of normal growth spurts. Radiographic evaluation of the skull often shows an enlarged sella as a result of the presence of a pituitary adenoma. The adenoma may result in hormonal deficiencies, such as hypothyroidism and hypoadrenocorticism, if the remaining normal pituitary gland tissue is compressed and destroyed. **McCune-Albright syndrome** (polyostotic fibrous dysplasia and *café au lait* pigmentation with associated endocrinologic disturbances; see p. 462) may account for as many as 20 percent of the cases of gigantism.

If the condition remains uncorrected for a prolonged period, extreme height (more than 7 feet tall) will be achieved and enlargement of the facial soft tissues, the mandible, and the hands and feet will become apparent. These changes often resemble those seen in **acromegaly** (discussed later). Another oral finding is true generalized macrodontia.

Treatment and Prognosis

Appropriate management of gigantism involves the surgical removal of the functioning pituitary adenoma, usually by a transsphenoidal approach. Radiation therapy may also be used.

The life span of patients with gigantism is usually markedly reduced. Complications associated with hypertension, peripheral neuropathy, osteoporosis, and pulmonary disease contribute to increased morbidity and mortality.

ACROMEGALY

Acromegaly is an uncommon condition characterized by the excess production of growth hormone after closure of the epiphyseal plates in the affected patient. Usually, this increase in growth hormone is due to a functional pituitary adenoma. The incidence is estimated to be approximately three to five new cases diagnosed per million population per year. The prevalence is believed to be 66 affected patients per million.

Clinical and Radiographic Features

Because most patients with acromegaly have a pituitary adenoma, symptoms related directly to the space-occupying mass of the tumor (Fig. 17–14) may be present. These symptoms include headaches, visual disturbances, and other signs of a brain tumor. Sometimes pressure atrophy of the residual normal pituitary by the adenoma results in diminished production of other pituitary hormones and causes other indirect endocrine problems. The direct effects of increased levels of growth

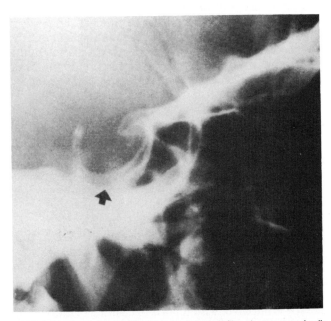

FIGURE 17–14. Acromegaly. This lateral skull film shows a markedly enlarged sella turcica (*arrow*) secondary to a pituitary adenoma, which is responsible for producing the excess growth hormone.

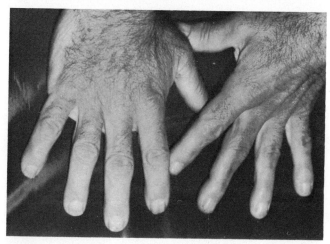

FIGURE 17–15. **Acromegaly**. Same patient as depicted in Figure 17–16, showing growth of the bones of the hands. (Courtesy of Dr. William Bruce.)

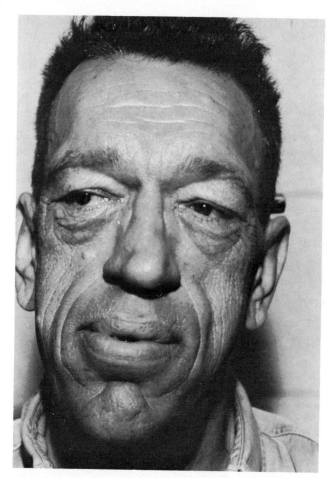

FIGURE 17–16. **Acromegaly**. This patient shows the typical coarse facial features. (Courtesy of Dr. William Bruce.)

hormone include a variety of problems, such as hypertension, heart disease, hyperhidrosis, arthritis, and peripheral neuropathy.

Renewed growth in the small bones of the hands and feet (Fig. 17–15) as well as in the membranous bones of the skull and jaws is typically observed. Patients may complain of gloves or hats becoming "too small." The soft tissue is also often affected, producing a coarse facial appearance (Fig. 17–16). Hypertrophy of the soft palatal tissues may cause or accentuate sleep apnea. Because these signs and symptoms are slow to develop and are vague at the onset, an average time of nearly 9 years elapses from the onset of symptoms to the diagnosis of disease. The average age at diagnosis is 42 years, and no sex predilection is seen.

From a dental perspective, these patients have mandibular prognathism as a result of the increased growth of the mandible (Fig. 17–17), which may cause apertognathia (anterior open bite). Growth of the jaws also may cause spacing of the teeth, resulting in diastema formation. Soft tissue growth often produces uniform macroglossia in affected patients.

Treatment and Prognosis

The treatment of a patient with acromegaly is typically directed at the removal of the pituitary tumor mass and the return of the growth hormone levels to normal. The most effective treatment with the least associated morbidity is surgical excision by a transsphenoidal approach. The prognosis for such a procedure is good, although a mortality rate of approximately 1 percent is still expected. The condition is usually controlled with this procedure, but patients with larger tumors and markedly elevated growth hormone levels are less likely to be controlled.

Radiation therapy may be used in some instances, but the return of the growth hormone levels to normal is not as rapid nor as predictable as with surgery. Because some

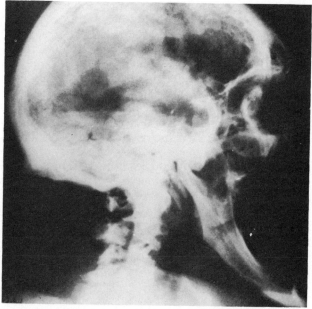

FIGURE 17–17. **Acromegaly**. This lateral skull film shows the dramatic degree of mandibular enlargement that may occur.

patients also experience hypopituitarism caused by radiation effects on the rest of the gland, some centers may offer radiation therapy as treatment only when surgery fails or is too risky. Pharmacotherapy with a somatostatin analogue (octreotide) may also help to control acromegaly when surgery is contraindicated and when the radiation therapy has not yet taken effect.

The prognosis for untreated patients is guarded, with an increased mortality rate compared with that of the general population. Hypertension, diabetes mellitus, coronary artery disease, congestive heart failure, respiratory disease, and colon cancer are seen with increased frequency in acromegalic patients, and each of these contributes to the increased mortality rate. Although treatment of the patient with acromegaly helps to control many of the other complicating problems and improves the prognosis, the life span of these patients still is shortened.

HYPOTHYROIDISM
(Cretinism; Myxedema)

Hypothyroidism is a condition that is characterized by decreased levels of thyroid hormone. When this decrease occurs during infancy, the resulting clinical problem is known as **cretinism**. If an adult has markedly decreased thyroid hormone levels for a prolonged period, deposition of a glycosaminoglycan ground substance is seen in the subcutaneous tissues, producing a nonpitting edema. Some call this severe form of hypothyroidism **myxedema**; others use the terms "myxedema" and "hypothyroidism" interchangeably.

Hypothyroidism may be classified as either *primary* or *secondary*. In primary hypothyroidism, the thyroid gland itself is in some way abnormal; in secondary hypothyroidism, the pituitary gland does not produce an adequate amount of thyroid-stimulating hormone (TSH), which is necessary for the appropriate release of thyroid hormone. Secondary hypothyroidism, for example, often develops after radiation therapy for brain tumors, resulting in unavoidable radiation damage to the pituitary gland. Most cases, however, represent the primary form of the disease.

Screening for this disorder is routinely carried out at birth, and the prevalence of congenital hypothyroidism in North America is approximately 1 in 4000 births. Usually, this is due to hypoplasia or agenesis of the thyroid gland. In adults, hypothyroidism is often caused by autoimmune destruction of the thyroid gland (known as **Hashimoto's thyroiditis**) or iatrogenic factors, such as radioactive iodine therapy or surgery for the treatment of hyperthyroidism. Because thyroid hormone is necessary for normal cellular metabolism, many of the clinical signs and symptoms of hypothyroidism can be related to the decreased metabolic rate in these patients.

Clinical Features

The most common features of hypothyroidism include such signs and symptoms as lethargy; dry, coarse skin;

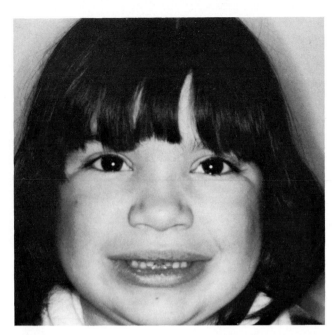

FIGURE 17–18. **Hypothyroidism**. The facial appearance of this 9-year-old child is due to the accumulation of tissue edema secondary to severe hypothyroidism.

swelling of the face (Fig. 17–18) and extremities; huskiness of the voice; constipation; weakness; and fatigue. The heart rate is usually slowed (*bradycardia*). Reduced body temperature (*hypothermia*) may be present, and the skin often feels cool and dry to the touch. In the infant, these signs may not be readily apparent, and the failure to grow normally may be the first indication of the disease.

With respect to the oral findings, the lips may appear thickened because of the accumulation of glycosamino-

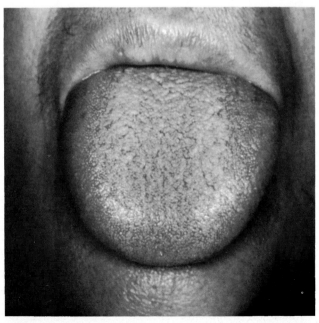

FIGURE 17–19. **Hypothyroidism**. The enlarged tongue (macroglossia) is secondary to edema associated with adult hypothyroidism (myxedema).

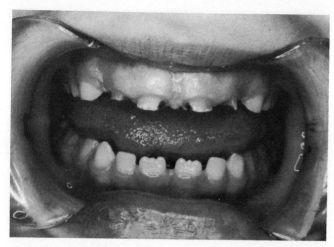

FIGURE 17–20. **Hypothyroidism**. Photograph of the same patient depicted in Figure 17–18. Note the retained deciduous teeth, for which the patient was initially referred.

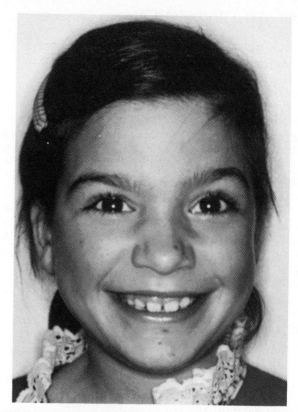

FIGURE 17–22. **Hypothyroidism**. Same patient depicted in Figure 17–18 after 1 year of thyroid hormone replacement therapy. Note the eruption of the maxillary permanent teeth.

glycans. Diffuse enlargement of the tongue occurs for the same reason (Fig. 17–19). If the condition develops during childhood, the teeth may fail to erupt, although tooth formation may not be impaired (Figs. 17–20 and 17–21).

Laboratory Findings

The diagnosis is made by assaying the free thyroxine (T_4) levels. If these levels are low, TSH levels are measured to determine whether primary or secondary hypothyroidism is present. With primary thyroid disease, TSH levels are elevated. With secondary disease caused by pituitary dysfunction, TSH levels are normal or borderline.

Treatment and Prognosis

Thyroid replacement therapy, usually with levothyroxine, is indicated for confirmed cases of hypothyroid-

ism. The prognosis is generally good for adult patients. If the condition is recognized within a reasonable time, the prognosis is also good for children. If the condition is not identified in a timely manner, however, permanent damage to the central nervous system may occur, resulting in mental retardation. For affected children, thyroid hormone replacement therapy often results in a dramatic resolution of the condition (Fig. 17–22).

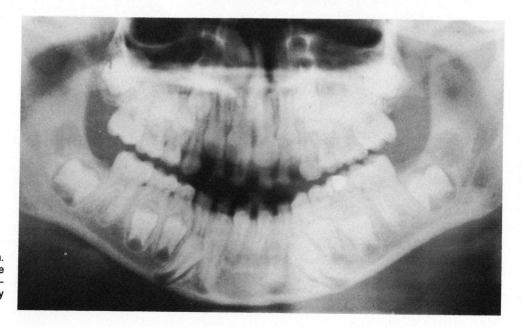

FIGURE 17–21. **Hypothyroidism**. Panoramic radiograph of the same patient in Figures 17–18 and 17–20. Note the unerupted, yet fully developed permanent dentition.

HYPERTHYROIDISM (Graves' Disease)

Hyperthyroidism is a condition caused by excess production of thyroid hormone. This excess production results in a state of markedly increased metabolism in the affected patient. Most cases (up to 85 percent) are due to **Graves' disease**, a condition that was initially described in the early 19th century. It is thought to be triggered by autoantibodies, which are directed against receptors for thyroid-stimulating hormone (TSH) on the surface of the thyroid cells. When the autoantibodies bind to these receptors, they seem to stimulate the thyroid cells to release inappropriate thyroid hormone.

Other causes of hyperthyroidism include hyperplastic thyroid tissue and thyroid tumors, both benign and malignant, which secrete inappropriate thyroid hormone. Similarly, a pituitary adenoma may produce TSH, which can then stimulate the thyroid to secrete excess thyroid hormone.

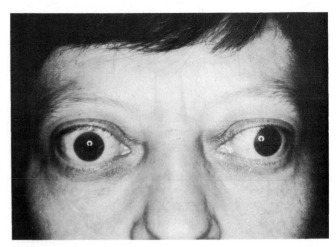

FIGURE 17–23. **Hyperthyroidism**. The prominent eyes are characteristic of the exophthalmos associated with Graves' disease.

Clinical Features

Graves' disease is five to ten times more common in women than in men and is seen with some frequency. It affects almost 2 percent of the female population. Graves' disease is most commonly diagnosed in patients during the third and fourth decades of life.

Most patients with Graves' disease present with diffuse thyroid enlargement. Many of the signs and symptoms of hyperthyroidism can be attributed to an increased metabolic rate caused by the excess thyroid hormone. Patients usually complain about nervousness, heart palpitations, heat intolerance, emotional lability, and muscle weakness. The following are often noted during the clinical evaluation:

- Weight loss despite increased appetite
- Tachycardia
- Excessive perspiration
- Widened pulse pressure (increased systolic and decreased diastolic pressures)
- Warm, smooth skin
- Tremor

Perhaps the most striking features of these patients, however, are the ocular manifestations. In the early stages of hyperthyroidism, patients have a characteristic stare with eyelid retraction and lid lag. With some forms of Graves' disease, protrusion of the eyes (*exophthalmos* or *proptosis*) develops (Fig. 17–23). This bulging of the eyes is due to an accumulation of glycosaminoglycans in the retro-orbital connective tissues.

Laboratory Findings

The diagnosis of hyperthyroidism is made by assaying free T_4 (thyroxine) and TSH levels in the serum. In affected patients, the T_4 levels should be elevated and the TSH concentration is typically depressed.

Histopathologic Features

Diffuse enlargement and hypercellularity of the thyroid gland are seen in patients with Graves' disease, typically with hyperplastic thyroid epithelium and little apparent colloid production. Lymphocytic infiltration of the glandular parenchyma is also often noted.

Treatment and Prognosis

Radioactive iodine (^{131}I) is perhaps the most effective means of therapy for most patients with Graves' disease. The thyroid gland normally takes up iodine from the blood stream because this element is a critical component of thyroid hormone. When radioactive iodine is given to a patient with Graves' disease, the thyroid gland quickly removes it from the blood stream and sequesters the radioactive material within the glandular tissue. The radioactivity then destroys the hyperactive thyroid tissue, bringing the thyroid hormone levels back to normal. Most of the radiation is received during the first few weeks because the half-life of ^{131}I is short.

Other techniques include drug therapy with agents that block the normal use of iodine by the thyroid gland. The two most widely used drugs in the United States are propylthiouracil and methimazole. At times, they are used prior to the radioactive iodine. Sometimes they may be administered chronically in the hope that a remission may be induced. In addition, a portion of the thyroid gland may be removed surgically, thereby reducing thyroid hormone production.

Drug therapy alone is often unsuccessful in controlling hyperthyroidism. Unfortunately, with radioactive iodine and surgery, the risk of hypothyroidism is relatively great, although thyroid hormone replacement therapy can be instituted if needed.

In a patient with uncontrolled hyperthyroidism, a definite risk exists with respect to an inappropriate release of large amounts of thyroid hormone at one time, resulting in a condition called a **thyroid storm**. A thyroid storm may be precipitated by infection, psychologic trauma, or stress. Clinically, patients may have delirium, an elevated temperature, and tachycardia. Such individuals should be hospitalized immediately because the mortality rate associated with thyroid storms is 20 to 40 percent. The clinician should be aware of the potential for this problem, and patients with hyperthyroidism should ideally have the condition under control prior to dental treatment.

HYPOPARATHYROIDISM

Calcium levels in extracellular tissues are normally regulated by parathyroid hormone (parathormone, PTH) in conjunction with vitamin D. If calcium levels drop below a certain point, the release of parathyroid hormone is stimulated. The hormone then acts directly on the kidney and the osteoclasts of the bone to restore the calcium to normal levels. In the kidney, calcium reabsorption is promoted, phosphate excretion is enhanced, and the production of vitamin D is stimulated, which increases the absorption of calcium from the gut. Osteoclasts are activated to resorb bone and thus liberate calcium.

If a reduced amount of PTH is produced, the relatively rare condition known as **hypoparathyroidism** results. Usually, hypoparathyroidism is due to inadvertent surgical removal of the parathyroid glands when the thyroid gland is excised for other reasons, but sometimes it is the result of autoimmune destruction of the parathyroid tissue. Rare syndromes, such as **DiGeorge syndrome** and the **endocrine-candidiasis syndrome**, may be associated with hypoparathyroidism.

Clinical Features

With the loss of parathyroid function, the serum levels of calcium drop, resulting in hypocalcemia. Often the patient with chronic hypoparathyroidism adapts to the presence of hypocalcemia and is asymptomatic unless situations that further reduce the calcium levels are encountered. Such situations include metabolic alkalosis, as seen during hyperventilation, when a state of tetany may become evident.

Chvostek's sign is an oral finding of significance, characterized by a twitching of the upper lip when the facial nerve is tapped just below the zygomatic process. A positive response suggests a latent degree of tetany. If the hypoparathyroidism develops early in life during odontogenesis, a pitting enamel hypoplasia as well as failure of tooth eruption may occur (Fig. 17–24). The presence of persistent oral candidiasis in a young patient may signal the onset of endocrine-candidiasis syndrome (see p. 168). Hypoparathyroidism may be only one of several endocrine deficiencies associated with this condition.

Laboratory Findings

Parathyroid hormone can be measured by means of a radioimmunoassay. If PTH levels are decreased in con-

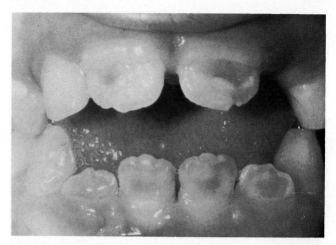

FIGURE 17–24. Hypoparathyroidism. Pitted enamel hypoplasia has affected the dentition of this patient, who had hypoparathyroidism while the teeth were forming.

junction with a decreased serum calcium concentration, elevated serum phosphate level, and normal renal function, a diagnosis of hypoparathyroidism can be made.

Treatment and Prognosis

Patients with hypoparathyroidism are usually treated with oral doses of a vitamin D precursor (ergocalciferol, or vitamin D_2). Additional supplements of dietary calcium may also be necessary to maintain the proper serum calcium levels. With this regimen, patients can often live a fairly normal life.

PSEUDOHYPOPARATHYROIDISM
(Albright Hereditary Osteodystrophy; Acrodysostosis)

The rare condition known as **pseudohypoparathyroidism** represents at least two disorders in which normal parathyroid hormone (PTH) is present in adequate amounts but the biochemical pathways responsible for activating the target cells are not functioning properly. The clinical result is a patient who appears to have hypoparathyroidism.

In the case of pseudohypoparathyroidism type Ia, a molecular defect of a specific intracellular binding protein known as Gs seems to prevent the formation of cyclic adenosine monophosphate (cAMP), a critical component in the activation of cell metabolism. Because other hormones also require binding with Gs to carry out their functions, patients have multiple problems with other endocrine organs and functions. This condition is usually inherited as an autosomal dominant trait.

With respect to pseudohypoparathyroidism type Ib, the problem is thought to be due to defective receptors for the parathyroid hormone on the surface of the target cells. For this reason, no other endocrine tissues or functions are affected. The mode of inheritance for type 1b is unclear.

Pseudohypoparathyroidism, type II, is characterized by the induction of cyclic AMP by PTH; however, a functional response by the cells is not invoked.

Clinical Features

Patients affected by pseudohypoparathyroidism type Ia have a characteristic array of features, which include mild mental retardation, obesity, round face, short neck, and markedly short stature. Mid-facial hypoplasia is also commonly observed. The metacarpals and metatarsals are usually shortened, and the fingers appear short and thick. Subcutaneous calcifications may be identified in some patients. Other endocrine abnormalities that are typically encountered include hypogonadism and hypothyroidism.

Patients with type Ib disease clinically appear normal, aside from their symptoms of hypocalcemia.

Dental manifestations of pseudohypoparathyroidism include generalized enamel hypoplasia, widened pulp chambers with intrapulpal calcifications, oligodontia, delayed eruption, and blunting of the apices of the teeth. The pulpal calcifications are often described as "dagger-shaped."

The diagnosis of pseudohypoparathyroidism is made on the basis of elevated serum levels of parathyroid hormone seen concurrently with hypocalcemia, hyperphosphatemia, and otherwise normal renal function. Characteristic clinical signs and endocrine disturbances distinguish the type Ia from type Ib forms of pseudohypoparathyroidism.

Treatment and Prognosis

Pseudohypoparathyroidism is managed by the administration of vitamin D and calcium. The serum calcium levels and urinary calcium excretion are carefully monitored. Because of individual patient differences, the medication may need to be carefully adjusted; however, the prognosis is considered to be good.

HYPERPARATHYROIDISM

Excess production of parathyroid hormone results in the condition known as **hyperparathyroidism**. Parathyroid hormone (PTH) normally is produced by the parathyroid glands in response to a decrease in serum calcium levels.

Primary hyperparathyroidism is the uncontrolled production of PTH, usually as a result of a parathyroid adenoma (80 to 90 percent of cases) or parathyroid hyperplasia (10 to 15 percent of cases). Infrequently (in less than 2 percent of cases), a parathyroid carcinoma may be the cause of primary hyperparathyroidism.

Secondary hyperparathyroidism develops when PTH is continuously produced in response to chronic low levels of serum calcium, a situation usually associated with chronic renal disease. The kidney processes vitamin D, which is necessary for calcium absorption from the gut. Therefore, in a patient with chronic renal disease, active vitamin D is not produced and less calcium is absorbed from the gut, resulting in lowered serum calcium levels.

Clinical and Radiographic Features

Most patients with primary hyperparathyroidism are older than 60 years of age. Women have this condition two to four times more often than men do.

Patients with the classic triad of signs and symptoms of hyperparathyroidism are described as having "stones, bones, and abdominal groans."

Stones refers to the fact that in these patients, particularly those with primary hyperparathyroidism, there is a marked tendency for renal calculi (kidney stones, nephrolithiasis) to develop because of the elevated serum calcium levels. Metastatic calcifications are also seen, frequently involving other soft tissues, such as blood vessel walls, subcutaneous soft tissues, the sclera, the dura, and the regions around the joints.

Bones refers to a variety of osseous changes that may occur in conjunction with hyperparathyroidism. One of the first clinical signs of this disease is seen radiographically as subperiosteal resorption of the phalanges of the index and middle fingers. Generalized loss of the lamina dura surrounding the roots of the teeth is also seen as an early manifestation of the condition (Fig. 17–25). Alterations in trabecular pattern characteristically develop next. A decrease in trabecular density and blurring of the normal trabecular pattern occur; often a "ground glass" appearance results.

With persistent disease, other osseous lesions develop, such as the so-called **brown tumor** of hyperparathyroidism. This lesion derives its name from the color of the tissue specimen, which is usually a dark reddish-brown because of the abundant hemorrhage and hemosiderin deposition within the tumor. These lesions appear radiographically as well-demarcated unilocular or multilocular radiolucencies (Fig. 17–26). They commonly affect the mandible, clavicle, ribs, and pelvis. They may be

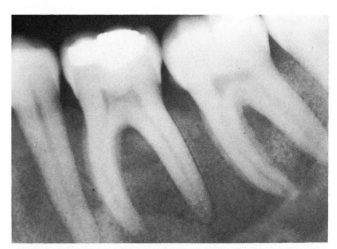

FIGURE 17–25. **Hyperparathyroidism.** This periapical radiograph reveals the "ground glass" appearance of the trabeculae as well as the loss of lamina dura in a patient with secondary hyperparathyroidism. (Courtesy of Dr. Randy Anderson.)

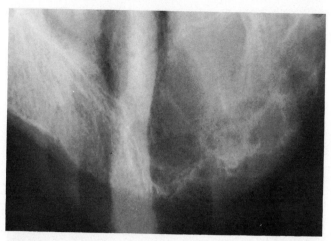

FIGURE 17–26. **Hyperparathyroidism**. This occlusal radiograph of the edentulous maxillary anterior region shows a multilocular radiolucency characteristic of a brown tumor of primary hyperparathyroidism. (Courtesy of Dr. Brian Blocher.)

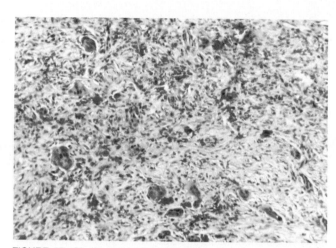

FIGURE 17–28. **Hyperparathyroidism**. This medium-power photomicrograph of a brown tumor of hyperparathyroidism shows a granulation tissue background that supports numerous multinucleated giant cells.

solitary but are often multiple, and longstanding lesions may produce significant cortical expansion (Fig. 17–27). Typically, the other osseous changes are observable if brown tumors are present. The most severe skeletal manifestation of chronic hyperparathyroidism has been called **osteitis fibrosa cystica**, a condition that develops from the central degeneration and fibrosis of longstanding brown tumors.

Abdominal groans refers to the tendency for the development of duodenal ulcers. In addition, changes in mental status are often seen, ranging from lethargy and weakness to confusion or dementia.

Histopathologic Features

The brown tumor of hyperparathyroidism is histopathologically identical to the **central giant cell granuloma** of the jaws, a benign tumor-like lesion that usually affects teen-agers and young adults (see p. 453). Both

lesions are characterized by a proliferation of exceedingly vascular granulation tissue, which serves as a background for numerous multinucleated osteoclast-type giant cells (Fig. 17–28). Some lesions may also show a proliferative response characterized by a parallel arrangement of spicules of woven bone set in a cellular fibroblastic background with variable numbers of multinucleated giant cells (Fig. 17–29). This pattern is often associated with secondary hyperparathyroidism related to chronic renal disease and has been called **renal osteodystrophy**.

Treatment and Prognosis

In *primary* hyperparathyroidism, the hyperplastic parathyroid tissue or the functional tumor must be removed surgically to reduce parathyroid hormone levels to normal.

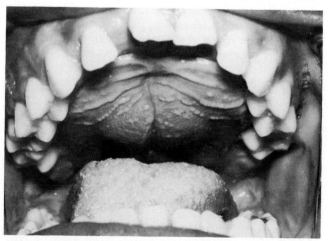

FIGURE 17–27. **Hyperparathyroidism**. Palatal enlargement is characteristic of the renal osteodystrophy associated with secondary hyperparathyroidism.

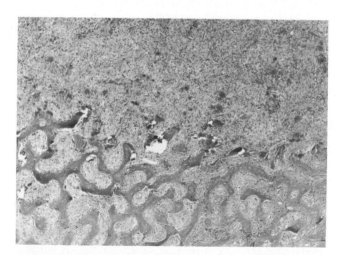

FIGURE 17–29. **Hyperparathyroidism**. This low-power photomicrograph shows the cellular granulation tissue with scattered multinucleated giant cells (*top*) and parallel spicules of woven bone (*bottom*). These features are characteristic of tissue changes seen in renal osteodystrophy.

Secondary hyperparathyroidism is not usually managed aggressively unless the patient has symptoms as a result of the renal calculi. Treatment with an active vitamin D metabolite may control the problem pharmacologically; however, renal transplantation usually restores the normal physiologic processing of vitamin D as well as phosphorus and calcium reabsorption and excretion.

HYPERCORTISOLISM
(Cushing's Syndrome)

Hypercortisolism is a clinical condition that results from a sustained increase in glucocorticoid levels. In most cases, this increase is due to corticosteroid therapy that is prescribed for other medical purposes. If the increase is caused by an endogenous source, such as an adrenal or pituitary (adrenocorticotropic hormone [ACTH]-secreting) tumor, the condition is known as **Cushing's disease**. This latter condition is rather rare and usually affects young adult women.

Clinical Features

The signs of Cushing's syndrome usually develop slowly. The most consistent clinical observation is weight gain, particularly in the central areas of the body. The accumulation of fat in the dorsocervical spine region results in a "buffalo hump" appearance; fatty tissue deposition in the facial area results in the characteristic rounded facial appearance known as "moon facies" (Fig. 17–30). Other common findings include:

- Red-purple abdominal striae
- Hirsutism
- Poor healing
- Osteoporosis
- Hypertension
- Mood changes (particularly depression)
- Hyperglycemia with thirst and polyuria
- Muscle wasting with weakness

Diagnosis

If the patient has been receiving large amounts of corticosteroids (greater than the equivalent of 20 mg of prednisone) on a daily basis for several months, the diagnosis is rather obvious, given the classic signs and symptoms described earlier. The diagnosis may be more difficult to establish in patients with a functioning adrenal cortical tumor or an ACTH-secreting pituitary adenoma. Evaluation of these patients should include the measurement of free cortisol in the urine and an assay of the effect of dexamethasone (a potent artificial corticosteroid) on the serum ACTH and cortisol levels. In an unaffected patient, the levels of free cortisol should be within normal limits, and the administration of an exogenous corticosteroid, such as dexamethasone, should suppress the normal level of ACTH, with a concomitant decrease in the cortisol levels. Because functioning tumors do not respond to normal feedback mechanisms, the anticipated

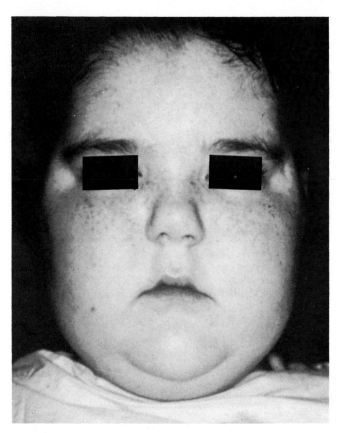

FIGURE 17–30. **Cushing's syndrome.** The rounded facial features ("moon facies") of this patient are due to the abnormal deposition of fat, which is induced by excess corticosteroid hormone. (Courtesy of Dr. George Blozis.)

decreases in ACTH and cortisol would not be seen in a patient with such a tumor.

Treatment and Prognosis

The clinician should be aware of the signs and symptoms of hypercortisolism in order to refer affected patients for appropriate endocrinologic evaluation and diagnosis. Once the diagnosis is established, if the cause is determined to be an adrenal or pituitary tumor, surgical removal of the lesion is the treatment of choice. In patients with unresectable tumors, drugs that inhibit cortisol synthesis, such as ketoconazole, metyrapone, or aminoglutethimide, may be used to help control the excess production of cortisol.

Most cases of hypercortisolism, however, are caused by systemic corticosteroid therapy for a variety of immunologic reasons, including treatment of autoimmune diseases and allogeneic transplant recipients. Certain strategies, such as the use of corticosteroid-sparing agents or alternate-day therapy, may minimize the corticosteroid dose needed. The goal should be for patients to use the lowest dose possible to manage immunologic disease.

In normal situations, cortisol is critical to the function of the body, particularly in dealing with stress. As the hormone is metabolized and serum levels drop, feedback to the pituitary gland signals it to produce ACTH, which stimulates the adrenal gland to produce additional cortisol. Unfortunately, therapeutic corticosteroids suppress the production of ACTH by the pituitary gland to the extent that the pituitary gland may not be able to produce ACTH in response to stress, and an acute episode of hypoadrenocorticism ("addisonian crisis") may be precipitated. Therefore, the clinician must be aware of the potential side effects of chronic high-dose corticosteroid use and must be able to adapt the treatment of the patient accordingly. For stressful dental and surgical procedures especially, it is often necessary to increase the corticosteroid dosage because of the greater need of the body for cortisol. Consultation with the physician who is managing the corticosteroid therapy is advised to determine to what extent the dosage should be adjusted.

ADDISON'S DISEASE
(Hypoadrenocorticism)

Insufficient production of adrenal corticosteroid hormones caused by the destruction of the adrenal cortex results in the condition known as **Addison's disease**, or **primary hypoadrenocorticism**. The incidence of new cases diagnosed in the Western Hemisphere is 40 to 50 per million population per year. The causes are diverse and include:

- Autoimmune destruction
- Infections (such as tuberculosis and deep fungal diseases, particularly in patients with acquired immunodeficiency syndrome [AIDS])
- Rarely, metastatic tumors, sarcoidosis, hemochromatosis, or amyloidosis

If the pituitary gland is not functioning properly, **secondary hypoadrenocorticism** may develop because of decreased production of ACTH, the hormone responsible for maintaining normal levels of serum cortisol.

Clinical Features

The clinical features of hypoadrenocorticism do not actually begin to appear until at least 90 percent of the glandular tissue has been destroyed. With gradual destruction of the adrenal cortex, an insidious onset of fatigue, irritability, depression, weakness, and hypotension is noted over a period of months. A generalized hyperpigmentation of the skin occurs, classically described as "bronzing." The hyperpigmentation is generally more prominent on sun-exposed skin and over pressure points, such as the elbows and knees; it is caused by increased levels of beta-lipotropin or ACTH, each of which can stimulate melanocytes. The patient usually complains of gastrointestinal upset with anorexia, nausea, diarrhea, weight loss, and a peculiar craving for salt.

The oral manifestations include diffuse or patchy, brown macular pigmentation of the oral mucosa caused by excess melanin production (Fig. 17–31; see Color Figure 118). Often the oral mucosal changes are the first manifestation of the disease, with the skin hyperpigmentation following. Sometimes the oral hypermelanosis

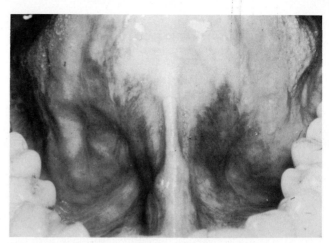

FIGURE 17–31. Addison's disease. Diffuse pigmentation of the floor of the mouth and ventral tongue in a patient with Addison's disease. See Color Plates. (Courtesy of Dr. George Blozis.)

may be difficult to distinguish from physiologic racial pigmentation, but a history of a recent onset of oral pigmentation should suggest the possibility of Addison's disease.

Laboratory Findings

The diagnosis of hypoadrenocorticism is confirmed by a rapid ACTH stimulation test and measurement of plasma ACTH levels. In primary hypoadrenocorticism, the plasma ACTH levels are high (>250 pg/mL). In secondary hypoadrenocorticism, the levels are low (0 to 20 pg/mL), as would be expected because the condition results from decreased ACTH production by the pituitary gland.

Treatment and Prognosis

Addison's disease is managed with corticosteroid replacement therapy. The physiologic dose of corticosteroid is considered to be approximately 5 mg of prednisone or its equivalent per day, usually given in divided doses. Because the body's need for corticosteroid hormones increases during stressful events, the patient must take this into account and increase the dosage accordingly. This adjustment may be necessary for certain dental and oral surgical procedures.

Prior to the availability of corticosteroids, the prognosis for patients with hypoadrenocorticism was poor, with most patients surviving less than 2 years. Today, however, with proper diagnosis and management, patients can expect to have a normal life span.

DIABETES MELLITUS

Diabetes mellitus is a common disorder of carbohydrate metabolism that probably has several causes, although the basic problem is one of either decreased production of insulin or tissue resistance to the effects of insulin. The net result of this abnormal state is an increase in the blood glucose level (*hyperglycemia*).

Diabetes mellitus is usually divided into two types:

- Insulin-dependent diabetes mellitus (IDDM), or type I or juvenile-onset diabetes
- Non–insulin-dependent diabetes mellitus (NIDDM), or type II or adult-onset diabetes

IDDM is characterized by a lack of insulin production. Patients usually present with severe hyperglycemia and ketoacidosis. Most patients with IDDM present with the disease during childhood, and they require exogenous insulin injections to survive.

NIDDM is sometimes more difficult to diagnose. It usually occurs in older, obese adults. Although hyperglycemia is present, ketoacidosis rarely develops. Furthermore, patients can produce some endogenous insulin. A few patients may take insulin to help control their disease; the insulin injections, however, are usually not necessary for the patient's survival.

With respect to epidemiology, in the United States diabetes mellitus affects approximately 3 percent of the population, or nearly 7 million people. About 650,000 new cases are diagnosed each year in the United States. Of these affected patients, most have NIDDM; only 7 to 10 percent have IDDM.

Diabetes is an important disease when we consider the many complications associated with it and the economic impact it has on society. One of the main complications of diabetes is *peripheral vascular disease*, a problem that results in kidney failure as well as ischemia and gangrenous involvement of the limbs. By some estimates, 25 percent of all new cases of kidney failure occur in diabetic patients. Diabetes is thus the leading cause of kidney failure in the United States. Each year 20,000 amputations are performed for the gangrenous complications of diabetes. This disease is the leading cause of lower limb amputations in the United States. Retinal involvement often results in blindness; thus, the leading cause of new cases of blindness in working-age adults in the United States is diabetes, with nearly 5000 people affected every year.

The cause of diabetes mellitus is essentially unknown, although evidence is accumulating that many cases of IDDM may be precipitated by a viral infection that triggers an autoimmune response, resulting in destruction of the pancreatic islet cells. NIDDM does not appear to have an autoimmune cause, however, because no destruction of the islet cells is seen microscopically. Instead, genetic abnormalities have been detected in patients with certain types of NIDDM, which may explain why the condition occurs so often in families. If one parent is affected by NIDDM, the chances of a child having the disorder is about 40 percent. Similarly, if one identical twin has NIDDM, the chances are 90 percent that the disease will also develop in the other twin.

Clinical Features

Although a complete review of the pathophysiology of diabetes mellitus is beyond the scope of this text, the clinical signs and symptoms of a patient with this disease are easier to understand with some basic knowledge of the process. The hormone insulin, produced by the beta cells of the pancreatic islets of Langerhans, is necessary for the uptake of glucose by the cells of the body. When insulin binds to its specific cell surface receptor, this sets into motion a cascade of intracellular molecular events that causes the recruitment of intracellular glucose-binding proteins, which facilitate the uptake of glucose by each cell.

Insulin-Dependent Diabetes Mellitus

Because patients with IDDM have a deficiency in the amount of insulin, glucose cannot be absorbed by the body's cells and it remains in the blood. Normal blood glucose levels are between 70 and 120 mg/dL; in diabetic patients, these levels are often between 200 and 400 mg/dL. Above 300 mg/dL, the kidneys can no longer reabsorb the glucose; therefore, it spills over into the urine. Because glucose is the main source of energy for the body, and since none of this energy can be used because glucose cannot be absorbed, the patient feels tired and lethargic. The body begins to use other energy sources, such as fat and protein, resulting in the production of ketones as a by-product of those energy consumption pathways. The patient often loses weight, despite increased food intake (*polyphagia*). With the hyperglycemia, the osmolarity of the blood and urine increases. The increased osmolarity results in frequent urination (*polyuria*) and thirst, which leads to increased water intake (*polydipsia*). Clinically, most patients with IDDM are younger (average age at diagnosis being 14 years), and they have a thin body habitus.

Non–Insulin-Dependent Diabetes Mellitus

By contrast, patients with NIDDM are usually older than 40 years of age at diagnosis, and 80 to 90 percent of them are obese. In this situation, it is thought that a decrease in the number of insulin receptors or abnormal postbinding molecular events related to glucose uptake results in glucose not being absorbed by the body's cells. Thus, patients are said to show "insulin resistance" because serum insulin levels are usually within normal limits or even elevated. If the hyperglycemia is taken into account, however, the amount of circulating insulin is typically not as much as would be present in a normal person with a similar level of blood glucose. Therefore, many of these patients are described as having a relative lack of insulin.

The symptoms associated with NIDDM are much more subtle in comparison to those seen with IDDM. The first sign of NIDDM is often detected with routine hematologic examination rather than any specific patient complaint. Ketoacidosis is almost never seen in patients with NIDDM. Nevertheless, many of the other complications of diabetes are still associated with NIDDM.

Complications

Many complications of diabetes mellitus are directly related to the *microangiopathy* caused by the disease. The microangiopathy results in occlusion of the small blood vessels, producing peripheral vascular disease. The resultant decrease in tissue perfusion results in ischemia. The ischemia predisposes the patient to infection, particularly severe infections such as gangrene. Another contributing factor is the impairment of neutrophil function, particularly neutrophil chemotaxis.

Amputation of the lower extremity often is necessary because of the lack of tissue perfusion and the patient's inability to cope with infection. Similar vascular occlusion may affect the coronary arteries (which places the patient at risk for myocardial infarction) or the carotid arteries and their branches (predisposing the patient to cerebrovascular accident, or stroke). When microvascular occlusion affects the retinal vessels, blindness typically results. Kidney failure is the outcome of renal blood vessel involvement. If the ketoacidosis is not corrected in IDDM, the patient may lapse into a diabetic coma.

The oral manifestations of diabetes mellitus are generally limited to patients with IDDM. Problems include periodontal disease, which occurs more frequently and progresses more rapidly than in normal patients. Healing after surgery may be delayed, and the likelihood of infection is probably increased. Diffuse, nontender, bilateral enlargement of the parotid glands, called **diabetic sialadenosis** (see p. 334), may be seen in patients with either IDDM or NIDDM. In uncontrolled or poorly controlled diabetic patients, a striking enlargement and erythema of the attached gingiva has been described (Fig. 17–32; see Color Figure 119). In addition, these patients appear to be more susceptible to **oral candidiasis** in its various clinical forms (see p. 163). **Erythematous candidiasis**, which presents as central papillary atrophy of the dorsal tongue papillae, is reported in up to 30 percent of these patients. **Zygomycosis** (see p. 175) may occur in patients with poorly controlled IDDM. An increased prevalence of **benign migratory glossitis** has also been associated with IDDM. **Xerostomia**, a subjective feeling of dryness of the oral mucosa, has been reported as a complaint in one third of diabetic patients. Unfortunately, studies that attempt to confirm an actual decrease in salivary flow rate in diabetic patients have produced conflicting results. Some studies show a decrease in salivary flow; some, no difference from normal; and some, an increased salivary flow rate.

Treatment and Prognosis

For patients with NIDDM, dietary modification may be the only treatment necessary. Usually, this consists of a reduction in the caloric value of the foods consumed, with the goal being weight loss. The dietary changes may need to be coupled with an oral hypoglycemic agent, such as tolbutamide, chlorpropamide, tolazamide, or glyburide. If these modalities do not control the blood glucose levels, treatment with insulin is necessary.

For patients with IDDM, injections of insulin are required to control blood glucose levels. Different types of insulin are marketed, each type having different degrees of duration and times of peak activity. Insulin was previously extracted primarily from beef and pork pancreata. In some patients, however, antibodies developed to this foreign protein and rendered the insulin useless. To overcome this problem, some pharmaceutical companies have developed brands of insulin that have the molecular structure of human insulin. This human insulin is produced by genetically engineered bacteria using recombinant DNA technology.

The patient's schedule of insulin injections must be carefully structured and monitored to provide optimal control of blood glucose levels. This schedule is carefully formulated by the patient's physician and takes into account such factors as the patient's activity level and the severity of the insulin deficiency. It is imperative that adequate dietary carbohydrates be ingested after the administration of the insulin; otherwise, a condition known as *insulin shock* may occur. If carbohydrates are not consumed after an insulin injection, the blood glucose levels may fall to dangerously low levels. The brain is virtually totally dependent on blood glucose as its energy source. If the blood glucose level drops below 40 mg/dL, the patient may go into shock. This condition may be treated by administration of sublingual dextrose paste, intravenous infusion of a dextrose solution, or injection of glucagon.

In summary, diabetes mellitus is a common, complex medical problem with many complications. The prognosis is guarded. Studies suggest that strict control of blood glucose levels results in a slowing of the development of the late complications of IDDM (e.g., blindness, kidney damage, and neuropathy) and reduces the frequency of these complications. Health care practitioners should be aware of the problems these patients may have and should be prepared to deal with them. Consultation with the patient's physician may be necessary, particularly for patients with IDDM who show poor blood glucose control, have active infections, or require extensive oral surgical procedures.

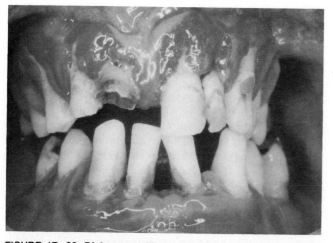

FIGURE 17–32. **Diabetes mellitus.** The diffuse, strikingly erythematous enlargement of the gingival tissues is an oral feature that has been identified in diabetic patients. See Color Plates.

HYPOPHOSPHATASIA

Hypophosphatasia is a rare metabolic bone disease that is thought to be inherited as an autosomal recessive trait. One of the first presenting signs may be the premature loss of the primary teeth, presumably caused by a lack of cementum on the root surfaces. In what probably represents the homozygous form, there are rather severe manifestations, and many of these patients are identified in infancy. The probable heterozygous form of the disease may appear in childhood or even adulthood, with variable degrees of expression. Generally, the younger the age of onset, the more severe the expression of the disease. The common factors in all types include:

- Reduced levels of the bone/liver/kidney isozyme of alkaline phosphatase
- Increased levels of blood and urinary phosphoethanolamine
- Bone abnormalities that resemble rickets

Most authorities believe that the decreased alkaline phosphatase levels probably are responsible for the clinically observed abnormalities. Alkaline phosphatase is thought to play a role in the production of bone, but its precise mechanism of action is unknown.

Clinical and Radiographic Features

Four types of hypophosphatasia are generally recognized, depending on the severity and the age of onset of the symptoms:

- Perinatal
- Infantile
- Childhood
- Adult

Perinatal Hypophosphatasia

The *perinatal* form has the most severe manifestations. It is usually diagnosed at birth, and the infant rarely survives for more than a few hours after birth. Death is due to respiratory failure. Marked hypocalcification of the skeletal structures is observed.

Infantile Hypophosphatasia

Babies affected by *infantile* hypophosphatasia may appear normal up to 6 months of age; after this time, they begin to show a failure to grow. Vomiting and hypotonia may develop as well. Skeletal malformations that suggest rickets are typically observed; these malformations include shortened, bowed limbs. Deformities of the ribs predispose these patients to pneumonia, and skull deformities cause increased intracranial pressure. Nephrocalcinosis and nephrolithiasis also produce problems for these infants. Radiographs show a markedly reduced degree of ossification with a preponderance of hypomineralized osteoid. If these infants survive, premature shedding of the deciduous teeth is often seen.

Childhood Hypophosphatasia

The *childhood* form is usually detected at a later age and has a wide range of clinical expression. One of the more consistent features is the premature loss of the primary teeth without evidence of a significant inflammatory response (Figs. 17–33 and 17–34). The deciduous incisor teeth are usually affected first and may be the only teeth involved. In some patients, this may be the only expression of the disease. The teeth may show enlarged pulp chambers in some instances, and a significant degree of alveolar bone loss may be seen. More severely affected patients may have open fontanels with premature fusion of cranial sutures. This early fusion occasionally leads to increased intracranial pressure and subsequent brain damage. The development of motor skills is often delayed.

Radiographically, the skull has the appearance of "beaten copper," and it shows uniformly spaced, poorly defined, small radiolucencies. This pattern may be due to areas of thinning of the inner cortical plate produced by the cerebral gyri.

Adult Hypophosphatasia

The *adult* form is typically mild. Patients often have a history of premature loss of their primary or permanent dentition, and many of these patients are edentulous. Stress fractures that involve the metatarsal bones of the feet may be a presenting sign of the condition, or an increased number of fractures associated with relatively minor trauma may alert the clinician to this disorder.

Diagnosis

The diagnosis of hypophosphatasia is based on the clinical manifestations as well as the finding of decreased levels of serum alkaline phosphatase and increased amounts of phosphoethanolamine in both the urine and the blood. Interestingly, as some patients grow older, serum alkaline phosphatase levels may approach normal.

Histopathologic Features

The histopathologic evaluation of bone sampled from a patient affected with the *infantile* form of hypophosphatasia shows abundant production of poorly mineralized osteoid. In the *childhood* or *adult* form, the bone may appear relatively normal or it may show an in-

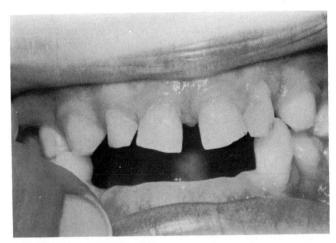

FIGURE 17–33. **Hypophosphatasia.** Premature loss of the mandibular anterior teeth. (Courtesy of Dr. Jim Bevans.)

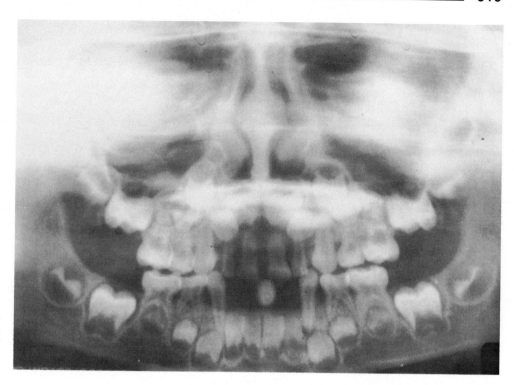

FIGURE 17–34. **Hypophosphatasia.** This panoramic radiograph shows the loss of the mandibular anterior teeth. (Courtesy of Dr. Jackie Banahan.)

creased amount of woven bone, which is a less mature form of osseous tissue.

The histopathologic examination of either a primary or permanent tooth that has been exfoliated from an affected patient often shows an absence or a marked reduction in the amount of cementum that covers the root's surface (Fig. 17–35). This reduced amount of cementum is thought to predispose to tooth loss because of the inability of periodontal ligament fibers to attach to the tooth and to maintain it in its normal position.

Treatment and Prognosis

The treatment of hypophosphatasia is essentially symptomatic because the lack of alkaline phosphatase

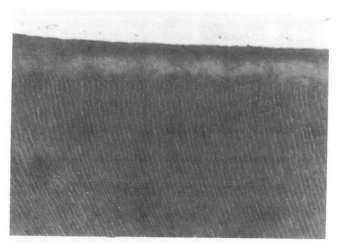

FIGURE 17–35. **Hypophosphatasia.** This medium-power photomicrograph of an exfoliated tooth shows no cementum associated with the root surface.

cannot be corrected. Attempts to treat this condition by infusing alkaline phosphatase have been unsuccessful, presumably because the enzyme functions within the cell rather than in the extracellular environment. Basically, fractures are treated with orthopedic surgery, followed by rehabilitation. Prosthetic appliances are indicated to replace missing teeth, but satisfactory results are not always possible because the alveolar bone is hypoplastic. Patients should also be provided with genetic counseling. As stated earlier, the prognosis varies with the onset of symptoms; the perinatal and infantile types are associated with a rather poor outcome. The adult form is usually compatible with a normal life span.

VITAMIN D–RESISTANT RICKETS
(Hereditary Hypophosphatemia)

After the use of vitamin D to treat rickets became widespread, it was recognized that some individuals with clinical features characteristic of rickets did not seem to respond to therapeutic doses of the vitamin. For this reason, this condition in these patients was called **vitamin D–resistant rickets.** Most cases of this rare condition appear to be inherited as an X-linked trait; therefore, males are affected more often than females. In the United States, this condition occurs at a frequency of 1 in 20,000 births. In addition to the rachitic changes, these patients are also hypophosphatemic and show a decreased capacity for reabsorption of phosphate from the renal tubules. The defect appears to be associated with the 1-alpha-hydroxylase system, which converts the relatively inactive vitamin D precursor, 25-hydroxycholecalciferol (calcifediol) to the active metabolite 1,25-dihydroxycholecalciferol (calcitriol) in the kidney.

Clinical Features

Patients with vitamin D–resistant rickets have a short stature. The upper body segment appears more normal, but the lower body segment is shortened. The lower limbs are generally shortened and bowed.

Laboratory investigation reveals hypophosphatemia with diminished renal reabsorption of phosphate and decreased intestinal absorption of calcium. This typically results in rachitic changes that are unresponsive to vitamin D (calciferol). With aging, ankylosis of the spine frequently develops.

From a dental standpoint, the teeth have large pulp chambers, with pulp horns extending almost to the dentino-enamel junction (Figs. 17–36 and 17–37). With attrition, the cuspal enamel is worn down to the level of the pulp horn, causing pulpal exposure and pulp death. The exposure is often so small that the periapical abscesses and gingival sinus tracts that develop seem to affect what appear to be otherwise normal teeth.

Histopathologic Features

The microscopic examination of an erupted tooth from a patient with vitamin D–resistant rickets usually shows markedly enlarged pulp horns. The dentin appears abnormal and is characterized by the deposition of globular dentin, which often exhibits clefting. The clefts may extend from the pulp chamber to the dentino-enamel

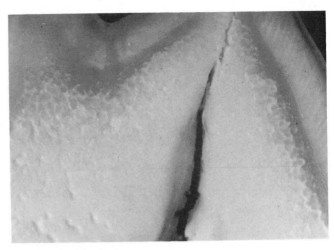

FIGURE 17–37. **Vitamin D–resistant rickets**. Ground section of the same tooth depicted in Figure 17–36. A pulp horn extends to the dentino-enamel junction. (Courtesy of Dr. Carl Witkop.)

junction. The pulp frequently is nonvital, presumably because of the bacterial contamination associated with the dentinal clefts.

Treatment and Prognosis

For a normal stature to develop, patients with vitamin D–resistant rickets usually need early treatment with calcitriol and multiple daily doses of phosphate. Endodontic therapy is necessary for the pulpally involved teeth. Although serum and urine calcium levels must be monitored carefully to prevent nephrocalcinosis with its potential for kidney damage, patients generally have a normal life span.

CROHN'S DISEASE (Regional Ileitis; Regional Enteritis)

Crohn's disease is an inflammatory, probably immunologically mediated, condition of unknown cause that primarily affects the distal portion of the small bowel and the proximal colon. It is now well established that the manifestations of Crohn's disease may be seen anywhere in the gastrointestinal tract, from the mouth to the anus. In addition, other extraintestinal sites, such as the skin, eyes, and joints, have also been identified. The oral lesions are significant because they may precede the gastrointestinal lesions in as many as 30 percent of the cases that have both oral and gastrointestinal involvement. It is interesting that the prevalence of Crohn's disease appears to be increasing for reasons that have not been determined.

Clinical Features

Most patients with Crohn's disease are teen-agers when the disease first becomes evident. Gastrointestinal signs and symptoms usually include abdominal cramping and pain, nausea, and diarrhea, occasionally accom-

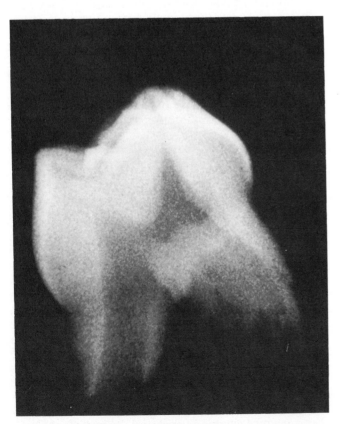

FIGURE 17–36. **Vitamin D–resistant rickets**. This radiograph of an extracted tooth shows a prominent pulp chamber with pulp horns extending out toward the dentino-enamel junction.

panied by fever. Weight loss and malnutrition may develop, which can lead to anemia, decreased growth, and short stature.

A wide range of oral lesions have been clinically reported in Crohn's disease; however, the abnormalities described are relatively nonspecific and may be associated with other conditions that cause **orofacial granulomatosis** (see p. 243). The more prominent findings include diffuse or nodular swelling of the oral and perioral tissues, a cobblestone appearance of the mucosa, and deep, granulomatous-appearing ulcers. The ulcers are often linear and develop in the buccal vestibule (Fig. 17–38). Soft tissue swellings that resemble denture-related fibrous hyperplasia may be seen, although the lesions occur in dentate individuals. Other manifestations that have been reported include metallic dysgeusia and aphthous-like oral ulcerations. The significance of the latter finding is uncertain because aphthous ulcerations are found rather frequently in the general population, including the same age group that is affected by Crohn's disease.

Histopathologic Features

Microscopic examination of tissue obtained from the intestine or from the oral mucosa should show non-necrotizing granulomatous inflammation within the submucosal connective tissue (Fig. 17–39). The severity of the granulomatous inflammation may vary tremendously from patient to patient and from various sites in the same patient. Therefore, a negative biopsy result at any one site and time may not necessarily rule out a diagnosis of Crohn's disease. As with the clinical lesions, the histopathologic pattern is relatively nonspecific, resembling orofacial granulomatosis. Special stains should be performed to rule out the possibility of deep fungal infection, tertiary syphilis, or mycobacterial infection.

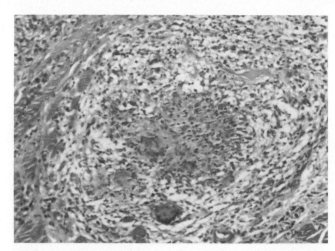

FIGURE 17–39. **Crohn's disease**. This medium-power photomicrograph of an oral lesion shows a non-necrotizing granuloma in the submucosal connective tissue.

Treatment and Prognosis

Most patients with Crohn's disease are initially treated medically with a sulfa-type drug (sulfasalazine), and some patients respond well to this medication. With moderate to severe involvement, systemic prednisone may be used and is often effective. Sometimes the disease cannot be maintained in remission by medical therapy, and complications develop that require surgical intervention. Complications may include bowel obstruction or fistula or abscess formation. If a significant segment of the terminal ileum has been removed surgically or is involved with the disease, injections of vitamin B_{12} may be necessary to prevent megaloblastic anemia secondary to the lack of ability to absorb the vitamin. Similar supplementation of iron and folate may also be required because of malabsorption.

PYOSTOMATITIS VEGETANS

Pyostomatitis vegetans is a relatively rare condition that has a controversial history. It has been associated in the past with diseases such as pemphigus or pyodermatitis vegetans. Most investigators today, however, believe that pyostomatitis vegetans is an unusual oral expression of inflammatory bowel disease, particularly **ulcerative colitis** or **Crohn's disease**. The pathogenesis of the condition, like that of inflammatory bowel disease, is poorly understood.

Clinical Features

Patients with pyostomatitis vegetans exhibit characteristic yellowish, slightly elevated, linear, serpentine pustules set on an erythematous oral mucosa. The lesions primarily affect the buccal and labial mucosa, soft palate, and ventral tongue (Figs. 17–40 [see Color Figure 120] to 17–42). These lesions have been called "snail-track" ulcerations, although in most instances the lesions are probably not truly ulcerated. Oral discomfort is variable

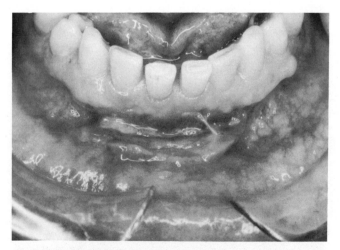

FIGURE 17–38. **Crohn's disease**. This patient has a linear ulceration of the mandibular vestibule. An adhesion between the alveolar and labial mucosae was caused by repeated ulceration and healing of the mucosa at this site.

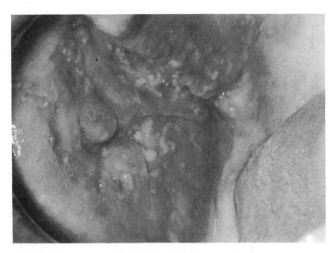

FIGURE 17–40. **Pyostomatitis vegetans**. The characteristic lesions are seen on the buccal mucosa, presenting as yellow-white, "snail-track" pustules. See Color Plates.

but can be surprisingly minimal in some patients. This variation in symptoms may be related to the number of pustules that have ruptured to form ulcerations. The oral lesions may appear concurrently with the bowel symptoms, or they may precede the intestinal involvement.

Histopathologic Features

A biopsy specimen of an oral lesion of pyostomatitis vegetans usually shows marked edema, causing an acantholytic appearance of the involved epithelium. This may be due to the accumulation of numerous eosinophils within the spinous layer, often forming intraepithelial abscesses. Subepithelial eosinophilic abscesses have been reported in some instances. The underlying connective tissue usually supports a dense mixed infiltrate of inflammatory cells that consists of eosinophils, neutrophils, and lymphocytes. Perivascular inflammation may also be present.

Treatment and Prognosis

Usually, the intestinal signs and symptoms of inflammatory bowel disease are of most concern for patients with pyostomatitis vegetans. Medical management of the bowel disease with sulfasalazine or systemic corticosteroids also produces clearing of the oral lesions (Fig. 17–43). Often the oral lesions clear within days after systemic corticosteroid therapy is begun, and they may recur if the medication is withdrawn.

UREMIC STOMATITIS

Patients who have either acute or chronic renal failure typically show markedly elevated levels of urea and other nitrogenous wastes in the blood stream. **Uremic stomatitis** represents a relatively uncommon complication of renal failure. In two series that included 562 patients with renal failure, only eight examples of this oral mucosal condition were documented. Nevertheless, for the

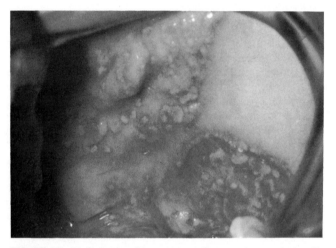

FIGURE 17–41. **Pyostomatitis vegetans**. Same patient as depicted in Figure 17–40 showing similar lesions distributed on the opposite buccal mucosa.

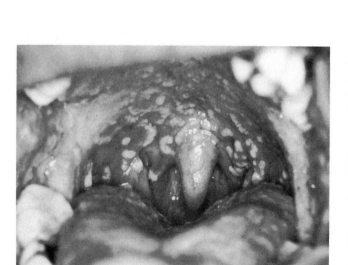

FIGURE 17–42. **Pyostomatitis vegetans**. These characteristic lesions involve the soft palate. (From Neville BW, et al. Pyostomatitis vegetans. Am J Dermatopathol 7:69–77, 1985.)

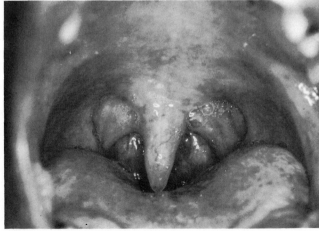

FIGURE 17–43. **Pyostomatitis vegetans**. Same patient as depicted in Figure 17–42 after 5 days of prednisone therapy. (From Neville BW, et al. Pyostomatitis vegetans. Am J Dermatopathol 7:69–77, 1985.)

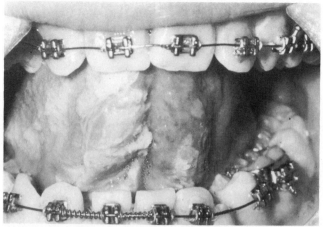

FIGURE 17-44. **Uremic stomatitis**. Ragged white plaques affect the ventral tongue and floor of the mouth. (From Ross WF III, Salisbury PL III. Uremic stomatitis associated with undiagnosed renal failure. Gen Dent 42:410-412, 1994.)

patients in whom uremic stomatitis develops, this can be a painful disorder. The cause of the oral lesions is unclear, but some investigators suggest that urease, an enzyme produced by the oral microflora, may degrade urea secreted in the saliva. This degradation results in the liberation of free ammonia, which damages the oral mucosa.

Clinical Features

Most cases of uremic stomatitis have been reported in patients with acute renal failure. The onset may be abrupt, with painful, white plaques or crusts distributed predominantly on the buccal mucosa, tongue, and floor of the mouth (Fig. 17-44). Patients complain of oral pain or a burning sensation with the lesions, and the clinician may detect an odor of ammonia or urine on the patient's breath.

Treatment and Prognosis

In some instances, uremic stomatitis may clear within a few days after renal dialysis (Fig. 17-45), although

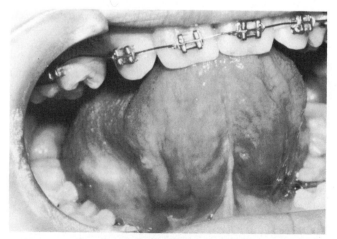

FIGURE 17-45. **Uremic stomatitis**. Same patient as depicted in Figure 17-44 after renal dialysis. (From Ross WF III, Salisbury PL III. Uremic stomatitis associated with undiagnosed renal failure. Gen Dent 42: 410-412, 1994.)

such resolution may take place over 2 to 3 weeks. In other instances, treatment with a mildly acidic mouth rinse, such as diluted hydrogen peroxide, seems to clear the oral lesions. For control of pain while the lesions heal, patients may be given palliative therapy with ice chips or a topical anesthetic, such as viscous lidocaine or dyclonine hydrochloride. Although renal failure itself is life-threatening, at least one example of a uremic plaque that presumably caused a patient's death has been recorded. This event was thought to have been due to the dislodging of the plaque with subsequent obstruction of the patient's airway.

REFERENCES

Mucopolysaccharidosis

Hopwood JJ, Morris CP. The mucopolysaccharidoses: Diagnosis, molecular genetics and treatment. Mol Biol Med 7:381-404, 1990.

Kinirons MJ, Nelson J. Dental findings in mucopolysaccharidosis type IV A (Morquio's disease type A). Oral Surg Oral Med Oral Pathol 70:176-179, 1990.

Nakamura T, et al. Rosette formation of impacted molar teeth in mucopolysaccharidoses and related disorders. Dentomaxillofac Radiol 21:45-49, 1992.

Nussbaum BL. Dentistry for the at-risk patient—mucopolysaccharidosis III (Sanfilippo syndrome): A nine-year case study. ASDC J Dent Child 57:466-469, 1990.

Lipid Reticuloendothelioses

Barton NW, et al. Replacement therapy for inherited enzyme deficiency—macrophage-targeted glucocerebrosidase for Gaucher's disease. N Engl J Med 324:1464-1470, 1991.

Beutler E. Gaucher disease. Blood Rev 2:59-70, 1988.

Beutler E, et al. Gaucher disease: Gene frequencies in the Ashkenazi Jewish population. Am J Hum Genet 52:85-88, 1993.

Blitzer MG, McDowell GA. Tay-Sachs disease as a model for screening inborn errors. Clin Lab Med 12:463-479, 1992.

Elleder M. Niemann-Pick disease. Pathol Res Pract 185:293-328, 1989.

Frenkel EP. Southwestern Internal Medicine Conference: Gaucher disease: A heterogeneous clinical complex for which effective enzyme replacement has come of age. Am J Med Sci 305:331-344, 1993.

Gravel RA, Triggs-Raine BL, Mahuran DJ. Biochemistry and genetics of Tay-Sachs disease. Can J Neurol Sci 18:419-423, 1991.

Levran O, Desnick RJ, Schuchman EH. Niemann-Pick disease: A frequent missense mutation in the acid sphingomyelinase gene of Ashkenazi Jewish type A and B patients. Proc Natl Acad Sci U S A 88:3748-3752, 1991.

Lustmann J, et al. Gaucher's disease affecting the mandible and maxilla: Report of a case. Int J Oral Maxillofac Surg 20:7-8, 1991.

Mankin HJ. Gaucher's disease: A novel treatment and an important breakthrough. J Bone Joint Surg (Br) 75-B:2-3, 1993.

Shiran A, et al. Increased risk of cancer in patients with Gaucher disease. Cancer 72:219-224, 1993.

Zevin S, et al. Adult-type Gaucher disease in children: Genetics, clinical features and enzyme replacement therapy. Q J Med 86:565-573, 1993.

Lipoid Proteinosis

Fleischmajer R, et al. Ultrastructure and composition of connective tissue in hyalinosis cutis et mucosae skin. J Invest Dermatol 82:252-258, 1984.

Konstantinov K, et al. Lipoid proteinosis. J Am Acad Dermatol 27:293-297, 1992.

Moy LS, et al. Lipoid proteinosis: Ultrastructural and biochemical studies. J Am Acad Dermatol 16:1193-1201, 1987.

Pierard GE, et al. A clinicopathologic study of six cases of lipoid proteinosis. Am J Dermatopathol 10:300-305, 1988.

Jaundice

Gordon SC. Jaundice and cholestasis. Postgrad Med 90:65–71, 1991.

Isselbacher KJ. Jaundice and hepatomegaly. *In*: Harrison's Principles of Internal Medicine, 12th ed. Edited by Wilson JD, et al. New York, McGraw-Hill, 1991, pp 264–269.

McKnight JT, Jones JE. Jaundice. Am Fam Physician 45:1139–1148, 1992.

Murtagh J. Jaundice. Austr Fam Physician 20:457–466, 1991.

Amyloidosis

Breathnach SM. Amyloid and amyloidosis. J Am Acad Dermatol 18:1–16, 1988.

Cohen AS, Connors LH. The pathogenesis and biochemistry of amyloidosis. J Pathol 151:1–10, 1987.

Cohen AS, Jones LA. Amyloidosis. Curr Opin Rheumatol 3:125–138, 1991.

Hachulla E, et al. Labial salivary gland biopsy as a reliable test for the diagnosis of primary and secondary amyloidosis: A prospective clinical and immunohistologic study in 59 patients. Arthritis Rheum 36:691–697, 1993.

Hawkins PN. Amyloidosis. Blood Rev 2:270–280, 1988.

Husby G. Nomenclature and classification of amyloid and amyloidoses. J Intern Med 232:511–512, 1992.

Johansson I, et al. Salivary hypofunction in patients with familial amyloidotic polyneuropathy. Oral Surg Oral Med Oral Pathol 74:742–748, 1992.

Raymond AK, Sneige N, Batsakis JG. Amyloidosis in the upper aerodigestive tracts. Ann Otol Rhinol Laryngol 101:794–796, 1992.

Vitamin Deficiency

Wilson JD. Vitamin deficiency and excess. *In*: Harrison's Principles of Internal Medicine, 12th ed. Edited by Wilson JD, et al. New York, McGraw-Hill, 1991, pp 434–442.

Iron-Deficiency Anemia

Brigden ML. Iron deficiency anemia: Every case is instructive. Postgrad Med 93:181–192, 1993.

Brown RG. Normocytic and macrocytic anemias. Postgrad Med 89:125–136, 1991.

Brown RG. Determining the cause of anemia. Postgrad Med 89:161–170, 1991.

Massey AC. Microcytic anemia. Differential diagnosis and management of iron deficiency anemia. Med Clin North Am 76:549–566, 1992.

Plummer-Vinson Syndrome

Bredenkamp JK, Castro DJ, Mickel RA. Importance of iron repletion in the management of Plummer-Vinson syndrome. Ann Otol Rhinol Laryngol 99:51–54, 1990.

Dantas RO, Villanova MG. Esophageal motility impairment in Plummer-Vinson syndrome: Correction by iron treatment. Dig Dis Sci 38:968–971, 1993.

Geerlings SE, Statius van Eps LW. Pathogenesis and consequences of Plummer-Vinson syndrome. Clin Invest 70:629–630, 1992.

Nagai T, Susami E, Ebihara T. Plummer-Vinson syndrome complicated by gastric cancer: A case report. Keio J Med 39:106–111, 1990.

Seitz ML, Sabatino D. Plummer-Vinson syndrome in an adolescent. J Adolesc Health 12:279–281, 1991.

Pernicious Anemia

Akinyanju OO, Okany CC. Pernicious anaemia in Africans. Clin Lab Haematol 14:33–40, 1992.

Colon-Otero G, Menke D, Hook CC. A practical approach to the differential diagnosis and evaluation of the adult patient with macrocytic anemia. Med Clin North Am 76:581–596, 1992.

Drummond JF, White DK, Damm DD. Megaloblastic anemia with oral lesions: A consequence of gastric bypass surgery. Oral Surg Oral Med Oral Pathol 59:149–153, 1985.

Greenberg M. Clinical and histologic changes of the oral mucosa in pernicious anemia. Oral Surg Oral Med Oral Pathol 52:38–42, 1981.

Hsing AW, et al. Pernicious anemia and subsequent cancer: A population-based cohort study. Cancer 71:745–750, 1993.

Loffeld BCAJ, van Spreeuwel JP. The gastrointestinal tract in pernicious anemia. Dig Dis 9:70–77, 1991.

Pituitary Dwarfism

Duck SC, et al. Subcutaneous growth hormone-releasing hormone therapy in growth hormone-deficient children: First year of therapy. J Clin Endocrinol Metab 75:1115–1120, 1992.

Kosowicz J, Rzymski K. Abnormalities of tooth development in pituitary dwarfism. Oral Surg Oral Med Oral Pathol 44:853–863, 1977.

Underwood LE, Van Wyk JJ. Normal and aberrant growth. *In*: Williams Textbook of Endocrinology. Edited by Wilson JD, Foster DW. Philadelphia, WB Saunders, 1992, pp 1079–1125.

Gigantism

Daughaday WH. Pituitary gigantism. Endocrinol Metab Clin North Am 21:633–647, 1992.

Underwood LE, Van Wyk JJ. Normal and aberrant growth. *In*: Williams Textbook of Endocrinology. Edited by Wilson JD, Foster DW. Philadelphia, WB Saunders, 1992, pp 1125–1127.

Acromegaly

Bates AS, et al. An audit of outcome of treatment in acromegaly. Q J Med 86:293–299, 1993.

Chew FS. Radiologic manifestations in the musculoskeletal system of miscellaneous endocrine disorders. Radiol Clin North Am 29:135–147, 1991.

Clayton RN. Modern management of acromegaly. Q J Med 86:285–287, 1993.

Cohen RB, Wilcox CW. A case of acromegaly identified after patient complaint of apertognathia. Oral Surg Oral Med Oral Pathol 75:583–586, 1993.

Frohman LA. Therapeutic options in acromegaly. J Clin Endocrinol Metab 72:1175–1181, 1991.

Molitch ME. Clinical manifestations of acromegaly. Endocrinol Metab Clin North Am 21:597–614, 1992.

Ron E, et al. Acromegaly and gastrointestinal cancer. Cancer 68:1673–1677, 1991.

Hypothyroidism

Constine LS, et al. Hypothalamic-pituitary dysfunction after radiation for brain tumors. N Engl J Med 328:87–94, 1993.

Larsen PR. Hypothyroidism and myxedema. *In*: Cecil Textbook of Medicine. Edited by Wyngaarden JB, Smith LH Jr, Bennett JC. Philadelphia, WB Saunders, 1992, pp 1260–1263.

Martinez M, Derksen D, Kapsner P. Making sense of hypothyroidism. Postgrad Med 93:135–145, 1993.

Mg'ang'a PM, Chindia ML. Dental and skeletal changes in juvenile hypothyroidism following treatment: Case report. Odonto-Stomatologie Tropicale 13:25–27, 1990.

Hyperthyroidism

Bahn RS, Heufelder AE. Pathogenesis of Graves' ophthalmopathy. N Engl J Med 329:1468–1475, 1993.

Caruso DR, Mazzaferri EL. Intervention in Graves' disease. Postgrad Med 92:117–134, 1992.

Davies TF. Graves' disease and its retroorbital aspects. Mt Sinai J Med 59:326–334, 1992.

Larsen PR. Graves' disease and other causes of hyperthyroidism. *In*: Cecil Textbook of Medicine. Edited by Wyngaarden JB, Smith LH Jr, Bennett JC. Philadelphia, WB Saunders, 1992, pp 1254–1260.

Perusse R, Goulet J-P, Turcotte J-Y. Contraindications to vasoconstrictors in dentistry: Part II: Hyperthyroidism, diabetes, sulfite sensitivity, cortico-dependent asthma, and pheochromocytoma. Oral Surg Oral Med Oral Pathol 74:687–691, 1992.

Hypoparathyroidism

Ahonen P, et al. Clinical variation of autoimmune polyendocrinopathy-candidiasis-ectodermal dystrophy (APECED) in a series of 68 patients. N Engl J Med 322:1829–1836, 1990.

Greenberg MS, et al. Idiopathic hypoparathyroidism, chronic candidiasis, and dental hypoplasia. Oral Surg Oral Med Oral Pathol 28:42–53, 1969.

Spiegel AM. Hypoparathyroidism. *In*: Cecil Textbook of Medicine. Edited by Wyngaarden JB, Smith LH Jr, Bennett JC. Philadelphia, WB Saunders, 1992, pp 1419–1420.

Walls AWG, Soames JV. Dental manifestations of autoimmune hypoparathyroidism. Oral Surg Oral Med Oral Pathol 75:452–445, 1993.

Pseudohypoparathyroidism

Brown MD, Aaron G. Pseudohypoparathyroidism: Case report. Pediatr Dent 13:106–109, 1991.

Faull CM, et al. Pseudohypoparathyroidism: Its phenotypic variability and associated disorders in a large family. Q J Med 78:251–264, 1991.

Potts JT. Diseases of the parathyroid gland and other hyper- and hypocalcemic disorders. *In*: Harrison's Principles of Internal Medicine, 12th ed. Edited by Wilson JD, et al. New York, McGraw-Hill, 1991, pp 1918–1919.

Hyperparathyroidism

Åkerström G, et al. Primary hyperparathyroidism: Aspects on pathophysiology, symptoms, and treatment. Surg Annu 23:133–155, 1991.

Deftos LJ, Parthemore JG, Stabile BE. Management of primary hyperparathyroidism. Annu Rev Med 44:19–26, 1993.

Hayes CW, Conway WF. Hyperparathyroidism. Radiol Clin North Am 29:85–96, 1991.

Mowschenson PM, Silen W. Developments in hyperparathyroidism. Curr Opin Oncol 2:95–100, 1990.

Silverman S Jr, et al. The dental structures in primary hyperparathyroidism. Studies in forty-two consecutive patients. Oral Surg Oral Med Oral Pathol 15:426–436, 1962.

Silverman S Jr, Ware WH, Gillooly C. Dental aspects of hyperparathyroidism. Oral Surg Oral Med Oral Pathol 26:184–189, 1968.

Solt DB. The pathogenesis, oral manifestations, and implications for dentistry of metabolic bone disease. Curr Opin Dent 1:783–791, 1991.

Cushing's Disease

Gabrilove JL. Cushing's syndrome. Compr Ther 18:13–16, 1992.

Tyrrell JB. Cushing's syndrome. *In*: Cecil Textbook of Medicine. Edited by Wyngaarden JB, Smith LH Jr, Bennett JC. Philadelphia, WB Saunders, 1992, pp 1284–1287.

Addison's Disease

Davenport J, et al. Addison's disease. Am Fam Physician 43:1338–1342, 1991.

Porter SR, et al. Chronic candidiasis, enamel hypoplasia, and pigmentary anomalies. Oral Surg Oral Med Oral Pathol 74:312–314, 1992.

Tyrrell JB. Adrenocortical hypofunction. *In*: Cecil Textbook of Medicine. Edited by Wyngaarden JB, Smith LH Jr, Bennett JC. Philadelphia, WB Saunders, 1992, pp 1281–1284.

Werbel, SS, Ober KP. Acute adrenal insufficiency. Endocrinol Metab Clin North Am 22:303–328, 1993.

Ziccardi VB, et al. Precipitation of an addisonian crisis during dental surgery: Recognition and management. Compend Contin Educ Dent 13:518–523, 1992.

Diabetes Mellitus

Cherry-Peppers G, Ship JA. Oral health in patients with type II diabetes and impaired glucose tolerance. Diabetes Care 16:638–641, 1993.

Cianciola LJ, et al. Prevalence of periodontal disease in insulin-dependent diabetes mellitus (juvenile diabetes). J Am Dent Assoc 104:653–660, 1982.

Geiss LS, et al. Surveillance for diabetes mellitus—United States, 1980–1989. MMWR Morb Mortal Wkly Rep 42:1–20, 1993.

Groop LC, et al. Association between polymorphism of the glycogen synthase gene and non-insulin-dependent diabetes mellitus. N Engl J Med 328:10–14, 1993.

Holdren RS, Patton LL. Oral conditions associated with diabetes mellitus. Diabetes Spectrum 6:11–17, 1993.

Lamey P-J, Darwazeh AMG, Frier BM. Oral disorders associated with diabetes mellitus. Diabetic Med 9:410–416, 1992.

Murrah VA. Diabetes mellitus and associated oral manifestations: A review. J Oral Pathol 14:271–281, 1985.

Nathan DM, et al. The effect of intensive treatment of diabetes on the development and progression of long-term complications in insulin-dependent diabetes mellitus. N Engl J Med 329:977–986, 1993.

Olefsky JM. Diabetes mellitus. *In*: Cecil Textbook of Medicine. Edited by Wyngaarden JB, Smith LH Jr, Bennett JC. Philadelphia, WB Saunders, 1992, pp 1291–1301.

Seppälä B, Seppälä M, Ainamo J. A longitudinal study on insulin-dependent diabetes mellitus and periodontal disease. J Clin Periodontol 20:161–165, 1993.

Smith RBW. Insulin dependent diabetes mellitus. N Z Med J 105:433–443, 1992.

Wang PH, Lau J, Chalmers TC. Meta-analysis of effects of intensive blood-glucose control on late complications of type I diabetes. Lancet 341:1306–1309, 1993.

Watanabe K. Prepubertal periodontitis: A review of diagnostic criteria, pathogenesis, and differential diagnosis. J Periodontal Res 25:31–48, 1990.

Wysocki GP, Daley T. Benign migratory glossitis in patients with juvenile diabetes. Oral Surg Oral Med Oral Pathol 63:68–70, 1987.

Zachariasen RD. Diabetes mellitus and xerostomia. Compend Contin Educ Dent 13:314–322, 1992.

Hypophosphatasia

Brenton DP, Krywawych S. Hypophosphatasia. Clin Rheum Dis 12:771–789, 1986.

Caswell AM, Whyte MP, Russell RGG. Hypophosphatasia and the extracellular metabolism of inorganic pyrophosphate: Clinical and laboratory aspects. Crit Rev Clin Lab Sci 28:175–232, 1991.

Chappie ILC, et al. Hypophosphatasia: A family study involving a case diagnosed from gingival crevicular fluid. J Oral Pathol Med 21:426–431, 1992.

El-Labban NG, Lee KW, Rule D. Permanent teeth in hypophosphatasia: Light and electron microscopic study. J Oral Pathol Med 20:352–360, 1991.

Fallon MD, et al. Hypophosphatasia: Clinicopathologic comparison of the infantile, childhood, and adult forms. Medicine 63:12–24, 1984.

Nangaku M, et al. Hypophosphatasia in an adult: A case report. Jpn J Med 30:47–52, 1991.

Vitamin D–Resistant Rickets

Archard HO, Witkop CJ. Hereditary hypophosphatemia (vitamin D-resistant rickets) presenting primary dental manifestations. Oral Surg Oral Med Oral Pathol 22:184–193, 1966.

Fadavi S, Rowold E. Familial hypophosphatemic vitamin D-resistant rickets: Review of the literature and report of case. ASDC J Dent Child 57:212–215, 1990.

Hanna JD, Niimi K, Chan JCM. X-linked hypophosphatemia: Genetic and clinical correlates. Am J Dis Child 145:865–870, 1991.

Scriver CR, Tenenhouse HS, Glorieux FH. X-linked hypophosphatemia: An appreciation of a classic paper and a survey of progress since 1958. Medicine (Baltimore) 70:218–228, 1991.

Crohn's Disease

Estrin HM, Hughes RW Jr. Oral manifestations in Crohn's disease: Report of a case. Am J Gastroenterol 80:352–354, 1985.

Farmer RG. Inflammatory bowel disease. *In*: Clinical Gastroenterology, 2nd ed. Edited by Achkar E, Farmer RG, Fleshler B. Philadelphia, Lea and Febiger, 1992, pp 337–348.

Frankel DH, Mostofi R, Lorincz AL. Oral Crohn's disease: Report of two cases in brothers with metallic dysgeusia and a review of the literature. J Am Acad Dermatol 12:260–268, 1985.

Plauth M, Jenss H, Meyle J. Oral manifestations of Crohn's disease: An analysis of 79 cases. J Clin Gastroenterol 13:29–37, 1991.

Rogers AI, Coelho-Borges S. Medical therapy in Crohn's disease. Postgrad Med 92:169–186, 1992.

Scully C, et al. Crohn's disease of the mouth: An indicator of intestinal involvement. Gut 23:198–201, 1982.

Pyostomatitis Vegetans

Ballo FS, Camisa C, Allen CM. Pyostomatitis vegetans: Report of a case and review of the literature. J Am Acad Dermatol 21:381–387, 1989.

Chan SWY, et al. Pyostomatitis vegetans: Oral manifestations of ulcerative colitis. Oral Surg Oral Med Oral Pathol 72:689–692, 1991.

Ficarra G, et al. Oral Crohn's disease and pyostomatitis vegetans: An unusual association. Oral Surg Oral Med Oral Pathol 75:220–224, 1993.

Neville BW, et al. Pyostomatitis vegetans. Am J Dermatopathol 7:69–77, 1985.

Thornhill MH, Zakrzewska JM, Gilkes JJH. Pyostomatitis vegetans: Report of three cases and review of the literature. J Oral Pathol Med 21:128–133, 1992.

VanHale HM, et al. Pyostomatitis vegetans: A reactive mucosal marker for inflammatory disease of the gut. Arch Dermatol 121:94–98, 1985.

Uremic Stomatitis

Halazonetis J, Harley A. Uremic stomatitis: Report of a case. Oral Surg Oral Med Oral Pathol 23:573–577, 1967.

Hovinga J, Roodvoets AP, Gaillard J. Some findings in patients with uraemic stomatitis. J Maxillofac Surg 3:124–127, 1975.

Larato DC. Uremic stomatitis: Report of a case. J Periodontol 46:731–733, 1975.

18

Facial Pain and Neuromuscular Diseases

BELL'S PALSY (Seventh Nerve Paralysis; Facial Paralysis)

Bell's palsy is an acute, unilateral paralysis of the facial musculature with no proven cause, although there is some speculation that it is associated with an abnormal immune response to reactivated herpes simplex virus (type I) in the geniculate ganglion. There is an unexplained seasonal variation; more cases are diagnosed in the spring and fall than in the summer and winter. Familial occurrences have been reported.

The disease can be triggered by a variety of events, including:

- Exposure to cold
- Local and systemic infections
- Tooth extraction
- Trauma or surgery to the seventh cranial nerve
- Ischemia of the nerve near the stylomastoid foramen

Additional manifestations in other sites are occasionally noted, usually in association with the **Melkersson-Rosenthal syndrome** (see p. 243), but also in **Lyme borreliosis** (Lyme peripheral facial palsy).

Clinical Features

People of all ages are susceptible to Bell's palsy, but middle-aged people are most frequently affected. Women are more often affected than men, and there is considerable variation in the severity of signs and symptoms.

The palsy is characterized by an abrupt loss of muscular control on one side of the face, resulting in an inability to smile, close the eye, wink, or raise the eyebrow on the affected side (Fig. 18–1). A few patients suffer from a prodromal pain of the affected side before the onset of paralysis. The paralysis may take several hours to become complete, but patients frequently awaken in the morning with a full-blown case.

The corner of the mouth usually droops, causing saliva to drool onto the skin. The eye usually waters, probably as a result of the inability to close the eyelid properly. There is also a mask-like appearance to the facial features on the affected side, and speech becomes slurred. Occasional patients experience a loss or alteration of taste.

Treatment and Prognosis

There is no effective treatment for Bell's palsy, although some patients have been helped by the use of histamine or other vasodilator medications. Topical ocular antibiotics may be required to prevent corneal ulceration in patients who cannot adequately close their eyelid.

Symptoms usually begin to slowly regress spontaneously within 1 to 2 months of onset; more severe cases take longer. Residual symptoms that remain after 1 year probably will remain indefinitely, and patients with dysfunctional taste that lasts more than 2 to 3 weeks are likely to retain symptoms longer than others. Recurrences are rare, except in Melkersson-Rosenthal syn-

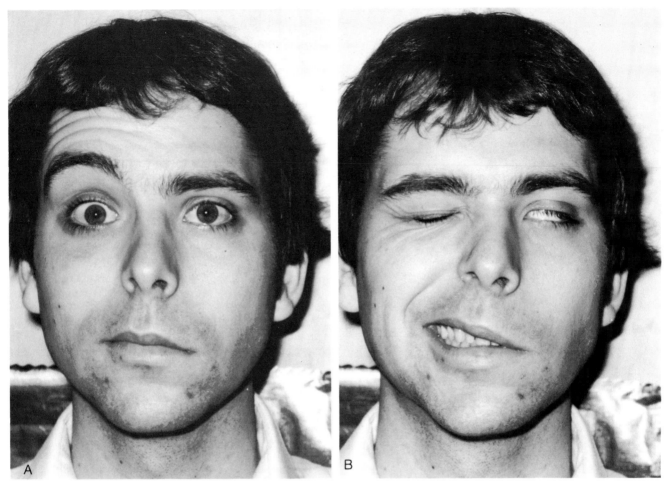

FIGURE 18–1. **Bell's palsy.** There is paralysis of the facial muscles on the patient's left side. In photograph A, the patient is trying to raise his eyebrows; in photograph B, he is attempting to close his eyes and make a smile. (Courtesy of Dr. Bruce B. Brehm.)

drome, but when they occur, the symptoms usually are no more severe than are those of the first attack.

TRIGEMINAL NEURALGIA (Tic Douloureux; Idiopathic Trigeminal Neuralgia)

Among the group of patients suffering from chronic facial pain is a subgroup for whom no cause can be found for the pain. These patients have no identifiable dental ailment (e.g., abscess or cracked tooth), head and neck tumor, injury, malformation of nerves, or infection, yet their pain exists. The term **neuralgia** is used for such unexplained peripheral nerve pain, and the head and neck area is one of the most common sites for such neuralgias (Table 18–1). Because facial neuralgias produce pain that often mimics pain of dental origin, the dental profession is frequently called on to rule out odontogenic or inflammatory causes.

Trigeminal neuralgia is by far the most frequently diagnosed form of neuralgia, annually afflicting more than 10,000 persons in the United States (4 in 100,000

persons each year). The disease is usually idiopathic, but occasional patients have intracranial tumors or vascular malformations that impinge on the nerve. Trigeminal neuralgia is usually an isolated disease; however, 4 percent of persons with the demyelinating disease **multiple sclerosis** have trigeminal neuralgia, and patients with **neuralgia-inducing cavitational osteonecrosis** (NICO) of the jaws (see p. 631) may have a pain so similar as to be indistinguishable from trigeminal neuralgia.

Table 18–1. TYPES OF FACIAL AND CERVICAL NEURALGIAS

Trigeminal neuralgia, idiopathic
Paratrigeminal neuralgia of Raeder
Idiopathic facial pain or neuralgia
Postherpetic facial neuralgia
Migrainous neuralgia
Vagoglossopharyngeal neuralgia
Superior laryngeal neuralgia
Geniculate neuralgia
Sphenopalatine ganglion neuralgia
Occipital neuralgia

Clinical Features

Trigeminal neuralgia characteristically affects individuals older than 40 years of age, although it may affect patients as young as 15. Women are affected slightly more often than men, and the right side is involved more often than the left. Although any branch of the trigeminal nerve may be involved, the ophthalmic division is affected in only 5 percent of cases. In 15 percent of patients, more than one branch is affected; 5 percent have bilateral involvement, although usually not at the same time.

The diagnosis necessitates that specific and strict criteria be met in each patient:

1. The onset of a pain "attack" is abrupt, often initiated by a light touch to a specific and constant trigger point.
2. The pain is extreme, paroxysmal, and lancinating.
3. The duration of a single pain "spasm" is less than 60 seconds, although the overall attack may consist of numerous repeating spasms of short duration.
4. For several minutes after an attack (the "refractory period"), additional attacks usually cannot be brought on by touching the trigger point.
5. The pain must be limited to the known distribution of one or more branches of the trigeminal nerve with no motor or sensory deficit in the affected area.
6. The pain is dramatically diminished, at least initially, with the use of carbamazepine.
7. Spontaneous remissions occur, often lasting more than 6 months, especially during the early phase of the disease.

If the pain pattern does not meet these criteria, a different diagnosis should be considered. When these criteria are not completely fulfilled, yet no other specific diagnosis fits the pattern, the pattern is usually designated by one of several allied terms, such as **atypical trigeminal neuralgia**, **atypical facial pain**, or **atypical facial neuralgia**.

In the early stages, the pain is rather mild and is described by the patient as a "twinge," dull ache, or burning sensation. There are long refractory periods of painlessness between painful attacks. With time, the attacks occur at more frequent intervals and the pain becomes much more severe. Patients may say that it is "like a lightning bolt" or a "hot ice pick jabbed into the face."

Although individual pains or pain spasms last only a few seconds, several of them may follow each other for up to 30 minutes of rapidly repeating volleys. Patients may clutch at the face and experience spasmodic contractions of the facial muscles during attacks, a feature that long ago led to the use of the term **tic douloureux** ("painful jerking") for this disease.

When a trigger zone is present, there are no visible distinguishing features. An attack may be brought on by a minimal stimulus, such as a strong breeze or a touch as light as a feather. The pain usually occurs immediately on stimulation of the trigger point, but it may begin as much as 60 seconds afterward. Trigger points are most frequently found on the nasolabial fold, the vermilion border of the lip, or the mid-facial and periorbital skin.

Intraoral trigger points are thought to be rare, but alveolar locations have been reported. Most investigators have not thoroughly evaluated the mouth for such points. The trigger points and the pain itself are so precisely localized in this disease that their arrest by local anesthetic blocking agents is considered to be diagnostic.

Histopathologic Features

There is no unique histopathologic characteristic to the nerves in trigeminal neuralgia, although the trigger points may show fibrosis and infiltration by small numbers of chronic inflammatory cells. Focal areas of myelin degeneration have been noted within the gasserian ganglia of a few patients whose specimens were examined by electron microscopy.

Treatment and Prognosis

The treatment of a patient with trigeminal neuralgia is varied and often unsuccessful. Injection of the nerve or the gasserian ganglion with irritating or caustic substances, such as alcohol or glycerin, has been tried with limited success, as has peripheral neurectomy. Anticonvulsant medications, such as phenytoin, are effective in many mild or early cases, but their effectiveness diminishes over time. More severe cases are often relieved by carbamazepine, but this drug may produce severe side effects and may not be tolerated indefinitely. The pain returns upon discontinuance of the medication.

Various neurosurgical procedures have also been effective in severe cases, for example:

- Severing the trigeminal sensory roots
- Microsurgical decompression of the trigeminal nerve found to be impinged on by a bony protuberance or a blood vessel
- Selective destruction of the sensory fibers of the nerve by crushing or by the application of heat (radiofrequency rhizotomy)

Most neurosurgical methods provide relief that averages 2 to 3 years for approximately two thirds of treated patients. Repeated surgical procedures are often necessary, however, and techniques that deliberately damage neural tissues leave the patient with a sensory deficit of the face, mouth, or both. After surgery, a patient may rarely have a combination of anesthesia and spontaneous pain of the facial skin (**anesthesia dolorosa**).

Because of the variable response to these treatment modalities, management of the patient with trigeminal neuralgia is difficult. Moreover, the seriousness of the disorder is underscored by the fact that some affected individuals resort to suicide as an escape from their pain.

GLOSSOPHARYNGEAL NEURALGIA
(Vagoglossopharyngeal Neuralgia)

Neuralgia of the ninth cranial nerve is similar in every way to trigeminal neuralgia except in the anatomic location of the pain. **Glossopharyngeal neuralgia** is a rare disease that occurs only once for every 100 cases of trigeminal neuralgia. The pain also may affect sensory areas supplied by the pharyngeal and auricular branches of the vagus nerve. As with trigeminal neuralgia, the cause is unknown.

Clinical Features

The age of onset for glossopharyngeal neuralgia is variable, from 15 to 85 years, but most cases arise after 40 years of age. There is no gender predilection, and fewer than 1 percent of affected persons have bilateral involvement.

The episodic pain in this neuralgia is sharp, intense, and lancinating. There is an abrupt onset and a short duration (30 to 60-second bursts that may repeat for 5 to 30 minutes). The pain may be precipitated by talking, chewing, swallowing, yawning, or touching a blunt instrument to the tonsil on the affected side, but a definite trigger zone is difficult to identify. The paroxysmal pain may be felt in the ear, infra-auricular area, tonsil, base of the tongue, posterior mandible, or lateral wall of the pharynx; however, the patient may have difficulty localizing the pain in the oropharynx. Because the pain is related to jaw movement, it may be difficult to differentiate it from that of temporomandibular joint dysfunction. Occasionally, the pain is only felt deeply in the ear (**tympanic plexus neuralgia**).

Patients frequently point to the neck immediately below the angle of the mandible as the site of greatest pain, but trigger points are not found on the external skin, except within the ear canal. The application of a topical anesthetic agent to the tonsillar fossa or external ear canal may be helpful in the diagnosis because it temporarily eliminates the triggering response. Rarely, syncope, seizures, arrhythmia, or cardiac arrest may accompany the paroxysmal pain, as may coughing or excessive salivation.

Histopathologic Features

Glossopharyngeal neuralgia is not usually associated with a recognizable histopathologic lesion. However, in occasional cases an intracranial or nasopharyngeal vascular malformation or neoplasm may irritate or place undue pressure on the glossopharyngeal nerve.

Treatment and Prognosis

About 80 percent of patients with glossopharyngeal neuralgia experience immediate pain relief when a topical anesthetic agent is applied to the tonsil and pharynx on the side of the pain. Because this relief lasts only 60 to 90 minutes, it is used more as a diagnostic tool and emergency measure than a long-term treatment. Repeated applications to a trigger zone for 2 or 3 days may extend the pain-free episode enough to allow the patient to obtain much needed rest and nutrition. Carbamazepine, phenytoin, or baclofen along with resection of the glossopharyngeal nerve may relieve the neuralgic pain

for a long period, but no therapy is considered to be uniformly effective or even adequate.

As in trigeminal neuralgia, this disease is subject to unpredictable remissions and recurrences. It is not unusual during the early years of the disease for remissions to last more than 6 months. Painful episodes are of varying severity but become generally more severe and frequent with time.

ATYPICAL FACIAL PAIN (Atypical Facial Neuralgia; Idiopathic Facial Pain; Atypical Trigeminal Neuralgia; Trigeminal Neuropathy)

Atypical facial pain describes a group of conditions characterized by vague, deep, poorly localized pain of the head and neck region. The use of this term as a diagnosis implies that identifiable causes of pain, such as other facial neuralgias, dental inflammation and trauma, sinus or parasinus inflammation, and tumors, have been ruled out. This is such a difficult diagnostic and therapeutic condition that patients travel from one health professional to another and receive many different diagnoses and treatments in a frustrated attempt to find relief. Patients sometimes have been described as being neurotic and obsessive-compulsive or anxious and depressed, with "little insight." Whether this is true or not, the strong emotional overtones of this condition make it difficult to distinguish functional (psychogenic) from organic pain.

Clinical Features

Atypical facial neuralgia or pain affects women more frequently than men and usually manifests itself during the third through sixth decades of life. The pain can be distinguished from trigeminal neuralgia by the following:

- Its continuous nature
- Its lack of paroxysm
- Its poor response to carbamazepine
- Its lack of trigger points
- Its nonanatomic distribution

The pain may be limited to a specific area of the face or alveolar arch but frequently is described as spreading toward the temples, the neck, or the occipital area. Patients have great difficulty describing the pain itself, but it may be represented as a deep, gnawing ache; an intense burning sensation; a pressure; or a sharp, lancinating pain. Bilateral involvement has been reported.

Periodic remissions are uncommon, and symptoms tend to become gradually more intense over time. Patients are irritable and fatigued because the pain keeps them awake at night, and most become depressed because of the constancy of the pain. One of the more constant features, and one that leads many clinicians to assume that they are dealing with a psychosomatic disease, is a remarkable lack of discomfort when the patient is distracted. Similarly, when asked to rate the degree of pain on a scale from 1 to 10, with 10 being the most severe pain imaginable, these patients often calmly state "9 or 10" and appear to be in no distress.

Treatment and Prognosis

Surgical intervention is not beneficial to patients with atypical facial pain. Patients are not benefited substantially by the drugs used for trigeminal neuralgia, such as carbamazepine and phenobarbital. Narcotic medications are generally ineffective. Clinicians instead concentrate on psychotherapy, behavior modification, and antidepressants to help patients to live with their pain. Although occasional cases of spontaneous remission are noted, most patients obtain little relief over time.

NEURALGIA-INDUCING CAVITATIONAL OSTEONECROSIS (NICO; Ratner Bone Cavity; Alveolar Cavitational Osteopathy; Roberts Bone Cavity)

A low-grade, non-suppurative, radiographically "invisible" osteomyelitis of the jaws has been described in at least some patients diagnosed with atypical facial pain or trigeminal neuralgia. Such jaw lesions have been reported under a number of different names, most recently **neuralgia-inducing cavitational osteonecrosis** (NICO).

The intraosseous NICO lesion closely resembles ischemic or aseptic necrosis of the long bones in its histopathologic and clinical presentations and, therefore, may result from poor vascular circulation of the bone marrow of the jaws. The cause is as yet unproven, however, and its relationship to facial neuralgias remains controversial. Whatever the cause, the local deficit does not seem to allow the affected jawbone to respond normally to routine dental or bone infections or to trauma, such as tooth extraction.

Clinical and Radiographic Features

NICO characteristically affects persons 40 to 60 years of age but has been diagnosed in patients aged from 18 to 84 years. Females are affected twice as frequently as males. Any alveolar site may be affected, but the third molar areas are most frequently involved. Approximately one third of patients have more than one alveolar site of involvement, and 10 percent have lesions in all four quadrants. Most affected sites have been edentulous for a number of years, and the lesions may be associated with a radiographically successful endodontic procedure. The average duration of neuralgia pain prior to a NICO diagnosis in the jaws is 6 years but ranges from a few months to more than 20 years.

NICO is almost always identified in patients with facial pain that mimics neuralgia, even to the point of occasionally possessing trigger points similar to those of trigeminal neuralgia. However, the trigger zones are usually intraoral, which is an unusual site for trigger zones of

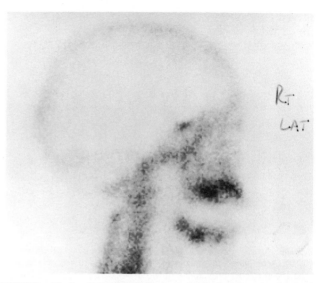

FIGURE 18-2. **Neuralgia-inducing cavitational osteonecrosis (NICO).** This technetium-99 bone scan reveals multiple sites of NICO involvement ("hot spots") 14 years after extraction of the entire dentition. None of the sites was visualized by periapical radiographs, panoramic radiographs, magnetic resonance imaging, computed tomography, or other forms of radioisotope bone scans. This scan also reveals involvement of the sphenoid bone.

trigeminal neuralgia. The site of involvement is best identified by searching for a small zone of hyperesthesia or normal pain response in an area otherwise anesthetized by a local anesthetic agent (the McMahon hyperesthesia/anesthesia test). Seldom are there visible alterations of the overlying mucosa.

The typical lesion is not visualized on panoramic radiographs, magnetic resonance imaging (MRI), computed tomography (CT), or any form of radioisotope bone scans, except technetium-99 scans. Many lesions present as "hot spots" with the latter technique (Fig. 18-2). Simple periapical radiographs appear to be the most sensitive imaging technique, but considerable diagnostic experience is required because the changes are subtle and may mimic a number of other entities. When visible, NICO lesions usually present as poorly demarcated, non-expansile radiolucencies, often with irregular vertical remnants of lamina dura associated with old extraction sites in the region (Fig. 18-3).

Histopathologic Features

Some NICO lesions present as a completely hollow or partially blood-filled bony cavity similar to that seen in traumatic bone cyst. In such cases, there is a scant connective tissue lining. More typically, surgically removed tissue is characterized by multifocal areas of apparent fatty degeneration and/or necrosis, often with pooled fat from destroyed adipose cells (oil cysts) and with marrow fibrosis (reticular fatty degeneration) (Fig. 18-4). Small numbers of chronic inflammatory cells may be present, but neutrophils are conspicuously missing. Deposition of calcific soaps, perhaps with incorporated chips of nonvi-

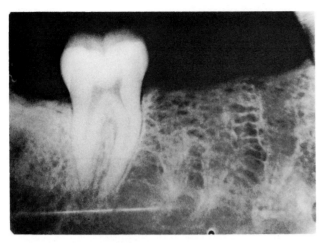

FIGURE 18-3. **Neuralgia-inducing cavitational osteonecrosis (NICO).** This periapical radiograph demonstrates the subtle loss of bone in a surgically proven site of NICO. Notice the fragmented lamina dura remnants, which are still visible 23 years after extraction of teeth in the area.

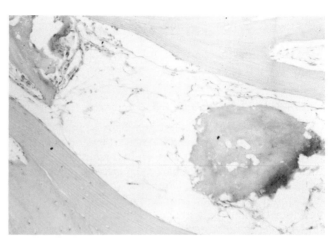

FIGURE 18-5. **Neuralgia-inducing cavitational osteonecrosis (NICO).** Photomicrograph showing smudged calcific debris and calcific "soapy" necrosis appearing as an isolated globular mass with little inflammation of the surrounding fatty marrow. This has been called "NICO bone" because of its uniqueness.

able bone may be seen, sometimes with minimal or no change in the surrounding fatty marrow (Fig. 18-5).

Most bony trabeculae appear at first glance to be viable, mature, and otherwise normal, but closer inspection demonstrates focal loss of osteocytes and variable microcracking (splitting along natural cleavage planes). The microscopic features are similar to those of ischemic or aseptic osteonecrosis of long bones, corticosteroid-induced osteonecrosis, and the osteomyelitis of caisson (deep-sea diver's) disease.

Treatment and Prognosis

Antibiotics may temporarily diminish the associated pain of NICO but are unlikely to cure it. The abnormal intrabony tissues usually must be surgically removed by decortication and curettage. Once they are removed, the defect frequently heals and the intense facial pain subsides dramatically or disappears completely. One third of

patients thus treated, however, experience no pain relief. Also, the disease has a strong tendency to recur or develop in additional jawbone sites. Often, a repetition of the same surgical procedure is necessary. A 70 percent overall "cure" rate (pain-free for an average of 5 years) has been reported, but additional studies are required for a corroboration of this figure.

CLUSTER HEADACHE (Migrainous Neuralgia; Sphenopalatine Neuralgia; Histaminic Cephalgia; Horton's Syndrome)

Cluster headache is an exquisitely painful affliction of the mid-face and upper face, particularly in and around the eye. It is a rare disease of unknown etiology. A vascular cause has been suggested, possibly mediated by abnormal hypothalamic function. It is termed "cluster" headache because the pain attacks occur over a period of a few weeks, followed by months of remission, only to recur again for a few weeks. Thus, the attacks seem to be "clustered" during these periods of disease activity.

Clinical Features

Cluster headache may occur at any age, although it usually affects persons in the third and fourth decades of life. There is a strong male predilection (a 6:1 male-to-female ratio).

The diagnosis of cluster headache is based on the medical history and clinical characteristics, which are distinctive. The pain is described as paroxysmal (abrupt onset) and intense, with a burning or lancinating quality and without a trigger zone. The attacks may last from 15 minutes to 3 hours and occur up to eight times daily (or on alternate days). The headaches occur in "cluster periods" that typically last for weeks; the intervening periods of remission usually last for months but may extend for years. The pain often begins at the same time in

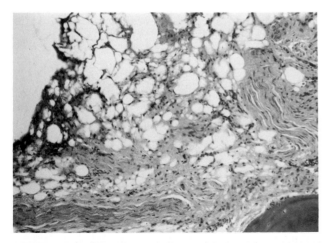

FIGURE 18-4. **Neuralgia-inducing cavitational osteonecrosis (NICO).** Photomicrograph showing marrow fibrosis, mild chronic inflammatory cell infiltration, and fatty degeneration of the marrow.

a given 24-hour period ("alarm clock" headaches), with most attacks beginning in the middle of the night. Consumption of alcohol may precipitate attacks in some patients.

The pain is almost always unilateral and usually involves the orbital, supraorbital, and temporal areas of the face. However, it may simulate a toothache or present as jaw pain in the anterior maxillary region. Because of this, patients may be inappropriately treated for dental pain with endodontic therapy or tooth extraction, which is thought to be successful when the pain subsequently resolves. When each successive "cluster" returns, the next tooth is treated, sometimes resulting in multiple, repeated episodes of unnecessary dental therapy.

Unlike true migraine headache, in which the patient feels a need to lie down and rest, a person with cluster headache characteristically feels a need to pace restlessly. In addition to the pain, these patients also may experience on the affected side such autonomic alterations as nasal stuffiness, tearing, facial flush, or congestion of conjunctival blood vessels ("red eye").

Treatment and Prognosis

The proper diagnosis is important to avoid sequential, unnecessary endodontic or extraction procedures for a patient with cluster headache. Systemic prednisone, ergotamine, lithium carbonate, indomethacin, methysergide maleate, and calcium channel blockers all provide some relief in some cases, and sumatriptan (agonistic to 5-HT_{1D} receptors) truncates the symptoms in 74 percent of cases. No single drug is, however, universally effective. Inhaling oxygen may abort impending attacks, and various surgical interventions have provided relief in some patients. Overall, only 50 percent of patients with cluster headaches benefit significantly and permanently with the available therapeutic modalities.

MIGRAINE (Migraine Syndrome; Migraine Headache)

Migraine is a common, severe, unilateral, recurring headache, possibly caused by the vasoconstriction of portions of the cerebral arteries. The vasoconstriction apparently leads to cerebral ischemia and is followed by a compensating vasodilation, with subsequent pain and cerebral edema. Many affected persons have a family history of migraine, sometimes with a clear autosomal dominant inheritance pattern. It is more frequently seen in professionals. Some authorities have suggested that stressful conditions, even dental trauma, may precipitate an attack.

Clinical Features

Migraine affects females twice as often as males, and women tend to experience more severe attacks than men. The disease is most prevalent in the third through fifth decades of life, but the first symptoms often begin at puberty.

The headache is usually confined to the temporal, frontal, and orbital areas, although occasional patients have pain in the parietal, postauricular, or occipital areas. The pain initially may be felt as a toothache, especially in the anterior maxilla. Symptoms may mimic those of sinusitis or allergic rhinitis. The pain is dull, with a superimposed throbbing, and is typically so severe as to be incapacitating.

Many patients experience prodromal neurologic symptoms or an "aura" before the actual headache pain. The aura may present as visual hallucination, "seeing sparks" (*scintillation*), temporary and partial blindness, partial or complete loss of light perception (*scotoma*), nausea, vertigo, lethargy, mental confusion, loss of the ability to express one's thoughts (*aphasia*), and/or unilateral facial paresthesia or weakness.

Migraine without an aura presents as a unilateral headache with a 5 to 20-minute gradual onset and a typical duration of 4 to 72 hours. The headache is described as pulsating, severe, and aggravated by physical activity; often the patient wants to lie down in a dark, quiet room. There is usually sensitivity to light (*photophobia*) and sensitivity to noise (*phonophobia*).

Migraine with aura also presents as an unilateral headache with a 5- to 20-minute gradual onset; usually, it lasts no more than 2 hours.

Treatment and Prognosis

The treatment of migraine includes a wide variety of medications. Severe attacks are frequently diminished by ergotamine tartrate, perhaps combined with caffeine, aspirin, acetaminophen, phenobarbital, and/or belladonna. Less severe attacks are treated prophylactically by other ergot compounds (e.g., methergine), beta-adrenergic agents (e.g., propranolol or metoprolol), calcium channel blockers (e.g., nifedipine or diltiazem), or serotonin (5-HT) antagonist drugs (e.g., methysergide or cyproheptadine). Some patients may be aided by simple pressure on the ipsilateral carotid artery. The headaches tend to become less severe and less frequent over time, with or without effective therapy.

TEMPORAL ARTERITIS (Giant Cell Arteritis)

Temporal arteritis is an idiopathic, multifocal vasculitis of cranial arteries, especially the superficial temporal arteries. The cause is unknown, although autoimmunity to the elastic lamina of the artery has been proposed.

The overall prevalence of temporal arteritis in the United States is 77 to 130 per 100,000 in people older than 50 years of age. The prevalence seems to be increasing over time, perhaps because the population is aging. No racial predilection is seen.

Clinical Features

Women are affected by temporal arteritis twice as often as men, and patients are usually 50 to 85 years of age (average, 70 years). The disease most frequently presents as a unilateral throbbing headache that is gradually replaced by an intense, aching, burning temporal and facial pain. The throbbing frequently coincides with the patient's heartbeat (systole). The superficial temporal artery is exquisitely sensitive to pressure and eventually appears erythematous, swollen, and tortuous. Most patients complain of pain during mastication, and the pain occasionally mimics a toothache. Significantly, ocular symptoms, such as loss of vision or retro-orbital pain, may be the first complaint.

Fever, malaise, fatigue, nausea, anorexia, vomiting, and earache may occur, perhaps as prodromal symptoms, and the erythrocyte sedimentation rate is usually elevated. Muscle aching and stiffness (*polymyalgia rheumatica*) frequently follow an acute attack. The affected artery may become thrombosed, after which it is palpated as a firm, pulseless cord.

Histopathologic Features

The diagnosis of temporal arteritis is confirmed by biopsy. At least a 1-cm portion of the affected vessel must be examined in several areas because the histopathologic changes tend to be segmental and can be missed if the specimen is too small. Involvement is characterized by chronic inflammation of the intima and tunica media, with narrowing of the lumen from edema and proliferation of the intima. Necrosis of the smooth muscle and elastic lamina is frequent. A variable number of foreign body–type multinucleated giant cells are mixed with macrophages, plasma cells, and lymphocytes. Thrombosis or complete occlusion of the lumen is not unusual.

Treatment and Prognosis

Temporal arteritis responds well to systemic corticosteroids; the symptoms subside within a few days. However, permanent loss of vision occurs in 25 to 50 percent of untreated patients. In occasional cases, vascular involvement is widespread throughout the body, a condition that may be fatal, even with corticosteroid therapy.

MYASTHENIA GRAVIS

Myasthenia gravis is an autoimmune disease that affects the acetylcholine receptors of muscle fibers and results in an abnormal and progressive fatigability of skeletal muscle. Defective neuromuscular transmission occurs, probably secondary to the coating of the acetylcholine receptors (AChR) by circulating antibodies to those receptors. Such antibodies are not normally found in humans; hence, the measurement of serum AChR antibody levels is an important diagnostic tool for this disease. The motor end plate itself is normal, and smooth and cardiac muscles are not affected.

Many patients demonstrate either thymus hyperplasia or an actual neoplasm (**thymoma**) of the thymus gland. Conversely, 75 percent of patients with thymomas have myasthenia gravis, and 90 percent have circulating AChR antibodies. Only rarely does myasthenia gravis affect more than one family member, but the infant of a mother with the disease may be affected for several weeks or months by antibodies that traverse the placenta.

Clinical Features

Myasthenia gravis is more common in females and can begin at any age. It presents as a subtle but progressive muscle weakness that is most frequently noticed first in the small muscles of the head and neck. This weakness may initially manifest as:

- An inability to focus the eyes (*extraocular muscular paresis*)
- Drooping eyelids (*ptosis*)
- Double vision (*diplopia*)
- Difficulty in chewing
- Difficulty in swallowing (*dysphagia*)
- Slurring of words (*dysarthria*)

Repeated muscle contractions, in particular, lead to progressively less power in the contracting muscle; hence, affected patients usually become weaker as the day progresses. The muscles of mastication may become so weak from eating a single meal that the jaws literally "hang open."

Histopathologic Features

The diagnosis of myasthenia gravis is based on the clinical symptoms, an elevated serum AChR antibody level, and improved strength after intravenous injection of edrophonium, a cholinesterase inhibitor. Degenerated muscle fibers are the only characteristic histopathologic feature, with fibers appearing much smaller than normal, having fewer nuclei, and showing a loss of the normal rounded cross-sectional appearance.

Treatment and Prognosis

The prognosis for myasthenia gravis is variable. Approximately 10 percent of patients never have more than weak extraocular muscles, but severe cases may progress, after months or years, to permanent muscular weakness and wasting of the neck, limbs, and trunk. Respiratory paralysis is a sometimes fatal complication.

The defective neuromuscular transmission can be partially reversed by cholinesterase inhibitors, such as edrophonium or neostigmine and its analogues, but thymectomy is the treatment of choice for all but the mildest cases. Spontaneous remission and complete, permanent recovery can occur, especially after thymectomy. Acute, generalized cases, however, do not respond well to any therapy; in such cases, death usually occurs within several months.

MOTOR NEURON DISEASE (Progressive Bulbar Palsy; Amyotrophic Lateral Sclerosis; Progressive Muscular Atrophy)

Motor neuron disease consists of a spectrum of overlapping motor nerve diseases that show a progressive degeneration of the motor nuclei of the cranial nerves, the anterior horn of the spinal cord, and the pyramidal tracts. Although the cause of these conditions is unknown in most cases, one hypothesis suggests that there may be a toxic accumulation of the excitatory amino acid neurotransmitter glutamate, which results in neuron death. A hereditary predisposition for one of the diseases, **amyotrophic lateral sclerosis (ALS)**, is sometimes seen (autosomal dominant trait with high penetrance) and a mutated gene on chromosome 21 has been identified in the familial form of that disease. Some authorities suggest trauma or slow viruses as important in the pathogenesis of motor neuron disease. The role of viruses is suggested by reported cases of progressive muscular atrophy that occur many years after an attack of paralytic poliomyelitis.

Motor neuron disease presents as three distinctive clinical syndromes with considerable overlapping of signs and symptoms:

- Progressive muscular atrophy
- Progressive bulbar palsy
- Amyotrophic lateral sclerosis (ALS)

All three entities entail progressive loss of muscle control and eventual atrophy of muscle; together, they affect approximately 5 of every 100,000 persons in the United States. There is some confusion over the appropriate terminology because some authors have used ALS to include all three disease syndromes.

Clinical Features

Progressive Muscular Atrophy

Progressive muscular atrophy occurs most frequently in childhood and affects males and females equally. It is characterized by progressive limb weakness and sensory disturbances, which result in difficulty in walking, leg pain, and paresthesia and atrophy of the feet and hands.

Progressive Bulbar Palsy

Progressive bulbar palsy typically affects children and young adults and demonstrates no gender predilection. It usually begins with a subtle but progressive difficulty in articulation or swallowing (dysphagia). Chronic hoarseness may develop. Attempts to swallow food produce bouts of choking and regurgitation, with liquids frequently thrown into the nasopharynx and nasal sinuses because of palatal paralysis. Atrophy of the facial muscles, tongue, and soft palate eventually occurs, as do weakness and spasticity of the limbs. There are no altered sensory perceptions.

Amyotrophic Lateral Sclerosis

Amyotrophic lateral sclerosis, commonly called **Lou Gehrig disease** (after a professional baseball player who died of the disease), affects males more frequently than females and begins to manifest itself in middle age. The disease typically presents as difficulty in walking, which is produced by bilateral and generalized leg stiffness. Occasionally, one leg is affected more than the other, forcing the patient to drag one leg behind the other. The physical examination reveals spastic quadriparesis, often with a remarkable increase in the tendon reflexes of all four limbs and with extensor plantar responses. Central reflexes, such as those of the abdomen, are not altered until late in the disease, and there are no alterations of the senses. Small, synchronous, subcutaneous muscle contractions (*fasciculation*) of the shoulders and thighs are another early symptom; muscle atrophy eventually develops at affected sites. Dysfunction of the muscles controlled by the medulla oblongata (*bulbar paralysis*) appears late in the disease, predominantly as spasticity and weakness.

Treatment and Prognosis

Although each of these conditions may have temporary remissions, the course of motor neuron disease is almost invariably fatal. Progressive bulbar palsy usually results in death from respiratory infection within 2 years of the diagnosis. Weakness of the bulbar muscles in ALS is the usual cause of death, typically within 2 to 5 years from the onset of symptoms. Progressive muscular atrophy typically leads to death within 4 to 6 years of symptom onset. The antiglutamate agent riluzole has shown some promise in slowing the progression of ALS and improving the survival in patients with disease of bulbar onset.

IDIOPATHIC BURNING TONGUE SYNDROME (Glossopyrosis; Glossodynia; Stomatopyrosis; Stomatodynia; Burning Mouth Syndrome)

Glossodynia refers to a painful or tender tongue; **glossopyrosis** refers to a burning sensation of the tongue. Although historically these were viewed as separate entities, many affected patients complain of both sensations. Various local and systemic factors are associated with both of these (Table 18–2), but most cases have no known cause. There is some evidence that abnormal levels of certain immunoglobulins, such as antinuclear antibody and rheumatoid factor, are found in the serum of more than 50 percent of affected patients. The signifi-

Table 18–2. LOCAL AND SYSTEMIC FACTORS REPORTEDLY ASSOCIATED WITH BURNING TONGUE SYNDROME (GLOSSOPYROSIS)

Local Factors	Systemic Factors
Xerostomia	Vitamin B deficiency
Chronic mouth breathing	Vitamin B_1 or B_2 deficiency
Chronic tongue thrust habit	Pernicious anemia (B_{12})
Chronic mechanical trauma	Pellagra (niacin deficiency)
Referred pain from teeth or tonsils	Folic acid deficiency
Trigeminal neuralgia	Diabetes mellitus
Atypical facial pain or neuralgia	Chronic gastritis or
Angioedema (angioneurotic edema)	regurgitation
Oral candidiasis	Chronic gastric hypoacidity
Temporomandibular dysfunction	Hypothyroidism
Oral submucous fibrosis	Mercurialism
Fusospirochetal infection	Estrogen deficiency
Contact stomatitis (allergy)	Psychosomatic disorder or
Trauma to lingual nerve	depression
	Acquired immunodeficiency
	syndrome (AIDS)

cance of this is not clear. The fact that most affected patients are postmenopausal woman has led to the common belief that estrogen deficit is the primary cause, but a strong correlation between the disorder and decreased blood levels of estrogen and/or progesterone has not been identified.

Idiopathic burning tongue syndrome is a common condition that affects approximately 2 percent of adults to some degree. No racial predilection is seen, and both problems occur in all socioeconomic groups.

Clinical Features

Glossodynia

Glossodynia characteristically affects middle-aged women. It is most often described as a sharp pain of the dorsal and lateral surfaces of the tongue, although other oral mucosal surfaces may also be affected. The onset is usually rapid and appears to the patient to be spontaneous. Affected areas are tender to palpation, sometimes exquisitely so. The tongue typically appears clinically normal, although erythema or pallor may be noted infrequently.

Burning Tongue Syndrome

Three-fourths of patients with burning tongue syndrome seen for evaluation are female, with an average age at diagnosis of 50 years. The onset in women usually occurs within 3 to 12 years after menopause. As with glossodynia, this disorder also has a typically spontaneous onset, although it may be gradual. The lingual dorsum has a burning sensation, often described as having been "burned with hot coffee." Ironically, the tip of the tongue may actually have an increased tolerance to heat. Close questioning often determines that additional oral membranes are similarly affected, especially the anterior hard palate and the lower lip mucosa and vermilion.

A persistent altered or diminished taste may accompany the burning sensation. The burning usually begins at midday and continues throughout the day or increases in intensity during the evening hours, but nightly remission during sleep is common. However, other patterns are also seen.

Most patients with burning tongue have no visible lingual changes. There is seldom a significant decrease in stimulated salivary output in tests, despite the frequent complaint of xerostomia. Salivary levels of various proteins, immunoglobulins, and phosphates may be elevated, and there may be a decreased salivary pH or buffering capacity.

As with other chronic pain disorders, affected patients frequently demonstrate psychologic dysfunction, usually depression, anxiety, or irritability. Such dysfunctions may disappear with resolution of the burning or painful tongue condition. This suggests that the psychologic component has resulted from the oral disorder rather than *vice versa*. However, it is possible that a portion of cases are psychosomatic in origin. In such cases, improvement in the clinical depression may reduce the lingual symptoms.

Treatment and Prognosis

If an underlying systemic or local cause (see Table 18–2) can be identified and corrected, of course, the lingual symptoms should disappear. The management of idiopathic cases is more difficult and frustrating. However, about two thirds of patients show at least some improvement of their symptoms when they take one of the mood-altering drugs; chlordiazepoxide is the most commonly used medication (5 to 10 mg three times daily).

The long-term prognosis for idiopathic burning tongue or mouth syndrome appears variable. Some patients experience a spontaneous or gradual remission of their condition, which may occur months or years after the onset of disease. However, many patients continue to experience symptoms throughout the rest of their lives. Even though the condition is chronic and may not always respond to therapy, patients should be reassured that it is benign and not a symptom of oral cancer.

DYSGEUSIA (Phantom Taste; Distorted Taste)

Dysgeusia is defined as a persistent aberrant taste. It is distinguished from the much more common deficiencies in olfactory (*hyposmia*, or *anosmia*) and taste (*hypogeusia*, or *ageusia*) perception seen in approximately 2 million adult Americans. Dysgeusias are less tolerated than simple deficiencies; this is attested to by the fact that they account for more than one third of all patient visits to the few available chemosensory research centers in the United States. The less noticeable loss of taste represents only 3 percent of visits to these centers, and almost all other visits are related to altered smell.

Most cases of dysgeusia are produced by or associated with an underlying systemic disorder or by radiation therapy to the head and neck region (Table 18–3). Trauma, tumors, or inflammation of the peripheral nerves of the gustatory system usually produce hypogeusia rather than dysgeusia and a transient alteration only. By way of contrast, relatively common upper respiratory infections produce a temporary and mild dysgeusia in almost one third of cases, although they seldom produce hypogeusia. Central nervous system neoplasms predominantly produce dysgeusia, not hypogeusia or ageusia, and gustatory hallucinations are fairly common during migraine headaches, Bell's palsy, or herpes zoster of the geniculate ganglion.

The perception of a particular taste depends on its concentration in a liquid environment; hence, persons with severe dry mouth may suffer from both hypogeusia and dysgeusia. Also, more than 200 drugs that can produce taste disturbances have been identified (see Table 18–4). Even without medication-induced alterations, approximately 40 percent of persons with clinical depression complain of dysgeusia. The clinician should be especially diligent in assessing local, intraoral causes of dysgeusia, such as periodontal or dental abscess, oral candidiasis, and routine gingivitis or periodontitis. The latter may produce a salty dysgeusia because of the high sodium chloride content of oozing crevicular fluids.

Clinical Features

In contrast to hypogeusia or the simple loss of taste discrimination, dysgeusia is promptly and distressingly discerned by affected individuals. The clinician must be certain that the patient's alteration is, in fact, a taste disorder rather than an olfactory one because 75 percent of "flavor" information (e.g., taste, aroma, texture, temperature, and irritating properties) is derived from smell. Abnormal taste function should be verified through formal taste testing by using standard tastants that are representative of each of the four primary taste qualities (e.g., sweet, sour, salty, and bitter) in a non-odorous solution. Additional electrical and chemical analysis of taste bud function is frequently required. Because this is outside the scope of most general practices, patients are typically referred to a chemosensory research center.

Affected patients may describe their altered taste as one of the primary ones, but many describe the new taste as metallic, foul, or rancid. The latter two are more likely to be associated with aberrant odor perception (*parosmia*) than with dysgeusia. The altered taste may require a stimulus, such as certain foods or liquids, in which case the taste is said to be distorted. If no stimulus is required, the dysgeusia is classified as a "phantom" taste.

Table 18–3. LOCAL AND SYSTEMIC FACTORS REPORTEDLY ASSOCIATED WITH ALTERED TASTE SENSATIONS (DYSGEUSIA)

Local Factors	Systemic Factors
Oral candidiasis	Vitamin A deficiency
Oral trichomoniasis	Vitamin B$_{12}$ deficiency
Desquamative gingivitis	Zinc deficiency
Oral galvanism	Nutritional overdose (zinc, vitamin A, pyridoxine)
Periodontitis or gingivitis	Food sensitivity or allergy
Chlorhexidine rinse	Sjögren's syndrome
Oral lichen planus	Anorexia, cachexia, bulimia
	Liver dysfunction
	Crohn's disease
	Cystic fibrosis
	Addison's disease
	Turner syndrome
	Alcoholism
	Psychosis or depression
	Pesticide ingestion
	Lead, copper, or mercury poisoning
	Temporal arteritis
	Migraine headaches
	Temporal lobe central nervous system tumor
	Nerve trauma, gustatory nerves
	Herpes zoster, geniculate ganglion
	Upper respiratory infection
	Chronic gastritis or regurgitation
	Systemic medications
	Bell's palsy
	Radiation therapy to head and neck

Table 18–4. EXAMPLES OF PHARMACEUTICAL AGENTS THAT MAY BE ASSOCIATED WITH ALTERED TASTE

Pharmaceutical Action	Examples
Anticoagulant	Phenindione
Antihistamine	Chlorpheniramine maleate
Antihypertensive or diuretic	Captopril, diazoxide, ethacrynic acid
Antimicrobial	Amphotericin B, ampicillin, griseofulvin, idoxuridine, lincomycin, metronidazole, streptomycin, tetracycline, tyrothricin
Antineoplastic or immunosuppressant	Doxorubicin, methotrexate, vincristine, azathioprine, carmustine
Antiparkinsonian agent	Baclofen, chlormezanone, levodopa
Antipsychotic or anticonvulsant	Carbamazepine, lithium, phenytoin
Antirheumatic	Allopurinol, colchicine, gold, levamisole, penicillamine, phenylbutazone
Antiseptic	Hexetidine and chlorhexidine
Antithyroid agent	Carbimazole, methimazole, thiouracil
Hypoglycemic	Glipizide, phenformin
Opiate	Codeine, morphine
Sympathomimetic	Amphetamines, phenmetrazine
Vasodilator	Oxyfedrine, bamifylline

Treatment and Prognosis

If an underlying disease or process is identified and successfully treated, the taste function should return to normal. For idiopathic cases of dysgeusia, there is no effective pharmacologic or surgical therapy; fortunately, however, many untreated cases gradually improve over time. For other patients, dysgeusia may significantly affect lifestyles and interpersonal relationships; this can lead to depression or anxiety or produce nutritional deficiencies from altered eating habits. The altered taste may be masked somewhat with the use of lozenges or chewing gums, but these are only temporarily effective.

AURICULOTEMPORAL SYNDROME (Frey Syndrome; Gustatory Sweating and Flushing)

The **auriculotemporal syndrome** develops as a result of injury to the auriculotemporal nerve. This nerve, in addition to supplying sensory fibers to the preauricular and temporal areas, carries parasympathetic fibers to the parotid gland and sympathetic vasomotor and sudomotor (sweat-stimulating) fibers to the preauricular skin.

Following parotid abscesses, trauma, mandibular surgery, or parotidectomy, the parasympathetic nerve fibers may be severed. In their attempt to re-establish innervation, these fibers occasionally become misdirected and regenerate along the sympathetic nerve pathways. From 5 to 30 percent of patients with parotidectomies may have auriculotemporal syndrome as a complication.

Clinical Features

The auriculotemporal syndrome presents with sweating, flushing, warmth, and occasionally pain in the preauricular and temporal areas during the enhanced salivary stimulation brought on by the chewing of food. After the initial nerve injury, a prodromal stage frequently occurs in which the preauricular area does not respond to local heat stimulus. Within 2 months to 2 years (average, 9 months), the sweating and flushing reaction commences and becomes steadily more severe for several months but remains constant thereafter.

To detect sweating, Minor's starch-iodine test may be used. A 1 percent iodine solution is painted on the affected area of the skin. This solution is allowed to dry and the area is then coated with a layer of starch. When the patient is given something to eat, the moisture of the sweat that is produced will mix with the iodine on the skin. This allows the iodine to react with the starch and produce a blue color (Fig. 18–6).

When flushing occurs, the local skin temperature may be raised 1 to 2°C. This may occur without sweating, especially in females. Pain, when present, is usually mild, and hypesthesia (hypoesthesia) or hyperesthesia is a common feature.

Related phenomena may accompany an operation or injury to the submandibular gland **(chorda tympani syndrome)** or the facial nerve proximal to the geniculate ganglion **(gustatory lacrimation syndrome)**. The chin and submental skin demonstrate sweating and flushing in the former. Chewing food in the latter syndrome produces abundant tear formation.

Treatment and Prognosis

Severing the auriculotemporal or glossopharyngeal nerve on the affected side inhibits or abolishes the sweating and flushing reaction of auriculotemporal syndrome, as do local atropine injections or scopolamine creams.

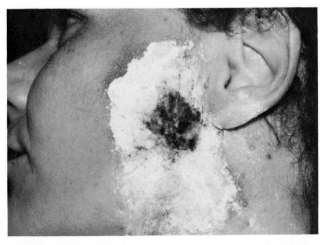

FIGURE 18–6. **Auriculotemporal (Frey) syndrome.** This patient received an injury to her auriculotemporal nerve during orthognathic surgery 3 years earlier. Notice the region of sweating detected during mastication by a color change of the starch in the Minor's starch-iodine test.

About 5 percent of patients experience spontaneous disappearance of the syndrome. Most cases are mild enough so that treatment is not required or sought by the patient.

OSTEOARTHRITIS (Degenerative Arthritis; Degenerative Joint Disease)

Osteoarthritis is a degenerative, destructive alteration of the joints. It represents 60 percent of all arthritis cases in humans and is responsible for more than 50 percent of all hip joint replacements in the United States. Until recently, osteoarthritis was thought to be the inevitable result of simple wear and tear on aging anatomic structures. It is now thought to have a strong inflammatory component as well, especially in small joints, such as the temporomandibular joint (TMJ), where there appears to be little association with the aging process.

Osteoarthritis of extragnathic joints is virtually unavoidable; 100 percent of people older than 50 years of age are affected to some extent. Even the TMJ is affected at the microscopic level in 40 percent of older adults and at the radiographic imaging level in 14 percent of older adults.

With advancing age, there may be a slower and less complete replacement of chondroblasts and chondrocytes in joint cartilage. The cartilage matrix (fibrocartilage in the case of the TMJ) possibly turns over less rapidly. This forces available fibers to work longer and become susceptible to fatigue. The matrix also holds less water and becomes desiccated and brittle. With continued joint use or "trauma," the surface fibers break down, and portions of the hyaline or fibrocartilage are destroyed. They often break away to expose underlying bone. The exposed bone then undergoes a dual process of degenerative destruction of the cortex, trabeculae, and marrow along with proliferation of new bone on the surface (exostoses and osteophytes).

Clinical and Radiographic Features

Extragnathic osteoarthritis usually involves multiple joints. These are typically the large weight-bearing joints, but the small bones of the hands also frequently are affected. The arthritis is characterized by a gradually intensifying deep ache and pain, which is usually worse in the evening than in the morning; however, at least some degree of morning joint stiffness and stiffness after inactivity is present in 80 percent of cases. The joint may become swollen and warm to the touch, rarely with erythema of the overlying skin. In the more serious cases, the joint eventually becomes so deformed that it limits motion. Degenerative changes are most likely to occur in the areas of greatest impact. Crepitation (crackling noise during motion) is a late sign of the disease.

These joint changes are also seen when the TMJ is affected, except that patients seldom experience stiffness of the TMJ. In addition, the muscles of mastication frequently exhibit tenderness because of the constant strain of "muscle guarding," i.e., attempting to keep the painful joint immobile.

With conventional radiography, joints affected by osteoarthritis demonstrate a narrowing or obliteration of the joint space, irregularity of the articular surface, flattening of the articular surface, sclerosis of bone immediately beneath the cartilage, osteolysis of underlying bone, surface bony protuberances or spurs (*osteophytes*), radiolucent subchondral cysts, and ossification within the synovial membrane (*ossicles*). More sensitive diagnostic techniques, such as CT scanning arthrography, MRI, and arthroscopy, reveal the same features but in much more detail; hence, they are able to identify earlier changes.

Histopathologic Features

The articulating surface of a joint affected by osteoarthritis has a diminished number of chondrocytes, is roughened, and contains variable numbers of vertical clefts; in older cases, these extend to the underlying bone. At surgery, the joint surface is noted to be proliferative in some areas (and produces osteophytes, for example) and degenerative in others. The latter bone is characterized by a loss of osteocytes, minimal osteoblastic or osteoclastic activity, fatty degeneration or necrosis of the marrow, infiltration by chronic inflammatory cells, and perhaps the formation of large degenerative "cysts" immediately beneath the articular cartilage (subchondral cysts). Inflammation of the surrounding synovial membrane results in a thickened membrane and, in some cases, metaplastic hyaline cartilage granules (chondral bodies), which may number in the hundreds within a single joint.

The TMJ is unique because of its fibrocartilage covering and its meniscus. The disk may be centrally destroyed, and there is little vertical clefting of the articular surface. All other features of TMJ osteoarthritis, however, are similar to those noted in other joints.

Treatment and Prognosis

The treatment of osteoarthritis is usually palliative and consists of analgesics for the pain and nonsteroidal anti-inflammatory agents for other symptoms and signs. Arthroplasty and joint replacement are often required for heavy weight-bearing joints and are occasionally used in the TMJ. Occlusal adjustment, orofacial physiotherapy, and the use of occlusal splints may reduce joint symptoms by relieving the pressure on the joint surfaces, and hot or cold packs may be helpful to relax involved muscles.

RHEUMATOID ARTHRITIS

Rheumatoid arthritis is a chronic, possibly autoimmune disorder characterized by a non-suppurative inflammatory destruction of the joints. It may result from a cross-reaction of antibodies generated against hemolytic streptococci or other microorganisms, or it may represent an antibody attack against bacterial cell walls or viral capsule fragments deposited within the synovium. The cause is still unknown in most cases. Some cases have a familial pattern, and there is at least a partial association with several histocompatibility (HLA) cell surface antigens.

This disease affects 3 percent of people in the United States to at least some degree, and approximately 200,000 new cases are diagnosed yearly. The TMJ eventually becomes involved in 75 percent of patients, although usually in a clinically insignificant manner.

In contrast to osteoarthritis (see previous topic), rheumatoid arthritis begins as an attack against the synovial membrane (*synovitis*). A reactive fibroblastic and macrophagic proliferation (*pannus*) from the synovium creeps onto the joint surface. This releases collagenases and other proteases, which destroy the cartilage and underlying bone. Attempted remodeling by the exposed bone results in a characteristic deformation of the joint.

Clinical and Radiographic Features

Rheumatoid arthritis affects women three times more frequently than men, although the condition in men is usually diagnosed at a somewhat younger age than in women (25 to 35 years of age versus 35 to 45 years, respectively). The onset and course of this disease are extremely variable. For many patients, never is more than one or two joints involved, and significant pain or limitation of motion may never develop. In others, their disease rapidly progresses to debilitating polyarthralgia.

Typically, the signs and symptoms become more severe over time and include swelling, stiffness, pain, joint deformity, and disability, with possible fibrous or bony fusion (ankylosis) of opposing articular surfaces. Periods of remission are often interspersed with periods of exacerbation. Symmetric involvement of the small joints of the hands and feet is almost always present, but it is not unusual for knees and elbows to be affected. The hip joint (a joint often affected by osteoarthritis) is the joint least affected by rheumatoid arthritis. Twenty percent of patients have firm, partially movable, nontender, *rheumatoid nodules* beneath the skin near the affected joint. These are pathognomonic for the disease.

Joints involved with rheumatoid arthritis have a characteristic "anvil" shape, with an irregular flattening of the central articular surface and a splaying of the lateral bone. Unlike the situation in osteoarthritis, narrowing of the joint space is seldom seen, except when ankylosis has occurred.

When present, TMJ involvement is usually bilateral; seldom are these joints affected early in the disease, however. The symptoms are seldom as severe as in other joints. Swelling is less obvious when the TMJs are affected, but more than 40 percent of affected TMJs demonstrate tenderness or stiffness of varying degrees.

The pain of TMJ rheumatoid arthritis is frequently not related to motion but rather to pressure on the joint. Clenching the teeth on one side produces pain of the contralateral joint. Similarly, subluxation or ankylosis is less frequent in the TMJs than in other joints, but gross destruction of the condylar heads may be so severe that mandibular micrognathia causes a receding chin and malocclusion. Permanent TMJ subluxation has been reported.

Radiographically, involved TMJs demonstrate a flattened condylar head with irregular surface features, an irregular temporal fossa surface, perhaps with remodeling of the fossa itself, and anterior displacement of the condyle. Several diagnostic techniques are available besides routine TMJ radiographs. CT, scanning arthrography, and arthroscopy are excellent tools for assessing TMJ damage. Thermography is commonly used in Europe to detect early disease. Ultrasonography is valuable for larger joints but has been little used in TMJ disease. Nuclear medicine scans that use scintoradiography have, in recent years, been largely replaced by MRI. The latter is sensitive and has rapidly become the diagnostic tool of choice for this disease.

Laboratory Values

Approximately 80 percent of patients with rheumatoid arthritis exhibit significant elevations of rheumatoid factor (RF), an autoantibody thought to be directed toward an altered host IgG antibody that is no longer recognized by the body as "self." In addition, antinuclear antibody (ANA) can be detected in about 50 percent of the patients with rheumatoid arthritis, although it is not diagnostically specific because it also may be associated with other autoimmune diseases. During active phases of the disease, almost all patients have an elevated erythrocyte sedimentation rate. In addition, some affected patients have mild anemia.

Histopathologic Features

Needle biopsy is the most popular technique for obtaining diagnostic synovial material, but aspiration and analysis of synovial fluid from the affected joint are frequently undertaken to rule out other forms of arthritis. These techniques are seldom used for TMJ involvement.

Microscopically, early cases of rheumatoid arthritis demonstrate hyperplasia of the synovial lining cells with hyperemia, edema, and perivascular lymphocytic and neutrophilic infiltration of the deeper portions of the membrane. Older lesions show continued and often severe synovial proliferation and edema. Typically, the membrane protrudes into the joint space as villi or finger-like projections. These projections occasionally undergo necrosis producing "rice bodies," small whitish villi fragments composed of cellular debris admixed with fibrin and collagen.

Hemorrhage and thrombosis of the joint space are common features of rheumatoid arthritis. Lymphocytes are numerous within the synovium; neutrophils are the predominant inflammatory cell in the synovial fluid. Cholesterol crystals are often noted in chronic cases. When the TMJ is severely involved, the meniscus is typically perforated or completely replaced by fibrous scar tissue.

Rheumatoid nodules or granulomas are characterized by moderately well-demarcated areas of amorphous, eosinophilic necrosis surrounded by a thick layer of mononuclear cells. The mononuclear cells closest to the amorphous center are typically large and palisaded. Neutrophils are frequently seen in the centers.

Treatment and Prognosis

There is no cure for rheumatoid arthritis, and current treatments strive only to suppress the process as much as possible. Drug therapy in early and mild cases consists of nonsteroidal anti-inflammatory agents, perhaps aided by occasional corticosteroid injections into the joint. The latter injections are used sparingly, however, because they have been occasionally associated with additional degenerative changes and fibrous ankylosis.

Many second-line medications are often required, and the wide variability in responses to these drugs typically results in an extended course of constantly changing doses and agents in an effort to achieve optimal relief. Systemic corticosteroids, gold injections, penicillamine, cyclophosphamide, and methotrexate are the commonly used second-line medications; all are associated with significant side effects. Severely damaged joints may have to be surgically replaced. The systemic nature of rheumatoid disease also requires an evaluation of extra-articular body functions.

TEMPOROMANDIBULAR JOINT DYSFUNCTION (TMD)

Pain and dysfunction of the TMJ are common and may result from a wide variety of etiologic factors, both traumatic and nontraumatic (Table 18–5). The syndrome of symptoms produced by these varied factors, however, has certain similarities and is collectively referred to as **temporomandibular joint dysfunction (TMD)**. The TMJ signs and symptoms in TMD include pain, altered mandibular function, and joint noises. The symptoms often vary over time because TMD frequently is a progressive disorder or continuum. Because of the extreme complexity of this disorder, the present discussion is limited to a brief overview of those facets of the disorder that are appropriate to the production of pain.

Before the inaccurate 1934 assumption by Costen that

Table 18–5. CLASSIFICATION OF TEMPOROMANDIBULAR DISORDERS

Muscular Disorders
Hyperactivity, spasm, and trismus
Inflammation (myositis)
Trauma
Myofascial pain and fibromyalgia
Atrophy or hypertrophy

Arthrogenic Disorders
Disc displacement (internal derangement)
Hypomobility of the disc (adhesions or scars)
Dislocation and subluxation
Arthritis
Infections
Metabolic disease (gout, chondrocalcinosis)
Capsulitis, synovitis
Ankylosis (fibrous, bony)
Fracture
Condylar hyperplasia, hypoplasia, aplasia
Neoplasia

a "closed bite" was the cause of TMD, little was known about the pathophysiology of the disease. Today, we accept the fact that the teeth, jaws, joint structures, and facial muscles are all parts of an integrated masticatory system and that all must be evaluated to arrive at the most specific diagnosis and management protocol.

The overall adult prevalence of facial and cervical pain and tenderness (which includes headache) from TMD is approximately 15 percent in the United States, but fewer than 1 percent of affected patients have severe symptoms.

Clinical and Radiographic Features

TMD is primarily seen in middle-aged women, but it may affect any age and either gender. Most patients have some degree of pain, which is the primary reason for seeking professional help. As expected, the pain is usually localized to the preauricular area but may radiate to the temporal, frontal, or occipital areas. It may present as headache, a ringing in the ears (*tinnitus*), earache (*otalgia*), or toothache.

Nonarthritic inflammatory disorders of the TMJ are typically characterized by continuous deep pain or ache. Normally, the pain is evoked by palpation of the affected joint or by mandibular movement, especially chewing or clenching. Many patients complain of headache with or without localized joint tenderness, and it is not unusual for headache, joint pain, and earache all to be present as a symptom triad. Both TMJs may be involved, at the same time or at differing times.

The pain may be associated more with the surrounding musculature and soft tissue than with the TMJ itself. Muscle splinting may lead to involuntary central nervous system (CNS)–induced muscular contractions (*myospasms*), or the muscle fibers themselves may become inflamed (*myositis*). The latter may result from protracted myospasms or, less commonly, from the spread of infection from nearby structures.

Myofascial trigger point pain appears to be unrelated to the other TMJ disorders. It is characterized by circumscribed regions within the muscle ("trigger points"), which elicit local or referred pain on palpation and may be a source of constant deep pain. In many instances, patients are aware only of the referred pain and not the trigger points themselves. The exact nature of the trigger points is not known, but they seem similar to small areas of myospasm and can, through their chronic nature, induce CNS excitatory effects.

Derangements of the condyle-meniscus complex are more often associated with dysfunction than with arthralgia. When present, the pain may be localized, nonspecific, or referred. It is often not a reliable finding for diagnostic purposes.

For TMD that results from internal joint damage or derangements, CT and MRI provide excellent diagnostic images of the TMJ, but transcranial or cephalometric radiographic techniques, which are much less detailed, are usually adequate and are more commonly used. The bone itself frequently appears normal, but a widened joint space, anteriorly displaced meniscus, or altered meniscus shape is a common finding. Irregularly altered joint surfaces, when present, may be related to arthritis or trauma.

Treatment and Prognosis

Therapies for TMD are numerous and depend on the exact pathogenesis of the pain. Because of the complex nature of TMD, it is beyond the scope of this text to give an in-depth discussion of the management of this problem, and the reader is referred to other texts that specifically deal with this disease.

In general, conservative treatments for TMD most frequently include simple rest or immobilization of the joint, application of cold (usually reserved for acute injuries) or heat, occlusal splints and adjustment, and physical therapy. Various medications have also been used for TMD, including:

- Aspirin
- Acetaminophen
- Other nonsteroidal anti-inflammatory agents
- Acetaminophen with codeine
- Centrally acting muscle relaxants, such as methocarbamol and chlorzoxazone
- Benzodiazepine derivatives, such as diazepam and chlordiazepoxide
- Glucocorticoids, such as cortisone and prednisone

Surgical intervention may be required in severely affected joints, especially those that involve internal meniscal derangements, condylar dislocation or fracture, ankylosis, and degenerative or developmental deformities.

TEMPOROMANDIBULAR JOINT ANKYLOSIS

Ankylosis refers literally to a "fusion" of body parts, in this case the opposing bony and cartilaginous components of a joint. The fusion can be fibrous or bony in nature — usually fibrous when the TMJ is involved. Joint infection, usually after trauma, accounts for 50% of all TMJ ankylosis cases, but 30 percent result from aseptic trauma to the joint. The remaining cases are idiopathic or produced by rheumatoid arthritis.

The ankylosis may be intra-articular or extra-articular. *Intra-articular* ankylosis is characterized by the destruction of the meniscus and the temporal fossa, thickening and flattening of the condylar head, and a narrowing of the joint space. Opposing joint surfaces then develop fibrous adhesions that inhibit normal movements and may become ossified. Fibrotic intra-articular ankylosis is the most common type seen in the TMJ, especially after trauma-induced hemorrhage (*hemarthrosis*). Osseous ankylosis is more likely with non-hemorrhagic infections of the joint.

Extra-articular involvement is less frequently seen and produces an external fibrous or osseous encapsulation with minimal destruction of the joint itself.

Clinical Features

TMJ ankylosis occurs predominantly in the first decade of life, and males and females are equally affected. Almost all cases are unilateral. The condition presents as a gradually worsening inability to open the jaws, with the mandible shifting toward the affected side on opening. Pain, tenderness, and malocclusion are not usually present.

In severe cases, there is almost complete immobilization of the mandible and the mandible may protrude forward as the excess tissues occupy the joint space. In very young children, unilateral micrognathia (**hemifacial microsomia**) may result from diminished growth on the affected side. Malocclusion may be severe in such cases.

Histopathologic Features

There is no specific histopathologic feature of TMJ ankylosis, except for an excessive amount of dense fibrous connective tissue or new bone formation. Intra-articular ankylosis demonstrates irregular destruction of cartilage and bone with a sparse lymphocytic infiltration.

Treatment and Prognosis

Surgical osteoplasty of the joint with removal of excessive fibrous or calcific tissues is the treatment of choice for TMJ ankylosis. For severe cases, complete joint replacement may be necessary.

REFERENCES

Bell's Palsy

Furuta Y, et al. Latent herpes simplex virus type 1 in human geniculate ganglia. Acta Neuropathol (Berl) 84:39–44, 1992.

Kuiper H, et al. Absence of Lyme borreliosis among patients with presumed Bell's palsy. Arch Neurol 49:940–943, 1992.

Morgan M, Nathwani D. Facial palsy and infection: The unfolding story. Clin Infect Dis 14:263–271, 1992.

Peitersen E. Natural history of Bell's palsy. Acta Otolaryngol (Stockh) 492(Suppl):122–124, 1992.

Sussman GL, Yang WH, Steinberg S. Melkersson-Rosenthal syndrome: Clinical, pathologic, and therapeutic considerations. Ann Allergy 69:187–194, 1992.

Trigeminal Neuralgia

Apfelbaum RI. Surgery for tic douloureux. Clin Neurosurg 31:351–368, 1984.

Brisman R. Trigeminal neuralgia and multiple sclerosis. Arch Neurol 44:379–381, 1987.

Burchiel KJ, et al. Long-term efficacy of microvascular decompression in trigeminal neuralgia. J Neurosurg 69:35–38, 1988.

Delfino U, Beltrutti DP, Clemente MS. Trigeminal neuralgia: Evaluation of percutaneous neurodestructive procedures. Clin J Pain 6:18–25, 1990.

Devor M. The pathophysiology and anatomy of damaged nerve. In: Textbook of Pain. Edited by Wall PD, Melzack R. New York, Churchill Livingstone, 1984, pp 49–64.

Fromm GH, Terrence CF, Maroon JCL. Trigeminal neuralgia—current concepts regarding etiology and pathogenesis. Arch Neurol 41:1204–1207, 1984.

Mokri B. Raeder's paratrigeminal syndrome: Original concept and subsequent deviations. Arch Neurol 39:395–399, 1982.

Rosenkopf KL. Current concepts concerning the etiology and treatment of trigeminal neuralgia. Cranio 7:312–318, 1989.

Sweet WH. The treatment of trigeminal neuralgia (tic douloureux). N Engl J Med 315:174–177, 1986.

Wilkins RH. Tic douloureux. Contemp Neurosurg 1:1–6, 1979.

Glossopharyngeal Neuralgia

Dandy WE. Glossopharyngeal neuralgia (tic douloureux): Its diagnosis and treatment. Arch Surg 15:198–214, 1927.

deMaragas JM, Kierland RR. The outcome of patients with herpes zoster. Arch Dermatol 75:193–196, 1957.

Donlon WC, Jacobson AL, Truta MP. Neuralgias. Otolaryngol Clin North Am 22:1145–1158, 1989.

Rushton JG, Stevens C, Miller RH. Glossopharyngeal (vagoglossopharyngeal) neuralgia: A study of 217 cases. Arch Neurol 38:201–205, 1981.

Stevens JC. Cranial neuralgias. J Craniomandib Disord 1:51–53, 1987.

Atypical Facial Pain

Brooke RI. Atypical odontalgia. Oral Surg Oral Med Oral Pathol 43:196–199, 1980.

Foster JB. Facial pain. Br Med J 4:667–669, 1969.

Gratt B, et al. Electronic thermography in the diagnosis of atypical odontalgia: A pilot study. Oral Surg Oral Med Oral Pathol 68:472–481, 1989.

Gregg JM. Studies of traumatic neuralgia in the maxillofacial region: Surgical pathology and neural mechanisms. J Oral Maxillofac Surg 48:228–237, 1990.

Hampf G, et al. Psychiatric disorders in orofacial dysaesthesia. Int J Oral Maxillofac Surg 16:402–407, 1987.

Kerr FWL. Atypical facial neuralgias; their mechanism as inferred from anatomic and physiologic data. Mayo Clin Proc 36:254–260, 1961.

Main JH, Jordan RC, Barewal R. Facial neuralgias: A clinical review of 34 cases. J Can Dent Assoc 58:752–755, 1992.

Marbach JJ, et al. Incidence of phantom tooth pain: An atypical facial neuralgia. Oral Surg Oral Med Oral Pathol 53:190–193, 1982.

Sessle BJ. The neurobiology of facial and dental pain: Present knowledge, future directions. J Dent Res 65:962–981, 1987.

Neuralgia-Inducing Cavitational Osteonecrosis

Bouquot J, Christian J. Long-term effects of jawbone curettage on the pain of facial neuralgia; treatment results in neuralgia-inducing cavitational osteonecrosis. Oral Surg Oral Med Oral Pathol 72:582, 1991.

Bouquot JE, et al. NICO (neuralgia-inducing cavitational osteonecrosis): Osteomyelitis in 224 jawbone samples from patients with facial neuralgias. Oral Surg Oral Med Oral Pathol 73:307–319, 1992.

Mankin HJ. Nontraumatic necrosis of bone (osteonecrosis). N Engl J Med 326:1473–1479, 1992.

McMahon RE, Adams W, Spolnik KJ. Diagnostic anesthesia for referred trigeminal pain: Part 1. Compendium 13:870–876, 1992.

Ratner EJ, et al. Jawbone cavities and trigeminal and atypical facial neuralgias. Oral Surg Oral Med Oral Pathol 48:3–20, 1979.

Roberts AM, Person P. Etiology and treatment of idiopathic trigeminal and atypical facial neuralgias. Oral Surg Oral Med Oral Pathol 48:298–308, 1979.

Cluster Headache

Brooke RI. Periodic migrainous neuralgia: A cause of dental pain. Oral Surg Oral Med Oral Pathol 46:511–516, 1978.

Campbell JK. Cluster headache. J Craniomandib Disord 1:27–33, 1987.

Campbell JK. Diagnosis and treatment of cluster headache. J Pain Symptom Manage 8:155–164, 1993.

Curless RG. Cluster headache in childhood. J Pediatr 101:393–395, 1982.

Di Sabato F, et al. Hyperbaric oxygen therapy in cluster headache. Pain 52:243–245, 1993.

Horton BT, MacLean AR, Craig WM. A new syndrome of vascular headache: Results of treatment with histamine: Preliminary report. Mayo Clin Proc 14:257–260, 1939.

Walling AD. Cluster headache. Am Fam Physician 47:1457–1465, 1993.

Migraine

Maxwell RE. Surgical control of chronic migrainous neuralgia by trigeminal gangliorhizolysis. J Neurosurg 57:459–466, 1982.

Moss RA. Oral behavioral patterns in common migraine. Cranio 5:196–202, 1987.

Olesen J. Some clinical features of acute migraine attack: An analysis of 750 patients. Headache 18:268–271, 1978.

Raskin NH. Headache, 2nd ed. New York, Churchill Livingstone, 1988.

Scheitler LE, Balciunas BA. Carotidynia. J Oral Maxillofac Surg 40:121–122, 1982.

Temporal Arteritis

Allen NB, Farmer JC. Giant cell arteritis and polymyalgia rheumatica. Ann Otol Rhinol Laryngol 96:373–379, 1987.

Bielory L, Ogunkoya A, Frohman LP. Temporal arteritis in blacks. Am J Med 86:707–708, 1989.

Fernandez-Herlihy L. Temporal arteritis: Clinical aids to diagnosis. J Rheumatol 15:1797–1801, 1988.

Gudmundsson M, et al. Plasma viscosity in giant cell arteritis as a predictor of disease activity. Ann Rheum Dis 52:104–109, 1993.

Scully C, et al. Necrosis of the lip in giant cell arteritis: Report of a case. J Oral Maxillofac Surg 51:581–583, 1993.

Myasthenia Gravis

Keeling CW. Myasthenia gravis. J Oral Surg 9:224–232, 1951.

Lopate G, Pestronk A. Autoimmune myasthenia gravis. Hosp Pract (Off Ed) 28:109–122, 1993.

Shah A, Lisak RP. Immunopharmacologic therapy in myasthenia gravis. Clin Neuropharmacol 16:97–103, 1993.

Zweiman B, Levinson AI. Immunologic aspects of neurological and neuromuscular diseases. JAMA 268:2918–2922, 1992.

Motor Neuron Disease

Bensimon G, et al. A controlled trial of riluzole in amyotrophic lateral sclerosis. N Engl J Med 330:585–591, 1994.

Fleck H, Surrow HB. Familial amyotrophic lateral sclerosis. NY State J Med 67:2368–2373, 1967.

Pradas J, et al. The natural history of amyotrophic lateral sclerosis and the use of natural history controls in therapeutic trials. Neurology 43:751–755, 1993.

Roller NW, et al. Amyotrophic lateral sclerosis. Oral Surg Oral Med Oral Pathol 37:46–52, 1974.

Rosen DR, et al. Mutations in Cu/Zn superoxide dismutase gene are associated with familial amyotrophic lateral sclerosis. Nature 362:59–62, 1993.

Swash M, Schwartz MS. What do we really know about amyotrophic lateral sclerosis? J Neurol Sci 113:4–16, 1992.

Idiopathic Burning Tongue Syndrome

Basker RM, Sturdee DW, Davenport JC. Patients with burning mouths: A clinical investigation of causative factors, including the climacteric and diabetes. Br Dent J 145:9–16, 1978.

Dutrée-Meulenberg RO, Kozel MM, van Joost T. Burning mouth syndrome: A possible etiologic role for local contact hypersensitivity. J Am Acad Dermatol 26:935–940, 1992.

Gorsky M, Silverman S Jr, Chinn H. Clinical characteristics and management outcome in the burning mouth syndrome. Oral Surg Oral Med Oral Pathol 72:192–195, 1991.

Grushka M, Sessle BJ. Burning mouth syndrome. Dent Clin North Am 35:171–184, 1991.

Maresky LS, van der Bijl, P, Gird I. Burning mouth syndrome: Evaluation of multiple variables among 85 patients. Oral Surg Oral Med Oral Pathol 75:303–307, 1993.

Mott AE, Grushka M, Sessle BJ. Diagnosis and management of taste disorders and burning mouth syndrome. Dent Clin North Am 37:33–71, 1993.

Rojo L, et al. Psychiatric morbidity in burning mouth syndrome: Psychiatric interview versus depression and anxiety scales. Oral Surg Oral Med Oral Pathol 75:308–311, 1993.

Tourne LP, Fricton JR. Burning mouth syndrome: Critical review and proposed clinical management. Oral Surg Oral Med Oral Pathol 74:158–167, 1992.

van der Waal I. The Burning Mouth Syndrome. Copenhagen, Munksgaard, 1990.

Yontchev E, Carlsson GE. Long-term follow-up of patients with orofacial discomfort complaints. J Oral Rehabil 19:13–19, 1992.

Dysgeusia

Amsterdam JD, et al. Taste and smell perception in depression. Biol Psychiatry 22:1481–1485, 1987.

Bartoshuk LM, et al. Taste and aging. J Gerontol 41:51–57, 1986.

Bradley RM. Effects of aging on the anatomy and neurophysiology of taste. Gerodontics 4:244–248, 1988.

Frank ME, Hettinger TP, Mott, AE. The sense of taste: Neurobiology, aging, and medication effects. Crit Rev Oral Biol Med 3:371–393, 1992.

Mott AE, Grushka M, Sessle BJ. Diagnosis and management of taste disorders and burning mouth syndrome. Dent Clin North Am 37:33–71, 1993.

Preti G, et al. Non-oral etiologies of oral malodor and altered chemosensation. J Periodontol 63:790–796, 1992.

Auriculotemporal Syndrome

Hays L. The Frey syndrome. Otolaryngol Head Neck Surg 90:419–425, 1982.

Hemenway WG. Gustatory sweating and flushing; the auriculotemporal—Frey's syndrome. Laryngoscope 70:84–90, 1960.

McGibbon BM, Paletta FX. Further concepts in gustatory sweating. Plast Reconstr Surg 49:639–642, 1972.

Zoller J, Maier H. Frey's syndrome secondary to a subcondylar fracture. Otolaryngol Head Neck Surg 108:751–753, 1993.

Osteoarthritis

Barrett AW, Griffiths MJ, Scully C. Osteoarthrosis, the temporomandibular joint, and Eagle's syndrome. Oral Surg Oral Med Oral Pathol 75:273–275, 1993.

DeBont LGM, et al. Osteoarthritis and internal derangement of the temporomandibular joint: A light microscopic study. J Oral Maxillofac Surg 44:634–643, 1986.

European Society of Osteoarthrology (ESOA). Joint destruction in arthritis and osteoarthritis: 19th Symposium of the ESOA. Agents Actions 39(Suppl):1–272, 1993.

Hollander AP, et al. Hypothesis: Cartilage catabolic cofactors in human arthritis. J Rheumatol 20:223–224, 1993.

Iacopino AM, Wathen WF. Craniomandibular disorders in the geriatric patient. J Orofacial Pain 7:38–53, 1993.

Kreutziger K, Mahan P. Temporomandibular degenerative joint disease. Oral Surg Oral Med Oral Pathol 40:165–182, 1975.

Pullinger AG, Seligman DA. TMJ osteoarthrosis: A differentiation of diagnostic subgroups by symptom history and demographics. J Craniomandib Disord 1:251–256, 1987.

Rheumatoid Arthritis

Chalmers IM, Blair GS. Rheumatoid arthritis of the temporomandibular joint. Q J Med 42:369–386, 1973.

Eriscon S, Lundberg M. Alterations in the temporomandibular joint at various stages of rheumatoid arthritis. Acta Rheum Scand 13:257–274, 1967.

Friedman MH, Weisberg J, Agus B. Diagnosis and treatment of inflammation of the temporomandibular joint. Semin Arthritis Rheum 12:44–51, 1982.

Harris ED. Pathogenesis of rheumatoid arthritis. Am J Med 80:4–10, 1986.

Larheim TA, Bjornland T. Arthrographic findings in the temporomandibular joint in patients with rheumatic disease. J Oral Maxillofac Surg 47:780–784, 1989.

Marbach JJ. Arthritis of the temporomandibular joints and facial pain. Bull Rheum Dis 27:918–921, 1976–1977.

Schumacher HR, Gall EP. Rheumatoid Arthritis: An Illustrated Guide to Pathology, Diagnosis, and Management. Philadelphia, JB Lippincott, 1988.

Solberg WK. Temporomandibular disorders: Management of problems associated with inflammation, chronic hypermobility and deformity. Br Dent J 16:421–428, 1986.

Zide MF, Carlton DM, Kent JN. Rheumatoid disease and related arthropathies: I. Systemic findings, medical therapy, and peripheral joint surgery. Oral Surg Oral Med Oral Pathol 61:119–125, 1986.

Temporomandibular Joint Dysfunction

Akerman S, Kopp S, Rohlin M. Histological changes in the temporomandibular joint from elderly individuals. Acta Odontol Scand 44:231–239, 1986.

Bell WE. Temporomandibular Disorders: Classification, Diagnosis, Management, 3rd ed. Chicago, Year Book Medical Publishers, 1990.

Burakoff RP, Kaplan AS. Temporomandibular disorders: Current concepts of epidemiology, classification, and treatment. J Pain Symptom Manage 8:165–172, 1993.

Costen JB. A syndrome of ear and sinus symptoms dependent upon disturbed function of the temporomandibular joint. Ann Otol Rhinol Laryngol 43:1–15, 1934.

Delfino JJ, Eppley BL. Radiographic and surgical evaluation of internal derangements of the temporomandibular joint. J Oral Maxillofac Surg 44:260–267, 1986.

Fricton JR, et al. Myofascial pain syndrome of the head and neck: A review of clinical characteristics of 164 patients. Oral Surg Oral Med Oral Pathol 60:615–623, 1985.

Greene CS, Laskin DM. Long-term evaluation of treatment for myofascial pain-dysfunction syndrome: A comparative analysis. J Am Dent Assoc 107:235–238, 1983.

Kaplan AS, Assael LA. Temporomandibular Disorders: Diagnosis and Treatment. Philadelphia, WB Saunders, 1991.

Kemper JT, Okeson JP. Craniomandibular disorders and headaches. J Prosthet Dent 49:702–705, 1983.

Lundh H, Westesson PL. Clinical signs of temporomandibular joint internal derangement in adults: An epidemiologic study. Oral Surg Oral Med Oral Pathol 72:637–641, 1991.

Okeson JP, Hayes DK. Long-term results of treatment for temporomandibular disorders: An evaluation by patients. J Am Dent Assoc 112:473–478, 1986.

Österberg T, et al. A cross-sectional and longitudinal study of craniomandibular dysfunction in an elderly population. J Craniomandib Disord 6:237–245, 1992.

Wright WJ Jr. Temporomandibular disorders: Occurrence of specific diagnoses and response to conservative management: Clinical observations. Cranio 4:150–155, 1986.

Temporomandibular Joint Ankylosis

Freedus MS, William DZ, Doyle PK. Principles of treatment of temporomandibular joint ankylosis. J Oral Surg 33:757–765, 1975.

Koorbusch GF, et al. Psoriatic arthritis of the temporomandibular joints with ankylosis. Oral Surg Oral Med Oral Pathol 71:267–274, 1991.

Munro IR, Chen YR, Park BY. Simultaneous total correction of temporomandibular joint reconstruction. J Oral Maxillofac Surg 44:520–533, 1986.

Rowe NL. Ankylosis of temporomandibular joint. J R Coll Surg Edinb 27:67–79, 1982.

Rowe NL. Ankylosis of the temporomandibular joint. Part 2. J R Coll Surg Edinb 27:167–173, 1982.

Rowe NL. Ankylosis of the temporomandibular joint. Part 3. J R Coll Surg Edinb 27:209–218, 1982.

Sarma UC, Dave PK. Temporomandibular joint ankylosis: An Indian experience. Oral Surg Oral Med Oral Pathol 72:660–664, 1991.

19

Forensic Dentistry

Edward E. Herschaft

Forensic dentistry, which is also referred to as *forensic odontology*, is the area of dentistry concerned with the correct management, examination, evaluation, and presentation of dental evidence in criminal or civil legal proceedings in the interest of justice. Thus, the forensic dentist must be knowledgeable in both dentistry and the law.

Classically, forensic dentistry can be considered a subspecialty of oral and maxillofacial pathology. This is analogous to the relationship in medicine between forensic pathology and pathology. The requirements of forensic dental field work, however, often demand an interdisciplinary knowledge of dental science. This has resulted in other dental specialists, and general dentists, joining oral and maxillofacial pathologists in providing legal authorities with dental expertise.

Regardless of background, forensic dentists assist legal authorities by preparing dental evidence in the following situations:

1. Management and maintenance of dental records that comply with legal requirements to document all unique dental information necessary to identify the patient and to reduce the potential for malpractice litigation.
2. Identification of human remains, through the comparison of antemortem and postmortem dental information, in cases that involve individual deaths, or multiple deaths in mass disasters.
3. Collection and analysis of patterned marks (bite marks) in inanimate material or injured tissue, which can be compared, and potentially matched, with a specific human or animal dentition.
4. Recognition of the signs and symptoms of child abuse and the dental health care worker's rights and responsibilities when reporting such abuse.
5. Presentation of dental evidence as an expert witness in identification, bite mark, child abuse, malpractice, and personal injury cases.

RECORD MANAGEMENT

The dental record is a legal document, owned by the dentist and containing all subjective and objective information about the patient. Initially, this information is secured when the patient's medical and dental history is obtained. Results of the physical examination of the dentition and supporting oral and paraoral structures are recorded.

In addition, the results of clinical laboratory tests, study casts, photographs, and radiographs become components of the record. With this data base, the dentist can develop a thorough assessment of all the patient's medical and dental problems. Subsequent documentation of this "problem list" facilitates the development of a plan of treatment and prognosis for the patient.

The treatment plan addresses the management of both systemic and oral problems. This can then be revised and updated periodically as problems resolve or as new ones develop. Supplemental material, such as dental laboratory authorizations, referral letters from other practitioners, statements of informed consent, written prescriptions, and insurance and financial statements, is also included and stored in the record.

The progress notes, a daily log of the actual treatment rendered, should contain information about the restorative and therapeutic procedures provided. Unusual physiologic and psychologic reactions and the patient's comments concerning therapy are entered in the record. Summaries of telephone conversations with patients, consultants, insurance company representatives, or legal authorities should be noted.

All entries should be signed or initialed by recording personnel. Changes in the record should be not erased but corrected by a single line drawn through the incorrect material. This permits the original entry to remain readable and removes any questions concerning fraudulent intent to alter recorded information.

These principles of record management describe a mechanism ensuring that dental information, which may be required to resolve a forensic problem, is properly maintained and retrievable. Additionally, records preserved in this manner are reliable evidenciary material if subpoenaed in peer review or malpractice litigation proceedings.

Time limits concerning how long records must be retained vary among the states. As a rule, states mandate that records be kept for 7 to 10 years. Federal legislation related to the problem of missing persons in the United States requires that records of pediatric dental patients be retained until the patient reaches the age of majority.

IDENTIFICATION

Legal situations often revolve around the establishment of a person's proper identity. The official who is responsible for establishing identification, determining the mode and manner of death, and issuing a death certificate is the coroner or medical examiner. The coroner is an elected official and, depending on the laws of each state, may not necessarily be a physician or have advanced training in death investigation. A medical examiner is an appointed official who is a pathologist specifically trained in forensic medicine.

A death certificate, identifying the decedent, is required before probation of a will, release of life insurance claims, or resolution of other affairs associated with the settlement of an estate. Criminal cases involving homicide, suicide, and fraudulent misidentification may also require the expertise of forensic dentists and other forensic scientists trained in identification techniques. These professionals act as consultants to the coroner or medical examiner and assist in this aspect of a death investigation.

Besides analysis of the teeth, the most common methods of identification include personal recognition, fingerprinting, physical anthropologic examination of bones, and serologic and genetic (DNA) comparison techniques. Each method has its advantages and disadvantages. However, all rely on the principle that identification is the positive correlation obtained by comparing known information about a suspect or victim with unique facts retrieved by physical examination of the suspect or victim.

Regardless of the method used to identify a decedent, the results of the antemortem and postmortem data comparison lead to one of the following situations:

1. *Positive identification.* There is sufficient uniqueness among the comparable items in the antemortem and postmortem data bases, and no major differences are observed.
2. *Presumptive (possible) identification.* There are commonalities among the comparable items in the antemortem and postmortem data bases; however, enough information may be missing from either source to prevent the establishment of a positive identification.
3. *Insufficient identification evidence.* There is insufficient supportive evidence available to compare and arrive at a conclusion based on scientific principles.
4. *Exclusion of identification evidence.* There are either explainable or unexplainable discrepancies among comparable items in the antemortem and postmortem data bases. This results in inconsistencies that prevent the establishment of any identification. Exclusion may be just as important as a determination of positive identification.

Personal Recognition

Personal recognition is the least reliable method used to identify an individual. It is often based on the visual identification of a decedent by a family member, friend, or acquaintance. This process assesses artifactual material, such as clothing, jewelry, keys, wallet contents, luggage, other personal effects, scars, and tattoos to determine an identification. Evidence in this type of identification can be accidentally or purposely exchanged between bodies. This can occur in mass disaster situations or when there is criminal intent to create a misidentification.

Even when a body is viewed shortly after death, distraught relatives can inadvertently misidentify the remains. After the occurrence of postmortem changes associated with soft tissue decomposition, burn artifact, or dismemberment, this method of identification may be precluded.

Fingerprinting

By the beginning of the 20th century, forensic science had recognized that the ridge-like patterns on the fingertips and palms are unique for each person. These friction ridges are genetically determined, and not even homozygous twins have the same pattern. A principal variation in the fingerprints of twins is that they appear as mirror images of each other. The variation in combinations of loops, arches, and whorls permits a scientific comparison of fingerprint records with the prints of an unidentified decedent.

Because the fingerprint pattern is inherited, it is a static characteristic and remains unchanged throughout life. This is an important advantage when one compares fingerprint identification with dental identification. The teeth and supporting structures have fluid characteristics. Dental patterns change as teeth erupt, exfoliate, decay, become restored, and, perhaps, are eventually extracted.

Unlike dental records, which are principally retained in private dental offices in North America, fingerprint information is maintained by governmental agencies. The Identification Division of the Federal Bureau of Investigation (FBI) contains approximately 200 million fingerprint records. The recent development of computerized automated fingerprint identification systems (AFISs) even permits input, matching, and retrieval of a single fingerprint image for identification.

Fingerprint nomenclature is standardized, and the same terminology is used by all fingerprint experts worldwide. This advantage is not observed in dental identification, in which numerous charting and tooth numbering systems are employed. Because soft tissues decompose after death, the fingerprint may not be retrievable. This is the principal disadvantage of fingerprint identification.

Physical Anthropologic Examination of Bones

Forensic anthropologists and forensic dentists often work together to resolve problems associated with identification. Both disciplines are concerned with analysis of calcified structures of the body—bones and teeth. This anatomic material can be used to determine the race, age, and sex of a person (Table 19–1).

In addition, the teeth can be studied clinically and radiographically to determine the age of the decedent on the basis of eruption patterns and calcification times. This information, combined with analysis of the calcification centers of the hand and wrist, can be used to determine the precise age of a person who is younger than 20 years of age.

Laboratory procedures used to determine the age of teeth include the study of variations in patterns of:

- Attrition
- Periodontal attachment
- Secondary dentin
- Cementum apposition
- Root resorption
- Transparency

This technique, developed by Gustafson in 1947, has recently been supplemented by a method that relies on an analysis of the rate of racemization of aspartic acid in enamel and dentin to determine an exact age. Often, anthropologic analysis is helpful in arriving at a presumptive identification based on these criteria.

Positive identification is achievable when the skull and facial bones are used as a foundation to reconstruct the facial soft tissues (Figs. 19–1 to 19–3). Three-dimensional computer images, computed tomographic (CT) images, and radiographs have been used in the replication of the face of a 5000-year-old person whose remains were removed from glacial ice on the Austrian-Italian border.

With a knowledge of the anatomic relationships between the skull and face, antemortem facial photographs or radiographs can be superimposed and matched with the skull. Prosthetic joint replacements, intraosseous implants, and radiographic signs of prior bone fracture are additional anthropologic findings that can be used to facilitate identification.

Serologic and Genetic (DNA) Comparison

A comparison of antigenic markers found on red blood cells and in body fluids of people who secrete these

Table 19–1. SKELETAL ANTHROPOLOGIC VARIATIONS ASSOCIATED WITH RACIAL AND SEXUAL CHARACTERISTICS OF THE SKULL

	Racial Characteristics		
	White	*Black*	*Asian/Native American*
Width	Narrow	Narrow	Broad
Height	High	Low	Intermediate
Profile	Straight	Prognathic	Intermediate
Orbit	Triangular/teardrop	Square	Circular
Nasal opening	Tapered	Wide	Rounded
Palate	Narrow	Wide	Intermediate

	Sexual Characteristics	
	Male	*Female*
Size	Large	Small
Glabellar (supraorbital) ridges	Pronounced	Not developed
Mastoid process	Large	Small
Occipital area	Pronounced muscle lines	Minimal muscle lines
Mandible	Larger, broader ramus	Smaller
Forehead	Steeper, slopes posteriorly	Rounded, more vertical

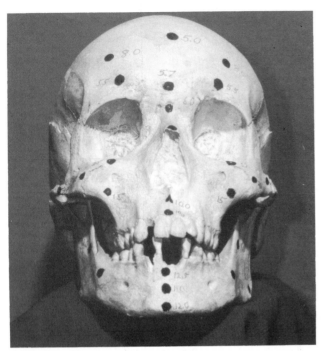

FIGURE 19-1. Reconstruction of the facial soft tissue uses predetermined, standard anthropologic thickness measurements for specific points around the face. These measurements are based on variables that are related to racial and sexual characteristics.

markers has traditionally been a source of exculpatory (exclusionary) evidence. This type of evidence is used to exclude a suspect or victim when negative results are achieved. Positive comparisons can only place the suspect or victim in a population of individuals who have similar serologic antigens.

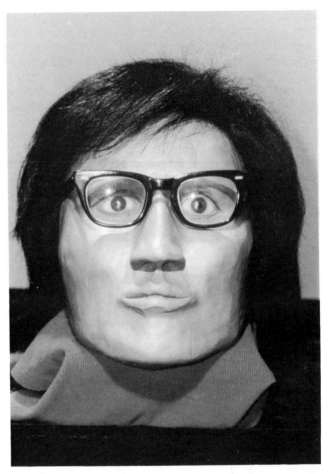

FIGURE 19-3. The width of the mouth is related to the interpupillary distance. The length and shape of the nose are determined by the relationship between the inferior and superior nasal spines. If known, the addition of a specific hair style, eyeglasses, and eye color can further individualize a facial reconstruction.

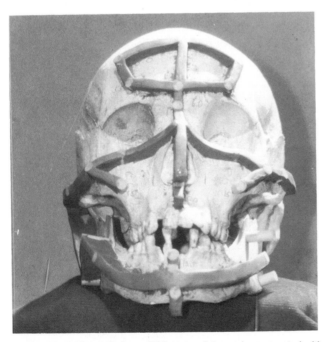

FIGURE 19-2. The soft tissue thickness points can be connected with sculpting clay or digitized on a computer screen. The ultimate result of these techniques is a recreation of the contour of the soft tissue features that permits a visual identification.

Antigenic substances A, B, and H of the ABO system; M, N, and S of the MN system; and various components of the rhesus (Rh) system and the Lewis system are accepted for medicolegal comparison. The ability to secrete the ABH antigens in saliva and other body fluids is genetically determined. More than 80 percent of people are secretors. With appropriate laboratory tests, even dried samples of fluid and blood can be analyzed for these markers.

Although each person is a unique individual by virtue of their DNA, it was not until 1986 that this "ultimate identification material" was employed in law enforcement. The laboratory techniques used to evaluate fragments of this genetic material are extremely accurate, precise, and reproducible. They are also advantageous because they permit analysis of small samples or of degraded evidence.

The U.S. Defense Department has initiated a policy of obtaining DNA samples on all military personnel. This DNA "fingerprint" would significantly reduce the possibility of another unknown soldier among future military casualties.

Despite the positive effects of DNA evidence in resolving questions of identity, the technique is not without controversy. Challenges have been made by population geneticists, concerned about random matching and variations among racial subgroups.

Dental Evaluation

Basic Principles

In identification cases, the principal advantage of dental evidence is that, like other hard tissue, it is often preserved indefinitely after death. Although the status of a person's teeth changes throughout life, the combination of decayed, missing, and filled teeth is measurable, reproducible, and comparable at any fixed point in time. Therefore, like the comparison of unique patterns in a fingerprint, a scientific, objective analysis of antemortem and postmortem dental variables is achievable.

The presence and position of individual teeth and the respective anatomic, restorative, and pathologic components provide the data base for the antemortem and postmortem comparison (Fig. 19–4). The pattern of the palatal rugae, ridges on the lip surface, and radiographic outline of the maxillary and frontal sinuses, are also considered unique. In addition, the legal community accepts the fact that dentists can recognize procedures that they have performed.

Problems associated with dental identification information are often related to acquiring and interpreting antemortem records. Most antemortem dental records are retrieved from private sector dental providers. However, dental records may be recovered from insurance carriers, dental schools, hospitals, clinics, state and fed-

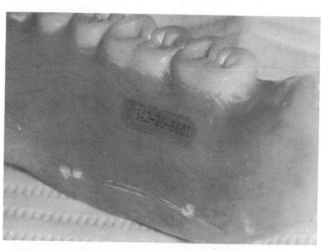

FIGURE 19–5. Denture identification is accomplished by inserting a typed name or code number (Social Security number, hospital patient number) in an area of the denture that will not interfere with the aesthetics of the prosthesis. This is performed in the laboratory during the final acrylic pack. This information can also be engraved in the framework of an all-metal appliance.

eral prisons, military files, and the FBI National Crime Information Center (NCIC).

To initiate a request for antemortem records, a putative (suspected) identification is required. Reports of missing and unidentified persons, obtained from law enforcement agencies, are the principal source for this material. Thousands of victims who cannot be identified by fingerprint methods remain unidentified because a putative identification has not been established.

The FBI-NCIC computer registry of missing and unidentified persons was established to help rectify this problem. This computer system maintains demographic, dental, and medical information on missing persons. It attempts to match these data with similar facts obtained from unidentified bodies. The latter information is submitted by various investigative and legal agencies. Potentially, the otherwise unidentifiable victims of random violence, serial homicides, and child abduction can now be identified without the need to determine a putative identification.

The Armed Forces, Department of Veterans Affairs, and many states require that identifying markings be placed on removable dental prostheses (Fig. 19–5). This policy is also supported by the American Dental Association. It is an attempt to provide a basis for identification among the substantial population of completely or partially edentulous individuals in the United States.

Identifying markings in dental prostheses are important because even if dental records of an edentulous person can be obtained, they may not reflect the current status of the ridges and alveolar bone. Commonly used information for identifying markings in removable dental prostheses includes the person's name, driver's license number, or Social Security number.

Even when a suspected identification is achieved, it may still be difficult to secure antemortem dental records. The family or acquaintances of the victim may not know where dental treatment was sought. Reviewing

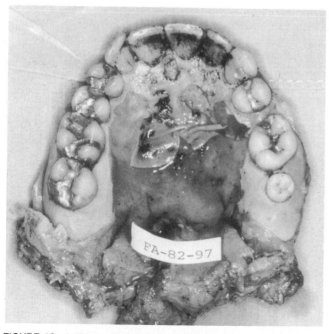

FIGURE 19–4. The combination of decayed, missing, and filled teeth, along with unique anatomic and pathologic findings, provides the data base for comparison in a dental identification. Note the microdont in the maxillary left quadrant.

the victim's canceled bank checks or medical deductions on tax records may be helpful in locating antemortem dental records in such cases.

Although records obtained from institutional or governmental dental facilities routinely indicate all restored teeth, this is not true of charts forwarded from private dentists. In these instances, previously restored teeth that have not been re-treated by the current dentist are often not charted. Therefore, in these records, the antemortem radiographs and progress notes become the principal sources for dental information.

Unfortunately, the nomenclature associated with dental charting systems is not standardized (Table 19–2). In 1984, the American Dental Association adopted the Universal Tooth Numbering System. This system is now used by all insurance companies, the Armed Forces, dental schools, and most dentists in the United States. This system should be used in all forensic dental cases at this time.

In the Universal Numbering System, a consecutive number from 1 to 32 is assigned to the adult dentition. It begins with the maxillary right third molar and ends with the mandibular right third molar. The deciduous dentition is identified by letters from A to T, beginning with the maxillary right deciduous second molar and ending with the mandibular right deciduous second molar. Thus, the quadrants are identified in a clockwise direction, beginning with the maxillary right.

Other tooth numbering methods include the Zsigmondy/Palmer System and the Federation Dentaire Internationale (FDI) Two-Digit System. Each uses a different coding technique to identify dental quadrants and specific teeth.

The Zsigmondy/Palmer System stresses the anatomic likeness of the eight tooth types in each symbolically identified dental quadrant. Homologous permanent teeth are assigned the same number from 1 to 8. Deciduous teeth are assigned letters A through E.

The FDI Two-Digit System is endorsed by the World Health Organization and is used in most developed countries except the United States and Canada. The first digit represents the quadrant. Quadrants 1 to 4 are assigned for permanent teeth; 5 to 8 represent quadrants for the primary dentition. As in the Universal Numbering System, the quadrants are identified in a clockwise direction, beginning with the maxillary right. The second digit designates the permanent tooth type from 1 to 8, or deciduous tooth type from 1 to 5.

Thus, in the Universal Numbering System, tooth 12 is the maxillary left first bicuspid. In the FDI Two-Digit System, tooth 12 (one-two) is the maxillary right lateral incisor. In the Zsigmondy/Palmer System, all lateral incisors are designated with a number 2 code. The position of a specific number 2 tooth is diagrammatically indicated by a symbolic quadrant.

Unless the forensic dentist knows which system has been used to encode the teeth in the antemortem record, all teeth should be referred to by their actual names. This will prevent errors because all dentists use the same anatomic nomenclature when referring to individual teeth.

Dental identification problems may be further compounded because dental radiographs can be mounted and viewed from right to left or vice versa. Radiographic duplicating film does not contain a raised dot to assist the dentist in orienting the film for mounting. This, too, can lead to transposition of dental evidence and potential misidentification based on an incorrect comparison.

With the advent of aesthetic materials for posterior restorations and the reduction in the incidence of caries, it may be difficult for the forensic dentist to determine whether restorations are present by simple visual assessment of the teeth. In addition, the postmortem dental evaluation is often performed in an autopsy room, temporary morgue, or funeral home. In these locations, proper lighting and access to dental instruments, which can facilitate analysis of the oral structures, are not readily available for detailed examination.

Often, there are additional demands for immediacy in providing a coroner, medical examiner, or other legal agent with the results of a dental identification. This further compounds the forensic dentist's technical and stress-related problems while performing the tasks related to this discipline. Because of the previous caveats, the forensic dentist should prepare an equipment kit (Table 19–3). The kit should be portable, containing instruments and supplies specifically required for the performance of dental procedures in an autopsy room environment.

Table 19–2. DENTAL NUMBERING SYSTEMS

Permanent Teeth

Maxillary Right / Mandibular Right	Maxillary Left / Mandibular Left

Universal Numbering System

1 2 3 4 5 6 7 8 9 10 11 12 13 14 15 16
32 31 30 29 28 27 26 25 24 23 22 21 20 19 18 17

Zsigmondy/Palmer System

8 7 6 5 4 3 2 1 | 1 2 3 4 5 6 7 8
8 7 6 5 4 3 2 1 | 1 2 3 4 5 6 7 8

Federation Dentaire International System

18 17 16 15 14 13 12 11 21 22 23 24 25 26 27 28
48 47 46 45 44 43 42 41 31 32 33 34 35 36 37 38 39

Deciduous Teeth

Universal Numbering System

A B C D E F G H I J
T S R Q P O N M L K

Alternate Universal Numbering System

4D 5D 6D 7D 8D 9D 10D 11D 12D 13D
29D 28D 27D 26D 25D 24D 23D 22D 21D 20D

Zsigmondy/Palmer System

E D C B A | A B C D E
E D C B A | A B C D E

Federation Dentaire International System

55 54 53 52 51 61 62 63 64 65
85 84 83 82 81 71 72 73 74 75

Table 19-3. A SUGGESTED INSTRUMENT KIT FOR FORENSIC IDENTIFICATION

Dental explorers	Scalpels and blades	Radiographic film
Dental mirrors	Cheek retractors	Tissue forceps
Bite blocks	ABFO no. 2 ruler	Tissue clamp
Tissue scissors	Bone mallet	Tongue clamp
Osteotome	Flashlight or head	Disclosing solution
Rubber air/water	lamp	Stryker saw
syringe	Single lens reflex	Gauze
Cotton swabs	camera	Film
Photographic mirrors	Case labels	Appropriate charts
Writing instruments	Rubber gloves	Masks
Periodontal probes		

Guidelines for Dental Identification

Although dental information can support the identification of a visually recognizable body, identification of dental remains is especially helpful when a decedent is skeletonized, decomposed, burned, or dismembered. Because each of these forensic situations presents the dentist with different technical problems, Body Identification Guidelines have been established by the American Board of Forensic Odontology (ABFO). The purpose of delineating these criteria is to assist dentists in comparing antemortem and postmortem dental information. Furthermore, the possibility of misidentification is reduced in both routine and mass disaster cases.

Under the Body Identification Guidelines, provisions are made for:

1. Examination of the postmortem dental remains in compliance with infection control and Occupational Safety and Health Administration (OSHA) requirements.
2. Examination of antemortem dental records.
3. Comparison of all dental and paradental information from the two data bases.
4. Development of a written report listing conclusions and an opinion regarding the strength of the identification (e.g., positive, presumptive, insufficient or, exculpatory).

Postmortem Examination

The postmortem dental evidence is gathered by photographic, radiographic, and charting techniques. All records should include the case number, date, demographic and anthropologic information, the name of the authority that is requesting the dental examination, the location of the examination, and the name of the examining dentist.

Photographs should be taken of full head and face views. Images of the occlusal planes of both dental arches and individual views of unusual pathologic, or restorative, findings are also obtained. A single-lens reflex 35-mm camera and appropriate electronic flash and lens systems for close-up photography should be used. Routinely, both color and black-and-white film is recommended for use in each case.

Dental impressions and jaw resection may also be required after the initial full head photographs have been obtained. If requested by the coroner or medical examiner, the dental specimens from the autopsy may have to be retained and preserved in a 10 percent formalin solution.

The guidelines for body identification recognize that the dentist and dental auxiliary personnel involved in performing forensic dental procedures do so at the request and direction of a legal authority, such as a coroner or medical examiner. Therefore, it is only with the permission of these individuals that techniques involving postmortem facial dissection or jaw resection are performed by the forensic dentist to achieve complete access to dental tissues.

These measures are used most often in decomposed, dismembered, or incinerated bodies to make postmortem dental charting and radiographic examination easier. Resection or soft tissue dissection may be necessary in visually recognizable bodies when the oral cavity is inaccessible because of rigor mortis.

When the jaws are removed with a reciprocating (Stryker) saw or osteotome and mallet, a Le Fort type 1 fracture of the maxilla is created. The dissection instruments are placed above the inferior nasal spine and malar processes to ensure that the apices of the maxillary teeth are not transected. Similarly, if the mandible is not removed by disarticulation, cuts into the mandibular rami should be high enough to prevent damage to impacted third molars.

While obtaining postmortem radiographic evidence, the forensic dentist may encounter technical obstacles that need to be addressed. Because all dental evidence may eventually be required to be relinquished in court, the use of double-pack intraoral radiographs permits the forensic dentist to retain a set of films.

Rigor mortis in partially decomposed bodies and charring of dental evidence in fourth-degree burn and cremation cases may prevent the positioning of intraoral periapical films. Occlusal films, 5×7 lateral plates, and panoramic radiographs are often used in these situations. With the coroner's or medical examiner's permission, the entire skull can be placed in a panoramic radiographic machine. This technique is useful in cremation cases, when dental evidence may be lost or compromised by the manipulation associated with oral dissection.

Fragmentation of dental structures in dismemberment cases and total loss of soft tissues in skeletonized remains necessitate alterations in routine radiation exposure settings. Generally, when radiographs of this type of material are taken, 10-mA and 65-kVp exposure settings are used. Because there is little or no soft tissue, standard exposure times or impulse settings are halved to prevent overexposure of the radiograph.

The maxilla can be split along the midsagittal suture, and each half can be placed horizontally on an occlusal film. This projection can be used to simulate antemortem panoramic radiographs or bitewing views. Similar exposures can be obtained from the mandible by mounting the jaw on the edge of a table or bracket tray and placing an occlusal film under the supporting half. Films of the opposite side of the arch are made by simply

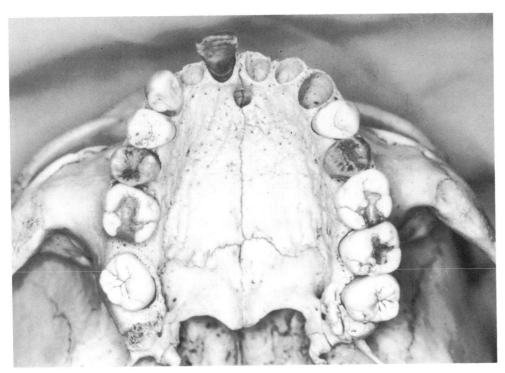

FIGURE 19–6. Postmortem tooth loss results in an alveolar socket with unfractured margins and no reossification. In this example, teeth 7, 9, 10, and 11 represent postmortem tooth loss. Tooth 2 is a result of antemortem loss. Teeth 4, 8, and 13 were found near the body and reinserted into their respective sockets.

flipping the mandible and repeating the exposure procedure.

The charting (odontogram) of the postmortem dentition should provide for situations in which teeth are missing after death. If such a discrepancy remains unexplained, it may preclude the positive identification of the body. Postmortem loss of teeth can be caused by scavenging animals or poor investigation of a crime or disaster scene. Environmental conditions at or around the time of death, such as tidal action in a salt-water drowning, can also contribute to perimortem loss of teeth. When teeth are lost in this manner, the crest of the alveolar bone remains intact. In addition, there is no reossification of the socket (Fig. 19–6). This pattern is inconsistent with what is observed after extraction of a tooth.

Postmortem tooth loss is associated with decomposition of the periodontal ligament. Thus, the tooth simply falls out when the body is moved by animals or during police recovery efforts. When this phenomenon occurs and is recognized, the charting abbreviation MPPA (Missing Postmortem, Present Antemortem) is used in that tooth's position in the dental odontogram.

Antemortem Record Examination

Antemortem records are usually obtained directly from the police, coroner, or medical examiner. Before accepting this evidence, the forensic dentist should determine that the records indicate the name of the person to be identified and the name and address of the submitting dentist. In addition, many jurisdictions require an evidence transfer document to be signed. This form indicates that the continuity of evidence has been maintained and specifies who is currently in possession of the material.

Several antemortem records of the same person may be submitted from different dental practices for comparison with postmortem dental evidence. It is not uncommon for the general dental records of a decedent and those obtained from the oral and maxillofacial surgeon, endodontist, orthodontist, and other dental specialty practices to be forwarded for forensic analysis.

Even if only one antemortem record is sent, the forensic dentist should rechart all information obtained from the radiographs, progress notes, and odontograms on a standardized form. This form should be identical to the one on which the postmortem information was documented. All of this material should be appropriately labeled as *the antemortem record*.

The use of computers in mass disaster situations accomplishes this same principle by entering all antemortem and postmortem dental information into the respective identification program. Besides making the comparison of records easier to manage, the creation of similar antemortem and postmortem analytic material is easier to present in court.

Comparison of Antemortem and Postmortem Records and Written Conclusions

After all dental information has been collected from the antemortem and postmortem data bases, it is compared for similarities and discrepancies. Comparison of dental evidence is unique among the techniques used to identify a decedent. A positive identification may still be established, even when some reconcilable discrepancies are observed.

Furthermore, the forensic dentist must routinely rely on the belief that premortem records are truly those of the person they are purported to represent. The latter problem is best exemplified by the controversy associated

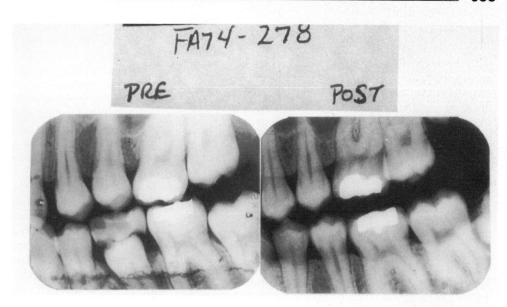

FIGURE 19–7. Antemortem and postmortem radiographs demonstrating the fluid, changing nature of dental information.

with the antemortem dental records used to identify the bodies of Adolph Hitler and Eva Braun. Until recently, there was uncertainty concerning the reliability of those records. This was based on the possibility that the records had been falsified to affect the misidentification of Hitler and his bride.

The case demonstrated in Figure 19–7 shows that all teeth, restorations, and anatomic structures are identical, except that deciduous tooth K is still present in the antemortem radiograph. Tooth number 20 is erupted in the postmortem film. This difference could not support a positive identification if it were a component of fingerprint or DNA evidence. The facts that the deciduous tooth has exfoliated and the permanent tooth erupted before death are acceptable discrepancies in comparable dental evidence.

Comparison of dental evidence is often complicated by the quality of the evidence submitted. The physical status of the postmortem dental material can be compromised when teeth have fractured or are avulsed secondary to trauma. Often, only fragments of the jaws may be presented for comparison.

Dental restorations can be separated from the teeth or melted in a fire. Acrylic melts below 540°C (1000°F), gold and amalgam melt by 870°C (1600°F), and porcelain can withstand temperatures above 1100°C (2010°F). Also, extreme temperature in a fire can cause the teeth to explode or appear shrunken.

The problems associated with incomplete antemortem records are compounded when radiographs are of poor quality. This is related to exposure and developing errors. Mischarted information in the antemortem record can also be considered a reconcilable discrepancy. This error often occurs when teeth have been extracted and adjoining teeth have moved into the position of the extraction site. Restorations may be inadvertently indicated on the wrong tooth when one is charting or entering information into the progress record.

Regardless of the difficulties encountered when dental evidence is compared, the final conclusions must be based on an objective analysis of the data presented. The conclusions must be supportable and defensible when they are presented under oath in a court of law.

Dentistry's Role in Mass Disaster Identification

The term "mass disaster" evokes images of a chaotic event, initiated by a destructive force, which results in multiple fatalities necessitating identification. Mass disasters can be classified as:

- Natural
- Accidental
- Criminal (e.g., serial homicide, bombings)

Each variety of mass disaster results in the death of multiple victims. However, the problems faced by the forensic dental team responsible for identifying the decedents may vary, depending on the type of mass disaster.

Natural Disasters

Natural mass disasters include earthquakes, tornadoes, hurricanes, volcanic eruptions, fire storms, and floods. These may occur over relatively short periods or may be protracted over days or weeks. Victims may be scattered throughout broad areas, extending for miles. In addition, many victims in natural disasters may be unknowns who cannot be presumptively identified. Transients, homeless individuals, and tourists who are visiting an area involved in a natural mass disaster are often difficult to identify.

In a natural disaster, the principal problem for the dental identification team is that the environmental infrastructure is often compromised. Dental offices containing antemortem records may be destroyed. Communication lines and roads are damaged, preventing the retrieval of any available antemortem records. All of these factors can delay or preclude the prompt identification of victims.

Accidents

Accidental mass disasters are most often associated with transportation accidents, fires, industrial accidents, and military accidents. These events usually occur over short periods. They are associated with closed populations, exemplified by the passengers on an airplane or a shift of workers in a mine. The airline has a list of individuals who are supposed to be on the plane. The mining company can document those who have reported for work. In these examples, the victims of accidents should logically come from the closed population. Therefore, antemortem records are first solicited from the families of these individuals.

Problems can be associated with the identification of victims of industrial and military accidents because these populations are often of similar age, may be ethnically similar, and may wear similar clothing. Military uniforms and protective industrial clothing decrease the potential use of personal recognition as an identification aid in these cases.

Criminal Disasters

Unlike natural and accidental mass disasters, criminal mass disasters may occur over extremely long periods (years) and wide ranges of territory (different cities or states). The remains of the victims of serial killers can be hidden, dismembered, and mutilated. Dental structures in these situations may not be available for postmortem review.

Law enforcement agencies are often unaware of the victims from other jurisdictions. Each agency may be investigating an individual homicide without recognizing a pattern of broader criminal involvement. Until the development of the FBI-NCIC computer registry, coordinated efforts at identification were hampered.

Responsibilities

Regardless of the type of mass disaster, the local coroner or medical examiner is ultimately responsible for performing the autopsy and identifying the victims. In accidents that involve modes of public transportation, the National Transportation Safety Board (NTSB) is empowered to investigate and determine the cause of the crash. Other agencies with jurisdiction at a disaster scene may represent local police, public safety, and funeral home personnel; members of the FBI fingerprint team; and the clergy.

The forensic dentists who are responsible for identification and their support personnel should also be organized into a team. Several state dental associations have developed, supplied, and trained such groups in preparation for emergencies requiring their expertise. Training sessions include mock mass disaster exercises. These drills can prepare the dental team members for dealing with the technical problems of mass disaster cases.

In addition, training sessions can be used to counsel the dental team and to inform members of the post-traumatic stress often associated with this type of forensic work. This delayed stress is a result of the sensory and psychologic insults encountered by the dentist who is dealing with human death on a large scale.

Working with the authorization of the coroner or medical examiner, a dental disaster team is responsible for antemortem record assembly and interpretation, postmortem physical and dental radiographic examination, and final comparison of dental information. These are the same principles used to establish an individual identification. Yet, when numerous victims need to be identified in a short time, problems of identification are compounded exponentially.

Dividing the team into subsections responsible for each of the three identification domains permits a division of labor among the team members. This reduces errors in identification, in that specific tasks in the identification process are assigned to separate subsections. A chain of command should be established, and the team leader is directly responsible to the coroner or medical examiner. This person is the only member of the team authorized to release the results of the dental identification process to appropriate investigative agencies.

The advent of computer software has assisted mass disaster dental identification teams in filing, storing, sorting, and matching bits of antemortem and postmortem information. Computer assistance has proved beneficial in disasters involving hundreds of victims. Commonly used programs include:

1. The FBI-NCIC program, based on the California Dental Identification System, developed by Dr. Norman Sperber and Dr. Robert Siegel.
2. CAPMI (Computer-Assisted Postmortem Identification), developed by Dr. Lewis Lorton of the U.S. Army Institute of Dental Research.
3. *ToothPics-MatchPics*, developed by Class I Inc., (Tempe, Ariz.).

Each of these systems is user-friendly, can be run on readily available and accessible hardware, is capable of networking, and relies on objective data entry. However, identification is the result of human thought processes. To arrive at correct conclusions on the basis of the evidence, individual dental team members must evaluate computer matches.

BITE PATTERN EVIDENCE

Basic Principles

Animal bites account for most bite injuries reported annually. Bites represent approximately 1 percent of all emergency visits that require medical attention. Of these, most are associated with dog bites. Animal bites may be observed post mortem when a body has not been buried or discovered quickly. Commonly, insect bites are made by ants and roaches, which leave pattern injuries that can be mistakenly interpreted as antemortem trauma. Postmortem bites from rats and scavenging dogs and cats are often avulsive and of narrower or smaller diameter than human bites.

Injuries caused by human bites are routinely related to

either aggressive or sexual behavior. Ironically, it is not uncommon for the perpetrator of an aggressive act to be bitten by the victim, as a means of self-defense. In children, biting is a form of expression that occurs when verbal communication fails. Biting injuries in children can result from playground altercations or sports competition. They are common among children who attend day care centers.

Self-inflicted bites are observed in **Lesch-Nyhan syndrome**. This is an X-linked, recessively transmitted disease manifesting—among other signs—insensitivity to pain and self-mutilation by chewing away the lips. This disease is rare, and self-inflicted bites are more commonly seen in adults and children who are victims of physical abuse or sexual assault. These individuals may bite their own forearms or hands in anguish or to prevent themselves from crying out while they are being traumatized.

Injuries resulting from animal or human bites may become septic or may progress to systemic infections. Secondary bacterial infections are more commonly associated with human bites than with animal bites. Infectious complications include tetanus, tuberculosis, syphilis, actinomycosis, and those related to streptococcal and staphylococcal organisms.

Viral complications, including hepatitis B virus, herpes simplex, and cytomegalovirus, have resulted from transmission through human bites. The human immunodeficiency virus (HIV) can also potentially be transmitted through the exchange of blood and saliva in a bite injury. The risk of seroconversion from this mode of HIV transmission, however, is believed to be extremely low.

Rabies is the most serious infectious complication that results from animal bites. It is often necessary to identify the specific offending animal for rabies control or potential litigation. This is not routinely done by matching the animal's teeth to the pattern injury. When humans bite, however, the marks left in injured tissue or inanimate objects are often analyzed and compared with the alleged perpetrator's dentition.

The concept of accepting evidence related to the analysis of patterns created by the dentition is relatively new to the United States justice system. However, the legal community has recognized tool mark and fingerprint pattern analysis as scientifically acceptable forensic disciplines for some time. The evidence presented by experts in these areas is accepted in the courts under the *Frye* standard and Federal Rules of Evidence. These are special rules that deal with the admissibility of scientific evidence.

The *Frye* test has three requirements that must be met for scientific evidence to be admissible:

1. The scientific principle must be recognizable.
2. The scientific principle must be sufficiently established.
3. The scientific principle must have gained acceptance in the discipline to which it belongs.

Further interpretation of the *Frye* standard by the legal community requires that the reliability of scientific evidence, which was gathered using correct scientific procedures, must also be established by expert testimony. The witness presenting the evidence must be qualified as an expert before giving an opinion on the material entered as evidence.

Not all courts in all states recognize the Federal Rules of Evidence. These rules differ from those described in the *Frye* test. They establish a paradigm for admissibility of scientific evidence that does not specifically require a general acceptance standard. Thus, under the Federal Rules of Evidence, more latitude is provided for judges to decide the admissibility, relevancy, and weight of scientific evidence in individual cases.

Because it is reasonable to consider the teeth as cutting or mashing tools, the basis for accepting bite pattern evidence can be supported on the same scientific principles used to evaluate tool marks. In addition, studies indicate that, like fingerprints, the human dentition is unique for each person. Variations in size, wear, and fractures; position in the dental arch; diastemata; and restored surfaces contribute to this principle.

Thus, bite mark evidence is admissible under the *Frye* standard and Federal Rules of Evidence. Although some legal experts believe the Federal Rules of Evidence provide better guidelines for admissibility decisions, no challenge to the scientific basis of bite mark evidence has been successful under either set of standards.

Characteristics of Bite Marks

To evaluate a pattern mark, its characteristics must be recognizable and distinguishable. Reasonably, the mark should be consistent with the face of the instrument from which it was generated. Specific teeth can create representative patterns that are recognizable. These individual marks are described as internal characteristics of the entire bite mark. Human incisors make rectangular marks. Depending on the amount of attrition observed on the cuspid's incisal edge, incisal surfaces of cuspids may be associated with points or triangular patterns. Bicuspid teeth are often associated with marks that resemble a "figure eight."

Class characteristics of a human bite mark are related to the shapes that are created when groups of teeth from both dental arches are impressed into a bitten surface. Round, ovoid, or elliptical patterns are usually observed, but variations may be associated with tapered, square, and U-shaped arches. When only one arch contacts a surface, a crescent pattern may be formed. The greatest dimensions of an adult human bite mark do not usually exceed 4 cm (Fig. 19–8).

Internal and class characteristics of bite patterns are generated by groups of specific teeth. The dynamics of occlusion and muscle function must also be accounted for when variations in internal and class characteristics of a bite mark are considered. Such variations can be caused by malocclusion, individual tooth mobility associated with periodontal disease, and movement of facial muscles during biting.

Class II malocclusion can cause the palatal surfaces of the maxillary anterior teeth, rather than their incisal edges, to contact the material being bitten. Shield-like imprints of the palatal surfaces are generated in the bite

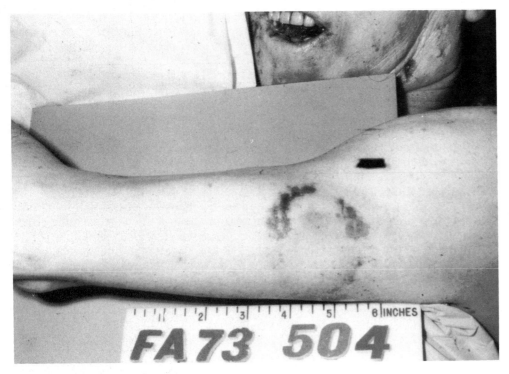

FIGURE 19–8. A bite mark pattern demonstrating the internal and class characteristics associated with impressions made by the human dentition. There is an ecchymotic area in the center of the ovoid pattern. This is not always related to the sucking action of a sexual bite. Therefore, this finding should not be overinterpreted to imply sexual intent on the part of the biter. The impressions made by the teeth of the mandibular arch are more delicate.

mark rather than the rectangular patterns routinely associated with these teeth.

Aberrant muscle forces associated with tongue thrusting can alter the way the teeth contact a bitten surface. Temporomandibular joint (TMJ) dysfunction can also contribute to variations in bite patterns. TMJ dysfunction can be associated with midline shifts or inability to achieve maximum opening while biting.

When bitten, many inanimate objects tend to act like dental impression material, retaining the marks of the teeth. This occurred in the first modern case in which bite mark evidence was accepted by an American court. The suspect's tooth marks, in a piece of hard cheese, were used to place him at the scene of a burglary and, ulti-

mately, to convict him of the crime. Additional cases have involved bite marks in other foods, chewing gum, paper toweling, and a roll of masking tape.

Unlike inanimate material, the skin is a dynamic tissue that can change after it is injured. Swelling, caused by the acute inflammatory response of the tissue, can distort and affect the interpretation of the pattern. Bleeding into the area of a bite mark can mask the pattern.

The age of an injury is the time elapsed from its infliction to the analysis of the damaged tissue. Reliable determination of the age of antemortem skin injuries requires histopathologic and histochemical analysis to relate the injury to the time of the alleged incident (Table 19–4). Color changes in the bitten tissue, associated with the

Table 19–4. HISTOPATHOLOGIC AND CLINICAL CHANGES USED TO MONITOR THE TIME ELAPSED (AGING) IN SKIN INJURIES ASSOCIATED WITH BITE MARKS

Time	Predominant Cellular Infiltrate and Deposits	Healing	Variable Clinical Color
Hours			
4–8	Polymorphonuclear leukocytes with a peripheral front		Red-blue-purple
12	Polymorphonuclear leukocytes		
16–24	Macrophages peak		Blue-black
24–36	Polymorphonuclear leukocytes peak	Peripheral fibroblasts	
Days			
1–3	Central necrosis		
3+	Hemosiderin		Green-blue
4		Collagen fibers	
4–5		Capillary growth	Brown yellow-green
6		Lymphocytes peak at periphery	
10–14		Granulation tissue	Tan-yellow

degradation of hemoglobin from lysed red blood cells, can be used only to estimate the time of occurrence.

Contusions and areas of ecchymosis are not unusual in bite marks made in living tissue. The absence of bleeding into the injury may imply that it was inflicted after death. Additional postmortem soft tissue changes that can affect the quality of a bite pattern injury and its eventual weight as evidence include lividity (caused by the settling of blood pigments in dependent body areas), decomposition, and embalming.

Bite marks from sexual attacks are commonly found on the neck, breasts, arms, buttocks, genitalia, and thighs. Axillary bites and bite patterns on the back, shoulder, penis, and scrotum are often associated with homosexual activity. Abused children may be bitten in areas of the face, particularly the cheek, ear, and nose. Assailants can also be bitten. The analysis of these bite pattern injuries is just as incriminating as those found on the victim of a violent act.

Guidelines for Bite Mark Analysis

In 1984 the American Board of Forensic Odontology established Guidelines for Bite Mark Analysis. This was done to create a scientific approach to the description of the bite mark, collection of evidence from suspect and victim, and subsequent analysis of the evidence.

The Guidelines do not mandate specific analytic methods for comparison. Through their careful use, however, the quality of the investigation and conclusions based on bite mark evidence follow customary procedures. Thus, with these Guidelines, it should be possible to determine the weight of bite mark evidence required to establish the validity of bite mark comparison.

Description of the Bite Mark

Demographic information (e.g., age, race, sex, name of the victim, examination date; referring agency; and case number) is obtained in cases involving both living and deceased victims. The names of the forensic dental examiner and referring agency contact person should also be included.

The location of the bite is then described. Attention is directed to the anatomic location, surface contour, and tissue characteristics of the bitten area. Underlying structures, such as bone or fat, may influence the analytic quality of the pattern injury. Relative skin mobility is also evaluated.

The shape, color, size, and type of injury are recorded. Metric measurements of the horizontal and vertical dimensions of the bite mark are determined. Irregularities and variations from the standard round, ovoid, and crescent shapes associated with human bite marks are noted. Injury types include abrasion, laceration, ecchymotic and petechial hemorrhage, incision, and avulsion. Artifactual injuries, such as proximate stab and bullet wounds, should be recorded because these may distort the pattern by separating anatomic cleavage lines of the skin (*Langer's lines*).

Evidence Collection

Examination of the Victim and Suspect

Both the victim and the suspect are examined, and evidence from each is gathered for comparative study and evaluation. Collection of evidence must be performed in a manner that protects the rights of the person who is providing the evidence and that permits the eventual acceptance of the evidence in court.

A standard health history and informed consent are obtained before any evidence recovery procedure regarding the suspect is performed. An intraoral and extraoral examination of the suspect is completed. This includes a dental charting, a soft tissue and tongue evaluation, and probing of the periodontium. Therefore, a knowledge of the suspect's medical history relative to systemic problems associated with cardiovascular disease, allergy, seizure disorder, or requirements for antibiotic prophylaxis is medicolegally important.

A search warrant, court order, or legal consent may be required before evidence is collected from a suspect. A specific list of the dentally related evidence desired should be recorded in the legal document. This list usually includes facial and oral photographs, impressions of the teeth, occlusal registrations and bite exemplars, and saliva samples. These documents protect the rights of the suspect against unreasonable search and seizure and provide for due process, as guaranteed by the Fourth and Fourteenth Amendments, respectively, to the Constitution.

Bite marks are considered similar to such physical evidence as fingerprint, hair, blood, semen samples, and sobriety tests. Therefore, this material is not protected under provisions of the Fifth Amendment, which deal with self-incrimination.

Photography

Ideally, standard photographic techniques include the use of a 35-mm single-lens reflex camera with a flat-field macro lens and electronic flash. Numerous photographs employing different camera positions, lighting, exposure settings, and types of film should be obtained. Orientation positions and close-up views with a reference scale are required. The scale should be positioned next to, and in the same plane as, the bite mark. The scale should be omitted from at least one view to document that no marks or other injuries have been hidden by the scale.

A reference scale permits the bite mark photographs to be measured and prepared as life-size (1:1) representations of the injury. They can then be compared with casts and other exemplars obtained from the suspect. The ABFO No. 2 reference ruler (Fig. 19–9) was developed by the American Board of Forensic Odontology for use in bite mark photography. This instrument contains two metric scales, an 18 percent color gray scale, circular symbols, and rectifying grids. Each of these components is used to account for potential photographic distortions, which can negate the value of the photographic evidence.

With living victims, serial pictures are taken over several days. This provides documentation of the color changes associated with healing of the wound. In addition, special photographic techniques, including the use

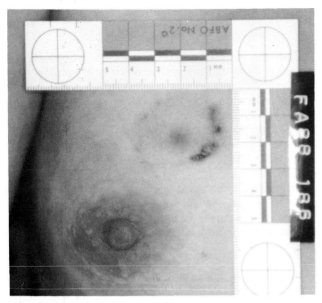

FIGURE 19-9. The American Board of Forensic Odontology ABFO No. 2 Reference Scale.

of reflective ultraviolet (UV) photography, can be used to identify latent images of the teeth. These may remain after the bite mark has clinically disappeared.

Reflective UV photography enhances the bite mark image by selectively identifying photoactive melanin pigment in the injured tissue. Variations in the amount of melanin in the traumatized tissue are observable. This is based on the fluorescence created when the skin is exposed to UV light in the 320- to 450-nm wavelength range. UV photography requires special films, illumination sources, or lens filters, such as the Wratten Filter No. 18A (visibly opaque glass filter), to work within the desired wavelengths. In addition, there may also be focusing problems associated with ultraviolet photography. The fact that this technique may permit recovery of latent evidence, even months after all clinical signs of a bite mark injury have disappeared, makes the effort worthwhile.

As stated previously, photographs of the suspect should involve the same attention to technical quality control. Extraoral, intraoral, and occlusal photographs are taken. Additional films of wax or acrylic test bites and measurements of maximum interincisal opening are also recorded.

Saliva Evidence

Collection of saliva trace evidence from the surface of the bite injury and a control skin surface of the victim is performed to identify blood group antigens. These samples can be used for comparison with saliva obtained from the suspect. A saliva sample should be collected on a cotton swab that has been moistened in sterile saline. The bite mark is rubbed with the cotton, which is then permitted to air-dry. After the sample dries, the cotton swab is placed in a test tube and refrigerated until it can be analyzed. The control sample is obtained from an area of the victim's skin surface that is not associated with the

bite. Because a victim may be bitten through the clothing, areas of garments that approximate a bite pattern injury should also be retained and evaluated for saliva.

Unfortunately, many victims of sexual abuse wash the area of a bite mark before reporting for treatment. Emergency room personnel should be trained to identify bite mark injuries and instructed not to wash or disinfect these areas until saliva evidence can be obtained.

Impressions and Study Casts

The Guidelines for Bite Mark Analysis deliberately do not dictate which impression materials should be used to create exemplars of a bite mark. Vinyl polysiloxanes are dimensionally stable impression materials that meet American Dental Association specifications, and are all acceptable. Hydrocolloid, polysulfide, polyether, and alginate materials are not recommended because of problems associated with long-term stability.

Orthopedic cast materials and non-exothermic resins have been used to create the rigid trays for bite mark impressions. All impression trays and study casts should be appropriately labeled. Originals are retained for presentation in court. Working casts and models should be duplicated from the original impression or master casts. It is recommended that master casts be poured in type IV stone, according to the manufacturer's specifications.

Tissue Samples

Tissue samples of a bite mark can be retained from decedents. With the permission of the medical examiner or coroner, the dermis and underlying muscle and adipose tissue can be removed for transillumination analysis. Prior to excision, an acrylic ring or stent must be secured within 1 inch of the borders of the injured tissue sample. This prevents shrinkage and distortion of the specimen when it is placed into a 4 percent formalin solution for fixation. The acrylic material is bound to the skin surface with cyanoacrylate and sutures (Fig. 19-10).

Evidence Analysis

The responsibility of comparing the photographs of the bite pattern injury with the dentition of the suspect rests with the forensic dentist. As an expert in the analysis of these patterns, this person objectively evaluates the evidence. The forensic dentist first determines whether the pattern is truly a result of biting or whether it is artifactual. Patterns of blood splatter around a wound or other tool marks unrelated to the teeth may be mistaken for bite marks.

Once it is established that the pattern is related to the teeth, it can be matched to the suspect's dentition for inclusionary or exclusionary purposes. An expert opinion is then made according to the results of the relationship of the bite pattern and suspect's teeth.

To accomplish these goals, the dentist uses numerous methods that have been accepted in the courts. Images of the bite mark and the teeth can be digitized in a computer. This information can then be enhanced and subsequently overlaid for matching purposes.

Clear overlays of the chewing surfaces of the teeth can be made by simply tracing these surfaces on a sheet of

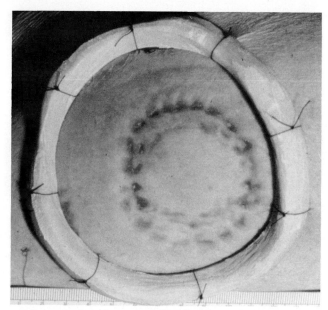

FIGURE 19–10. An experimental bite pattern injury on a cadaver. This bite mark has had an acrylic stent glued and sutured around its circumference before dissection and fixation in 4 percent formalin. (Courtesy of Dr. E. Steven Smith.)

transparent acetate. Placing the incisal edges of the study casts on the glass of an office photocopier and duplicating on special paper achieves the same end. A similar effect is obtained by placing an opaque powder, like barium sulfate, into wax or acrylic test bites, and by obtaining radiographs of these exemplars. All of these overlays are then superimposed over the bite mark for comparison (Figs. 19–11 and 19–12).

In court, bite mark evidence must be able to withstand legal challenges based on its scientific validity and the credibility of the expert witness who presents the evidence. This is true regardless of the techniques used to retrieve, compare, and determine a conclusion based on the evidence. When the Guidelines for Bite Mark Analysis are used, such challenges can be minimized.

CHILD ABUSE AND NEGLECT

Epidemiology and Classification

Child abuse is the non-accidental, physical, mental, emotional, or sexual trauma; exploitation; or neglect endured by a child younger than 18 years of age while under the care of a responsible person, such as a parent, sibling, baby sitter, teacher, or other person acting *in loco parentis*. Approximately 2 million cases of child abuse are reported annually in the United States; 2000 to 4000 cases result in death. Victims and their abusers come from all racial, ethnic, religious, socioeconomic, and educational backgrounds.

Reports concerning the distribution of cases among the different types of abuse vary widely. Up to 70 percent of the cases may be the result of physical trauma. Some studies relate 15 to 25 percent of the cases to sexual abuse and 50 percent to neglect. Neglective abuse is subclassified by the caretaker's neglect of the child's medical, dental, and safety needs; physical well-being; or education. Intentional drugging or poisoning and failure to thrive are additional types of maltreatment classified as abusive.

Many abusive individuals were themselves abused as children. Criminal charges are often lodged against an abusing caretaker. It is recognized, however, that counseling, psychologic, and emotional support can also help to stabilize a dysfunctional family unit.

Signs and Symptoms

Regardless of the overall statistical variations in subclassification of this problem, the dentist is most likely to encounter physical and sexual abuse and health care and safety neglect among pediatric dental patients. Of the

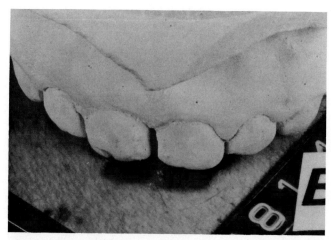

FIGURE 19–11. An overlay of the maxillary cast of a suspect's dentition on a photograph of a bite pattern injury. Note the diastema between the central incisor teeth. The distal incisal surfaces of the lateral incisor teeth are not in the plane of occlusion.

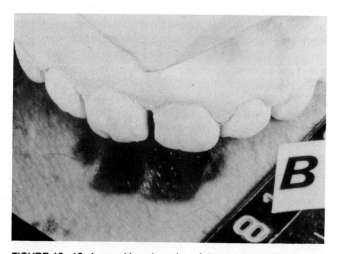

FIGURE 19–12. A repositioned overlay of the maxillary cast of a suspect's dentition on a photograph of a bite pattern injury (same case as depicted in Fig. 19–11). The drag marks, diastema space, and mesial contact points of the lateral incisor teeth become apparent in the pattern. (From Nuckles DB, Herschaft EE, Whatmough LN. Forensic odontology in solving crimes: Dental techniques and bite-mark evidence. Gen Dent 42:210–214, 1994.)

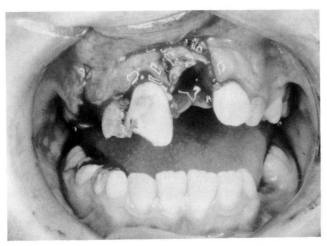

FIGURE 19-13. An avulsed tooth, a fractured tooth, and a torn labial frenum associated with oral facial injuries in physical child abuse.

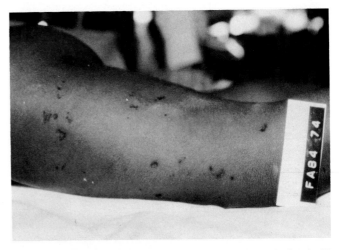

FIGURE 19-14. Multiple circular ulcerated injuries are associated with intentional burns from a cigarette. When a child is accidentally burned by a cigarette, only one elliptical ulcer is observed.

children who are physically abused, 50 percent manifest orofacial injuries (Fig. 19-13). These are unexplained injuries that are inappropriately reported by the caretaker or inconsistent with the history provided. Abusive trauma to the face and mouth includes:

1. Laceration of the labial or lingual frenum, which results from a blow to the lip or forceful feeding.
2. Repeated fracture or the avulsion of teeth.
3. Zygomatic arch and nasal fractures.
4. Bilateral contusions of the lip commisures from the placement of a gag.

Pattern injuries can be associated with the semicircular or crescent shape of bite marks. Other instruments that contact the skin may leave parallel linear patterns; these include injuries made by a hanger, strap, belt, or ruler. Multiple parallel lines are associated with finger marks after an open-handed slap. Multiple round, circular, punched-out, or ulcerated areas are caused by intentional burning with a cigarette or cigar. Loop patterns are created by electrical cord, rope, and wire (Figs. 19-14 and 19-15).

Other characteristics of child abuse injuries are related to their multiplicity and repetitive nature. They often appear in various stages of resolution. Some injuries are acute; others are healing or even scarred. Therefore, the dentist should examine the skin of the pediatric dental patient. Suspicion of abuse is increased when the child appears overdressed for seasonal conditions; this may be done in an attempt to mask or hide the physical signs of abuse.

By adulthood, 10 percent of men and 25 percent of women are the victims of sexual abuse. Oral infections associated with sexually transmitted diseases (STDs) are obviously a sign of sexual abuse when they are observed in a minor. Erythematous or petechial lesions of the palate or ulceration of the sublingual area should be noted because these findings can result from the physical trauma associated with performing fellatio or cunnilingus (see p. 224).

Among siblings, "milk bottle caries" is a sign of neglective abuse and indicates the caretaker's inattention to the dental needs of the children. The dentist may become aware of other abusive behavior by a responsible caretaker. This can involve refusal or delay in seeking treatment for serious medical or dental problems, abandonment, refusal to cooperate with planned treatment, and failure to return to the same physician or dentist for treatment.

The Role of Dentistry in Recognizing and Reporting Child Abuse

Awareness of the signs and symptoms of child abuse should be a goal for any dentist who treats children. As a component of the dental relicensure process, New York State requires documentation of continuing education credits in the area of child abuse recognition and the dental professional's responsibility to report such cases.

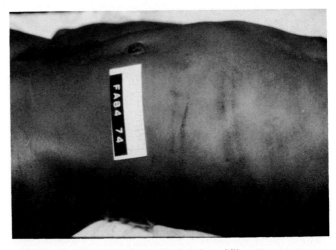

FIGURE 19-15. Parallel linear ("railroad track") patterns are associated with blows to the skin with such straight-edged objects as a belt, a hangar, an electrical cord, and a ruler.

By statute, all states require that dental personnel, other health care professionals, teachers, and day care employees report suspected cases of child abuse. The agency to whom the report is made varies among the different jurisdictions. Commonly, the police, social service, child welfare, or family services departments are the governmental offices designated to accept reports.

When a report is made in good faith, the dentist is immune from any counterprosecution or civil liability that might stem from a false report. Failure to report is considered a misdemeanor in most states. In addition, the dentist may be subject to license revocation or malpractice litigation by failing to make a report.

When a dentist determines that a report of child abuse should be made, documentation of the physical evidence to support the charge is mandatory. All evidence is collected according to the principles described for identification and bite mark cases. Descriptions of the injuries and their locations, supporting photographs and radiographs, and information stating the basis for suspicion of abuse are included in the report. When abuse is considered, parental consent is not required to obtain appropriate physical evidence.

THE DENTIST AS AN EXPERT WITNESS

Observational, or lay, witnesses testify only to the facts known to them. They are referred to as witnesses of fact. Such witnesses are permitted to make inferences about physical facts based on ordinary experience. The witness of fact is not entitled to present hearsay evidence related by another person.

The judicial system recognizes that people with a scientific background or specialized field of study that is admissible under the *Frye Rule* or Federal Rules of Evidence can provide the courts with analyses or explanations relative to that discipline. The facts and opinions offered by such a witness are beyond the scope of information that could be expected to be provided by a lay person or witness of fact. A witness who is qualified to testify under this standard is acknowledged as an "expert."

Members of the dental profession are experts. They are qualified to testify by the judge, who bases his or her opinion on educational background, dental and forensic expertise, publications, and other professional qualifications. Dentists who have additional training in one of the dental specialties may be called on to present specific information from that discipline.

Dental experts assist attorneys, judges, and ultimately juries (the triers of fact) in understanding the scope and complexities of dental science and practice in relation to questions of law. The dentist should not become an advocate for either side in a case but should strive to be an educator and friend of the court.

As experts, dentists may be required to testify in civil litigation cases that involve the following situations:

1. *Malpractice based on negligence.* This includes battery (e.g., extraction of the wrong tooth); misdiagnosis; and failure to diagnose, refer, or inform. All of these actions fall outside the standard of care for the profession.
2. *Personal injury.* Temporomandibular joint damage or dental trauma suffered in vehicular, home, sports, recreational, and work-related accidents fall under this category.
3. *Dental fraud.* Charging for materials or procedures that were not used or performed are examples of fraud.
4. *Identification of mass disaster victims.*

In criminal court, dental expertise is requested in identification of homicide victims and in bite mark and child abuse cases.

Dentists are often unfamiliar with, and may be intimidated by, the adversarial nature of courtroom procedure and protocol. When presenting evidence, the dental expert should remember that his or her role in the legal process is to help the jury understand the dental issues in the case. To this end, and as a scientist, the dental expert witness should present the evidence confidently, accurately, and objectively, relating information in nontechnical terms.

When cross-examined by the opposing attorney, the dental expert witness should remain composed and confident. As an expert, the dentist has the right to refer to records and exemplars prepared for the case. The dentist is entitled to read and review any books or articles proffered by the opposing attorney with the intent of discrediting the testimony.

Pretrial preparation is required if the dental expert and the attorney who has retained his or her services are to develop the evidence to be presented in court. Both must be aware of the strengths and weaknesses of the material and decide how best to provide the jury with this information. Adequate time must be allotted to prepare exhibits for court. It is also advantageous to attempt to determine the position that will be taken by dental experts called by the opposing side.

SUMMARY

Each practitioner has a responsibility to understand the forensic implications associated with the practice of his or her profession. This understanding should include more than ethics and jurisprudence, which were traditionally the only aspects of a dentist's knowledge of the law. Appreciation of forensic dental problems permits clinicians to maintain legally acceptable records and assist legal authorities in the identification of victims of disasters and crimes.

The pursuit of justice in cases of rape and child abuse often relies on dental testimony to interpret bite pattern injuries. New photographic techniques, computer software development, and laboratory and clinical procedures have permitted forensic dentists to provide objective, scientific evidence in these types of cases.

The legal community's reliance on the dental profession to continue to provide expertise in civil and criminal proceedings ensures that forensic dentistry will remain a viable component of the forensic sciences.

REFERENCES

Averill DC. Manual of Forensic Odontology, 2nd ed. Burlington, Vt., American Society of Forensic Odontology, 1991.

Barsley RE. Forensic and legal issues in oral diagnosis. Dent Clin North Am 37:143–144, 1993.

Barsley RB, et al. Forensic dentistry: The general dentist's responsibilities. *In*: Clark's Clinical Dentistry. Vol 1. Edited by Hardin JF. Philadelphia, JB Lippincott, 1992.

Child Abuse Prevention Act (PL93-247). DHEW Publication 78-30137, 1978; 42 USCS Section 5106 g (4) (1988).

Commission on Life Sciences of the National Research Council. DNA Technology in Forensic Science. Washington, DC, National Academy Press, 1992.

Cottone JA, Standish SM. Outline of Forensic Dentistry. Chicago, Year Book Medical Publishers, 1982.

da Fonseca MA, Feigal RJ, ten Bensel RW. Dental aspects of 1248 cases of child maltreatment on file at a major county hospital. Pediatr Dent 14:152–157, 1992.

Doyle v State, 159 Tex. C. R. 310, 263 S W. 2d 779, January 20, 1954.

Epstein JB, Scully C. Mammalian bites: Risk and management. Am J Dent 5:167–172, 1992.

Frair J, West MH. Ultraviolet forensic photography. Kodak Tech Bits 2:311, 1989.

Gorlin RJ, Cohen MM, Levin LS. Syndromes of the Head and Neck, 3rd ed. New York, Oxford University Press, 1990.

Hyzer WG, Krauss TC. The bitemark standard reference scale ABFO No. 2. J Forensic Sci 33:498–506, 1988.

Jakush J. Forensic dentistry. J Am Dent Assoc 119:355–368, 1989.

Moenssens AA, Inbau FE, Starrs JE. Scientific Evidence in Criminal Cases, 3rd ed. Mineola, N.Y., The Foundation Press, 1986.

Peck S, Peck L. A time for change of tooth numbering systems. J Dent Educ 57:643–647, 1993.

Pitluck HM. Bite mark case management and legal considerations update. Presented at the 41st Annual Meeting of the American Academy of Forensic Sciences, Las Vegas, February 15, 1989.

Roberts D. The iceman: Lone voyager from the copper age. National Geographic 183:36–67, 1993.

Sanger RG, Bross DC. Clinical Management of Child Abuse and Neglect: A Guide for the Professional. Chicago, Quintessence Publishing, 1984.

Smith ES, Rawson RD. Proceedings of the First National Symposium on Dentistry's Role and Responsibility in Mass Disaster Identification. Chicago, American Dental Association, 1988.

Spitz WU. Spitz and Fischer's Medicolegal Investigation of Death: Guidelines for the Application of Pathology to Criminal Investigation, 3rd ed. Springfield, Ill, Charles C Thomas, 1993.

Standish SM, Stimson PG, eds. Forensic dentistry: Legal obligations and methods of identification for the practitioner. Dent Clin North Am 21:1–196, 1977.

Vale GL, Cogan JL, Suchey JM. Forensic dentistry: Investigation of the Los Angeles airport disaster. J Calif Dent Assoc 19:20–26, 1991.

Vale GL, et al. Guidelines for bite mark analysis. J Am Dent Assoc 112:383–386, 1986.

Warnick AJ. Forensic Dental Identification Team Manual. Detroit, Michigan Dental Association, 1989.

Yoshino M, Seta S. Personal identification of the human skull: Superimposition and radiographic techniques. Forensic Sci Rev 1:24–42, 1989.

Zarkowski P. Bite mark evidence: Its worth in the eyes of the expert. J Law Ethics Dent 1:47–57, 1988.

Appendix

Differential Diagnosis of Oral and Maxillofacial Diseases

The most important aspect of patient care is the accurate diagnosis of the patient's disease. Unfortunately, the clinical presentation of many disease processes can be strikingly similar, despite their vast differences in etiology and pathogenesis. Because treatment and, ultimately, prognosis are based on the diagnosis, the diagnostic process is critical in optimal patient management. This Appendix provides some guidelines for expediting and facilitating the diagnostic process from a clinical perspective.

The first step in gathering information is the acquisition of a thorough history of the disease process. This typically includes such items as the onset, severity, location, duration, character, and course of the signs and symptoms being experienced by the patient. Additional information regarding medical, social, and family history may be necessary. With this information, the clinician often can start the process of formulating a list of possible diagnoses, even before performing an examination.

The information obtained during the clinical examination is also very important because many lesions have characteristic appearances. By evaluating these characteristics in conjunction with the patient's history, often the clinician can narrow the list of diagnostic possibilities. This list, known as a *differential diagnosis*, essentially includes possible pathologic entities, usually ranked in order from most likely to least likely.

DEFINITIONS

To better describe the appearances of lesions and communicate these features to our colleagues, the clinician should be familiar with the following terms:

Macule. A focal area of color change which is not elevated or depressed in relation to its surroundings.

Papule. A solid, raised lesion which is less than 5 mm in diameter.

Nodule. A solid, raised lesion which is greater than 5 mm in diameter.

Sessile. Describing a tumor or growth whose base is the widest part of the lesion.

Pedunculated. Describing a tumor or growth whose base is narrower than the widest part of the lesion.

Papillary. Describing a tumor or growth exhibiting numerous surface projections.

Verrucous. Describing a tumor or growth exhibiting a rough, warty surface.

Vesicle. A superficial blister, 5 mm or less in diameter, usually filled with clear fluid.

Bulla. A large blister, greater than 5 mm in diameter.

Pustule. A blister filled with purulent exudate.

Ulcer. A lesion characterized by loss of the surface epithelium and frequently some of the underlying connective tissue. It often appears depressed or excavated.

Erosion. A superficial lesion, often arising secondary to rupture of a vesicle or bulla, that is characterized by partial or total loss of the surface epithelium.

Fissure. A narrow, slit-like ulceration or groove.

Plaque. A lesion that is slightly elevated and is flat on its surface.

Petechia. A round, pinpoint area of hemorrhage.

Ecchymosis. A non-elevated area of hemorrhage, larger than a petechia.

Telangiectasia. A vascular lesion caused by dilatation of a small, superficial blood vessel.

Cyst. A pathologic epithelium-lined cavity, often filled with liquid or semi-solid contents.

Unilocular. Describing a radiolucent lesion having a single compartment.

Multilocular. Describing a radiolucent lesion having several or many compartments.

By using these terms, the clinician can describe the characteristics of lesions efficiently and uniformly. Applying these clinical descriptors to the lesions also can help to categorize them with respect to the differential diagnosis. By adding such additional characteristics as prevalence, patient race or nationality, patient age at diagnosis, patient gender, and sites of predilection, the clinician can hone the differential diagnosis list considerably.

HOW TO USE THIS APPENDIX

This Appendix is designed to help the clinician formulate a differential diagnosis by organizing and categorizing disease entities according to their most prominent or identifiable clinical features. Under each "clinical feature" heading is a list of lesions with that clinical feature as a prominent component. Diseases are listed according to estimated frequency relative to similar diseases or lesions.

The most common lesions are marked with triple asterisks (***); rare lesions are marked with a single asterisk (*). Such estimated frequency indicators should not be compared between lists; they are intended only for the single differential diagnosis list in which they occur.

Clinical features that most readily distinguish the lesions are listed with each disease process in order to help focus the clinician's search for the most accurate diagnosis. Finally, the corresponding page number in the book is provided for each disease entity so that the reader can refer to the text for a more detailed discussion.

Index to the Appendix: Differential Diagnosis Lists

Part 5

Pathology of Teeth   *Page*

Part 1

Mucosal and Soft Tissue Pathology: Color Changes

FREQUENCY OF OCCURRENCE	LESION OR CONDITION	COMMENTS OR SPECIAL CHARACTERISTICS	PAGE NO.
	A. WHITE LESIONS: CAN BE SCRAPED OFF		
***	White coated tongue	May be scraped off slightly, with difficulty	—
***	Pseudomembranous candidiasis	"Milk curd" or "cottage cheese" appearance; may leave red base when rubbed off	163
***	Morsicatio	Surface may appear to be peeling off	211
**	Thermal burn	Example: pizza burn	215
**	Sloughing traumatic lesion	Example: cotton roll "burn"	217
**	Toothpaste or mouthwash reaction	Filmy whiteness; leaves normal appearing mucosa when rubbed off	249
**	Chemical burn	Example: aspirin burn secondary to direct application for toothache	216
*	Secondary syphilis	Mucous patch; may be only partially scraped off	146
*	Diphtheria	Gray-white pseudomembrane of oropharynx	145
	B. WHITE LESIONS: CANNOT BE SCRAPED OFF		
***	Linea alba	Buccal mucosa along occlusal plane	211
***	Leukoedema	Primarily in blacks; milky-white alteration of buccal mucosa bilaterally; disappears when stretched	7
***	Leukoplakia	May show benign hyperkeratosis, epithelial dysplasia, or invasive carcinoma	280
***	Tobacco pouch keratosis	Usually in mandibular vestibule; associated with use of snuff or chewing tobacco	288
***	Actinic cheilosis	Pale, gray-white, scaly alteration of lower lip; usually in older men with history of chronic sun exposure; precancerous	293

Continued   667

FREQUENCY OF OCCURRENCE	LESION OR CONDITION	COMMENTS OR SPECIAL CHARACTERISTICS	PAGE NO.
	B. WHITE LESIONS: CANNOT BE SCRAPED OFF *Continued*		
***	Lichen planus	Wickham's striae; typically bilateral on buccal mucosa	572
***	Morsicatio	Most common on anterior buccal mucosa, labial mucosa, and lateral border of tongue; exhibits ragged surface	211
***	White coated tongue	Diffuse involvement of dorsal tongue	—
**	Nicotine stomatitis	Usually associated with pipe smoking; occurs on hard palate	291
*	Hairy leukoplakia	Usually lateral border of tongue; rough surface with vertical fissures; usually associated with HIV infection	202
*	Hyperplastic candidiasis	Most commonly affects anterior buccal mucosa	167
*	Lupus erythematosus	Most common on buccal mucosa; may mimic lichen planus or leukoplakia; associated skin lesions usually present	580
*	Skin graft	History of previous surgery	—
*	Submucous fibrosis	More common in South Asia; associated with betel nut chewing	291
*	White sponge nevus	Hereditary; onset in childhood; generalized lesions, especially buccal mucosa	542
*	Hereditary benign intraepithelial dyskeratosis	Hereditary; onset in childhood; generalized lesions, especially buccal mucosa; ocular involvement possible	543
*	Pachyonychia congenita	Hereditary; onset in childhood; most common on dorsal tongue and areas of trauma; nail, palmar, and plantar changes also present	545
*	Dyskeratosis congenita	Hereditary; onset in childhood; dystrophic nail changes	545
*	Tertiary syphilis	Syphilitic glossitis	146
*	Uremic stomatitis	Renal failure	622
	C. WHITE AND RED LESIONS		
***	Erythema migrans	Geographic tongue; continually changing pattern; rarely involves other oral mucosal sites	569

FREQUENCY OF OCCURRENCE	LESION OR CONDITION	COMMENTS OR SPECIAL CHARACTERISTICS	PAGE NO.
***	Candidiasis	White component may be rubbed off	163
***	Lichen planus	Atrophic or erosive forms; Wickham's striae; typically bilateral on buccal mucosa	572
**	Burns	Examples: pizza burn, aspirin burn, other chemical burns; white component may be rubbed off	215
**	Actinic cheilosis	Pale, gray-white and red alteration to lower lip; usually in older men with history of chronic sun exposure	293
**	Nicotine stomatitis	Usually associated with pipe smoking; occurs on hard palate	291
**	Erythroleukoplakia	Usually shows epithelial dysplasia or carcinoma	284
**	Cinnamon reaction	Related to cinnamon-flavored gum; typically on buccal mucosa and lateral tongue	251
*	Lupus erythematosus	Most common on buccal mucosa; may mimic lichen planus or leukoplakia; associated skin lesions usually present	580
*	Scarlet fever	Secondary to β-hemolytic streptococcal infection; strawberry/raspberry tongue	144
*	Verruciform xanthoma	Most common on gingiva and hard palate; surface may be papillary	267

D. RED LESIONS

***	Pharyngitis	Examples: strep throat, viral pharyngitis	143
***	Traumatic erythema	Caused by local irritation	—
***	Denture sore mouth	Denture-bearing palatal mucosa	166
***	Erythematous candidiasis	Example: central papillary atrophy (median rhomboid glossitis)	165
***	Erythema migrans	Geographic tongue (cases with absence of white borders); continually changing pattern; rarely involves other mucosal sites	569
***	Angular cheilitis	Erythema and cracking at labial commissures	166
**	Thermal burns	Example: caused by hot liquids	215
**	Erythroplakia	Usually shows epithelial dysplasia or carcinoma	288

Continued

FREQUENCY OF OCCURRENCE	LESION OR CONDITION	COMMENTS OR SPECIAL CHARACTERISTICS	PAGE NO.
	D. RED LESIONS *Continued*		
*	Anemia	Atrophic, red tongue; can be due to pernicious anemia, iron-deficiency anemia, hypovitaminosis B	604
*	Hemangioma	Develops in younger patients; may blanch; may show bluish hue	390
*	Lupus erythematosus	Usually with associated skin lesions	580
*	Scarlet fever	Secondary to β-hemolytic streptococcal infection; strawberry/raspberry tongue	144
*	Plasma cell gingivitis	Allergic reaction usually related to flavoring agents	126
*	Radiation mucositis	Patient currently undergoing radiotherapy	218
	E. PETECHIAL, ECCHYMOTIC, AND TELANGIECTATIC LESIONS		
***	Nonspecific trauma	History of injury to lesional site	—
**	Upper respiratory infections	Soft palate petechiae	—
*	Infectious mononucleosis	Soft palate petechiae; tonsillitis and/or pharyngitis may be present	190
*	Idiopathic thrombocytopenic purpura	Areas of trauma; gingival bleeding possibly present	425
*	Trauma from fellatio	Posterior palatal petechiae or ecchymosis	224
*	Hemophilia	Hereditary; childhood onset; gingival bleeding may be present	417
*	Leukemia	Caused by secondary thrombocytopenia; gingival bleeding may be present	427
*	Hereditary hemorrhagic telangiectasia	Multiple, pinhead-sized telangiectasias; possible history of nosebleeds or gastrointestinal bleeding	550
*	CREST syndrome	Multiple, pinhead-sized telangiectasias; **C**alcinosis cutis, **R**aynaud's phenomenon, **E**sophageal motility defect, **S**clerodactyly, **T**elangiectasias	586
	F. BLUE AND/OR PURPLE LESIONS		
***	Varicosities	Especially after 45 years of age; most common on ventral tongue and lips	13

FREQUENCY OF OCCURRENCE	LESION OR CONDITION	COMMENTS OR SPECIAL CHARACTERISTICS	PAGE NO.
***	Submucosal hemorrhage	Also see Appendix List, Part 1, E. (previous topic) Petechial, Ecchymotic, and Telangiectatic Lesions	223
***	Amalgam tattoo	Most common on gingiva; blue-gray; radiopaque amalgam particles sometimes discovered on radiographs	225
***	Mucocele	Especially on lower labial mucosa; typically pale blue; cyclic swelling and rupturing often exhibited	322
**	Eruption cyst	Overlying an erupting tooth	496
**	Salivary duct cyst	Usually pale blue	325
**	Hemangioma	Usually reddish-purple; may blanch under pressure; onset in younger patients	390
**	Ranula	Pale blue, fluctuant swelling of lateral floor of mouth	323
**	Kaposi's sarcoma	Especially in AIDS patients; usually purple; most common on palate and maxillary gingiva	203
*	Nasopalatine duct cyst	Midline of anterior palate	25
*	Salivary gland tumors	Especially mucoepidermoid carcinoma and pleomorphic adenoma; usually pale blue; most common on posterior lateral palate	Ch. 11
*	Gingival cyst of the adult	Most common in mandibular bicuspid-cuspid region	503
*	Blue nevus	Most common on hard palate	279
*	Malignant melanoma	Most common on hard palate and maxillary gingiva; may show mixture of deep blue, brown, black, and other colors	312

G. BROWN, GRAY, AND/OR BLACK LESIONS

***	Racial pigmentation	Most common on attached gingiva in darker-complexioned patients	—
***	Amalgam tattoo	Most common on gingiva; usually slate-gray to black; opaque amalgam particles may be found on radiographs	225
***	Black/brown hairy tongue	Discoloration and elongation of filiform papillae	12

Continued

FREQUENCY OF OCCURRENCE	LESION OR CONDITION	COMMENTS OR SPECIAL CHARACTERISTICS	PAGE NO.
	G. BROWN, GRAY, AND/OR BLACK LESIONS *Continued*		
**	Melanotic macule	Brown; most common on lower lip	274
**	Smoker's melanosis	Most common on anterior facial gingiva	228
**	Non-amalgam tattoos	Example: graphite from pencil	225
*	Melanocytic nevus	Most common on hard palate; can be flat or raised	276
*	Malignant melanoma	Most common on hard palate and maxillary gingiva; may show mixture of deep blue, brown, black, and other colors	312
*	Drug ingestion	Examples: chloroquine, chlorpromazide, minocycline; especially on hard palate	229
*	Peutz-Jeghers syndrome	Freckle-like lesions of vermilion and perioral skin; intestinal polyps; hereditary	550
*	Addison's disease	Chronic adrenal insufficiency; associated with bronzing of skin	615
*	Neurofibromatosis	*Café au lait* pigmentation; cutaneous neurofibromas	381
*	McCune-Albright syndrome	*Café au lait* pigmentation; polyostotic fibrous dysplasia; endocrine disorders	462
*	Heavy metal poisoning	Typically along marginal gingiva; e.g., lead, bismuth, silver	227
*	Melanotic neuroectodermal tumor of infancy	Anterior maxilla; destroys underlying bone	385

H. YELLOW LESIONS

***	Fordyce granules	Sebaceous glands; usually multiple submucosal papules on buccal mucosa or upper lip vermilion	5
**	Superficial abscess	Example: parulis from nonvital tooth	109
**	Accessory lymphoid aggregate	Most common in oropharynx and floor of mouth; may exhibit orange hue	416
**	Lymphoepithelial cyst	Most common on lingual and palatine tonsils, and floor of mouth; may be yellowish-white	33
**	Lipoma	Most common on buccal mucosa; soft to palpation	376

FREQUENCY OF OCCURRENCE	LESION OR CONDITION	COMMENTS OR SPECIAL CHARACTERISTICS	PAGE NO.
*	Jaundice	Generalized discoloration, especially involving soft palate and floor of mouth; sclera usually affected also	598
*	Verruciform xanthoma	Most common on gingiva and hard palate; surface may be rough or papillary	267
*	Pyostomatitis vegetans	"Snail-track" pustules; associated with inflammatory bowel disease	621

Part 2

Mucosal and Soft Tissue Pathology: Surface Alterations

FREQUENCY OF OCCURRENCE	LESION OR CONDITION	COMMENTS OR SPECIAL CHARACTERISTICS	PAGE NO.
A. VESICULOEROSIVE AND ULCERATIVE LESIONS: ACUTE (SHORT-DURATION AND SUDDEN-ONSET)			
***	Traumatic ulcer	Mild to moderate pain; history of local trauma	213
***	Aphthous stomatitis	Extremely painful; may be single or multiple; non-keratinized movable mucosa; often recurs	236
***	Recurrent herpes labialis	Vermilion and labial skin; begins as multiple vesicles; often recurs	181
**	Primary herpetic gingivostomatitis	Fever and malaise; children and young adults; multiple vesicles; gingiva consistently affected	181
**	Varicella (chickenpox)	Associated with skin eruption; few oral vesicles and ulcers; usually in children	186
**	Acute necrotizing ulcerative gingivitis (ANUG)	Painful destruction of gingival papillae; fetid odor; mostly in teen-agers and young adults	124
**	Mucosal burns	Chemical or thermal	215
**	Recurrent intraoral herpes simplex	Gingiva or hard palate (except in immunocompromised); focal cluster of vesicles and shallow ulcers	181
**	Allergic reactions	Example: Caused by topical medications or dental materials; erythema and vesicles	247
**	Erythema multiforme	Predominantly in children and young adults; multiple blisters and ulcers; often crusting, hemorrhagic lip lesions; may have associated "target" skin lesions or involvement of ocular and genital mucosa (Stevens-Johnson syndrome)	567
**	Herpangina	Especially in children; multiple small ulcers on soft palate and tonsillar pillars	193

674

FREQUENCY OF OCCURRENCE	LESION OR CONDITION	COMMENTS OR SPECIAL CHARACTERISTICS	PAGE NO.
*	Herpes zoster	Unilateral involvement along nerve distribution; usually middle-aged and older adults; painful vesicles and ulcers	188
*	Hand-foot-and-mouth disease	Especially in children; multiple vesicles and ulcers; associated vesicles on hands and feet	193
*	Necrotizing sialometaplasia	Usually posterior lateral hard palate; prior swelling may be present; deep crater-like ulcer; may be only minimal pain	335
*	Anesthetic necrosis	Usually at site of palatal injection	222
*	Primary syphilis	Chancre at site of inoculation; usually painless with clean ulcer bed	146
*	Behçet's syndrome	Aphthous-like ulcers; genital ulcers and ocular inflammation	239

B. VESICULOEROSIVE AND ULCERATIVE LESIONS: CHRONIC (LONG-DURATION)

FREQUENCY OF OCCURRENCE	LESION OR CONDITION	COMMENTS OR SPECIAL CHARACTERISTICS	PAGE NO.
***	Erosive lichen planus	Associated with white striae; usually in middle-aged and older adults; most common on buccal mucosa and gingiva ("desquamative gingivitis")	572
**	Squamous cell carcinoma	Usually in middle-aged and older adults; usually indurated and may have rolled border; may be painless	295
**	Cicatricial (mucous membrane) pemphigoid	Most common in middle-aged and older women; most commonly presents as a "desquamative gingivitis"; may involve ocular and genital mucosa	563
**	Traumatic granuloma	Solitary, non-healing ulcer	213
*	Lupus erythematosus	May have associated red and white change; usually with skin involvement	580
*	Pemphigus vulgaris	Usually in middle-aged and older patients; multiple oral blisters and ulcers usually precede skin lesions	559
*	Deep fungal infections	Examples: histoplasmosis, blastomycosis; may be painless	Ch. 6
*	Tuberculosis	Associated mass may be present; may be painless	150
*	Sarcoidosis	May be associated with erythematous macules or plaques; may be painless	241

Continued

FREQUENCY OF OCCURRENCE	LESION OR CONDITION	COMMENTS OR SPECIAL CHARACTERISTICS	PAGE NO.
*	Epidermolysis bullosa	Hereditary (except epidermolysis bullosa acquisita); onset in infancy and childhood; multiple skin and oral blisters or ulcers in areas of trauma; may result in extensive scarring	556
*	Pyostomatitis vegetans	Yellowish "snail-track" pustules; associated with inflammatory bowel disease	621
*	Wegener's granulomatosis	Usually palatal ulceration and destruction; associated lung and kidney involvement may be present; may show "strawberry gingivitis"	245
*	Midline lethal granuloma	Palatal lymphoma with ulceration and destruction of underlying bone; may be painless	439
*	Noma	Gangrenous necrosis secondary to acute necrotizing ulcerative gingivitis; usually in malnourished children or immunocompromised individuals	155
*	Tertiary syphilis	Gumma; associated mass may be present; may be painless; may perforate palate	146

B. VESICULOEROSIVE AND ULCERATIVE LESIONS: CHRONIC (LONG-DURATION) *Continued*

C. PAPILLARY GROWTHS: FOCAL OR DIFFUSE

FREQUENCY OF OCCURRENCE	LESION OR CONDITION	COMMENTS OR SPECIAL CHARACTERISTICS	PAGE NO.
***	Hairy tongue	Usually brown or black discoloration; hyperkeratotic elongation of filiform papillae on posterior dorsal tongue	12
***	Papilloma	Can be white or pink; most common on soft palate and tongue; usually pedunculated	259
***	Inflammatory papillary hyperplasia	Usually involves midportion of hard palate beneath denture	367
**	Verruca vulgaris	Common wart; especially in younger patients; most common on labial mucosa	262
**	Leukoplakia (some variants)	Examples: proliferative verrucous leukoplakia, granular or nodular leukoplakia	280
**	Squamous cell carcinoma	Examples with papillary surface changes	295
*	Hairy leukoplakia	Usually lateral border of tongue; rough surface with vertical fissures; usually associated with HIV infection	202

FREQUENCY OF OCCURRENCE	LESION OR CONDITION	COMMENTS OR SPECIAL CHARACTERISTICS	PAGE NO.
*	Giant cell fibroma	Usually in children and young adults; most common on gingiva	363
*	Verruciform xanthoma	Most common on gingiva and hard palate	267
*	Verrucous carcinoma	Especially in older patients with long history of snuff or chewing tobacco use; especially in mandibular vestibule and buccal mucosa; may be white or red	304
*	Condyloma acuminatum	Venereal wart; broad-based lesions with blunted projections; frequently multiple	263
*	Focal epithelial hyperplasia	Usually multiple, flat-topped papular lesions; usually in children; most common in Native Americans and Inuits (Eskimos); color may vary from normal to white	265
*	Keratosis follicularis	Most commonly presents as pebbly appearance of hard palate; associated crusty, greasy skin lesions; hereditary	548
*	Acanthosis nigricans (malignant type)	Most commonly presents as generalized pebbly alteration of upper lip; pigmented, pebbly skin changes in flexural areas; associated gastrointestinal malignancy	587

Part 3

Mucosal and Soft Tissue Pathology: Masses or Enlargement

FREQUENCY OF OCCURRENCE	LESION OR CONDITION	COMMENTS OR SPECIAL CHARACTERISTICS	PAGE NO.
	A. SOFT TISSUE MASSES (LUMPS AND BUMPS): LOWER LIP		
***	Mucocele	Typically pale blue; often exhibits cyclic swelling and rupturing; labial mucosa only	322
***	Irritation fibroma	Usually normal in color	362
**	Squamous cell carcinoma	Tumor with rough, granular, irregular surface; usually on vermilion border	295
*	Other mesenchymal tumors	Examples: hemangioma, neurofibroma, lipoma	Ch. 12
*	Salivary duct cyst	May be bluish; labial mucosa only	325
*	Salivary gland tumor	Usually mucoepidermoid carcinoma	Ch. 11
*	Keratoacanthoma	Volcano-shaped mass with central keratin plug; rapid development; vermilion border only	270
	B. SOFT TISSUE MASSES (LUMPS AND BUMPS): UPPER LIP		
**	Irritation fibroma	Usually normal in color	362
**	Salivary gland tumor	Usually canalicular adenoma (older than age 40) or pleomorphic adenoma (younger than age 40)	Ch. 11
**	Salivary duct cyst	May be bluish	325
*	Minor gland sialolith	Small, hard submucosal mass; may be tender	326
*	Other mesenchymal tumors	Examples: hemangioma, neurofibroma, neurilemoma	Ch. 12
*	Nasolabial cyst	Fluctuant swelling of lateral labial vestibule	23
	C. SOFT TISSUE MASSES (LUMPS AND BUMPS): BUCCAL MUCOSA		
***	Irritation fibroma	Usually normal in color; along occlusal plane	362

FREQUENCY OF OCCURRENCE	LESION OR CONDITION	COMMENTS OR SPECIAL CHARACTERISTICS	PAGE NO.
**	Lipoma	May be yellow; soft to palpation	376
**	Mucocele	Typically pale blue; often exhibits cyclic swelling and rupturing	322
*	Hyperplastic lymph node	Usually buccinator node; movable submucosal mass	416
*	Other mesenchymal tumors	Examples: hemangioma, neurofibroma	Ch. 12
*	Squamous cell carcinoma	Tumor with rough, granular, irregular surface	295
*	Salivary gland tumor	Pleomorphic adenoma and mucoepidermoid carcinoma most common	Ch. 11

D. SOFT TISSUE MASSES (LUMPS AND BUMPS): GINGIVA/ALVEOLAR MUCOSA

***	Parulis	Fistula from nonvital tooth	109
***	Epulis fissuratum	Ill-fitting denture	365
***	Pyogenic granuloma	Usually red, ulcerated, easily bleeding; increased frequency in pregnant women	371
***	Peripheral ossifying fibroma	May be red or normal in color; may be ulcerated	374
**	Peripheral giant cell granuloma	Reddish-purple; frequently ulcerated	373
**	Irritation fibroma	Usually normal in color	362
*	Squamous cell carcinoma	Tumor with rough, granular, irregular surface	295
*	Metastatic tumors	May be painful and destroy bone	410
*	Gingival cyst of the adult	Most common in mandibular bicuspid-cuspid region; may be blue	503
*	Traumatic neuroma	Edentulous mandible in mental foramen area; often painful to palpation	377
*	Kaposi's sarcoma	Especially in AIDS patients; usually purple	203
*	Peripheral odontogenic tumors	Example: peripheral ameloblastoma	519
*	Congenital epulis	Usually in females; especially anterior maxilla	388
*	Melanotic neuroectodermal tumor of infancy	Anterior maxilla; destroys underlying bone; may be pigmented	385
*	Other mesenchymal tumors	Examples: hemangioma, neurofibroma	Ch. 12

FREQUENCY OF OCCURRENCE	LESION OR CONDITION	COMMENTS OR SPECIAL CHARACTERISTICS	PAGE NO.
	E. SOFT TISSUE MASSES (LUMPS AND BUMPS): FLOOR OF MOUTH		
**	Ranula/mucocele	Typically a pale blue, fluctuant swelling	323
**	Sialolith	Usually hard mass in submandibular duct; may be associated with tender swelling of affected gland; radiopaque mass	326
**	Squamous cell carcinoma	Tumor with rough, granular, irregular surface	295
**	Lymphoepithelial cyst	Small, yellow-white submucosal lesion	33
*	Epidermoid or dermoid cyst	Midline yellow-white submucosal lesion	30
*	Salivary gland tumors	Especially mucoepidermoid carcinoma	Ch. 11
*	Mesenchymal tumors	Examples: lipoma, neurofibroma, hemangioma	Ch. 12
	F. SOFT TISSUE MASSES (LUMPS AND BUMPS): TONGUE		
***	Irritation fibroma	Usually normal in color; most common on margins of tongue	362
**	Squamous cell carcinoma	Tumor with rough, granular, irregular surface	295
**	Mucocele	Usually anterior ventral surface; usually bluish or clear color	322
*	Granular cell tumor	Dome-shaped; usually on dorsum of tongue	387
*	Other mesenchymal tumors	Examples: lymphangioma, hemangioma, neurofibroma, osseous choristoma	Ch. 12
*	Pyogenic granuloma	Usually red, ulcerated, easily bleeding	371
*	Salivary gland tumors	Especially mucoepidermoid carcinoma and adenoid cystic carcinoma	Ch. 11
*	Lingual thyroid	Usually posterior midline of dorsal surface; usually in women	10
	G. SOFT TISSUE MASSES (LUMPS AND BUMPS): HARD OR SOFT PALATE		
***	Palatal abscess	Associated with nonvital tooth	109
***	Leaf-like denture fibroma	Pedunculated hyperplastic growth beneath ill-fitting denture	366
**	Salivary gland tumors	Especially pleomorphic adenoma, mucoepidermoid carcinoma, adenoid	Ch. 11

FREQUENCY OF OCCURRENCE	LESION OR CONDITION	COMMENTS OR SPECIAL CHARACTERISTICS	PAGE NO.
		cystic carcinoma, polymorphous low-grade adenocarcinoma; may have bluish hue	
**	Kaposi's sarcoma	Usually purple; may be multiple; usually associated with AIDS	203
**	Nasopalatine duct cyst	Fluctuant swelling of anterior midline palate	25
*	Other mesenchymal tumors	Examples: irritation fibroma, hemangioma, neurofibroma	Ch. 12
*	Squamous cell carcinoma	Tumor with rough, granular, irregular surface; occasionally arises from maxillary sinus	295
*	Mucocele/salivary duct cyst	Usually has bluish hue	322
*	Lymphoma	Often boggy and edematous; may have bluish hue; may be bilateral	431
*	Melanocytic nevus/melanoma	Usually pigmented	276
*	Necrotizing sialometaplasia	Early-stage lesion; often associated with pain or paresthesia	335
*	Adenomatoid hyperplasia of minor salivary glands	—	335

H. SOFT TISSUE MASSES (LUMPS AND BUMPS): MULTIPLE LESIONS

**	Kaposi's sarcoma	Usually purple lesions of palate and maxillary gingiva; usually associated with AIDS	203
**	Neurofibromatosis	Oral and skin neurofibromas; *café au lait* skin pigmentation	381
*	Focal epithelial hyperplasia	Usually flat-topped papular lesions; usually in children; most common in Native Americans and Inuits (Eskimos); color may vary from normal to white	265
*	Amyloidosis	Pale, firm deposits, especially in tongue; periocular cutaneous lesions frequently present; most often associated with multiple myeloma	599
*	Granulomatous diseases	Examples: sarcoidosis, Crohn's disease, leprosy	241
*	Multiple endocrine neoplasia, type III	Mucosal neuromas of lips and tongue; adrenal pheochromocytomas; medullary thyroid carcinoma; marfanoid body build	384

Continued

FREQUENCY OF OCCURRENCE	LESION OR CONDITION	COMMENTS OR SPECIAL CHARACTERISTICS	PAGE NO.

H. SOFT TISSUE MASSES (LUMPS AND BUMPS): MULTIPLE LESIONS *Continued*

FREQUENCY OF OCCURRENCE	LESION OR CONDITION	COMMENTS OR SPECIAL CHARACTERISTICS	PAGE NO.
*	Tuberous sclerosis	Small fibroma-like growths on gingiva; angiofibromas of face; epilepsy; mental retardation	553
*	Multiple hamartoma syndrome	Cowden syndrome; small fibroma-like growths on gingiva; multiple hamartomas of various tissues; breast cancer in affected women	555

I. SOFT TISSUE MASSES (LUMPS AND BUMPS): MIDLINE NECK LESIONS

FREQUENCY OF OCCURRENCE	LESION OR CONDITION	COMMENTS OR SPECIAL CHARACTERISTICS	PAGE NO.
**	Thyroid gland enlargement	Examples: goiter, thyroid tumor	—
*	Thyroglossal duct cyst	May move up and down with tongue motion	31
*	Dermoid cyst	Soft and fluctuant	30
*	Plunging ranula	Soft and compressible	323

J. SOFT TISSUE MASSES (LUMPS AND BUMPS): LATERAL NECK LESIONS

FREQUENCY OF OCCURRENCE	LESION OR CONDITION	COMMENTS OR SPECIAL CHARACTERISTICS	PAGE NO.
***	Reactive lymphadenopathy	Secondary to oral and maxillofacial infection; often tender to palpation	416
**	Epidermoid cyst	Soft and movable	29
**	Lipoma	Soft mass	376
**	Infectious mononucleosis	Fatigue; sore throat; tender lymph nodes	190
**	Metastatic carcinoma	Deposits from oral and pharyngeal carcinomas; usually indurated and painless; may be fixed	301
**	Lymphoma	May be unilateral or bilateral; usually painless; Hodgkin's and non-Hodgkin's types	429
*	Salivary gland tumors	Arising from submandibular gland or tail of parotid gland	Ch. 11
*	Submandibular sialadenitis	Example: secondary to sialolithiasis	327
*	Cervical lymphoepithelial cyst	Soft and fluctuant; most common in young adults	32
*	Granulomatous diseases	Examples: sarcoidosis, tuberculosis	241
*	Cat-scratch disease	History of exposure to cat	157
*	Cystic hygroma	Infants; soft and fluctuant	395

FREQUENCY OF OCCURRENCE	LESION OR CONDITION	COMMENTS OR SPECIAL CHARACTERISTICS	PAGE NO.
*	Plunging ranula	Soft and compressible	323
*	Other mesenchymal tumors	Examples: neurofibroma, carotid body tumor	Ch. 12

K. GENERALIZED GINGIVAL ENLARGEMENT

FREQUENCY OF OCCURRENCE	LESION OR CONDITION	COMMENTS OR SPECIAL CHARACTERISTICS	PAGE NO.
***	Hyperplastic gingivitis	Examples: associated with puberty, pregnancy, diabetes	122
**	Drug-related gingival hyperplasia	Examples: phenytoin, calcium-channel blockers, cyclosporine; may be fibrotic	129
*	Gingival fibromatosis	May be hereditary; onset in childhood	132
*	Leukemic infiltrate	Usually boggy and hemorrhagic	427
*	Wegener's granulomatosis	"Strawberry" gingivitis; may have palatal ulceration and destruction; lung and kidney involvement	245
*	Scurvy	Vitamin C deficiency	601

Part 4

Radiographic Pathology

FREQUENCY OF OCCURRENCE	LESION OR CONDITION	COMMENTS OR SPECIAL CHARACTERISTICS	PAGE NO.
A. UNILOCULAR RADIOLUCENCIES: PERICORONAL LOCATION			
***	Hyperplastic dental follicle	<5 mm in thickness	495
***	Dentigerous cyst	>5 mm in thickness	493
**	Eruption cyst	Bluish swelling overlying erupting tooth	496
**	Odontogenic keratocyst	—	497
*	Orthokeratinizing odontogenic cyst	—	500
*	Ameloblastoma	Especially unicystic type	512
*	Ameloblastic fibroma	Usually in younger patients	525
*	Adenomatoid odontogenic tumor	Usually in anterior region of jaws; most often with maxillary canine; usually in teen-agers	529
*	Calcifying odontogenic cyst	Gorlin cyst	506
*	Carcinoma arising in dentigerous cyst	Mostly in older adults	510
*	Intraosseous mucoepidermoid carcinoma	Mostly in posterior mandible	351
*	Other odontogenic lesions	Examples: calcifying epithelial odontogenic tumor, odontogenic myxoma, central odontogenic fibroma	Ch. 15
B. UNILOCULAR RADIOLUCENCIES: PERIAPICAL LOCATION			
***	Periapical granuloma	Nonvital tooth	102
***	Periapical cyst	Nonvital tooth	105
**	Periapical cemental dysplasia (early)	Especially in black females; usually apical to mandibular anteriors; teeth are vital	464
*	Periapical scar	Usually endodontically treated tooth with destruction of cortical plate	104
*	Dentin dysplasia, type I	Multiple periapical granulomas or cysts; shortened, malformed roots	87

FREQUENCY OF OCCURRENCE	LESION OR CONDITION	COMMENTS OR SPECIAL CHARACTERISTICS	PAGE NO.
		C. UNILOCULAR RADIOLUCENCIES: OTHER LOCATIONS	
***	Developing tooth bud	Within alveolar bone	—
**	Lateral radicular cyst	Nonvital tooth; lateral canal	106
**	Nasopalatine duct cyst	Between and apical to maxillary central incisors; palatal swelling may occur	25
**	Lateral periodontal cyst	Especially in mandibular bicuspid-cuspid region	504
**	Residual (periapical) cyst	Edentulous area	107
**	Odontogenic keratocyst	—	497
**	Central giant cell granuloma	Especially in anterior mandible	453
**	Stafne bone defect	Angle of mandible below mandibular canal	21
*	Cemento-osseous dysplasia	Early stage; usually in young adult and middle-aged black women; usually in mandible	464
*	Central ossifying fibroma	Early-stage lesion	469
*	Ameloblastoma	Especially unicystic type	512
*	Other odontogenic cysts and tumors	Examples: ameloblastic fibroma, central odontogenic fibroma, calcifying odontogenic cyst	Ch. 15
*	Langerhans cell disease	"Histiocytosis X"; usually in children or young adults	451
*	Melanotic neuroectodermal tumor of infancy	Anterior maxilla; may be pigmented	385
*	Median palatal cyst	Clinical midline swelling of hard palate	27
*	Neurilemoma/neurofibroma	Usually associated with mandibular nerve	379
		D. MULTILOCULAR RADIOLUCENCIES	
***	Odontogenic keratocyst	—	497
***	Ameloblastoma	Especially in posterior mandible; often associated with impacted tooth	512
**	Central giant cell granuloma	Especially in anterior mandible	453
*	Ameloblastic fibroma	Especially in younger patients	525
*	Odontogenic myxoma	"Cobweb" trabeculation	536
*	Central odontogenic fibroma	—	533

Continued

FREQUENCY OF OCCURRENCE	LESION OR CONDITION	COMMENTS OR SPECIAL CHARACTERISTICS	PAGE NO.
	D. MULTILOCULAR RADIOLUCENCIES *Continued*		
*	Calcifying epithelial odontogenic tumor	Often associated with impacted tooth	522
*	Orthokeratinized odontogenic cyst	Often associated with impacted tooth	500
*	Lateral periodontal cyst (botryoid type)	Especially in mandibular bicuspid-cuspid region	505
*	Calcifying odontogenic cyst	Especially in cases with minimal or no calcifications; often associated with impacted tooth	506
*	Central hemangioma/arteriovenous malformation	Especially in younger patients; may have honeycombed radiographic appearance; may pulsate	478
*	Aneurysmal bone cyst	Especially in younger patients	459
*	Cherubism	Hereditary; onset in childhood; multiple quadrants involved	456
*	Hyperparathyroidism (brown tumor)	Usually elevated serum calcium levels	612
*	Intraosseous mucoepidermoid carcinoma	Usually in posterior mandible	351
*	Fibrous dysplasia	Very rarely on panoramic films of mandibular lesions	461
	E. RADIOLUCENCIES: POORLY DEFINED OR RAGGED BORDERS		
***	Periapical granuloma or cyst	Nonvital tooth	102
***	Hematopoietic bone marrow defect	Especially edentulous areas in posterior mandible; more common in females	447
**	Osteomyelitis	Usually painful or tender	114
*	Traumatic bone cyst	Mandibular lesion that scallops up between roots of teeth; usually in younger patients	458
*	Metastatic tumors	Painful; paresthesia; usually in older adults	489
*	Osteoradionecrosis	History of radiation therapy; painful	220
*	Multiple myeloma	May be painful; in older adults	437
*	Primary intraosseous carcinomas	Odontogenic or salivary origin	520
*	Osteosarcoma	Often painful; usually in young adults	482
*	Chondrosarcoma	—	485
*	Ewing's sarcoma	Almost always in children	487

FREQUENCY OF OCCURRENCE	LESION OR CONDITION	COMMENTS OR SPECIAL CHARACTERISTICS	PAGE NO.
*	Other primary bone malignancies	Examples: fibrosarcoma, lymphoma	481
*	Desmoplastic fibroma of bone	Especially in younger patients	480
*	Massive osteolysis	Phantom (vanishing) bone disease	448
*	NICO (neuralgia-inducing cavitational osteonecrosis)	Local or referred pain	631

F. RADIOLUCENCIES: MULTIFOCAL OR GENERALIZED

***	Cemento-osseous dysplasia	Early-stage lesion; usually in black females; usually in mandible	464
**	Nevoid basal cell carcinoma syndrome	Odontogenic keratocysts	501
**	Multiple myeloma	Painful; in older adults; "punched-out" lesions	437
*	Cherubism	Usually multilocular; onset in childhood; hereditary	456
*	Hyperparathyroidism	Multiple brown tumors	612
*	Langerhans cell disease	"Histiocytosis X"; in children and young adults; teeth "floating in air"	451

G. RADIOPACITIES: WELL-DEMARCATED BORDERS

***	Torus or exostosis	Associated with bony surface mass	17
***	Retained root tip	Remnants of periodontal ligament usually seen	—
***	Condensing osteitis	Usually at apex of nonvital tooth	117
***	Idiopathic osteosclerosis	Most commonly associated with roots of posterior teeth; no apparent inflammatory etiology	447
**	Pseudocyst of the maxillary sinus	Homogeneous, dome-shaped relative opacity rising above bony floor of maxillary sinus	231
**	Odontoma, compound	Tooth-like structures with thin, radiolucent rim at junction with surrounding bone; may prevent eruption of teeth; more common in anterior segments of jaws	531
**	Odontoma, complex	Amorphous mass with thin, radiolucent rim at junction with surrounding bone; may prevent eruption of teeth; more common in posterior segments of jaws	531

Continued

FREQUENCY OF OCCURRENCE	LESION OR CONDITION	COMMENTS OR SPECIAL CHARACTERISTICS	PAGE NO.
\multicolumn{4}{c}{G. RADIOPACITIES: WELL-DEMARCATED BORDERS *Continued*}

FREQUENCY OF OCCURRENCE	LESION OR CONDITION	COMMENTS OR SPECIAL CHARACTERISTICS	PAGE NO.
**	Cemento-osseous dysplasia	Late-stage lesions; especially in middle-aged and older black women; usually in mandible	464
**	Soft tissue radiopacity superimposed on bone	Examples: sialoliths, calcified nodes, pheboliths, bullet fragments, shotgun pellets, amalgam tattoos (Also see Appendix List, Part 4, Q, p. 690)	—
*	Intraosseous foreign body	—	—
*	Osteoma	Associated with bony surface mass	472
*	Enamel pearl	Furcation area of molar tooth	72
*	Osteoblastoma/osteoid osteoma/cementoblastoma	Late-stage lesions	473

H. RADIOPACITIES: POORLY DEMARCATED BORDERS

FREQUENCY OF OCCURRENCE	LESION OR CONDITION	COMMENTS OR SPECIAL CHARACTERISTICS	PAGE NO.
**	Cemento-osseous dysplasia	Late-stage lesions; especially in middle-aged and older black women; usually in mandible	464
**	Condensing osteitis	Usually at apex of nonvital tooth	117
**	Sclerosing osteomyelitis	May be painful	116
**	Fibrous dysplasia	"Ground glass" appearance; onset usually in younger patients	461
*	Paget's disease of bone	"Cotton wool" appearance; late-stage lesions; in older patients	449
*	Proliferative periostitis	"Onion-skin" cortical change; in younger patients; often associated with nonvital tooth	118
*	Osteosarcoma	May have "sunburst" cortical change; frequently painful; usually in young adults	482
*	Chondrosarcoma	—	485

I. RADIOPACITIES: MULTIFOCAL OR GENERALIZED

FREQUENCY OF OCCURRENCE	LESION OR CONDITION	COMMENTS OR SPECIAL CHARACTERISTICS	PAGE NO.
**	Florid cemento-osseous dysplasia	Late-stage lesions; especially in middle-aged and older black women; usually in mandible	467
**	Idiopathic osteosclerosis	—	447
*	Paget's disease of bone	"Cotton wool" appearance; late-stage lesions; in older patients; more common in maxilla	449

FREQUENCY OF OCCURRENCE	LESION OR CONDITION	COMMENTS OR SPECIAL CHARACTERISTICS	PAGE NO.
*	Gardner syndrome	Multiple osteomas; epidermoid cysts; gastrointestinal polyps with high tendency toward malignant transformation; hereditary	473
*	Polyostotic fibrous dysplasia	"Ground glass" appearance; onset usually in younger patients; may be associated with *café au lait* skin pigmentation and endocrine abnormalities (Albright syndrome)	461
*	Osteopetrosis	Hereditary; recessive form may be associated with secondary osteomyelitis, visual and hearing impairment	444

J. MIXED RADIOLUCENT/RADIOPAQUE LESIONS: WELL-DEMARCATED BORDERS

***	Developing tooth	—	—
**	Cemento-osseous dysplasia	Intermediate-stage lesions; especially in middle-aged black women; usually in mandible	464
**	Odontoma	Compound or complex type; in younger patients; may prevent eruption of teeth	531
*	Central ossifying fibroma	—	469
*	Ameloblastic fibro-odontoma	Usually in children	527
*	Adenomatoid odontogenic tumor	Usually in anterior region of jaws; most often with maxillary canine; usually in teen-agers	529
*	Calcifying epithelial odontogenic tumor	Pindborg tumor; often associated with impacted tooth; may show "driven-snow" opacities	522
*	Calcifying odontogenic cyst	Gorlin cyst; may be associated with odontoma	506
*	Osteoblastoma/osteoid osteoma	Intermediate-stage lesion; usually in younger patients; often painful	473
*	Cementoblastoma	Intermediate-stage lesion; attached to tooth root	476

K. MIXED RADIOLUCENT/RADIOPAQUE LESIONS: POORLY DEMARCATED BORDERS

**	Osteomyelitis	With sequestrum formation or with sclerosing type; often painful	114
*	Metastatic carcinoma	Especially prostate and breast carcinomas; may be painful	489
*	Osteosarcoma/chondrosarcoma	May be painful	482

FREQUENCY OF OCCURRENCE	LESION OR CONDITION	COMMENTS OR SPECIAL CHARACTERISTICS	PAGE NO.
	L. MIXED RADIOLUCENT/RADIOPAQUE LESIONS: MULTIFOCAL OR GENERALIZED		
**	Florid cemento-osseous dysplasia	Intermediate-stage lesions; especially in middle-aged black women; usually in mandible	467
*	Paget's disease of bone	In older patients; more common in maxilla	449
	M. UNIQUE RADIOGRAPHIC APPEARANCES: "GROUND GLASS" (FROSTED GLASS) RADIOPACITIES		
*	Fibrous dysplasia	Onset usually in younger patients	461
*	Hyperparathyroidism	May cause loss of lamina dura	612
	N. UNIQUE RADIOGRAPHIC APPEARANCES: "COTTON WOOL" RADIOPACITIES		
**	Cemento-osseous dysplasia	Especially in middle-aged black women; usually in mandible	464
*	Paget's disease of bone	In older patients; more common in maxilla	449
*	Gardner syndrome	Multiple osteomas; epidermoid cysts; gastrointestinal polyps with high tendency toward malignant transformation; hereditary	473
*	Gigantiform cementoma	Hereditary; facial enlargement may be present	468
	O. UNIQUE RADIOGRAPHIC APPEARANCES: "SUNBURST" RADIOPACITIES		
*	Osteosarcoma	Often painful; usually in young adults	482
*	Intraosseous hemangioma	Especially in younger patients	478
	P. UNIQUE RADIOGRAPHIC APPEARANCES: "ONION-SKIN" RADIOPACITIES		
*	Proliferative periostitis	In younger patients; often associated with nonvital tooth; best seen with occlusal radiograph	118
*	Ewing's sarcoma	In young children	487
*	Langerhans cell disease	"Histiocytosis X"; usually in children or young adults	451
	Q. SOFT TISSUE RADIOPACITIES		
***	Amalgam tattoo	Markedly radiopaque; associated with surface discoloration	225

FREQUENCY OF OCCURRENCE	LESION OR CONDITION	COMMENTS OR SPECIAL CHARACTERISTICS	PAGE NO.
**	Other foreign bodies	Examples: bullet fragments, shotgun pellets	—
**	Sialolith	Glandular pain may be present while patient is eating	326
**	Calcified lymph nodes	Example: tuberculosis	150
**	Phlebolith	May occur in varicosities or hemangiomas	14
*	Tonsillolith	—	145
*	Soft tissue osteoma/chondroma	Most common on tongue	400
*	Calcinosis cutis	May be seen with systemic sclerosis (especially CREST syndrome)	586
*	Myositis ossificans	Reactive calcification in muscle	—

Part 5

Pathology of Teeth

FREQUENCY OF OCCURRENCE	LESION OR CONDITION	COMMENTS OR SPECIAL CHARACTERISTICS	PAGE NO.
A. HYPERDONTIA (EXTRA TEETH)			
***	Idiopathic supernumerary teeth	Mesiodens, paramolar, distomolar	60
**	Cleft lip and palate	Extra lateral incisor or canine	1
*	Gardner syndrome	Osteomas and gastrointestinal polyps	473
*	Cleidocranial dysplasia	Hypoplastic or missing clavicles; failure of tooth eruption	445
B. HYPODONTIA (MISSING TEETH)			
***	Idiopathic oligodontia	Missing third molars, lateral incisors	60
**	Cleft lip and palate	Missing lateral incisor or canine	1
*	Hereditary hypohidrotic ectodermal dysplasia	Cone-shaped teeth	541
*	Incontinentia pigmenti	Cone-shaped teeth	547
*	Radiotherapy during childhood	Stunted tooth development	221
C. MACRODONTIA (LARGER THAN NORMAL TEETH)			
**	Fusion	Joining of two tooth germs	65
**	Gemination	Incomplete splitting of a tooth germ	65
*	Idiopathic macrodontia	—	64
*	Facial hemihyperplasia	Affected side only; nondental tissues also enlarged	34
*	Gigantism	Abnormally tall stature	606
D. MICRODONTIA (SMALLER THAN NORMAL TEETH)			
***	Supernumerary teeth	Mesiodens; fourth molars	60
***	Peg-shaped lateral incisors	Cone-shaped teeth	64

692

FREQUENCY OF OCCURRENCE	LESION OR CONDITION	COMMENTS OR SPECIAL CHARACTERISTICS	PAGE NO.
**	Dens invaginatus	Cone-shaped teeth; tendency for pulpal death and periapical pathosis	70
**	Cleft lip and palate	Lateral incisor or canine	1
*	Idiopathic microdontia	Usually generalized	64
*	Hereditary hypohidrotic ectodermal dysplasia	Cone-shaped teeth; sparse, blond hair; diminished sweating	541
*	Radiotherapy during childhood	Stunted tooth development	221
*	Congenital syphilis	Hutchinson's incisors	148
*	Hypopituitarism	Associated dwarfism	605

E. MALFORMED CROWN

FREQUENCY OF OCCURRENCE	LESION OR CONDITION	COMMENTS OR SPECIAL CHARACTERISTICS	PAGE NO.
***	Mesiodens and other supernumeraries	Cone-shaped teeth or microdont	60
**	Environmental enamel hypoplasia	Examples: high fever during tooth development	44
**	Peg-shaped lateral incisors	Cone-shaped teeth	64
**	Dens invaginatus	Cone-shaped teeth; tendency toward pulpal death and periapical pathosis	70
**	Turner's tooth	Infection or trauma to associated primary tooth	45
**	Fusion or gemination	"Double" tooth	65
*	Talon cusp	Extra cusp on lingual of anterior tooth	68
*	Dens evaginatus	Extra cusp on occlusal of premolar tooth	69
*	Amelogenesis imperfecta	Hereditary defect in enamel formation	79
*	Dentinogenesis imperfecta	Fracturing away of enamel due to hereditary defect in dentin formation; gray-yellow opalescent teeth; calcified pulp chambers	84
*	Regional odontodysplasia	Poor tooth formation in a focal area; "ghost teeth"	90
*	Congenital syphilis	Hutchinson's incisors; mulberry molars	148
*	Vitamin D–resistant rickets	Hereditary condition; high pulp horns	619
*	Renal osteodystrophy	Abnormal calcium and phosphate metabolism	613
*	Hypoparathyroidism	Possible associated endocrine-candidiasis syndrome	611

Continued

FREQUENCY OF OCCURRENCE	LESION OR CONDITION	COMMENTS OR SPECIAL CHARACTERISTICS	PAGE NO.
	E. MALFORMED CROWN *Continued*		
*	Pseudohypoparathyroidism	—	611
*	Epidermolysis bullosa	Hereditary blistering skin disease	556
*	Radiotherapy during childhood	Stunted tooth development	221
	F. ENAMEL LOSS AFTER TOOTH FORMATION		
***	Caries	—	—
***	Trauma	Fractured tooth	—
***	Attrition	Physiologic loss of tooth structure	48
***	Abrasion	Pathologic loss of tooth structure	48
**	Erosion	Chemical loss of tooth structure	48
*	Dentinogenesis imperfecta	Hereditary defect in dentin formation; poor junction between enamel and dentin	84
*	Amelogenesis imperfecta	Hereditary defect in enamel formation; especially hypocalcified types	79
	G. EXTRINSIC STAINING OF TEETH		
***	Tobacco	Black or brown	55
***	Coffee, tea, and cola drinks	Brown or black	55
**	Chromogenic bacteria	Brown, black, green, or orange	55
	H. INTRINSIC DISCOLORATION ("STAINING") OF TEETH		
***	Aging	Yellow-brown; less translucency	—
***	Death of pulp	Gray-black; less translucency	96
**	Fluorosis	White; yellow-brown; brown; mottled	47
**	Tetracycline	Yellow-brown; yellow fluorescence	57
**	Internal resorption	"Pink tooth of Mummery"	51
*	Calcific metamorphosis	Yellow	98
*	Dentinogenesis imperfecta	Blue-gray; translucent	84
*	Amelogenesis imperfecta	Yellow-brown	79

FREQUENCY OF OCCURRENCE	LESION OR CONDITION	COMMENTS OR SPECIAL CHARACTERISTICS	PAGE NO.
*	Congenital erythropoietic porphyria	Yellow; brown-red; red fluorescence	56
*	Erythroblastosis fetalis	Yellow; green	56
*	Heavy metal exposure	Especially bismuth and lead; various colors	53

I. ABNORMALLY SHAPED ROOTS

***	External root resorption	Secondary to infection, cyst, tumor	51
***	Dilaceration	Abnormal curvature	76
**	Hypercementosis	Excessive cementum production	75
**	Accessory roots	—	78
**	Concrescence	Joining of teeth by cementum	65
**	Taurodontism	Enlarged pulp chambers; shortened roots	74
**	Enamel pearl	Ectopic enamel in furcation	72
*	Benign cementoblastoma	Tumor attached to root	476
*	Radiotherapy during childhood	Stunted root development	221
*	Dentinogenesis imperfecta	Shortened roots; obliterated pulps	84
*	Dentin dysplasia, type I	Shortened, pointed roots ("rootless teeth"); obliterated pulps; periapical pathosis	87

J. ENLARGED PULP CHAMBER OR CANAL

**	Internal resorption	Secondary to caries or trauma	51
**	Taurodontism	Enlarged pulp chambers; shortened roots	74
*	Dentinogenesis imperfecta, type III	"Shell teeth"	84
*	Regional odontodysplasia	"Ghost teeth"	90
*	Vitamin D–resistant rickets	High pulp horns	619
*	Hypophosphatasia	—	617
*	Dentin dysplasia, type II	"Thistle-tube" pulps; pulp stone formation	88

K. PULPAL CALCIFICATION

***	Pulp stones	Asymptomatic radiographic finding	101
***	Secondary dentin	Response to caries	98

Continued

FREQUENCY OF OCCURRENCE	LESION OR CONDITION	COMMENTS OR SPECIAL CHARACTERISTICS	PAGE NO.
	K. PULPAL CALCIFICATION *Continued*		
**	Calcific metamorphosis	Pulpal obliteration secondary to aging or trauma	98
*	Dentinogenesis imperfecta	Pulpal obliteration by excess dentin	84
*	Dentin dysplasia, type I	Pulpal obliteration by excess dentin; "chevron"-shaped pulp chambers	87
*	Dentin dysplasia, type II	Pulpal obliteration of primary teeth; pulp stones in permanent teeth	88
	L. THICKENED PERIODONTAL LIGAMENT		
***	Periapical abscess	Focal thickening at apex of nonvital tooth; painful, especially on percussion of involved tooth	109
***	Current orthodontic therapy	—	—
**	Increased occlusal function	—	—
*	Systemic sclerosis (scleroderma)	Generalized widening	583
*	Sarcoma or carcinoma infiltration	Especially osteosarcoma; localized to teeth in area of tumor	482
	M. GENERALIZED LOSS OF LAMINA DURA		
*	Hyperparathyroidism	Calcium removed from bones; bone may have "ground glass" appearance	612
*	Osteomalacia	Vitamin D deficiency in adults	602
*	Paget's disease of bone	"Cotton wool" change hides lamina dura	449
*	Fibrous dysplasia	"Ground glass" change hides lamina dura	461
	N. PREMATURE EXFOLIATION OF TEETH		
***	Trauma	Avulsed tooth	—
**	Juvenile periodontitis	Premature alveolar bone loss	136
**	Immunocompromised states	AIDS, leukemia, chemotherapy	198
**	Diabetes mellitus	Increased susceptibility to infection and severity of periodontitis	615
*	Osteomyelitis	Bone destruction loosening teeth	114
*	Cyclic or chronic neutropenia	Increased susceptibility to infection; premature alveolar bone loss	423

FREQUENCY OF OCCURRENCE	LESION OR CONDITION	COMMENTS OR SPECIAL CHARACTERISTICS	PAGE NO.
*	Langerhans cell disease	"Histiocytosis X"; eosinophilic granuloma; premature alveolar bone loss	451
*	Dentin dysplasia, type I	"Rootless teeth"	87
*	Regional odontodysplasia	"Ghost teeth"	90
*	Papillon-Lefèvre syndrome	Palmar and plantar hyperkeratosis; premature periodontitis	138
*	Down syndrome	Premature periodontitis	134
*	Hypophosphatasia	Lack of cementum production in primary teeth	617
*	Scurvy	Vitamin C deficiency	601

Index

Note: Page numbers in *italics* indicate figures; those followed by t indicate tables.